INFECTIOUS DISEASES OF CHILDREN

INFECTIOUS DISEASES OF CHILDREN

SAUL KRUGMAN, M.D.
Professor of Pediatrics, New York University School of Medicine;
formerly Chairman, Department of Pediatrics,
Director of Pediatrics, Bellevue Hospital Center, and
Director of Pediatrics, University Hospital,
New York, New York

SAMUEL L. KATZ, M.D.
Wilburt C. Davison Professor and formerly Chairman,
Department of Pediatrics, Duke University School of Medicine,
Durham, North Carolina

ANNE A. GERSHON, M.D.
Professor of Pediatrics, Columbia University
College of Physicians and Surgeons,
New York, New York

CATHERINE M. WILFERT, M.D.
Professor of Pediatrics and Microbiology,
Duke University School of Medicine,
Durham, North Carolina

NINTH EDITION

with 172 illustrations and 22 color illustrations in 9 plates

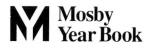 **Mosby Year Book**

St. Louis Baltimore Boston Chicago London Philadelphia Sydney Toronto

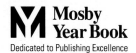

**Mosby
Year Book**
Dedicated to Publishing Excellence

Editor: Stephanie Manning
Assistant Editor: Jane Petrash
Project Manager: Peggy Fagen
Production: Suzanne C. Fannin
Book and Cover Design: Gail Morey Hudson

NINTH EDITION

Printed in the United States of America

Mosby–Year Book, Inc. Company
11830 Westline Industrial Drive, St. Louis, Missouri 63146

International Standard Book Number 0-8016-5754-7

92 93 94 95 96   GW/MY   9 8 7 6 5 4 3 2

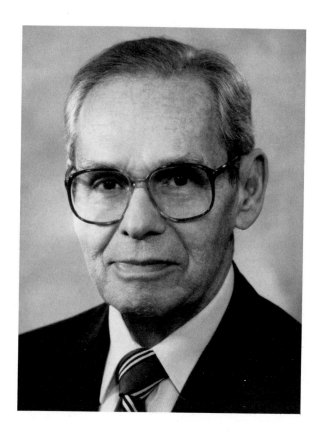

To

SAUL KRUGMAN

with admiration and affection from his fellow authors and editors
who salute him on 45 years of contributions to
Pediatrics and Infectious Diseases

CONTRIBUTORS

WILLIAM BORKOWSKY, M.D.

Associate Professor of Pediatrics
Director, Infectious Diseases and Immunology
Department of Pediatrics
New York University
New York, New York

KENNETH BOYER, M.D.

Associate Professor of Pediatrics
Department of Pediatrics
Rush Medical School
Chicago, Illinois

THOMAS G. CLEARY, M.D.

Professor of Pediatrics
Department of Pediatrics
University of Texas Medical School
Houston, Texas

DENNIS A. CLEMENTS, M.D., Ph.D.

Assistant Professor
Department of Pediatrics
Duke University Medical Center
Durham, North Carolina

SAMUEL P. GOTOFF, M.D.

Professor of Pediatrics
Department of Pediatrics
Rush Medical College
Chicago, Illinois

MARGARET R. HAMMERSCHLAG, M.D.

Professor
Department of Pediatrics and Medicine
State University of New York
Health Science Center at Brooklyn
Brooklyn, New York

EDWARD L. KAPLAN, M.D.

Professor of Pediatrics, School of Medicine
Professor, Division of Epidemiology
School of Public Health
University of Minnesota
Minneapolis, Minnesota

BEN Z. KATZ, M.D.

Infectious Disease Division
Children's Memorial Hospital
Chicago, Illinois

JEROME O. KLEIN, M.D.

Professor of Pediatrics
Boston University School of Medicine;
Director, Division of Pediatric Infectious Diseases
Boston City Hospital
Boston, Massachusetts

KEITH M. KRASINSKI, M.D.

Associate Professor of Pediatrics
Department of Pediatrics
New York University Medical Center
New York, New York

PHILIP LaRUSSA, M.D.

Assistant Professor of Pediatrics
Department of Pediatrics
College of Physicians and Surgeons
Columbia University
New York, New York

LINDA L. LEWIS, M.D.

Infectious Disease Section
National Cancer Institute
National Institutes of Health
Bethesda, Maryland

GEORGE H. McCRACKEN, Jr., M.D.

Professor of Pediatrics
The University of Texas Southwestern Medical
Center at Dallas
Dallas, Texas

RIMA McLEOD, M.D.

Attending Physician
Michael Reese Hospital and Medical Center;
Professor of Medicine,
The University of Illinois at Chicago;
Department of Medicine—Infectious Diseases
University of Chicago
Chicago, Illinois

MARIAN E. MELISH, M.D.

Professor of Pediatrics
Tropical Medicine and Medical Microbiology;
Chief of Infectious Diseases
Department of Pediatrics
John A. Burns School of Medicine of the University
of Hawaii at Manoa
Honolulu, Hawaii

GEORGE MILLER, M.D.

J.F. Enders Professor of Pediatrics Infectious
Diseases;
Professor of Epidemiology and Molecular
Biophysics and Biochemistry
Departments of Pediatrics, Epidemiology, and
Public Health, and Molecular Biophysics and
Biochemistry
Yale University School of Medicine
New Haven, Connecticut

EDWARD A. MORTIMER, Jr., M.D.

Professor of Epidemiology and Pediatrics
Department of Epidemiology and Biostatistics
Case Western Reserve University
Cleveland, Ohio

JOHN D. NELSON, M.D.

Professor of Pediatrics
Department of Pediatrics
The University of Texas Southwestern Medical
Center at Dallas
Dallas, Texas

JAMES C. NIEDERMAN, M.D., D.Sc.

Clinical Professor of Medicine and Epidemiology
Department of Internal Medicine and
Epidemiology
Yale University School of Medicine
New Haven, Connecticut

LARRY K. PICKERING, M.D.

David R. Park Professor of Pediatrics
Director, Infectious Diseases
Department of Pediatrics Vice-Chairman for
Research
The University of Texas Medical School at Houston
Houston, Texas

PHILIP A. PIZZO, M.D.

Chief of Pediatrics
Head, Infectious Disease Section
National Cancer Institute
National Institutes of Health;
Professor of Pediatrics
Uniformed Services University for Health Sciences
Bethesda, Maryland

ALICE PRINCE, M.D.

Associate Professor of Clinical Pediatrics
College of Physicians and Surgeons
Columbia University
New York, New York

SARAH A. RAWSTRON, M.B.B.S.

Assistant Professor of Pediatrics
Department of Pediatrics
State University of New York
Health Science Center at Brooklyn
Brooklyn, New York

XAVIER SÁEZ-LLORENS, M.D.

Assistant Professor of Pediatrics
School of Medicine
Universidad de Panama; Pediatrics Infectious
Disease Service
Division of Clinical Investigation
Department of Pediatrics
Hospital del Niño
Panama City, Panama

PAUL A. SHURIN, M.D.

Associate Professor of Clinical Pediatrics
Department of Pediatrics
Columbia University College of Physicians and
Surgeons
New York, New York

DAVID P. SPEERT, M.D.

Head, Division of Infectious and Immunological
Diseases
Professor, Department of Pediatrics
University of British Columbia
Vancouver, British Columbia
Canada

EMMANUEL B. WALTER, Jr., M.D.

Associate, Department of Pediatrics
Duke University
Durham, North Carolina

RUSSELL E. WARE, M.D., Ph.D.

Assistant Professor of Pediatrics
Division of Hematology/Oncology
Department of Pediatrics
Duke University Medical Center
Durham, North Carolina

JACQUELINE WISNER, M.D.

Departments of Medicine, Microbiology, and
Immunology
Michael Reese Hospital and Medical Center
The University of Illinois and the University of
Chicago
Chicago, Illinois

PREFACE

The goals of this book have changed little since its first publication in 1958, edited in collaboration with the late Dr. Robert Ward. The preface to that initial edition stated that "the purpose of this book is to provide a concise and handy description of certain common infectious diseases of children. It is written primarily for pediatricians, general practitioners, and medical students who deal with children." We have resisted strenuously the temptation to enlarge the volume to become an encyclopedia covering extensively all aspects of all infectious diseases. This is done very well by a number of other more voluminous textbooks. Our goal has been to maintain this book as a handy, concise, practical reference used readily in the office, in the clinic, in the emergency room, and in the ward library.

This ninth edition has seen an augmentation of the numbers of contributors and authors. The four editors of the eighth edition have enlisted the support of talented colleagues who have brought their personal knowledge and experience to new chapters and to revisions of older ones. Infections caused by *Haemophilus influenzae* have merited the designation of a separate chapter as we enter a phase of successful immunization and the anticipation that invasive disease caused by this virulent organism may in the next few years become as rare in highly immunized populations as polio has become since the early editions of this textbook. Although it has not been proven that Kawasaki syndrome is an infectious disease, its epidemiology and clinical manifestations warrant its tentative inclusion under this rubric and therefore a new chapter has been added. We have always included rickettsial diseases among our topics, but the most prevalent tick-borne infection in recent years has become Lyme disease, which is now included with the rickettsial diseases in a new chapter on tick-borne infections.

In addition to acquired immunodeficiency syndrome (AIDS), which found its way for the first time into our eighth edition, the rapidly increasing numbers of children who are immunocompromised by other illnesses, medications, or suppression for the acceptance of organ or bone marrow transplants has prompted us to include a new chapter on infections in immunocompromised children. Although erythema infectiosum (fifth disease) had earned a few pages in previous editions, the great expansion in our knowledge of parvovirus B-19 and its effects has resulted in an expanded chapter including the new information relating to arthritis, aplastic crises in patients with chronic hemolytic anemias, and transmission of infection to the fetus. The virus responsible for roseola infantum (exanthem subitum) has been identified as human herpesvirus type 6 (HHV-6). New agents and new mechanisms of pathogenesis have been discovered for gastroenteritis. Viral hepatitis has been expanded with the identification of hepatitis virus C and E. To cover all the agents currently classified under the rubric "sexually transmitted diseases" (STD) is a monumental task that has been redone for this edition.

The foregoing as well as other additions and revisions have been integrated into the text to make it as current as possible at the time of publication. The cooperation of the publishers in bringing the book to press in a relatively short span is deeply appreciated by the authors and will be enormously helpful to the readers. Nevertheless, there will undoubtedly be new developments that emerge even in that hiatus of a few months, so the well-informed reader will continue to use this text as a base for clinical problem-solving but look beyond to journals and consultants for information not yet "in press." The editors remain deeply grateful to their respected colleagues who have added so much to this ninth edition.

Saul Krugman, M.D.
Samuel L. Katz, M.D.
Anne A. Gershon, M.D.
Catherine M. Wilfert, M.D.

CONTENTS

COLOR PLATES

1

ACQUIRED IMMUNODEFICIENCY SYNDROME

WILLIAM BORKOWSKY
CATHERINE M. WILFERT

An outbreak of community-acquired *Pneumocystis carinii* pneumonia (PCP) was recognized in California and New York in 1980. Simultaneously, Kaposi's sarcoma occurred at 50 times the expected rate in male homosexuals. These events combined to define an immunodeficiency syndrome never before described. In addition, this syndrome soon was observed in intravenous drug users, recipients of standard blood products (both male and female), and non-drug-using female sex partners of individuals with the disease.

In 1982 an "acquired immunodeficiency syndrome (AIDS)" was recognized in children (Centers for Disease Control, 1982) and was described in New Jersey (Oleske et al., 1983), New York (Rubinstein et al., 1983), San Francisco (Ammann et al., 1983), and Miami (Scott et al., 1984). By 1987 AIDS had become the ninth leading cause of death for children between the ages of 1 and 4 years in the United States (Kilbourne, Buehler, and Rogers, 1990) and the third leading cause of death for black children and Hispanic children of this age in New York and New Jersey. The total number of cases of AIDS in children less than 13 years of age reported to the Centers for Disease Control (CDC) by the end of 1990 exceeded 2500. It is estimated that five to 10 times as many children may be infected by the agent that causes AIDS but have not yet fulfilled the clinical criteria established by the CDC for reporting the disease. AIDS has also become the seventh leading cause of death for adolescents and young adults (ages 15 to 24 years). It in-

creased 100-fold between 1981 and 1987 (The Final Report of the Secretary's Work Group, 1988), and it is anticipated that this infection will be the leading cause of death for these populations by 1991. The most rapid increase in acquisition of human immunodeficiency virus infection is occurring in persons reporting that their risk behavior is heterosexual contact with an infected person. In 1989 as compared to 1988, a 36% increase in AIDS attributable to heterosexual transmission occurred (Oxtoby, 1991). In the same year an increase of 38% in reported pediatric AIDS cases occurred (Oxtoby, 1991; Fig. 1-1). Thus the acquisition of infection by heterosexual contact is reflected in the occurrence of AIDS in children who have acquired infection perinatally.

In less than a decade a previously unknown disease has ascended to become the single most important communicable disease in the United States and many other nations. Although pediatric HIV infection comprises only 2% of the total number of reported cases of AIDS in the United States, the rapid increase in reported cases in children and its emergence as a cause of death in young infants and children is clear.

ETIOLOGY

The causative agents of AIDS were isolated from the blood of patients and were described in both France (Barre-Sinoussi et al., 1983) and the United States (Gallo et al., 1984; Levy et al., 1984). They were referred to as the *lymphadenopathy-associated viruses (LAV)*, the *hu-*

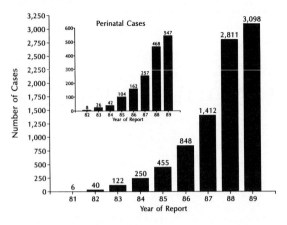

Fig. 1-1. AIDS in women of reproductive age (15 to 44 years) compared to perinatally acquired AIDS in children by year of report in United States through December 1989. (From Oxtoby MJ: In Pizzo P, Wilfert CM, editors. Pediatric AIDS. Baltimore: Williams & Wilkins, 1991.)

man T cell lymphotrophic viruses (HTLV-III), and the AIDS-related retroviruses (ARV) by the respective groups. By consensus, these agents now are termed the *human immunodeficiency viruses (HIVs)*. These enveloped RNA viruses are in the lentivirus subfamily of retroviruses and are 80 to 120 nm in diameter. Characteristics of HIV that resemble those of lentiviruses include (1) the long incubation period; (2) the ability to establish latent or persistent infection; (3) the ability to produce immune suppression; (4) tropism to lymphoid cells, particularly macrophages; (5) the ability to affect the hematopoietic system; (6) tropism to the central nervous system (CNS); and (7) the ability to produce cytopathic effects observed in appropriate cell types (Bryant and Ratner, 1991). The major targets of HIV include CD4-antigen–bearing cells, including helper T cells, monocytes and macrophages, Langerhans' cells, and glial cells of the CNS. HIV has also been reported as capable of infecting non-CD4–bearing cells such as enterocytes and certain neuronal cells.

HIV has a cylindrical eccentric core, or nucleoid, that contains the diploid RNA genome (Fig. 1-2). A nucleic acid–binding protein and reverse transcriptase are associated with the genome. Nucleocapsid structure is completed by the capsid antigen (p24), which encloses the nucleoid components. Surrounding the core of the virus is p17, the matrix antigen, which lines the

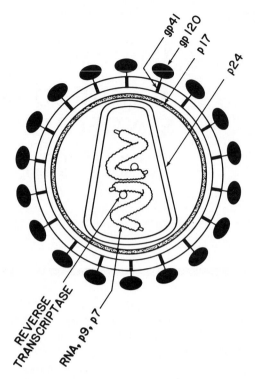

Fig. 1-2. Schematic representation of the morphological structure of HIV-1. ENV gene products, gp120 and gp41; gag gene products, p24, p17, p9, and p7; pol gene product, RT.

inner surface of the envelope. Knoblike projections formed by the envelope glycoprotein, gp120, are on the surface of the virus. An associated intermembranous portion of envelope, gp41, anchors the gp120 component. The lipid bilayer of the viral particle is derived from the host cell plasma membrane as the virus buds from the cell. A portion of the gp120 domain of the envelope binds to the CD4 molecule of human cells with high affinity, and a segment of the gp41 plays a crucial role in the fusion of the viral envelope with the host cell (Fig. 1-3).

After viral entry and uncoating, the reverse transcriptase characteristic of all retroviruses produces double-stranded virally encoded DNA that enters the nucleus and integrates randomly in the host genome by using the long-terminal-repeat (LTR) segments that flank the other genes of the virus. The virus is then in a latent state in which it may remain indefinitely. A variety of stimuli, including antigens, mitogens, ultraviolet light, heat shock, hypoxia, and proteins derived from other viruses, are capable of ini-

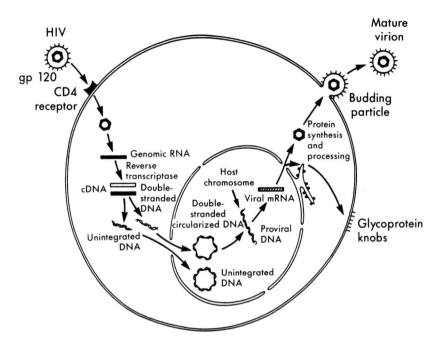

Fig. 1-3. The life cycle of the human immunodeficiency virus. (From Pizzo P, Wilfert CM, editors. Pediatric AIDS. Baltimore: Williams & Wilkins, 1991.)

tiating the transcription of HIV messenger RNA, which is first translated into complex spliced messages. These encode a group of regulatory molecules that ultimately govern the production of HIV messenger RNA capable of producing full-length transcripts and the associated structural proteins. The ribonucleoprotein core buds from the cellular membrane and acquires a coat of viral envelope glycoprotein and the lipid bilayer from the host cell. A viral enzyme (protease) completes the maturation of the virion by cleaving specific internal core components.

The individual isolates of HIV-1 from different persons vary a great deal. There is also considerable variation between sequential isolates obtained from the same person. HIV can spread from cell to cell independent of release of virus from the cell. This spread may occur through the fusion or syncytial formation of an infected cell with uninfected cell(s).

PATHOGENESIS

HIV infection in children is characterized by an incubation period or asymptomatic interval that is much shorter than it is in adults. The inevitable consequence of infection with the HIV is profound immunosuppression, which leaves the host susceptible to the development of infections and neoplasms.

T4 cells

The depletion of helper T cells (CD4) in symptomatic patients has been noted since 1981. HIV is capable of causing a profound cytopathic affect in T4 cells in vitro. However, only a small proportion of cells are infected with the virus, and not all are killed. Uninfected cells also die or are dysfunctional, perhaps mediated by the binding of gp120 to CD4 and thus interfering in its essential association with major histocompatibility complex (MHC) class II molecules. The virus is capable of establishing latency or a low level of replication in some cells.

T4 cell depletion is due in part to direct virus-induced damage, and there is some indication that "memory" helper T cells are more selectively depleted than "virgin" cells. The budding of large numbers of virus particles disrupting the external cell membrane contributes to destruction of the cell by creating osmotic disequilibrium. HIV replication results in the accumulation of a number of foreign products, including viral DNA, RNA, and core proteins, which may interfere with normal cellular function and contribute to death of the cell. Syncytia or multi-nucleated giant cells are observed in vitro with HIV replication. Such syncytia can form when CD4 molecules of uninfected T4 cells bind to the gp120 expressed on the surface of HIV-infected T4 cells. It is unknown whether syncytial formation contributes to cell death.

The functional abnormalities of T4 cells from HIV-infected individuals are numerous despite the fact that the virus is present in only a small percentage of circulating T4 cells. These abnormalities include (1) defective helper interaction with B cells for immunoglobulin production; (2) defective proliferative responses to antigenic stimuli; (3) diminished expression of interleukin (IL-2) receptors; and (4) defective lymphokine production in response to antigenic stimuli, particularly of IL-2 and gamma interferon. These defects would be expected to predispose infected persons to infections with intracellular pathogens.

In the course of a normal immune response the CD4 molecule binds to the class II MHC molecules on the surface of an antigen-presenting immune cell. However, the CD4 molecule binds to gp120 of HIV with a greater affinity than for its normal ligand (class II MHC molecules). This high-affinity binding of gp120 to CD4 may contribute to the impaired T-cell responses and may also be the basis of autoimmune reactions destroying T4 cells. The gp41 of the virus possesses a region of homology with the class II MHC molecule. Anti-gp41 HIV antibodies from AIDS patients can react with class II MHC antigens and may therefore be involved in cytotoxicity or complement-mediated cell killing of uninfected target cells carrying only the class II MHC molecule.

Antibody-dependent cellular cytotoxicity (ADCC) may contribute to cell death of both infected cells and uninfected cells. If an uninfected T4 cell binds free gp120 to its surface, the cell can be mistakenly identified as infected and subsequently be destroyed by ADCC or by gp120-specific, CD4-positive cytotoxic T cells.

Monocyte and macrophage

HIV also infects cells of the monocyte-macrophage lineage. The virus is not cytopathic to these cells but may interfere in their ability to present antigens to helper T cells. Intact virus particles may replicate to high numbers in these cells and may also be disseminated to tissues such as the brain, spinal cord, lung, bone marrow, liver, heart, and gut where soluble virus products may produce organ dysfunction. Alternatively, the virus may be borne to tissues wherein they replicate directly, thereby producing cell damage. These infected cells may also produce increased quantities of IL-1, IL-6, prostaglandins, and other molecules that may affect adjacent cell functions.

B cells

Spontaneously infected B cells have not been observed in vivo, although some B lymphocytes bear CD4 on their surface and can be infected in vitro. Nevertheless, HIV infection results in profound effects on B cell function. In vitro the HIV envelope has induced polyclonal B cell activation (Pahwa et al., 1985). It may also produce increased IL-6 production by other cells with resulting hypergammaglobulinemia. In spite of the observed hypergammaglobulinemia that commonly is seen, both primary and secondary antibody responses to some antigens may be impaired (Bernstein et al., 1985), contributing to the high incidence of infection with common bacterial pathogens. The B-cell impairment often is observed in association with impaired T-cell responses to the same antigens (Borkowsky et al., 1987), and these findings are correlated with a poorer clinical outcome (Blanche et al., 1986).

Although neutrophils are not directly infected by HIV, autoimmune neutropenias have been observed, and neutrophil dysfunction has been described (Roilides et al., 1990). This defect may contribute to the immunodeficiency-related infections that occur.

PATHOLOGY

The primary pathological effects of HIV infection are seen in the lymphoreticular system in which marked cell depletion is the end-stage pathology. HIV probably infects the epithelial cells of the thymus, and thymitis has been described. This initial inflammatory response is characterized by multinucleated giant cells in the medulla of the thymus or by diffuse lymphoplasmocytic or lymphomononuclear infiltrates of the cortex and medulla. These changes precede the involution noted in end-stage disease. The involution is characterized by depletion of lymphocytes, loss of corticomedullary differentiation, and microcystic dilation of Hassall's corpuscles (Joshi, 1991). In a few instances a reduction of Hassall's corpuscles has also been described, and this constellation is termed *dysinvolution*. The severe effects of the virus on the thymus of the young infant or fetus may contribute to the more rapid progression of the immunological compromise. It is likely that thymic dysfunction continues to contribute to illness in adult life.

Lymphoproliferation in lymph nodes, the gastrointestinal tract, and lungs is seen. Multinucleated giant cells are present. Late in the disease, lymph nodes are depleted of lymphocytes in the paracortex, ultimately progressing to marked lymphocyte depletion of the entire lymph node. Atrophic changes of the spleen, appendix, and Peyer's patches are also described in late stages. The pathological features in the brain include atrophy, sclerosis, microglial nodules, and necrosis with or without an inflammatory cell infiltrate, loss of myelin, vasculitis, and calcification of vessels and basal ganglia (Sharer, Cho, and Epstein, 1985; Sharer et al., 1986). The virus has been localized by in situ hybridization in macrophages, microglia, and giant cells and less frequently in glial cells and neurons (Shaw et al., 1985; Stoler et al., 1986). Opportunistic infections and malignancies of the CNS are infrequently seen in children.

Pathological findings associated with a broad spectrum of infectious agents, including *P. carinii* in the lungs, *Candida* of the mucous membranes, *Mycobacterium avium-intracellulare* of almost all tissues, and cryptosporidia of the gastrointestinal tract, are seen in biopsy and autopsy specimens. Viruses that are common causes of infection include herpes simplex, cytomegalovirus, Epstein-Barr virus, and varicella-zoster virus (VZV).

Other findings of undetermined pathogenesis appear frequently in tissue examinations. Dilated cardiomyopathy is observed with microscopic hypertrophy of myocardial fibers, focal vacuolation, interstitial edema, small foci of fibrosis, and endocardial thickening. Unusually sparse inflammatory infiltrates are seen.

Clinically important renal disease is accompanied by microscopic findings of focal segmental glomerulosclerosis and mesangial proliferative glomerulonephritis (Connor et al., 1988).

Immunoglobulin and complement deposits are evident by immunofluorescence. It is speculated that circulating immune complexes may be contributing to the pathogenesis of the renal disease. P24 antigen has been demonstrated by in situ hybridization in tubular and glomerular epithelial cells in renal biopsy specimens of adults.

A variety of neoplastic disorders, including lymphoma, Kaposi's sarcoma (rarely), and leiomyosarcoma of the gastrointestinal tract, have been described. Longer survival of children may result in more frequent occurrence of malignancies.

Pathological studies of placentas are relevant because most pediatric HIV infection is acquired by maternal-to-infant transmission. Studies in Africa demonstrated chorioamnionitis in placentas of women who delivered infected babies. These women had more advanced disease, and it is not possible to determine whether this inflammatory response is a result of secondary infections or a direct consequence of the severity of the HIV infection. The detection of HIV in the placenta does not predict whether an infant has acquired infection. Recovering HIV from placental tissue has been difficult, but HIV has been found in placentas by in situ hybridization (Chandwani, 1991) and by the polymerase chain reaction (PCR) (Andiman and Modlin, 1991). HIV has been demonstrated in placental macrophages (Hofbauer cells) in fetal villi. These cells could serve either as a barrier to HIV or as a means of fetal HIV infection.

LABORATORY DIAGNOSIS

Antibody to HIV can be measured accurately and is the mainstay of laboratory diagnosis of HIV infection in adults, in children perinatally infected who are more than 15 months of age, and in children of any age who have acquired HIV infection through transfusion or blood products. Enzyme-linked immunosorbent assay (ELISA) and Western blot assays measure antibodies to the major structural proteins or antigens of the virus and are commercially available. A positive ELISA must be confirmed by a second determination plus a positive Western blot assay on the same specimen to reduce the rate of false positives to approximately 1 in 100,000.

Since all newborns receive maternal antibodies during the latter part of pregnancy through the placenta, any infant born to a mother with antibodies to HIV will also test positive, regardless of whether actually infected with HIV. The titer of maternal antibodies is often in the range of several million. Since the half-life of IgG1, the predominant maternally transmitted immunoglobulin, is approximately 3 to 4 weeks, maternally derived anti-HIV antibody may persist for up to 15 or more months. Consequently, the standard antibody assays for HIV may be misleading for the diagnosis of HIV infection in the infant less than 18 months of age.

Assays that measure IgM, IgA, and IgG4 subclass HIV-specific antibodies are currently in development and may facilitate the serological diagnosis of HIV infection in young infants between 2 months and 1 year of age. The specific IgA antibody tests hold the most promise and may be useful for infants from 2 to 6 months of age.

HIV can be grown in tissue culture from the majority of HIV-infected adults and children. HIV is detected in peripheral blood mononuclear cells and as cell-free virus in plasma and cerebrospinal fluid. These cultures may prove positive as early as 3 days after initiation but may require as much as 4 to 6 weeks for the diagnosis of low levels of virus. Early experience with attempts to isolate HIV from newborn or cord-blood lymphocytes suggests that no more than half of infected children will be culture positive for HIV at this early period. The HIV recovery rate increases substantially during the ensuing months, and almost all can be diagnosed by culture within the first 6 months of life.

HIV core (p24) antigen can be detected in body fluids by ELISA. This antigen appears early after HIV infection and then often becomes undetectable, associated with the appearance of anti-p24 antibody in most infected adults. The antigen reappears as the HIV infection progresses and can be found with increasing frequency in more symptomatic individuals. This antigen can be found in more than half of HIV-infected infants during the first year of life but in substantially fewer babies during the first months of life and in only 10% of infected newborns (Borkowsky et al., 1989). The measurement of p24 antigen may also help identify the 10% of HIV-infected hypogammaglobulinemic children who are anti-HIV ELISA negative (Borkowsky et al., 1987).

One of the most promising diagnostic techniques is the polymerase chain reaction (PCR). PCR is the method by which the viral DNA can be amplified a million times. Virus culture and PCR detection of virus DNA in infant blood appear to be equally sensitive as tests to diagnose infection of the infant. The CDC, in collaboration with the New York City Department of Health and several New York hospitals, has reported an evaluation of the use of PCR in early diagnosis of infection in infants born to HIV-infected mothers (Rogers et al., 1989). Eight of 20 infants who ultimately met the CDC definition of HIV infection had detectable HIV DNA in the neonatal period. Eleven infants developed CDC-defined AIDS in the first 1½ years of life, and seven of these 11 had been found positive by PCR in the newborn period. Twenty of the 22 infected infants had positive PCR for HIV by 6 months of age.

PCR can be used to evaluate infants who have catabolized maternal antibody. In the studies from the CDC, infants who lost maternal antibody and remained antibody negative were repeatedly PCR negative. The technical problems with PCR relate to the extreme sensitivity of the test. If there is the smallest amount of contaminating DNA in the material tested, it can be amplified and give either ambiguous or false-positive results. The test can be completed in 1 to 2 days.

Other nonspecific laboratory parameters that may be helpful in the diagnosis of infection include immunological measurements. The classic hallmark of infection is a low CD4 cell count and an altered CD4:CD8 ratio. Age-appropriate normal values must be used for comparison (Table 1-1). Elevated serum immunoglobulin levels are characteristic of infection. A minority (approximately 10%) of children may have hypogammaglobulinemia.

Other promising assays for detection of infant infection use the measurement of antibody production by the infant. Several approaches to measure infant production of antibody have been used. Peripheral blood lymphocytes have been harvested and stimulated with pokeweed mitogen or Epstein-Barr virus and the supernatant fluids tested for the production of specific HIV antibody. Alternatively, peripheral blood mononuclear cells have been placed into cell culture wells containing HIV antigens. Using labeled antihuman globulin, the cells producing

Table 1-1. Age-adjusted CD4+ lymphocyte parameters for normal, healthy children and adults

	Age				
	1-6 mo.	*7-12 mo.*	*13-24 mo.*	*25-74 mo.*	*Adults*
Number tested	106	28	46	29	327
Absolute CD4+ count					
Median (cells/mm³)	3211	3128	2601	1668	1027
5-95 percentile (cells/mm³)	1153-5285	967-5289	739-4463	505-2831	237-1817
Percentage CD4+ cells					
Median (%)	51.6	47.9	45.8	42.1	50.9
5-95 percentile (%)	36.3-67.1	32.8-63.0	31.2-60.4	32.2-52.0	34.7-67.1
CD4:CD8 ratio					
Median	2.2	2.1	2.0	1.4	1.7
5-95 percentile	0.9-3.5	0.8-3.4	0.6-3.4	0.7-2.1	0.4-3.0

From MMWR 1991; 40:1-13 (March 15).

antibody will be identified by "spots" in the wells. Maternal IgA antibody does not cross the placenta, so the presence of HIV-specific antibody of this subclass describes an infant who is infected. Detection of specific IgA antibody is being evaluated as a means of making an early diagnosis of HIV infection in young infants, and it has been demonstrated by 6 months of age in cohorts of infected infants.

In summary, despite the advances in diagnostic methodology, accurate detection of the infected infant requires continued evaluation.

EPIDEMIOLOGY AND NATURAL HISTORY

More than 215,000 cases of AIDS had been reported to the World Health Organization as of January 31, 1990. More than half the cases were reported from the United States alone. However, in some African and Caribbean cities 5% to 20% of pregnant women are HIV seropositive. Bidirectional heterosexual transmission has been well documented. Unfortunately, studies have been too small to compare the relative efficiency of transmission from men to women vs. women to men. The reported rates of infection in sexual partners are given in Table 1-2.

Sexual transmission is the major mode of spread of HIV-1 infection in most developing countries. The role of heterosexual transmission is steadily increasing in the United States. Peri-

Table 1-2. Reported rates of HIV infection of sexual partners

Partner	Acquisition rate by female partner (%)	Acquisition rate by male partner (%)
Hemophiliac	9.2	NA
Bisexual	26.0	NA
Transfusion recipient	19.7	14.8
Intravenous drug user	47.8	50.0

From Quinn TC, Ruff A, Halsey N: In Pizzo P, Wilfert C, editors. Pediatric AIDS. Baltimore: Williams & Wilkins, 1991.

natal transmission parallels the heterosexual transmission because a substantial proportion of these infected persons are women of reproductive age. The male-to-female ratio of reported AIDS approaches 1 when heterosexual transmission of infection predominates, and the percentage of pediatric AIDS cases increases dramatically (Table 1-3) with this ratio.

The CDC has been responsible for conducting a comprehensive series of blinded HIV seroprevalence surveys performed on heel-stick samples from newborns. As of October 1990, the highest seroprevalence rates were in the District of Columbia (0.97%), New York State (0.66%)— with a rate of 1.25% in New York City, New

Table 1-3. Reported pediatric AIDS in relation to reported male:female ratios of AIDS

Country	Male:female ratio	Pediatric cases (%)
Bahamas	1.8	19
French Guiana	1.5	15
Jamaica	3.1	12
Haiti	2.3	6
Trinidad	4.6	6
Brazil	11.1	4
United States	10.7	2

From Quinn TC, Ruff A, Halsey N: In Pizzo P, Wilfert CM, editors. Pediatric AIDS. Baltimore: Williams & Wilkins, 1991.

Jersey (0.49%), and Florida (0.49%) (Oxtoby, 1991). A number of Southeastern states, including North Carolina, Tennessee, Georgia, Louisiana, and Texas, had seroprevalence rates of 0.5 to 1.9 per 1,000 women. These data suggest that the Southeast is an area with increasing seroprevalence rates in women, and the geographical distribution of HIV infection has continued to enlarge.

The risk factors associated with the development of AIDS among women are also risk factors for the transmission of AIDS to infants and children. They include (1) intravenous drug use, which is an admitted risk behavior in 50% of infected women in the United States; (2) heterosexual contact with a person who is HIV infected, which is the risk behavior for 40% of infected women in the United States (two thirds of the partners are admitted intravenous drug users; sexual exposure in prepubertal children may occur in the context of childhood sexual abuse [Gutman et al., 1991]); and (3) receiving blood products (whole blood and its components, including clotting factor concentrates). Although the screening of blood products for HIV antibody as of May 1984 has largely eliminated any transmission of HIV by blood products in the United States, such transmission continues to plague developing countries and countries such as Russia and Romania.

In the United States a reported 59% of pediatric perinatally acquired AIDS cases are among black children, and 26% are among Hispanic children, a rate 21 and 13 times that in white children, respectively (Oxtoby, 1991). Minority populations are disproportionately infected. In the U.S. population lower socioeconomic status is also disproportionately represented.

Perinatal infection

Approximately 87% of all AIDS reported in children less than 13 years of age is attributed to perinatally acquired infection. The principal risk factor for pediatric HIV infection is having a mother with HIV infection.

It is unknown whether HIV infection is transmitted predominantly in utero or during parturition. HIV transmission probably can occur by more than one mechanism. There is evidence that in utero infection occurs, based on the recovery of HIV in cell culture from fetuses that have been aborted between 9 and 20 weeks of gestation (Sprecher et al., 1986; Kashkin et al., 1988; Jovais et al., 1985; DiMaria et al., 1986). These and other observations suggest that a portion of the cohort found to be infected perinatally is infected in utero. Nevertheless, virtually all newborns of HIV-infected mothers are born without obvious signs of clinical or immunological abnormalities. Studies performed worldwide have found that 15% to 30% of children born to infected women will prove to be infected with HIV, even in the absence of breast-feeding. Yet half of this group cannot be shown to have evidence of HIV infection at birth using current virological, immunological, and molecular biological techniques. Thus it remains likely that some HIV transmission is occurring at the time of parturition, similar to that of the model of hepatitis B transmission.

Data suggest that maternal HIV infection results in lower birth weights for infants born to these women. Many of the studies have been complicated by the high rate of drug use in HIV-I seropositive women, and infants born to cocaine- or heroin-using women have significantly lower birth weights and higher mortality rates than non-drug-using women (Selwyn et al., 1989). Studies in developing nations have been free of the confounding effects of drug use, but women having babies in these nations have more advanced disease. In both Africa and Haiti the birth weights of infants born to HIV-I–seropositive women are significantly lower than the birth weights of infants born to seronegative women (Ryder et al., 1989; Halsey et al., 1990). In addition, the mortality rates in both Africa and Haiti are higher in infants born to seropositive women. This may be due to an increased exposure to other infectious agents and/or to decreased accessibility of medical care. Mortality rates in infants born to HIV-negative women are substantially higher in these areas than in developed nations, and it is apparent that HIV and AIDS are increasing the overall perinatal mortality rate.

Several recent reports (Devash et al., 1990; Goedeart et al., 1989; Rossi, 1989) have suggested that the frequency of perinatal HIV transmission is decreased in those women who have antibodies directed at gp120. More specifically, women with antibody (particularly of "high affinity") to the third variable region (V3 loop) of the HIV envelope were far less likely to transmit HIV to their offspring. Unfortunately there has been a great deal of disagreement about the actual site recognized by these antibodies. There have also been discrepant findings when shared sera were analyzed by these and independent investigators. Thus continued study of a role for maternal antibody in altering transmission of virus to the infant is essential.

The majority of infected children become symptomatic during the first 6 months of life, with the development of lymphadenopathy as the initial finding. Some HIV-infected children will develop a severe failure to thrive and/or encephalopathy during their first year of life. A recent prospective study confirms estimates that 80% of infected infants developed clinical disease within 24 months of birth (Hutto et al., 1991).

Children who survive the first year of life are likely to develop one or several of the HIV-related syndromes that may not be recognized as associated with HIV by the treating physician.

Transfusion and coagulation factor acquired disease

Approximately one half (or 10,000) of the persons with hemophilia are seen regularly in treatment facilities. The largest cohort study reported to date indicates that the prevalence of HIV antibodies in those with severe factor VIII deficiency is 76.5%, in those with moderate dis-

ease, 46.3%, and in those with mild disease, 25.4% (Eyster, 1991). In a smaller population of persons with Christmas disease (factor IX deficiency) the prevalence is 41.9% in those with severe disease, 26.9% in those with moderate disease, and 8.3% in those with mild disease (Eyster, 1991). The cumulative 8-year AIDS incidence is 13.3% ($\pm$5.3%) when the HIV infection was acquired between the ages of 1 and 17 years. The cumulative 8-year incidence is 26.8% ($\pm$6.4%) when infection was acquired between ages 18 and 34 and 43.7% ($\pm$16.4%) when infection was acquired between ages 35 and 70 (Goedeart et al., 1989).

For children who acquire infection by transfusion, the incubation period is uncertain. It has been estimated that the median incubation period is at least 41 months for those children acquiring infection before the age of 13 years (Eyster, 1991).

Adolescents

The absolute number of cases of AIDS among adolescents 13 to 19 years of age is smaller than that reported in children less than 13 years of age, but this number underestimates acquisition of this infection in teenagers. The incubation period is sufficiently long that adolescents who have acquired infection may not become ill until an older age (i.e., in their twenties and thirties). The steady rate of increase of reported AIDS in adolescents has paralleled that recorded in adults and children.

Eighty percent of the total number of adolescents with AIDS are male (Gayle and D'Angelo, 1991). However, the cumulative male-to-female ratio has declined from 4:1 to 3:1. This reflects an 80% increase in the number of female cases reported between 1987 and 1988 (Gayle and D'Angelo, 1991). Black and Hispanic adolescents are disproportionately represented among persons with AIDS. These populations represent only 14% and 8%, respectively, of the 1980 U.S. population between the ages of 13 and 19 years, but 36% of adolescents with AIDS are black, and 18% are Hispanic (Gayle and D'Angelo, 1991).

Transmission in adolescents results from transmission by the same routes as for adults. Initially, the largest proportion of reported adolescent AIDS cases were comprised of those

AIDS-INDICATIVE DIAGNOSES IN THE 1987 CDC REVISED SURVEILLANCE DEFINITION FOR AIDS

Multiple or recurrent bacterial infections*

Candidiasis of the trachea, bronchi, or lungs*

Candidiasis of the esophagus†‡

Coccidioidomycosis, disseminated or extrapulmonary*

Cryptococcosis, extrapulmonary†

Cryptosporidiosis, chronic intestinal†

Cytomegalovirus disease (other than liver, spleen, nodes) onset at >1 month of age†

Cytomegalovirus retinitis (with loss of vision)†‡

HIV encephalopathy*

Chronic herpes simplex ulcer (>1 month duration) or pneumonitis or esophagitis, onset at >1 month of age†

Histoplasmosis, disseminated or extrapulmonary*

Isosporiasis, chronic intestinal (>1 month duration)*

Kaposi's sarcoma†‡

Lymphoid interstitial pneumonitis†‡

Lymphoma, primary brain†

Lymphoma (Burkitt's or immunoblastic sarcoma)*

Mycobacterium avium complex or *Mycobacterium kansasii*, disseminated or extrapulmonary†

Mycobacterium tuberculosis or acid-fast infection (species not identified), disseminated or extrapulmonary*

Pneumocystis carinii pneumonia†‡

Progressive multifocal leukoencephalopathy†

Toxoplasmosis of brain, onset at >1 month of age†‡

Wasting syndrome caused by HIV*

From MMWR 1987; 36:225-230, 235.

* Requires laboratory evidence of HIV infection (1987 addition).

† If indicator disease is diagnosed definitively (e.g., by biopsy or culture) and there is no other cause of immunodeficiency, laboratory documentation of HIV infection is not required.

‡ Presumptive diagnosis of indicator disease is accepted if there is laboratory evidence of HIV infection (1987 addition).

mm^3 have been observed in 90% of reported cases of PCP younger than 12 months (CDC, 1991). PCP occurs in children 1 to 2 years old when CD4 counts are <750/mm^3 and in children 2 to 6 years old when CD4 counts are <500/mm^3. These values reflect the higher numbers of CD4 cells normally present in young children. Thus prophylaxis for PCP can be empirically based on the CD4 values (see Treatment).

In children multiple or recurrent serious bacterial infections are included as a prominent manifestation of AIDS. Two or more serious infections in a 2-year period meet the case definition of AIDS in a young HIV-seropositive infant. When AIDS was first identified in children, bacteremia appeared to occur in almost half of the children who were diagnosed. More recent estimates of the frequency of bacteremia suggest that it occurs less frequently. This decrease may in part be attributable to the ability to diagnose HIV infection before such severe complications bring a child to medical attention. Children less than 2 years old have an evolving ability to identify polysaccharide antigens. Thus even normal infants are susceptible to pathogens such as pneumococcus and *Haemophilus influenzae* type b. Children with HIV infection are just as susceptible, and with their compromised immune system, susceptibility is prolonged. Hypergammaglobulinemia is a common development in children with HIV infection because of polyclonal activation of B cells. These antibodies are largely nonspecific, and children do not recognize antigens or respond well as their disease progresses. Thus elevated IgG levels in these children indicate an abnormal host and one that is functionally antibody deficient.

The major bacterial diseases in HIV-infected children are bacteremia and sepsis, but meningitis, cellulitis, wound infection, gastroenteritis, and pneumonia also occur frequently. A primary focus of infection is not uniformly identified in bacteremic children; more than half may have no known focus. Several reports (Krasinski et al., 1988; Bernstein et al., 1985) have indicated that *Streptococcus pneumoniae* is the most common pathogen in bacteremic disease and is reported in approximately 30% of infections. A recent National Institute of Child Health and Human Development (NICHD) study has estimated that pneumococcal bacteremia in untreated symptomatic patients occurs at a rate of 37 per 1,000 patients per year. Infections with *Haemophilus influenzae*, *Salmonella* species, staphylococci, and a variety of other encapsulated organisms have been reported. Unfortunately, many of these children have had community- and hospital-acquired gram-negative bacteremias.

Upper respiratory infections, including sinusitis and otitis media, are very common. Recurrent episodes of these infections are frequent sources of chronic fever and require vigorous antibiotic therapy. Chronic sinusitis may require prolonged intravenous antibiotic therapy or aggressive surgical drainage.

Chronic pneumonitis

Lymphoid interstitial pneumonitis (LIP), or pulmonary lymphoid hyperplasia, is a common occurrence and was reported in 28% of children with AIDS in 1988 and 1989. LIP usually is diagnosed in children with perinatally acquired HIV infection who are more than 1 year of age. It often begins as an asymptomatic pulmonary infiltrate but can progress to severe pulmonary compromise with superimposed complications of disease such as pneumonia or congestive heart failure. The chronic illness and hypoxemia can be similar to that with chronic bronchiectasis. Children with LIP tend to have a longer survival time than children with PCP or encephalopathy. The entity frequently is associated with parotitis, hypergammaglobulinemia, and lymphadenopathy. A possible adult equivalent of LIP has been described and appears to occur exclusively in individuals with a particular HLA class II haplotype (Itescu et al., 1989).

Encephalopathy and myelopathy

CNS involvement is frequent in children with HIV infection. Studies reporting children with advanced HIV disease suggest that up to 60% of them will have neurological manifestations (Belman et al., 1988; Epstein et al., 1986). Approximately 40% of the children may develop progressive encephalopathy, resulting in the loss of developmental milestones or subcortical dementia. Other neurological findings include impaired brain growth, generalized weakness with pyramidal signs, pseudobulbar palsy, ataxia, seizures, myoclonus, and extrapyramidal rigidity. However, some preliminary natural history studies suggest that progressive encephalopathy may be present in a smaller proportion (i.e., 9% to 20%) of children (European Collaborative Study, 1988; Blanche et al., 1989; Mok et al., 1987). These children were observed to a mean

age of 18 months and included those with mild and asymptomatic disease. It has also been reported that approximately 25% of children have an encephalopathy that does not progress (Epstein et al., 1988). Although the manifestations of CNS involvement with HIV may vary considerably, it is agreed that the virus does infect the CNS and that the young infant with an immature CNS is uniquely susceptible to damage, resulting in an array of developmental deficits and neurological abnormalities such as spastic paraparesis.

In addition to the harmful effects of HIV infection per se on the CNS, HIV-infected children can develop additional CNS complications, including neoplasm, stroke, and infections with other pathogenic organisms.

Wasting syndrome and diarrhea

The gastrointestinal tract is also a source of invasive pathogens, and children with HIV infection sustain symptomatic infections with the common bacterial organisms such as *Salmonella*, *Shigella*, *Campylobacter*, and *Clostridium difficile*. *Salmonella* species occur more commonly than in normal children and cause invasive disease. Relapse of symptomatic illness has been reported. Adult studies have suggested that ceftriaxone may be more successful in eradicating *Salmonella* than more commonly used forms of therapy such as ampicillin or trimethoprim-sulfamethoxazole (Rolston et al., 1989).

Gastrointestinal tract infections with protozoal organisms are usually of short duration in normal persons. However, in persons with a compromised immune system such as children with AIDS, the clinical course often is protracted. *Cryptosporidium*, *Isospora belli*, *Giardia lamblia*, and *Microsporidium* infection have been reported in AIDS patients. Cryptosporidia are probably the most common parasitic causes of diarrhea in adult AIDS patients and have produced similar chronic disease, although less frequently, in children.

Failure to thrive, or the HIV wasting syndrome, may be due to a complex array of infectious agents, including HIV. HIV-infected adult patients have malabsorption even when no opportunistic infections are present. HIV infection can be associated with abnormal small bowel mucosa, and the histology varies from normal to villous atrophy with crypt hypoplasia. HIV RNA has been demonstrated in macrophages and lymphocytes in the lamina propria of intestinal biopsies (Fox et al., 1989; Nelson et al., 1988). A child may have acute diarrhea, chronic nonspecific diarrhea, and/or failure to thrive.

In addition to these problems, HIV-infected individuals apparently are in a hypermetabolic state, which probably increases normal caloric and fluid requirements.

Opportunistic infections

Opportunistic infections are a common complication in HIV-infected children but are somewhat different from those in adults. Oral *Candida* infection is extremely common in immunocompetent infants because they may acquire the organism as early as parturition. It is thought that 80% of infants are colonized by 4 weeks of age (Russell and Lay, 1973). It is estimated that 15% to 40% of children with HIV infection have oral candidiasis. In the normal child oral *Candida* infection is often mild and readily treated. *Candida* infection in children with HIV infection appears as oral mucosal candidiasis, gingivostomatitis, and periodontitis. Although it may respond initially to simple therapy such as oral nystatin solution, the hallmark of HIV infection is the persistence of *Candida*. Children are likely to have diminished numbers of CD4 cells at this time. This infection may extend to the esophagus and/or the larynx. Esophageal candidiasis is an indicator disease of AIDS, and it can occur without obvious oral pharyngeal candidiasis. Disseminated candidiasis is an unusual occurrence in HIV-infected children.

Infections with agents of the *Herpesvirus* group, including herpes simplex viruses, cytomegalovirus, and varicella-zoster virus (VZV), are among the reported manifestations of HIV infection in children. These are ubiquitous pathogens of children, and their ability to establish latency and the potential to induce severe infections in immunocompromised hosts are manifest as both severe and chronic infection in children with HIV infection.

Infection with both *Mycobacterium tuberculosis* and organisms of the *Mycobacterium avium-intracellulare* complex has increased dramatically because of the AIDS epidemic. The latter have been more numerous in adults with AIDS but are being appreciated with increasing frequency as the lives of children with HIV infection are prolonged.

Hematological syndromes

Although cervical lymphadenopathy is a very nonspecific sign, the presence of axillary and inguinal nodes in a young infant should arouse suspicion of HIV infection. Hepatosplenomegaly may accompany the lymphadenopathy. CD4+ cell numbers may remain normal at this time.

The most common abnormality is microcytic or normocytic anemia, which occurs even with elevated erythropoietin levels. Thrombocytopenia resulting from the clearance of immune-complex–coated platelets by the reticuloendothelial system occurs in approximately 10% of patients. This syndrome can be differentiated from idiopathic thrombocytopenic purpura (ITP) by the presence of complement on the platelet surface but may respond to standard therapies effective in treating ITP. Treatment with antiviral medications that inhibit HIV replication may be the treatment of choice for this disorder. Lupus anticoagulants are seen in HIV-infected adults and are probably also found in HIV-infected children.

Hepatitis syndrome

Liver transaminases and alkaline phosphatase are often elevated in HIV-infected children. Hyperbilirubinemia occurs infrequently. Although this hepatitis may be due to infection with secondary pathogens or may be a hypersensitivity reaction to drugs such as trimethoprim-sulfamethoxazole, it is often intrinsic to HIV infection alone. HIV can replicate in hepatoma cell lines and can be found in liver macrophages. Chronic hepatitis B infection is usually milder in HIV-infected immunocompromised individuals than in those not infected, reaffirming the belief that chronic active hepatitis is immunologically mediated.

Renal syndrome

Some children with HIV infection may present with a rapidly progressive glomerulopathy. Light microscopy demonstrates focal segmental glomerulosclerosis and mesangial glomerulonephritis (Connor et al., 1988). Immunoglobulin and complement deposits are evident by immunofluorescence. It is speculated that circulating immune complexes may contribute to the disease. HIV p24 antigen has been demonstrated by in situ hybridization in tubular and glomerular epithelial cells in renal biopsy specimens of adults. The increased production of IL-6, a lymphokine associated with other glomerulopathies, may also play a role in pathogenesis.

Cardiac syndrome

Abnormalities, including poor myocardial contractility, may occur early in children with HIV disease without obvious clinical consequences. The progression of this disease and the occurrence of myocarditis, pericardial effusion, and the effects of LIP on function of the right side of the heart may ultimately produce congestive heart failure. Secondary agents such as cytomegalovirus, enteroviruses, and *M. avium-intracellulare* may contribute to this syndrome. HIV RNA has been found in macrophages infiltrating myocardial tissue in children with this disorder.

Malignancies

Although Kaposi's sarcoma is the most common neoplasm in adults with AIDS, it occurs very rarely in children. Lymphoreticular malignancies are being reported with increasing frequency in both HIV-infected adults and children. These tumors can appear as both Hodgkin's and non-Hodgkin's lymphomas. The latter is most often a B-cell malignancy (e.g., Burkitt's lymphoma) but may also be a T-cell lymphoma. The lymphomas may be discrete or disseminated and commonly present in the CNS. The risk for developing them is increased in individuals who have lived with fewer than 50 CD4 + cells/mm^3 for more than 2 years.

Leiomyosarcomas and progressive giant papillomas also may be seen rarely.

DIFFERENTIAL DIAGNOSIS

HIV infection can both mimic a host of other disorders and predispose an individual to them. These disorders include the following:
1. Maturational immunodeficiency of newborns, resulting in neonatal sepsis and severe infection with herpesviruses
2. Congenital infections, with associated lymphadenopathy and hepatosplenomegaly
3. Congenital immunodeficiency states
   a. Severe combined immunodeficiency
   b. DiGeorge syndrome
   c. Wiskott-Aldrich syndrome
   d. Agammaglobulinemia or hypogammaglobulinemia
   e. Ataxia telangiectasia
   f. Neutrophil defects in mobility or killing
   g. Chronic mucocutaneous candidiasis
4. Inflammatory bowel diseases
5. Hereditary encephalopathies and neuropathies
6. ITP
7. Chronic allergies with sinusitis, otitis, and dermatitis
8. Cystic fibrosis or α-1-antitrypsin deficiency
9. Primary lymphoreticular malignancy

TREATMENT
Specific retroviral therapy

The ideal goal of treatment would be to eradicate all virus-infected cells and cure the infection. This is not currently feasible. Available therapeutic agents suppress viral multiplication and improve or reverse some of the symptoms, improving the quality and duration of life.

Azidothymidine (AZT), or zidovudine, has been approved for use in children. The recommended dosage for children is 180 mg/m^2 administered every 6 hours. Studies in adult populations suggest that lower dosages (as little as 60 mg/m^2) may be comparable in effectiveness. Pediatric studies to test this hypothesis are in progress. AZT increases the rate of the patient's growth, decreases p24 antigen levels in the serum and cerebrospinal fluid, and produces a decrease in the serum immunoglobulin levels (McKinney et al., 1991). AZT also improves the neurobehavioral status of children with HIV infection. The survival of AZT-treated children with AIDS appears longer than that of historical controls. Prolonged use of AZT probably will be limited by bone marrow toxicity to erythroid and myeloid elements. Some of the toxicity can be modified by dose reduction. The emergence of AZT-resistant HIV isolates after 6 to 12 months of therapy is also a potential barrier to prolonged therapy with AZT as a single agent.

Other nucleoside derivatives, including dideoxyinosine (DDI) and dideoxycytidine (DDC), are being evaluated in adults and children. Early experience with DDI in children suggests that clinical and immunological improvement occurs in a dose-related fashion (Butler et al., 1991). DDI has been approved for use in children and adults who do not tolerate or have failed AZT

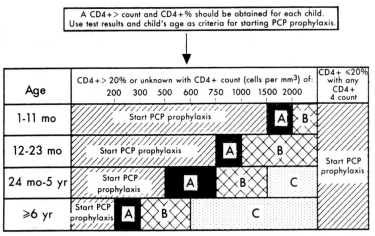

A CD4+> count and CD4+% should be obtained for each child.
Use test results and child's age as criteria for starting PCP prophylaxis.

A: No prophylaxis recommended at this time; recheck CD4+ count in 1 month.

B: No prophylaxis recommended at this time; recheck CD4+ count at least every 3-4 months.

C: No prophylaxis recommended at this time; recheck CD4+ count at least every 6 months.

Fig. 1-5. Recommendations for initiation of PCP prophylaxis for children 1 month of age or older who are (1) HIV infected, (2) HIV seropositive, or (3) less than 12 months old and born to an HIV-infected mother. (From MMWR 1991; 40:1-14, [March 15].)

therapy. Peripheral neuropathy and pancreatitis are recognized toxicities of DDI.

Studies of the recombinant molecule CD4 in adults have failed to reveal any therapeutic benefit. All therapeutic studies with soluble CD4 have been discontinued. Studies with the CD4-IgG molecule are ongoing.

Adjunctive therapies

Antiparasitic therapy. Recommendations recently have been made for prophylaxis of HIV-seropositive infants against *P. carinii* infection (MMWR, 1991). These guidelines are summarized in Fig. 1-5 and the boxes on p. 17 and depend on normal CD4 numbers in infants, the safety of available therapy, and problems of the early diagnosis of HIV infection in young infants.

Children with acute PCP should be treated with parenteral trimethoprim-sulfamethoxazole or parenteral pentamidine. Recent evidence suggests that the introduction of corticosteroid therapy early in this infection in adults helps preserve residual pulmonary function in those who recover.

Immunomodulators. A recent placebo vs. in-travenous immunoglobulin (IVIG) trial conducted by the NICHD reported no difference in survival time but did report a decrease in the number of bacterial infections in children with CD4 counts greater than 400/mm^3 who received IVIG. Most of these children did not receive retroviral therapy, and trimethoprim-sulfamethoxazole for prevention of PCP was progressively administered over the duration of the trial. It is not possible to assess the effect of these variables on the outcome of the trial. The single most common pathogen was *S. pneumoniae*, which caused 19 bacteremias in 16 children. An ongoing study is comparing the effect of IVIG to placebo in AZT-treated HIV-infected children. The comparative efficacy of IVIG to that of prophylactic antibiotics has not been studied.

Antifungals. Effective therapy for mucocutaneous candidal disease requires the use of ketoconazole or clotrimazole troches. The relative efficacy of newer drugs such as oral fluconazole is being evaluated. Disseminated candidal disease can occur in the absence of neutropenia and requires treatment with parenteral amphotericin B. Cryptococcal pneumonia and menin-

RECOMMENDED REGIMEN FOR PCP PROPHYLAXIS (see box at right for alternative regimens)

Trimethoprim-sulfamethoxazole (TMP-SMX): 150 mg TMP/m²/day with 750 mg SMX/m²/day given orally in divided doses twice a day three times per week on consecutive days (e.g., Monday, Tuesday, Wednesday). When starting TMP-SMX prophylaxis:
- Obtain baseline complete blood count (CBC), differential count, platelet count.
- Monitor CBC, differential count, platelet count monthly.
- Monitor CD4+ count at least every 3 months.

NOTE: Any child who has had an episode of PCP **should be started on PCP prophylaxis** regardless of age or CD4+ count. From MMWR 1991;40:1-14(March 15).

DRUG REGIMENS

Recommended regimen (children ≥1 month of age)
Trimethoprim-sulfamethoxazole (TMP-SMX):
150 mg TMP/m²/day with 750 mg SMX/m²/day given orally in divided doses twice a day (b.i.d.) three times per week on consecutive days (e.g., Monday, Tuesday, Wednesday)
Acceptable alternative TMP-SMX dosage schedules:
150 mg TMP/m²/day with 750 mg SMX/m²/day given orally **as a single daily dose** three times per week on consecutive days (e.g., M, T, W)
150 mg TMP/m²/day with 750 mg SMX/m²/day orally divided b.i.d. and **given 7 days/week**
150 mg TMP/m²/day with 750 mg SMX/m²/day given orally divided b.i.d. and given three times per week on **alternate days** (e.g., M, W, F)

Alternative regimens, if TMP-SMX not tolerated
Aerosolized pentamidine (≥5 years of age): 300 mg given via Respirgard II inhaler monthly
Dapsone (≥1 month of age): 1 mg/kg (not to exceed 100 mg) given orally once daily
If neither aerosolized pentamidine nor dapsone is tolerated, some clinicians use **intravenous pentamidine** (4 mg/kg) given every 2 or 4 weeks

From MMWR 1991;40:1-14(March 15).

gitis require parenteral treatment with amphotericin, followed by lifelong suppressive maintenance therapy with fluconazole.

Antivirals. HIV-infected children may develop overwhelming or chronic secondary viral infections. VZV may produce disseminated disease and death, or it may result in a necrotizing ulcerating skin lesion. Varicella-zoster immune globulin (VZIG) should be used prophylactically to prevent or modify VZV infection when a known exposure occurs in a child susceptible to varicella. Intravenous acyclovir therapy may be used to modify VZV infection. Prolonged high-dose oral acyclovir therapy may be required to heal and prevent exacerbations of the skin ulcers (Jura et al., 1989).

Measles produces a fulminating and often fatal disease in HIV-infected children (Krasinski et al., 1988). Gammaglobulin may modify the clinical appearance of the disease but has not prevented measles. All HIV-infected children, even if vaccinated, should receive gamma globulin if a known exposure to measles occurs. Some limited experience with ribavirin, given parenterally, has suggested that it may be an effective antimeasles agent.

Respiratory syncytial virus (RSV) infection in the HIV-infected infant results in delayed eradication of this respiratory pathogen. It also produces a modified clinical picture, with only the rare occurrence of wheezing and the more common appearance of pneumonia (Chandwani et al., 1990). Aerosolized ribavirin has not been systematically studied in this situation.

Immunizations

HIV-seropositive and infected children should receive all of their recommended childhood immunizations. Inactivated poliovirus vaccine should be substituted for oral poliovirus vaccine in both the children and their household contacts who are receiving vaccine, although this may not be possible in developing nations. In particular, HIV-seropositive infants should receive measles, mumps, and rubella vaccines. Studies done in Africa have shown that protection attributable to vaccine in these children is substantial but less than that achieved in healthy children (Oxtoby et al., 1988).

General nutrition

Many of the children with HIV infection are unable to sustain a positive nutritional balance. Protein and caloric support can be provided with tube feedings and/or total parenteral nutrition.

MEDICAL MANAGEMENT

Infants born to HIV-seropositive women should be identified so they can receive optimal medical care. Access to care is of critical importance. Ideally, identification of infected women would occur before or during pregnancy so that they too could receive optimal medical care. The recommendation by the U.S. Public Health Service is for seropositive women not to breast-feed because of the undefined risk of viral transmission in the postpartum period. However, in developing nations the benefits of breast-feeding clearly are more important than the small risk of transmission of the virus, and those women should breast-feed their infants. The care of HIV-seropositive infants in the first year of life is very much the same as that for healthy infants. However, these infants should have a CD4 count and HIV culture done every 1 to 3 months if possible. Depending on the resources available, a PCR should be done when the viral culture is done. The supportive care provided to children known to be seropositive is of critical importance. The response to an unknown febrile illness or the suspicion that pulmonary disease may be PCP can be life saving for these infants. Finally, the institution of *Pneumocystis* prophylaxis is probably the single most important lifesaving part of their medical management at the present time. It is possible that early administration of retroviral therapy may provide even greater benefit than its administration to symptomatic children; thus infected infants must be identified as early as possible.

PROGNOSIS

The epidemiological and circumstantial data suggest that there are two groups of children who have different responses to HIV infection. The first group, which presents with illness during the first year of life, has a more rapid progression of disease and death. Other infants may

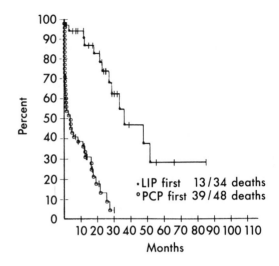

Fig. 1-6. Kaplan-Meier plots of survival for children diagnosed with *Pneumocystis carinii* pneumonia (PCP) or lymphocytic interstitial pneumonitis (LIP) as presenting illness. (From Connor E: Personal communication, 1991.)

Table 1-4. Perinatal HIV infection

Diagnosis	Rogers* AIDS	Scott† Onset of illness	ACTU‡
Median age at diagnosis (mo)	9	8	10
Overall survival from time of diagnosis (mo)	9.4	38	30
Survival (mo)			
<1 yr at diagnosis	6.5	24.8	20
>1 yr at diagnosis	19.7	>60	48

*Rogers et al., 1987. 307 children; 244 perinatal.
†Scott et al., 1989. 172 perinatal.
‡Conner, 1991. Summary of AIDS Clinical Trial Unit (ACTU). 11 centers 1979-1987; 234 perinatal (includes 49 transfused at <2 months of age).

be infected in the first year but present with symptoms later; they appear to have a more sustained course of illness. Computer modeling based on reported AIDS cases suggests that approximately 8% of HIV-infected children will develop AIDS per year (Auger et al., 1988). Defining the incubation period as the time to development of AIDS has produced current estimates that the median age at diagnosis of AIDS will be longer than 3 years and perhaps as long as 5 years. These numbers are derived from mathematical calculations based on reported AIDS in infants (Oxtoby, 1991). The reported mortality rate for children with HIV infection or AIDS from several different studies is depicted in Table 1-4. The children reported by the CDC had reached the diagnosis of AIDS. Those children reported in the other two studies were retrospectively evaluated to note the onset of symptoms. The median survival time calculated from the onset of symptoms is longer than the median survival time calculated from the diagnosis of AIDS.

The diagnosis of PCP in an HIV-infected child carries a poor prognosis in contrast to a diagnosis of LIP. The survival rate after diagnosis of PCP or LIP is shown in Fig. 1-6 from a retrospective analysis of 269 children (Connor, 1991). The survival curves represent the two extremes of outcome.

Although the current survival statistics are grim, the improved methods for early HIV diagnosis, coupled with earlier implementation of primary and adjunctive therapies, including prophylactic measures, should dramatically improve future prognoses.

REFERENCES

Ammann AJ, Cowan MJ, Wara DW, et al. Acquired immunodeficiency in an infant: possible transmission by means of blood products. Lancet 1983;1:956-958.

Andiman WA, Modlin JF. Vertical transmission. In Pizzo P, Wilfert CM (eds). Pediatric AIDS. Baltimore: Williams & Wilkins, 1991.

Auger I, Thomas P, DeGruttola V, et al. Incubation periods for pediatric AIDS patients. Nature 1988:336;575-577.

Barre-Sinoussi F, Cherman JC, Rey F, et al. Isolation of a T-lymphotrophic retrovirus from a patient at risk for acquired immunodeficiency syndrome (AIDS). Science 1983;220:868-871.

Belman AL, Diamond G, Dixon D, et al. Pediatric acquired immunodeficiency syndrome: neurologic syndromes. Am J Dis Child 1988;149:29-35.

Bernstein LJ, Bye MR, Rubinstein A. Prognostic factors and life expectancy in children with acquired immunodeficiency syndrome and *Pneumocystis carinii* pneumonia. Am J Dis Child 1989;143:775-778.

Bernstein LJ, Krieger BZ, Novick B, et al. Bacterial infection in the acquired immunodeficiency syndrome of children. Pediatr Infect Dis 1985;4:472-475.

Bernstein LJ, Ochs HD, Wedgwood RJ, Rubinstein A. Defective humoral immunity in pediatric acquired immunodeficiency syndrome. J Pediatr 1985;107:352-357.

Blanche S, Le Deist F, Fischer A, et al. Longitudinal study of 18 children with perinatal LAV/HTLV III infection: attempt at prognostic evaluation. J Pediatr 1986;109:965-970.

Blanche S, Rouziouz C, Moscato ML, et al. A prospective study of infants born to mothers seropositive for human immunodeficiency virus type 1. N Engl J Med 1989;320:1643-1648.

Blanche S, Tardieu M, Duliege AM, et al. Longitudinal study of 94 symptomatic infants with perinatally acquired human immunodeficiency virus infection. Evidence for a bimodal expression of clinical and biological symptoms. Am J Dis Child 1990;144:1210-1215.

Borkowsky W, Krasinski K, Paul D, et al. Human immunodeficiency virus infections in infants negative for anti-HIV by enzyme linked immunoassay. Lancet 1987;1:1168-1171.

Borkowsky W, Krasinski K, Paul D, et al. Human immunodeficiency virus core protein antigenemia in children with HIV infection. J Pediatr 1989;114:940-945.

Boue F, Pons JC, Keros L, et al. Risk for HIV-1 perinatal transmission vary with the mother's stage of HIV infection. Abstract Th.C. 44, p 144, Vol 1. Sixth International Conference on AIDS, 1990.

Broliden PA, Moschese V, Fjungren K, et al. Diagnostic implication of specific immunoglobulin G patterns of children born to HIV infected mothers. AIDS 1989;3:577-82.

Bryant ML, Ratner L. Biology and molecular biology of HIV. In Pizzo P, Wilfert CM (eds). Pediatric AIDS. Baltimore: Williams & Wilkins, 1991.

Butler KM, Husson RN, Balis FM, et al. Dideoxyinosine in children with symptomatic human immunodeficiency virus infection. N Engl J Med 1991;324:137-144.

Centers for Disease Control. Unexplained immunodeficiency and opportunistic infections in infants—New York, New Jersey, California. MMWR 1982;31:665-667.

Centers for Disease Control. Update: acquired immunodeficiency syndrome—United States, 1989. MMWR 1990;39:81-86.

Centers for Disease Control. *Pneumocystis carinii* pneumonia prophylaxis in children. MMWR, 1991:40:1-14.

Chandwani S, Borkowsky W, Krasinski K, et al. Respiratory syncytial virus infections in human immunodeficiency virus infected children. J Pediatr 1990;117:251-254.

Chandwani S, Greico A, Mittal K, et al. Pathology and human immunodeficiency virus expression in placentas of seropositive women. J Infect Dis 1991; 163:1134-1138.

Connor E. Personal communication, 1991.

Connor E, Gupta S, Joshi V, et al. Acquired immunodeficiency syndrome—associated renal disease in children. J Pediatr 1988;113:38-44.

Devash Y, Calvetti TA, Wood DG, et al. Vertical transmission of human immunodeficiency viruses correlated with the absence of high affinity/avidity maternal antibodies to the GP 120 principal neutralizing domain. Proc Natl Acad Sci USA 1990;87:3445-3449.

Di Maria H, Courpotin C, Rouzioux C, et al. Transplacental transmission of human immunodeficiency virus. Lancet 1986;2:215-216.

Epstein LG, Sharer LR, Goudsmit J. Neurologic and neuropathological features of HIV infection in children. Ann Neurol 1988;23:S19-S23.

Epstein LG, Sharer LR, Oleski JM, et al. Neurologic manifestations of human immunodeficiency virus infection in children. Pediatrics 1986;78:678-687.

European Collaborative Study. Mother to child transmission of HIV infection. Lancet 1988;2:1039-1042.

European Collaborative Study. Children born to women with HIV-1 infection: natural history and risk of transmission. Lancet 1991;337:253-260.

Eyster ME. Transfusion and coagulation factor acquired disease. In Pizzo P, Wilfert CM (eds). Pediatric AIDS. Baltimore: Williams & Wilkins, 1991.

Felowyn PA, Schoenbaun EE, Davenny K, et al. Prospective study of human immunodeficiency virus infection and pregnancy outcomes in intravenous drug users. JAMA 1989;261:1289-1294.

Final Report of the Secretary's Work Group on Pediatric HIV Infection and Disease. Washington, DC: Department of Health and Human Services, November 18, 1988.

Fox CH, Kotler D, Tierney A, et al. Detection of HIV-1 RNA in the lamina propria of patients with AIDS in GI disease. J Infect Dis 1989;159:467-471.

Gallo RC, Salahuddin SZ, Popovic M, et al. Frequent detection and isolation of cytopathic retroviruses (HTLV-3) from patients with AIDS and at high risk for AIDS. Science 1984;224:500-503.

Gayle HD, D'Angelo LJ. The epidemiology of AIDS and HIV infection in adolescents. In Pizzo P, Wilfert CM (eds). Pediatric AIDS. Baltimore: Williams & Wilkins, 1991.

Goedert JJ, Kessler CM, Alerdort LM, et al. A prospective study of human immunodeficiency virus type 1 infection and the development of AIDS in subjects with hemophilia. N Engl J Med 1989a;321:1141-1148.

Goedert JJ, Mendez H, Drummond JE, et al. Mother to infant transmission of human immunodeficiency virus type 1: association with prematurity or low anti-gp 120. Lancet 1989b;2:1351-1354.

Gutman LT, St.-Claire K, Weedy C, et al. Human immunodeficiency virus transmission by sexual abuse. Am J Dis Child 1991; 145:137-141.

Halsey NA, Boulos R, Holt E, et al. Transmission of HIV-1 infections from mothers to infants and babies. Impact on childhood mortality and malnutrition. JAMA 1990; 264:2088-2092.

Hutto C, Parks WP, Lai S, et al. A hospital-based prospective study of perinatal infection with human immunodeficiency virus type 1. J Pediatr 1991;118:347-353.

Itescu S, Brancato LJ, Winchester R. A sicca syndrome in HIV infection: association with HLA-DR5 and CD8 lymphocytosis. Lancet 1989;2:466-468.

Joshi, Vijai V. Pathologic findings association with HIV infection in children. In Pizzo P, Wilfert CM (eds). Pediatric AIDS. Baltimore: Williams & Wilkins, 1991.

Jovais E, Koch MA, Schafer A, et al. LAV/HTLV-III in a 20-week fetus (letter). Lancet 1985;2:1129.

Jura E, Chadwick E, Joseph S, et al. Varicella-zoster virus infections in children infected with human immunodeficiency virus. Pediatr Infect Dis 1989;8:586-590.

Kashkin JM, Shliozberg J, Lyman WD, et al. Detection of human immunodeficiency virus (HIV) in human fetal tissues. Pediatr Res 1988;23(part 2):355A.

Kilbourne B, Buehler J, Rogers M. AIDS as a cause of death in children, adolescents, and young adults (letter). Am J Public Health 1990;80:499-500.

Krasinski K, Borkowsky W, Bonk S, et al. Bacterial infections in human immunodeficiency virus infected children. Pediatr Infect Dis 1988;7:323-328.

Levy JA, Hoffman AD, Kramer SM, et al. Retroviruses from San Francisco patients with AIDS. Science 1984;225:840-842.

Martin N, Wara D, Levy J, et al. Abstract TH.C. 46, p 145, Vol 1. Sixth International Conference on AIDS, 1990.

McKinney RE, Maha MA, Conner EM, et al. A multicentered trial of oral zidovudine in children with advanced human immunodeficiency virus disease. N Engl J Med 1991. In press.

Mok JG, Gianquinto C, Derossi A, et al. Infants born to mothers seropositive for human immunodeficiency virus: preliminary findings from the multicenter European study. Lancet 1987;1:1164-1168.

Nelson JA, Wiley CA, Reynolds-Kohler C, et al. Human immunodeficiency virus detected in bowel epithelium from patients with gastrointestinal symptoms. Lancet 1988;1:259-262.

Oleske J, Minnefor A, Cooper R, et al. Immune deficiency in children. JAMA 1983;249:2345-2349.

Oxtoby MJ. Perinatally acquired HIV infection. In Pizzo P, Wilfert CM (eds). Pediatric AIDS. Baltimore: Williams & Wilkins, 1991.

Oxtoby MS, Mvula M, Ryder R, Baende E, et al. Measles and measles immunity in African children with HIV (abstract 1353). Los Angeles: Interscience Conference on Antimicrobial Agents and Chemotherapy, 1988.

Pahwa S, Pahwa R, Saxinger C, et al. Influence of the human T-lymphotropic virus/lymphadenopathy virus on functions of human lymphocytes: evidence for immunosuppressive effects and polyclonal B-cell activation by banded viral preparations. Proc Natl Acad Sci USA 1985;82:8198-8202.

Parks WP. In Nicholas SW, Sondheimer DL, Willoughby AD, et al. Human immunodeficiency virus infection in childhood, adolescence, and pregnancy: a status report and national research agenda. Pediatrics 1989;83:293-308.

Phair J, Munoz A, Detels R, et al. The risk of *Pneumocystis carinii* pneumonia among men infected with human immunodeficiency virus type 1. N Engl J Med 1990; 322:161-165.

Pizzo PA, Butler K, Balis F, et al. Dideoxycytidine alone and in an alternating schedule with zidovudine in children with symptomatic human immunodeficiency virus infection. J Pediatr 1990;117:799-808.

Quinn TC, Ruff A, Halsey N. Special considerations for developing nations. In Pizzo P, Wilfert CM (eds). Pediatric AIDS. Baltimore: Williams & Wilkins, 1991.

Rogers MF, Ou CY, Rayfield M, et al. Use of the polymerase chain reaction for early detection of the proviral sequences of human immunodeficiency virus in infants born to seropositive mothers. N Engl J Med 1989;320:1649-1654.

Rogers MF, Thomas PA, Starcher ET, et al. AIDS in children: report of the CDC national surveillance 1982-1985. Pediatrics 1987;79:1008-1014.

Roilides E, Mertins S, Eddy J, et al. Impairment of neutrophil chemotactic and bactericidal function in children infected with HIV-1 and partial reversal after in vitro exposure to granulocyte-macrophage colony stimulating factor. J Pediatr 1990;117:531-540.

Rolston K, Rodriquez S, Mansell P. Therapy of salmonella infection in AIDS patients (abstract). Montreal: 5th international conference on AIDS, June 1989.

Rossi P, Moschese V, Broliden PA, et al. Presence of maternal antibodies to human immunodeficiency virus 1 envelope glycoprotein gp120 epitopes correlates with the uninfected status of children born to seropositive mothers. Proc Natl Acad Sci USA 1989;86:8055-8058.

Rubinstein A, Sicklick M, Gupta A, et al. Acquired immunodeficiency with reversed T4/T8 ratios in infants born to promiscuous and drug-addicted mothers. JAMA 1983;249:2350-2356.

Russell C, Lay K. Natural history of *Candida* species of the yeast in the oral cavities of infants. Arch Oral Biol 1973;18:957-962.

Ryder RW, Nsaw W, Hassigs E, et al. Perinatal transmission of the human immunodeficiency virus type 1 to infants of seropositive women in Zaire. N Engl J Med 1989; 320:1637-1642.

Scott GB, Buck BE, Leterman JG, et al. Acquired immunodeficiency syndrome in infants. N Engl J Med 1984; 310:76-81.

Scott GB, Hutto C, Makuch RW, et al. Survival in children with perinatally acquired human immunodeficiency virus type 1 infection. N Engl J Med 1989;321:1791-1796.

Selwyn PA, Schoenbaum EE, Davenny K, et al. Prospective study of human immunodeficiency virus infection and pregnancy outcomes in intravenous drug users. JAMA 1989;261:1289-1294.

Sharer LR, Epstein LG, Cho ES, et al. Pathologic features of AIDS encephalopathy in children: evidence for LAV/HTLV-III infection of brain. Hum Pathol 1986;17:271-284.

Sharer LR, Cho ES, Epstein LG. Multinucleated giant cells and HTLV/III in AIDS encephalopathy. Hum Pathol 1985;16:760.

Shaw GM, Harper ME, Hahn BH, et al. HTLV/III infection of brains of children and adults with AIDS encephalopathy. Science 1985;227:117-182.

Sprecher S, Soumenkoff G, Puissant F, Degueldre M. Vertical transmission of HIV in 15-week fetus. Lancet 1986;2:288-289.

Stoler MH, Skinta, Benn S, et al. Human T-cell lymphotrophic virus type 3 infection of the central nervous system. A preliminary in situ analysis. JAMA 1986;256:2360-2364.

Uetmann MH, Belman WL, Ruff HA, et al. Developmental abnormalities in infants and children with acquired immune deficiency syndrome (AIDS) and AIDS related complex. Dev Med Child Neurol 1985;27:563-571.

Weiblen B, McIntosh K, Pelton S, et al. Detection of IgA HIV antibodies for diagnosis of HIV infected infants. Abstract S.B. 206, p 131. Sixth International Conference on AIDS, 1990.

2

BOTULISM IN INFANTS

Since the first case report in 1976 (Pickett et al.) describing two infants with a clinical illness attributed to in vivo formation of *Clostridium botulinum* toxin, more than 800 similar cases have been found among infants in the United States. Although most of the cases initially came from California, almost all states have now reported patients with infantile botulism. California, Utah, Arizona, Hawaii, and Pennsylvania have the highest rates. Additional reports have come from Canada, Europe, Asia, South America, and Australia. These infants have had constipation followed in varying degrees by lethargy, weakness, difficult feeding, general floppiness, descending paralysis, and oculomotor dysfunction; some progress to life-threatening respiratory failure. The detection of clostridial organisms and specific toxin in the infants' stools has led to the term *infant botulism*, in contrast with the more frequently recognized form of botulism, which is a "food poisoning" resulting from ingestion of food contaminated by preformed toxin.

ETIOLOGY

C. botulinum organisms, serotypes A and B, have been isolated from feces of affected infants. The same fecal specimens contained the specific toxin of the botulinal serotype (Midura and Arnon, 1976). Toxin has rarely been detected in serum samples. Apparently, ingested vegetative cells or spores germinate in the infant gastrointestinal tract and release their neurotoxin, which causes the clinical manifestations. *C. botulinum* toxin binds to the synaptic membrane of cholinergic nerves and prevents the release of acetylcholine, blocking neuromuscular synaptic transmission and resulting in autonomic dysfunction and flaccid paralysis. No evidence has been found that these infants ingested preformed toxin, the usual mechanism for botulism of adults and older children. Those factors that permit the sequence of toxin formation in the infant gastrointestinal tract are not yet defined. Of the seven distinct serotypes of *C. botulinum* (A to G), types A and B have been responsible for 90% of cases of botulism in infants.

PATHOLOGY

Because nearly all identified patients have recovered after provision of supportive therapy, no published autopsy studies are available. However, an investigation of postmortem specimens from 280 California infants who died in the first year of life revealed *C. botulinum* organisms and/or toxin in 10 infants (Arnon et al., 1981). Nine of the 10 deaths had been classified as resulting from sudden infant death syndrome (SIDS). Among the SIDS infants with positive *C. botulinum* organisms and/or toxin, the study reported intrathoracic organ petechiae, alveoli and airways filled with frothy fluid, and extramedullary hepatic erythropoiesis. Arnon et al. have postulated that infant botulism may be one cause of SIDS.

EPIDEMIOLOGICAL FACTORS

The age of patients at onset has ranged from 1 week to 11 months, and there has been no sex predilection. Seventy percent of the affected in-

---

INITIAL FEATURES OF CLINICAL HISTORY AND PHYSICAL FINDINGS IN INFANT BOTULISM

Constipation	Hypotonia
Floppiness	Ptosis
Decreased activity	Pupillary dilatation
Poor sucking	Facial paresis
Slow feeding	Ophthalmoplegia
Weakness	Decreased gag reflex
Poor cry	Shallow respirations
Loss of head control	Decreased deep tendon reflexes

---

fants have been predominantly breast-fed (Morris et al., 1983). There was an interesting association of the type B cases in California with the use of honey as a carbohydrate source in infant feeding (Arnon et al., 1979), and up to 27% of subsequent patients had been fed honey before their illness. The full extent of the disease is not yet known, but it is safe to assume that many mild cases continue to go unrecognized. Less severely affected infants with moderate hypotonia, transient feeding difficulties, and failure to thrive are not hospitalized and escape detection because stool cultures and toxin assays are not performed. In association with their study of a possible relationship between infant botulism and SIDS, Arnon et al. (1978) pointed out the similar age distribution curves of patients with the two conditions in the first 6 months of life.

CLINICAL MANIFESTATIONS

Constipation (no spontaneous stools for 3 or more days) has been the initial manifestation in most cases. Within a few days this may be followed by lethargy, poor sucking, slow feeding, feeble cry, weakness, loss of head and neck control, generalized floppiness, swallowing difficulties, pooling of oral secretions, and in some, respiratory arrest. On examination there is loss of muscle tone and diminished deep tendon reflexes. Additional cranial nerve findings may include ptosis, sluggish pupillary light reflexes, decreased extraocular motility, lack of facial movement, and decreased gag reflex (Berg, 1977; Long et al., 1985; Long, 1985; Spila, 1989). The symptoms and signs have been variable in degree and duration, responding spontaneously

over a period ranging from 10 days to 8 weeks. The most serious complication has been respiratory arrest, occurring in nearly one half of hospitalized patients within the first 2 to 5 days. For this reason, admission to an intensive care unit where prompt respiratory support can be provided is crucial. Recovery has been gradual and complete, but rare relapses have been observed. The only deaths reported have been caused by respiratory arrests.

The box above lists a number of the relevant clinical features and findings.

DIAGNOSIS

The clinical suspicion of infant botulism should lead to diagnostic studies initiated while supportive care is underway (Hatheway and McCroskey, 1987). Electromyography may demonstrate a somewhat characteristic pattern of brief, low-amplitude, overabundant motor reaction potentials (Clay et al., 1977). Confirmation of precise diagnosis requires demonstration of *C. botulinum* and/or heat-labile botulinal toxin in the patient's stool. Appropriate reference laboratories are available (state health department or Centers for Disease Control) if local facilities are unable to perform the isolation and identification techniques. Midura and Arnon (1976) have described the appropriate tests and their application to fecal specimens.

DIFFERENTIAL DIAGNOSIS

Other conditions considered on the initial presentation of these infants have included sepsis, poliomyelitis, myasthenia gravis, brain tumor, failure to thrive, drug or chemical poisoning, metabolic disorders, infantile polyneuropathy,

Werdnig-Hoffmann disease, Reye's syndrome, congenital myopathy, and Leigh's disease. With appropriate cultures and screening tests to exclude many of the others, a specific diagnosis should be achieved. Cerebrospinal fluid and peripheral blood studies in infant botulism have been normal.

TREATMENT

The difficulties that may arise in handling oropharyngeal secretions and the unpredictability of sudden respiratory arrests require the level of supportive care usually available only in an intensive care unit. If the infant's course is a prolonged one, supplementary nutritional support also will become essential (Schreiner et al., 1991). No advantage has been demonstrated from the use of antitoxin, antibiotics, or cholinomimetic drugs. Infants treated with antibiotics have continued to excrete organisms and toxins for weeks after clinical recovery. The use of aminoglycoside antibiotics is specifically contraindicated because they may augment neuromuscular blockade and produce respiratory arrest (L'Hommedieu et al., 1979; Santos, Swenson, and Glasgow, 1981).

PREVENTION

Although the prevention of infantile botulism is not clearly defined, avoiding known food sources of *C. botulinum* spores during the first year of life is epidemiologically justified. This would entail the discontinuation of honey and corn syrup as sources of calories and sweeteners for infant feeding.

REFERENCES

Arnon SS, Damus K, Chin J. Infant botulism. epidemiology of and relation to sudden infant death syndrome. Epidemiol Rev 1981;3:45-66.

Arnon SS, et al. Intestinal infection and toxin production by *Clostridium botulinum* as one cause of sudden infant death syndrome. Lancet 1978;1:1273.

Arnon SS, et al. Honey and other environmental risk factors for infant botulism. J Pediatr 1979;94:331.

Berg BO. Syndrome of infant botulism. Pediatrics 1977; 59:322.

Clay SA, et al. Acute infantile motor disorder: infantile botulism? Arch Neurol 1977;34:236.

Hatheway CL, McCroskey LM. Examination of feces and serum for diagnosis of infant botulism in 336 patients. J Clin Microbiol 1987;25:2334.

L'Hommedieu C, Stough R, Brown L, et al. Potentiation of neuromuscular weakness in infant botulism by aminoglycosides. J Pediatr 1979;95:1965.

Long SS. Epidemiologic study of infant botulism in Pennsylvania: report of the infant botulism study group. Pediatrics 1985;75:928.

Long SS, Gajewski JL, Brown LW, Gilligan PH. Clinical, laboratory and environmental features of infant botulism in southeastern Pennsylvania. Pediatrics 1985;75:935.

Midura TF, Arnon SS. Infant botulism. Identification of *Clostridium botulinum* and its toxins in faeces. Lancet 1976;2:934.

Morris JG Jr, Snyder JD, Wilson R, Feldman RA. Infant botulism in the United States: an epidemiologic study of cases occurring outside of California. Am J Public Health 1983;73:1385-1388.

Pickett J, et al. Syndrome of botulism in infancy: clinical and electrophysiologic study. N Engl J Med 1976;295:770.

Santos JI, Swensen P, Glasgow LA. Potentiation of *Clostridium botulinum* toxin by aminoglycoside antibiotics: clinical and laboratory observations. Pediatrics 1981; 68:50-54.

Schreiner MS, Field E, Ruddy R. Infant botulism: a review of 12 years' experience at the Children's Hospital of Philadelphia. Pediatrics 1991;87:159.

Spila JS, Shaffer N, Hargrett-Bean N, et al. Risk factors for infant botulism in the United States. Am J Dis Child 1989;143:828.

3

CYTOMEGALOVIRUS INFECTIONS

Infections of newborn infants caused by human cytomegalovirus (CMV) were first recognized in the latter part of the nineteenth century. It was believed they were caused by a protozoan or represented a form of syphilis, and the salivary glands were believed the major pathological site. By the 1950s it was known the clinical signs and symptoms of the congenital viral infection in infants were hepatosplenomegaly, thrombocytopenia, jaundice, intracerebral calcifications, chorioretinitis, poor growth, and eventual development of microcephaly and mental retardation. These infants were said to have "cytomegalic inclusion disease" or infection with "salivary gland virus" since by then the causative agent had been isolated in tissue culture and identified (Rowe et al., 1956; Smith, 1956; Weller et al., 1957). In 1960 Weller, Hanshaw, and Scott proposed the term *cytomegalovirus infection* for the illness since it better reflected the nature of the disease. It was then thought that CMV infection of infants was rare, but it is now known it is not uncommon and that infants with obvious CMV infection represent the proverbial "tip of the iceberg." Devastating congenital CMV infections, however, are unusual; a far greater number of inapparent infections are acquired in the perinatal period because of maternal shedding of CMV in genital secretions and breast milk. Recent studies of the epidemiology of CMV infections in the United States reveal that 1% to 2% of newborns and 5% to 25% of pregnant women harbor occult infections with CMV.

Another significant cause of morbidity and mortality due to CMV occurs in the immunosuppressed host, in particular in patients with an underlying malignancy, those who have had organ transplantation, and persons with co-existing human immunodeficiency virus (HIV) infection. Infections in immunologically normal hosts beyond the newborn period are frequent but are also usually without symptoms or sequelae. Thus, as with many other agents whose initial association was with only a limited clinical syndrome, CMV has emerged as a ubiquitous virus with host interactions ranging over the full spectrum of health and disease.

ETIOLOGY

Despite initial confusion concerning the cause of cytomegalic inclusion disease, some investigators suspected this illness was caused by a virus long before the agent itself was identified. Similarities observed in pathological specimens between cytomegalic inclusion cells (Goodpasture and Talbot, 1921) and those in herpetic lesions (von Glahn and Pappenheimer, 1925) are remarkable in the light of modern evidence classifying CMV in the herpesvirus group. Smith in 1954 was the first to carry out serial propagation of murine CMV in mouse tissue cultures, following which human CMV was isolated (Rowe et al., 1956; Smith, 1956; Weller et al., 1957). Subsequently, it became possible to develop serological tests to delineate a broader understanding of the epidemiology of this common viral infection.

Cytomegalovirus is a DNA virus, the genome of which is the largest of the human herpesviruses. Virions (Fig. 3-1) consist of an inner core with a diameter of 65 nm, an icosahedral capsid composed of 162 capsomeres with a diameter of 110 nm, a tegument, and an envelope with a diameter of 200 nm. Virions are similar in appearance to those of the other human herpesviruses exemplified by herpes simplex virus (HSV). The CMV genome, however, is large and more complex than that of HSV. CMV DNA encodes for a number of structural viral proteins and glycoproteins and also many nonstructural viral proteins. Replication of CMV occurs in a regulated sequence with immediate early (α) genes controlling subsequent transcription and translation of early (β) and late (γ) gene products (Merigan and Resta, 1990; Plotkin et al., 1990). The envelope glycoproteins, which are antigenic, are believed to play an important role in generating immune responses on the part of the infected host, and undoubtedly they also play roles in viral infectivity (Plotkin et al., 1990). In addition, nonstructural antigens induced by immediate early genes also play an important role in immune stimulation in CMV infection (Kozinowski et al., 1987).

A great many strains of human CMV exist; it has been possible to distinguish between them both by analyzing their DNA with restriction enzyme technology and antigenically (Chou, 1989a,b). There is extensive homology between strains, however, so that, although reinfections with CMV may occur, primary infection may provide at least partial immunity against other strains (Plotkin et al., 1990). Viral antigens may be identified in infected cells by immunological means such as fluorescent-labeled antibody assays. Cultivation of CMV in human fibroblasts reveals characteristic cytomegaly with nuclear and cytoplasmic inclusions containing viral antigenic structures.

In the cell human CMV causes both permissive infections, in which viral progeny are produced, and abortive infections, in which there are no progeny but there is DNA replication and formation of some viral antigens. Although CMV also causes oncogenic transformation in some tissue culture systems (Heggie et al., 1986), no specific malignancies of humans have been related to this virus.

All of the herpesviruses share the charac-

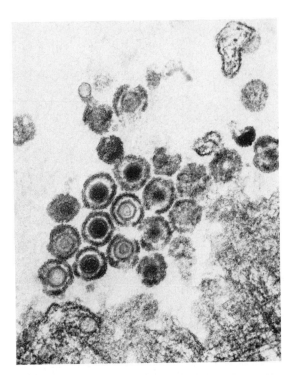

Fig. 3-1. A group of negatively stained cytomegalovirus particles propagated in human lung fibroblasts. The core, a typical hexagonal capsid (actually icosahedral in three dimensions) of a herpesvirus surrounded by a tegument and double-layered envelope, can be seen. (× 155,000.) (Courtesy Janet D Smith, PhD.)

teristic of causing latent infection as well as primary infection and reinfections. The site of latency of CMV probably is one or more cells of lymphoid origin and possibly granulocytes (Merigan and Resta, 1990). The virus has been detected in mononuclear blood cells from healthy seropositive donors (Schrier, et al., 1985; Spector and Spector, 1985) and may be inadvertently transmitted by blood transfusions. It has been postulated that CMV that is latent in white blood cells may account for transmission of the virus by organ transplantation (Merigan and Resta, 1990). In general, primary infections with CMV are potentially more serious than secondary infections, although this is not necessarily so in highly immunocompromised hosts.

PATHOGENESIS

The natural history of CMV infections is exceedingly complicated, with the possibility

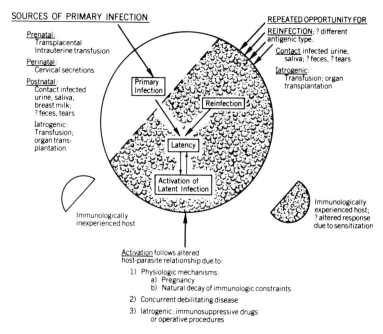

Fig. 3-2. Natural history of human cytomegalovirus infection. (From Weller TH: N Engl J Med 1970; 285:203.)

of primary infection, reactivation of latent infection, and reinfection with a new strain of virus. These potential events are diagrammed in Fig. 3-2.

Primary infection

A susceptible (immunologically inexperienced) host may be infected during the prenatal, perinatal, or postnatal period. Prenatal, or congenital, infection presumably is acquired transplacentally. Viremia during pregnancy may be the most common source of prenatal CMV infection. Perinatal infection probably is caused by exposure to CMV-infected cervical secretions. The presence of CMV in cervical secretions is well documented (Alexander, 1967; Diosi et al., 1967).

Postnatal infections most commonly are acquired by contact with various secretions known to be infected with CMV such as urine, semen, saliva, and tears (Lang and Hanshaw, 1969; Lang and Kummer, 1975). The exact route of postnatal transmission is unknown; it may be by the oral route, the respiratory route, or both. Breast milk is a recognized vector for transmission of CMV to infants despite the presence of maternal CMV antibody. Acqui-

sition of CMV by the infant from breast milk has been associated with prolonged viral shedding, but rarely do symptoms occur. Sexual transmission of CMV is probably a major route of spread in adult life (Chandler, et al., 1985). Day-care settings in which there are many children in diapers who may be teething and drooling are also recognized as foci for potential spread of CMV to other children, their parents, and the staff (Adler, 1988a, 1988b; Pass et al., 1986). Other sources of postnatal CMV infection include transfusions with CMV-infected blood and transplantation of organs that harbor the virus (Yeager, Jacobs, and Clark, 1972; Yeager et al., 1981; Whitley et al., 1976; Stagno et al., 1981; Meyers, Flournoy, and Thomas, 1986; Merigan and Resta, 1990).

Secondary infection: reactivation of and reinfection with CMV

Hosts with prior immunological experience with CMV may be exposed to exogenous or endogenous sources of infection. Reactivation of latent CMV infection may stem from various physiological, pathological, or iatrogenic mechanisms such as pregnancy, concurrent malignancy, and/or transplantation with concomitant administration of immunosuppressive therapy. The frequent detection of IgM antibodies in healthy individuals suggests that reactivation infections with CMV occur often in immunocompetent individuals (McEvoy and Adler, 1989). CMV infections in seropositive individuals may also be secondary to reinfection with a new strain of virus (Huang et al., 1980). In a study of women attending a clinic for sexually transmitted diseases, four of eight (50%) were infected with more than one strain of CMV as evidenced by analysis of viral DNAs by restriction enzymes. Two were simultaneously shedding different strains of CMV from different body sites (Chandler et al., 1987). Simultaneous viral shedding of two different strains of CMV in other healthy persons (McFarlane and Koment, 1986) and in immunocompromised persons (Spector et al., 1984; Chou, 1986) has also been reported. Finally, more than one strain of CMV can establish latent infection in one host, and new viral strains may emerge due to recombination of these strains (Chou, 1989a).

Since secondary infection with CMV is possible due either to reactivation of latent virus or to reinfection, it is obvious that immunity to this virus is often only partial. Therefore it is not surprising that seropositive women may transmit a congenital CMV infection to their offspring. Stagno et al. (1977b) found that intrauterine infection with CMV occurred in 3.4% of seropositive mothers. The birth of a second *symptomatic* congenitally infected infant to one mother, however, is exceedingly rare, which probably reflects at least partial immunity to CMV in most seropositive women (Ahlfors et al., 1981).

In a study of 3,712 pregnant women reported by Stagno et al. (1982) approximately one third were seronegative and had no evidence of prior experience with CMV before pregnancy. Infants with *symptomatic* CMV infection were born only to women in this group. Some women who had been seropositive before pregnancy gave birth to congenitally infected infants, but their babies were asymptomatic at birth and also at 1 year of age. An extension of this study (Stagno et al., 1986) involving 16,218 pregnant women confirmed the importance of gestational *primary* infection as a risk factor for development of symptomatic congenital CMV infection in the infant. The risk to the infant was greatest when mater-

nal infection occurred in the first half of pregnancy. There was a 30% to 40% rate of transmission of CMV in utero for women with primary CMV infection. Although there were fewer seronegative results among women from low-income than from high-income families, women in low-income families were more likely to experience a primary infection during pregnancy than women from high-income families.

The rates of CMV excretion by seropositive women increase in the later months of pregnancy. One factor in the failure of immune mothers to restrict spread of CMV to their infants despite the presence of positive antibody titers may be the specific impairment of cell-mediated immunity to CMV (Rola-Pleszczynski et al., 1977; Reynolds et al., 1979; Starr et al., 1979). On the other hand, since fetal infection is not invariably the result of depressed maternal cellular immunity to CMV, the exact role of cellular immunity in modulating transmission of congenital infection is unclear (Faix et al., 1983). Possibly antibody affords the infant some protection from the adverse effects of the virus. Clinically apparent maternal CMV infections in which there is a greater viral burden are more likely to result in transmission of CMV to the fetus (Alford, Hayes, and Britt, 1988).

PATHOLOGY

The histological lesion of CMV infection is characterized by enlarged cells that contain intranuclear and cytoplasmic inclusion bodies. The intranuclear inclusion body appears reddish purple after being stained with hematoxylin and eosin and is surrounded by a halo, the so-called "owl's eye" appearance. The paranuclear cytoplasmic inclusion or dense body is more granular and more basophilic in appearance.

Inclusion-bearing cells may be widely disseminated in the rare fatal infection. Involvement of almost every tissue and organ in the body has been described. Infection of the kidneys and lungs may induce chronic interstitial nephritis and pneumonitis, with focal areas of infiltration of mononuclear cells in the interstitial tissue. In the liver focal areas of necrosis may occur. The brain may show necrotizing granulomatous lesions and extensive calcifications in congenital infections (Fig. 3-3), and the liver and spleen may display evidence of extramedullary hematopoiesis. In patients with acquired immunodeficiency syndrome (AIDS) the retina, gastrointestinal tract (especially the colon), and lungs are most frequently invaded by CMV. In AIDS patients CMV may be isolated from even more body sites than in transplant patients (Ho, 1990). In patients with colitis caused by CMV the presence of inclusion bodies and thrombi in endothelial cells in the submucosa and muscle wall indicative of vasculitis has been observed (Tatum, et al., 1989).

CLINICAL MANIFESTATIONS

The clinical manifestations of congenital and postnatal CMV infections cover a broad spectrum. Both types of infection may range from an asymptomatic process associated with viruria

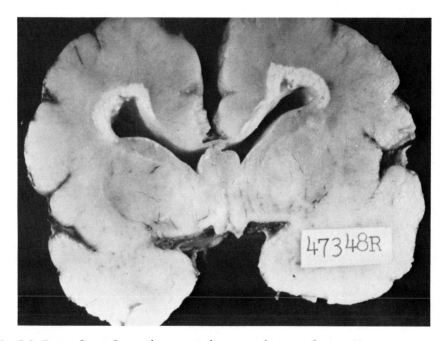

Fig. 3-3. Brain of an infant with congenital cytomegalovirus infection. Note extensive periventricular necrosis and calcification.

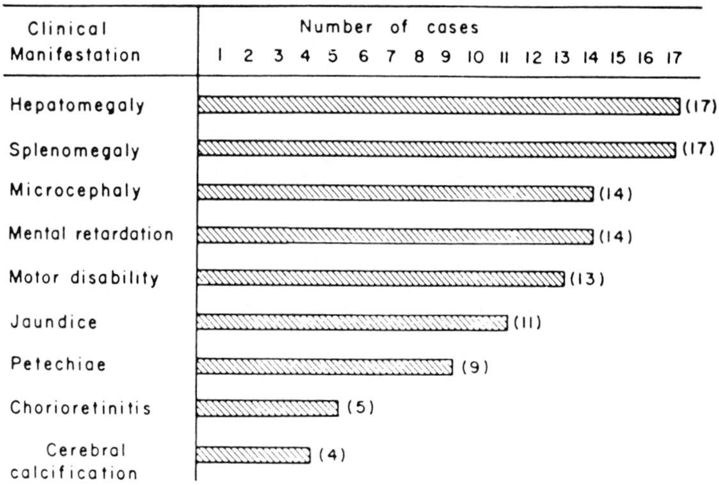

Clinical Manifestation	Number of cases 1 2 3 4 5 6 7 8 9 10 11 12 13 14 15 16 17
Hepatomegaly	▨▨▨▨▨▨▨▨▨▨▨▨▨▨▨▨▨ (17)
Splenomegaly	▨▨▨▨▨▨▨▨▨▨▨▨▨▨▨▨▨ (17)
Microcephaly	▨▨▨▨▨▨▨▨▨▨▨▨▨▨ (14)
Mental retardation	▨▨▨▨▨▨▨▨▨▨▨▨▨▨ (14)
Motor disability	▨▨▨▨▨▨▨▨▨▨▨▨▨ (13)
Jaundice	▨▨▨▨▨▨▨▨▨▨▨ (11)
Petechiae	▨▨▨▨▨▨▨▨▨ (9)
Chorioretinitis	▨▨▨▨▨ (5)
Cerebral calcification	▨▨▨▨ (4)

Fig. 3-4. Clinical features in 17 infants with congenital cytomegalovirus infection. (From Weller TH and Hanshaw JB: N Engl J Med 1962;266:1233.)

and presence of specific antibody to a severe widely disseminated disease involving virtually every organ in the body. The great majority of CMV infections, however, are totally inapparent.

Congenital infection

The typical clinical manifestations of severe generalized CMV infection are listed in Fig. 3-4, the skull roentgenogram of such a child with congenital CMV is shown in Fig. 3-5, and a child

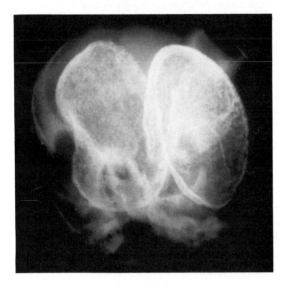

Fig. 3-5. Skull roentgenogram demonstrating massive intracranial calcifications of a 1-week-old infant with severe congenital cytomegalovirus infection.

with severe congenital CMV is shown in Fig. 3-6. This fulminating illness is characterized by jaundice, hepatosplenomegaly, and a petechial rash; it occurs several hours or days after birth in a newborn infant who usually is premature. Early onset of lethargy, respiratory distress, and convulsive seizures may be followed by death at any time from a few days to many years later.

In infants who survive, jaundice may subside in as few as 2 weeks, or it may persist for months. The hemorrhagic phenomena subside rapidly. The hepatosplenomegaly may increase for the first 2 to 4 months and persist for a prolonged period. Chorioretinitis is common.

Laboratory findings usually include anemia and thrombocytopenia. The cerebrospinal fluid (CSF) may show pleocytosis and increased concentration of protein. Roentgenograms of the skull may reveal cerebral calcifications (Fig. 3-6). The virus can be isolated from many body fluids, including urine, blood, and saliva. Examination of a *fresh* urine specimen sometimes reveals the inclusion bodies in cells in the urinary sediment. Recovery of virus is a more sensitive technique than cytology, which on occasion may give repeatedly negative results in the presence of large quantities of virus isolated from the urine.

As indicated in Fig. 3-4, many affected infants have severe neurological sequelae. Mental retardation and motor disability are common. In many infants microcephaly either is present at

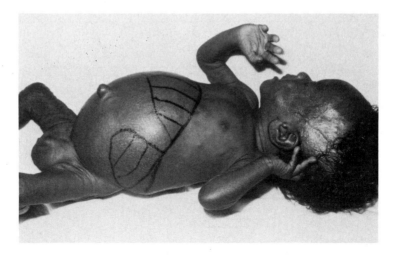

Fig. 3-6. Four-month-old child with symptomatic congenital infection manifesting severe failure to thrive, hepatitis with hepatosplenomegaly, bilateral inguinal hernias, and micropenis. (From Stagno S: Curr Prob Pediatr 1986;16:646.)

birth or becomes apparent in a few months. Other manifestations of cerebral damage include spasticity, diplegia, epileptiform seizures, and blindness. An excellent review by Hanshaw (1970) includes a summary of cerebral, ocular, and extraneural abnormalities associated with congenital CMV infection of 260 infants from birth to 12 months of age. These defects may occur singly or in combination.

Deafness, which may become increasingly apparent with increasing age of the child, is a major sequela of congenital CMV infection (Stagno et al., 1977a; Peckham et al., 1987). A study by Stagno et al. (1977a) reported on 10 patients with sensorineural hearing loss caused by congenital CMV, seven of whom had been clinically well at birth. The defect was bilateral and moderate to profound in 8 of the 10, and it was progressive in 2. Immunofluorescent studies of the inner ear in the infants who died revealed widespread viral invasion of cochlear structures.

In contrast to rubella virus, CMV is believed to have only weak teratogenic capabilities. Reported structural abnormalities caused by congenital CMV infection include inguinal hernia in males, abnormalities of the first brachial arch, hypoplasia or agenesis of central nervous system (CNS) structures, and defects of enamel of primary dentition (Reynolds, et al., 1986). Malformations associated with CMV infection probably are mainly the result of tissue necrosis rather than interference in organogenesis.

Extensive overt disease presenting in the neonatal period as just described is by far the exception in congenital CMV infection. More than 95% of congenitally infected infants are totally asymptomatic in the neonatal period (Alford, et al., 1975). Approximately 90% have benign infections that remain inapparent; many result from secondary maternal CMV infection caused by reactivation of latent virus or reinfection with CMV during pregnancy. Even the majority of CMV-infected infants whose mothers had primary CMV infections during early pregnancy never develop sequelae.

Approximately 10% of asymptomatic congenitally infected infants whose mothers presumably had primary CMV infection during pregnancy will develop sequelae such as deafness and mental retardation (Stagno et al., 1986). Since transmission from mother to fetus occurs in only approximately 40% of women, the risk

of having a child damaged by CMV even after a primary infection during pregnancy is very low—less than 5%. Moderate-to-profound bilateral sensorineural deafness and increased school failure rates associated with low intelligence quotients in 15% to 20% of children congenitally infected with CMV have been observed (Reynolds et al., 1974; Hanshaw et al., 1975; Stagno et al., 1977a). Unfortunately, there is still no reliable, widely available means to identify these high-risk infants prospectively.

Perinatal infection

Infants may be infected at the time of birth, despite the presence of maternal CMV antibody, by passage through the maternal cervix where secretions harbor reactivated CMV. Perinatal infections, although common, are considered of little significance; approximately 2% to 5% of all newborn infants are so infected. The infants develop viruria at approximately 1 month of age, but they remain asymptomatic. All are seropositive both before and during infection.

Infants may also be infected after birth from either a maternal or nonmaternal source. Maternally derived infections usually are contracted through breast milk, presumably by lymphocytes infected with latent CMV. These infections usually are not accompanied by symptoms or sequelae.

On the other hand, when CMV is acquired by a seronegative infant from a nonmaternal source, a severe infection may occur. Yeager, Jacobs, and Clark (1972) described two low-birth-weight infants with CMV infections believed to have been acquired from blood transfusions. Subsequently, Yeager (1974) determined that CMV infections occurred in 19 of 77 (25%) of high-risk infants who were transfused and in only seven of 74 (11%) of those who were not. It is now recognized that premature infants who were seropositive to CMV at birth but whose transplacental maternal antibodies have waned over time are also at increased risk to acquire severe CMV infections.

Others have also reported CMV infections in small premature infants who had received multiple blood transfusions in the first week of life (Ballard et al., 1979). At approximately 6 weeks of age they developed hepatosplenomegaly, gray pallor, respiratory deterioration, lymphocytosis with atypical lymphocytes, and thrombocytopenia. Of 14 such infants, three died. Prospective studies indicated that these infants had acquired CMV infection in the intensive care nursery, most likely as a result of multiple blood transfusions (mean of 21 separate blood units per infant). Unpasteurized banked breast milk is also a potential source of such infection, especially for low-birth-weight infants.

Acute respiratory disease with cough, pneumonitis, and abnormalities of pulmonary function and chest roentgenogram have been ascribed to CMV infection in young infants; often this occurs in conjunction with other pathogens such as *Chlamydia trachomatis* or *Ureaplasma urealyticum* (Brasfield et al., 1987). According to a study of 32 infants and 32 matched controls, CMV infection of low-birth-weight infants may also play a role in subsequent development of bronchopulmonary dysplasia (Sawyer et al., 1987). Intestinal infection by CMV in young infants has also been associated with symptoms of an acute surgical abdomen (Kosloske et al., 1988). It is unknown whether these syndromes are the result of perinatal infection or postnatal infection or both.

Postnatal infection

Postnatal CMV infection in children and infection in adults are usually inapparent and asymptomatic. The clinical manifestations, when present, may be associated with specific involvement of the liver and with a mononucleosis-like syndrome.

Evidence of a relationship between a spontaneously occurring illness resembling infectious mononucleosis and CMV was reported by Kääriäinen et al. (1966a). A significant rise of antibodies to CMV was described in four adult patients and one child, all of whom had a negative heterophil agglutination test. Illness in the four adults was characterized by fever lasting 2 to 5 weeks, cough, headache or pain in the back or limbs, a large number of atypical lymphocytes in the peripheral blood, and abnormal liver function tests. There was no exudative pharyngitis or lymphadenopathy. A 22-month-old child exhibited fever, migratory polyarthritis in the knees, fingers, and toes, a maculopapular skin rash, and pneumonia. The pneumonia and arthritis cleared completely, and the child was well 2 months after discharge from the hospital. None of 19 control patients with heterophil-positive infectious mononucleosis showed a significant rise in titer of antibodies to CMV.

Subsequently, it was recognized that this syndrome could also follow blood transfusion (Kääriäinen et al., 1966b). An illness resembling infectious mononucleosis with fever, rubelliform rash, atypical lymphocytes, and a negative heterophil antibody test was reported in a 28-year-old woman 3 weeks after open heart surgery during which she received fresh blood from 14 donors. CMV was isolated from the urine 40 days after onset of illness, and the antibody titer rose from a titer of less than 1:4 at onset to 1:512 on the fortieth day. Moreover, a significant rise in antibodies to CMV was demonstrated in the absence of clinical manifestations of disease in eight of 20 successive patients after open-heart surgery associated with fresh blood transfusions (Kääriäinen et al., 1966a, 1966b). These findings were confirmed by Lang and Hanshaw (1969), who also recognized the association of the syndrome with transfusion of fresh but not stored blood and implicated the leukocytes in viral transmission.

A more recent study is that of Horwitz et al. (1986), who reported 82 previously healthy individuals with a mononucleosis-like syndrome caused by CMV. None of these patients had received recent blood transfusions. These investigators emphasized the difficulty of making an accurate diagnosis in these patients, many of whom were initially thought to have serious diverse entities such as leukemia, systemic lupus erythematosus, and autoimmune hemolytic anemia.

CMV infection has been implicated as a trigger for autoimmunity leading to type I diabetes in children (Pak et al., 1988). Using a molecular probe, CMV DNA was identified in the lymphocytes of 22% of 59 children within 1 month of diagnosis of diabetes and in only 2.6% of 38 control subjects, suggesting that persistent CMV infections may be involved in the pathogenesis of some cases of diabetes.

Systemic overt disease caused by CMV is more likely to occur in immunocompromised persons than in those who are immunologically normal. These infections are well recognized in patients who have had organ transplantation, who are being treated for malignant disease, or who have infection with HIV. These patients may manifest fever, lymphadenopathy, hepatitis, pneumonia, gastritis, colitis, arthralgia, arthritis, encephalopathy, retinitis, and leukopenia. Risk factors for infection in seronegative patients are transplantation with an organ from a seropositive donor and blood transfusion (including granulocytes) from a seropositive individual.

The presence of acute graft-vs.-host disease is a significant risk factor for both CMV-seronegative and CMV-seropositive patients. In general, the severity of CMV infection is higher in seronegatives than in seropositives, but highly immunocompromised CMV seropositive patients may become ill because of reactivation of or reinfection with CMV. Receipt of antithymocyte globulin (OKT3 antibodies) is an additional risk factor for infection (Meyers et al., 1986; Singh et al., 1988; Pollard, 1988). In patients with AIDS, CMV has been the cause of colitis, encephalitis, pneumonia, and progressive retinitis leading to blindness (Drew, 1988). In leukemic children, CMV infection has been reported to cause fever, pneumonia, and chorioretinitis (Cox and Hughes, 1975).

A growing body of clinical and experimental evidence indicates that CMV is itself immunosuppressive (Grundy, 1990). Patients with CMV mononucleosis have depressed in vitro cell-mediated immune responses to mitogens and other antigens (Ho, 1981). The virus also depresses natural killer cell activity and T cell proliferation in vitro (Schrier et al., 1986). In a series of 49 recipients of heart transplants the incidence of pulmonary bacterial and *Pneumocystis* infections was higher in 11 patients with primary CMV infection after transplantation than in 19 patients with evidence of CMV infection before transplantation (Rand, Pollard, and Merigan, 1978). It is also possible that CMV may contribute to the immunosuppression in patients with HIV infection. Although it was suspected at one time that primary CMV infections in childhood might predispose children to serious bacterial infections, this has not been substantiated (Adler, 1988a).

The effects of CMV on the immune system, however, are far from simple. Despite its being thought that CMV is immunosuppressive, its frequent association with graft rejection in transplanted patients has led to the hypothesis that CMV plays a significant role in this process. Interestingly in this regard, the virus enhances both cytoplasmic and surface expression of HLA class I antigens in vitro (Grundy et al., 1988), and it also induces a variety of autoantibodies (Grundy, 1990). It remains controversial, however, as to whether CMV plays a central role in triggering rejection or is simply activated as a result of prophylaxis or treatment of rejection (Grundy, 1990; Merigan and Resta, 1990).

DIAGNOSIS

Serious infection with CMV should be strongly considered in a newborn infant with enlargement of the liver and spleen, jaundice, petechial rash, microcephaly, thrombocytopenia, and cerebral calcifications. Microcephaly, mental retardation, and motor disability may become evident in older infants.

In older children and adults the possibility of CMV infection should be kept in mind (1) in instances of pneumonia in immunocompromised patients or in those with chronic debilitating diseases such as malignant tumors and leukemia, (2) in unexplained liver disease, (3) in illnesses similar to infectious mononucleosis in which heterophil antibody tests are normal, (4) in febrile patients who have received organ transplants, and (5) in those patients with risk factors for HIV infection or those with AIDS (Scott et al., 1984).

The diagnosis of CMV disease may be extremely difficult to make with certainty. It is helpful to analyze tissue (e.g., from a lung biopsy) for the presence of viral invasion. Isolation of CMV in tissue culture and/or histological, immunological, or molecular evidence of the presence of virus from tissue (or fluid) presumed infected may be diagnostic. However, CMV may be a bystander or coexist with other pathogens and may not necessarily cause disease even if its presence is documented, since shedding of CMV by apparently healthy persons can occur.

It is often useful for diagnostic purposes to perform serological analyses for detection of CMV antibodies such as complement fixation, indirect immunofluorescence anticomplement assay, or enzyme linked immunosorbent assay (ELISA) in addition to attempts to detect the virus (Drew, 1988). Antibody titers to CMV, however, are known to fluctuate even in the absence of disease, making interpretation of results of antibody titers very difficult (Waner et al., 1973). In some patients a negative antibody

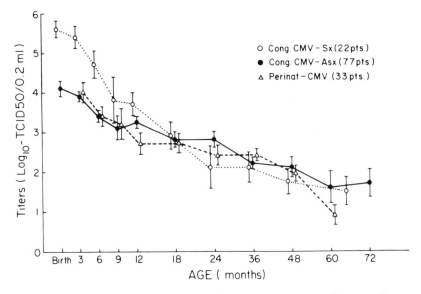

Fig. 3-7. Quantitative assessment of cytomegalovirus excretion in subjects with congenital symptomatic *(open circles)*, congenital asymptomatic *(closed circles)*, and perinatal *(triangles)* infections. (From Stagno S et al: Semin Perinatol 1983;7:34-42.)

test may be helpful in ruling out CMV infection.

As indicated in Fig. 3-7, CMV may persist in urine for prolonged periods of time. Urinary excretion of CMV by 99 congenitally infected infants, of whom 22 were symptomatic, and 33 perinatally infected infants is shown in Fig. 3-7 (Stagno et al., 1983). Symptomatic congenitally infected infants shed the greatest amount of virus, an observation that may have diagnostic implications in selected situations. Infants with perinatal infections usually began to shed the virus between 4 to 8 weeks of age; in one such infant shedding began at 3 weeks of age. Practically speaking, therefore, culture of urine for CMV during the first 2 weeks of life is necessary to distinguish between congenital and perinatal infection. Since prolonged viral shedding by all infected infants is the rule, diagnosis of congenital infection by urine culture may be problematic. A positive culture is conclusive in the newly born infant with obvious symptoms of CMV infection and no evidence of other congenital infections. Urinary shedding of CMV in infants with other congenital infections has been documented (Florman et al., 1973). Diagnosis of CMV in the infant who is asymptomatic at birth but later manifests developmental problems, statistically the most likely situation, is virtually impossible because congenital infection cannot be distinguished from postnatal CMV infection by urine culture after the neonatal period. Isolation of CMV from a site such as CSF is considered significant, although rather unusual (Jamison and Hathorn, 1978).

Antibody titers to CMV may also be difficult to interpret. Specific IgM has been detected in sera from healthy patients who presumably are experiencing an asymptomatic episode of viral reactivation (McEvoy and Adler, 1989), and IgG titers may also increase significantly without disease (Waner et al., 1973). There are few differences in titers from babies with congenital and perinatal infections. Interestingly, however, levels of specific IgG antibodies in maternal and infant sera are higher in babies with clinically apparent CMV infection with multiple system involvement than in babies with subclinical CMV infection (Britt and Vugler, 1990).

Presumably any specific IgM present in an infant's serum is diagnostic of infection, but the methodology is often questioned. An indirect immunofluorescence test for CMV IgM, described by Hanshaw et al., (1968), was positive only in infants with congenital CMV infections. This test has yielded false-positive and false-negative results in some other laboratories, however, and it is not generally available. A radio-immunoassay (RIA) for CMV IgM has been developed and tested by Griffiths et al. (1982a and b). These investigators found CMV IgM in 17 of 17 (100%) infants with symptomatic CMV infections; however, 66 of 76 (87%) infants with asymptomatic infections also had detectable CMV IgM.

With this same assay, primary and recurrent maternal CMV infections were studied since only mothers with primary CMV developed CMV IgM. CMV IgM was detected by RIA in 16 of 29 (55%) women with primary CMV and in none of 18 women with recurrent infection. It was thus possible to identify high-risk pregnancies and infants with a high likelihood of symptomatic congenital CMV (Griffiths et al., 1982a, 1982b). Unfortunately, however, it is unlikely that this test will ever become widely available because of technical difficulties involved in the assay. More data, in addition, are required to confirm that IgM develops only in primary CMV infection. The observation that CMV-specific IgM is detectable in more than 90% of homosexual men suggests that, as has been found for other herpesvirus infections, IgM is produced in secondary as well as primary infections and therefore is not a specific indicator for primary infection except in the newborn infant (Drew, 1988).

An ELISA procedure for CMV IgM has been developed. Data thus far suggest that it compares favorably with RIA but only in serum obtained beyond the neonatal period (Demmler et al., 1986a). Other studies have found that, although CMV IgM may be detected by ELISA in congenitally infected infants, this test is less sensitive and specific than RIA (Stagno et al., 1985). Since some ELISA results are reported as an optical density reading rather than as a titer, it is necessary to check with the laboratory for the range of normal values.

Diagnosis of CMV syndromes other than congenital infection may be suggested by detection of virus in urine or other body fluids by molecular techniques. CMV has been detected in clinical samples using DNA hybridization (Chou and Merigan, 1983; Spector and Spector, 1985; Schrier, Nelson, and Oldstone, 1985; Jenson and Robert, 1987). Although low levels of CMV DNA can be detected in urine from some patients with asymptomatic shedding of virus, those with disease caused by CMV excrete much

greater quantities of virus; therefore this assay may identify patients with illness caused by CMV (Chou and Merigan, 1983). With this same technique, CMV has also been detected in buffy coat cells from bone marrow transplant patients (Spector et al., 1983). In this study DNA hybridization was more sensitive than culture of buffy coat for CMV, which often yielded negative results on patients who obviously were infected with CMV. In older patients, including AIDS patients in whom CMV pneumonia was suspected, bronchiolar lavage specimens have been useful for diagnosis of CMV (Stover et al., 1984, Springmeyer et al., 1986; Drew, 1988). The major advantage of DNA hybridization procedures, however, is the rapidity with which results can be reported rather than sensitivity. These techniques, moreover, are usually only available on a research basis.

Another molecular test for demonstration of CMV, currently available almost entirely on a research basis, is polymerase chain reaction (PCR). With this methodology, minute amounts of viral nucleic acid are specifically amplified and then detected with molecular probes. Although highly subject to the possibility of nonspecificity, when performed carefully, PCR has been highly successful in rapid identification of CMV in urine from congenitally infected newborns (Demmler et al., 1988). Although available currently only as a research test, it is predicted that with time this assay may become clinically very useful for diagnosis.

In most hospitals culture for CMV is performed in the diagnostic virology laboratory, and amplification methods for viral growth in tissue culture are used to speed the time for identification of CMV. Amplification procedures include centrifugation of the inoculum into tissue culture cells and early identification of positive cultures by staining with fluorescent-labeled monoclonal antibodies after several days of incubation (Alpert et al., 1985; Drew, 1988). Thus a positive culture may be reported within days rather than weeks. The presence of high titers of virus in clinical specimens shortens the interval necessary for viral growth, which is also correlated with significant CMV infection; thus a rapid report of a positive culture may be indicative of CMV infection rather than asymptomatic viral shedding.

In summary, although diagnosis of CMV *infection* may not be difficult, proving that the virus is actually causing a *disease* is more problematic. In general, a significant increase in CMV antibody titer and/or positive IgM determination associated with evidence of viral invasion or excretion in urine or other body fluids, if accompanied by symptoms consistent with CMV infection, is considered presumptive evidence of CMV-induced disease.

DIFFERENTIAL DIAGNOSIS

In children CMV infection may be confused with various forms of hepatitis, Epstein-Barr virus (EBV) infections, and toxoplasmosis. Congenital symptomatic CMV infection must be distinguished from a variety of infections and diseases that are characterized by jaundice, hepatosplenomegaly, and purpura in the neonatal period.

Congenital toxoplasmosis

The clinical picture of congenital toxoplasmosis is remarkably similar to that of generalized congenital CMV. Both are characterized by jaundice, hepatosplenomegaly, chorioretinitis, and cerebral calcifications. Petechial and purpuric eruptions, which are common in patients with symptomatic congenital CMV infections, are rare with toxoplasmosis. When toxoplasmosis involves the CNS, elevated protein levels and pleocytosis often are detected in CSF, findings much less frequently associated with CMV infections. The precise diagnosis is established by serological evidence of congenital toxoplasmosis or virological and serological evidence of CMV infection.

Congenital rubella syndrome

The consequences of fetal infection with rubella virus during the first trimester of pregnancy, which in the aggregate has been termed the *congenital rubella syndrome*, include features also seen in infants with CMV such as hepatosplenomegaly, jaundice, petechial and purpuric rashes, thrombocytopenia, microcephaly, abnormalities of long bones on x-ray film, and mental retardation (Jenson and Robert, 1987). The diagnosis of the congenital rubella syndrome, suggested by a history of maternal infection in the first 3 to 4 months of pregnancy, should be confirmed by virological and serological evidence.

Erythroblastosis fetalis

The jaundice, purpura, and lethargy in an infant with erythroblastosis fetalis are associated with a positive Coombs' test. The serum alanine aminotransferase (ALT) activity, which is increased in patients with CMV hepatitis, is within normal limits in those with erythroblastosis fetalis. A similar syndrome with prominent congestive heart failure and edema is also caused by parvovirus B19 infection (see Chapter 18).

Disseminated herpes simplex virus infection

Skin lesions, which may be found in 80% of babies with perinatal HSV infection, are rare in CMV infection. Cerebral calcifications generally have not been observed in patients with perinatal HSV, but a few cases have been reported. Isolation of HSV or detection of HSV antigens in skin lesions or other tissues is usually required to confirm a diagnosis of HSV.

Sepsis of the newborn

Sepsis of the newborn may be characterized by lethargy, jaundice, and hepatomegaly. A blood culture usually reveals the causative organism.

Congenital syphilis

Congenital syphilis, which is becoming much more common in the United States, can be differentiated from CMV infection by serological tests and roentgenographic evidence of syphilitic osteitis.

EPIDEMIOLOGICAL FACTORS

CMV infections are worldwide in distribution. Virological and serological studies have contributed to knowledge of the epidemiology of CMV infection. Surveys of unselected newborn infants in the United States and England have revealed a startling 1% to 2% incidence of viruria, indicative of congenital infection. Surveys of virus shedding in pregnant women from various countries have revealed incidences ranging from 1.9% to 5.6%. Based on an estimate of 3.5 million births each year, therefore, it could be estimated that 70,000 infants with CMV infection are born each year in the United States. Approximately 10%, or 7,000, will eventually manifest symptoms such as deafness and varying degrees of mental retardation. These findings suggest that CMV infection is the most common congenital infection of humans.

The incidence of CMV infection is related to age, geographical location, and economic status. Serological evidence of CMV infection increases with advancing age, reaching levels of 80% in various parts of the world. In general, infection is acquired at an earlier age by children who live under crowded, unhygienic conditions that may be prevalent in slum areas, institutions for mentally retarded children, and day-care centers with more than 20 children.

The epidemiology of CMV infection in the United States apparently is changing as more and more children of middle and upper socioeconomic status are placed in day care and since breast-feeding is becoming more common in our society. Both would tend to increase the incidence of CMV infections in young children and to increase the incidence of disease in seronegative adults with whom they have contact (Yow et al., 1987). In a study of 1,989 pregnant women of middle to upper socioeconomic status seropositivity was associated with nonwhite race, less than 16 years of education, being breast-fed in infancy, presence of children in the home, and being more than 30 years of age (Walmus et al., 1988). In the large study by Stagno et al. (1986) 65% of young women of upper socioeconomic status and 23% of young women of lower socioeconomic status lacked detectable antibodies against CMV. The incidence of primary CMV during pregnancy was higher in women from low-income families than in upper middle class women (Stagno et al., 1986). In this large study the annualized rate of primary CMV infection was 6.8% in the former and 2.5% in the latter.

The incidence of symptomatic congenital CMV infection is greater in highly industrialized countries than in developing nations. Acquisition of CMV in girls may be thought of as a natural form of immunization that later prevents symptomatic CMV infection in offspring.

Intrauterine transmission of CMV after primary infection is thought to occur in approximately 40% of cases (Stagno et al., 1986). More than 35% of postpartum women excrete reactivated CMV in breast milk, vaginal secretions, urine, or saliva. Approximately 20% of breast-fed infants become infected with CMV (Stagno et al., 1983).

Infection of children in day-care centers in the United States is very common. Variables concerning whether infection will occur include the number of children in the center, their age, and the time spent in the setting. After an 18-month interval, approximately 50% of seronegative children below the age of 3 years who are in a day-care center with more than 50 children will be infected. In children in day care who are 12 to 36 months of age the rate of excretion of CMV is very high—between 25% and 100% (Adler, 1988a, 1988b). No data are available on transmission for children who are cared for in smaller groups. CMV has been isolated from many potential sources of spread such as saliva, urine, toys, hands, and diapers (Demmler et al., 1987; Adler, 1988a, 1988b).

It is likely that there is significant transmission of CMV from infants and small children. Taber et al. (1985) noted that an important risk factor for maternal acquisition of CMV was an infected child in the home. Pass et al. (1986) observed an increased incidence of CMV infection among 67 parents whose children attended day care. In this study susceptible parents whose children were infected had an infection rate of 30%. If only parents whose children were less than 18 months old were analyzed, the parental infection rate increased to 45%. There were no CMV infections in 21 parents whose children were in day care and not shedding CMV nor in 21 children cared for at home. Other observers have also found that the risk of parental infection, particularly maternal, is increased as a result of exposure to infected children; in some cases transmission has been proven since the virus isolated from both parent and child has been identical on analysis of DNA (Spector and Spector, 1982; Pass et al., 1987; Adler, 1988a, 1988b). Although infection at day care is not particularly harmful to children, their parents may become infected as a result, which may have serious consequences if the mother is pregnant.

Whether hospital workers are at increased risk to become infected by CMV from their patients is difficult to assess. One study of the risks of 122 seronegative pediatric health care workers acquiring a primary CMV infection revealed an annual attack rate of approximately 3%, similar to that of young women in the community (Dworsky et al., 1983a). This low risk of nosocomial transmission in nurses exposed to patients who were shedding CMV was confirmed by Balfour and Balfour (1986). However, another study of 842 female employees in a pediatric hospital revealed that 5 of 45 (10.9%) intensive care nurses, 2 of 11 (18.2%) intravenous team nurses, and 3 of 81 (3.7%) ward nurses seroconverted to CMV after 1 year (Friedman et al., 1984).

During a 2-year period Demmler et al. (1987) investigated patient-to-caretaker, patient-to-patient, and caretaker-to-patient transmission of CMV in two pediatric settings, a chronic care unit and a neonatal nursery. In 2 years of study 2 of 69 (3%) nurses in the neonatal nursery seroconverted, and none of the nurses in the chronic care facility seroconverted. Of 188 personnel and 630 patients, there was one instance of possible patient-to-patient spread and one instance of patient-to-caretaker spread. Analysis of CMV isolates by restriction enzymes revealed that one additional presumed instance of patient-to-caretaker spread was actually a case of spread from husband to wife (Demmler et al., 1986b). This observation illustrates a significant point: the source of transmission cannot be identified by antibody assays; viral isolates taken from both the presumed source and the secondary case in question must have identical DNA before it can be concluded that transmission actually occurred. Using this criterion, it can be said that nosocomial transmission of CMV from a patient to a hospital worker has yet to be proven, although on occasion undoubtedly it occurs.

The development of restriction endonuclease "fingerprinting" techniques has made it possible to prove various transmissions of CMV and thus clarify routes of transmission. For example, transmission from mother to fetus has been documented (Huang et al., 1980; Wilfert et al., 1982; Pass et al., 1987; Adler, 1988a, 1988b), as has transmission from infant to mother (Spector and Spector, 1982; Dworsky et al., 1984; Pass et al., 1987; Adler, 1988). Nosocomial transmission from infant to infant has been demonstrated (Demmler et al., 1987; Spector, 1983), although it apparently is an unusual phenomenon (Adler et al., 1986). Transmission among infants in a day-care setting has been proven (Adler, 1985; Murph et al., 1986; Adler, 1988b), as has transmission from husband to wife (Demmler et al., 1987).

On the other hand, three medical staff personnel known to have been exposed to a patient with CMV were shown to have been infected with CMV from a different source (Wilfert et al., 1982; Yow et al., 1982; Dworsky et al., 1984). Data from one of these cases are shown in Fig. 3-8. A pregnant physician who contracted CMV while caring for a baby with CMV had her pregnancy terminated. As indicated in Fig. 3-8, DNA of the CMV isolated from the physician-mother and her fetus were similar but different from the DNA isolated from the presumed index case, indicating that the source of the physician's infection was not her patient.

There is increasing evidence for iatrogenic CMV disease in certain individuals. Some of these infections are undoubtedly reactivation

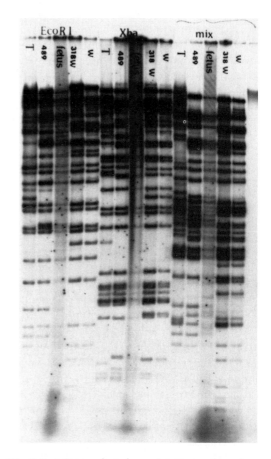

Fig. 3-8. DNA analysis by restriction endonucleases obtained from *T*, Towne (control) strain of CMV; *489*, mother's cytomegalovirus (CMV); *fetus*, fetal CMV; *318W* and *W*, CMV of index case. Fetus and 489 are similar but different from 318W and W.

syndromes that occur when immunosuppressive drugs are given to patients for underlying malignancy or organ transplantation. Others are primary infections caused by transfusions containing white blood cells harboring latent CMV or by transplantation of a kidney from a CMV-seropositive donor into a CMV-seronegative recipient (Ho et al., 1975). Although the risk of CMV infection in renal transplant patients is higher when the recipient is seronegative, infection may also occur in seropositives (Chou, 1986). The risk of acquiring CMV from transfusion rises as increasing units of transfused blood and numbers of donors are used (Adler, 1983).

PROGNOSIS

Infants who survive generalized severe congenital CMV infection usually have significant neurological sequelae such as microcephaly, mental retardation, and motor disability. Of 16 patients followed by Weller and Hanshaw (1962), only two failed to show residual damage. Of 34 patients with congenital symptomatic CMV infections followed for 9 months to 14 years, 10 died, 16 (47%) had microcephaly, 14 (41%) had mental retardation, 7 (21%) had hearing loss, 8 (24%) had neuromuscular disorders, and 5 (15%) had chorioretinitis or optic atrophy (Pass et al., 1980). No strains of CMV with a predilection to cause neurological damage have been identified (Griller et al., 1988).

The many infants who have symptomatic congenital CMV infection may show no effects until later childhood when some manifest hearing loss and school failure (Reynolds et al., 1974; Hanshaw et al., 1975; Stagno et al., 1977a). Current studies suggest this may occur in as many as 10% of congenitally infected children. With approximately 3.5 million births annually in the United States, this could involve 3,500 to 7,000 school children each year. Interestingly, a follow-up study of 32 children with symptomatic congenital CMV infection showed no correlation between the sequela of deafness and low intelligence (Conboy et al., 1987). On the other hand, chorioretinitis, in particular, but also microcephaly and neurological abnormalities manifested by 1 year of age were all associated with development of severe mental retardation. These investigators have stressed, therefore, the wide range of possible outcomes of primary congenital infection that may not be generally appreciated. They have pointed out, for example, that an infant with hepatosplenomegaly, thrombocytopenia, jaundice, prematurity, and hearing loss might be expected to attain intellectual and developmental outcomes that are nearly normal.

Infants infected in the perinatal period rarely if ever manifest sequelae, with the exception of seronegative premature infants inadvertently infected with CMV by blood or banked breast milk containing latent virus. The long-term prognosis for these particular infants is unknown.

Evaluation of the prognosis of CMV infection in immunocompromised patients, including older children, is often complicated by the underlying condition and its therapy.

Transplant patients who acquire CMV may develop illnesses caused directly by CMV such as pneumonia, retinitis, and bacterial, protozoal, and fungal superinfections. In a series of 545 individuals who had undergone bone marrow transplantation, CMV infection occurred in approximately one third of seronegative patients and in two thirds of seropositive patients (Meyers et al., 1986). In general, however, the prognosis is better in patients who are seropositive at the time of infection than in those who are seronegative. Pneumonia caused by CMV carries a very high case/fatality ratio, although recently, with the availability of ganciclovir and high-titered immune globulin, the prognosis has improved somewhat.

The long-term prognosis of CMV infection in HIV-infected infants, including those with congenital or perinatal infections with both viruses, is not known, nor is it known whether congenital infection with one of these viruses predisposes to infection with the other. Similarly, the long-term prognosis of HIV-infected children infected with CMV in early infancy, as might occur in a day-care setting, has not been determined.

PREVENTION

A number of approaches to prevention of severe CMV infections in immunocompromised patients are being explored. They include active and passive immunization and administration of antiviral compounds on a prophylactic basis. It is conceivable that one day a vaccine will be used to prevent congenital CMV infection as is done to prevent congenital rubella.

Experimental live CMV vaccines are being

evaluated by various investigators. Studies by Plotkin et al. (1976) have revealed that it is possible to prepare a live CMV vaccine that is well tolerated and antigenic. Questions that have been raised about a live CMV vaccine include (1) the degree of its attenuation, (2) its potential to become oncogenic, (3) its potential to induce a persistent infection, (4) the duration of immunity, and (5) whether it will protect against disease.

Placebo-controlled studies in 91 renal transplant patients indicated that although infection was not prevented by prior immunization, illness caused by CMV was modifed in those immunized in comparison to those who received a placebo (Plotkin et al., 1984). Immunized patients do not excrete vaccine-type CMV in their urine, and it is believed that the vaccine virus does not cause latent infection (Plotkin et al., 1984, 1985; Plotkin and Huang, 1985). Studies in healthy human volunteers have indicated that the vaccine is attenuated in comparison to wild-type strains of CMV and that prior inoculation with the vaccine strain prevents disease after challenge with wild-type virus (Plotkin et al., 1985; Plotkin et al., 1987). A subunit glycoprotein CMV vaccine that would avoid the theoretical problems of viral latency is also being evaluated currently (Plotkin et al., 1990).

Several approaches to prevention of CMV infection may be taken in low-birth-weight hospitalized infants. Breast-fed infants may be given milk from only their own mothers, frozen or pasteurized banked human breast milk, or a prepared formula (Stagno et al., 1980; Dworsky et al., 1983b). Unfortunately, any cellular immunity present in milk that is theoretically of potential benefit to the infant will be destroyed along with the virus by pasteurization or freezing. The infectivity of CMV is lost after freezing (except at very low temperatures such as $-70°$ C) or heating to 62° C (pasteurization).

Probably the most important method of prevention of CMV in low-birth-weight infants is by transfusion with blood that does not contain latent CMV. One approach is to transfuse these infants with blood from CMV-seronegative donors; another is to use frozen deglycerolized red blood cells (Yeager et al., 1981; Adler, 1983). Unfortunately, infection with CMV cannot be prevented by transfusion of saline-washed red blood cells, which are much simpler to prepare (Demmler et al., 1986c). Identification of potentially CMV-infected donor blood by DNA hybridization has not proven successful (Jackson et al., 1987). Although it has been possible to identify blood that is unlikely to transmit CMV by testing it for the presence of CMV IgM antibodies, the assay is neither generally available nor consistently accurate and therefore is impractical (Lambertson et al., 1988).

Although only CMV-seronegative infants are at risk, most hospitals do not test babies for CMV antibodies. Appropriate preventive measures therefore are best carried out for all low-birth-weight infants unless CMV antibody determinations are performed.

Hyperimmune globulin has been found to reduce the incidence of severe CMV infections in some studies of bone marrow transplant patients (Meyers et al., 1983; Condie and O'Reilly, 1984) but not in others (Bowden et al., 1986). Hyperimmune globulin decreased the incidence of CMV disease in approximately two thirds of renal transplant patients in controlled studies (Snydman et al., 1987). Treated patients also experienced fewer fungal and bacterial superinfections. Hyperimmune globulin has been approved for use by the Food and Drug Administration (FDA) and is commercially available. Administration of acyclovir (ACV) on a prophylactic basis decreases the incidence of serious CMV infections in renal transplant patients (Balfour et al., 1989).

Performing serological screening of women to determine if they are susceptible to CMV and therefore at risk to have a primary infection during pregnancy is controversial. Those who advocate testing point out that knowledge of susceptibility is helpful for counseling, particularly for women at increased risk of infection such as those with small children in day care or hospital workers (Walmus et al., 1988). Women who are seropositive against CMV may be reassured. In contrast, however, Pass et al. (1987) and Adler (1988a, 1988b) have emphasized the difficulties of diagnosis of maternal infection, the futility of trying to prevent CMV infection in susceptibles, and the problem of deciding whether to continue a pregnancy if CMV is diagnosed. Until a means of prevention of CMV is developed, serological screening of pregnant women for antibodies to CMV is probably of little use. At this time, experts seem to agree that there is not enough information to indicate the exact risk of CMV infection to the infant; therefore termination of pregnancy, even if a primary maternal infection is documented during the first trimester, is not recommended (Stagno et al., 1986; Adler, 1988a, 1988b).

THERAPY

Specific therapy is not indicated for normal hosts. Whether specific therapy could improve the outcome of congenital infection is not known.

In immunocompromised patients nonspecific measures such as decreasing the dosage of immunosuppressive drugs is recommended if possible (Pollard, 1988). Fortunately, CMV infections in immunocompromised patients apparently are less severe since the introduction of cyclosporine (Pollard, 1988). CMV immunoglobulin in conjunction with ganciclovir has been used to treat CMV pneumonia (Reed et al., 1988).

The drug ganciclovir, which is structurally similar to ACV but has greater activity against CMV, has been used with some success to treat severe CMV infections in immunocompromised patients. The drug has been licensed in the United States for treatment of severe CMV infections such as those that occur in renal transplant patients and patients with AIDS. Although most of the studies of this drug have been uncontrolled, it appears that, in general, patients with retinitis and colitis caused by CMV respond well, but the outcome in those with pneumonia is less positive (Collaborative DHPG Study Group, 1986; Keay, Bissett, and Merigan, 1987; Laskin et al., 1987; Lim et al., 1988). Often the virological response is more prominent than the clinical response. Latent infection with CMV is neither cured nor prevented; the drug is not curative. Iatrogenically immunosuppressed patients who have had organ transplantation seem to respond better than patients with underlying AIDS (Keay, Bissett, and Merigan, 1987; Laskin et al., 1987). In patients with AIDS, CMV relapses are common after therapy so that longterm administration of ganciclovir is required. The recommended therapeutic dose of ganciclovir is 7.5 mg/kg/day intravenously (IV); 5 mg/ kg IV five to seven times per week is recommended for maintenance dosage. Reported adverse effects include neutropenia and leukopenia. Zidovudine (AZT) and gancyclovir cannot be administered simultaneously because of drug toxicity. Other approaches in immunocompromised patients include administration of foscarnet for CMV retinitis in HIV-infected patients and interferon.

REFERENCES

Adler SP. Transfusion-associated cytomegalovirus infections. Rev Infect Dis 1983;5:977-993.

Adler SP. The molecular epidemiology of cytomegalovirus transmission among children attending a day care center. J Infect Dis 1985;152:760-768.

Adler SP. Cytomegalovirus transmission among children in day care, their mothers and caretakers. Pediatr Infect Dis 1988a;7:279-285.

Adler SP. Molecular epidemiology of cytomegalovirus: viral transmission among children attending a day care center, their parents, and caretakers. J Pediatr 1988b;112:366-372.

Adler SP, Baggett J, Wilson M, et al. Molecular epidemiology of cytomegalovirus in a nursery: lack of evidence for nosocomial transmission. J Pediatr 1986;108:117-123.

Ahlfors D, Harris S, Ivarsson S, et al. Secondary maternal cytomegalovirus infection causing symptomatic congenital infection. N Engl J Med 1981;305:284.

Alexander ER. Maternal and neonatal infection with cytomegalovirus in Taiwan. Pediatr Res 1967;1:210.

Alford CA, Hayes K, Britt W. Primary cytomegalovirus infection in pregnancy: comparison of antibody responses to virus-encoded proteins between women with and without intrauterine infection. J Infect Dis 1988;158:917-924.

Alford CA Jr, Reynolds DW, Stagno S. Current concepts of chronic perinatal infections. In Gluck L (ed.) Modern perinatal medicine. Chicago: Year Book Medical Publishers, 1975.

Alpert G, Mazeron M-C, Colimon R, Plotkin S. Rapid detection of human cytomegalovirus in the urine of humans. J Infect Dis 1985;152:631-633.

Balfour CL, Balfour HH Jr. Cytomegalovirus is not an occupational risk for nurses in renal transplant and neonatal units: results of a prospective surveillance study. JAMA 1986;256:1909-1914.

Balfour HH, Chace BA, Stapleton JT, et al. A randomized placebo-controlled trial of oral acyclovir for the prevention of cytomegalovirus disease in recipients of renal allografts. N Engl J Med 1989;320:1381-1387.

Ballard RA, Drew WL, Hufnagle KG, et al. Acquired cytomegalovirus infection in preterm infants. Am J Dis Child 1979;133:482.

Bowden RA, Sayers M, Fluornoy N, et al. Cytomegalovirus immune globulin and seronegative blood products to prevent primary cytomegaloviurs infection after bone marrow transplantation. N Engl J Med 1986;314:1006-1010.

Brasfield DM, Stagno S, Whitley RJ, et al. Infant pneumonitis associated with cytomegalovirus, *Chlamydia*, *Pneumocystis*, and *Ureaplasma*: follow up. Pediatrics 1987;79:76-83.

Reed EC, Bowden RA, Dandliker PS, et al. Treatment of cytomegalovirus pneumonia with gancyclovir and intravenous cytomegalovirus immunoglobulin in patients with bone marrow transplants. Ann Intern Med 1988;109:783-788.

Reynolds DW, Dean PH, Pass RF, Alford CA. Specific cell-mediated immunity in children with congenital and neonatal cytomegalovirus infection and their mothers. J Infect Dis 1979;140:493-499.

Reynolds DW, Stagno S, Alford C. Congenital cytomegalovirus infection. In Reynolds DW, Stagno S, Alford C (eds). Teratogen update: environmentally induced birth defect risks. New York:Alan R Liss, 1986, pp 93-95.

Reynolds DW, Stagno S, Stubbs G, et al. Inapparent congenital cytomegalovirus infection with elevated cord IgM levels. Causal relation with auditory and mental deficiency. N Engl J Med 1974;290:291-296.

Rola-Pleszczynski M, Frenkel L, Fuceillo DA, et al. Specific impairment of cell-mediated immunity in mothers of infants with congenital infection due to cytomegalovirus. J Infect Dis 1977;135:386-391.

Rowe WP, et al. Cytopathogenic agent resembling human salivary gland virus recovered from tissue cultures of human adenoids. Proc Soc Exp Biol Med 1956;92:4181.

Sawyer MH, Edwards DK, Spector SA. Cytomegalovirus infection and bronchopulmonary dysplasia in premature infants. Am J Dis Child 1987;141:303-305.

Schrier RD, Nelson JA, Oldstone MBA. Detection of human cytomegalovirus in peripheral blood leucocytes in a natural infection. Science 1985;230:1048-1051.

Schrier RD, Rice GPA, Oldstone MBA. Suppression of natural killer cell activity and T cell proliferation by fresh isolates of human cytomegalovirus. J Infect Dis 1986;153:1084-1091.

Scott GB, Buck BE, Leterman JG, et al. Acquired immunodeficiency syndrome in infants. N Engl J Med 1984;310:76-81.

Singh N, Dummer JS, Kusne S, et al. Infections with cytomegalovirus and other herpesviruses in 121 liver transplant recipients: transplantation by donated organ and the effect of OKT3 antibodies. J Infect Dis 1988;158:124-131.

Smith MG. Propagation of salivary gland virus of the mouse in tissue cultures. Proc Soc Exp Biol Med 1954;86:435.

Smith MG. Propagation in tissue cultures of a cytopathogenic virus from human salivary gland virus (SGV) disease. Proc Soc Exp Biol Med 1956;92:424.

Snydman DR, Werner BG, Heize-Lacey B, et al. Use of cytomegalovirus immune globulin to prevent cytomegalovirus disease in renal transplant recipients. N Engl J Med 1987;317:1049-1054.

Spector SA. Transmission of cytomegalovirus among infants in hospital documented by restriction-endonuclease-digestion analyses. Lancet 1983;1:378-381.

Spector SA, Hirata KK, Neuman TR. Identification of multiple cytomegalovirus strains in homosexual men with acquired immunodeficiency syndrome. J Infect Dis 1984;150:953-956.

Spector SA, Rua LA, Spector DH, et al. Rapid diagnosis of CMV viremia in bone marrow transplant patients by DNA-DNA hybridization (abstract 914). Las Vegas: Twenty-Third Interscience Conference in Antimicrobial Agents and Chemotherapy, 1983.

Spector SA, Spector DH. Molecular epidemiology of cytomegalovirus infections in premature twin infants and their mother. Pediatr Infect Dis 1982;1:405-409.

Spector SA, Spector DH. The use of DNA probes in studies of human cytomegalovirus. Clin Chem 1985;31:1514-1520.

Springmeyer SC, Hackman RC, Holle R, et al. Use of bronchoalveolar lavage to diagnose acute diffuse pneumonia in the immunocompromised host. J Infect Dis 1986;154:604-610.

Stagno S, Brasfield DM, Brown MB et al. Infant pneumonitis associated with cytomegalovirus, chlamydia, pneumocystis, and ureaplasma: a prospective study. Pediatrics 1981;68:322-329.

Stagno S, Pass R, Cloud G, et al. Primary cytomegalovirus infection in pregnancy. Incidence, transmission to fetus, and clinical outcome. JAMA 1986;256:1904-1908.

Stagno S, Pass RF, Dworsky ME, et al. Congenital cytomegalovirus infection. The relative importance of primary and recurrent maternal infection. N Engl J Med 1982;306:945-949.

Stagno S, Pass R, Dworsky M, et al. Congenital and perinatal cytomegalovirus infections. Semin Perinatol 1983;7:31.

Stagno S, Reynolds D, Amos CS, et al. Auditory and visual defects resulting from symptomatic and subclinical congenital cytomegaloviral and toxoplasma infections. Pediatrics 1977a;59:699-678.

Stagno S, Reynolds DW, Huang ES, et al. Congenital cytomegalovirus infection. Occurrence in an immune population. N Engl J Med 1977b;296:1254-1258.

Stagno S, Reynolds DW, Pass RF, Alford CA. Breast milk and the risk of cytomegalovirus infection. N Engl J Med 1980;302:1073-1076.

Stagno S, Tinker M, Elrod C, et al. Immunoglobulin M antibodies detected by enzyme-linked immunosorbent assay and radioimmunoassay in the diagnosis of cytomegalovirus infections in pregnant women and newborn infants. J Clin Micro 1985;31:930-935.

Starr SE, Tolpin MD, Friedman HM, et al. Impaired cellular immunity to cytomegalovirus in congenitally infected children and their mothers. J Infect Dis 1979;140:500-505.

Stover DE, Zaman MB, Hajdu SI, et al. Bronchoalveolar lavage in the diagnosis of diffuse pulmonary infiltrates in the immunosuppressed host. Ann Intern Med 1984;101:1-7.

Taber LH, Frank Al, Yow MD, et al. Acquisition of cytomegaloviral infections in families with young children: a serologic study. J Infect Dis 1985;151:948-952.

Tatum ET, Sun PC, Cohn DJ. Cytomegalovirus vasculitis and colon perforation in a patient with the acquired immunodeficiency syndrome. Pathology 1989;21:235-238.

von Glahn WC, Pappenheimer AM. Intranuclear inclusions in visceral disease. Am J Pathol 1925;1:445.

Walmus BF, Yow MD, Lester JW, et al. Factors predictive of cytomegalovirus immune status in pregnant women. J Infect Dis 1988;157:172-177.

Waner JL, Weller TA, Kevy SV. Patterns of cytomegalovirus complement fixing antibody activity: a longitudinal study of blood donors. J Infect Dis 1973;127:538-543.

Weller TH, Hanshaw JB. Virologic and clinical observations on cytomegalic inclusion disease. N Engl J Med 1962;26:1233.

Weller TH, Hanshaw JB, Scott DE. Serologic differentiation of viruses responsible for cytomegalic inclusion disease. Virology 1960;12:130.

Weller TH, Macaulay JC, Craig JM, et al. Isolation of intranuclear inclusion agents from infants and illnesses resembling cytomegalic inclusion disease. Proc Soc Exp Biol Med 1957;94:4.

Whitley RJ, Brasfield D, Reynolds DW, et al. Protracted pneumonitis in young infants associated with perinatally acquired cytomegaloviral infection. J Pediatr 1976;89:16-22.

Wilfert CM, Huang ES, Stagno S. Restriction endonuclease analysis of cytomegalovirus deoxyribonucleic acid as an epidemiologic tool. Pediatrics 1982;70:717-721.

Yeager AS. Transfusion-acquired cytomegalovirus infection in newborn infants. Am J Dis Child 1974;128:478-483.

Yeager AS, Grumet FC, Hafleigh EB, et al. Prevention of transfusion-acquired cytomegalovirus infections in newborn infants. J Pediatr 1981;98:281-287.

Yeager AS, Jacobs H, Clark J. Nursery-acquired cytomegalovirus infection in two premature infants. J Pediatr 1972;81:332-335.

Yow MD, Lakeman AD, Stagno S, et al. Use of restriction enymes to investigate the source of a primary cytomegalovirus infection in a pediatric nurse. Pediatrics 1982;70:713-716.

Yow MD, White N, Taber L, et al. Acquisition of cytomegalovirus infection from birth to 10 years: a longitudinal serologic study. J Pediatr 1987;110:37-42.

4

DIPHTHERIA

Diphtheria is a preventable acute disease caused by *Corynebacterium diphtheriae*. The microorganism produces an exotoxin that is responsible for the resulting illness. The disease is characterized clinically by a sore throat and a membrane that may cover the tonsils, pharynx, and larynx. Diphtheria is so rare today in developed areas of the world that it is considered of little importance and is neglected as a differential diagnosis. Nevertheless, it is still prevalent in many developing countries, and importation of cases may occur.

HISTORY

The recognition of diphtheria as a disease probably dates back to the second century. It was in 1826, however, that Bretonneau named the illness *la diphthérite* and accurately described the clinical manifestations. He distinguished scarlet fever from diphtheria and identified membranous croup as a form of diphtheria.

The diphtheria bacillus was discovered by Klebs in 1883 and was isolated in pure culture by Löffler. It was called the Klebs-Löffler bacillus, and its etiological relationship to the disease was demonstrated in 1884. Roux and Yersin in 1888 showed that the bacillus produced an exotoxin that was responsible for the various clinical manifestations of the disease such as myocarditis and neuritis. In 1890 von Behring showed that the toxin stimulated the production of antitoxin. Subsequently, in 1894 Roux and Martin used horses for the production of antitoxin that was used for treatment. In the same

year von Behring used toxin neutralized by antitoxin to induce immunity in animals and man. A large-scale immunization program to protect children was initiated by Park in 1922. Finally, in 1923 Ramon showed that formalin-treated toxin, currently known as *toxoid*, was superior to toxin-antitoxin as an immunizing agent. A century of progress culminated in 1923 in the development of a safe and effective vaccine capable of preventing the disease.

ETIOLOGY

C. diphtheriae is the only major human pathogen of the corynebacterial group. These organisms are taxonomically related to the mycobacteria and *Nocardia*.

Morphology

C. diphtheriae organisms are slender gram-positive rods that measure 2 to 4 μm by 0.5 to 1 μm. When grown on suboptimal media, the bacteria are pleomorphic. The cells vary in diameter, and the ends are broader than the center, producing a typical club-shaped appearance. A beaded or bandlike appearance is produced by the metachromatic granules, which are accumulations of polymerized polyphosphates. The bacteria appear in palisades or as individual cells at sharp angles to each other as a result of cell division.

Cultural characteristics

C. diphtheriae is an aerobe requiring complex media for isolation and characterization. Potassium tellurite medium selectively inhibits a number of potentially contaminating organisms and allows three colony types of *C. diphtheriae*—gravis, mitis, and intermedius—to be distinguished. No constant relationship exists between colonial type and disease severity.

C. diphtheriae is an antigenically heterogeneous species with a large number of serological types. The different colonial types reflect cell-surface differences. Heat-labile K antigens, which are proteins of the superficial cell wall, are responsible for type specificity. These multiple-surface antigens are probably the reason the host can be colonized by *C. diphtheriae* despite previous experience with the organism.

The heat stable O antigen is a group antigen common to the corynebacteria parasitic to man. The O antigen is a polysaccharide containing arabinogalactans and is responsible for cross-reactivity with mycobacteria and *Nocardia*.

Colonization of mucous membranes can be accomplished by both toxogenic and nontoxogenic strains. The organisms have a toxic glycolipid, a cord factor, considered necessary for virulence.

The most important characteristic of the diphtheria bacillus is its ability to produce an exotoxin both in vivo and in vitro (Collier 1975; Murphy, 1978). This toxin is responsible for many of the serious clinical manifestations of the disease. It is extremely unstable and is easily destroyed by heat (75° C for 10 minutes), light, and aging. Toxin is produced only by strains of *C. diphtheriae* that are lysogenic for a bacteriophage carrying the *tox* gene (Freeman 1953; Parsons, 1955). Thus a person may harbor *C. diphtheriae* and acquire one of many phages that convert the bacterium to a toxin producer. Toxin production does not require lytic growth of the phage. The tox gene confers an advantage in survival both to the phage and to *C. diphtheriae* in the human host.

In vitro diphtheria toxin is maximally produced when there is a limited amount of iron present. When adequate iron is present, a repressor-iron complex binds to the phage tox gene and prevents toxin formation. When the iron concentration is lowered, dissociation of the repressor complex from the tox gene occurs, and toxin is produced.

The toxin is synthesized on membrane-bound polysomes and is released extracellularly as a single inactive precursor polypeptide chain. Cleavage exposes the active enzymatic site of toxin, and the biologically active toxin consists of two functionally distinct polypeptides, A and B, linked by a disulfide bond. Fragment B is unstable, is not enzymatically active, and is required for attachment of the activated toxin molecule to receptors of sensitive host cells. All human cells have receptor sites, which may be glycoproteins for fragment B, and the binding is rapid and irreversible. The attachment of B is necessary for penetration of fragment A into the cell. Both A and B are necessary for cytotoxicity.

Diphtheria toxin receptors on cell membranes appear to concentrate in a "coated pit," and toxin penetrates cells by endocytosis. This enfolding and vesicular formation provides access of the toxin to the interior of the cell. The subsequent natural acidification of the endosome containing the toxin results in passage of toxin across the membrane of the endosome to the cytosol. Species such as mice and rats are resistant to toxin but have plasma membrane receptors for the toxin. However, the transport process is defective, and toxin cannot reach the cytosol of the cell.

Fragment A is extremely stable, enzymatically active, and responsible for the toxic effects, which are achieved by inhibition of cellular protein synthesis. Fragment A inactivates elongation factor 2 (EF-2), which is a protein common to all eukaryotic cells. This protein is essential for translocation of peptidyl transfer RNA on ribosomes. An unusual amino acid named *diphthamide* is the single site on EF-2 that is adenosine 5′-diphosphate (ADP)-ribosylated.

PATHOGENESIS AND PATHOLOGY

Virulent diphtheria bacilli lodge in the nasopharynx of susceptible persons. As bacterial growth takes place in the secretions and epithelial debris, the toxin is elaborated and absorbed by the local mucous membrane. The toxic effect on the cells causes tissue necrosis, which provides the environment for growth of the organism and production of more toxin.

In addition to the necrosis, an inflammatory and exudative reaction is induced by the toxin. The necrotic epithelial cells, leukocytes, red blood cells, fibrinous material, diphtheria bacilli, and other bacterial inhabitants of the na-

by a variable amount of cervical adenitis, and in severe cases the marked swelling produces a so-called "bull-neck" appearance.

The course of the illness depends in large part on the severity of the toxemia. The temperature remains either normal or slightly elevated, but the pulse is disproportionately rapid. In mild cases the membrane sloughs off between the seventh and tenth days, and the patient has an uneventful recovery. In moderately severe cases convalescence is slow, with the course frequently complicated by myocarditis and neuritis (see Complications). Severe cases are characterized by increasing toxemia manifested by severe prostration, striking pallor, rapid thready pulse, stupor, coma, and death within 6 to 10 days.

Laryngeal diphtheria

Laryngeal diphtheria most often develops as an extension of pharyngeal involvement. Occasionally, however, it may be the only manifestation of the disease. The illness is ushered in by fever, hoarseness, and cough, which develops a barking quality. Increasing obstruction of the airway by the membrane is manifested by inspiratory stridor followed by suprasternal, supraclavicular, and subcostal retractions. The membrane may extend downward to involve the entire tracheobronchial tree.

The clinical picture of laryngeal diphtheria is dominated by the consequences of the mechanical obstruction to the air passages caused by the membrane, congestion, and edema. In mild cases or in those modified by antitoxin therapy the airway remains patent, and the membrane is coughed up between the sixth and tenth days. A sudden acute and fatal obstruction may occur in a mild case in which a partially detached piece of membrane blocks the airway. In very severe cases there is increasing obstruction followed by progressive hypoxia, which is manifested by restlessness, cyanosis, severe prostration, coma, and death.

Signs of toxemia are minimal in primary laryngeal involvement because toxin is poorly absorbed from the mucous membrane of the larynx. In most instances, however, the laryngeal involvement is associated with tonsillar and pharyngeal diphtheria. Consequently, the clinical manifestations are those of both obstruction and severe toxemia.

Unusual types of diphtheria

Diphtheritic infections occasionally develop in sites other than the respiratory tract. Cutaneous, conjunctival, aural, and vulvovaginal infections may occur (Belsey, 1975). The typical skin lesion is an ulcer with sharply demarcated edges and a membraneous base. The conjunctival lesion primarily involves the palpebral surface, which is reddened, edematous, and membranous. Involvement of the external auditory canal is usually manifest by a persistent purulent discharge. Vulvovaginal lesions are usually ulcerative and confluent.

DIAGNOSIS

An early diagnosis of diphtheria is essential because delay of administration of antitoxin may impose a serious and preventable risk to the patient. Accurate bacteriological confirmation by means of culture requires a minimum of 15 to 20 hours; smears are not reliable. Consequently, the initial diagnosis, as a basis for therapy, must be made on clinical grounds alone. Occasionally, a rapidly executed blood smear and heterophil antibody test may point to a diagnosis of infectious mononucleosis and obviate the need for antitoxin.

Bacteriological diagnosis

An accurate diagnosis of diphtheria is made by the demonstration of diphtheria bacilli cultured from material obtained from the site of infection. Care should be exercised in taking the culture. The swab should be rubbed firmly over the lesion or, if possible, should be inserted beneath the membrane. The physician must notify the laboratory that diphtheria is suspected to have correct media used. A Löffler slant, a blood agar plate, and a tellurite plate should be streaked with the swab. The slant and plates should be placed in the incubator without delay. After incubation, the organisms on the plates should be identified by an experienced person.

Diphtheria bacilli that are isolated on culture should be tested for toxigenicity by means of a virulence test. Two guinea pigs are inoculated intracutaneously with a broth suspension of the test microorganisms; one of the animals should be pretreated with diphtheria antitoxin. If the bacilli are toxigenic, an inflammatory lesion will appear at the site of inoculation in the untreated animal in 24 hours, and it will become necrotic in 72 hours. The antitoxin-treated animal will show no skin reaction.

DIFFERENTIAL DIAGNOSIS

The differential diagnosis of diphtheria varies with the particular anatomical site of involvement. In all types of possible diphtheria the patient's immunization history would provide helpful information for the physician.

Nasal diphtheria

The following may simulate nasal diphtheria.

Foreign body in the nose. The condition caused by a foreign body in the nose frequently is confused with nasal diphtheria. It is characterized by a secondary infection with a persistent, profuse nasal discharge that may at times be bloody. The diagnosis is made by examination with a nasal speculum that reveals evidence of either a foreign body or a diphtheritic type of membrane.

Rhinorrhea. Rhinorrhea caused by a common cold or a sinus or adenoid infection may be distinguished from nasal diphtheria by the absence of a membrane and, generally, by the absence of a bloody discharge.

Tonsillar and pharyngeal diphtheria

The following diseases may resemble tonsillar and pharyngeal diphtheria.

Acute streptococcal membranous tonsillitis. During the first few days of this disease the patient usually appears more acutely ill, the temperature is higher, and the membrane usually is confined to the tonsil. The recovery of streptococci on culture and the dramatic response to penicillin therapy within 24 hours usually establish the diagnosis.

Infectious mononucleosis. This disease commonly is characterized by membranous tonsillitis and splenomegaly in addition to the lymphadenopathy. A blood smear showing a large percent of abnormal lymphocytes and a positive heterophil antibody test (p. 92) are helpful diagnostic aids.

Nonbacterial membranous tonsillitis. Nonbacterial membranous tonsillitis is a common pediatric entity of varying etiologies. The illness is characterized by fever, sore throat, membranous tonsillitis, and a 4- to 10-day course that is not affected by antimicrobial therapy. The white blood cell count is usually low or normal, and cultures from throat specimens reveal normal bacterial flora. This syndrome has been reported as a manifestation of adenovirus infection and acquired toxoplasmosis. Other agents may be responsible for this disease.

Primary herpetic tonsillitis. The lesions of herpes simplex may occasionally coalesce on the tonsil and produce a pseudomembrane. This is usually accompanied by herpetic involvement of other portions of the mucous membrane.

Thrush. Thrush may also simulate a diphtheritic membrane. However, the absence of constitutional symptoms and presence of lesions on the buccal mucosa and tongue usually clarify the diagnosis.

Posttonsillectomy faucial membranes. These membranes have an alarming resemblance to the membranes of diphtheria. It is clear the patient has had surgery, and the lesions are usually stationary and do not spread.

Laryngeal diphtheria

The following diseases and conditions may simulate laryngeal diphtheria.

Infectious croup. Infectious croup is a term that describes two types of acute obstructive laryngitis of which diphtheria is the least common today; the most common type is caused by a virus (p. 352). The absence of a membrane and a negative culture for bacterial pathogens suggest the possibility of viral croup.

Spasmodic croup. Spasmodic croup, or acute subglottic edema, may also simulate laryngeal diphtheria. It appears suddenly, usually at night, and clears up by morning. The condition tends to recur for 1 or 2 nights.

Epiglottitis. The second most common type of obstructive lower airway diseases is caused by *Haemophilus influenzae* type b. This condition has a typical clinical picture characterized by sudden onset of high fever, drooling because of pain when swallowing, and dyspnea caused by supraglottic obstruction. The epiglottis is markedly swollen and beefy red. This characteristic physical finding establishes the diagnosis, which is confirmed by positive blood and/or throat culture for *H. influenzae* type b.

Foreign body in larynx. If there is a history of aspiration, there is no difficulty in diagnosing the condition caused by a foreign body in the larynx. Frequently, however, aspiration is not witnessed. A history of sudden choking and coughing spells suggests the diagnosis. The presence of the object is usually detected by laryngoscopic and roentgenographic examination.

COMPLICATIONS

Since the advent of antimicrobial therapy, the incidence of secondary bacterial complications has been significantly reduced. Penicillin, which is recommended for eradication of the diphtheria bacillus, prevents the occurrence of secondary streptococcal infections. The most common and most serious complications are those caused by the effect of the toxin on the heart and central nervous system (CNS).

Myocarditis

Myocarditis occurs frequently as a complication of severe diphtheria, but it may also follow milder forms of the disease (Sayers, 1958). The more extensive the local lesion and the more delayed the institution of antitoxin therapy, the more frequently myocarditis occurs. In most instances the cardiac manifestations appear during the second week of the disease. Occasionally, myocarditis may be noted as early as the first week and as late as the sixth week of the disease.

Diminution in intensity of the first heart sound or arrhythmia during the course of diphtheria is usually indicative of myocardial involvement. Abnormal electrocardiographic findings confirm this impression, including elevation of the ST segment, prolongation of the PR interval, and evidence of heart block. The myocarditis may be followed by cardiac failure.

Neuritis

Neuritis also is generally a complication of severe diphtheria. The manifestations of neuritis have the following characteristics: (1) they appear after a variable latent period; (2) they are predominantly bilateral with motor rather than sensory involvement; and (3) they usually clear completely.

Paralysis of soft palate. Soft-palate paralysis is the most common manifestation of diphtheritic neuritis. It occurs during the third week and is characterized by a nasal quality to the voice and nasal regurgitation. The paralysis usu-ally subsides completely within 1 to 2 weeks.

Ocular palsy. This palsy usually occurs during the fifth week and is characterized by paralysis of the muscles of accommodation, causing blurring of vision. Less commonly there may be involvement of the extraocular muscles, causing strabismus. Involvement of the lateral rectus muscle, causing an internal squint, is most common.

Paralysis of diaphragm. Paralysis of the diaphragm may occur between the fifth and seventh weeks as a result of neuritis of the phrenic nerve. Death will occur if mechanical respiratory aids are not used.

Paralysis of limbs. Limb paralysis may occur between the sixth and tenth weeks. The absence of deep tendon reflexes, bilateral symmetrical involvement, and the presence of an elevated level of spinal fluid protein make this complication clinically indistinguishable from the Guillain-Barré syndrome.

PROGNOSIS

Before the turn of the century the mortality rate of diphtheria was 30% to 50%. The advent of diphtheria antitoxin in 1894 and the beginning of large-scale active immunization programs in 1922 were followed by a dramatic reduction in the mortality rate to less than 5%.

In spite of the low fatality rate, the prognosis in the individual case of diphtheria must be extremely guarded. Sudden death may be caused by a variety of unpredictable events such as (1) the sudden complete obstruction of the airway by a detached piece of membrane, (2) the development of myocarditis and heart failure, and (3) the late occurrence of respiratory paralysis caused by phrenic nerve involvement. Patients who survive myocarditis or neuritis generally recover completely. Occasionally, however, diphtheritic myocarditis may be followed by permanent damage to the heart.

The prognosis in a particular case depends on a variety of factors pertaining to the disease, the host, and the environment.

IMMUNITY
Passive immunity

Passive immunity may be acquired either by transplacental transfer of antibody from an immune mother or by parenteral inoculation with diphtheria antitoxin. Congenitally acquired passive immunity persists for approximately 6 months. Protection after injection of diphtheria antitoxin disappears after 2 to 3 weeks.

Active immunity

Active immunity may be induced either by an attack of diphtheria or, more commonly today, by inoculations with diphtheria toxoid. The toxin is more toxic than immunogenic; thus more reliable immunity is produced by toxoid injections. Persons having diphtheria therefore should be immunized. Recurrent attacks of the disease are not unusual. Some individuals show evidence of immunity probably acquired as a result of an inapparent infection. Immunization with diphtheria toxoid can be relied on to prevent serious or fatal disease. The widespread and routine immunization of infants and children has had a profound effect on the immune status of the population at large (Nelson et al., 1978; Sheffield et al., 1978). Fully immunized individuals have antibody to toxin but do not have antibody to the organism and may become nasopharyngeal carriers or, uncommonly, may develop mild disease (Munford et al., 1974).

EPIDEMIOLOGICAL FACTORS

Diphtheria is worldwide in distribution. The extensive use of diphtheria toxoid since World War II has been associated with a striking decline to fewer than five reported cases annually in the United States. It is believed that antitoxin levels of ≥ 0.01 unit/ml are protective. The highest seasonal incidence occurs during the autumn and winter months. The age incidence is dependent on the immune status of the population. In most areas in which infants and children are routinely immunized, the disease is becoming relatively more common in adults because antibody levels may no longer be protective in intervals of greater than 10 years without a booster dose of vaccine. Most reports of recent outbreaks of diphtheria confirm the predominance of the disease among the poor, who have limited access to health care facilities (Marcuse and Grand, 1970). The fatalities usually occur among unimmunized children.

Diphtheria is acquired by contact with an ill person with the disease or with an asymptomatic carrier of the organism. The microorganisms are disseminated by the acts of coughing, sneezing, or even talking. Milkborne epidemics have been reported. Fomites play a small part in the spread of the disease.

TREATMENT
Antitoxin therapy

Diphtheria antitoxin must be given promptly and in adequate dosage. Any delay increases the possibility that myocarditis, neuritis, or death may occur.

During an infection, diphtheria toxin may be present in three forms: (1) circulating or unbound; (2) bound to the cells; or (3) internalized in cytoplasm. Antitoxin will neutralize circulating toxin and may affect bound toxin but will not affect internalized toxin, which is bound to EF-2.

The precise dose and route of administration of antitoxin will be determined by the location and extent of the membrane, the degree of toxemia, and the duration of the illness. The patient's age and weight are of no consequence. The dosages shown in Table 4-1 are recommended for the various types of diphtheria.

If a patient is sensitive to horse serum, the indications for the diphtheria antitoxin should be reevaluated because of this potential risk. If the antitoxin is administered, it can be given as described in Tables 4-2 and 4-3. Signs of acute anaphylaxis call for the immediate intravenous injection of 0.2 to 0.5 ml of 1:1000 epinephrine solution.

Table 4-1. Dosage of antitoxin recommended for various types of diphtheria

Type of diphtheria	Dosage (units)	Route
Anterior nasal	10,000-20,000	Intramuscular
Tonsillar	15,000-25,000	Intramuscular or intravenous
Pharyngeal	20,000-40,000	Intramuscular or intravenous
Laryngeal	20,000-40,000	Intramuscular or intravenous
Combined types	40,000-50,000	Intravenous
Late cases	40,000-60,000	Intravenous

Table 4-2. Intradermal, subcutaneous, intramuscular route of desensitization to serum

Dose number*	Route of administration†	Dilution of serum in normal saline	Amount of injection (ml)
1	ID	1:1,000	0.1
2	ID	1:1,000	0.3
3	SC	1:1,000	0.6
4	SC	1:100	0.1
5	SC	1:100	0.3
6	SC	1:100	0.6
7	SC	1:10	0.1
8	SC	1:10	0.3
9	SC	1:10	0.6
10	SC	Undiluted	0.1
11	SC	Undiluted	0.2
12	IM	Undiluted	0.6
13	IM	Undiluted	1.0

From Report of the Committee on Infectious Diseases: Am Acad Pediatr 1988, p. 37.
*Administer consistently at 15-minute intervals.
†ID, intradermal; SC, subcutaneous; IM, intramuscular.

Table 4-3. Intravenous route of desensitization to serum

Dose number*	Dilution of serum in normal saline	Amount of injection (ml)
1	1:1,000	0.1
2	1:1,000	0.3
3	1:1,000	0.6
4	1:100	0.1
5	1:100	0.3
6	1:100	0.6
7	1:10	0.1
8	1:10	0.3
9	1:10	0.6
10	Undiluted	0.1
11	Undiluted	0.2
12	Undiluted	0.6
13	Undiluted	1.0

From Report of the Committee on Infectious Diseases: Am Acad Pediatr 1988, p. 37.
*Administer at 15-minute intervals.

Antibacterial therapy

Penicillin and erythromycin are effective against most strains of diphtheria bacilli. Penicillin is usually the preferred drug and may be given as aqueous procaine penicillin G, 300,000 units or 600,000 units intramuscularly once daily for children weighing <10 kg or >10 kg, respectively. Patients who are sensitive to penicillin should be given erythromycin in a daily dosage of 40 mg per kilogram of body weight for 14 days. The maximum dose is 2 gm/day. Antimicrobial therapy is not a substitute for antitoxin therapy but should be given as supplementary and generally is continued until three consecutive cultures are negative for *C. diphtheriae*. Since the treatment may be prolonged, penicillin may be given orally instead of parenterally. Eradication of the organism should be documented by culture.

Supportive treatment

Bed rest is more important in the management of diphtheria than in most other infectious diseases. It should be enforced for at least 12 days because of the possibility of complicating myocarditis. The patient's activity subsequently will be guided by the results of the daily physical examinations, the serial electrocardiograms, and the presence or absence of complications. Steroid therapy did not prevent myocarditis or neuritis in one controlled trial (Thisyakorn, et al., 1984).

Laryngeal diphtheria. In addition to requiring antitoxin, penicillin, and other supportive measures, patients with laryngeal diphtheria require special treatment for the relief of obstruction to breathing. Intubation and/or tracheostomy may be necessary.

Treatment of complications

Myocarditis and neuritis are the most important complications requiring therapy.

Myocarditis. In general, the management of diphtheritic myocarditis and its sequelae is the same as that used for any other type of acute myocardial damage. Bed rest and inactivity may be beneficial. Sudden death caused by myocardial failure may be precipitated by excessive activity. The administration of digitalis is controversial; however, it should not be withheld if there is evidence of cardiac decompensation.

Diphtheritic neuritis. Palatal and pharyngeal paralysis may be complicated by aspiration because of the tendency for regurgitation and difficulty in swallowing. Under these circumstances gastric or duodenal intubation is indicated.

Treatment of diphtheria carriers

A carrier is an individual who has no symptoms and harbors virulent diphtheria bacilli in the nasopharynx. The eradication of these microorganisms may be extremely difficult and occasionally impossible. The following measures are recommended for use in sequence until the culture becomes negative:

Procaine penicillin: 600,000 units daily for 4 days

Penicillin: 200,000 units orally four times daily for 4 days

Erythromycin: 40 mg per kilogram of body weight per day for 1 week

Occasionally, an undetected foreign body in the nose may be responsible for persistence of a carrier state.

ISOLATION AND QUARANTINE
Care of patient

The patient is infective until diphtheria bacilli can be no longer cultured from the site of the infection. The duration of this infective period is variable. After the acute stage of the disease has subsided, three consecutive negative cultures are usually required before the patient is released from isolation.

Care of exposed persons

Intimate contacts should be cultured and kept under surveillance for 7 days. Cultures of nose and throat specimens should be done. Symptomatic previously immunized contacts should be given a booster dose of diphtheria toxoid if they have not received a dose of vaccine in 5 years. Children with positive cultures should be treated with antibiotics. Asymptomatic contacts who are unimmunized or whose immunization status is unknown should receive antibiotics (erythromycin, 40 mg/kg/day × 7 days or benzathine penicillin 600,000, 1.2 × 10^6 units intramuscularly, depending on weight, < 30 kg, > 30 kg). They should be cultured after prophylaxis and have active immunization initiated. Contacts who cannot be kept under surveillance should receive benzathine penicillin and one dose of age-appropriate vaccine, depending on their immunization history.

PREVENTIVE MEASURES

The dramatic decline in the incidence of diphtheria subsequent to 1922 can be attributed for the most part to mass immunization programs and routine immunization of infants and children. The following guidelines for the use of the currently licensed vaccine are from the recommendations of the Immunization Practices Advisory Committee (ACIP), MMWR 1991;40: RR-10, 1-28.

PREPARATIONS USED FOR VACCINATION

Diphtheria and tetanus toxoids are prepared by formaldehyde treatment of the respective toxins and are standardized for potency according to the regulations of the U.S. Food and Drug Administration. The limit of flocculation (Lf) content of each toxoid (quantity of toxoid as assessed by flocculation) may vary among different products. The concentration of diphtheria toxoid in preparations intended for adult use is reduced because adverse reactions to diphtheria toxoid are apparently directly related to the quantity of antigen and to the age or previous vaccination history of the recipient, and because a smaller dosage of diphtheria toxoid produces an adequate immune response among adults.

Pertussis vaccine is a suspension of inactivated *B. pertussis* cells. Potency is assayed by comparison with the U.S. standard pertussis vaccine in the intracerebral mouse protection test. The protective efficacy of pertussis vaccines for humans has been shown to correlate with this measure of vaccine potency.

Diphtheria and tetanus toxoids and pertussis vaccine, as single antigens or various combinations, are available as aluminum-salt-adsorbed preparations. Only tetanus toxoid is available in nonabsorbed (fluid) form. Although the rates of seroconversion are essentially equivalent with either type of tetanus toxoid, the adsorbed toxoid induces a more persistent level of antitoxin antibody. The following preparations are currently available in the United States:

1. Diphtheria and Tetanus Toxoids and Pertussis Vaccine Adsorbed (DTP) and Diphtheria and Tetanus Toxoids Adsorbed (DT) (for pediatric use) are for use among infants and children <7 years of age. Each 0.5-mL dose is formulated to contain 6.7-12.5 Lf units of diphtheria toxoid, 5 Lf units of tetanus toxoid, and ≤16 opacity units of pertussis vaccine. A single human immunizing dose of DTP contains an estimated 4-12 protective units of pertussis vaccine.
2. Tetanus and Diphtheria Toxoids Adsorbed for Adult Use (Td) is for use among persons ≥7 years of age. Each 0.5-mL dose is formulated to contain 2-10 Lf units of tetanus toxoid and ≤2 Lf units of diphtheria toxoid.
3. Pertussis Vaccine Adsorbed (P),* Tetanus Toxoid (fluid), Tetanus Toxoid Adsorbed (T), and Diphtheria Toxoid Adsorbed (D)† (for pediatric use), are single-antigen products for use in special instances when combined antigen preparations are not indicated.

Work is in progress to study the effectiveness of improved acellular pertussis vaccines that have reduced adverse reaction rates. Currently, several candidate vaccines containing at least one of the bacterial components thought to provide protection are undergoing clinical trials. Candidate antigens include filamentous hemagglutinin, lymphocytosis promoting factor (pertussis toxin), a recently identified 69-kiloDalton outer-membrane protein (pertactin), and agglutinogens. In published studies, some of these vaccines are less prone to cause common adverse reactions than the current whole-cell preparations, and they are immunogenic. Whether their clinical efficacy among infants is equivalent to that of the whole-cell preparations remains to be established.

VACCINE USAGE

The standard, single-dose volume of each of DTP, DT, Td, single-antigen adsorbed preparations of pertussis vaccine, tetanus toxoid, and diphtheria toxoid, and of the fluid tetanus toxoid is 0.5 mL. Adsorbed preparations should be administered intramuscularly (IM). Vaccine administration by jet injection may be associated with more frequent local reactions.

Primary vaccination
Children 6 weeks through 6 years old (up to the seventh birthday)

Table 4-4 details a routine vaccination schedule for children <7 years of age. One dose of DTP should be given IM on four occasions–the first three doses at 4- to 8-week intervals, beginning when the infant is approximately 6 weeks-2 months old; customarily, doses of vaccine are given at 2, 4, and 6 months of age. Individual circumstances may warrant giving the first three doses at 6, 10, and 14 weeks of age to provide protection as early as possible, especially during pertussis outbreaks. The fourth dose is given approximately 6-12 months after the third dose to maintain adequate immunity during the preschool years. This dose is an integral part of the primary vaccinating course. If a contraindication to pertussis vaccination exists (see Precautions and Contraindications), DT should be substituted for DTP as outlined (see Special Considerations).

Children ≥7 years of age and adults

Table 4-5 details a routine vaccination schedule for persons ≥7 years of age. Because the severity of pertussis decreases with age, and because the vaccine may cause side effects and adverse reactions, pertussis vaccination has not been recommended for children after their seventh birthday or for adults. For primary vaccination, a series of three doses of Td should be given IM; the second dose is given 4-8 weeks after the first and the third dose 6-12 months after the second. Td rather than DT is the preparation of choice for vaccination of all persons ≥7 years of age because side effects from higher doses of diphtheria toxoid are more common than they are among younger children.

Interruption of primary vaccination schedule

Interrupting the recommended schedule or delaying subsequent doses does not lead to a reduction in the level of immunity reached on completion of the primary series.

---

*Distributed by the Division of Biologic Products, Michigan Department of Public Health. Contact Dr. Robert Myers, Chief, Division of Biologic Products, Bureau of Laboratories and Epidemiological Services, Michigan Department of Public Health, Lansing, Michigan 48909 (telephone: 517-335-8120).

†Distributed in the United States by Sclavo, Inc.

shown in Table 4-6. The frequencies of local reactions and fever are substantially higher with increasing numbers of doses of DTP vaccine, while other mild-to-moderate systemic reactions (e.g., fretfulness, vomiting) are substantially less frequent.

Concern about the possible role of pertussis vaccine in causing neurologic reactions has been present since the earliest days of vaccine use. Rare but serious acute neurologic illnesses, including encephalitis/encephalopathy and prolonged convulsions, have been anecdotally reported following receipt of whole-cell pertussis vaccine given as DTP vaccine. Whether pertussis vaccine causes or is only coincidentally related to such illnesses or reveals an inevitable event has been difficult to determine conclusively for the following reasons: a) serious acute neurologic illnesses often occur or become manifest among children during the first year of life irrespective of vaccination; b) there is no specific clinical sign, pathological finding, or laboratory test which can determine whether the illness is caused by the DTP vaccine; c) it may be difficult to determine with certainty whether infants <6 months of age are neurologically normal, which complicates assessment of whether vaccinees were already neurologically impaired before receiving DTP vaccine; and d) because these events are exceedingly rare, appropriately designed large studies are needed to address the question.

To determine whether DTP vaccine causes serious neurologic illness and brain damage, the National Childhood Encephalopathy Study (NCES) was undertaken during 1976-1979 in Great Britain. This large case-control study attempted to identify every patient with serious, acute, childhood, neurologic illness admitted to a hospital in England, Scotland, and Wales. A total of 1,182 young children 2-36 months of age was identified. Excluding those with infantile spasms, an illness shown in a separate analysis not to be attributable to DTP vaccine, 30 of these children (18 with prolonged convulsions and 12 with encephalitis/encephalopathy) had received DTP vaccine within 7 days of the reported onset of their neurologic illness. Analysis of the data from these patients and from age-matched control children showed a significant association (odds ratio = 3.3; 95% confidence interval 1.7-6.5) between the development of serious acute neurologic illness and receipt of DTP vaccine. Most of these events were prolonged seizures with fever. The attributable risk for all neurologic events was estimated to be 1:140,000 doses of DTP vaccine administered. These 30 children were followed up for at least 12 months to determine whether they had neurologic sequelae. Seven of these children presumed to have been previously normal neurologically had died or had subsequent neurologic impairment. A causal relation between receipt of DTP vaccine and

Table 4-6. Adverse events* occurring within 48 hours of DTP vaccinations

Event	Frequency†
Local	
redness	1/3 doses
swelling	2/5 doses
pain	1/2 doses
Systemic	
fever ≥ 38 C (100.4 F)	1/2 doses
drowsiness	1/3 doses
fretfulness	1/2 doses
vomiting	1/15 doses
anorexia	1/5 doses
persistent, inconsolable crying (duration ≥3 hours)	1/100 doses
fever ≥40.5 C (≥105 F)	1/330 doses
collapse (hypotonic-hyporesponsive episode)	1/1,750 doses
convulsions (with or without fever)	1/1,750 doses

*From Cody CL, Baraff LJ, Cherry JD, et al., 1981.
†Rate per total number of doses regardless of dose number in DTP series.

permanent neurologic injury was suggested. The estimated attributable risk for DTP vaccine was 1:330,000 doses with a wide confidence interval.

The methods and results of the NCES have been thoroughly scrutinized since publication of the study. This reassessment by multiple groups has determined that the number of patients was too small and their classification subject to enough uncertainty to preclude drawing valid conclusions about whether a causal relation exists between pertussis vaccine and permanent neurologic damage. Preliminary data from a 10-year follow-up study of some of the children studied in the original NCES study also suggested a relation between symptoms following DTP vaccination and permanent neurologic disability. However, details are not available to evaluate this study adequately, and the same concerns remain about DTP vaccine precipitating initial manifestations of pre-existing neurologic disorders.

Subsequent studies have failed to provide evidence to support a causal relation between DTP vaccination and either serious acute neurologic illness or permanent neurologic injury. These include: a) the 1979 Hospital Activity Analysis of the North West Thames Study in England, in which the hospital records of approximately 17,000 children who each received three doses of DTP vaccine were compared with records of 18,000 children who each received three doses of DT vaccine; b) a 1974-1983 case-cohort study of children in the Group Health Cooperative of Puget Sound who received a total of 106,000 doses of DTP vaccine; and c) a 1974-1984 cohort study of 38,171 Medicaid children in Tennessee who received 107,154 doses of DTP vaccine. An additional study in Denmark of approximately 150,000 children (554 of which had epilepsy) demonstrated no relation between the age at onset of epilepsy and the scheduled age of administration of DTP vaccine. Although each of these studies individually contained too few subjects to provide definitive conclusions, taken together they stand in contrast to the original NCES findings. A recent study performed in 1987-1988 in Washington and Oregon of neurologic illness among children did not provide evidence of a significantly increased risk of all serious acute neurologic illnesses within 7, 14, or 28 days of DTP vaccination. However, as a pilot effort, this study had limited power to detect significantly increased risks for individual conditions.

The NCES was the basis of prior ACIP statements suggesting that on rare occasions DTP vaccine could cause brain damage. However, on the basis of a more detailed review of the NCES data as well as data from other studies, the ACIP has revised its earlier view and now concludes:

1. Although DTP may rarely produce symptoms that some have classified as acute encephalopathy, a causal relation between DTP vaccine and permanent brain damage has not been demonstrated. If the vaccine ever causes brain damage, the occurrence of such an event must be exceedingly rare. A similar conclusion has been reached by the Committee on Infectious Diseases of the American Academy of Pediatrics, the Child Neurology Society, the Canadian National Advisory Committee on Immunization, the British Joint Committee on Vaccination and Immunization, the British Pediatric Association, and the Institute of Medicine.
2. The risk estimate from the NCES study of 1 : 330,000 for brain damage should no longer be considered valid on the basis of continuing analyses of the NCES and other studies.

In addition to these considerations, acute neurologic manifestations related to DTP vaccine are mainly febrile seizures. In an individual case, the role of pertussis vaccine as a cause of serious acute neurologic illness or permanent brain damage is impossible to determine on the basis of clinical or laboratory findings. Anecdotal reports of DTP-induced acute neurologic disorders with or without permanent brain damage can have one of several alternate explanations. Some instances may represent simple coincidence because DTP is administered at a time in infancy when previously unrecognized underlying neurological and developmental disorders first become manifest. Some patients may have short-lived seizures with prompt recovery, and these events represent the first seizure of a child with underlying epilepsy. When epilepsy has its onset in infancy, it is frequently associated with severe mental retardation and developmental delay. These conditions become apparent over a period of several months. The known febrile and other systemic effects of DTP vaccination may stimulate or precipitate inevitable symptoms of underlying central-nervous-system disorders, particularly since DTP may be the first pyrogenic stimulus an infant receives. When children who experience acute, severe central-nervous-system disorders in association with DTP vaccination are studied promptly and carefully, an alternate cause is often found.

Among a subset of NCES children with infantile spasms, both DTP and DT vaccination appeared either to precipitate early manifestations of the condition or to cause its recognition by parents. This and other studies suggest that neither vaccine causes this illness.

Approximately 5,200 infants succumb to sudden infant death syndrome (SIDS) in the United States each year. Because the peak incidence of SIDS for infants is between 2 and 3 months of age, many instances of a close temporal relation between SIDS and receipt of DTP are to be expected by simple chance. Only one methodologically rigorous study has suggested that DTP vaccine might cause SIDS. A total of four deaths were reported within 3 days of DTP vaccination, compared with 1.36 expected deaths. However, these deaths were unusual in that three of the four occurred within a 13-month interval during the 12-year study. These four children also tended to be vaccinated at older ages than their controls, suggesting that they might have other unrecognized risk factors for SIDS independent of vaccination. In contrast, DTP vaccination was not associated with SIDS in several larger studies performed in the past decade. In addition, none of three studies that examined unexpected deaths among infants not classified as SIDS found an association with DTP vaccination.

Claims that DTP may be responsible for transverse myelitis, other more subtle neurologic disorders (such as hyperactivity, learning disorders and infantile autism), and progressive degenerative central-nervous-system conditions have no scientific basis. Furthermore, one study indicated that children who received pertussis vaccine exhibited fewer school problems than those who did not, even after adjustment for socioeconomic status.

Recent data suggest that infants and young children who have ever had convulsions (febrile or afebrile) or who have immediate family members with such histories are more likely to have seizures following DTP vaccination than those without such histories. For those with a family history of seizures, the increased risks of seizures occurring within 3 days of receipt of DTP or 4-28 days following receipt of DTP are identical, suggestiong that these histories are non-specific risk factors and are unrelated to DTP vaccination.

Rarely, immediate anaphylactic reactions (i.e., swelling of the mouth, breathing difficulty, hypotension, or shock) have been reported after receipt of preparations containing diphtheria, tetanus, and/or pertussis antigens. However, no deaths caused by anaphylaxis following DTP vaccination have been reported to CDC since the inception of vaccine-adverse-events reporting in 1978, a period during which more than 80 million doses of publically purchased DTP vaccine were administered. While substantial underreporting exists in this passive surveillance system, the severity of anaphylaxis and its immediacy following vaccination suggest that such events are likely to be reported. Although no causal relation to any specific component of DTP has been established, the occurrence of true anaphylaxis usually contraindicates further doses of any one of these components. Rashes that are macular, papular, petechial, or urticarial and appear hours or days after a dose of DTP are frequently antigen-antibody reactions of little consequence or are due to other causes such as viral illnesses, and are unlikely to recur following subsequent injections. In addition, there is no evidence for a causal relation between DTP vaccination and hemolytic anemia or thrombocytopenic purpura.

REPORTING OF ADVERSE EVENTS

The U.S. Department of Health and Human Services has established a new Vaccine Adverse Event Reporting System (VAERS) to accept all reports of suspected adverse events after the administration of any vaccine, including but not limited to the reporting of events required by the National Childhood Vaccine Injury Act of 1986. The telephone number to call for answers to questions and to obtain VAERS forms is 1-800-822-7967.

The National Vaccine Injury Compensation Program, established by the National Childhood Vaccine Injury Act of 1986, requires physicians and other health-care providers who administer vaccines to maintain permanent vaccination records and to report occurrences of certain adverse events to the U.S. Department of Health and Human Services. These requirements took effect March 21, 1988. Reportable events include those listed in the Act for each vaccine and events specified in the manufacturer's vaccine package insert as contraindications to further doses of that vaccine.

REDUCED DOSAGE SCHEDULES OR MULTIPLE SMALL DOSES OF DTP

The ACIP recommends giving only full doses (0.5 mL) of DTP vaccine; if a specific contraindication to DTP exists, the vaccine should not be given.

Concern about adverse events following pertussis vaccine has led some practitioners to reduce the volume of DTP vaccine administered to <0.5mL/dose in an attempt to reduce side effects. No evidence exists to show that this decreases the frequency of uncommon severe adverse events, such as seizures and hypotonic-hyporesponsive episodes. Two studies have reported substantially lower rates of local reactions with the use of one half the recommended dose (0.25mL) compared with a full dose. However, a study among preterm infants showed that the incidence of side effects was unaltered when a reduced dosage of DTP vaccine was used. Two studies also showed substantially lower pertussis agglutinin responses after the second and third half-doses, although in one of the studies the differences were small. These investigations used pertussis agglutinins as a measure of clinical protection; however, agglutinins are not satisfactory measures of protection against pertussis disease. Further, no evidence exists to show that the low screening dilution used (1:16) indicates protection. Currently, no reliable measures of efficacy other than clinical protection exist. Other evidence against the use of reduced doses comes from earlier studies of DTP vaccine preparations with potencies equivalent to that of half-doses of current vaccine. The risk of pertussis for exposed household members who received these lower potency vaccines was approximately twice as high as the risk of pertussis for those who received vaccines as potent as full doses of current vaccine (29% compared with ≤14%).

The use of an increased number of reduced-volume doses of DTP in order to equal the total volume of the five recommended doses of DTP vaccine is not recommended. Whether this practice reduces the likelihood of vaccine-related adverse events is unknown. In addition, the likelihood of a temporally associated but etiologically unrelated event may be enhanced by increasing the number of vaccinations.

SIMULTANEOUS ADMINISTRATION OF VACCINES

The simultaneous administration of DTP, oral poliovirus vaccine (OPV), and measles-mumps-rubella vaccine (MMR) has resulted in seroconversion rates and rates of side effects similar to those observed when the vaccines are administered separately. Simultaneous vaccination with DTP, MMR, OPV, or inactivated poliovirus vaccine (IPV), and *Haemophilus* b conjugate vaccine (HbCV) is also acceptable. The ACIP recommends the simultaneous administration of all vaccines appropriate to the age and previous vaccination status of the recipient, including the special circumstance of simultaneous administration of DTP, OPV, HbCV, and MMR at ≥15 months of age.

PRECAUTIONS AND CONTRAINDICATIONS
General considerations

The decision to administer or delay DTP vaccination because of a current or recent febrile illness depends largely on the severity of the symptoms and their etiology. Although a moderate or severe febrile illness is sufficient reason to postpone vaccination, minor illness such as mild upper-respiratory infections with or without low-grade fever are not contraindications. If ongoing medical care cannot be assured, taking every opportunity to provide appropriate vaccinations is particularly important.

Children with moderate or severe illnesses with or without fever can receive DTP as soon as they have recovered. Waiting a short period before administering DTP vaccine avoids superimposing the adverse effects of the vaccination on the underlying illness or mistakenly attributing a manifestation of the underlying illness to vaccination.

Routine physical examinations or temperature measurements are not prerequisites for vaccinating infants and children who appear to be in good health. Appropriate immunization practice includes asking the parent or guardian if the child is ill, postponing DTP vaccination for those with moderate or severe acute illnesses, and vaccinating those without contraindications or precautionary circumstances.

When an infant or child returns for the next dose of DTP, the parent should always be questioned about any adverse events that might have occurred following the previous dose.

A history of prematurity generally is not a reason to defer vaccination. Preterm infants should be vaccinated according to their chronological age from birth.

Immunosuppressive therapies—including irradiation, antimetabolites, alkylating agents, cytotoxic drugs, and corticosteroids (used in greater than physiologic doses)—may reduce the immune response to vaccines. Short-term (<2-week) corticosteroid therapy or intra-articular, bursal, or tendon injections with corticosteroids should not be immunosuppressive. Although no specific studies with pertussis vaccine are available, if immunosuppressive therapy will be discontinued shortly, it is reasonable to defer vaccination until the patient has been off therapy for 1 month; otherwise, the patient should be vaccinated while still on therapy.

Special considerations for preparations containing pertussis vaccine

Precautions and contraindications guidelines that were previously published regarding the use of pertussis vaccine were based on three assumptions about the risks of pertussis vaccination that are not supported by available data: a) that the vaccine on rare occasions caused acute encephalopathy resulting in permanent brain damage; b) that pertussis vaccine aggravated preexisting central-nervous-system disease; and c) that certain nonencephalitic reactions are predictive of more severe reactions with subsequent doses. In addition, children from whom pertussis vaccine was withheld were thought to be well protected by herd immunity, a belief that is no longer valid. The current revised ACIP recommendations reflect better understanding of the risks associated not only with pertussis vaccine but also with pertussis disease.

Contraindications

If any of the following events occur in temporal relationship to the administration of DTP, further vaccination with DTP is contraindicated (see Table 4-7):

1. An immediate anaphylactic reaction. The rarity of such reactions to DTP is such that they have not been adequately studied. Because of uncertainty as to which component of the vaccine might be responsible, no further vaccination with any of the three antigens in DTP should be carried out. Alternatively, because of the importance of tetanus vaccination, such individuals may be referred for evaluation by an allergist and desensitized to tetanus toxoid if specific allergy can be demonstrated.
2. Encephalopathy (not due to another identifiable cause). This is defined as an acute, severe central-nervous-system disorder occurring within 7 days following vaccination, and generally consisting of major alterations in consciousness, unresponsiveness, generalized or focal seizures that persist more than a few hours, with failure to recover within 24 hours. Even though causation by DTP cannot be established, no subsequent doses of pertussis vaccine should be given. It may be desirable to delay for months before administering the balance of the doses of DT necessary to complete the primary schedule. Such a delay allows time for the child's neurologic status to clarify.

Precautions (warnings)

If any of the following events occur in temporal relation to receipt of DTP, the decision to give subsequent doses of vaccine containing the pertussis component should be carefully considered (Table 4-

Table 4-7. Contraindications and precautions to further DTP vaccination

---

Contraindications

An immediate anaphylactic reaction.

Encephalopathy occurring within 7 days following DTP vaccination.

Precautions

Temperature of ≥40.5 C (105 F) within 48 hours not due to another identifiable cause.

Collapse or shock-like state (hypotonic-hyporesponsive episode) within 48 hours.

Persistent, inconsolable crying lasting ≥3 hours, occurring within 48 hours.

Convulsions with or without fever occurring within 3 days.

---

7). Although these events were considered absolute contraindications in previous ACIP recommendations, there may be circumstances, such as a high incidence of pertussis, in which the potential benefits outweigh possible risks, particularly because these events are not associated with permanent sequelae. The following events were previously considered contraindications and are now considered precautions:

1. Temperature of ≥40.5 C (105 F) within 48 hours not due to another identifiable cause. Such a temperature is considered a precaution because of the likelihood that fever following a subsequent dose of DTP vaccine also will be high. Because such febrile reactions are usually attributed to the pertussis component, vaccination with DT should not be discontinued.

2. Collapse or shock-like state (hypotonic-hyporesponsive episode) within 48 hours. Although these uncommon events have not been recognized to cause death nor to induce permanent neurological sequelae, it is prudent to continue vaccination with DT, omitting the pertussis component.

3. Persistent, inconsolable crying lasting ≥3 hours, occurring within 48 hours. Follow-up of infants who have cried inconsolably following DTP vaccination has indicated that this reaction, though unpleasant, is without long-term sequelae and not associated with other reactions of greater significance. Inconsolable crying occurs most frequently following the first dose and is less frequently reported following subsequent doses of DTP vaccine. However, crying for >30 minutes following DTP vaccination can be a predictor of increased likelihood of recurrence of persistent crying following subsequent doses.

Children with persistent crying have had a higher rate of substantial local reactions than children who had other DTP-associated reactions (including high fever, seizures, and hypotonic-hyporesponsive episodes), suggesting that prolonged crying was really a pain reaction.

4. Convulsions with or without fever occurring within 3 days. Short-lived convulsions, with or without fever, have not been shown to cause permanent sequelae. Furthermore, the occurrence of prolonged febrile seizures (i.e, status epilepticus*), irrespective of their cause, involving an otherwise normal child does not substantially increase the risk for subsequent febrile (brief or prolonged) or afebrile seizures. The risk is significantly increased (p = 0.018) only among those children who are neurologically abnormal before their episode of status epilepticus. Accordingly, although a convulsion following DTP vaccination has previously been considered a contraindication to further doses, under certain circumstances subsequent doses may be indicated, particularly if the risk of pertussis in the community is high. If a child has a seizure following the first or second dose of DTP, it is desirable to delay subsequent doses until the child's neurologic status is better defined. By the end of the first year of life, the presence of an underlying neurologic disorder has usually been determined, and appropriate treatment instituted. DT vaccine should not be administered before a decision has been made about whether to restart the DTP series. Regardless of which vaccine is given, it is prudent also to administer acetaminophen, 15 mg/kg of body weight, at the time of vaccination and every 4 hours subsequently for 24 hours.

Vaccination of infants and young children who have underlying neurologic disorders

Infants and children with recognized, possible, or potential underlying neurologic conditions present a unique problem. They seem to be at increased risk for the appearance of manifestations of the underlying neurologic disorder within 2-3 days after vaccination. However, more prolonged manifestations or increased progression of the disorder, or exacerbation of the disorder have not been recognized. In addition, most neurologic conditions in infancy and young childhood are associated with evolving, changing neurological findings. Functional abnormalities are often unmasked by progressive neurologic development.

---

*Any seizure lasting >30 minutes or recurrent seizures lasting a total of 30 minutes without the child fully regaining consciousness.

Thus, confusion over the interpretation of progressive neurologic signs may arise when DTP vaccination or any other therapeutic or preventive measure is carried out.

Protection against diphtheria, tetanus, and pertussis is as important for children with neurologic disabilities as for other children. Such protection may be even more important for neurologically disabled children. They often receive custodial care or attend special schools where the risk of pertussis is greater because DTP vaccination is avoided for fear of adverse reactions. Also, if pertussis affects a neurologically disabled child who has difficulty in handling secretions and in cooperating with symptomatic care, it may aggravate preexisting neurologic problems because of anoxia, intracerebral hemorrhages, and other manifestations of the disease. Whether and when to administer DTP to children with proven or suspected underlying neurologic disorders must be decided on an individual basis. Important considerations include the current local incidence of pertussis, the near absence of diphtheria in the United States, and the low risk of infection with *Clostridium tetani*. On the basis of these considerations and the nature of the child's disorder, the following approaches are recommended:

1. **Infants and children with previous convulsions.** Infants and young children who have had prior seizures, whether febrile or afebrile, appear to be at increased risk for seizures following DTP vaccination than children and infants without these histories. A convulsion within 3 days of DTP vaccination in a child with a history of convulsions may be initiated by fever caused by the vaccine in a child prone to febrile seizures, may be induced by the pertussis component, or may be unrelated to the vaccination. As noted earlier, current evidence indicates that seizures following DTP vaccination do not cause permanent brain damage. Among infants and children with a history of previous seizures, it is prudent to delay DTP vaccination until the child's status has been fully assessed, a treatment regimen established, and the condition stabilized. It should be noted, however, that delaying DTP vaccination until the second 6 months of life will increase the risk of febrile seizures among persons who are predisposed. When DTP or DT is given, acetaminophen, 15 mg/kg, should also be given at the time of the vaccination and every 4 hours for the ensuing 24 hours.

2. **Infants as yet unvaccinated who are suspected of having underlying neurologic disease.** It is prudent to delay initiation of vaccination with DTP or DT (but not other vaccines) until further observation and study have clarified the child's neurologic status and the effect of treatment. The decision as to whether to begin vaccination with DTP or DT should be made no later than the child's first birthday.

3. **Children who have not received a complete series of vaccine and who have a neurologic event occurring between doses.** Infants and children who have received ≥ one dose of DTP and who experience a neurologic disorder (e.g., a seizure, for example) not temporally associated with vaccination, but before the next scheduled dose, present a special management challenge. If the seizure or other disorder occurs before the first birthday and before completion of the first three doses of the primary series of DTP, further doses of DTP or DT (but not other vaccines) should be deferred until the infant's status has been clarified. The decision whether to use DTP or DT to complete the series should be made no later than the child's first birthday, and should take into consideration the nature of the child's problem and the benefits and possible risks of the vaccine. If the seizure or other disorder occurs after the first birthday, the child's neurologic status should be evaluated to ensure that the disorder is stable before a subsequent dose of DTP is given. (See the following #4.)

4. **Infants and children with stable neurologic conditions.** Infants and children with stable neurologic conditions, including well-controlled seizures, may be vaccinated. The occurrence of single seizures (temporally unassociated with DTP) do not contraindicate DTP vaccination, particularly if the seizures can be satisfactorily explained. Parents of infants and children with histories of convulsions should be informed of the increased risk of postvaccination seizures. Acetaminophen, 15 mg/kg, every 4 hours for 24 hours, should be given to children with such histories to reduce the possibility of postvaccination fever.

5. **Children with resolved or corrected neurologic disorders.** DTP vaccination is recommended for infants with certain neurologic problems, such as neonatal hypocalcemic tetany or hydrocephalus (following placement of a shunt and without seizures), that have been corrected or have clearly subsided without residua.

Vaccination of infants and young children who have a family history of convulsion or other central nervous system disorders

A family history of convulsions or other central nervous disorders is not a contraindication to pertussis vaccination. Acetaminophen should be given at the time of DTP vaccination and every 4 hours for 24 hours to reduce the possibility of postvaccination fever.

Preparations containing diphtheria toxoid and tetanus toxoid

The only contraindication to tetanus and diphtheria toxoids is a history of a neurologic or severe hypersensitivity reaction following a previous dose. Vaccination with tetanus and diphtheria toxoids is not known to be associated with an increased risk of convulsions. Local side effects alone do not preclude continued use. If an anaphylactic reaction to a previous dose of tetanus toxoid is suspected, intradermal skin testing with appropriately diluted tetanus toxoid may be useful before a decision is made to discontinue tetanus toxoid vaccination. In one study, 94 of 95 persons with histories of anaphylactic symptoms following a previous dose of tetanus toxoid were nonreactive following intradermal testing and tolerated further tetanus toxoid challenge without incident. One person had erythema and induration immediately following skin testing, but tolerated a full IM dose without adverse effects. Mild, nonspecific skintest reactivity to tetanus toxoid, particularly if used undiluted, appears to be fairly common. Most vaccinees develop inconsequential cutaneous delayed hypersensitivity to the toxoid.

Persons who experienced Arthus-type hypersensitivity reactions or a temperature of >103 F (39.4 C) following a prior dose of tetanus toxoid usually have high serum tetanus antitoxin levels and should not be given even emergency doses of Td more frequently than every 10 years, even if they have a wound that is neither clean nor minor.

If a contraindication to using tetanus toxoid-containing preparations exists for a person who has not completed a primary series of tetanus toxoid immunization and that person has a wound that is neither clean nor minor, *only* passive immunization should be given using tetanus immune globulin (TIG). (See Tetanus Prophylaxis in Wound Management).

Although no evidence exists that tetanus and diphtheria toxoids are teratogenic, waiting until the second trimester of pregnancy to administer Td is a reasonable precaution for minimizing any concern about the theoretical possibility of such reactions.

Misconceptions concerning contraindications to DTP

Some health-care providers inappropriately consider certain conditions or circumstances as contraindications to DTP vaccination. These include the following:

1. Soreness, redness, or swelling at the DTP vaccination site or temperature of ≥40.5C(105 F).

2. Mild, acute illness with low-grade fever or mild diarrheal illness affecting an otherwise healthy child.
3. Current antimicrobial therapy or the convalescent phase of an acute illness.
4. Recent exposure to an infectious disease.
5. Prematurity. The appropriate age for initiating vaccination among the prematurely born infant is the usual chronological age from birth. Full doses (0.5 mL) of vaccine should be used.
6. History of allergies or relatives with allergies.
7. Family history of convulsions.
8. Family history of SIDS.
9. Family history of an adverse event following DTP vaccination.

PREVENTION OF DIPHTHERIA AMONG CONTACTS OF A DIPHTHERIA PATIENT
Identification of close contacts

The primary purpose of contact investigation is to prevent secondary transmission of *C. diphtheriae* and the occurrence of additional diphtheria cases. Only close contacts of a patient with culture-confirmed or suspected* diphtheria should be considered at increased risk for acquiring secondary disease. Such contacts include all household members and other persons with a history of habitual, close contact with the patient, as well as those directly exposed to oral secretions of the patient. Identification of close contacts of a diphtheria patient should be promptly initiated.

Cultures and antimicrobial prophylaxis

All close contacts (regardless of their vaccination status) should have samples taken for culture, receive prompt antimicrobial chemoprophylaxis, and be examined daily for 7 days for evidence of disease. Awaiting culture results before administering antimicrobial prophylaxis to close contacts is not warranted. The identification of carriers among close contacts may support the diagnosis of diphtheria for a patient whose cultures are negative either because of prior antimicrobial therapy or because of other reasons. Antimicrobial prophylaxis should consist of either an IM injection of benzathine penicillin (600,000 units for persons <6 years old and 1,200,000 units for those ≥6 years old) or a 7- to 10-day course of oral erythromycin (children: 40 mg/kg/day; adults: 1 g/day). Erythromycin may be slightly more effective, but IM benzathine penicillin may be preferred, because it

---

*For example, a patient for whom the decision has been made to treat with diphtheria antitoxin. Antitoxin can be obtained either from a manufacturer (Connaught Labs, Inc., or Sclavo, Inc.) or the Division of Immunization, CDC (telephone: 404-639-2888).

avoids possible noncompliance with a multi-day oral drug regimen. The efficacy of antimicrobial prophylaxis in preventing secondary disease is presumed but not proven. Identified carriers of *C. diphtheriae* should have follow-up cultures done after they complete antimicrobial therapy. Those who continue to harbor the organism after either penicillin or erythromycin should receive an additional 10-day course of oral erythromycin and follow-up cultures.

Immunization
Active

All household and other close contacts who have received <three doses of diphtheria toxoid or whose vaccination status is unknown should receive an immediate dose of a diphtheria toxoid-containing preparation and should complete the primary series according to schedule (Tables 4-4 and 4-5). Close contacts who have completed a primary series of ≥three doses and who have not been vaccinated with diphtheria toxoid within the previous 5 years should receive a booster dose of a diphtheria toxoid-containing preparation appropriate for their age.

Passive

The only preparation available for passive immunization against diphtheria is equine diphtheria antitoxin. Even when close surveillance of unvaccinated close contacts is impossible, use of this preparation is not generally recommended because of the risks of allergic reaction to horse serum. Immediate hypersensitivity reactions occur among approximately 7%, and serum sickness among 5% of adults receiving the recommended prophylactic dose of equine antitoxin. The risk of an adverse reaction to equine antitoxin must be weighed against the small risk that an unvaccinated household contact who receives chemoprophylaxis will contract diphtheria. No evidence exists to support any additional benefit of diphtheria antitoxin use for contacts who have received antimicrobial prophylaxis. If antitoxin is to be used, 5,000-10,000 units IM—after appropriate testing for sensitivity—at a site different from that of the toxoid injection is the dosage usually recommended. Diphtheria antitoxin is unlikely to impair the immune response to simultaneous administration of diphtheria toxoid, but this has not been adequately studied.

A serum specimen collected from a patient with suspected diphtheria (before antitoxin therapy is initiated) may be helpful in supporting the diagnosis of diphtheria if a level of diphtheria antitoxin below that considered to be protective (i.e., <0.01 IU/mL) can be demonstrated. Such testing may be particularly helpful with a patient for whom antimicrobial therapy had been initiated prior to obtaining diphtheria cultures.

Cutaneous diphtheria

Cases of cutaneous diphtheria generally are caused by infections with nontoxigenic strains of *C. diphtheriae*. If a toxigenic *C. diphtheriae* strain is isolated from a cutaneous lesion, investigation and prophylaxis of close contacts should be undertaken, as with respiratory diphtheria. If a cutaneous case is known to be due to a nontoxigenic strain, routine investigation or prophylaxis of contacts is not necessary.

TETANUS PROPHYLAXIS IN WOUND MANAGEMENT

Chemoprophylaxis against tetanus is neither practical nor useful in managing wounds. Wound cleaning, debridement when indicated, and proper immunization are important. The need for tetanus toxoid (active immunization), with or without TIG (passive immunization), depends on both the condition of the wound and the patient's vaccination history (Table 4-8; see also Precautions and Contraindications). Rarely has tetanus occurred among persons with documentation of having received a primary series of toxoid injections.

A thorough attempt must be made to determine whether a patient has completed primary vaccination. Patients with unknown or uncertain previous vaccination histories should be considered to have had no previous tetanus toxoid doses. Persons who had military service since 1941 can be considered to have received at least one dose. Although most people in

Table 4-8. Summary guide to tetanus prophylaxis in routine wound management, 1991

History of adsorbed tetanus toxoid (doses)	Clean, minor wounds		All other wounds*	
	TD(†)	TIG	Td(†)	TIG
Unknown or < three	Yes	No	Yes	Yes
≥ Three(§)	No(¶)	No	No(**)	No

*Such as, but not limited to, wounds contaminated with dirt, feces, soil, and saliva; puncture wounds; avulsions; and wounds resulting from missiles, crushing, burns and frostbite.

†For children <7 years old; DTP (DT, if pertussis vaccine is contraindicated) is preferred to tetanus toxic alone. For persons ≥7 years of age, Td is preferred to tetanus toxoid alone.

§If only three doses of *fluid* toxoid have been received, then a fourth dose of toxoid, preferably an adsorbed toxoid, should be given.

¶Yes, if >10 years since last dose.

**Yes, if >5 years since last dose. (More frequent boosters are not needed and can accentuate side effects.)

the military since 1941 may have completed a primary series of tetanus toxoid, this cannot be assumed for each individual. Patients who have not completed a primary series may require tetanus toxoid and passive immunization at the time of wound cleaning and debridement (Table 4-8).

Available evidence indicates that complete primary vaccination with tetanus toxoid provides long-lasting protection ≥ 10 years for most recipients. Consequently, after complete primary tetanus vaccination, boosters—even for wound management—need be given only every 10 years when wounds are minor and uncontaminated. For other wounds, a booster is appropriate if the patient has not received tetanus toxoid within the preceding 5 years. Persons who have received at least two doses of tetanus toxoid rapidly develop antitoxin antibodies.

Td is the preferred preparation for active tetanus immunization in wound management of patients ≥ 7 years of age. Because a large proportion of adults are susceptible, this plan enhances diphtheria protection. Thus, by taking advantage of acute health-care visits, such as for wound management, some patients can be protected who otherwise would remain susceptible. For routine wound management among children <7 years of age who are not adequately vaccinated, DTP should be used instead of single-antigen tetanus toxoid. DT may be used if pertussis vaccine is contraindicated or individual circumstances are such that potential febrile reactions following DTP might confound the management of the patient. For inadequately vaccinated patients of all ages, completion of primary vaccination at the time of discharge or at follow-up visits should be ensured (Tables 4-4 and 4-5).

If passive immunization is needed, human TIG is the product of choice. It provides protection longer than antitoxin of animal origin and causes few adverse reactions. The TIG prophylactic dose that is currently recommended for wounds of average severity is 250 units IM. When tetanus toxoid and TIG are given concurrently, separate syringes and separate sites should be used. The ACIP recommends the use of only adsorbed toxoid in this situation.

PROPHYLAXIS FOR CONTACTS OF PERTUSSIS PATIENTS

Spread of pertussis can be limited by decreasing the infectivity of the patient and by protecting close contacts. To reduce infectivity as quickly as possible, a course of oral erythromycin (children: 40 mg/kg/day; adults: 1g/day) or trimethoprim-sulfamethoxazole (children: trimethoprim 8 mg/kg/day, sulfamethoxazole 40 mg/kg/day; adults: trimethoprim 320 mg/day, sulfamethoxazole 1,600 mg/day) is recom-

mended for patients with clinical pertussis. Antimicrobial therapy should be continued for 14 days to minimize any chance of treatment failure. It is generally accepted that symptoms may be ameliorated when effective therapy is initiated during the catarrhal stage of disease. Some evidence suggests erythromycin therapy can alter the clinical course of pertussis when initiated early in the paroxysmal stage.

Erythromycin or trimethoprim-sulfamethoxazole prophylaxis should be administered for 14 days to all household and other close contacts of persons with pertussis, regardless of age and vaccination status. Although data from controlled clinical trials are lacking, prophylaxis of all household members and other close contacts may prevent or minimize transmission. All close contacts <7 years of age who have not completed the four-dose primary series should complete the series with the minimal intervals (Table 4-4). Those who have completed a primary series but have not received a dose of DTP vaccine within 3 years of exposure should be given a booster dose.

Prophylactic postexposure passive immunization is not recommended. The use of human pertussis immune globulin neither prevents illness nor reduces its severity. This product is no longer available in the United States.

REFERENCES

Belsey MA. Skin infections and the epidemiology of diphtheria: acquisition and persistence of C. diphtheriae infections. Am J Epidemiol 1975;102:197.

Collier RJ: Diphtheria toxin: mode of action and structure. Bacteriol Rev 1975;39:54.

Fisher CM, Adams RD. Diphtheritic polyneuritis. A pathological study. J Neuropathol Exp Neurol 1956;15:243.

Freeman VJ, Morse U. Further observations on the change of virulence of bacteriophage infected avirulent strains of Corynebacterium diphtheriae. J Bacteriol 1953;63:407.

Klebs E. Ueber Diphtheria. Verh Cong Inn Med 1883; 2:139.

Loffler FAJ. Untersuchungen uber die Bedeutung der Mikroorganismen fuer die Entstehung die Diphtherie beim Menschen, bei der Taube und beim Kalbe. Mitt ADK Gesundheits 1884;2:451.

Marcuse EK, Grand G. Epidemiology of diphtheria in San Antonio, Tex., 1970. JAMA 1973;224:305.

Munford RS, Ory HW, Brooks GF, Feldman RS. Diphtheria deaths in the United States, 1959-1970. JAMA 1974;229: 1890.

Murphy JR, et al: Evidence that the regulation of diphtheria toxin production is directed at level of transcription. J Bacteriol 1978;135:511.

Nelson LA, et al. Immunity to diphtheria in an urban population. Pediatrics 1978;61:703.

Park WH, Zingher A. Active immunization in diphtheria and treatment by toxin-antitoxin. JAMA 1914;63:859.

Parsons EI. Induction of toxigenicity in nontoxigenic strains of *C. diphtheriae* with bacteriophages derived from nontoxigenic strains. Proc Soc Exp Biol Med 1955;90:91.

Sayers EC. Diphtheritic myocarditis with permanent heart damage. Ann Intern Med 1958;48:146.

Sheffield FW, et al. Susceptibility to diphtheria. Lancet 1978;1:428.

Tasman A, et al. Importance of intravenous injection of diphtheria antisera. Lancet 1958; 1:1299.

Thisyakorn U, Wongvanich J, Kampeng V. Failure of corticosteroid therapy to prevent diphtheritic myocarditis or neuritis. Pediatr Infect Dis 1984;3:126.

5

ENTEROVIRAL INFECTIONS

Human illnesses caused by enteroviruses have certain features in common such as a predilection for the central nervous system (CNS) and meninges. The various clinical manifestations range in severity from paralytic poliomyelitis and fatal myocarditis to very mild or inapparent infections. Many enteroviruses have clinical manifestations. A great deal of them overlap in the spectrum of illness induced. No single clinical syndrome is restricted to only one viral type.

HISTORY

Sporadic cases of paralytic disease are as old as recorded history. The term *poliomyelitis* was derived from the Greek for gray marrow of the spinal cord and the Latin (*-itis*) for inflammation. The anterior horn location of the involved cells in the spinal cord contributed the designation *anterior*. The first isolation of poliovirus was achieved in 1908 by the intracerebral inoculation of CNS tissue into susceptible monkeys. In 1949 Enders, Weller, and Robbins reported their classic experiments on the cultivation of poliovirus in tissue cultures of nonneural human cells.

The histories of the other enteroviruses are relatively recent. In 1948 Dalldorf and Sickles isolated an agent from the stool of a patient with paralytic illness from Coxsackie, New York. Subsequently, a large group of antigenically related viruses has been designated *Coxsackie A* and *Coxsackie B*. Isolation of echoviruses was accomplished from fecal specimens and frequently

from patients without overt disease. The echovirus name is an acronym: *E*, enteric; *C*, cytopathic; *H*, human, *O*, orphan. They have been associated with a wide variety of illnesses and are no longer "orphans." Since 1969 new enteroviruses have been assigned "enterovirus numbers" rather than being designated Coxsackie viruses or echoviruses.

ETIOLOGY

Enteroviruses were so named because of their natural habitat within the gastrointestinal tract. The enterovirus genus (see box) of the picornavirus family consists of six major groups; polioviruses; echoviruses; coxsackieviruses group A; coxsackieviruses group B; the new enterovirus serotypes 68 to 71; and hepatitis A virus. All of these agents infect and multiply in the gastrointestinal tract.

Enteroviruses are 30 nm particles composed of a single-stranded RNA genome with a protein coat of icosahedral symmetry. The viruses are indistinguishable morphologically, are stable at pH 3, and resist inactivation by ether. Assignment of a virus to one of these groups is based on chemical properties, differences in growth in tissue culture systems, pathogenicity for various strains of laboratory animals, and serological reactivity.

The RNA of enteroviruses is infectious, is a positive single strand, and therefore serves as the messenger RNA for the replication cycle of the virus. This messenger RNA codes for a polyprotein containing the amino acid sequence for

HUMAN ENTEROVIRUSES

Polioviruses	Serotypes 1, 2, and 3
Echoviruses	Serotypes 1-9, 11-27, 29-34*
Coxsackie A virus	Serotypes 1-22, 24†
Coxsackie B virus	Serotypes 1-6
Enteroviruses	Serotypes 68-71 (enterovirus 72)
Hepatitis A virus	

*Echovirus 10 currently is classified as reovirus type 1, whereas echovirus 28 is classified as human rhinovirus 1A.
†Coxsackie A23 currently is classified as echovirus 9.

all structural proteins of the virus. All enteroviruses code for four proteins (VP1, VP2, VP3, and VP4), which constitute the capsid of the virus and are derived by cleavage of the precursor polyprotein. Experiments examining the antigenic relationship of poliovirus strains by immunoprecipitation and neutralization of virus with monoclonal antibodies suggest that the four capsid proteins contain the antigens that determine the serotype of the virus strain.

Virus neutralization by antibody is complex, and infected persons generate a number of different antibodies to each infecting enterovirus. Antibody can act by reducing the infective efficiency of the particle itself (Icenogle et al., 1983), and a single antibody particle can neutralize a polio virion (Wetz et al., 1986). Alternatively, antibody can cause aggregation of viral particles by cross-linking them, thus reducing the number of infectious particles without altering the intrinsic infectivity of the particle. Mosser, Leipee, and Rueckert (1989) have examined the neutralization of poliovirus 1 using 15 neutralizing monoclonal antibodies. All antibodies that neutralize strongly do so by interaction with one site on the particle that contains a projecting portion of VP3. Neutralization sites are generally hypervariable areas projecting from the surface. It has been proposed that antibody must be able to bind by both arms to sites on one particle to reduce the infectivity of a single particle. Thus the location and symmetry of the site on the virion surface are determinants of neutralization. Antibodies to a second site that contains a portion of VP1 and VP2 neutralize by aggregation, which would occur because the two antibody arms more efficiently find this site on adjacent particles. This too is determined by the location and symmetry of the site. The neutral-

ization sites vary with different enteroviruses, but the general principles apply.

One or more of the capsid proteins is responsible for specific virus-cell interaction. The specificity of the interaction of a viral protein with a cell receptor most likely determines the tissue tropism of enteroviruses.

Rhinovirus (another genus of the picornavirus family) attachment to cells has been delineated better than that of the enteroviruses, but the similarities of picornaviruses render the data relevant to enteroviruses. A single small molecule (i.e., a specific fab fragment to cellular receptor) can effectively block a virus' binding to the cell (Colonno et al., 1989). This rhinovirus cell receptor has been isolated (Tomassini and Colonno, 1986) and is the intercellular adhesion molecule (ICAM-1) found on human and higher primate cells, thus determining the host range. A deep canyon exists on the surface of the rhinovirus capsid and on other picornaviruses. This canyon contains the attachment site on VP1 that is highly conserved and not accessible to antibody (Colonno et al., 1988). It is thought that the slope of the canyon can then define the accessibility of the viral receptor-protein. The viral attachment site therefore is not directly accessible to antibody. Thus a single conserved attachment site can function for different serotypes. The accessible neutralizable sites are therefore different from the attachment site of the virus.

PATHOGENICITY FOR ANIMALS

Grouping of enteroviruses requires mention of their pathogenicity for various species of animals. Coxsackie A viruses grow poorly in cell cultures, whereas newborn mice provide a more reliable system for their detection. The distinction between Coxsackie groups A and B depends on the pathological lesions produced in mice. Group A viruses cause generalized myositis and flaccid paralysis. Group B viruses cause focal myositis and typical lesions in the infrascapular fat pad and brain. Myocarditis, endocarditis, hepatitis, and necrosis of the acinar tissue of the pancreas can also be produced by group B viruses. Freshly isolated polioviruses and echoviruses are not pathogenic for mice. However, a strain (Lansing) of poliovirus type 2 has been adapted to these rodents, and laboratory strains of echovirus 9 have produced disease in mice. Changes in amino acids 93 to 103 in VP1 of poliovirus type 2 correlate with neurovirulence in mice (LaMonica et al., 1987).

PATHOGENESIS AND PATHOLOGY OF ENTEROVIRAL INFECTIONS

Enteroviruses gain entry to the host through the mouth. The virus establishes infection in the oropharynx and portions of the gastrointestinal tract where multiplication subsequently occurs. The virus then gains access to adjacent lymph nodes and the bloodstream. With echovirus 9 infections, viremia occurs up to 5 days before onset of symptoms (Yoshioka and Horstmann, 1962). The incubation period of enterovirus infections is usually 1 to 5 days. During the initial replication of virus within the gastrointestinal tract, there may be no overt illness or a nonspecific febrile illness.

Enteroviruses can multiply in peripheral white blood cells in vitro, although there are too few data to make broad generalizations. Gnann et al. (1979) showed echovirus 33 multiples in peripheral mononuclear white blood cells, specifically in monocytes. Other studies suggest that these viruses might also replicate in lymphocytes.

Virus invasion of other tissues such as the meninges or the myocardium typically occurs 7 to 10 days after initial exposure to the virus, resulting in the classic biphasic illness such as occurs with poliovirus. Enteroviruses may be excreted in the stool for as long as 6 to 8 weeks after onset of illness. Virus is present for a shorter time in the oropharynx, usually detected only during the first 5 to 7 days of illness.

Most Coxsackie and echovirus infections are transient and nonfatal; therefore limited histological information is available. The pathogenic

changes of poliovirus in the CNS are most prominent in the spinal cord, medulla, pons, and midbrain. Initially, cytoplasmic alterations in the Nissl substance of the motor neurons occur, followed by nuclear changes and pericellular infiltration of polymorphonuclear and mononuclear cells. The end result is neuronal destruction.

Fatal newborn infection with enteroviruses has shown nonspecific but extensive damage of the infected tissues. Echovirus infections are associated with hepatic necrosis and evidence of disseminated intravascular coagulation in multiple organs. If the patient has lived long enough, the liver may then show cirrhosis as opposed to the acute process.

CLINICAL ILLNESS

The broad spectrum of clinical disease produced by the enteroviruses overlaps among groups. A list of the various syndromes is in Table 5-1. Several illnesses suspected of being caused by enteroviruses but lacking definitive proof include diabetes mellitus, dermatomyositis, and congenital hydrocephalus. The more common manifestations associated with infection are discussed briefly.

Febrile illness

The great majority of infections with enteroviruses produce no specific clinical manifestations. Although the portal of entry is the gastrointestinal tract, enteroviruses are not frequently responsible for gastroenteritis. In young children undifferentiated febrile illness, nonspecific malaise, and myalgias frequently are associated with enterovirus infections. There is nothing unique about this type of clinical presentation. A prospective study of newborn infants in Rochester, New York, demonstrated that during a typical enterovirus season, as many as 13% of infants acquired infection with these viruses during the first month of life (Jenista et al., 1984). Although four fifths of these patients were asymptomatic, most of the symptomatic infants were admitted to the hospital because they were suspected of having bacterial sepsis. An estimate of the frequency of enteroviral infection of very young infants based on these observations suggests that in the first month of life seven infections per 1,000 live births occur during the months of seasonal prevalence of these agents. Reported enteroviral disease indicates morbidity is highest in infancy.

Table 5-1. Clinical manifestations of enterovirus infections

Clinical syndrome	Virus implicated				
		Coxsackie			Enteroviruses
	Polio	A	B	ECHO	68 to 71
Asymptomatic infection	X*	X	X	X	
Nonspecific febrile illness	X	X	X	X	
Respiratory disease		X	X	X	
Exanthems		X	X	X	
Enanthems		X			
Pleurodynia			X		
Orchitis					
Myocarditis			X		
Pericarditis			X	X	
Aseptic meningitis and meningoencephalitis	X	X	X	X	X
Disseminated neonatal infection			X	X	
Transitory muscle paresis	X	X	X	X	
Paralytic disease	X	X	X	X	X
Hemorrhagic conjunctivitis		X			X

*X, may be due to multiple serotypes.

Congenital and neonatal infections

Transplacental and neonatal transmission have been demonstrated with Coxsackie B viruses, resulting in a serious disseminated disease that may include hepatitis, myocarditis, meningoencephalitis, and adrenal cortical involvement (Kibrick and Benirschke, 1958). Coxsackie viruses have also been established as a cause of acute myocarditis of infants. Isolation of Coxsackie B3, B4, and A16 viruses from the myocardium and/or intestine of newborn infants was first reported in the late 1950s (van Creveld and deJager, 1956). The onset of illness is sudden, with loss of appetite, vomiting, coughing fits, cyanosis, and dyspnea. Pneumonia caused by these viruses may be prominent in the early illness. Marked pallor and tachycardia are characteristic features, with rapid decompensation. The heart and liver become enlarged. No cardiac murmur is heard as a rule. The electrocardiogram shows evidence of severe myocardial damage. In fatal cases the infant shows a gray pallor, goes rapidly into severe prostration and circulatory collapse, and dies. In those who survive recovery may be equally rapid.

The heart is grossly enlarged and pale; it is dilated and sometimes hypertrophied. Microscopic examination shows myocarditis of varying extent, with little or no evidence of involvement of the pericardium or endocardium. The valves are normal, and the myocardium shows a diffuse cellular infiltration between the muscle fibers. The striations are distinct in some areas, and others show degeneration and necrotic fibers. The infiltration consists of polymorphonuclear leukocytes, lymphocytes, eosinophils, plasma cells, and reticulum cells. The brain of one patient showed focal areas of cellular infiltration and degeneration of glial tissue and ganglion cells (Fig. 5-1).

Specific etiology and diagnosis are established by virus isolation. Infants infected in the newborn period with echoviruses have died with hepatic necrosis as the predominant feature of disseminated infection (Modlin, 1980). Serological studies have suggested that maternal antibody protects infants from severe disease, although the infants can acquire infection as documented by viral excretion (Modlin et al., 1981). Delivery must not be induced if a pregnant woman near term is suspected of having an enteroviral infection so that maternal antibody formation and subsequent transplacental transmission can occur. When poliovirus infections were common, examples of virus transmission from infected mother to fetus were reported to result in the birth of paralyzed infants.

Heart   Liver

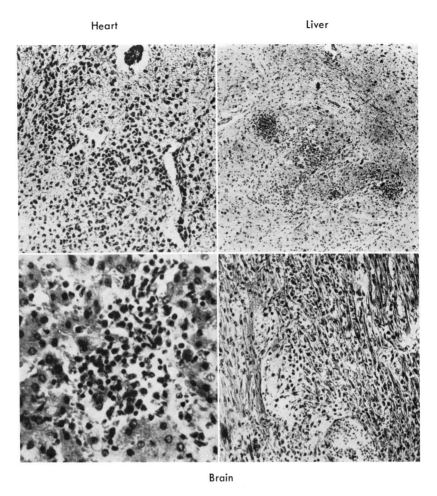

Brain

Fig. 5-1. Histologic appearance of the heart, liver, and brain in Coxsackie virus infection, showing diffuse and focal cellular infiltration. (From van Crevald S, de Jager H: Ann Pediatr 1956; 187:100.)

Respiratory disease

Mild upper respiratory tract illness has been associated with several of the Coxsackie and echo viruses. Very few cases of pneumonia have been attributed to Coxsackie virus infection.

Hemorrhagic conjunctivitis

A pandemic of acute hemorrhagic conjunctivitis was ascribed to enterovirus 70 and occurred from 1969 to 1971 in Africa, Southeast Asia, Japan, and India. The second epidemic in 1981 reached the Americas. Coxsackie A24 has also been implicated in this syndrome. Severe subconjunctival hemorrhage creates a noticeable and alarming sign. The patient also has swelling, redness, congestion, tearing, and pain in the eye. The prognosis is excellent, with complete recovery in approximately 1 week. Unusually,

polio-like motor paralysis has accompanied the conjunctivitis (Wadia et al., 1983).

Exanthems and enanthems

Various enteroviruses (particularly echoviruses 9 and 16, Coxsackie A2, A4, A9, and A16, and Coxsackie B3, B4, and B5) have been associated with large outbreaks of febrile rash disease. Younger children are more likely to develop exanthems, which vary widely in their characteristics. Macular and maculopapular eruptions indistinguishable from rubella have been observed with a number of Coxsackie viruses and echoviruses. Petechiae have accompanied some rashes, especially with echovirus 9. The presence of virus has been demonstrated in the skin lesions themselves.

Hand-foot-and-mouth disease

Hand-foot-and-mouth disease is characterized by fever and a vesicular eruption involving chiefly the buccal mucosa and tongue and less frequently the palate, gums, and lips; a maculopapular rash appears on the hands and feet, becomes vesicular, is interdigital on the dorsum of hands and feet, and involves the palms and soles. Robinson, Doane, and Rhodes (1957) first described this syndrome and its cause as Coxsackie virus A16. Subsequent reports have confirmed these observations and have added Coxsackie viruses A5 and A10 as other etiological agents.

Herpangina

Herpangina is most commonly associated with Coxsackie virus A infections and is characterized by sudden onset with high fever lasting from 1 to 4 days. Loss of appetite, sore throat, and dysphagia are common, and vomiting or abdominal pain occurs in approximately 25% of cases. The hallmark of the infection lies in the throat. Minute vesicles or, if these have ruptured, small punched-out ulcers appear on the anterior pillars of the fauces, the tonsils, the uvula, the pharynx, and the edge of the soft palate. The gray-white vesicles are 1 to 2 mm in diameter with red areolae. The lesions enlarge for 2 to 3 days, and the areolae become more intensely red; later, shallow gray-yellow ulcerations not more than 5 mm in diameter appear. The general and local symptoms disappear in 4 to 6 days, and recovery is complete. Different serotypes of the echovirus and Coxsackie groups can cause identical clinical pictures, so viral isolation is necessary to identify the specific etiological agent. Herpangina is easily confused with herpetic gingivostomatitis (p. 178). Herpangina is likely to occur during the summer or early fall and may also be epidemic, whereas herpes simplex infections occur sporadically in any season. The distinguishing features of herpes simplex infections are swollen red gums, involvement of the buccal mucosa, and the confluent character of the lesions.

Pleurodynia

Pleurodynia is also called *epidemic pleurodynia*, *epidemic myalgia*, *Bornholm disease*, and *devil's grip*. It is an acute disease caused chiefly by various group B Coxsackie viruses, although occasionally group A viruses may be implicated. The onset is sudden, with severe paroxysmal thoracic pain that is pleuritic in type. The pain is described as stabbing, knifelike, smothering, catching, or like being caught in a vise. It may be most severe in the substernal region, simulating coronary artery disease. Approximately one fourth of the patients have prodromal symptoms beginning 1 to 10 days before the onset of pain and consisting of headache, malaise, anorexia, and vague muscular aches. Abdominal pain occurs in addition to chest pain in approximately 50% of patients. Cough is either nonproductive or productive of a small amount of sputum and aggravates the pain. In most instances if anorexia, nausea, vomiting, and diarrhea accompany the chest pain, they are of short duration.

Fever ranges from 37.2° to 40° C (99° to 104° F). It may last from 1 to 14 days, with the average 3½ days. A pleural friction rub may be heard in approximately one fourth of the patients. Tenderness and splinting may be found in the upper abdomen, in the periumbilical area, and on the right side more often than on the left. The tenderness apparently most often is superficial, suggesting involvement of the muscle wall rather than that of deeper structures. Laboratory findings, including a roentgenogram of the chest, are normal in most cases, but pleural effusions may be observed.

Orchitis

Although viral orchitis most often is due to mumps, it has accompanied infections with the Coxsackie B viruses.

Myocarditis and pericarditis

Isolated myocarditis and/or pericarditis in older children and adults may result from Coxsackie B or echovirus infections. The spectrum has ranged from benign, self-limited pericarditis to severe, chronic, fatal myocardial disease. Pathogenesis of myocardial disease has been studied extensively in animal models. Coxsackie B viruses are those most commonly implicated, but infectious virus has not been isolated from myocardial tissue in children and adults, possibly because, in part, the tissue was obtained late in the illness. It has been suggested that myocardial disease is a result of viral infection and of the host immune response to the infection. Coxsackie B–specific RNA sequences in endomyocardial biopsy samples of acute and healed myocarditis have been reported (Bowles et al., 1986). Persistence of the viral genome must be confirmed and the mechanism investigated. In murine models, lytic T cells contribute to cell damage but are not essential for elimination of virus. T-cell–depleted mice have less severe myocarditis than mice with normal T-cell function. In some mice strains, antibodies against myocytes are a mediator of tissue damage. In humans the relative contributions of cell-mediated and humoral-mediated damage are not known.

Meningitis-encephalitis

The clinical manifestations of enteroviral CNS infection are not specific. The onset can be gradual or abrupt, and the predominant symptoms include fever, headache (when a child is old enough to report it), malaise, and signs of meningeal irritation. Temperatures as high as 40° C can be recorded, and fever usually lasts for 3 to 5 days. Infants less than 1 year of age often lack meningeal signs. Although the child may have an altered sensorium, focal neurological findings are rare. Severe illness may be accompanied by seizures, particularly in the youngest infants. A prospective concurrent case-controlled study of infants with viral meningitis has undergone preliminary analysis. Modlin (personal communication) has reported no discernible neurological sequelae attributable to enterovirus meningitis. Occasionally, paralytic illness indistinguishable from poliomyelitis occurs due to nonpolio enteroviruses. The spectrum of illness includes motor weakness and encephalitis. Most patients with enteroviral meningitis recover so that pathological descriptions are based on only a few cases. There is inflammation of the meninges with perivascular inflammatory cell infiltration. The most acute process is likely to have a predominance of polymorphonuclear cells, whereas mononuclear cells become predominant after relatively few days.

The physician's assessment of the CNS inflammatory response is based primarily on the laboratory findings in the cerebrospinal fluid (CSF). The CSF shows a leukocyte cell count ranging from none to several thousand cells/mm³. Most often the cell count is less than 500. It is common to have a polymorphonuclear cell predominance early in the illness. Cases of viral meningitis with onset of symptoms averaging 1½ days before initial lumbar puncture showed from 68% to

86% polymorphonuclear cells (Feigin and Shackelford, 1973). A second lumbar puncture done after 6 to 8 hours revealed a shift to mononuclear cell predominance in 87% of patients. The rapid shift to lymphocyte predominance during a matter of hours is unusual in bacterial meningitis even with antimicrobial therapy (Feigin and Shackelford, 1973).

The total protein content of the CSF is often within normal limits, but it may be elevated, even markedly so, in a small percentage of the patients. Glucose content of CSF is usually normal, but it may be diminished (<50% of a simultaneous serum glucose or <40 mg/dl) in enteroviral CNS infection (Singer et al., 1980).

Patients with agammaglobulinemia are unable to eradicate enteroviruses from the CNS (Wilfert et al., 1977; McKinney et al., 1987). Infections have persisted for longer than a decade. Relentless progressive deterioration in CNS function occurs, frequently accompanied by seizures, transient hemiparesis, and an altered sensorium. Symptoms and signs may wax and wane, but progressive loss of function ultimately is associated with focal defects or cortical atrophy on computed tomographic scan. The final phase of illness is characterized by a dermatomyositis syndrome, with virus present in blood and many other tissues (McKinney et al., 1987).

Poliomyelitis

Poliovirus infections range from asymptomatic poliomyelitis to paralytic illness. The ratio of inapparent infection to paralytic infection variously is estimated as 100:1 to 850:1. Even with overt infection, most persons have a mild and brief illness, starting abruptly and lasting from a few hours to a few days. The illness is characterized by fever, uneasiness, sore throat, headache, nausea, anorexia, vomiting, and pain in the abdomen; one or more of these symptoms may occur. Except for slight redness of the throat, there usually are no physical findings, and there are no signs of involvement of the CNS. This may be the entire self-limited illness. These nonspecific symptoms may also occur as the initial presentation of aseptic meningitis or paralytic disease.

Nonparalytic poliomyelitis. Nonparalytic poliomyelitis (meningitis) is characterized by many of the same features just listed and by pain and stiffness of the neck, back, and legs. Headache

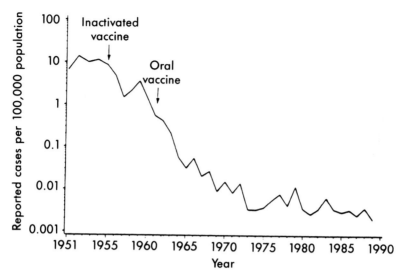

Fig. 5-2. Poliomyelitis (paralytic) by year in United States, 1951 to 1989. (From Centers for Disease Control: MMWR 1990; 38:135.)

is more severe, the temperature is higher, and the patient is sicker than with minor illness. Hyperesthesia and sometimes paresthesia may occur. The CSF shows a pleocytosis with a slight predominance of polymorphonuclear leukocytes, with subsequent increase in the proportion of lymphocytes. The protein level is slightly elevated. As the protein level rises later in illness, the cell count declines.

Paralytic disease. Poliovirus infection, especially type 1, is responsible for most of the paralytic disease caused by enteroviruses. Occasional cases of transient paralysis and muscle weakness have been noted with other enteroviruses, particularly the Coxsackie B agents. Enteroviruses 70 and 71 have been associated with paralytic disease and encephalitis (Shindarov et al., 1979; Wadia et al., 1983). Three of five children with enterovirus 71 paralysis had residual weakness and muscle wasting (Hayward et al., 1989). With classic paralytic polio, there is a 2- to 6-day incubation period with an initial nonspecific febrile illness. This period probably coincides with early replication of virus in the pharynx and gastrointestinal tract.

With the subsequent hematogenous spread of virus, CNS involvement may result in meningitis and anterior horn cell infection. From 1% to 4% of susceptible patients infected with polioviruses develop CNS involvement. The spectrum of paralytic disease is enormously variable and may involve the denervation of an isolated muscle group or extensive denervation and paralysis of all extremities. Characteristically, the picture is one of asymmetrical distribution, with the lower extremities more frequently involved than the upper. Large muscle groups are more often affected rather than the small muscles of the hands and feet. Involvement of cervical and thoracic segments of the spinal cord may result in paralysis of the muscles of respiration. Infection of cells in the medulla and cranial nerve nuclei results in bulbar polio with compromise of the respiratory and vasomotor centers.

Studies have indicated that tonsillectomy and adenoidectomy within a month of infection predispose to paralytic poliomyelitis including bulbar involvement. Strenuous exercise and fatigue occurring at the onset of the major illness have often been followed by severe paralysis. Intramuscular injections of vaccines, especially combinations of diphtheria, tetanus, and pertussis, have been associated with subsequent paralysis in the injected extremity. With the return of the patient's temperature to normal, the progress of paralysis ceases, and the subsequent weeks and months reveal a varying spectrum of recovery ranging from full return of function to significant residual paralysis. Atrophy of involved muscles becomes apparent after 4 to 8 weeks. Recovery may be exceedingly slow, and its full extent cannot be judged for 6 to 18 months.

Bulbar poliomyelitis. Bulbar poliomyelitis is characterized by damage to the motor nuclei of the cranial nerves and other vital zones in the medulla concerned with respiration and circulation. It may occur in the absence of clinically recognized involvement of the spinal cord. Bulbar poliomyelitis is potentially the most life-endangering form. The incidence of bulbar involvement varies from 5% to 10% of the total number of paralytic cases. In a Minnesota group of 107 cases cranial nerve nuclei were affected in descending frequency, with the tenth nerve affected in 90%, seventh in 66%, eleventh in 37%, sixth and twelfth in 14%, third in 11%, and fifth in 9%.

The most ominous form of bulbar poliomyelitis results from spread of infection to the respiratory and vasomotor centers. Damage to the respiratory center causes breathing to become irregular in rhythm and depth. Respirations are shallow and are associated with periods of apnea. The pulse rate and temperature increase. The blood pressure, at first elevated, may drop rapidly to shock levels. The patient becomes confused, delirious, and comatose, and then respiration stops. When the vasomotor center is involved, the pulse becomes extremely rapid, irregular, and difficult to palpate. The blood pressure fluctuates from high to low levels with a small pulse pressure.

On clinical grounds it is impossible to distinguish nonparalytic and preparalytic poliomyelitis from aseptic meningitis of another cause. Paralytic poliomyelitis has been confused with infectious polyneuritis, or Guillain-Barré syndrome. Since the striking decrease in incidence of poliomyelitis in the postvaccine era, the most commonly recognized causes of aseptic meningitis are Coxsackie viruses and ECHO viruses.

In the United States in the vaccine era fewer than 10 paralytic cases of poliomyelitis are reported per year. The majority are associated with receipt of attenuated vaccine or contact with a vaccinee. The differential diagnosis should consider paralysis caused by other enteroviruses, Guillain-Barré syndrome, and transverse myelitis.

Some patients who had paralytic illness develop new neuromuscular symptoms years later. Some of these patients develop new muscular weakness and have lymphocytic infiltrates in biopsied muscle. The pathogenesis is not understood.

EPIDEMIOLOGY

The epidemiology of all human enteroviruses is quite similar. The pattern is most clearly defined for the polioviruses because paralytic disease has been identifiable. As early as 1916, the epidemiological features were defined on the basis of an outbreak that occurred that year in New York City. These principles were (1) that poliomyelitis is exclusively a human infection, transmitted from person to person; (2) that the infection is far more prevalent than is apparent from the incidence of clinically recognized cases; (3) that the most important sources of infection are asymptomatic or mild illnesses escaping recognition; and (4) that an epidemic of one to three recognized cases per 1,000 infects the general population to such an extent that the outbreak declines spontaneously.

Enteroviruses have a worldwide distribution, with increased prevalence during the warm months of the year in temperate climates. In the United States some variation in geographical distribution of infections may be due to importation of viruses from other countries. Epidemics occur between May and October in the United States and other areas of the Northern temperate zone, but sporadic infections are identified throughout the year. The seroepidemiology of enteroviral infections, including polio and hepatitis A viruses, demonstrates an increased transmission of infection at a young age among persons of lower socioeconomic status. Crowded living conditions and poor hygiene enhance the fecal-to-oral transmission of these agents. Since 1985 in the United States surveillance data on isolates obtained from March through May have been used to predict the serotypes that will predominate from July to December.

Enteroviral illness is most commonly reported in children 1 to 4 years of age. The infections may occur more frequently in infants, and recognition and reporting of disease may reflect an enhanced concern over any illness at that age. Nevertheless, when specific outbreaks occur within a community, persons of all ages may be infected.

A 2- to 5-year periodicity has been observed with Coxsackie B infection, perhaps related to the limited number of serotypes. These agents cause outbreaks of disease when a newly susceptible population is present in the community. When a specific virus circulates frequently, younger infants who have not been exposed previously are more likely to be susceptible and develop disease. Perhaps the numerous serotypes of echoviruses have a broader range of age-related attack rates because a given serotype circulates through a community less often. It is unlikely that any individual would encounter all serotypes of enteroviruses in childhood.

The clinical epidemiology of these infections suggests that respiratory excretion of virus is not as important a means of spread as is fecal-to-oral transmission. Intimate human contact is important in transmission of virus, and communicability within households is greatest between children. Diapered infants apparently are more efficient disseminators of infection than other individuals. In the current era of day-care centers and nursery school it already has been shown that hepatitis A virus is transmitted in this setting and, if present, is transmitted to virtually all children in the nursery. It is likely that outbreaks of infection caused by other enteroviruses are also occurring in these facilities.

Community outbreaks of enteroviral infection can spread to hospital nurseries. A newborn who acquires a virus from his mother or from nursery personnel may spread it throughout the nursery. The viruses can be introduced into intensive care units by patients or personnel. Recognition of such infections imposes a need to institute isolation precautions such as cohorting of infants and personnel to minimize spread of infection.

IMMUNITY

Enteroviruses induce secretory and humoral antibody responses. The humoral responses initially are predominantly IgM antibodies, followed by IgA and IgG antibodies that persist for months to years. Coproantibodies, primarily IgA, have been studied as a response to administration of poliovirus vaccines or to natural infection. Local secretory immunoglobulin A production occurs at the site of contact of the virus with lymphoid cells. Development of type-specific antibody provides lifelong protection against clinical illness caused by the same agents. Local reinfection of the gastrointestinal tract may occur, but this is accompanied by an abbreviated period of viral replication without clinical illness.

In experimental poliovirus infection specific IgG antibody-producing cells and measurable antibodies can be demonstrated in areas of the CNS where virus is replicating. Local CNS antibody production is independent of systemic humoral antibody production. Although specific CNS enteroviral antibodies are probably produced primarily within the CNS, some passive transfer of serum antibody to the CSF may occur as permeability is increased by inflammation. Evidence for the extreme importance of CNS antibody is deduced from agammaglobulinemic patients who are unable to eliminate enteroviruses from the CNS. Administration of extraordinarily large quantities of parenteral globulin or plasma with specific antibody is necessary to achieve measurable antibody levels in the CSF (Weiner et al., 1979).

Cellular immunity against enteroviral infection is not well defined. Circulating peripheral white blood cells have been a source of viral isolation during acute illness. Recognition of virus by lymphocytes occurs in experimental models using Coxsackie viruses. The abnormal response of some children with immunodeficiency disease to infection with attenuated polioviruses may offer further insights to immune processes normally stimulated by enterovirus infection.

DIAGNOSIS

The clinical illnesses in some instances may permit a presumptive diagnosis of enterovirus infection. However, as shown in Table 5-1, the spectrum of illness is wide. The time of the year may be helpful. In temperate zones enteroviral infections occur most often in the summer and early autumn. Specimens for viral isolation should be obtained early in the course of illness. The CSF of patients with viral meningitis and/or meningoencephalitis has been a rich source of enteroviruses except for the three polio types. Materials such as pleural and pericardial fluid should also be cultured when available.

Specific etiological diagnosis of enteroviral disease has been dependent on demonstration of the enterovirus by cell culture techniques. Viral culture has been the most sensitive means of detecting virus because of the amplification in cell culture. Unfortunately, most of the Coxsackie A viruses grow poorly in cell cultures, and only newborn mice provide a reliable system for detection of these agents. Various primate and human epithelial cell cultures support replication of most of the enteroviruses, with cytopathic effects revealing their presence. However, no single cell-culture system permits replication of all numbers of the enterovirus groups, and a period of days is needed to detect virus. The specimens submitted most often for attempted viral isolations are nasopharyngeal swabs and stool specimens. An enterovirus may be excreted in fecal material for several weeks after the onset of clinical illness. Recovery of an enterovirus from the throat or stool of the patient does not in itself establish it as the etiological agent of the illness observed. The temporal association of illness, viral recovery, and an antibody rise specific to that agent provide firmer evidence of a causative relationship.

A potentially useful and more practical approach to diagnosis would be the demonstration of viral antigen in clinical specimens, especially CSF. It would be ideal if antigen could be detected by a method capable of providing a specific diagnosis within hours. Recent work has demonstrated the feasibility of detecting enterovirus RNA by hybridization or polymerase chain reaction (PCR) assays using cell-culture–grown virus. Rotbart (1989) and Hyypia et al. (1984) demonstrated the feasibility of a nucleic acid probe (cDNA) to detect many serotypes of enteroviruses. Rotbart demonstrated the conservation of sequences at the 5′ end of the genome, and Hyypia showed similar conservation of sequences in the 3′ end of the genome. CSF was used for development of the optimal experimental system. Combinations of probes containing both conserved regions detected polioviruses 1, 2, and 3, echoviruses 2, 4, 6, and 11, Coxsackie viruses A9 and A16, and Coxsackie viruses B1 and B6. The assay could detect from 10^2 to 10^5 50% tissue culture infectious doses of virus (TCID50). Not many studies quantitate infectious virus in the CSF, but reports suggest 10^0 to 10^4 TCID50 are present (Wilfert and Zeller, 1984). The number of RNA molecules present may be greater than the number of infectious virions. A small clinical trial suggested the probes were not sufficiently sensitive or specific (Rotbart, 1989). The use of RNA probes and PCR provide an approach to increase the sensitivity of the detection system, and studies are currently in progress. Such assays may be very helpful in elucidating the pathogenesis of known and putative enterovirus diseases.

Acute and convalescent serum samples obtained 7 to 21 days apart help define quantitative changes in antibody titers. Complement fixation, viral neutralization, immunoprecipitation, enzyme-linked immunosorbent assay (ELISA), and in a few instances, hemagglutination inhibition are the available techniques for assaying enterovirus antibodies. Neutralizing antibodies are type specific, whereas complement fixation demonstrates group-reactive antibodies. If specific polypeptides are available for ELISA tests, serotype-specific antibodies can be measured to a single serotype. There may be shared antigens among many serotypes, which could provide a means to recognize many serotypes of enteroviruses (Romero et al., 1986). In the course of a lifetime humans sustain multiple infections, occult or overt, with a variety of enteroviruses. IgM serology for Coxsackie B viruses has had some clinical use (Bell et al., 1986; Dorries and Meulen, 1983; McCartney et al., 1986). A specific infection elicits the production of antibody specific to that virus type but also may prompt an anamnestic response demonstrated by an increase in group-reactive antibody and by parallel rises in antibodies to serotypes of some of the other enteroviruses previously encountered. The concomitant serological rises in heterologous antibody titer create problems with serological surveys, rendering the complement fixation test inadequate to define a specific infection. In the absence of the recovery of a virus the problem of seeking specific antibody rises against the whole genus of enteroviruses remains. Thus the complexity of serology makes the serological diagnosis of these infections impractical. The isolation of a specific virus provides the opportunity for assessment of the patient's antibody against his own viral agent. Identification of an enterovirus during an outbreak makes it possible to assess the sera of patients for the presence of antibody to that serotype. Serological diagnosis by virus neutralization is a convenient but cumbersome epidemiological tool for diagnosis in epidemic settings.

TREATMENT

There is no specific treatment for poliomyelitis. There is no evidence that the administration of immune serum globulin changes the course of events once signs of the illness have appeared. In fact, most patients already have specific antibodies in the early stages of illness.

The amount of physical activity early in the major illness seems to correlate with the incidence and severity of subsequent paralysis. The management of individual patients with paralytic poliomyelitis in all of its complex details requires the collaboration of the physician and the physical therapist.

In patients who have difficulty in swallowing, with involvement of either the medullary centers or muscles of respiration, the preservation of a clear airway is vital. Respiratory support may include the use of oxygen, endotracheal intubation, and respiratory-assisted ventilation. The nurse contributes enormously to the physical needs of the patients and help maintain the patient's morale.

There are experimental drugs with in vitro and in vivo (animal) activity against enteroviruses. They have not yet been tested in humans.

PREVENTION

Because there currently is no specific treatment for enterovirus infections, efforts have focused on means of prevention. The multiple antigenic types and the usual self-limited course of most echovirus and Coxsackie virus infections have resulted in little stimulus to the development of vaccines, but recent recognition of morbidity in infants may stimulate further thought about vaccines and therapy. The story of the poliovirus vaccines, however, has been one of the most exciting and rewarding sagas in microbiological history.

Enders and colleagues' tissue culture techniques lent themselves to the propagation in vitro of sufficient amounts of relatively pure poliovirus so that controlled formaldehyde inactivation could be used to produce a noninfectious virus that retained its antigenicity (Enders et al., 1949). Salk and his colleagues pursued this line of research and by 1954 were able to embark on a field trial that established the efficacy of an inactivated poliovirus vaccine in the prevention of paralytic disease. The vaccine was widely used in the United States during the 5 years from 1956 through 1960. The results were dramatic. Ten thousand to twenty thousand cases of paralytic disease decreased to 2,000 to 3,000 reported annually with the widespread use of Salk vaccine.

By the early 1960s a second vaccine was available. Strains of poliovirus that Sabin had selected and studied in his laboratory were proven attenuated for monkey and man. Ingestion of these strains resulted in intestinal infection and viral excretion so that humoral and gastrointestinal tract immunity developed without any illness. This vaccine could be administered more readily (by the oral route) and the multiplication in the gastrointestinal tract more closely mimicked natural infection. These advantages led to its replacing the injectable Salk vaccine. Over the first 5 years of the 1960s more than 400 million doses of oral vaccine were distributed in the United States. At the same time, trials also were successfully conducted in European nations, Japan, and other countries. The use of oral vaccine in this country was accompanied by a further decrease in the annual reported polio cases (Fig. 5-2) so that beginning in 1966 fewer than 100 cases have been reported each year. From 1980 through 1988 a total of 81 cases of paralytic polio have been reported. In less than 20 years a disease that had claimed thousands of victims annually and that had been the source of indescribable community anxiety was reduced to a rarity.

In the complex processes of development, commercial production, and widespread use of polio vaccines, a number of unexpected events transpired that merit consideration. After the highly successful field trials of 1954, commercial manufacture of the Salk-type vaccine was licensed. Within a few weeks of its use, paralytic disease was observed in April through June of 1955 among children in California and Idaho who had received some of the first lots of commercial vaccine manufactured by the Cutter Laboratories. By the time this occurrence had been fully investigated and resolved, it was learned that there were 204 cases of vaccine-associated disease. Seventy-nine were among children who had received the vaccine, 105 were among their family contacts, and 20 were in community contacts. Nearly three quarters of the cases were paralytic, and there were 11 deaths. The agent isolated from these patients was type

1 poliovirus. Laboratory tests on vaccine revealed viable virulent type 1 poliovirus in seven of 17 lots (Nathanson and Langmuir, 1963). Revisions of the federal regulations governing the steps in vaccine manufacture were promulgated and implemented to prevent recurrence of such a tragic episode.

Manufacturers faced further difficulties in maintaining the fine balance between the complete elimination of the infectious live virus from the production process and the retention of effective antigenicity of the inactivated components. A number of lots of vaccine subsequently were proven to be poorly antigenic for type 3 poliovirus. As a result, when community polio outbreaks occurred among well-immunized groups, there were "breakthroughs" with paralytic disease, especially caused by type 3 virus, in previously immunized subjects. Such an outbreak was studied in 1959 in Massachusetts where an analysis of polio cases revealed that 47% (62 of 137) of the patients had previously received three or more inoculations of inactivated vaccine (Berkovich et al., 1961).

In the United States almost all current immunization is performed with the oral attenuated product. A number of European countries, especially those in Scandinavia, have adhered to the use of inactivated polio vaccine (IPV). Their record of achievement in the control of polio had been parallel to that of this country until 1984. From August 1984 through January 1985 nine cases of paralytic poliomyelitis and one case of aseptic meningitis caused by wild-type virus occurred in Finland. Widespread polio virus circulation was documented throughout the country by isolation of poliovirus type 3 from asymptomatic family members and sewage. Seven of the 10 patients had received three to five doses of inactivated vaccine, one person received one dose, and two persons, ages 31 and 48 years, had not been immunized (Centers for Disease Control, 1986). The IPV vaccine in use in Finland produced lower levels of antibodies to poliovirus 3 than to types 1 and 2. More potent IPV is available and now in use. However, persons immunized only with IPV can excrete polioviruses for longer periods and in larger quantities because of the absence of gastrointestinal tract immunity (Onorata et al., 1991). This may facilitate community circulation of polioviruses. An essential question is whether a person previously vaccinated with IPV with waning humoral immunity and lacking gastrointestinal immunity is again at risk of paralytic disease because virulent virus can multiply in the gastrointestinal tract and produce viremia before an anamnestic humoral response to virus can occur.

The marked decrease in paralytic disease caused by "wild" polioviruses has disclosed a small but significant number of cases of oral vaccine recipients who have developed paralytic illness in temporal association with the ingestion of vaccine. Paralytic episodes have also been reported among susceptible family or community contacts of the vaccine recipients. Fewer than 10 cases per year of paralytic disease are identified in the United States. A small portion of these patients are immunodeficient children, particularly those with congenital hypogammaglobulinemia. Increased neurovirulence (i.e., reversion) has been documented after viral replication in the gastrointestinal tract. It is now thought that attenuation of virus is largely due to base changes in the 5′ noncoding region and in the encoding region for VP3, although it is not yet known how these changes produce attenuation (Minor et al., 1989). It is probable that comparable changes in polioviruses types 1 and 2 contribute to attenuation.

Monovalent oral polio vaccine (MOPV) was used extensively until 1964 when it was supplanted by trivalent vaccine (TOPV). With MOPV the estimated risk of vaccine-associated illness in recipients was 0.19 per million doses distributed. With TOPV the overall figure of risk to recipients and their contacts is one case per 2.5 million doses of vaccine distributed. The calculated risk of paralysis is one case per 520,000 doses with the first dose of vaccine and one case per 12.3 million with subsequent doses (Nkowane et al., 1987).

The achievements with poliovirus vaccination have been impressive in the United States, Canada, and most of Europe, Australia, and some Asian and African nations. Paralytic poliomyelitis is declining consistently and substantially in the Western hemisphere, with only three wild-type isolates reported in the first 32 weeks of 1990. However, polio remains an endemic disease in many tropical lands. It is premature therefore to relax the use of poliovirus vaccination in those parts of the world where disease

Table 5-2. Routine poliomyelitis immunization schedule summary, 1981*

Dose	OPV age/interval	IPV age/interval
Primary 1	Initial visit, preferably 6-12 weeks of age	Initial visit, preferably 6-12 weeks of age
Primary 2	Interval of 6-8 weeks	Interval of 4-8 weeks
Primary 3	Interval of ≥6 weeks, customarily 8-12 months	Interval of 4-8 weeks
Primary 4		Interval of 6-12 months
Supplementary	4-6 years of age† (school entry)	4-6 years of age† (school entry)
Additional supplementary		Interval of every 5 years‡

*Important details are in the text.

†If the third primary dose of OPV is administered on or after the fourth birthday, a fourth (supplementary) dose is not required. If the fourth primary dose of IPV is administered on or after the fourth birthday, a fifth (supplementary) dose is not required at school entry.

‡Supplementary doses are recommended every 5 years after the last dose until the 18th birthday or unless a complete primary series of OPV has been completed.

has been nearly eradicated. The possibility of the inadvertent introduction of virulent virus is omnipresent.

The following guidelines for the use of currently licensed vaccine(s) are extracted from the recommendations of the Immunization Practices Advisory Committee (ACIP) of the USPHS as reported in the *Morbidity and Mortality Weekly Report* of January 29, 1982, and that of December 11, 1987.

Poliovirus vaccines

Two types of poliovirus vaccines are currently licensed in the United States: Oral Polio Vaccine (OPV)* and Inactivated Polio Vaccine (IPV).†

Routine immunization
Rationale for choice of vaccine

Although IPV and OPV are both effective in preventing poliomyelitis, OPV is the vaccine of choice for primary immunization of children in the United States when the benefits and risks for the entire population are considered. OPV is preferred because it induces intestinal immunity, is simple to administer, is well accepted by patients, results in immunization of some contacts of vaccinated persons, and has a record of having essentially eliminated disease associated with wild polioviruses in this country. The choice of OPV as the preferred polio vaccine in the United States has also been made by the Committee on Infectious Diseases of the American Academy of

Pediatrics and a special expert committee of the Institute of Medicine, National Academy of Sciences.

Prospective vaccinees or their parents should be made aware of the polio vaccines available and the reasons why recommendations are made for giving specific vaccines at particular ages and under certain circumstances. Furthermore, the benefits and risks of the vaccines for individuals and the community should be stated so that vaccination is carried out among persons who are fully informed.

Recommendations for infants, children, and adolescents
Primary immunization (Table 5-2)

OPV: For infants, children, and adolescents through secondary school age (generally up to age 18) the primary series of OPV consists of 3 doses. In infancy the primary series is integrated with DTP vaccination, and the first dose is commonly given at 6-12 weeks of age. At all ages the first 2 doses should be separated by at least 6, and preferably 8, weeks. The third dose is given at least 6 weeks, customarily 8-12 months, after the second dose. In high-risk areas, an additional dose of OPV is often given within the first 6 months of life. Breast feeding does not interfere with successful immunization.

IPV: The primary series consists of 4 doses of vaccine; volume and route of injection are specified by the manufacturer. In infancy, the primary schedule is usually integrated with DTP vaccination, as with OPV. Three doses can be given at 4- to 8-week intervals; the fourth dose should follow 6-12 months after the third.

All children should complete primary immunization before entering school, preferably with all OPV or all IPV. If, however, a combination of IPV and

---

*Official name: Poliovirus vaccine, live, oral, trivalent.

†Official name: Poliomyelitis vaccine.

OPV is used, a total of 4 doses constitutes a primary series.

Supplementary immunization

OPV: Before entering school, all children who previously received primary immunization with OPV (3 doses) in early childhood should be given a fourth dose. However, if the third primary dose is administered on or after the fourth birthday, a fourth (supplementary) dose is not required. The additional dose will increase the likelihood of complete immunity in the small percentage of children who have not previously developed serum antibodies to all 3 types of polioviruses. The need for supplementary doses after 4 doses of OPV has not been established, but children considered to be at increased risk of exposure to poliovirus (as noted below under recommendations for adults) may be given a single additional dose of OPV.

IPV: Before entering school, all children who previously received primary immunization with either IPV alone or a combination of IPV and OPV (a total of 4 doses) in early childhood should be given at least 1 dose of OPV or 1 additional dose of IPV. However, if the fourth primary dose is administered on or after the fourth birthday, a fifth (supplementary) dose is not required at school entry. Use of a primary series of OPV would eliminate the need for subsequent booster doses of IPV. Children who received primary immunization with IPV should obtain a booster dose of IPV every 5 years until the age of 18 years, unless a primary series of OPV is given. The need for such supplementary doses after the 5 basic doses of the currently available IPV product has not been firmly established. Further experience may lead to alteration of this recommendation.

Children incompletely immunized

Polio vaccination status should be reevaluated periodically, and those who are inadequately protected should complete their immunizations.

OPV: To help assure seroconversion to all 3 serotypes of poliovirus, completion of the primary series of 3 doses of OPV is recommended. Time intervals between doses longer than those recommended for routine primary immunization do not necessitate additional doses of vaccine. Individuals who received only 1 dose of each of the monovalent OPVs in the past should receive 2 doses of trivalent OPV at least 6 weeks apart. One dose of each monovalent OPV (poliovirus types 1, 2, and 3) is at least equivalent to 1 dose of trivalent OPV.

IPV: Regulations for vaccine licensure adopted since 1968 require a higher potency IPV than was previously manufactured. Four doses of IPV administered after 1968 are considered a complete primary series. As with OPV, time intervals between doses longer than those recommended for routine primary immunization do not necessitate additional doses.

Incompletely immunized children who are at increased risk of exposure to poliovirus (as noted below under recommendations for adults) should be given the remaining required dose or, if time is a limiting factor, at least a single dose of OPV.

Recommendations for adults

Routine primary poliovirus vaccination of adults (generally those 18 years old or older) residing in the United States is not necessary. Most adults are already immune and also have a very small risk of exposure to poliomyelitis in the United States. Immunization is recommended for certain adults who are at greater risk of exposure to wild polioviruses than the general population, including:

1. travelers to areas or countries where poliomyelitis is epidemic or endemic;
2. members of communities or specific population groups with disease caused by wild polioviruses;
3. laboratory workers handling specimens which may contain polioviruses;
4. health-care workers in close contact with patients who may be excreting polioviruses.

For individuals in the above categories, polio vaccination is recommended as detailed below.

Unvaccinated adults

For adults at increased risk of exposure to poliomyelitis, primary immunization with IPV is recommended whenever this is feasible. IPV is preferred because the risk of vaccine-associated paralysis following OPV is slightly higher in adults than in children. Three doses should be given at intervals of 1-2 months; a fourth dose should follow 6-12 months after the third.

In circumstances where time will not allow at least 3 doses of IPV to be given before protection is required, the following alternatives are recommended:

1. If less than 8, but more than 4, weeks are available before protection is needed, 2 doses of IPV should be given at least 4 weeks apart.
2. If less than 4 weeks are available before protection is needed, a single dose of OPV is recommended.

In both instances, the remaining doses of vaccine should be given later at the recommended intervals, if the person remains at increased risk.

Incompletely immunized adults

Adults who are at increased risk of exposure to poliomyelitis and who have previously received less than a full primary course of OPV or IPV should be given the remaining required doses of either vaccine, regardless of the interval since the last dose and the type of vaccine previously received.

Adults previously given a complete primary course of OPV or IPV

Adults who are at increased risk of exposure to poliomyelitis and who have previously completed a primary course of OPV may be given another dose of OPV. The need for further supplementary doses has not been established. Those adults who previously completed a primary course of IPV may be given a dose of either IPV or OPV. If IPV is used exclusively, additional doses may be given every 5 years, but their need also has not been established.

Unimmunized or inadequately immunized adults in households in which children are to be given OPV

Adults who have not been adequately immunized against poliomyelitis with OPV or IPV are at a very small risk of developing OPV-associated paralytic poliomyelitis when children in the household are given OPV. About 4 such cases have occurred annually among contacts since 1969, during which time about 24 million doses of OPV were distributed yearly. (See Adverse reactions.)

Because of the overriding importance of ensuring prompt and complete immunization of the child and the extreme rarity of OPV-associated disease in contacts, the Committee recommends the administration of OPV to a child regardless of the poliovirus-vaccine status of adult household contacts. This is the usual practice in the United States. The responsible adult should be informed of the small risk involved. An acceptable alternative, if there is strong assurance that ultimate, full immunization of the child will not be jeopardized or unduly delayed, is to immunize adults according to the schedule outlined above before giving OPV to the child.

Precautions and contraindications
Pregnancy

Although there is no convincing evidence documenting adverse effects of either OPV or IPV on the pregnant woman or developing fetus, it is prudent on theoretical grounds to avoid vaccinating pregnant women. However, if immediate protection against poliomyelitis is needed, OPV is recommended.

Immunodeficiency

Patients with immune-deficiency diseases, such as combined immunodeficiency, hypogammaglobulinemia, and agammaglobulinemia, should not be given OPV because of their substantially increased risk of vaccine-associated disease. Furthermore, patients with altered immune states due to diseases such as leukemia, lymphoma, or generalized malignancy, or

with immune systems compromised by therapy with corticosteroids, alkylating drugs, antimetabolites, or radiation should not receive OPV because of the theoretical risk of paralytic disease. OPV should not be used for immunizing immunodeficient patients and their household contacts; IPV is recommended. Many immunosuppressed patients will be immune to polioviruses by virtue of previous immunization or exposure to wild-type virus at a time when they were immunologically competent. Although these persons should not receive OPV, their risk of paralytic disease is thought to be less than that of naturally immunodeficient individuals. Although a protective immune response to IPV in the immunodeficient patient cannot be assured, the vaccine is safe and some protection may result from its administration. If OPV is inadvertently administered to a household-type contact of an immunodeficient patient, close contact between the patient and the recipient of OPV should be avoided for approximately 1 month after vaccination. This is the period of maximum excretion of vaccine virus. Because of the possibility of immunodeficiency in other children born to a family in which there has been 1 such case, OPV should not be given to a member of a household in which there is a family history of immunodeficiency until the immune status of the recipient and other children in the family is documented.

Adverse reactions
OPV

In rare instances, administration of OPV has been associated with paralysis in healthy recipients and their contacts. Other than efforts to identify persons with immune-deficiency conditions, no procedures are currently available for identifying persons likely to experience such adverse reactions. Although the risk of vaccine-associated paralysis is extremely small for vaccinees and their susceptible, close, personal contacts, they should be informed of this risk.

IPV

No serious side effects of currently available IPV have been documented. Since IPV contains trace amounts of streptomycin and neomycin, there is a possibility of hypersensitivity reactions in individuals sensitive to these antibiotics.

Case investigation and epidemic control

Each suspected case of poliomyelitis should prompt an immediate epidemiologic investigation, including an active search for other cases. If evidence implicates wild poliovirus and there is a possibility of transmission, a vaccination plan designed to contain spread should be developed. If evidence implicates vaccine-derived poliovirus, no vaccination plan need be developed, as no outbreaks associated with vaccine virus have been documented to date. Within an epidemic area, OPV should be provided for all persons over 6 weeks of age who have not been completely immunized or whose immunization status is unknown, with the exceptions noted above under immunodeficiency.

Poliomyelitis prevention: enhanced-potency inactivated poliomyelitis vaccine—supplementary statement

The supplementary statement provides information on and recommendations for the use of inactivated poliovirus vaccine (IPV) of enhanced potency.* The Immunization Practices Advisory Committee (ACIP) believes that, in the United States, polio immunization should rely primarily on oral poliovirus vaccine (OPV), with selected use of enhanced-potency IPV as specified in this document. However, this subject should be reviewed on a continuing basis, and an extensive review of polio vaccines and potential vaccine policies will take place during 1988. General recommendations on poliomyelitis prevention, including the use of and schedules for OPV, are found in the current ACIP recommendations.

Enhanced-potency IPV. A method of producing a more potent IPV with greater antigenic content was developed in 1978 and led to the newly licensed IPV, which is produced in human diploid cells. Results of studies from several countries have indicated that a reduced number of doses of IPV produced with this technique can immunize children satisfactorily. A clinical trial of two preparations of enhanced-potency IPV was completed in the United States in 1984. Children received three doses of one of the enhanced-potency IPVs at 2, 4, and 18 months of age. In spite of the presence of maternal antibodies in the majority of the infants at the time of the first dose, 99%-100% of the children were seropositive for all three poliovirus types at 6 months of age (2 months after their second dose). The percentage of seropositive children did not rise or fall significantly during the 14-month period following the second dose, a result that confirms that seroconversion had occurred in almost all children.

Vaccine usage

Indications. Persons with a congenital immune deficiency disease, such as agammaglobulinemia; an acquired immune deficiency disease, such as acquired immunodeficiency syndrome (AIDS); or an altered immune status as a result of other diseases or immunosuppressive therapy are at increased risk for paralysis associated with OPV. Therefore, if polio im-

munization is indicated, these persons and their household members and other close contacts should receive IPV rather than OPV. Although a protective immune response following receipt of enhanced-potency IPV cannot be assured, some protection may be provided to the immunocompromised patient. Available data on children previously diagnosed with asymptomatic human immunodeficiency virus (HIV) infection do not suggest that they are at increased risk of adverse consequences from OPV. However, for such persons, use of IPV rather than OPV is prudent since family members may be immunocompromised because of AIDS or HIV infection and may be at increased risk for paralysis from contact with an OPV virus.

Schedules. The primary series for enhanced-potency IPV consists of three 0.5-ml doses administered subcutaneously. The interval between the first two doses should be at least 4 weeks, but preferably 8 weeks. The third dose should follow in at least 6 months, but preferably nearer to 12 months. A primary series can be started as early as 6 weeks of age, but preferably at 2 months of age. Although studies have not been conducted, young children should receive the third dose along with diphtheria, tetanus, pertussis vaccine (DTP), and measles, mumps, rubella vaccine (MMR) at 15 months of age, if possible.

A primary series of polio vaccine usually consists of enhanced-potency IPV alone or OPV alone. However, a combination of both vaccines totalling three doses and separated by appropriate intervals constitutes a primary series. If enhanced-potency IPV is administered to persons with a previously incomplete series of conventional IPV, a final total of four doses of polio vaccine is necessary for a primary series.

All children who received a primary series of enhanced-potency IPV or of a combination of polio vaccines should be given a booster dose before entering school, unless the final dose of the primary series was administered on or after the fourth birthday. The need for routinely administering additional doses is unknown at this time.

For unvaccinated adults at increased risk of exposure to poliovirus, a primary series of enhanced-potency IPV is recommended. While the responses of adults to a primary series have not been studied, the recommended schedule for adults is two doses given at a 1- to 2-month interval and a third dose given 6 to 12 months later. If less than 3 months but more than 2 months are available before protection is needed, three doses of enhanced-potency IPV should be given at least 1 month apart. Likewise, if only 1 to 2 months are available, two doses of enhanced-potency IPV should be given at least 1 month apart. If less than 1 month is available, a single dose of either OPV or enhanced-potency IPV is recommended.

*Poliovirus Vaccine Inactivated, which is manufactured by Connaught Laboratories Ltd., will be distributed by Connaught Laboratories Inc. beginning in March 1988.

Adults who are at increased risk of exposure and have had (1) at least one dose of OPV, (2) fewer than three doses of conventional IPV, or (3) a combination of conventional IPV and OPV totalling fewer than three doses should receive at least one dose of OPV or enhanced-potency IPV. Additional doses needed to complete a primary series should be given if time permits.

Adults who are at increased risk of exposure and who have previously completed a primary series with any one or combination of polio vaccines can be given a dose of OPV or enhanced-potency IPV.

Side effects and adverse reactions. Available data indicate that the rate of adverse reactions in the kidney cells of monkeys receiving enhanced-potency IPV are low and that the reactions are not different from those following administration of a placebo. The recently licensed human diploid cell-derived vaccine was not compared to a placebo. Rates of local adverse events following its use are similar to rates found in controlled studies using vaccine derived from the kidney cells of monkeys. There is no evidence that conventional IPV causes any serious side effects. Consequently, serious side effects are not expected to occur with enhanced-potency IPV. This conclusion can be confirmed only with postmarketing surveillance.

Precautions and contraindications. Vaccine administration should not be postponed because of minor illnesses, such as mild upper-respiratory infections. Generally, however, persons with severe febrile illnesses should not be vaccinated until they have recovered.

REFERENCES

Bell EJ, McCartney RA, Basquill D, Chaudhuri AKR. Antibody capture ELISA for the rapid diagnosis of enterovirus infections in patients with aseptic meningitis. J Med Virol 1986;19:213-217.

Berkovich S, Pickering JE, Kibrick S. Paralytic poliomyelitis in Massachusetts, 1959. A study of the disease in a well vaccinated population. N Engl J Med 1961;264:1323.

Bowles NE, Olsen EG, Richardson PJ, Archard LC. Detection of Coxsackie B virus specific RNA sequences in myocardial biopsy samples from patients with myocarditis and dilated cardiomyopathy. Lancet 1986; May 17:1120-1122.

Centers for Disease Control. MMWR update: poliomyelitis outbreak—Finland, 1984-85. 1986;35:82-86.

Centers for Disease Control. MMWR summary of notifiable disease, US 1989-1990. MMWR 1990;38:35.

Colonno RJ, Abraham G, Tomassini E. Molecular and biochemical aspects of human rhinovirus attachment to cellular receptors. In molecular aspects of picornavirus infection and detection. In Semler BC, Ehrenfeld E (eds). Washington, DC: American Society for Microbiology, 1989, p 169-178.

Colonno RJ, Condra JH, Mizutami S, et al. Evidence for the direct involvement of the rhinovirus canyon in receptor binding. Proc Natl Acad Sci USA 1988;85:5449-5453.

Dalldorf G, Sickless GM. An unidentified filtrable agent isolated from the faces of children with paralysis. Science 1948;108:61-62.

Dorries R, Meulen VT. Specificity of IgM antibodies in acute human coxsackievirus B infections, analysed by indirect solid phase enzyme immunoassay and immunoblot technique. J Gen Virol 1983;64:159-167.

Enders JF, Weller TH, Robbins FC. Cultivation of the Lansing strain of poliomyelitis virus in cultures of various human embryonic tissues. Science 1949;109:85.

Feigin RD, Shackelford PG. Value of repeat lumbar puncture in the differential diagnosis of meningitis. N Engl J Med 1973;289:571.

Gnann JW, Hayes EC, Smith JZ, et al. Echovirus 33 replication in human peripheral white blood cells. J Med Virol 1979;3:291.

Hayward JC, Gillespie SM, Kaplan KM, et al. Outbreak of poliomyelitis like paralysis associated with enterovirus 71. Pediatr Infect Dis 1989;8:611-616.

Hyypia TP, Stalhandske R, Vainionpaa R, Pettersson U. Detection of enteroviruses by spot hybridization. J Clin Microbiol 1984;19:436-438.

Icenogle J, Shcwin H, Duke G et al. Neutralization of poliovirus Rey a monoclonal antibody: kinetics and stoichiometry. Virology 1983;127:412-425.

Jenista JA, Powell KR, Menegus MA. Epidemiology of neonatal enterovirus infection. J Pediatr 1984;104:685.

Kibrick S, Benirschke K. Severe generalized disease (encephaloheptomyocarditis) occurring in the newborn period and due to infection with Coxsackie virus, group B. Evidence of intrauterine infection with this agent. Pediatrics 1958;22:857.

LaMonica N, Kupsky WJ, Raczaniello VR. Reduced mouse neurovirulence of poliovirus type 2 Lansing antigenic variants selected with monoclonal antibodies. Virology 1987;161:429-37.

McCartney RA, Banatvala JE, Bell EJ. Routine use of antibody capture ELISA for the serological diagnosis of coxsackie B virus infections. J Med Virol 1986;19:205-212.

McKinney RE, Katz SL, Wilfert CM. Chronic enteroviral meningoencephalitis in agammaglobulinemic patients. Rev Infect Dis 1987:2;334-356.

Minor, PD, Dunn G, Phillips JA, et al. Attenuation and reversion of the Sabin type 3 vaccine strain. Molecular aspects of picornavirus infection and detection. In BC Semler, Ehrenfeld E (eds). Washington, DC: American Society for Microbiology, 1989.

Modlin JF. Fatal echovirus 11 disease in premature neonates. Pediatrics 1980;66:775.

Modlin JF, Polk BF, Horton P, et al. Perinatal echovirus infection: risk of transmission during a community outbreak. N Engl J Med 1981;305:368.

Mosser AG, Leipee DM, Rueckert RR. Neutralization of picornaviruses: support for the pentamer bridging hypothesis. Molecular aspects of picornavirus infection and detection. In Semler BC, Ehrenfeld E (eds). American Society of Microbiology, 1989, Washington, DC: p 155-167.

Nathanson N, Langmuir AD. The Cutter incident, I, II, III. Am J Hyg 1963;78:16-81.

Nkowane BM, Wassilak SG, Orenstein WA, et al. Vaccine associated paralytic poliomyelitis US: 1973 through 1984. JAMA 1987;257:1335-1340.

Onorata IM, Modlin JF, McBeam AM et al. Mucosal immunity induced by enhanced potency inactivated and oral polio vaccines. J Infect Dis 1991;163:1-6.

Robinson CR, Doane FW, Rhodes AJ. Report of an outbreak of febrile illness with pharyngeal lesions and exanthem, Toronto summer 1957: isolation of group A Coxsackie virus. Can Med Assoc J 1957;79:615.

Romero JR, Putnak JR, Wimmer E. The use of poliovirus proteins VP3 and 2C as group antigens for the detection of enteroviral infections by indirect immunofluorescence (abstract 967). Pediatr Res 1986;20:319A.

Rotbart HA. Human enterovirus infections: molecular approaches to diagnosis and pathogenesis. In molecular aspects of picornavirus infection and detection. In Semler BC, Ehrenfeld E (eds). Washington, DC: American Society for Microbiology, 1989.

Shindarov LM, Chumakov MP, Voroshilova MK, et al. Epidemiological, clinical and pathomorphological characteristics of epidemic poliomyelitis-like disease caused by enterovirus 71, J Hyg Epidemiol Microbiol Immunol 1979;23:284-295.

Singer JI, Mauer PR, Riley JP, et al. Management of central nervous system infections during an epidemic of enteroviral aseptic meningitis. J Pediatr 1980;96:559.

Tomassini JE, Colonno RJ. Isolation of a receptor protein involved in attachment of human rhinorviruses. J Virol 1986;58:290-295.

Van Creveld S, de Jager H. Myocarditis in newborns caused by Coxsackie virus. Clinical and pathological data. Ann Pediatr 1956;187:100-112.

Wadia NH, Katrak SM, Misra VP, et al. Polio-like motor paralysis associated with acute hemorrhagic conjunctivitis in an outbreak in 1981 in Bombay, India: clinical and serologic studies. J Infect Dis 1983;147:660.

Weiner LS, Howell JT, Langford MP, et al. Effects of specific antibodies on chronic Echovirus Type 5 encephalitis in a patient with agammaglobulinemia. J Infect Dis 1979;140:858.

Wetz K, Willingmann P, Zeichhardt H, Habermehl KO. Neutralization of poliovirus by polyclonal antibodies requiring binding of a single IgG molecule per virion. Arch Virol 1986;11:207-220.

Wilfert CM, Buckley RH, Rosen FS, et al. Persistent enterovirus infections in agammaglobulinemia. In Schlessinger D (ed) Microbiology 1977, Washington, DC: American Society for Microbiology, 1977, p 488.

Wilfert CM, Zeller J. Enterovirus diagnosis. In de la Maza L, Peterson EM (ed). Medical virology IV: proceedings of the 1984 International symposium on Medical Virology. London: Lawrence Erlbaum Associates.

Yoshioka I, Horstmann DM. Viremic infection due to echovirus type 9. N Engl J Med 1962;262:224.

6

EPSTEIN-BARR VIRUS INFECTIONS

GEORGE MILLER
BEN Z. KATZ
JAMES C. NIEDERMAN

The Epstein-Barr virus (EBV) was discovered in the 1960s in cell lines derived from African Burkitt lymphomas (Epstein et al., 1964). Today this virus is well recognized as the etiologic agent of infectious mononucleosis. Extensive virological and serological evidence also implicates EBV as the cause of various lymphoproliferative disorders such as large cell lymphomas and lymphocytic interstitial pneumonia in immunosuppressed patients (Andiman et al., 1985). EBV has also been regularly associated with two malignant conditions in patients who are not otherwise globally immunodeficient: African (endemic) lymphoma, or Burkitt's lymphoma, and nasopharyngeal carcinoma. Recently, there has been increasing evidence of an association of EBV with Hodgkin's disease (Mueller et al., 1989; Weiss et al., 1989) and with certain autoimmune disorders such as Sjogren's syndrome (Fox et al., 1986).

INFECTIOUS MONONUCLEOSIS

Infectious mononucleosis is the typical, symptomatic, primary EBV infection seen in the otherwise healthy host. Infectious mononucleosis is an acute infectious disease occurring predominantly in older children and young adults. It is characterized clinically by fever, exudative or membranous pharyngitis, generalized lymphadenopathy, and splenomegaly. Characteristically the peripheral blood shows an absolute increase in the number of atypical lymphocytes, and the serum has a high titer of heterophil antibody. Specific EBV antibodies are detected early in the illness and persist for years thereafter.

History

Infectious mononucleosis was first described as "glandular fever" by Pfeiffer in 1889. The term *infectious mononucleosis* was used by Sprunt and Evans (1920) in their description of hematological changes in six young adults with a clinical syndrome characterized by a mononuclear leukocytosis. A diagnostic serological test based on the association of heterophil antibody and mononucleosis was described by Paul and Bunnell (1932). This nonspecific test was made more specific by the development of differential absorption tests by Davidsohn (1937) (Table 6-1) and considerably simpler and more rapid (but occasionally less specific) by the more recent slide tests. The association of infectious mononucleosis with EBV was described by Henle, Henle, and Diehl (1968) three decades later, 4 years after the virus was discovered.

Etiology

Although discovery of the causative agent of infectious mononucleosis eluded the efforts of competent investigators for many years, the assumption was that it was a virus. A report by Henle, Henle, and Diehl (1968) provided evidence of a relationship between the herpesvirus now known as EBV and infectious mononucleosis.

In 1968 Niederman et al. detected antibodies against EBV in patients with infectious mono-

Table 6-1. Heterophil antibody reactions in normal and infectious mononucleosis (IM) sera

In the presence of:	Agglutination of sheep red blood cells after absorption with:	
	Guinea pig kidney cells	Beef red blood cells
Some normal human sera	−	+
Most IM sera	+	−

nucleosis by means of an indirect immunofluorescence test. In 24 patients with infectious mononucleosis, antibodies that were absent in pre-illness specimens appeared early in the disease, rose to peak levels within a few weeks, and remained at high levels during convalescence. These antibodies were distinct from heterophil antibodies.

Subsequent studies by Niederman et al. in 1970 and Sawyer et al. in 1971 provided additional evidence indicating that EBV is the cause of infectious mononucleosis. The evidence that supports this concept is as follows: (1) EBV antibody is absent before onset of illness, appears during illness, and persists for many years thereafter; (2) clinical infectious mononucleosis occurs only in persons lacking antibody, and it fails to occur when antibody is present; (3) EBV has been isolated from the pharynx and saliva of infectious mononucleosis patients during their illness and for many months thereafter (Miller et al., 1973); and (4) cultured lymphocytes from patients who have had infectious mononucleosis will form continuous cell lines in vitro that contain the EBV genome and EBV antigens.

EBV is a member of the herpesvirus group. Mature infectious particles are 150 to 200 nm in diameter, with a lipid-containing envelope surrounding an icosahedral nucleocapsid. The genome is composed of approximately 172,000 base pairs of double-stranded DNA. The entire nucleotide sequence of one strain is known (Baer et al., 1984). Within the viral particle the genome is linear; within latently infected cells the genome is a circular extrachromosomal plasmid (Adams and Lindahl, 1975). In some cells EBV DNA also is integrated into the host cell chromosome (Matsuo et al., 1984).

In vitro the virus has a narrow host range, infecting B lymphocytes of human or other primate origin. However, in vivo the virus can be found in epithelial elements of the buccal mucosa, salivary glands, tongue, and ectocervix and in the epithelial cells of nasopharyngeal carcinoma. Within the mouth both parotid ductal epithelium and oropharyngeal squamous epithelial cells harbor EBV DNA and are sites of viral replication and release (Morgan et al., 1979; Sixbey et al., 1984; Wolf et al., 1984).

A number of viral antigens have been characterized, including viral capsid antigen (VCA), EB nuclear antigen (EBNA), membrane antigen (MA), and an early antigen (EA) complex of a diffuse component (D) and a restricted component (R). Each of these antigen systems is composed of a number of distinct viral gene products. For example, there are at least six different EBNA genes. Antibodies to these different antigen systems can be demonstrated by a variety of techniques, including indirect immunofluorescence, immunoblotting, and enzyme-linked immunosorbent assay (ELISA).

Pathology

The generalized nature of infectious mononucleosis becomes apparent when the pathological aspects of the disease are studied. Grossly, there may be diffuse enlargement of the lymphoid tissues manifested by lymphadenopathy, splenomegaly, and pharyngeal lymphoid hyperplasia. Histologically, focal mononuclear infiltrations involve lymph nodes, spleen, tonsils, lungs, heart, liver, kidneys, adrenal glands, central nervous system (CNS), and skin. Bone marrow hyperplasia develops regularly, and in some instances small granulomas are present.

The lymphoid hyperplasia of infectious mononucleosis is not diagnostic; it can be seen in other conditions. Most of the hyperplasia involves T cells in the paracortical areas of the lymph node; however, in some instances there may be pronounced hyperplasia of B cells in the germinal follicle. The lymphoid hyperplasia is thought to consist of several distinct components. A few proliferating B cells are infected by EBV; they represent less than 0.1% of the circulating mononuclear cells in the acute phase of uncomplicated infectious mononucleosis. Other proliferating B cells may be "polyclonally activated" by the EBV infection but may not themselves contain EBV. The majority of the proliferating cells, represented by the atypical lymphocytes present in the blood, are reactive T cells, usually CD8 positive, and natural killer (NK) cells; they are not EBV-infected B lymphocytes (Pattengale, Smith, and Perlin, 1974). The proliferating T cells induce generalized lymph node hyperplasia and infiltrate many organs.

Thus it is the immune response against the virus that provides much of the pathology seen in acute infectious mononucleosis. Purtilo (1981) has called these atypical lymphocytes "combatants in an immune struggle." Some of these cells, cytotoxic T cells, have the specific ability to eliminate EBV-infected B cells (Svedmyr and Jondal, 1975). Others suppress activation of EBV-infected B cells (Tosato et al., 1979). There are also NK cells that nonspecifically eliminate EBV-infected cells (De Waele et al., 1981). Antibodies, especially neutralizing antibodies, may play a role in limiting acute infectious mononucleosis as well. These antibodies may limit the spread of extracellular virus and also participate in antibody-dependent cellular cytotoxicity (ADCC). It has been proposed that when this complex and finely tuned immunoregulatory mechanism fails, chronic or fatal EBV infection results. For example, if cytotoxic or suppressor T cells fail to eliminate infected B cells, excessive lymphoproliferation may occur. If, on the other hand, NK and/or cytotoxic T-cell activity is excessive, extensive B-cell death with resultant agammaglobulinemia may result (Andiman, 1984).

In the normal individual the extensive lymphoproliferation subsides, but the virus nevertheless persists in a latent state in the lymphoid compartment. Approximately one in a million peripheral blood mononuclear cells harbors EBV in the healthy EBV-seropositive individual (Rocchi et al., 1977).

Epidemiology

Although EBV infection is worldwide in distribution, clinical infectious mononucleosis is observed predominantly in developed countries, principally among adolescents and young adults. Seroepidemiological surveys have revealed a gradual acquisition of antibody with age so that 50% to 90% of persons show a positive antibody reaction by young adult life. The overall incidence of clinical infectious mononucleosis is approximately 50 per 100,000 persons per year in the general population of the United States; however, the incidence of mononucleosis in susceptible college students is approximately 5,000 per 100,000 persons, 100 times higher than in the general population (Niederman et al., 1970). The total EBV infection rate in college students is estimated as at least twice as high (approximately 12,000 per 100,000 yearly), indicating that as many subclinical infections occur as overt infections. The so-called subclinical infections may be truly inapparent infections or atypical EBV-induced disease such as thrombocytopenia, hemolytic anemia, pneumonitis, and/or rash (Andiman, 1979; Andiman et al., 1981).

The epidemiological factors that have a significant effect on the host response to EBV infection include age, socioeconomic status, and geographical location. In general, infection during infancy and childhood probably will be inapparent, perhaps because of the immaturity of the immunological responses of children (Sumaya, 1977). Clinical infectious mononucleosis is more common in adolescents and young adults (Evans et al., 1968). In developing countries of the world where sanitation is poor, exposure to EBV occurs at a very early age. In these countries most older children and adolescents are immune to the virus. Therefore infectious mononucleosis is rare. In the United States infection generally occurs at an early age mainly in individuals in low socioeconomic groups who live in crowded conditions with poor hygiene.

Many seroepidemiological studies have confirmed the well-known fact that infectious mononucleosis is not highly contagious, even in family settings. Henle and Henle (1970) found evidence of spread in three of eight families (37.5%), and Fleischer et al. (1981) found spread in seven of 36 susceptible contacts (19%). However, EBV infection appears to spread more efficiently under the conditions that exist in certain day-care nurseries (Pereira et al., 1969) and orphanages (Tischendorf et al., 1970).

The most likely modes of transmission are oral-salivary spread in children and close intimate contact (kissing) in young adults (Hoagland, 1955; Evans, 1960). Cell-free infectious virus is carried in saliva (Morgan et al., 1979).

Prolonged pharyngeal excretion of EBV for periods up to several months after clinical infectious mononucleosis has been demonstrated (Miller et al., 1973; Niederman et al., 1976). Approximately 15% to 20% of immune individuals excrete EBV in saliva at any one point in time. Patients undergoing immunosuppression have an increased frequency (>50%) of oropharyngeal excretion (Strauch et al., 1974). If the saliva is concentrated, up to 100% of normal individuals may shed the virus (Yao et al., 1985). Thus the virus may never be truly "latent" in oropharyngeal elements but, instead, may produce a chronic, low-grade, productive infection. The infection can also be transmitted by transfusion of blood that is contaminated with EBV-infected lymphocytes (Gerber et al., 1969; Blacklow et al., 1971).

Clinical manifestations

The incubation period has been estimated as 4 to 6 weeks on the basis of contact infections (Hoagland, 1984). After blood transfusion heterophil-positive infectious mononucleosis developed 5 weeks later (Blacklow et al., 1971; Turner et al., 1972).

The disease may begin abruptly or insidiously with headache, fever, chills, anorexia, and malaise, followed by lymphadenopathy and severe sore throat. The clinical picture is extremely variable in both severity and duration. The disease in children is generally mild; in adults it is more severe and has a more protracted course.

Fever. The temperature usually rises to 39.4° C (103° F) and gradually falls over a variable period, averaging 6 days. In a severe case it is not unusual for temperatures to hover between 40° and 40.6° C (104° and 105° F) and to persist for 2 weeks or more. Children are more likely to have low-grade fever or may be afebrile.

Lymphadenopathy. Shortly after onset of illness, the lymph nodes rapidly enlarge to a variable size of approximately 1 to 4 cm. The nodes are typically tender, tense, discrete, and firm.

Any chain of lymph nodes may become enlarged, but the cervical group is most commonly involved. In addition, the following nodes are commonly affected: axillary, inguinal, epitrochlear, popliteal, mediastinal, and mesenteric. Massive mediastinal lymph node enlargement has been observed. Mesenteric lymphadenopathy frequently has been confused with acute appendicitis. Lymph node enlargement gradually subsides over a period of days or weeks, depending on the severity and extent of involvement.

Splenomegaly. Moderate enlargement of the spleen occurs in approximately 50% of cases. In rare instances enlargement may be followed by rupture, causing hemorrhage, shock, and death if it is not recognized. Rutkow (1978) reviewed 107 reports of splenic rupture in patients with infectious mononucleosis and concluded that only 18 ruptures were truly spontaneous; most followed trauma.

Tonsillopharyngitis. Sore throat is one of the cardinal symptoms of the disease. The tonsils are usually enlarged and reddened, and more than 50% develop exudate. Thick grayish-white, shaggy membranous tonsillitis is a common finding and may persist for 7 to 10 days. During the first week small petechiae are present on the palate in approximately one third of patients. In the past many patients referred to physicians with "diphtheria" because of the appearance of the throat proved to have infectious mononucleosis.

The triad of lymphadenopathy, splenomegaly, and exudative pharyngitis in a febrile patient is typical but not pathognomonic of infectious mononucleosis. Other manifestations of the disease include hepatitis, skin eruptions, pneumonitis, myocarditis, pericarditis, and CNS involvement.

Hepatitis. Liver involvement occurs relatively frequently in patients with infectious mononucleosis. Hepatomegaly is present in 10% to 15% of cases, but moderately abnormal hepatic isoenzymes are found in more than 80% of patients tested. Frank jaundice develops in less than 5% of cases and is usually mild; however, hyperbilirubinemia is reported in 25% of patients. Hepatitis may provoke such symptoms as anorexia, nausea, and vomiting.

Skin manifestations. In some cases of infectious mononucleosis that are well documented clinically and serologically, the incidence of dermatitis is 3% to 19% (Bernstein, 1940; Contratto, 1944; Milne, 1945; Press et al., 1945; McCarthy and Hoagland, 1964). The rash, when present, is usually located on the trunk and arms; rarely, it may present solely as palmar dermatitis (Petrozzi, 1971). It appears during the first few days of illness, lasts 1 to 6 days, and is erythematous, macular, and papular or morbilliform. Sometimes urticarial or scarlatiniform eruptions are seen (Press et al., 1945; McCarthy and Hoaglad, 1964; Cowdrey and Reynolds, 1969). Occasionally, cold-induced urticaria and acrocyanosis may be associated with infectious mononucleosis (Tyson and Czarny, 1981; Barth, 1981; Dickerman et al., 1980). Rarely, the rash may be petechial, vesicular, or hemorrhagic, but other more common and more serious causes of such rashes should be sought before they are ascribed to infectious mononucleosis.

In 1967 Pullen et al., and Patel nearly simultaneously observed an increased incidence of skin rashes in patients with infectious mononucleosis who were given ampicillin. The copper-colored rash begins 5 to 10 days after the drug is begun, mainly over the trunk. It then develops into an extensive, generalized (including the palms and soles), macular and papular pruritic eruption. It can last up to a week, with desquamation persisting for several more days. At its peak, the rash is confluent over exposed areas and pressure points and more marked extensor surfaces. A faint macular rash sometimes is seen on the palatal and buccal mucosae. This rash may also be seen with the administration of ampicillin derivatives such as amoxicillin (Mulroy, 1973) and other penicillins such as methicillin (Fields, 1980). This rash does not represent a long-lasting hypersensitivity to ampicillin; the drug may be used again once the infectious mononucleosis has subsided (Nazareth et al., 1972; Levene and Baker, 1968; McKenzie et al., 1976; Bjorg et al., 1975).

Pneumonitis. A small percentage of patients with infectious mononucleosis develop a cough that is paroxysmal in type, with a clinical picture and roentgenograms indistinguishable from those of atypical pneumonia. Pleural effusion also may develop. Hilar adenopathy is often observed in patients with extensive lymphoid hyperplasia in the course of infectious mononucleosis.

Central nervous system involvement. During the past three decades there have been increasing numbers of reports of CNS involvement in patients with infectious mononucleosis. These manifestations have been observed in the adult age group and also in children. The neurological syndromes have included aseptic meningitis, encephalitis, infectious polyneuritis (Guillain-

Barré syndrome), Bell's palsy, transverse myelitis, acute cerebellar ataxia, and CNS lymphoma (Cleary et al., 1980; Schiff et al., 1982; Grose et al., 1975).

CASE 1. A 10-year-old black boy with generalized lymphadenopathy, splenomegaly, typical blood picture, and positive heterophil antibody titer developed encephalitis during the course of his infection. He had headache, vomiting, and drowsiness that progressed to stupor. The cerebrospinal fluid showed pleocytosis with a predominance of lymphocytes and an elevated protein level. His sensorium gradually improved, and he made an uneventful recovery.

CASE 2. A 12-year-old white girl with a classic picture of infectious mononucleosis developed weakness of both lower and upper extremities, with absent reflexes. Spinal fluid findings showed albuminocytological dissociation characteristic of the Guillain-Barré syndrome. There were no cells, and the protein value was 300 mg/dl. The paralysis cleared completely within 6 weeks. The diagnosis of infectious mononucleosis was confirmed by a typical blood smear and positive heterophil antibody test.

In general, the neurological manifestations depend on the site of involvement, which may be anywhere in the CNS. The majority of patients recover completely, although fatalities have been associated with encephalitis.

Complications

Rupture of the spleen. Rupture of the spleen is a serious but, fortunately, rare complication of infectious mononucleosis. It has been attributed to an extensive lymphocytic and mononuclear cell infiltrate that presumably causes stretching and weakening of the capsule and trabeculae. Consequently, minor trauma to the splenic area or sudden increases in intraabdominal pressure may precipitate rupture. In rare instances it may be a spontaneous development caused by progressive intrasplenic hyperplasia. The presence of this complication should be suspected in any patient who suddenly develops abdominal pain on the left side and signs of peritoneal irritation, hemorrhage, and shock (Rutkow, 1978).

Hematological complications. The development of epistaxis, petechial and ecchymotic skin lesions, and hematuria suggests a rare complication of infectious mononucleosis. Low platelet counts, prolonged bleeding time, and poor clot retraction confirm the diagnosis of thrombocytopenic purpura. Recovery is the rule (Clarke and Davies, 1964). Other rare hematological complications include hemolytic anemia, aplastic anemia, agranulocytosis, and agammaglobulinemia (Grierson and Purtilo, 1987).

A rare acute hemophagocytic syndrome resembling malignant histiocytosis in infants and children has been linked to EBV infection (Wilson et al., 1981). Patients may present with fever, hepatosplenomegaly, pancytopenia, and disseminated intravascular coagulation; hemophagocytosis is found on examination of bone marrow. The mortality rate ranges from 30% to 40%. Overall the syndrome is poorly understood except that it is associated with EBV and with many other infections. Some of these patients apparently are immunodeficient (McKenna et al., 1981; Purtilo et al., 1982).

Cardiac complications. Electrocardiographic changes during the course of infectious mononucleosis have been reported in adults. These are usually the only manifestations of cardiac involvement. However, there have been several reports of pericarditis and myocarditis characterized by severe chest pain and typical electrocardiographic findings (Hudgins, 1976; Butler et al., 1981).

Orchitis. Orchitis may occur rarely in association with infectious mononucleosis. In one case report (Ralston et al., 1960) the testicular involvement was bilateral; in another report (Wolnisty, 1962) it was unilateral. The orchitis subsided in 2 to 4 weeks.

Diagnosis

The diagnosis of infectious mononucleosis is usually made on the basis of (1) suggestive clinical features, (2) typical blood picture, (3) positive heterophil agglutination antibody test, and (4) ancillary laboratory findings such as specific serology to EBV antigens. Younger children may have EBV infection with symptoms not characteristic of infectious mononucleosis and with negative heterophil antibody titers. In such in-

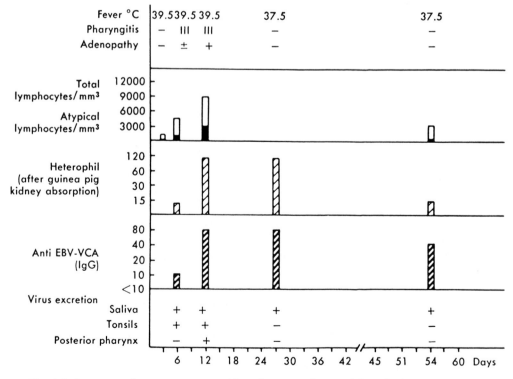

Fig. 6-1. Sequence of symptoms, atypical lymphocytosis, heterophil antibody, EBV antibody (anti-EBV–VCA), and EBV oral excretion in a patient with mononucleosis seen early in the illness. (From Niederman JC et al: N Engl J Med 1976; 294:1355.)

stances measurement of specific EBV serology is required for diagnosis. The diagnosis can be confirmed by the specific tests for various antibodies against EBV antigens (Evans et al., 1975; Rapp and Hewetson, 1978). Examination and test results from a patient with mononucleosis seen early in the illness are illustrated in Fig. 6-1.

Clinical features. A history of fever associated with the triad of lymphadenopathy, exudative pharyngitis, and splenomegaly should suggest infectious mononucleosis as a diagnostic possibility. The following laboratory tests are not specific but are helpful in establishing the diagnosis.

Blood tests. An absolute increase in the number of atypical lymphocytes is a characteristic finding during some stages of the disease. In a blood smear these cells usually represent 10% or more of the field. These so-called Downey cells vary markedly in size and shape. With Wright's stain the cytoplasm is dark blue and vacuolated, presenting a foamy appearance; the nucleus is round, bean shaped, or lobulated and contains no nucleoli. The white blood cell count is variable. During the first week of the disease there may be leukopenia, but commonly there is leukocytosis with a predominance of lymphocytes. The white blood cell count may be so elevated that the presence of leukemia is suspected. In an occasional immunodeficient patient infectious mononucleosis does progress to frank leukemia; in this instance all the primitive blasts in the circulation are EBV-transformed B cells (Robinson et al., 1980).

Atypical lymphocytes are not specific for infectious mononucleosis. They may be observed in a variety of clinical entities, including infectious hepatitis, rubella, primary atypical pneumonia, allergic rhinitis, asthma, and other diseases. Morphologically, the atypical cells in these conditions are indistinguishable from those seen in infectious mononucleosis. However, there is a quantitative difference; in infectious mononucleosis there are usually more than 10% atypical cells in contrast to the other conditions in which the percentage is usually less.

Heterophil antibodies. The heterophil antibodies were the first serological markers discovered that could reasonably confirm the diagnosis of infectious mononucleosis. Heterophil antibody tests are still used more frequently than any of the virus-specific assays. Most sera of patients with infectious mononucleosis cause sheep red blood cells to agglutinate after they have been absorbed with guinea pig kidney antigens but not after absorption with beef red blood cells. The reverse is often true of normal sera (see Table 6-1). The heterophil antibody responsible for this differential absorption in infectious mononucleosis is principally of the IgM class, appears during the first or second week of illness, and disappears gradually over 3 to 6 months. In a group of 166 patients studied by Niederman (1956) the heterophil antibody test was positive in 38% during the first week, in 60% during the second week, and in approximately 80% during the third week after onset of symptoms.

Sheep cell agglutinins are not specific for infectious mononucleosis. They occur in a number of other conditions such as serum sickness, viral hepatitis, rubella, leukemia, and Hodgkin's disease. Low titers can also be demonstrated in the serum of some normal persons. Usually the absorption tests serve to distinguish these agglutinins from the heterophil antibodies of infectious mononucleosis. In general, the agglutinin titer is higher in patients with infectious mononucleosis than in those with other conditions; an unabsorbed heterophil antibody titer above 1:128 and 1:40 or greater after absorption is considered significant.

A rapid slide test using equine red blood cells stabilized by formaldehyde has been evaluated as a diagnostic test for infectious mononucleosis. In 1965 Hoff and Bauer reported a high degree of correlation with the standard heterophil antibody test. They described the following advantages: (1) low incidence of false reactions, (2) high degree of specificity for infectious mononucleosis antibody, and (3) great rapidity (2 minutes) and ease of performance. This rapid test is a valuable diagnostic aid in clinical practice. Other rapid slide tests have become available, using the same principle of the absorbed heterophil agglutination but using equine or bovine erythrocytes that are citrated or formalinized. All have shown a high index of positive correlation with the standard Paul-Bunnell test results (Rapp and Hewetson, 1978).

Antibody titers to specific EBV antigens. Although infectious mononucleosis occurs only in previously seronegative individuals, IgG antibody to the VCA may already be detectable early

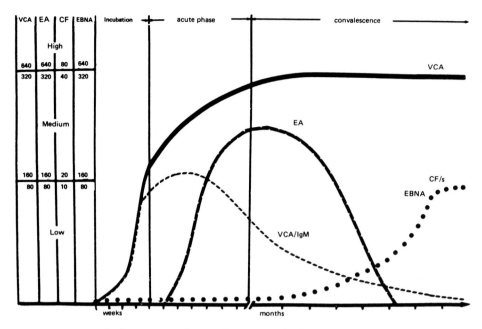

Fig. 6-2. EBV antibody response during the course of infectious mononucleosis. *EA*, Early antigen; *VCA*, viral capsid antigen; *EBNA*, EB nuclear antigen; *CF*, complement fixation test. (From de Thé G: In Klein G: Viral oncology, New York: Raven Press, 1980, p 775.)

in the course of the illness. The acute illness may be diagnosed if VCA-specific IgM is present in serum, but this assay is difficult to perform and may yield false-positive reactions because of rheumatoid factors in blood. It is only available on a research basis. VCA-IgM responses disappear after several months, whereas VCA-IgG levels persist for life. Antibodies to EA complexes, associated with viral replication, are present in 70% to 80% of patients during acute disease and usually disappear after 6 months. Recent studies indicate that antibody to the component of the EA complex may be detectable in healthy individuals for years after having infectious mononucleosis (Horwitz et al., 1985). Antibody to the nuclear antigen (EBNA) appears more slowly, taking from 1 to 6 months to become detectable. The antibody response to EB nuclear antigen one (EBNA-1) is more delayed (Niederman and Miller, 1986). Testing acute and convalescent sera for titer rises to EBNA-1 is a useful diagnostic procedure. Thus a positive anti-VCA titer and a negative anti-EBNA titer are diagnostic of a primary EBV serological response such as occurs in infectious mononucleosis. All late convalescent sera from healthy individuals contain EBNA antibodies. A diagram showing the sequence of development and persistence of these antibodies to EBV is shown in Fig. 6-2.

Detection of the virus. Biologically active virus can be isolated from saliva, peripheral blood, or lymphoid tissue by means of its ability to immortalize cultured human lymphocytes, usually from umbilical-cord blood. Occasionally, lymphoid cell lines can be grown directly from blood or lymph nodes. This assay is time-consuming (6 to 8 weeks) and requires specialized tissue-culture facilities that are not generally available.

Viral antigens representative of the latent life cycle of the virus can be found in lymphoid tissues, in nasopharyngeal carcinoma tumors, and occasionally in the peripheral blood if the level of leukoviremia is high enough. During the acute phase of mononucleosis, approximately 1% or less of the circulating peripheral blood lymphocytes contain an EBNA.

The most specific method of demonstrating EBV in pathological material is nucleic acid hybridization. Three general techniques have been used: (1) Southern hybridization, which is capable of distinguishing the specific portions of EBV DNA that are present in the lesions; (2) in situ hybridization, which identifies the cells that contain EBV DNA; and (3) polymerase chain reaction (PCR). Probes for nucleic acid detection methods are made from cloned EBV DNA fragments prepared by recombinant DNA techniques or from synthetic oligonucleotides. The probes are labeled by radioactive or nonisotopic methods.

The sensitivity of the Southern hybridization technique under the best conditions is approximately 10^5 EBV genomes, more often approximately 10^6 genomes. This sensitivity is sufficient to detect EBV DNA in nasopharyngeal carcinoma, Burkitt's lymphoma, and polyclonal lymphomas, all of which contain many copies of EBV DNA in each cell. However, it is not sensitive enough to detect EBV DNA regularly in peripheral blood of mononucleosis patients, in which only a few cells harbor EBV DNA. The PCR is highly sensitive; it can detect approximately 10^4 genomes or less; therefore in most cases of acute infectious mononucleosis EBV DNA can be detected in the blood by PCR. Nucleic acid hybridization methods can be used as a rapid assay for salivary excretion of EBV.

Southern hybridization can determine whether patients are infected with the same or different viruses (Katz et al., 1988). Probes from regions of the genome near the termini provide additional information about whether the EBV is monoclonal or multiclonal (Raab-Traub and Flynn, 1986). Furthermore, the same probes can distinguish between latent and lytically replicating forms of EBV DNA. Using these techniques, it recently has been found that many EBV-associated lymphoproliferative diseases contain lytically replicating forms of EBV DNA (Katz et al., 1990).

Differential diagnosis

Infectious mononucleosis is a notorious mimic of many other diseases. Lymphadenopathy, splenomegaly, and exudative tonsillitis are common manifestations of a number of entities. The following conditions are often confused with infectious mononucleosis.

Streptococcal tonsillitis or pharyngitis. This condition is suggested by fever, sore throat, exudative tonsillitis, and cervical adenitis. An increase in the number of polymorphonuclear leukocytes, positive culture from a throat swab specimen, and prompt therapeutic response to penicillin all point to a streptococcal cause.

Diphtheria. The membranous tonsillitis of infectious mononucleosis frequently resembles diphtheria. The diagnosis is confirmed by positive culture.

Blood dyscrasias. Blood dyscrasias, particularly leukemia, are suggested by the lymphadenopathy, splenomegaly, and increase in number of peripheral blood atypical lymphocytes. Laboratory tests, including bone marrow aspiration, establish the true diagnosis.

Rubella. Rubella is commonly associated with a 2- to 4-day period of malaise and lymphadenopathy preceding the appearance of the rash. Rubella has a milder course, and frequently there is a history of exposure. A definite diagnosis of rubella can be established by evidence of a rise in the level of specific antibodies.

Measles. Measles, which is less frequently confused with infectious mononucleosis, is easily identified by the pathognomonic Koplik's spots. In doubtful cases a diagnosis of measles can be confirmed by demonstration of a rise in the level of measles antibodies.

Viral hepatitis. This disease may be clinically indistinguishable from infectious mononucleosis with jaundice. Specific serological tests can confirm a diagnosis of hepatitis A, B, or C.

Cytomegalovirus infection. A mononucleosis-like syndrome characterized by fever, splenomegaly, and atypical lymphocytes occurs in some patients with acute cytomegalovirus infection. These patients have a negative heterophil-agglutination determination and no evidence of recent EBV infection.

Acquired toxoplasmosis with lymphadenopathy. Toxoplasmosis infection may be clinically indistinguishable from infectious mononucleosis. It is characterized by generalized lymphadenopathy, chiefly of the cervical group, and occasionally by pharyngeal involvement and exanthem. The differentiation is based on the EBV and toxoplasma antibody determination.

In addition to simulating the diseases just described, infectious mononucleosis with its protean manifestations may simulate Hodgkin's disease, scarlet fever, secondary syphilis, typhoid fever, rickettsial diseases, and many others.

Prognosis

In general, the prognosis for patients with infectious mononucleosis is excellent. Severe cases may be followed by long periods of asthenia. Neurological complications, although rare, may cause serious sequelae or death. Spontaneous rupture of the spleen, which also is very rare, is fatal if it is not recognized and treated promptly. Deaths reported in infectious mononucleosis have resulted from CNS complications, splenic rupture, secondary bacterial infection in neutropenic patients, myocarditis, and disseminated lymphoproliferative disease.

Treatment

Infectious mononucleosis is a self-limited disease, and treatment is chiefly supportive. Antimicrobial drugs are not effective and do not alter the course of the infection. Bed rest is indicated in the acute stage of the disease. Aspirin can usually control the pain or discomfort caused by the enlarged lymph nodes and pharyngeal involvement. In severe cases codeine or meperidine (Demerol) may be required.

Corticosteroid therapy has been reported to have a beneficial effect. Symptoms referable to the throat and enlarged lymph nodes improve within 24 hours of corticosteroid therapy in many instances. In a well-controlled study of 132 patients with severe uncomplicated mononucleosis, Bender (1967) observed a significant decrease in the duration of fever; it persisted for an average of 1.4 days in the 66 corticosteroid-treated patients as compared with 5.6 days in the 66 matched control patients. Steroids may be considered for treatment of severe cases characterized by severe hematological complications, marked toxemia, progressive tonsillary enlargement leading to airway encroachment, and evidence of neurological or hematological complications. Steroids are not recommended for treatment of mild cases of infectious mononucleosis because the long-term effects of intervention on the normal immune response to EBV are unknown.

Contact sports should be avoided until the patient's spleen size has returned to normal. Spontaneous rupture of the spleen requires immediate surgery. Transfusions, treatment for shock, and splenectomy are lifesaving measures.

Acyclovir has minimal effects on the symptoms of mononucleosis and is not routinely used in the treatment of patients with the disease. There are anecdotal reports of the use of acyclovir in the treatment of EBV-associated post-transplantation lymphoma and of other lymphoproliferative disorders in immunocompromised hosts, but the efficacy of the drug is not documented in controlled clinical trials (Hanto et al., 1982).

Acyclovir acts on the lytic (but not the latent) phase of EBV replication. It inhibits viral DNA synthesis (represented by linear DNA), leading to virion production, but it has no effect on the number of latent (circular) genomes (Colby et al., 1980). Acyclovir inhibits the EBV DNA polymerase. The drug is presumably preferentially incorporated into viral DNA through the action of the EBV thymidine kinase.

When given to patients with infectious mononucleosis, acyclovir reduces the level of oropharyngeal viral replication during the period of administration (Ernberg and Andersson, 1986). However, after cessation of treatment, replication returns to previously high levels. During acyclovir treatment there is little or no reduction in the number of EBV-infected B cells found in the peripheral circulation.

OTHER EBV-ASSOCIATED DISEASES
X-linked lymphoproliferative syndrome: Duncan's disease

A spectrum of clinical manifestations of EBV infections in patients with recognized or presumed immunological impairment has been reported. Severe and often fatal infectious mononucleosis, X-linked lymphoproliferative disease (XLP), with death occurring after 1 or 2 weeks from hemorrhage, hepatic failure, or bacterial superinfection, was described in kindred males by Bar et al. in 1974 and Purtilo et al. in 1977. This sex-linked recessive genetic disorder has variable phenotypic expression. Boys who survive EBV infection may subsequently develop a variety of hematological complications such as agammaglobulinemia, hypergammaglobulinemia, agranulocytosis, aplastic anemia, and malignancy. The mean age of 100 of these boys at death was approximately 6 years (Purtilo et al., 1982). The underlying problem probably is variable immunodeficiency to EBV under the control of a defective lymphoproliferative control locus (XLC) on the X chromosome. In children who develop monoclonal B-cell neoplasms or fatal infectious mononucleosis, failure to control proliferation of B cells by NK cells, cytotoxic T cells, and antibodies may be occurring. In contrast, agammaglobulinemia, agranulocytosis, and aplastic anemia may be secondary to destruction of antibody-forming B cells by EBV or an excescessive suppressor T-cell response or both (Purtilo et al., 1977). This disease may be difficult to diagnose because many patients have low or undetectable serological responses to EBV despite infection. Many such patients experience lymphocytosis; EBV DNA can be shown in tissues by molecular hybridization techniques.

Rarely, cases of classic infectious mononucleosis in apparently normal girls have evolved into monoclonal or polyclonal lymphomas (Robinson et al., 1980; Abo et al., 1982). These patients presumably have undiagnosed immunoregulatory disorders with an abnormal immune response to EBV, which results in chronic or malignant disease following primary EBV infection.

EBV infections in transplant patients

A variety of EBV-associated lymphoproliferative syndromes varying from mononucleosis-like syndromes with benign outcomes to fatal disseminated lymphoproliferation and frank lymphomas have been described in patients who have received kidney, heart, bone marrow, liver, or thymus transplants under cover of immunosuppressive therapy.

At least three factors are thought to contribute to the pathogenesis of these lymphoproliferative syndromes: (1) the dose, duration, and number of immunosuppressive drugs, particularly cyclosporin A; (2) whether the patient is undergoing primary or reactivated EBV infection; and (3) the use of antibody to T cells as an immunosuppressive agent to maintain the graft or, in the case of bone marrow transplantation, to prevent graft-vs.-host disease (Martin et al., 1984). Use of monoclonal anti–T-cell antibodies is often associated with lymphomas arising in donor cells, which can be detected with markers such as a sex chromosome or mitochondrial DNA polymorphism (Schubach et al., 1982). Chronic antigenic stimulation caused by the engrafted cells is thought to play a role in pathogenesis of EBV-associated lymphomas in recipients of allogeneic transplants; however, EBV-associated B-cell lymphomas recently have been described in recipients of autologous marrow transplant as well (Ho et al., 1985, 1988).

The posttransplant lymphoproliferative lesions display the same latent EBV gene products observed in B cells immortalized in vitro. Thus they differ from those of Burkitt's lymphoma both in histology and in the spectrum of expression of EBV latent gene products.

Hanto et al. (1981) estimated an incidence of 1% (12 per 1,119) lymphomas and other lymphoproliferative disorders among recipients of renal transplants. The incidence of lymphomas among heart transplant patients in the Stanford series was 5% (9 per 182). The frequency of lymphomas in patients with transplantation of other organs is not known. Nucleic acid hybridization is the principal technique used to demonstrate an association of EBV with these tumors.

The relative risk imposed by one or another immunosuppressive regimen such as antilymphocyte antibodies or cyclosporin A is not yet defined in precise epidemiological terms. There is anecdotal evidence that discontinuation of cyclosporin A therapy is accompanied by remission of the lymphoproliferative disease (Starzl et al., 1984).

Apparently the risk of EBV-associated lymphoproliferative disease among persons receiving an organ transplant who experience primary EBV infection during transplantation or shortly thereafter is increased (Ho et al., 1985). There is serological and virological evidence for reactivation of latent EBV in conjunction with immunosuppressive therapy (Strauch et al., 1974). Such reactivation may also be associated with a spectrum of clinical manifestations, including benign or fatal lymphoproliferative disorders or nonBurkitt nonHodgkin's lymphomas (Ho et al., 1988).

EBV-associated diseases in AIDS patients

Acquired immunodeficiency syndrome (AIDS) patients develop three different EBV-associated lesions: (1) lymphomas, (2) lymphocytic interstitial pneumonitis (LIP), and (3) oral "hairy" leukoplakia of the tongue (Greenspan et al., 1984, 1985; Conant, 1987).

Lymphomas. AIDS predisposes to EBV-associated lymphomas of several histological types, including classic Burkitt's lymphoma with its associated chromosome abnormality. However many cases of Burkitt's lymphoma occurring in AIDS patients do not contain EBV (as is generally true of Burkitt's lymphoma outside the endemic regions) (Subar et al., 1988). Several other types of EBV-associated lymphomas, including CNS lymphoma and diffuse poly- or oligoclonal B-cell lymphoma found in extranodal sites such as the gut, are common complications of AIDS.

Lymphocytic interstitial pneumonitis. LIP is a polyclonal lymphoproliferative process (Joshi et al., 1987) seen mainly in children with AIDS. The occurrence of LIP correlates with lymphoproliferative activity (i.e., lymphadenopathy and parotitis) elsewhere in the body. It initially is seen as a subacute or chronic pulmonary process (e.g., with dyspnea on exertion and clubbing) rather than as acute pneumonitis. It is characterized by a reticulonodular pattern on chest radiography (Rubinstein et al., 1986). Histologically, lung biopsies of these lesions reveal mature lymphoid follicle formation in the lung, including germinal centers, and infiltration with plasmacytoid cells. Up to 80% of the lesions are associated with EBV DNA (Andiman et al., 1985), and patients, when compared to matched controls, often have evidence of a primary or reactivated EBV serological response (Katz et al., 1990). LIP may regress with acyclovir treatment or a low dose of corticosteroids given every other day (Pahwa, 1988). The lesion tends to worsen concomitant with other pulmonary infections.

Oral hairy leukoplakia. Oral hairy leukoplakia, which resembles thrush, is seen principally on the lateral surface of the tongues of homosexual men with AIDS. Pathologically, the lesions resemble flat warts. Lytic EBV DNA replication and production of mature virions have been documented within the epithelial cells of these lesions, which regress with acyclovir treatment (Greenspan et al., 1985; Resnick et al., 1988).

CNS lymphoma. One of the most serious CNS complications of EBV infection is the occurrence of CNS lymphoma. It is due to proliferation of EBV-infected B cells in an immunologically privileged site. It occurs infrequently in otherwise healthy individuals but is more common in immunosuppressed patients with AIDS or organ transplants (Hochberg et al., 1983).

Burkitt's lymphoma

Epidemiology. Burkitt's lymphoma is a disease with striking epidemiological features that first led to its recognition. In endemic areas Burkitt's lymphoma is the most common childhood cancer, and it may reach an incidence of eight to 10 cases per 100,000 people per year. In Burkitt's original series of cases the mortality rate was high—approximately 80% within the first year after diagnosis. However, the tumor is sensitive to chemotherapy, and recent series have described a first-year mortality rate of 20%.

Burkitt's lymphoma occurs throughout the world. There are, however, high-incidence areas such as part of equatorial East Africa and New Guinea. Areas with extremely high incidences are in the hot, wet, rural lowlands. In these areas malaria infection is universal, occurs very early in life, and is transmitted throughout the year; areas of Africa that are nearby but do not have holoendemic malaria as a result of malaria eradication campaigns do not have high rates of Burkitt's lymphoma. The disease is sporadic in all parts of the world, but in certain areas such as Malaysia, Colombia, and Brazil the incidence is intermediate.

The median age of patients with Burkitt's lymphoma is remarkably constant within the endemic areas. For example, in Uganda, Nigeria, Ghana, and New Guinea the median age is from 7.7 to 9.2 years. Where the tumors occur in lower incidence or sporadically, the patients are slightly older. In America the median age of 20 patients was 10½ years. However, Burkitt's lymphoma has been described in adults over the age of 30.

Association with EBV. The association of Burkitt's tumor with EBV is based on two types of findings: (1) demonstration of EBV genomes in the majority of tumors from endemic areas and (2) serological relationships. More than 90% of Burkitt's lymphoma biopsy specimens from Africa contain EBV DNA. A rare tumor in the endemic area that is histologically compatible with Burkitt's lymphoma fails to demonstrate the viral genome. In Burkitt's lymphoma occurring outside the endemic area, EBV DNA is associated with approximately 20% of the tumors, and the remainder are genome negative.

Several seroepidemiological findings indicate a relationship between Burkitt's lymphoma and EBV. In a prospective study of 42,000 children from the West Nile District of Uganda, it was determined that children who developed Burkitt's lymphoma were infected with the virus months to years before onset of the tumor (de Thé et al., 1978). Their antibody titers to capsid antigen were approximately twofold higher than those of the controls (matched for age) who did not develop Burkitt's lymphoma. Once the disease appears, Burkitt's lymphoma patients have considerably higher (approximately tenfold) antibody titers to capsid and early antigens than do children without the tumor. Seroepidemiological studies show that in the endemic area EBV infections are acquired at a very early age and are readily transmitted. The phenomenon of elevated EBV antibody titers is not regularly seen in patients with other lymphomas, although patients with Hodgkin's disease have slightly higher titers than normal. This elevation in antibody is present before the diagnosis of Hodgkin's lymphoma (Mueller et al., 1989).

The association of elevated EBV antibody titers with Burkitt's lymphoma is most pronounced in the endemic areas. Outside the endemic areas patients with Burkitt's lymphoma seem to fall into two categories: (1) those whose tumors contain EBV DNA and who develop elevated EBV antibodies and (2) those whose tumors are genome negative and who may be infected with the virus but do not develop high antibody titers.

Clinical features. In approximately 60% of children, Burkitt's lymphoma is seen initially as a unilateral swelling of the jaw. Characteristically, the jaw tumors are the presenting sign in younger children. Abdominal masses are the first sign in older children.

Jaw tumors are less frequently seen in patients with Burkitt's lymphoma outside the endemic areas of Africa. Only rarely does the tumor present as hepatosplenomegaly or enlargement of peripheral lymph nodes. Leukemic involvement of the bone marrow is also an infrequent initial clinical manifestation. Occasionally, the tumor may become recognized because of signs of CNS involvement such as paraplegia, cranial nerve paralysis, or meningeal irritation.

Since the tumor is rapidly growing, the clinical history is usually short. Some of the clinical features of the disease result from rapid tumor growth and the breakdown and release of intracellular metabolites. Thus complications include azotemia, hyperuricemia, hyperkalemia, and lactic acidosis.

Chromosome abnormalities. Burkitt's lymphomas regularly contain abnormalities of those chromosomes that contain immunoglobulin genes and chromosome 8q24, which is the locus for the c-*myc* proto-oncogne (Leder et al., 1976). The cytogenetic abnormalities occur in both the endemic and sporadic forms of the tumor, independent of their geographical location. The translocations are found whether or not EBV is associated with the tumor. The chromosomal abnormalities are not detected in peripheral blood lymphocytes of Burkitt's lymphoma or in lymphoblastoid cells lines derived from Burkitt's lymphoma patients. They have been found only in the malignant cells, not in hematopoietic stem cells. The most common abnormality, t(8;14), which is seen in approximately 75% of cases, is a reciprocal translocation between the long arm of chromosome 8 (24q) and the long arm of chromosome 14 (32q) bearing the heavy-chain locus. Variant translocations involve the c-*myc* gene on 8q24 and the genes for light chains on chromosome 2p11 (the kappa chain) and 22q11 (the lambda chain) (Lenoir et al., 1982).

Nasopharyngeal carcinoma

Association with EBV. The association of EBV with nasopharngeal carcinoma, an epithelial cell malignancy, is strong. EBV DNA is regularly found in all cases of undifferentiated nasopharyngeal carcinoma and recently has been detected in differentiated forms of the carcinoma as well (Raab-Traub et al., 1987). On the basis of the structure of EBV episomes, which can vary in size as a result of different numbers of the EBV terminal repeats, it has been determined that a single clone of EBV is associated with each tumor (Raab-Traub and Flynn, 1986). This finding implies that EBV DNA has been associated with the progenitor of the tumor cell from the time of tumor initiation, although it does not prove that EBV induced the transformation event. There is, furthermore, a convincing serological association between EBV and nasopharyngeal carcinoma: the sera of patients with the carcinoma have IgA antibodies to a variety of EBV latent and replicative antigens (Neel et al., 1983). Such antibodies rarely are found in the serum of healthy persons. A similar association has been found between EBV and several other carcinomas believed derived from embryonic branchial cleft remnants such as carcinomas derived from the thymus, parotid, palatine tonsil, and supraglottic region of the larynx (Leyvraz et al., 1985; Brichacek et al., 1983, 1984).

In China where there is a high incidence of nasopharyngeal carcinoma, mass serological screening for serum IgA antibody to the EBV capsid antigen has been undertaken (Henle and

Henle, 1976). The frequency of IgA antibody among 150,000 people studied was approximately 1%. Approximately 20% of those persons with elevated IgA anti-VCA who were biopsied had nasopharyngeal carcinoma. The use of serological screening for IgA antibody accompanied by nasopharyngeal examination and radiological examination, including computerized tomography scans, has been useful in diagnosis of nasopharyngeal carcinoma at treatable stages of the disease.

Clinical features. The presenting symptoms of nasopharyngeal carcinoma depend on the location of the primary tumor within the nasopharynx. In approximately half the cases the presenting sign is a cervical mass resulting from spread to regional lymph nodes. Other symptoms may include nasal obstruction, postnasal discharge, or epistaxis or may even include symptoms attributable to obstruction of the eustachian tube such as impairment of hearing, tinnitus, or otitis media. If there has been local spread, the patient may present with cranial nerve involvement, headache, or trismus resulting from involvement of jaw muscles. Occasionally, initial symptoms result from obstruction of the paranasal sinuses. Nasopharyngeal carcinoma may metastasize to the skeleton, especially the spine, and to the liver, lung, skin, and peripheral lymph nodes.

Congenital infection

Occasional infants with birth defects believed secondary to congenital EBV infection have been described. One infant manifested bilateral congenital cataracts, cryptorchidism, hypotonia, and mild micrognathia. A "celery stalk" appearance of long bones was noted radiologically, similar to that seen with congenital rubella (Goldberg et al., 1981). A report by Icart et al. (1981) described more than 700 pregnant women with serological evidence of EBV infection during pregnancy. Their pregnancies were three times more likely to result in early fetal death, premature labor, or delivery of an infant who would become ill. Until further data are available, however, it is difficult to know whether these associations are real or coincidental. One prospective study of 4,063 pregnant women during 4,108 gestations failed to show any intrauterine EBV infections (Fleischer and Bologonese, 1984).

Chronic active EBV infections and chronic fatigue syndrome

Rarely, patients with the chronic fatigue syndrome have a true chronic active infection with EBV. In these patients there are numerous objective clinical and laboratory findings, which include pneumonitis, hepatitis, uveitis, and a variety of hematological abnormalities such as neutropenia, eosinophilia, and thrombocytopenia (Schooley et al., 1986; Straus, 1988). These patients have prolonged severe relapsing courses, occasionally with a fatal outcome. In some instances death has been associated with respiratory failure caused by interstitial pneumonitis; in other instances it has been linked with diffuse T-cell lymphomas that were associated with EBV DNA (Jones et al., 1988). The pathogenesis of this syndrome is not clear, but it possibly is due to increased EBV replication. Patients with the severe form of chronic active infection often have extremely high levels of antibody to the EBV replicative antigens VCA and EA. Characteristically, these patients have low or absent antibody to the EBNAs. Some of these patients have selective absence of antibody to EBNA-1 (Miller et al., 1987).

Several families have been described in which the syndrome of "chronic mononucleosis" has occurred in several members (Joncas et al., 1984). One hypothesis is that mechanisms involved in the restriction of viral replication are deficient, either at the cellular level or at the immune level. A deficiency of killer cells that participate in ADCC has been suggested. That it is difficult to identify transforming virus in the saliva of some of the patients has prompted the alternative hypothesis that they are infected with nontransforming of lytic EBV variants.

More commonly, patients have a "neuromyasthenic," "polymyalgic," or "chronic fatigue" syndrome (Holmes et al., 1988). In most instances EBV is not the probable causative agent of this syndrome, although some patients have elevations of antibody titers to EAs and a few lack antibody to EBNA-1 (Jones et al., 1985). The symptoms include fatigue, chronic pharyngitis, tender lymph nodes, headaches, myalgia, and arthralgias. The symptoms are recurrent and prolonged, but no fatalities have been described. The natural history is variable.

REFERENCES

Abo W, Takada K, Kamada M, et al. Evolution of infectious mononucleosis into EVB carrying monoclonal malignant lymphoma. Lancet 1982;1:1272-1275.

Adams A, Lindahl T. Epstein-Barr virus genomes with properties of circular DNA molecules in carrier cells. Proc Natl Acad Sci USA 1975;72:1477-1481.

Andiman WA. The Epstein-Barr virus and EB virus infections in childhood. J Pediatr 1979;95:171-182.

Andiman WA. Epstein-Barr virus-associated syndromes: a critical reexamination. Pediatr Infect Dis 1984;3:198-203.

Andiman WA, Eastman R, Martin K, et al. Opportunistic lymphoproliferations associated with Epstein-Barr viral DNA in infants and children with AIDS. Lancet 1985;1390-1393.

Andiman WA, Markowitz RI, Horstmann DM. Clinical, virologic, and serologic evidence of Epstein-Barr virus infection in association with childhood pneumonia. J Pediatr 1981;99:880-886.

Baer R, Bankier AT, Biggin MD, et al. DNA sequence and expression of the B95-8 Epstein-Barr virus genome. Nature 1984;310:207-211.

Bar RS. DeLor CJ. Clauben KP, et al. Fatal infectious mononucleosis in a family. N Engl J Med 1974;290:363-367.

Barth JH: Infectious mononucleosis (glandular fever) complicated by cold agglutinins, cold urticaria and leg ulceration. Acta Dermatol Venereol (Stockh) 1981;61:451.

Bender CE. The value of corticosteroids in the treatment of infectious mononucleosis. JAMA 1967;199:97.

Bernstein A. Infectious mononucleosis. Medicine 1940; 19:85-159.

Bjorg M, et al. Temporary skin reactions to penicillins during the acute stage of infectious mononucleosis. Scand J Infect Dis 1975;7:21-28.

Blacklow NR, et al. Mononucleosis with heterophile antibodies and EB virus infection. Acquisition by an elderly patient in a hospital. Am J Med 1971;51:549-52.

Brichacek B. Hirsch I. Sibl O. et al. Association of some supraglottic laryngeal carcinomas with EB virus. Int J Cancer 1983;32:193-197.

Brichacek B, Hirsch I, Sibl O, et al. Presence of Epstein-Barr virus DNA in carcinomas of the palatine tonsil. J Natl Cancer Inst 1984;72:809-815.

Butler T, Pastore J. Simon G, et al. Infectious mononucleosis myocarditis. J Infect 1981;3:172-175.

Clarke BF, Davies SH. Severe thrombocytopenia in infectious mononucleosis. Am J Med Sci 1964;248:703-708.

Cleary TG, Henie W, Pickering LK. Acute cerebellar ataxia associated with Epstein-Barr virus infection. JAMA 1980;243:148-149.

Colby BM, Shaw JE, Elion GB, Pagano JS. Effect of acyclovir [9-(2-hydroxyethoxymethyl)guanine] on Epstein-Barr virus DNA replication. J Virol 1980;34:560-568.

Conant MA. Hairy leukoplakia. A new disease of the oral mucosa. Arch Dermatol 1987;123:585-587.

Contratto AN. Infectious mononucleosis: a study of one-hundred and ninety-six cases. Arch Intern Med 1944; 73:449-459.

Cowdrey SC, Reynolds JS. Acute urticaria in infectious mononucleosis. Ann Allergy 1969;27:182.

Davidsohn I. Serologic diagnosis of infectious mononucleosis. JAMA 1937;108:289.

de Thé G, Geser A, Day NE, et al. Epidemiological evidence for causal relationship between Epstein-Barr virus and Burkitt's lymphoma from Ugandan prospective study. Nature 1978;274:756-761.

De Waele M, Thielemans C, Van Camp BKG. Characterization of immunoregulatory T cells in EBV-induced infectious mononucleosis by monoclonal antibodies. N Engl J Med 1981;304:460-462.

Dickerman JD, et al. Infectious mononucleosis initially seen as cold-induced acrocyanosis: association with auto-anti-M and anti-I antibodies. Am J Dis Child 1980;134:159.

Epstein MA, Achong BG, Barr YM. Virus particles in cultural lymphoblasts from Burkitt's lymphoma. Lancet 1964;1:702-703.

Ernberg I, Andersson J. Acyclovir efficiently inhibits oropharyngeal excretion of Epstein-Barr virus in patients with acute infectious mononucleosis. J Gen Virol 1986; 67:2267-2272.

Evans AS. Infectious mononucleosis in University of Wisconsin students. Report of five-year investigation. Am J Hyg 1960;71:342.

Evans AE, Niederman J, Cenabre LC, et al. A prospective evaluation of heterophile and Epstein-Barr virus-specific IgM antibody tests in clinical and subclinical infectious mononucleosis: specificity and sensitivity of the tests and persistence of antibody. J Infect Dis 1975;132:546.

Evans AS, Niederman JC, McCollum RW. Seroepidemiologic studies of infectious mononucleosis with EB virus. Engl J Med 1968;279:1121-1127.

Fields DA. Methicillin rash in infectious mononucleosis (letter). West J Med 1980;133:521.

Fleisher G, Bologonese R. Epstein-Barr virus infections in pregnancy: a prospective study. J Pediatr 1984;104:374-379.

Fleisher GR, Pasquariello PS, Warren WS, et al. Intrafamilial transmission of Epstein-Barr virus infections. J Pediatr 1981;98:16-19.

Fox RI, Pearson G, Vaughan JH. Detection of Epstein-Barr virus-associated antigens and DNA in salivary gland biopsies from patients with Sjogren's syndrome. J Immunol 1986;137:3162-3168.

Gerber P, Walsh JN, Rosenblum EN, Purcell RH. Association of EB-virus infection with the post-perfusion syndrome. Lancet 1969;1:593-596.

Goldberg GN, Fulginiti VA, Ray CG, et al. In utero EBV (infectious mononucleosis) infection. JAMA 1981;246: 1579-1581.

Greenspan D, et al. Oral "hairy" leucoplakia in male homosexuals: evidence of association with both papillomavirus and a herpes-group virus. Lancet 1984;2:831-34.

Greenspan JS, Greenspan D, Lennette ET, et al. Replication of Epstein-Barr virus within the epithelial lesions of oral "hairy" leukoplakia, and AIDS-associated lesion. N Engl J Med 1985;313:1564-1571.

Grierson H, Purtilo DT. Epstein-Barr virus infections in males with X-linked lymphoproliferative syndrome. Ann Intern Med 1987;106:538-545.

Grose C, Henle W, Henle G, Feorino PM. Primary Epstein-Barr virus infections in acute neurologic diseases. N Engl J Med 1975;292:392.

Hanto DW, Frizzera G, Gajl-Peczalska KJ, et al. Epstein-Barr virus-induced B-cell lymphoma after renal transplantation: acyclovir therapy and transition from polyclonal to monoclonal B-cell proliferation. N Engl J Med 1982;306:913-918.

Hanto DW, Frizzera G, Purtilo DT, et al. Clinical spectrum of lymphoproliferative disorders in renal transplant recipients and evidence for the role of the Epstein-Barr virus. Cancer Res 1981;41:4253-4261.

Henle G, Henle W. Observations on childhood infections with the Epstein-Barr virus. J Infect Dis 1970; 121:303.

Henle G, Henle W. Epstein-Barr virus-specific IgA serum antibodies as an outstanding feature of nasopharyngeal carcinoma. Int J Cancer 1976;17:1-7.

Henle G, Henle W, Diehl V. Relation of Burkitt's tumor-associated herpes-type virus to infectious mononucleosis. Proc Natl Acad Sci USA 1968;59:94.

Ho M, Jaffe R, Miller G, et al. The frequency of Epstein-Barr virus infection and associated lymphoproliferative syndrome after transplantation and its manifestations in children. Transplantation 1988;45:719-727.

Ho M, Miller G, Atchison RW, et al. Epstein-Barr virus infections and DNA hybridization studies in posttransplantation lymphoma and lymphoproliferative lesions: the role of primary infection. J Infect Dis 1985;152:876-886.

Hoagland RJ. The transmission of infectious mononucleosis. Am J Med Sci 1955;229:262.

Hoagland RJ. The incubation period of infectious mononucleosis. Am J Public Health 1984;54:1699-1705.

Hochberg FH, Miller G, Schooley RJ, et al. Central-nervous system lymphoma related to Epstein-Barr virus. N Engl J Med 1983;309:745-748.

Hoff G, Bauer S. A new rapid slide test for infectious mononucleosis. JAMA 1965;194:351.

Holmes GP, et al. Chronic fatigue syndrome: a working case definition. Ann Intern Med 1988;108:387-389.

Horwitz CA et al. Long term serological follow-up of patients for Epstein-Barr virus after recovery from infectious mononucleosis. J Infect Dis 1985;151:1150-1153.

Hudgins JM. Infectious mononucleosis complicated by myocarditis and pericarditis. JAMA 1976;235:2626.

Icart J, Didier J, Dalens M, et al. Prospective study of Epstein-Barr virus (EBV) infection during pregnancy. Biomedicine 1981;34:160-163.

Joncas JH, Ghibu F, Blagdon M, et al. A familial syndrome of susceptibility to chronic active Epstein-Barr virus infection. Can Med Assoc J 1984;130:280-285.

Jones JF, Ray CG, Minnich LL, et al. Evidence for active Epstein-Barr virus infection in patients with persistent, unexplained illnesses: elevated anti-early antigen antibodies. Ann Intern Med 1985;102:1-7.

Jones JF, Shurin S, Abramowsky C, et al. T-cell lymphomas containing Epstein-Barr viral DNA in patients with chronic Epstein-Barr virus infections. N Engl J Med 1988;318:733-741.

Joshi VV, Kauffman S, Oleske JM, et al. Polyclonal polymorphic B-cell lymphoproliferative disorder with prominent pulmonary involvement in children with acquired immune deficiency syndrome. Cancer 1987;59:1455-1462.

Katz BZ, Berkman AB, Shapiro ED. Serologic evidence of active Epstein-Barr virus infection in the EBV-associated lymphoproliferative disorders of AIDS (abstract 422). Presented at the 30th Interscience Conference on Antimicrobial Agents and Chemotherapy, Atlanta GA, October 22, 1990.

Katz BZ, Niederman JC, Olson BA, Miller G. Fragment length polymorphisms among independent isolates of Epstein-Barr virus from immunocompromised and normal hosts. J Infect Dis 1988;157:299-308.

Katz BZ, Raab-Traub N, Miller G. Latent and Replicating forms of Epstein-Barr virus DNA in lymphomas and lymphoproliferative diseases. J Infect Dis 1989;160:589-598.

Leder P, Battery J, Lenoir G, et al. Translocations among antibody genes in human cancer. Science 1976;222:765-771.

Lenoir G, Preud'homme JL, Bernheim A, Berger R. Correlation between immunoglobulin light chain expression and variant translocation in Burkitt's lymphoma. Nature 1982;298:474-476.

Levene G, Baker H. Drug reactions: ampicillin and infectious mononucleosis. Br J Dermatol 1968;80:417-421.

Leyvraz S, Henle W, Chahinian AP, et al. Association of Epstein-Barr virus with thymic carcinoma. N Engl J Med 1985;312:1296-1299.

Martin PJ, Shulman HM, Schubach WH, et al. Fatal EBV-associated proliferation of donor B cells following treatment of acute graft-versus-host-disease with a murine monoclonal anti-T cell antibody. Ann Intern Med 1984;101:310.

Matsuo T, Heller M, Petti L, et al. Persistence of the entire Epstein-Barr virus genome integrated into human lymphocyte DNA Science 1984:226:1322-1325.

McCarthy JT, Hoagland RJ. Cutaneous manifestations of infectious mononucleosis. JAMA 1964;187:153-154.

McKenna RW, Risdall RJ, Brunning RD. Virus associated with hemophagocytic syndrome. Hum Pathol 1981; 12:395-398.

McKenzie H et al. IgM and IgG antibody levels to ampicillin in patients with infectious mononucleosis. Clin Exp Immunol 1976;26:214-221.

Miller G, Grogan E, Rowe D, et al. Selective lack of antibody to a component of EB nuclear antigen in patients with chronic active Epstein-Barr virus infection. J Infect Dis 1987;156:26-35.

Miller G, Niederman JC, Andrews LL: Prolonged oropharyngeal excretion of Epstein-Barr virus after infectious mononucleosis. N Engl J Med 1973;288:229.

Milne J: Infectious mononucleosis. N Engl J Med 1945; 233:727.

Morgan DG, Miller G, Neiderman JC, et al. Site of Epstein-Barr virus replication in the oropharynx. Lancet 1979; 2:1154-1157.

Mueller N, Evans A, Harris NL, et al. Hodgkin's disease and Epstein-Barr virus: altered antibody pattern before diagnosis. N Engl J Med 1989;320:689-695.

Mulroy R: Amoxicillin rash in infectious mononucleosis (letter): Br Med J 1973;1:554.

Nazareth I, et al. Ampicillin sensitivity in infectious mononucleosis—temporary or permanent? Scand J Infect Dis 1972;4:229-230.

Neel HB, Pearson GR, Weiland LH, et al. Application of Epstein-Barr virus serology to the diagnosis of staging of North American patients with nasopharyngeal carcinoma. Otolaryngol Head Neck Surg 1983;91:255-262.

Niederman JC. Heterophil antibody determination in a series of 166 cases of infectious mononucleosis listed according to various stages of the disease. Yale J Biol Med 1956;28:629.

Niederman JC, Evans AS, Subrahmanyan MS, McCollum RW. Prevalence, incidence and persistence of EB virus antibody in young adults. N Engl J Med 1970;282:361.

Niederman JC, McCollum RW, Henle G, Henle W. Infectious mononucleosis: clinical manifestations in relation to EB virus antibodies. JAMA 1968;203:205.

Niederman JC, Miller G. Kinetics of the antibody response to BamHI-K nuclear antigen in uncomplicated infectious mononucleosis. J Infect Dis 1986;154:346-349.

Niederman JC, et al. Infectious mononucleosis: Epstein-Barr-virus shedding in saliva and oropharynx. N Engl J Med 1976;294:1355.

Pahwa S. Human immunodeficiency virus infection in children: nature of immunodeficiency, clinical spectrum and managment. Pediatr Infect Dis J 1988;7:61-71(suppl).

Patel BM. Skin rash with infectious mononucleosis and ampicillin. Pediatrics 1967;40:910-911.

Pattengale PK, Smith RW, Perlin E. Atypical lymphocytes in acute infectious mononucleosis. Identification by multiple T and B lymphocyte markers. N Engl J Med 1974;291:1145.

Paul JR, Bunnell WW. The presence of heterophile antibodies in infectious mononucleosis. Am J Med Sci 1932;183:90.

Pereira MS, Blake JM, Macrae AD. EB virus antibody at different ages. Br Med J 1969;4:526.

Petrozzi JW. Infectious mononucleosis manifesting as a palmar dermatitis. Arch Dermatol 1971;104:207.

Pfeiffer E. Dreusenfieber. Jahrb Kinderheilkd 1889;29:257.

Press JH, et al. Infectious mononucleosis: a study of 96 cases. Ann Intern Med 1945;22:546.

Pullen H, Wright N, Murdock, JMcC: Hypersensitivity reactions to antimicrobial drugs in infectious mononucleosis. Lancet 1967;2:1176.

Purtilo DT. Malignant lymphoproliferative diseases induced by Epstein-Barr virus in immunodeficient patients, including X-linked, cytogenetic, and familial syndromes. Cancer Genet Cytogenet 1981;4:251-268.

Purtilo DT, DeFlorio D, Hutt LM, et al. Variable phenotypic expression of an X-linked recessive lymphoproliferative syndrome. N Engl J Med 1977;297:1077-1081.

Purtilo DT, Sakamoto K, Barnabei V, et al. Epstein-Barr virus-induced diseases in boys with the X-linked lymphoproliferative syndrome (XLP). Am J Med 1982;73:49-56.

Raab-Traub N, Flynn K. The structure of the termini of the Epstein-Barr virus as a marker of clonal cellular proliferation. Cell 1986;47:883-889.

Raab-Traub N, Flynn K, Pearson G, et al. The differentiated form of nasopharyngeal carcinoma contains Epstein-Barr virus DNA. Int J Cancer 1987;39:25-29.

Ralston LS, Saiki AK, Powers WT. Orchitis as a complication of infectious mononucleosis. JAMA 1960;173:1348.

Rapp CE Jr, Hewetson JF. Infectious mononucleosis and the Epstein-Barr virus. Am J Dis Child 1978;132:78.

Resnick L, Herbst JS, Ablashi DV, et al. Regression of oral hairy leukoplakia after orally administered acyclovir therapy. JAMA 1988;259:384-388.

Robinson JE, Brown N, Andiman W, et al. Diffuse polyclonal B-cell lymphoma during primary infection with Epstein-Barr virus. N Engl J Med 1980;302:1293-1297.

Rocchi G, et al. Quantitative evaluation of Epstein-Barr-virus-infected mononuclear peripheral blood leukocytes in infectious mononucleosis. N Engl J Med 1977;296:132.

Rubinstein A, Morecki R, Silverman B, et al. Pulmonary disease in children with acquired immune deficiency syndrome and AIDS-related complex. J Pediatr 1986;108:498-503.

Rutkow IM. Rupture of the spleen in infectious mononucleosis. Arch Surg 1978;113:718.

Sawyer RN, Evans AS, Niederman JC, McCollum RW. Prospective studies of a group of Yale University freshmen. I. Occurrence of infectious mononucleosis. J Infect Dis 1971;123:263.

Schiff J, et al. Cell-associated Epstein-Barr virus in the cerebrospinal fluid of a patient with meningo-encephalitis complicating infectious mononucleosis. Yale J Biol Med 1982;55:59-63.

Schooley RT, Carey RW, Miller G, et al. Chronic Epstein-Barr virus infection associated with fever and interstitial pneumonitis. Clinical and serologic features and response to antiviral chemotherapy. Ann Intern Med 1986;636-643.

Schubach WH, Hackman R, Neiman PE, et al. A monoclonal immunoblastic sarcoma in donor cells bearing Epstein-Barr virus genomes following allogeneic marrow grafting for acute lymphoblastic leukemia. Blood 1982;60:180-187.

Sixbey JW, Nedrud JG, Raab-Traub N, et al. Epstein-Barr virus replication in oropharyngeal epithelial cells. N Engl J Med 1984;310:1225-1230.

Sprunt TP, Evans FA. Mononuclear leukocytosis in reaction to acute infections ("infectious mononucleosis"). Bull Johns Hopkins Hosp 1920;31:410.

Starzl TE, Nalesnik MA, Porter KA, et al. Reversibility of lymphomas and lymphoproliferative lesions developing under cyclosporin-steroid therapy. Lancet 1984;17:583-587.

Strauch B, Siegel N, Andrews LL, Miller G. Oropharyngeal excretion of Epstein-Barr virus by renal transplant recipients and other patients treated with immunosuppressive drugs. Lancet 1974;1:234.

Straus SE, The chronic mononucleosis syndrome. J Infect Dis 1988;157:405-412.

Subar M, Neri A, Inghirami G, et al: Frequent c-*myc* oncogene activation and infrequent presence of Epstein-Barr virus genome in AIDS-associated lymphoma. Blood 1988;72:667-671.

Sumaya CV. Primary Epstein-Barr virus infections in children. Pediatrics 1977;59:16.

Svedmyr E, Jondal M. Cytotoxic effector cells specific for B cell lines transformed by EBV are present in patients with infectious mononucleosis. Proc Natl Acad Sci USA 1975;7:1622-1626.

Tischendorf P, et al. Development and persistence of immunity to Epstein-Barr virus in man. J Infect Dis 1970;122:401.

Tosato G, Magrath I, Koski I, et al. Activation of suppressor T cells during Epstein-Barr-virus-induced infectious mononucleosis. 1979;301:1133-1137.

Turner AR, MacDonald RN, Cooper BA. Transmission of infectious mononucleosis by transfusion of pre-illness plasma. Ann Intern Med 1972;77:751-753.

Tyson CJ, Czarny D. Cold-induced urticaria in infectious mononucloeosis. Med J Aust 1981;1:33.

Weiss LM, Movabhed LA, Warnke RA, Sklar J. Detection of Epstein-Barr viral genomes in Reed-Sternberg cells of Hodgkin's disease. N Engl J Med 1989;320:502-506.

Wilson ER, Malluh A, Stagno S, et al. Fatal Epstein-Barr virus-associated hemophagocytic syndrome. J Pediatr 1981;98:260-262.

Wolf H, Haus M, Wilmes E. Persistence of Epstein-Barr virus in the parotid gland. J Virol 1984;51:795-798.

Wolnisty C. Orchitis as a complication of infectious mononucleosis: report of a case. N Engl J Med 1962;266:88.

Yao QY, Rickinson AB, Epstein MA. A re-examination of the Epstein-Barr virus carrier state in healthy seropositive individuals. Int J Cancer 1985;35:35-42.

7

ACUTE GASTROENTERITIS

THOMAS G. CLEARY
LARRY K. PICKERING

Acute infectious gastroenteritis is one of the most common infectious disease syndromes of humans, ranking second to acute respiratory tract infections as a worldwide cause of morbidity. In developing areas of the world diarrhea is a significant cause of death in infants. It has been estimated that up to 15% of children in developing nations die of diarrhea before 3 years of age. The usual clinical syndrome is characterized by various combinations of nausea, vomiting, abdominal cramps, and diarrhea. Fever may or may not be present. The causative agent is most often bacteria, virus, or protozoa (see box, p. 106). Bacterial and viral causes of diarrhea and *Giardia lamblia* are reviewed in this chapter.

BACTERIAL GASTROENTERITIS

Bacterial agents associated with diarrhea that are discussed in this chapter include *Escherichia coli*, *Salmonella*, *Shigella*, *Campylobacter jejuni*, *Yersinia enterocolitica*, and *Vibrio cholerae*. Staphylococcal gastroenteritis is presented in Chapter 27. Some of these bacterial pathogens are identifiable in the microbiology laboratory, whereas others require a more specialized facility for identification. Fluid replacement and appropriate specific therapy may favorably alter the course of illness.

Etiology

Escherichia coli. The *E. coli* bacterium was named for Escherich, a pediatrician who isolated

Portions of this chapter are incorporated from the eighth edition of this text, authored by Catherine M. Wilfert.

it in 1885. *E. coli* are common inhabitants of the intestine and ordinarily cause no clinical symptoms. The organism is a gram-negative bacillus, measuring 2 to 3 μm long and 0.6 μm wide. The bacilli may form chains, and most strains are motile. This facultatively anaerobic organism grows on media routinely used in microbiology laboratories. The optimal temperature for growth is 37° C; it is killed at a temperature of 60° C for 30 minutes. Although isolation of *E. coli* is not difficult, recognition of pathogenic strains is complex because of the multiple factors that enable this organism to cause disease. Specific recognition of pathogenic strains is readily accomplished only in research laboratories; therefore laboratory confirmation of gastrointestinal (GI) tract disease caused by *E. coli* is not generally available.

In 1951 *E. coli* organisms were shown as serologically heterogeneous by Kauffman, who divided the species into various somatic groups. In addition to the cell wall, O (somatic) antigens, H (flagellar) antigens, and K (capsular) antigens also were identified. The serotype is a chromosomally determined characteristic and is stable. Serogroups have been shown to correlate with disease production in infants, despite the inability to demonstrate a universal virulence factor.

E. coli strains that cause diarrhea are currently grouped according to their pathogenic mechanism(s). The provisional classification includes enterotoxigenic *E. coli* (ETEC), enteroinvasive *E. coli* (EIEC), enteropathogenic *E. coli* (EPEC), enterohemorrhagic *E. coli*

105

ETIOLOGY OF ACUTE GASTROENTERITIS

Bacteria
Escherichia coli
Salmonellae
Shigellae
Campylobacter jejuni
Vibrio cholerae
Other vibrios
Yersinia enterocolitica
Clostridium difficile
Aeromonas hydrophila
Plesiomonas shigelloides

Viruses
Rotavirus
Enteric adenovirus (types 40 and 41)
Small, round enteric viruses
    Astroviruses
    Caliciviruses
    Norwalk and Norwalk-like virus
    Parvovirus
Coronaviruses
Others
    Pestivirus
    Breda virus

Protozoa
Giardia lamblia
Cryptosporidium
Entamoeba histolytica
Isospora belli
Microsporidia
Strongyloides stercoralis

(EHEC), and enteroadherent (or auto agglutinating) *E. coli* (EAEC) (Table 7-1).

Enterotoxigenic E. coli. ETEC are those organisms that produce plasmid-encoded enterotoxins. Although belonging to specific serogroups, these organisms are not identified by serotyping. The heat-labile enterotoxin (LT) and heat-stable enterotoxin (ST) produced by ETEC are compared to Shiga toxin in Table 7-3. LT, like cholera toxin, activates adenylate cyclase, resulting in increased production of cyclic adenosine monophosphate (cAMP). The toxin is detectable in tissue culture or by immunological tests. ST activates guanylate cyclase, with a resulting increase in cyclic guanosine monophosphate (cGMP). Many of the ETEC strains possess specific adhesion factors enabling them to colonize the small intestine. Such colonization factor antigens (e.g., CFA-1 and CFA-2) contribute to disease production by these toxigenic bacteria. Colonization factors are visualized by electron microscopy as filamentous structures that often resemble fimbriae.

Enteroinvasive E. coli. A second group of *E. coli*, the EIEC, produce GI tract disease by their ability to penetrate and multiply within the intestinal epithelial cells. These enteroinvasive *E. coli* resemble shigellae in this respect. Although these *E. coli* tend to fall into certain serological groups, serotyping to identify disease caused by these organisms and of shigellae are dependent on a transmissible plasmid. Demonstration of the enteroinvasive quality of the organism is possible by tissue culture tests or by the Sereny test, which is the production of keratoconjunctivitis in the guinea pig eye after inoculation of the organism into the conjunctival space.

Enteropathogenic E. coli. All *E. coli* that cause diarrhea originally were called *enteropathogenic E. coli* when it was realized that certain serotypes could be associated with disease. The terminology has evolved as the pathogenic mechanisms have been elucidated so that enteropathogenic *E. coli* currently refers only to those organisms that cause disease but do not produce LT or ST, do not have the genes coding for these toxins, and are not enteroinvasive. EPEC has caused diarrhea in volunteers. Pathophysiological studies have shown some of these organisms adhere to the microvilli of the rabbit ileum. In vitro adherence to HEp-2 cells is a correlate of their ability to adhere in vivo. Biopsies of human intestine show that the brush border of the small intestine is effaced, and the organisms are densely adherent. This ability to adhere apparently also is associated with the presence of a plasmid that is different from that necessary for the invasive qualities of EIEC mentioned previously. Two classes of EPEC can be distinguished by adherence patterns in tissue culture and by gene probe for this characteristic (EAF probe). The precise mechanism of adherence and diarrhea remains uncertain.

Enterohemorrhagic E. coli. In 1983 a previously unrecognized class of *E. coli* was described (Riley et al., 1983). The major virulence trait was production of one of several toxins closely related to Shiga toxin. The *E. coli* that produce these toxins are called *enterohemorrhagic E. coli* or *verotoxin-producing E. coli* (VTEC).

Table 7-1. *E. coli* associated with diarrhea

Classification	Pathogenic mechanism	Common sero groups (somatic antigens)

Enterotoxigenic *E. coli* (ETEC)	Enterotoxins causing fluid loss
	   Heat stable (ST)
	   Heat labile (LT) (cholera-like)
	Adhesins
	Colonization factor antigens
		6, 8, 15, 20, 25, 27, 63, 78, 80, 85, 115, 128ac, 139, 148, 153, 159, 167

Enteroinvasive *E. coli* (EIEC)	Invasion of intestinal cells Invasion plasmid is closely related to invasion plasmid of shigellae	28ac, 29, 124, 136, 143, 144, 152, 164, 167
Enteropathogenic *E. coli* (EPEC)	Adhesins	Class I (EAF +): 55, 86, 111, 119, 125, 126, 127, 128ab, 142 Class II (EAF −): 18, 44, 112, 114

Enterohemorrhagic *E. coli* (EHEC)	Protein synthesis inhibiting toxins
	   Shigalike toxin I (VT1)
	   Shigalike toxin II (VT2)
	   Shigalike toxin II variants
		157 (most common), 26, 111, others

Enteroadherent *E. coli* (EAEC)	Adhesins	Not determined

VT, Verotoxin; *EAF*, EPEC adherence factor.

The most common EHEC serotype is *E. coli* O157:H7, although approximately 50 serotypes that produce Shigalike toxins (SLT-I and/or SLT-II) have been recognized. Shortly after the recognition of this class of *E. coli*, it was demonstrated that the distinctive gastroenteritis (hemorrhagic colitis) associated with these organisms was frequently complicated by development of classic hemolytic uremic syndrome (HUS) (Cleary, 1988). Although other causes for HUS exist, it appears that nearly all cases of HUS are the result of EHEC infection.

Enteroadherent *E. coli*. This recently recognized group of pathogens, EAEC, is not yet well characterized either mechanistically or clinically. The major virulence trait thus far defined is the ability of these cells to adhere to HEp-2 cells in tissue culture in a distinctive way.

Vibrio cholerae. *V. cholerae* is a gram-negative curved bacillus with a single flagellum responsible for its motility. The name *Vibrio* is derived from the organism's movement, which is apparent as a vibration in wet preparations. There are two major somatic antigenic types of the organism (Inaba and Ogawa) and two biotypes (classic and El Tor) that may cause disease. All clinical isolates of *V. cholerae* 01 from the United States have been biotype El Tor, serotype Inaba. These strains were isolated from people who had consumed contaminated raw and undercooked shellfish from the Gulf of Mexico or who had acquired the strain in South America where an epidemic of cholera was occurring.

V. cholerae elaborates a heat-labile enterotoxin in alkaline growth conditions. The toxin production of this organism is coded by chromosomal DNA (see Table 7-2). This toxin has provided a wealth of information about the structure and function of enterotoxins and about the pathogenesis of diarrheal diseases. This protein exotoxin activates adenylate cyclase and catalyzes the formation of cyclic AMP, resulting in the secretion of fluid into the lumen of the GI tract. The toxin has two component parts, one of which (B) binds to a receptor, GM_1 ganglioside, present on the surface of intestinal cells. The second part of the toxin (A) penetrates the cell and must gain access to the interior to catalyze the adenosine diphosphate (ADP) ribosylation of a guanosine triphosphate (GTP)-binding protein. This results in activation of adenylate cyclase and conversion of adenosine triphosphate (ATP) to cAMP. The increased concentration of intracellular cAMP activates electrolyte transport isosmotically with water from the extracellular fluid to the lumen of the GI tract. Secretion then exceeds fluid absorption.

Table 7-2. Diarrhea-associated toxins

Characteristics of organism toxin	V. cholerae cholera toxin	E. coli labile toxin	E. coli stable toxin	Shiga toxin (SLT-I, II, IIv)
Molecular weight (MW)	84,000	73,000	2,000	71,000
Immunogenic	Yes	Yes	No	Yes
Genetic control of toxin	Chromosomal	Plasmid	Plasmid	Phage
Multimeric protein (A and B subunits)	Yes	Yes	No	Yes
A and B synthesized separately and then associated	Yes	Yes		Yes
B subunit binds to cell	Yes	Yes		Yes
Cell receptor	GM_1, ganglioside	GM_1, ganglioside	100,000 MW protein (not GM_1)	Galactose α1-4, galactose β1-4, glucose ceramide (Gb$_3$)
Internalization	By noncoated surface microinvaginations	By noncoated surface microinvaginations	?	By receptor-mediated endocytosis through coated pits
Subunit with enzymatic activity	Yes	Yes		Yes
Intracellular target site	Inner surface plasma membrane	Inner surface plasma membrane	Inner surface plasma membrane	Cytosol
Action	Modification of plasma membrane enzymes	Modification of plasma membrane enzymes	Modification of plasma membrane enzymes	Cleaves adenine residue from 28S ribosomal RNA
Enzyme affected	Activation of adenylate cyclase	Activation of adenylate cyclase	Activation of guanylate cyclase	Blocks attachment site for EF-1– dependent aminoacyl tRNA binding
Mode of action	NAD-dependent ADP ribosylation of GTP-binding component of adenylate cyclase		?	A1 catalyzed inactivation of the 28S ribosomal subunit
Site of action	Small intestine epithelium	Small intestine epithelium	Small intestine epithelium	Small and large intestine
Physiological action	↓ Absorption ↑ Secretion	↓ Absorption ↑ Secretion	↓ Absorption ↑ Secretion	Probably causes fluid loss through injury to enterocytes with decreased absorption

Increased cAMP also inhibits the transport of sodium and chloride from the lumen of the gut across the brush border and into the cell; that is, absorption is decreased as membrane permeability in the villus cell is diminished. Glucose-coupled sodium and water transport into cells occurs by an independent mechanism that is unaltered. Thus oral electrolyte solution can still be absorbed from the intestine.

Salmonellae. Salmonellae are gram-negative, motile aerobic bacilli that do not ferment lactose and sucrose but produce acid when using glucose, maltose, and mannitol. All human species except *Salmonella typhi* produce gas with fermentation. Salmonellae currently are classified into three species: *S. enteritidis*, *S. typhi*, and *S. choleraesuis*. There are more than 1,700 serobiotypes of *S. enteritidis*, which are typed by their heat-stable (O), or somatic, antigens and heat-labile (H), or flagellar, antigens. *S. typhi* and *S. choleraesuis* each have only one serobiotype. Salmonellae frequently are given names of places (e.g., *S. newport*) in which outbreaks occurred. Serogrouping may be useful epidemiologically and is generally done by state health laboratories. Biotype *S. typhimurium* is responsible for approximately 20% to 30% of all reported infections in the United States each year, but virtually any serotype can cause human disease. *S. typhi* is a pathogen only of humans and, in contrast to all other salmonellae, is not harbored by other animal species.

Shigellae. In 1896 Shiga isolated a gram-negative nonmotile bacillus from patients studied in an epidemic of dysentery in Japan and presented evidence for the causal relationship to the microorganism that was later named for him. Four years later Flexner studied cases of dysentery in the Philippines and reported the detection of an organism very similar to Shiga's bacillus. Today there are four main groups of *Shigella* organisms responsible for diarrhea. Each group comprises a number of types that are distinguished by biochemical and serological criteria: group A, *S. dysenteriae;* group B, *S. flexneri;* group C, *S. boydii;* and group D, *S. sonnei.* Group D accounts for 60% to 80% of the episodes of shigellosis in the United States.

The human GI tract is the natural habitat of shigellae. They are slender, motile, gram-negative bacilli that ferment glucose but not lactose and do not produce hydrogen sulfide. They are isolated on an agar media such as MacConkey's, which allows selection of non-lactose-fermenting organisms. They are best cultured from fresh stool obtained early in illness and plated soon after collection. However, volunteer studies have shown that stool culture may be negative in patients with symptomatic shigellosis. *S. dysenteriae* produces a protein synthesis–inhibiting toxin (shigatoxin) (Bartlett et al., 1986). Other shigellae make little or no shigatoxin, although EHEC (described previously) always make a toxin either essentially identical to shigatoxin (SLT-I) or less closely related (SLT-II). Experimentally, shigatoxin causes hemorrhagic fluid secretion in the jejunum of animals and is a cytotoxin in cell culture.

Yersinia enterocolitica. The genus *Yersinia* includes *Y. pestis*, *Y. pseudotuberculosis*, and *Y. enterocolitica*. *Y. enterocolitica* has emerged as a significant pathogen of the GI tract of humans. These organisms are small pleomorphic gram-negative bacilli with rounded ends. They are motile at 22° C and are nonlactose fermenters, but they do ferment sucrose and split urea. Five biotypes and 34 serotypes of *Y. enterocolitica* inhabit the GI tract of many animals and birds and survive in fresh water. The laboratory usually must be alerted to the possibility that this organism is being considered so that appropriate selective media can be used.

Campylobacter. Species of *Campylobacter* are recognized as one of the most important causes of acute bacterial diarrhea throughout the world. *C. jejuni* is the most frequently identified species, but others, including *C. coli*, *C. laridis*, *C. hyointestinalis*, and *C. upsalienais*, have also been associated with diarrhea in humans. In most laboratories *C. coli* is identified as *C. jejuni*. *C. fetus* is an uncommon cause of disease in humans, but when infection occurs, this organism produces fever and bacteremia, usually in immunocompromised hosts and neonates. *C. fetus* are bacilli (1.5 to 5 μm × 0.2 to 0.5 μm) that are motile with a polar flagellum. They do not ferment or oxidize carbohydrates. A selective medium and growth conditions of reduced oxygen tension are necessary for optimal growth of the organisms from stool.

Other bacteria. Other microorganisms implicated less often as causes of gastroenteritis include *Clostridium difficile, Aeromonas hydro-*

phila, Plesiomonas shigelloides, and *Vibrio parahaemolyticus.*

Giardia lamblia. *G. lamblia* is a flagellate protozoan that exists in trophozoite and cyst forms. The cyst form is the infectious form (Pickering and Engelkirk, 1988). After its ingestion, each cyst produces two trophozoites, which penetrate the mucous gel layer and attach to the intestinal epithelium of the duodenum and proximal jejunum. As detached trophozoites pass through the GI tract, they encyst to form smooth, oval-shaped cysts, which are passed in feces. The exact mechanism of disease production is unknown.

Epidemiology

Bacterial enteropathogens are transmitted by the fecal-oral route. Transmission often occurs through contaminated food or water, allowing the organisms to multiply. A large inoculum is necessary for virtually all these bacteria, ranging from estimates of 10,000 to millions of organisms. Shigellae (and perhaps EHEC) are the exceptions, with 10 to 100 organisms transmitting infection. *S. typhi* and *Shigella* are inhabitants of only the human GI tract, whereas the other organisms have animal hosts and can be introduced to humans by contact with contaminated materials.

ETEC cause disease primarily in infants less than 18 months of age in developing nations and in adult travelers (Gorbach et al., 1975). Occasional outbreaks of disease have been associated with contaminated water. EPEC cause outbreaks of disease, especially in infants in nurseries through contaminated instruments, health personnel, or other aspects of the environment. EIEC are an uncommon cause of infantile diarrhea and are more often transmitted through contaminated food. EHEC are recognized increasingly as a cause of sporadic diarrhea, with a few endemic foci having a high risk. EAEC have been recognized in the developing world both in children and in travelers to those locales.

Cholera has occurred in devastating worldwide pandemics, with perpetual endemic disease occurring in India and Bangladesh. An epidemic of cholera began in Peru in January of 1991 and has subsequently spread to several other countries in Latin America. Cases have been identified in the United States over the past decade and are related to eating shellfish in the Gulf of Mexico or from travel to South America. Ratios of inapparent infection to clinical disease vary from an estimated 4:1 to 36:1. Carriage and excretion of the organism usually last several weeks but may last longer. Thus quarantine of symptomatic cases does not curtail spread. In endemic areas cholera is a disease of childhood, although infants less than 1 year are usually spared. When epidemics reach previously uninfected countries, all ages are infected.

Humans usually ingest *Salmonella* from contaminated food, with meat and poultry products heading the list. Organisms are present on the surface of meat; thus any conditions favoring multiplication enhance the possibility of disease production. The animals are infected and perpetuate the infection among themselves, easily contaminating other animals during transport. An estimated 2 million cases of *Salmonella* gastroenteritis occur per year in the United States. Nosocomial transmission within hospitals, nursing homes, and institutions results from cross contamination involving personnel, equipment, and aerosol. In those areas where sewage disposal and water purification are inadequate, enteric infections are frequent and the likelihood of spread is enhanced.

Shigella and *S. typhi* are exclusively human pathogens, and communicability of disease depends on human fecal material transmitting infection either through person-to-person contact or through food and water. The highest incidence of *Shigella* is in infants 1 to 4 years of age. Large outbreaks of infection usually are related to contaminated food or water.

Campylobacter jejuni. The reservoir of *C. jejuni* is the GI tract of wild and domestic animals. Most farm animals, meat sources, poultry carcasses, and many pet dogs and cats, especially the young, harbor this organism. Transmission occurs from ingestion of contaminated meat, unpasteurized milk, or contaminated water. Person-to-person spread occurs, and outbreaks have been reported.

Yersinia enterocolitica. *Y. enterocolitica* causes a spectrum of illness that includes gastroenteritis and affects all age groups. Some geographical variation in recognized disease in the United States occurs for reasons that are not clear. Outbreaks of disease have been traced to contaminated food. The reservoirs of these organisms are probably animals, but this is less well documented than some of the other pathogens described.

Giardia lamblia. G. *lamblia* is a common cause of enteritis and is found with increased frequency in homosexual men, children in day-care centers, and travelers to endemic areas. It has been found in 4% to 70% of patients with acquired immunodeficiency syndrome (AIDS) in the United States (Quinn et al., 1983; Smith et al., 1988; Pickering and Engelkirk, 1988; Laughon et al., 1988; Janoff et al., 1988) and in patients with AIDS from Europe (Connolly et al., 1989). Transmission occurs through the fecal-oral route by passage of infectious cysts from person to person or through ingestion of contaminated food or water.

Pathogenesis and pathology

The GI tract has a number of nonimmunological defense mechanisms that help form a barrier against infection. The indigenous flora are present in numbers up to 10^{11} organism per gram of stool in the large bowel. Competition for substrate plus other environment alterations such as decreased pH or production of antibacterial substances probably contribute to which organisms succeed in causing disease. Antibiotics alter growth of indigenous flora and may contribute to successful colonization by pathogens.

Secretions such as saliva and mucin may diminish bacterial adherence to epithelial cells both mechanically and by competition at receptor sites. Normal peristalsis expels organisms that are not adherent. Gastric acid inhibits growth of many bacteria such as salmonellae. Lysozyme and bile salts are also in the GI tract and can hinder growth of many bacteria. Immunological defense mechanisms include secretory IgA, the production of which is dependent on antigen exposure to the local intestinal surface. The secretory piece of IgA increases resistance of these antibodies to proteases; thus this class of antibody best withstands the environment of the lumen of the bowel. Antibody binds toxins and bacteria, thus preventing adsorption, and may be bactericidal in combination with complement and lysozyme.

Malabsorption or profuse watery isotonic diarrhea is caused by dysfunction of the small intestine. Some organisms (V. *cholerae* is the prototype) cause profuse malabsorption because of the effects of their enterotoxins on intestinal cells. In other instances such as dysentery the colon and/or terminal ileum are invaded by bacteria. Shigellae comprise the prototype of invasive organisms causing dysentery. The mucosal invasion and disruption are visible as ulcerations and result in the presence of blood and pus in stool. The symptoms of dysentery include painful cramps and tenesmus.

Bacterial pathogens must be able to adhere in the intestinal mucosa to cause disease, establishing the adhesins of the bacteria as a critical part of virulence. The flagellum of V. *cholerae* appears to have adhesins responsible for adherence to the brush border (Attridge and Rowley, 1983). The organism produces a soluble protease capable of hydrolyzing mucin, which may facilitate adsorption. This organism does not destroy the brush border or invade cells, and no histological lesions are observed.

E. coli cause disease by several mechanisms as described previously. Approximately 40% to 50% of ETEC produce only ST, 30% to 40% produce ST and LT, and 20% to 30% produce only LT. Disease may be produced by either or both enterotoxins produced by ETEC and the stool is watery and often of large volume.

The EIEC and shigellae must also adhere to mucosal cells. These virulent organisms induce their own uptake by epithelial cells. They penetrate the mucosa and multiply in enterocytes of the large intestine. The exudative response of neutrophils and mononuclear cells is apparent microscopically. The superficial ulcerations of the mucosa and submucosa heal with formation of granulation tissue.

The adherent but noninvasive EPEC colonize the small intestine by undefined receptors. The in vitro adherence to HEp-2 cells by these organisms is mediated by nonfimbrial adhesins. The mechanism of disease production by these organisms is unknown. Pathologically, clusters of organisms adhere to the brush border of the epithelium. The villi are blunted, and hypertrophy of the crypts occurs. Some EPEC and EAEC likely will be reclassified in the future as understanding of their mechanisms increases.

The toxins of EHEC have been called shigalike toxin 1 (SLT-I) (or verotoxin 1 [VT1]), and shigalike toxin 2 (SLT-II) (or verotoxin 2 [VT2]). SLT-II is immunologically distinct from SLT-I but is genetically and mechanistically closely related. Other closely related variant toxins, some of which have been studied extensively, also exist. These toxins work like shigatoxin produced by S. *dysenteriae* 1.

To cause disease salmonellae must adhere to

and then penetrate the mucosal cells by endocytosis (mucosal translocation) before reaching the lamina propria. Bacterial proliferation occurs in the lamina propria and mesenteric nodes. The penetration is rapid, and macrophage engulfment without killing has been demonstrated. The terminal ileum and cecum are maximally involved, and neutrophilic inflammation is apparent in these locations. Peyer's patches and the mesenteric nodes may be enlarged. Salmonellae seem to survive in an intracellular location, gain access to the reticuloendothelial system, and are thus protected from antibody and some antibiotics. This intracellular location may contribute to prolonged carriage and excretion of the organism.

Although several enterotoxins are produced by various salmonellae, their role in disease is not well defined. Water and electrolyte transport abnormalities accompany experimental *Salmonella* infections. The tissue invasion places the organism in position to enter the lymphatic and/or the vascular system with access to the reticuloendothelial system. Involvement of tissues outside the GI tract is an unusual occurrence. *S. typhi*, on the other hand, elicits a mononuclear cell response in the lamina propria. *S. typhi* traverses the mucosa and is more likely to cause bacteremia than other *Salmonella* species.

C. jejuni and *Y. enterocolitica* produce a dysentery syndrome and are similar to shigellae. Pathologically, they generally mimic the mucosal translocation and bacterial proliferation in nodes and lamina propria described for *Salmonella* species. An enterotoxin that has an action similar to cholera toxin and LT of ETEC has been described for *C. jejuni*. A stable toxin has been produced in vitro at 26° C to 30° C by *Y. enterocolitica*. Both organisms must invade the mucosa, and the features contributing to their virulence have not yet been fully delineated.

Clinical manifestations

Escherichia coli. ETEC are an important cause of diarrhea in infants of developing nations. When a cause is determined, one half of the cases of traveler's diarrhea in adults is attributable to ETEC. The severity varies from mild to severe, with up to 10 to 20 stools per day. An inoculum of a million or more organisms produces disease with an incubation period of several days in adults. Disease is self-limited,

lasting 3 to 5 days in a normal host, but severe dehydration may occur in infants. The disease is a malabsorptive diarrhea with watery stools without blood or white blood cells, and low-grade fever may be present.

EIEC produce dysentery with blood and pus in the stools. Onset of fever, nausea, cramps, and tenesmus may be rapid. The clinical manifestations are similar to those produced by shigellae. EIEC disease is uncommon in infants.

EPEC characteristically infect infants and have caused numerous outbreaks of acute and chronic infantile enteritis. These organisms are of particular importance in tropical countries and developing nations with crowding and poor hygiene. Frequent, green, slimy stools are produced, usually without blood or fecal leukocytes.

EHEC produce an illness that begins with nausea, vomiting, abdominal pain, and watery diarrhea that progresses to bloody diarrhea over several days. Only 10% of patients have fever as part of this syndrome. This afebrile bloody diarrhea syndrome is called hemorrhagic colitis. Although this is the most distinctive presentation for EHEC, nonspecific watery diarrhea and asymptomatic infections also occur. Classic hemolytic-uremic syndrome (HUS) follows EHEC enteritis in approximately 10% of patients; however, in a few outbreaks the incidence has approached 50%. Infection is usually foodborne, with meat or unpasteurized dairy products implicated, but EHEC can also be spread by person-to-person contact, suggesting that it is a low-inoculum disease.

EAEC have been recognized primarily in children in the developing world as a cause of both acute and chronic diarrhea. Data suggest that these organisms may be common enteropathogens of early childhood.

Cholera. Contaminated food or water transmits *V. cholerae*. Over a million organisms are necessary to infect humans unless achlorhydria is present, in which case 100 to 10,000 organisms will cause infection. After a brief incubation period, usually 2 to 3 days (range, 6 hours to 5 days), there is the sudden onset of profuse, painless, watery diarrhea. Severe cases may be characterized by rapid fluid loss in excess of 20 L per 24 hours. Profound shock and death can occur within a day if fluid replacement is not instituted.

The acutely ill patient usually appears in a

shocklike state, with soiling of clothes by the excessive fecal discharge. The feces are usually clear, without odor and contain flecks of mucus that impart a "rice-water" appearance. Vomiting without nausea, described as effortless, usually follows the onset of diarrhea. The skin of the hands has a characteristic appearance, resembling wrinkled "washer-woman's hands." Fever, if present, is low grade, or the patient may develop hypothermia.

Salmonellae. Infection with salmonellae may cause one of four types of clinical syndrome: (1) acute gastroenteritis, which is most common; (2) enteric fever; (3) septicemia with or without localized infections; and (4) inapparent infection and carrier state. The clinical manifestations of these syndromes often overlap.

Gastroenteritis. Food poisoning is by far the most common manifestation of *Salmonella* infection, with more than 200,000 cases reported yearly in the United States. The infection varies in severity from mild to extremely severe forms. The onset of symptoms may vary from a few to 72 hours after the ingestion of contaminated food. The illness is due to infection, not ingestion of preformed toxin. Nausea, vomiting, and diarrhea are associated with severe abdominal cramps. Fever and prostration may be pronounced. Chills and feelings of weakness are common. The stools are numerous and may contain mucus, pus, and blood. Such cases are clinically indistinguishable from other causes of bacillary dysentery. Bloody diarrhea is observed often in young children but rarely in adults. Physical findings are scant. Rose spots and meningismus sometimes are present. The spleen is seldom enlarged. In approximately one half of the patients the temperature falls to normal within 1 or 2 days, and recovery is uneventful. In others the disease may last 1 week or more. Protracted or recurrent diarrhea occurs and may represent secondary consequences of mucosal invasion and destruction of the epithelium. In very severe infections the patient may be in shock with cyanosis, hypothermia, and circulatory collapse, which precedes death.

In some cases the gastroenteric type of infection is followed by the septicemic syndrome or by signs of localization. Metastatic foci are more likely to occur in patients with sickle cell disease, infants less than 6 months of age, or an immunocompromised person such as one with AIDS.

The leukocyte count is usually 10,000 to 15,000/μl, with a slight increase in number of polymorphonuclear cells. The leukopenia found in the enteric fever type of infection is seldom seen in the gastroenteric form. Positive blood cultures are more frequent in infants less than 6 months of age and are occasionally found in older persons, especially in ones with severe infections. Stool cultures almost always yield salmonellae during the acute phase of the disease and often for weeks to months thereafter. Symptoms subside despite continued colonization with the organism.

Enteric fever. Although infections caused by salmonellae of various types constitute a serious public health problem, those caused by *S. typhi* have become relatively infrequent in the United States. For example, the number of cases of typhoid fever reported in the United States during the last two decades rarely exceeded 500 per year.

The onset of symptoms of typhoid fever in most cases is gradual, with fever, headache, malaise, and loss of appetite. The typical course in an adult is illustrated in Fig. 7-1. The temperature rises in a steplike manner during 2 to 7 days to an average of approximately 40° C (104° F) and characteristically remains at this level for 3 to 4 weeks in the absence of specific antimicrobial therapy. The pulse rate is slow relative to the fever. Diarrhea is present in some patients, although constipation may persist throughout the infection. Either manifestation may be accompanied by abdominal tenderness, distention, and pain. In the early stages of illness discrete rose-colored spots may be scattered over the trunk, especially the abdomen. The spleen is enlarged in most patients. Severely ill patients may become delirious or stuporous. The white blood cell count as a rule shows leukopenia.

Typhoid fever in the first 2 years of life exhibits certain differences from the clinical course seen in adults. The diagnosis in infancy is often made by the chance isolation of *S. typhi* from stools or blood. The disease may resemble bacillary dysentery. The onset is often abrupt, with high fever, vomiting, convulsions, and meningeal signs. The slow pulse rate is not a frequent finding. Rose spots are seen less commonly than in adults. Leukocytosis is the rule, and the white blood cell count may be as high as 20,000 to

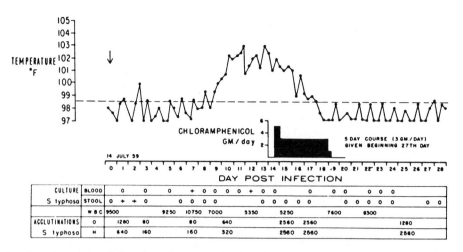

		0	1	2	3	4	5	6	7	8	9	10	11	12	13	14	15	16	17	18	19	20	21	22	23	24	25	26	27	28
CULTURE	BLOOD	0		0		0		+	0	0	0	0		+	0	0			0				0	0		0	0	0		
S typhosa	STOOL	0	+	+	0			0	0	0	0			0	0	0	0			0	0	0	0	0				0		0
	W B C	9500					9250		10750	7000			5350			5250				7600		8300								
ACCLUTINATIONS	O		1280	80			80			640					2560	2560							1280							
S typhosa	H		640	160			160			320					2560	2560							2560							

Fig. 7-1. Summary of the clinical course of induced typhoid fever in an adult volunteer. Therapy consisted of two 5-day courses of chloramphenicol separated by a 1-week interval. (From Hornick RB, et al: N Engl J Med 1970; 283:686.)

25,000/μl, but neutrophils rarely exceed 60% to 70%. The spleen is usually palpable. The course of the disease is short, rarely persisting more than 2 weeks. Although previously the mortality rate in infancy was high (12.5%), probably as a result of dehydration, deaths currently are not common when appropriate therapy is administered.

Salmonellae other than *S. typhi* may produce a disease with all the manifestations of typhoid fever, including persistent fever, GI tract symptoms, rose spots, leukopenia, and positive cultures of blood, stool, and urine specimens.

Septicemia with or without localized infection. Salmonellae are also responsible for a disease characterized by intermittent fever, chills (in adults), anorexia, and loss of weight. The characteristic features of typhoid are absent. Stool cultures are usually negative, although blood cultures yield the causative organism. A focus of infection is identified in approximately one fourth of the patients with bacteremia. The acute focal process may be directly or indirectly connected with the GI tract, causing appendicitis, cholecystitis, peritonitis, or salpingitis. Hematogenous spread of organisms may result in foci of infection in the brain, skin, lungs, spleen, middle ear, bone, or joints. Meningitis is caused by a variety of *Salmonella* types and occurs principally in young infants, with a high morbidity rate. The urinary tract can also be infected.

Osteomyelitis and pyarthrosis are caused by many serotypes. Almost any bone may be involved, but the long bones, spine, and ribs are most commonly affected. Pneumonia occurs, usually is accompanied by a high temperature, and often terminates fatally. This manifestation occurs almost exclusively in elderly patients, many of whom suffer from unrelated medical problems.

Inapparent infection and the carrier state. Asymptomatic infection with salmonellae occurs in an estimated 0.2% of people as documented by positive stool cultures in the absence of clinical illness. Some of these persons have had known contact with symptomatic persons or are being investigated because of a recognized source of contaminated food. Persons who have been infected usually excrete organisms for weeks to months. Carriers of *S. typhi* may excrete organisms for years.

Shigellae. The classic clinical picture of bacillary dysentery is characterized by severe abdominal pain, tenesmus, and constitutional symptoms with frequent stools containing mucus, pus, and blood. Patients with moderately severe disease may have an abrupt onset with fever, abdominal pain, vomiting, and then diarrhea. Stools occur seven to 12 times daily, are watery, green, or yellow, and contain mucus and undigested food. Disease may progress with development of all of the features of dysentery. Acute symptoms may persist for 7 to 10 days, and meningismus, delirium, and convulsions may accompany *Shigella* dysentery. Morbidity and mortality usually result from severe dehydration. The worst illness occurs most frequently at the extremes of life—in young infants, in the elderly, and in debilitated persons. Mild infection with transient diarrhea is a common manifestation of *Shigella* infection. Persons with this mild infection have watery diarrhea or loose stools for a few days, with mild or absent constitutional symptoms.

Campylobacter jejuni. *C.jejuni* may produce bloody diarrhea or watery diarrhea or may be excreted without producing symptoms. Infected individuals may manifest diarrhea, abdominal pain, chills, and fever. Blood, mucus, and fecal leukocytes may be present in stool, resembling the illness produced by *Shigella*. The incubation period is 1 to 7 days. Organisms may be excreted for 2 to 3 weeks in untreated persons.

Yersinia enterocolitica. Diarrhea is the most common manifestation of *Y. enterocolitica* infection and is usually watery or malabsorptive in character. However, infection with these organisms can produce a dysentery syndrome, and systemic signs such as arthritis or erythema nodosum occur. To some extent, signs and symptoms are age related in that infants more commonly manifest the infection as febrile diarrhea. Older children and adolescents have acute mesenteric adenitis and/or ileitis and may have findings suggestive of appendicitis. Adults have diarrhea with fever, enterocolitis, arthritis, and erythema nodosum. Acute bacteremia with metastatic foci, including the liver and spleen, occurs in elderly adults or immunocompromised hosts.

Giardia lamblia. Clinical symptoms in individuals infected with *Giardia* include an acute diarrheal illness characterized by nausea, bloating, and abdominal cramps. More rarely and especially in immunocompromised individuals, there may be a chronic illness manifested by a protracted, intermittent, frequently debilitating diarrhea (Pickering and Engelkirk, 1988). The malabsorption and anorexia that occur can result in significant weight loss and failure to thrive.

Diagnosis and differential diagnosis

The bacteria presented and the viruses enumerated in the latter part of this chapter, plus *G. lamblia*, *Entamoeba histolytica*, *Cryptospor-idium*, *Isospora belli*, Microsporidia, and *Strongyloides stercoralis* comprise the most common causative agents of GI tract infection. The age of the patient, life-style, geographical setting, and broad classification of symptoms provide the clinical framework for establishing the cause. Examination of stool for the presence of leukocytes and/or blood provides insight into whether the organism is invasive. Laboratory culture can detect *V. cholerae*, *Salmonella*, *Shigella*, *Campylobacter*, and *Y. enterocolitica*. Laboratory confirmation of *E. coli*–associated disease is not generally accessible because detection of toxins or invasive properties requires cell culture, animal models, or other specific assays. Serotyping of *E. coli* in diarrheal outbreaks in infants is potentially helpful for recognition of EPEC but probably provides epidemiological insights of an outbreak more effectively than diagnostic help with a single infant. The most common EHEC, *E. coli* O157:H7, should be suspected if non-sorbitol-fermenting *E. coli* are present; confirmation in a local public health laboratory is necessary.

S. typhi frequently is detected in blood cultures during the first 2 weeks of illness, and when enteric fever is suspected, blood and bone marrow for culture must be obtained. In patients not from endemic areas serological tests may be helpful if they are positive, as they will be in approximately two of three patients. Usually a single agglutinin titer of 1:320 or greater for antibody to the O antigen alerts the physician to consider typhoid. Recent vaccination, infection with another *Salmonella*, or liver disease may give false-positive agglutinins.

Most clinical microbiology laboratories now include Campy BAP and Butzler's media, or Skirrow's medium for culture of stool at 42° C in a low oxygen, high carbon dioxide environment for *C.jejuni*. However, since this practice is not universal, the physician must be aware of the available laboratory facilities.

V. cholerae presents diagnostic problems in the United States where it is an uncommon pathogen. The unprepared laboratory may miss the diagnosis, so it is essential that the clinician suspect the diagnosis, alert the laboratory, and thus increase the likelihood of a correct diagnosis. *V. cholerae* grows rapidly on certain alkaline-enrichment media such as thiosulfate citrate bile salts sucrose (TCBS) agar, which has a pH greater than 6.0. The organisms can be distinguished from other enteric bacteria on TCBS agar since they form characteristic opaque yellow colonies.

Similarly, to culture *Y. enterocolitica*, laboratory personnel must be alerted to use specific conditions and/or media to facilitate growth and recognition of this organism.

Prognosis

The prognosis is largely dependent on the age and nutritional status of the patient and the presence of an underlying disease. The vast majority of gastroenteritis is self-limited with no complications and complete recovery. The very young, the aged, and those with protein-calorie malnutrition or underlying disease are at risk for complications and/or prolonged illness. Overall, fatality from any of these agents seldom exceeds 1% when health care delivery is adequate. Those with meningitis or endocarditis caused by *Salmonella* have a much higher mortality rate.

Complications

The severity of acute bacterial gastroenteritis is correlated best with fluid and electrolyte loss and the extent of dehydration. Most of these infections are self-limited and localized to the GI tract. The availability of fluid replacement has altered the morbidity and mortality rates of cholera. Extracellular volume depletion secondary to the intestinal loss of isotonic fluid, acidosis secondary to bicarbonate loss in stool, and hypokalemia secondary to fecal potassium loss are the major deficits during cholera. Abnormalities in renal function occur secondary to the initial deficits, and renal failure has even occurred as a result of hypovolemia and shock. Replacement fluids have diminished the morbidity rate for all diarrheal illnesses, and specific antibiotics have contributed to effective therapy of several of these entities. In developing nations in which nutrition is poor, diarrheal illnesses often contribute to protein-calorie malnutrition, growth failure, and susceptibility to additional pathogens.

Salmonella suppurative foci such as meningitis, pyarthrosis, and osteomyelitis occur infrequently. The patient may have an altered mental status, with a spectrum of effects including delirium, stupor, and aphasia. It is important to ascertain if direct invasion of the central nervous system (CNS) has occurred in the presence of such signs and symptoms. Fortunately, GI tract perforation and hemorrhage are extremely rare even with *S. typhi*, primarily because infections are treated. These complications characteristically occur after 2 weeks of untreated disease. Relapse may occur in 15% to 20% of treated *S. typhi* patients and does so usually within 10 to 18 days of stopping antibiotics. Chronic carriage of *S. typhi* has been attributed to chronic infection of the gallbladder.

Although the pathogenesis of Reiter's syndrome is not clear, it has been observed in association with *Salmonella, Campylobacter, Yersinia,* and *Shigella* infections.

Unusually *Y. enterocolitica* can cause chronic and recurrent enteric symptoms, which respond to antibiotic therapy. Septicemic illness is potentially severe and has occurred in immunocompromised hosts. The nonsuppurative arthritis is usually self-limited and normally lasts a few months.

Immunity

ETEC must be able to adhere to the mucosa to elaborate their toxins and produce disease. Immunization of animals with organisms bearing fimbrial adherence antigens but not elaborating toxin produces protection to homologous organisms that do elaborate toxin. Apparently, local antibody directed at fimbrial (attachment) factors prevents disease by blocking attachment. A series of epidemiological observations in humans supports the concept of acquired immunity: (1) breast milk can confer passive protection to an infant's GI tract; (2) that the disease primarily affects infants in the endemic areas suggests that immunity is acquired; and (3) adults from areas in which organisms are endemic have less disease than travelers from nonendemic areas. Challenge and rechallenge studies in adult volunteers have corroborated the epidemiological findings with the demonstration of homologous immunity against disease. However, the asymptomatic subjects shed organisms in the same quantity and for the same period of time, suggesting that antibodies are not bactericidal. Despite these data, it is still appreciated that a person can experience diarrhea caused by ETEC more than once. Several colonization factors already are known, each inducing only homologous antibodies; this is one explanation for several episodes of disease. The LT elaborated by various human *E. coli* is believed to be the same. Serum antibody to LT is easily measured as is GI tract antibody to toxin after natural infection; thus an explanation for repeated disease is needed. It is known that ST toxin is a poor immunogen, and no local IgA antibodies can be measured with infection. Organisms often elaborate both LT and ST, so repeated disease could be due to ST. Finally, it is also becoming apparent that adherence is more complex than the single protein CFAs. Multiple factors contribute to adherence.

Enteroinvasive *E. coli* have surface antigens that cross-react with those of shigellae and are essential for virulence. Local (secretory IgA) antibody develops within the first week of illness and is probably protective against disease. Circulating antibodies also develop, but it is doubtful that they contribute to protection.

V. cholerae stimulate a complex series of responses on the part of the host. Humoral IgM and IgG bactericidal antibodies can be measured, wane over the months following infection, and correlate in general with resistance to cholera. Systemic antibody to cholera toxin is also demonstrable but without any correlation with resistance to infection. It has been suggested that local antibody both to toxin and to the organism is important in protecting the host. Breast milk diminishes occurrence of disease, but infants still may be colonized. Whole killed organisms used as parenteral vaccine provide suboptimal protection, with development of humoral immunity to the organism without local antibody to either organism or toxin. Similarly, parenteral administration of toxoid provides no GI protection by production of only humoral antibodies against toxin. Challenge and rechallenge studies in adults demonstrate that immunity can be induced; measurable local antibody to toxin and to humoral vibriocidal and antitoxin antibodies occurs.

General control measures

Interruption of the intestinal-oral circuit is essential for diminishing transmission of enteric pathogens. Individual patients should be isolated during the illness. Strict handwashing should be initiated as well as appropriate processing or disposal of contaminated materials.

For those pathogens such as *S. typhi* and *Shi-gella* species that are exclusively human pathogens, the incidence of disease can be diminished by (1) sanitary disposal of human feces, (2) purification and protection of water supplies, (3) pasteurization of milk and milk products, (4) strict sanitary supervision of preparation and serving of all foods, (5) proper refrigeration of food and milk, and (6) exclusion of persons with diarrhea from handling food.

Reducing the spread of enteric pathogens where animal reservoirs play an important role is more complex. Any food or drink contaminated with organisms can transmit infection. Animal reservoirs are probably responsible for the majority of human *Salmonella* infections in the United States. Poultry and milk products often are implicated, either directly or indirectly, with contamination of meat-processing areas, markets, or kitchens. By-products of the meat packing industry (e.g., fertilizer or bone meal) perpetuate infection in animals. Prevention of *Salmonella* infections in humans depends on interrupting transmission. The task of controlling salmonellosis among animals and preventing the spread of infection to people is enormous. Continued surveillance is needed to identify and to eliminate the multiple sources of infection.

Treatment

Infants, children, and adults with gastroenteritis require fluid replacement. Oral hydration with fluid containing carbohydrates and electrolytes has significantly reduced the morbidity and mortality from diarrheal disease. Hospitalization is usually not necessary unless a fluid deficit of ≥5% has occurred and rehydration cannot be provided through oral solutions. *V. cholerae* causes the most rapid losses, and replacement may be an emergency. Since glucose-coupled electrolyte and water transport across the epithelium are unaltered by the various toxins, it is possible to replace fluids orally. Replacement fluids should not be prepared by parents without medical supervision, for there is a tendency to think that if a little salt is good, a lot is better. Hypernatremia is thus a risk of inappropriately prepared fluid and electrolyte solutions. Fluid replacement using the World Health Organization (WHO) formulation, mixed and used as recommended, is preferred. Premixed fluid and electrolyte replacement solutions are also

Table 7-3. Antimicrobial therapy for organisms causing gastroenteritis

Organism	Antimicrobial agent
Escherichia coli:	
EPEC, ETEC, EIEC	Trimethoprim-sulfamethoxazole (TMP-SMX)
EHEC, EAEC	Uncertain
Salmonella gastroenteritis	None (ampicillin, TMP-SMX, chloramphenicol, ceftriaxone, or cefotaxime for other sites of infection)
Salmonella typhi	Chloramphenicol, TMP-SMX, ampicillin, cefotaxime, or ceftriaxone
Shigellae	TMP-SMX or nalidixic acid for resistant strains or ciprofloxacin for resistant strains if patient is more than 17 years of age
Vibrio cholerae	Tetracycline if patient is more than 9 years of age; TMP-SMX if less than 9 years of age
Yersinia enterocolitica	TMP-SMX, tetracycline, or aminoglycoside
Campylobacter jejuni	Erythromycin

available and are preferable if cost is not an issue.

Drugs such as motility inhibitors or analgesics are not recommended because they do not alter the fluid loss and in some situations have been implicated in prolongation and exacerbation of symptoms (Dupont and Hornick, 1973).

It is well documented that specific antimicrobial therapy (Table 7-3) alters the course of typhoid and *Shigella* infections. Additionally the period of time shigellae are excreted is shortened; therefore communicability is lessened. In contrast, the course of infections of salmonellae, other than *S. typhi*, is not altered by antibiotics, and excretion of the organisms may be prolonged by their use. Routine antibiotic therapy is not of benefit. Many experts recommend therapy for infants and immunocompromised patients with *Salmonella* gastroenteritis with appropriate antimicrobial agents because of the risk of dissemination of organisms. It is hoped that therapy during the acute gastroenteritis phase will provide protection while the patient develops an immune response to the organism, thereby diminishing the risk of bacteremia. Patients with *Salmonella* infections in sites other than the GI tract should also be treated with parenteral antimicrobial agents.

V. cholerae, ETEC, and *C. jejuni* infections are all treated with antibiotics when the patient is symptomatic and the organism has been identified. Excretion of the organism is shortened, and therapy may alter the disease. Toxins attach to epithelial cells and generally penetrate membranes. It appears that their effects are perma-

nent; that is, the epithelial cell must be sloughed before effects will cease. Thus antibiotics may stop organisms from elaborating toxin but do not immediately alter symptoms. At present, it is unclear whether antibiotics decrease the severity of illness or complications with *Y. enterocolitica*, EHEC, and EAEC.

Specific antimicrobial therapy often is administered empirically to the febrile, dehydrated individual with gastroenteritis. Table 7-3 lists the organisms and drugs used for therapy. Trimethoprim-sulfamethoxazole (TMP-SMX) has been effective in treating *Shigella* infections and diarrhea associated with *E. coli*. Therefore, when the physician feels obligated to treat the child with diarrhea, electing to use an absorbable compound such as TMP-SMX or ampicillin has a better chance of being effective against the entire spectrum of pathogens. Children with resistant strains of *Shigella* can be treated with nalidixic acid or ceftriaxone, whereas adults respond to ciprofloxacin or norfloxacin. Suspicion of *S. typhi* or *V. cholerae* in areas in which these infections are endemic would affect the choice of drug. If the stool culture yields *C. jejuni*, erythromycin is the drug of choice and should be given early in the course of disease. Therapy for patients with diarrhea caused by *Y. enterocolitica* has not been demonstrated as beneficial.

Confirmation of infection by *G. lamblia* depends on demonstration of cysts or trophozoites by microscopic examination of stool, duodenal aspirate, or biopsy material. Stools may be examined fresh or preferably after preservation in formalin or polyvinyl alcohol and subsequent trichrome iron hematoxylin staining. Formalin-ether or zinc sulfate flotation concentration techniques may increase the yield. Rapid diagnostic tests that detect *Giardia* antigens in stool specimens also are available (Knisley et al., 1989).

Quinacrine (Atabrine), metronidazole (Flagyl), and furazolidone (Furoxone) are specific therapeutic agents for patients with *G. lamblia*. Furazolidone (6 mg/kg/day in four doses orally for 7 days, maximum of 400 mg/day) is the only drug that is available in liquid suspension for use in young children (Pickering and Engelkirk, 1989).

Metronidazole is not approved for treatment of patients with giardiasis in the United States, but it is widely used. Quinacrine has frequent toxic side effects, including yellow discoloration of skin and sclerae, nausea and vomiting, toxic psychosis, and exfoliative dermatitis. Both metronidazole and quinacrine have an unpleasant taste that precludes ingestion by children. Relapse is common in immunocompromised patients, and therapy in these individuals may need prolongation.

Immunization

Vibrio cholerae. Parenterally inoculated, killed whole cell vaccine has been available for years. This vaccine stimulates high titers of serum vibriocidal antibodies, but it does not induce antibodies to toxin. In an individual previously primed by GI tract contact with *V. cholerae*, the vaccine also produces an anamnestic response in GI tract IgA directed against the O antigen. In field trials homologous protection by vaccine has been induced for approximately 1 year, with vaccine efficacy approximately 70%. Local GI tract immunity against the organism and against the toxin should provide a better, less reactogenic immunogen. Using recombinant DNA technology, an "attenuated" *V. cholerae* organism that lacks the genes for production of the A and B subunits of toxin was created. A plasmid containing the B subunit gene was then constructed and inserted. Thus a candidate live *V. cholerae* vaccine containing all the cell-wall antigens necessary for adherence and the capacity to produce only the B subunit of toxin has been engineered (Levine et al., 1984). In theory it could provide ideal local immunity

without toxicity. Initial trials have demonstrated a vaccine efficacy of 90% to rechallenge with virulent organisms.

Enterotoxigenic Escherichia coli. Humans produce serum IgM and secretory IgA antibodies to the homologous O antigen of an infecting strain of ETEC. These antibodies do not prevent adherence of the organism or action of the toxin. Experience with ETEC in animals has greatly advanced the understanding of the disease and its prevention. The disease can be prevented by blocking adherence of organisms; for human ETEC infections this requires delineation of all the critical colonizing factors because only homologous immunity is produced. Purified fimbriae (CFA-2), given orally, has produced a local IgA response that primed the recipient. Later a parenteral inoculation of CFA-2 was given to stimulate a humoral and secretory immune response.

Any effective immunogen should induce a local antibody response to LT and ST. Since ST is a poor immunogen, such approaches as conjugation of the ST toxoid to the B (receptor) subunit of LT are being investigated.

Salmonella typhi. A live attenuated oral typhoid vaccine has become available. This vaccine is the stable mutant of *S. typhi* strain Ty21a. It lacks an enzyme, UDP-galactose-4-epimerase, that normally converts UDP-glucose to UDP-galactose. Since galactose is essential for its lipopolysaccharide, absence of the enzyme forces the organism to use exogenous galactose, thereby accumulating galactose-1-phosphate and UDP-galactose. In the presence of galactose these organisms lyse spontaneously. The results of field trials have shown that infections were reduced by approximately 70% in high-risk areas during the 4 years after vaccination. Although the older inactivated vaccines are still available, the new vaccine is preferred for all those who must be vaccinated, with the exception of those with immunodeficiency, including persons with AIDS. Side effects are minimal with the attenuated vaccine, unlike the inactivated vaccines, which often produce severe systemic and local adverse reactions.

Shigella. No vaccine currently is available for *Shigella*. Various attenuated organisms were tested in the 1960s and 1970s without demonstration of consistent efficacy; however, work is ongoing.

group A rotaviruses most frequently occurs in children 6 months to 24 months of age. Incidence rates in community-based and day-care center studies in this age group range from 0.2 to 0.8 episodes per child per year (Kapikian et al., 1976; Brandt et al., 1979). Rotaviruses cause up to 50% of the episodes of diarrhea requiring hospitalization and are common causes of outbreaks in children in day-care centers and hospitals (Bartlett et al., 1988). Serotypes 1 and 3 are the most frequently isolated serotypes from children with rotavirus diarrhea in the United States. Rotaviruses can be excreted for several days before and for up to 10 days after diarrhea occurs, with the quantity of virus highest early in the course of illness. Transmission occurs through the fecal-oral route. The incubation period ranges from 1 to 3 days.

Both types 40 and 41 of enteric adenovirus apparently are widespread and cause endemic diarrhea and outbreaks of diarrhea in hospitals, orphanages, and day-care centers. These viruses infect children more than adults (Kotloff et al., 1989), with antibody prevalence studies showing more than 50% of children are seropositive by the third to fourth year of life. Infection appears to occur all year. The mode of transmission is fecal-oral, and the incubation period lasts from 3 to 10 days.

Epidemic gastroenteritis caused by the Norwalk group of viruses may affect an entire community. Outbreaks have involved school-age children, family contacts, and adults. Roughly one third of the identified outbreaks of gastroenteritis may be attributed to a Norwalklike agent. Outbreaks have occurred at all times of the year, and antibody surveys suggest that the agent is worldwide in distribution. Transmission of Norwalk virus occurs as a result of ingestion of contaminated food (shellfish, salads, and cake frosting) or water and by person-to-person spread. In the less-developed nations antibody is detected in early childhood. In the United States antibody usually develops during late adolescence and early adulthood.

Astrovirus has been associated with diarrhea worldwide and has been linked to outbreaks of diarrhea in schools, pediatric wards, and nursing homes. Illness occurs mainly in children and the elderly. More than 80% of adults have antibodies against the virus. Astrovirus may account for 3% of hospital admissions for diarrhea.

Antibodies to calicivirus have been demon-strated in virtually all children by the age of 5 years. Studies in day-care centers showed that calicivirus-associated diarrhea and asymptomatic infection are both widespread. Human calicivirus infections occur year-round as a result of fecal-oral transmission. This virus may be a cause of foodborne outbreaks of gastroenteritis. The incubation period is approximately 4 days.

Coronaviruses are unlikely causes of diarrhea within the first year of life. They have been visualized more commonly in the diarrheal stools of older children and young adults. The prolonged excretion of virus makes it difficult to assess the role of these agents in the etiology of gastroenteritis.

Pathogenesis and pathology

Rotavirus is excreted in extraordinarily high concentrations early in the course of the illness, with as many as 10^{11} particles per gram of feces. Rotaviral particles have been visualized by electron microscopy in intestinal epithelial cells, aspirated duodenal secretions, and feces of infected persons. Morphologically, shortening and blunting of the villi of the duodenum and upper small intestine accompany acute illness. The microvilli of the absorptive cells are distorted, and other cells have swollen mitochondria. Rotavirus particles infect the mature enterocytes located in the middle and upper villous epithelium. This destruction of the mature enterocyte is associated with a decrease in the surface area of the intestine and decreased production of one or more mucosal disaccharidases. The destroyed infected cells are replaced by immature cells, resulting in a deficit in glucose-facilitated sodium transport. Diarrhea then results from decreased absorption secondary to the altered ion transport. Complete recovery has been confirmed by biopsy as early as 4 weeks after the episode of diarrhea. There is no evidence of infection outside the GI tract by these viruses, although associated respiratory tract symptoms are common and liver involvement has been demonstrated in immunodeficient mice and humans.

The Norwalk-like group of agents are also transmitted by the fecal-oral route. Infected volunteers have had detectable virus in their stools during the first 72 hours after the onset of illness. Infection with these agents results in delayed gastric emptying, although the gastric mucosa is morphologically normal. Microscopic broadening and blunting of the villi in the jejunum are apparent. The mucosa remains histologically intact, but there is a mononuclear cell infiltration. Viruses have not yet been detected in involved mucosal cells. Small intestinal enzyme studies showed decreased amounts of the enzymes measured. The incubation period is approximately 48 hours.

Clinical manifestations

Acute infections caused by rotavirus are characterized by an abrupt onset of watery diarrhea that is not characteristically associated with blood or mucus in the stool. The mean duration of illness in immunocompetent hosts is 5 to 7 days, but chronic infection can occur in immunodeficient children, and disease can be more severe in malnourished hosts. Vomiting is often present before or after onset of diarrhea. Dehydration and metabolic acidosis are common and may necessitate hospitalization. Rotaviruses are responsible for at least one half of the cases of infantile diarrhea requiring hospitalization. There is evidence that rotavirus may cause liver damage, especially in immunodeficient hosts. In children in day-care centers asymptomatic infections represent up to 50% of all rotavirus infections. Recurrent infections are common in children in day-care and in other settings in which exposure is frequent.

Enteric adenoviruses cause diarrhea that lasts 6 to 9 days and may be associated with emesis and fever. The diarrhea is watery without blood or fecal leukocytes. Persistent lactose intolerance has been reported.

Roughly one third of identified outbreaks of gastroenteritis can be attributed to a Norwalk-like agent. The outbreaks have occurred in schools, recreation camps, cruise ships, and nursing homes and after ingestion of inadequately cooked contaminated shellfish or contaminated water. Although respiratory tract symptoms are unusual in patients with Norwalk infections, the rapidity of spread suggests the possibility of aerosolization of virus. Most patients who sustain these infections have nausea, vomiting, and abdominal cramps, and approximately half of them have associated diarrhea. Fever and chills are less common. The symptoms last from 12 to 24 hours, and the incubation period apparently is approximately 48 hours. Usually stools are not bloody and do not contain mucus or lymphocytes. Transient lymphopenia has been observed in volunteers challenged with these agents.

Diarrhea caused by astroviruses usually occurs in children and in the elderly, with disease rarely becoming manifest in older adults. Symptoms include low-grade fever, malaise, and watery diarrhea that usually last 3 days. Vomiting is uncommon. Cow's milk intolerance has been reported after the infection. The incubation period is 1 to 4 days.

The clinical symptoms produced by calicivirus are similar to those produced by rotavirus. Asymptomatic infection is common. Viral excretion usually lasts less than 1 week.

Diagnosis and differential diagnosis

The clinical differentiation of viral from bacterial gastroenteritis is often difficult. Various epidemiological factors such as season and age may be helpful, but laboratory support is needed to substantiate a clinical diagnosis. The most widely used assays for detection of a viral enteropathogen are electron microscopy, immune electron microscopy, enzyme-linked immunosorbent assay (ELISA), latex agglutination, gel electrophoresis, and culture of the virus. Different assays currently are used for each virus. Commercially available assays are available only for detection of rotavirus and enteric adenoviruses.

For detection of rotavirus in stool specimens, the original diagnostic technique of electron microscopy is still used as the single method available to identify all of the viral pathogens, including group A and non–group A rotavirus. The ELISA and latex agglutination assays are more generally available and detect group A rotaviruses. As a general rule, latex agglutination tests have shown as high a specificity but a lower sensitivity when compared to ELISA (Dennehy et al., 1988). Electropherotyping is a valuable means of studying the epidemiology of rotavirus infection but is not used as a diagnostic test. Oligonucleotide probes and polymerase chain reaction (PCR) tests are currently being evaluated (Gouvea et al., 1990). Serological assays for total antibody to rotavirus or serotype-specific response are useful to substantiate an infection but are not useful diagnostic tests during the acute course of an infection.

Electron microscopy initially was used to detect enteric adenoviruses, but commercially available assays that use monoclonal antibodies incorporated into ELISA techniques are now available. Enteric adenoviruses can be cultivated in special cell lines. Restriction enzyme analysis is the definitive method used for classifying individual isolates.

Electron microscopy is used to detect Norwalk-like viruses in stool. Immune electron microscopy and radioimmunoassay are not generally available. Specific coating of the particle with antibody must be observed if the immune response is being assessed. Radioimmunoassay is more efficient than immune electron microscopy because it can detect both soluble antigens and particulate antigens. This test is dependent on the availability of appropriate high-titered serum from volunteers.

Astroviruses grow in human embryonic kidney cells in the presence of trypsin. Electron microscopy, immune electron microscopy, and immunofluorescence of cell culture can be used as detection methods. A monoclonal antibody-based ELISA has been developed (Herman et al., 1990).

Caliciviruses can be detected in stools by electron microscopy. Both immune electron microscopy and ELISA are more sensitive techniques but are not readily available.

Complications

Severe dehydration as a consequence of vomiting and diarrhea is the major complication of viral gastroenteritis, especially in young infants or elderly debilitated adults.

Prognosis

In general, the prognosis with any of these viral infections of the GI tract is excellent. The illness is self-limited and usually lasts a matter of days.

Immunity

After rotavirus infection a systemic rise in IgA, IgM, and IgG occurs, as does a rise in secretory IgA. Newborns asymptomatically infected with rotavirus appear to have less severe disease after a reexposure to rotavirus later in life than children with no early exposure. The role of preexisting homotypic and heterotypic serum and secretory antirotavirus antibodies in the prevention of systemic rotavirus infection is under in-

vestigation. Protective immunity to rotavirus is most probably directed against VP7 and/or VP4. It appears the humoral antibody response in humans may be homotypic in infants and small children and heterotypic in older children and adults with a previous exposure. The role of cell-mediated immunity in rotavirus infection is being evaluated.

Specific antibody has been demonstrated in colostrum and milk for as long as 9 months of lactation. In nurseries where rotavirus infection has been endemic, breast-fed infants seem to acquire infection less often than formula-fed infants. Those who are infected excrete less virus and are less often symptomatic. Antibodies in human colostrum and milk are capable of neutralizing rotavirus in vitro. Weaning from breast milk in developing nations is temporally associated with onset of the diarrhea-malnutrition cycle.

Immunity to the Norwalk-like virus is a puzzling feature of the infections that they cause. Challenge of volunteers will produce disease in some persons and not in others. Repeat challenge with a homologous virus within several months of the original infection will not produce clinical illness. Subsequent challenge 2 to 4 years later produces disease in the same volunteers who had symptomatic illness with the first contact with the virus. Those individuals who were asymptomatic and did not acquire infection with the first contact did not do so with subsequent challenge. Those individuals who acquire clinical infection have demonstrable antibody that wanes but rises after a subsequent challenge a short time later. Volunteers who fail to develop illness have no demonstrable antibody. Individuals who develop illness have higher mean antibody titers in jejunal fluid than do those who remain well. Neither serum nor local intestinal antibody correlates with resistance to Norwalk virus challenge. Thus those individuals who have demonstrable serum antibody are at risk for symptomatic infection. These findings are not understood, but it is possible that some individuals are resistant to these viruses because of genetically determined factors.

Treatment

The general principles of rehydration therapy are the same as those described for bacterial gastroenteritis. There is no specific antiviral therapy for any of the viral enteropathogens.

Preventive measures

Appropriate hygiene and frequent handwashing are necessary for interruption of the fecal-oral spread of these agents. Careful food preparation measures must be enforced to reduce spread by contaminated food and water.

Prevention of rotavirus infection would be a major contribution in reduction of the morbidity from gastroenteritis. To achieve effective immunization, immunity within the GI tract is probably a necessity. Various approaches to immunization are being considered. Reassortant viruses containing the gene from the human rotavirus-encoding VP7 and the remaining 10 genes from an animal rotavirus are being studied.

REFERENCES

Attridge SR, Rowley D. The role of the flagellum in the adherence of *V. cholerae*. J Infect Dis 1983;147:864-872.

Bartlett AV III, Reves RR, Pickering LK. Rotavirus in infant-toddler day care centers: epidemiology relevant to disease control strategies. J Pediatr 1988; 113:435-441.

Bartlett AV, Prado D, Cleary TG, Pickering LK. Production of shigatoxin and other enterotoxins by serogroups of *Shigella*. J Infect Dis 1986;154:996-1002.

Bhan MK, Raj P, Levine MM, et al. Enteroaggregative *E. coli* associated with persistent diarrhea in a cohort of rural children in India. 1989;159:1061-1064.

Bishop RF, Davidson GP, Holmes IH, Ruck BJ. Evidence for viral gastroenteritis. N Engl J Med 1973;289:1096.

Blaser MJ, Reller LB. *Campylobacter* enteritis. N Engl J Med 1981; 305:1444-1452.

Brandt CD, Kim HW, Rodriguez WJ et al. Adenovirus and pediatric gastroenteritis. J Infect Dis 1985;151:437-443.

Brandt CD, Kim HW, Rodriguez WJ, et al. Comparative epidemiology of two rotavirus serotypes and other viral agents associated with pediatric gastroenteritis. Am J Epidemiol 1979;110(3):243-54.

Clausen CR, Christie DL. Chronic diarrhea in infants caused by adherent enteropathogenic *E. coli*. J Pediatr 1982; 100:358-61.

Cleary TG. Cytotoxin producing *E. coli* and the hemolytic uremic syndrome. Pediatr Clin North Am 1988; 30:485-501.

Connolly GM, Shanson D, Hawkins DA, et al. Noncryptosporidial diarrhoea in human immunodeficiency virus (HIV) infected patients. Gut 1989;30:195-200.

Dennehy PH, Gauntlett DR, Tente WE. Comparison of nine commercial immunoassays for the detection of rotavirus in fecal specimens. J Clin Microbiol 1988;26:1630-1634.

Dolin R, et al. Biological properties of Norwalk agent of acute infectious nonbacterial gastroenteritis. Proc Soc Exp Biol Med 1972;140:578.

DuPont HL, Hornick RB. Adverse effects of Lomotil therapy in shigellosis. JAMA 1973;226:1525.

Eidels L, Proia RL, Hart DA. Membrane receptors for bacterial toxins. Microbiol Rev 1983;47:596-620.

Estes MK, Cohen J. Rotavirus gene structure and function. Microbiol Rev 1989;53:410-449.

Fekety R. Recent advances in management of bacterial diarrhea. Rev Infect Dis 1983;5:246-257.

Goldschmidt MC, DuPont JL. Enteropathogenic *Escherichia coli:* lack of correlation of serotype with pathogenicity. J Infect Dis 1976;133:153.

Gorbach SL, Khurana CM. Toxigenic *Escherichia coli:* a cause of infantile diarrhea in Chicago. N Engl J Med 1971;287:791.

Gorbach SL, et al. Travelers' diarrhea and toxigenic *Escherichia coli*. N Engl J Med 1975;292:933.

Gouvea V, Glass RI, Woods P, et al. Polymerase chain reaction amplification and typing of rotavirus nucleic acid from stool specimens. J Clin Microbiol 1990; 28:276-282.

Grady GF, Keusch GT. Pathogenesis of bacterial diarrheas. N Engl J Med 1971;285:831.

Green KY, Taniguchi K, Mackow ER, et al. Homotypic and heterotypic epitope-specific antibody responses in adult and infant rotavirus vaccines: implications for vaccine development. J Infect Dis 1990;161:667-679.

Gutman LT, et al. An inter-familial outbreak of *Yersinia enterocolitica* enteritis. N Engl J Med 1973;288:1372.

Herrman JE, Nowak NA, Perron-Henry DM et al. Diagnosis of astrovirus gastroenteritis by antigen detection with monoclonal antibodies. J Infect Dis 1990; 161:226-229.

Holmgren J. Actions of cholera toxin and the prevention and treatment of cholera. Nature 1981;292:413.

Hornick RB, et al. Typhoid fever: pathogenesis and immunologic control. N Engl J Med 1970;283:686, 739.

Janoff EN, Smith PD, Blaser MJ. Acute antibody responses to *Giardia lamblia* are depressed in patients with AIDS. J Infect Dis 1988;157:798-804.

Kapikian AZ, et al. Visualization by immune electronmicroscopy of a 27-nm particle associated with acute infectious non-bacterial gastroenteritis. J Virol 1972;10:1075.

Kapikian AZ, et al. Reovirus-like agent in stools: association with infantile diarrhea and development of serologic tests. Science 1974;185:1049.

Kapikian AZ, et al. Human reovirus-like agent as the major pathogen associated with "winter" gastroenteritis in hospitalized infants, young children and their contacts. N Engl J Med 1976;294:965.

Karmali MA, Fleming PC. *Campylobacter* enteritis in children. J Pediatr 1979;94:527.

Karmali MA, Petric M, Steele BT, Lin C. Sporadic cases of haemolytic uremic syndrome associated with faecal cytotoxin and cytotoxin producing *E. coli* in stools. Lancet 1983;1:619-620.

Knisley CV, Engelkirk PG, Pickering LK, et al. Rapid detection of *Giardia* antigen in stool using enzyme immunoassays. Am J Clin Pathol 1989;91:704-708.

Kotloff KL, Losonsky GA, Morris JG, et al. Enteric adenovirus infection and childhood diarrhea: an epidemiologic study in three clinical settings. Pediatrics 1989; 84:219-225.

Laughon BE, Druckman DA, Vernon A, et al. Prevalence of enteric pathogens in homosexual men with and without acquired immunodeficiency syndrome. Gastroenterology 1988;94:984-993.

Levine MM, Berquist EJ, Nalin DR, et al. *E. coli* strains that cause diarrhea but do not produce heat-labile or heat stable enterotoxins are non-invasive. Lancet 1978;1:1119-1122.

Levine MM, Black RE, Clements ML, et al. Duration of infection derived immunity to cholera. J Infect Dis 1981;143:818-820.

Levine MM, Black RE, Clements ML, et al. Evaluation in humans of attenuated *V. cholerae* El Tor Ogawa strain Texas State-SR as a live oral vaccine. Infect Immunol 1984;43:515-522.

Levine MM, Edelman R. Enteropathogenic *E. coli* of classic serotypes associated with infant diarrhea: epidemiology and pathogenesis. Epidemiol Rev 1984;6:31-51.

Levine MM, Kaper JB, Black RE, Clements ML. New knowledge on pathogenesis of bacterial enteric infections as applied to vaccine development. Microsci Rev 1983;47:510-550.

Levine MM, Nalin DR, Hoover DL, et al. Immunity to ETEC. Infect Immunol 1979;23:729-736.

Levine WC, Stephenson WT, Craun GF. Waterborne disease outbreaks 1986-1988. MMWR 1990;39:1-14.

Mathewson JJ, Oberhelman RA, DuPont HL, et al. Enteroadherent *E. coli* as a cause of diarrhea among children in Mexico. J Clin Microbiol 1987;25:1917-1919.

Matson DO, Estes MK, Burns JW, et al. Serotype variation of human group A rotaviruses in two regions of the United States. J Infect Dis 1990;162:605-614.

Matson DO, Estes MK, Tanaka T, et al. Asymptomatic human calicivirus infection in a day care center. Pediatr Infect Dis J 1990;9:180-186.

Novak R, Feldman S. Salmonellosis in children with cancer: review of 42 cases. Am J Dis Child 1979;133:298.

Okada S, Sekine S, Andol T, et al. Antigenic characterization of small, round-structured viruses by immune electron microscopy. J Clin Microbiol 1990;28:1244-1248.

O'Ryan ML, Matson DO. Viral gastroenteritis pathogens in the day care center setting. Semin Pediatr Infect Dis 1990;1:252-262.

O'Ryan ML, Matson DO, Estes MK, et al. Molecular epidemiology of rotavirus in children attending day care centers in Houston. J Infect Dis 1990;162:810-816.

Pai CH, Sorger S, Lackman L. *Campylobacter* gastroenteritis in children. J Pediatr 1979;94:589.

Pickering LK, Engelkirk PG. *Giardia lamblia*. Pediatr Clin North Am 1988;35:565-567.

Pickering LK, Bartlett AV, Reves RR, et al. Asymptomatic excretion of rotavirus before and after rotavirus diarrhea in children in day care centers. J Pediatr 1988;112:361-365.

Pickering LK, DuPont HL, Olarte J. Single-dose tetracycline therapy for shigellosis in adults. JAMA 1978;239:853.

Prasad BVV, Burns JW, Mariette E, et al. Localization of VP4 neutralization sites in rotavirus by three dimensional cryoelectron microscopy. Nature 1990;343:476-479.

Quinn TC, Stamm WE, Goodnell SE, et al. The polymicrobial origin of intestinal infections in homosexual men. N Engl J Med 1983;309:75 582.

Riley IW, et al. Hemorrhagic colitis associated with a rare *E. coli* serotype. N Engl J Med 1983;308:681-685.

Robins-Browne RM, Levine MM, Rowe B, Gabriel EM. Failure to detect conventional enterotoxins in classical enteropathogenic (serotyped) *E. coli* strains of proven pathogenicity. Infect Immunol 1982;138:798-801.

Rudoy RC, Nelson JD. Enteroinvasive and enterotoxigenic *Escherichia coli*: occurrence in acute diarrhea of infants and children. Am J Dis Child 1975;129:688.

Sack DA, Sack RB. A test for enterotoxigenic *Escherichia coli*. Infect Immunol 1975;11:334.

Saphra I, Winter JW. Clinical manifestations of salmonellosis in man. An evaluation of 7,779 human infections identified at the New York Salmonella Center. N Engl J Med 1957;256:1128.

Schriber DS, Blacklow NR, Trier JS. The mucosal lesion of the proximal small intestine in acute infections non-bacterial gastroenteritis. N Engl J Med 1973;288:1318.

Scragg JN, Rubidge CJ, Applebaum PC. *Shigella* infection in African and Indian children with special reference to septicemia. J Pediatr 1978;93:796.

Shore EG, et al. Enterotoxin-producing *Escherichia coli* and diarrheal disease in adult travelers: a prospective study. J Infect Dis 1974;129:577.

Smith PD, Lane HC, Gill VJ, et al. Intestinal infections in patients with the acquired immunodeficiency syndrome (AIDS). Etiology and response to therapy. Ann Intern Med 1988;108:328-333.

Snow J. On the mode of communication of cholera-1855. In Snow on cholera. A reprint of two papers by John Snow. New York; Hofner, 1965.

Thomas DD, Knoop FC. The effect of calcium and prostaglandin inhibitors on the intestinal fluid response to heat stable enterotoxin of *E. coli*. J Infect Dis 1982;145:141-147.

Thomas DD, Knoop FC. Effect of heat-stable enterotoxin of *E. coli* on cultured mammalian cells. J Infect Dis 1983;147:450-459.

Thorén A, Wolde-Mariam T, Stintzing G, et al. Antibiotics in the treatment of gastroenteritis caused by enteropathogenic *E. coli*. J Infect Dis 1980;141:27-31.

Tyrrell DAJ, Bynoe MC. Cultivation of a novel type of common cold virus in organ cultures. Br Med J 1965;1:1467-1470.

Tyrrell DAJ, Kapikian AZ (eds). Virus infections of GI tract. New York; Marcel Dekker, Inc, 1982.

Ulshen MH, Rollo JL. Pathogenesis of *E. coli* gastroenteritis in man-another mechanism. N Engl J Med 1980;302:99-101.

Vaughan M. Cholera and cell regulation. Hosp Pract 1982;June:145-152.

Walter WA. Host defense mechanisms in GI tract. Pediatrics 1976;57:901-916.

Walker WA, Isselbacher KJ. Intestinal antibodies. N. Engl J Med 1977;297:767-775.

Yolken RH, et al. Epidemiology of human rotavirus types 1 and 2 as studied by enzyme-linked immunosorbent assay. N Engl J Med 1978;229:1156.

8

HAEMOPHILUS INFLUENZAE TYPE B

DENNIS A. CLEMENTS

Haemophilus influenzae type b (HIB) is a small, pleomorphic, nonmotile gram-negative bacterium that is a natural parasite only of humans. Its name derives from the mistaken idea by Pfeiffer in 1892 that it was responsible for the influenza pandemic plus the fact that it requires two factors from blood for growth. *H. influenzae* is divided easily into encapsulated forms that cause invasive disease (discussed in this chapter) and unencapsulated forms, which Pfeiffer had identified in the airways of those dying from influenza. The unencapsulated forms typically cause mucosal disease (otitis media, bronchitis, and conjunctivitis) except in aged, immunosuppressed, malnourished, or premature individuals, in whom they may cause invasive disease.

HIB has been the most common bacterial cause of meningitis in children in countries in which nationwide reporting of diseases has been established (see box, p. 128). In 1978 HIB was estimated to have caused 46% of all bacterial meningitis (10,000 cases) in the United States, regardless of age. In addition, it caused an equal number of other invasive diseases such as buccal and periorbital cellulitis, pneumonia, arthritis, epiglottitis, and pericarditis. This disease burden is equivalent to that caused by paralytic polio in the United States in the 1950s (Cochi et al., 1988).

ETIOLOGY

HIB organisms are gram-negative coccobacilli or filamentous rods, hence the descriptive term *pleomorphic*. They grow on chocolate agar on which they have a glistening, semi-transparent appearance. They are further identified by the requirement for X (hemin or other porphyrins) and V (coenzyme nicotinamide-adenine dinucleotide) factors for growth on blood agar. A more sensitive test for the X factor requirement is to test the ability of *H. influenzae* to convert delta aminolevulinic acid to porphyrin. Other tests such as the production of indole from tryptophan and the detection of β-galactosidase (ONPG test) activity are also useful in discriminating *H. influenzae* from other *Haemophilus* species.

A more rapid method of identifying type b organisms is to use type b antiserum on a slide with the unidentified organism. If agglutination does not occur, the organism is not type b. However, if agglutination does occur, it is possible the organism is type b. False-positive results are frequent because of cross-reactivity of antigens and because of autoagglutination by nontypeable strains.

Another method for selective identification of type b organisms is to use antiserum agar as described by Michaels et al. (1975). A suitable clear nutrient agar is prepared containing hyperimmune HIB antiserum. When this selective medium is inoculated with appropriate specimens, a halo of agglutination is observed around each HIB colony after 24 to 48 hours. This is a very sensitive method for detecting colonization and also allows for a quantitative assay.

A BRIEF HISTORY

1892: Pfeiffer erroneously identified *Haemophilus influenzae* as the causative agent in the lungs of patients dying during the influenza pandemic.

1930: Margaret Pittman described six serotypes (a-f) of encapsulated *Haemophilus influenzae* based on antigenic differences in their capsular polysaccharides.

1935: Fothergill and Wright described an inverse relationship between the age of HIB disease patients and the serum level of bactericidal antibody against *Haemophilus influenzae* type b (HIB).

1944: Alexander demonstrated that hyperimmune sera protected rabbits against developing meningitis when inoculated with HIB.

1950: The use of chloramphenicol markedly decreased the mortality rate from infection caused by HIB.

1970: Schneerson purifed the HIB polysaccharide capsule component polyribosyl-ribitol phosphate (PRP) for use as a vaccine immunogen.

1974: Peltola demonstrated that PRP was immunogenic in children more than 18 months of age in a vaccine trial of 100,000 children in Finland.

1984: Käyhty reported a 90% protective vaccine efficacy in children older than 18 months in the 1974 Finnish HIB trial.

1985: PRP vaccine was licensed in the United States to be given to children more than 2 years of age.

1980s: PRP was conjugated with various proteins to increase its immunogenicity in children less than 18 months of age.

1985-1987: A controlled trial of PRP-D given in the first 6-12 months of life in Finland was shown to be protective.

1987: PRP-D was licensed for use in the United States in children who had reached 18 months of age.

1990: HIB-OC and PRP-OMP were licensed for use in children as young as 2 months of age in the United States.

Typeable and nontypeable *H. influenzae* can be divided into biotypes by the presence or absence of three enzyme activities: urease, ornithine decarboxylase, and reduction of indole from tryptophan (Kilian, 1976). This system divides *H. influenzae* organisms into eight (1 through 8) groups, but 90% of type b organisms are biotype 1; hence this system has proved of little epidemiological use for type b organisms. Unencapsulated *H. influenzae* organisms, however, show a much wider distribution of biotypes, and this technique is more useful in epidemiological studies of nontypeable disease.

The polysaccharide capsule of *H. influenzae* is an important virulence factor. The type b capsule consists of a repeating polymer of five carbon sugar units of ribose and ribitol phosphate. The cell envelope includes lipo-oligosaccharide (LOS) and other membrane proteins (OMP). Pili or fimbriae extend from the outer membrane, but their presence is variable. They appear to mediate the attachment of HIB to epithelial cells, which is essential to establish colonization but perhaps disadvantageous in the blood.

H. influenzae was invariably sensitive to ampicillin until the early 1970s when resistance resulting from the production of a plasmid-mediated β-lactamase was first described, and at present 15% to 50% of HIB isolates are β-lactamase producers, depending on geographical location (Wenger et al., 1990). Resistance to chloramphenicol because of plasmid-mediated chloramphenicol acetyltransferase production has also been described.

There has been keen interest in the last 10 years in determining which subtypes of HIB cause invasive disease. This has been explored in the United States by Barenkamp et al. (1983). They reported that a high proportion of cases (84%) of invasive HIB disease is caused by only a few OMP subtypes (1H, 44%; 3L, 28%; and 1L, 12%), but there was no specificity of disease by subtype. They also reported that subtype prevalence varies over time. Subtype 2L accounted for 22% of cerebrospinal fluid (CSF) and blood isolates during the years 1977 to 1980 but only 4% in 1981 to 1982. From Holland, van Alphen et al. (1987) documented that 80% to 90% of HIB organisms causing invasive disease in Europe are OMP subtype 3L (van Alphen subtype 1) and that 83% of the isolates from Iceland are subtype 2L (van Alphen subtype 2). Recently, Takala et al. (1989) reported that one subtype (van Alphen 1c), which has been rarely isolated elsewhere, causes very little epiglottitis in Finland compared to meningitis. Thus there is suggestive evidence that virulence may vary with OMP subtype.

Attempts have also been made to categorize HIB isolates by LOS typing because LOS subtypes are more varied, possibly increasing their value as an epidemiological tool. Unfortunately, LOS patterns of individual isolates are unstable during storage, and in the animal model LOS expression by an individual clone may vary, depending on environmental conditions.

Newer techniques such as multilocus enzyme electrophoresis and clonotyping attempt to identify HIB isolates by differences in single enzyme loci or DNA sequence changes, respectively. Most isolates with the same enzyme electrophoretic pattern belong to the same OMP subtype and LOS subtypes, suggesting homogeneity of isolates. Musser et al. (1988) showed that HIB strains could be separated into three genetic groups, or "clonotypes," each of which is associated with a restricted group of OMP subtypes, suggesting limited clonal ancestry of HIB. One clonotype was predominant in Europe, but all three were found in the United States.

PATHOGENESIS

HIB, a natural infection only in humans, is spread by respiratory secretions. However, most colonized children do not become ill, and carriage alone does not necessarily induce an antibody response. Type b strains may persist in the airway for prolonged periods, thus increasing the opportunity for transmission. Animal models indicate that, in the minority in whom disease occurs, invasion through the mucosa into the blood is facilitated by mucosal damage (e.g., viral infection, trauma) and/or increased numbers of mucosal organisms. After penetration into the bloodstream, they are protected from phagocytosis by their capsules and multiply while disseminating to the meninges, epiglottis, or synovial surfaces. The patient may become symptomatic at any time after bacteremia occurs. The predilection of HIB for causing epiglottitis is not understood.

CLINICAL MANIFESTATIONS

Meningitis. The pathology of meningitis is discussed in Chapter 14. HIB appears to have more associated subdural effusions than other causes of bacterial meningitis. The slow resolution of these effusions, some of which may be empyema, has led to debate about the length of time these patients should be treated and whether surgical intervention is necessary. The persistence of bacterial cell products (particularly LOS) in the subdural space is thought responsible for prolonged fever in some of these patients.

Cellulitis. Buccal cellulitis occurs principally in children less than 18 months of age and may be related to bottle feeding. It can appear overnight in an otherwise healthy child. It often has a violaceous hue, or it can appear erysipeloid. HIB often can be cultured from the blood or a saline aspirate of the cheek. Due consideration should be given to whether the child might have another focus of infection, particularly if blood cultures are positive. Other bacterial causes must be considered, particularly in the older child or if there is an associated facial abrasion.

Orbital cellulitis (Fig. 8-1) can be a medical emergency. It is usually an extension of ethmoid sinusitis. If there is proptosis of the eye or paralysis of eye movement, decompression of the

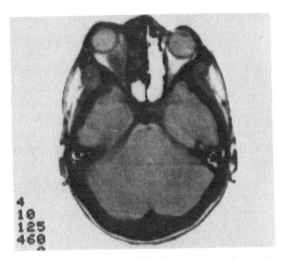

Fig. 8-1. Computed tomographic scan of a child with orbital cellulitis. Proptosis of the eye and involvement of deeper structures are evident.

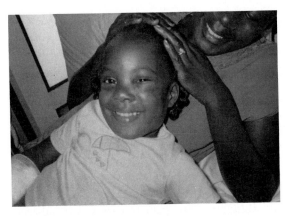

Fig. 8-2. Child recovering from a case of HIB preseptal (periorbital) cellulitis.

orbit is mandatory. This disease must be distinguished from preseptal, or periorbital, cellulitis (Fig. 8-2), which is cellulitis of the eyelid and contiguous structures that does not compromise the blood supply or the movement of the eye (Goldberg et al., 1978).

Epiglottitis. The epiglottis with HIB is acutely edematous and erythematous. HIB can often be cultured from the surface of the pharynx and from the blood. Some investigators believe there may be an allergic component to this disease, which accounts for the extremely rapid course (as few as 4 to 6 hours) during which it often manifests. Children appear toxic, but more strikingly they hold their heads forward, trying to keep their airway patent. A short period of intubation with appropriate antibiotic treatment reverses this process quickly.

Septic arthritis. HIB is a leading cause of septic arthritis in the young child. It is clinically indistinguishable from the disease caused by *Staphylococcus aureus*. Large joints, the hip in particular, are involved. Providing adequate drainage is important when large joints are affected, both for organism identification and for healing. Latex agglutination tests may be positive on fluid from the joint space. If the child is very young, the presence of contiguous osteomyelitis must be considered.

Pneumonia. The incidence of pneumonia caused by HIB is unknown. Many children probably are inadvertently treated when they are given antibiotics for other upper respiratory illnesses such as otitis media or sinusitis. Children with documented meningitis, pericarditis, or epiglottitis may have pneumonia as well. A definitive diagnosis is hampered in many cases because of the inability to obtain a positive diagnosis. One British study suggested that a positive HIB latex agglutination test in children with pneumonia may not be accurate (Isaacs, 1989). Thus many children in the past may have been falsely assumed to have HIB pneumonia. HIB cultured from the blood in a patient with clinical or roentgenographic pneumonia can be considered confirmatory. It has been reported that as many as 90% of patients with HIB pneumonias will have a pleural reaction and effusion.

Pericarditis. Although infrequent, pericarditis caused by HIB is frightening because of its rapidity of onset and lack of clinical symptoms. Respiratory distress in a child who is toxic and has a normal chest x-ray is often the only symptom. The child may have underlying pneumonia or meningitis, and this disease process has occurred while the child was receiving antibiotic treatment. Echocardiography followed by pericardiocentesis and appropriate antibiotic therapy is indicated. Copious pericardial exudate often persists for several days after therapy is initiated.

Bacteremia. Children who appear toxic but have no focus of infection may have HIB bacteremia, which is diagnosed with a positive blood culture.

DIAGNOSIS

The isolation of HIB from a sterile body site

is the diagnosis of choice in all diseases. HIB bacteremia, for instance, is always diagnosed with the isolation of HIB from the blood. However, there are limitations to this otherwise optimal gold standard. Occasionally, a child may be given an antibiotic for treatment of a less severe disease before manifesting clinical meningitis. If the clinical history is compatible with meningitis and there are CSF changes (low sugar, high protein, and increased number of neutrophils) and a positive CSF latex agglutination test for HIB, most would agree that the child should be assumed to have HIB meningitis. If the CSF latex agglutination test is negative, however, even if the urinary antigen test is positive, it is unlikely that this patient should be considered to have HIB meningitis if HIB does not grow from the CSF. If HIB grows from the CSF culture and the CSF is otherwise benign, it should be assumed that the child has HIB meningitis and that the disease was detected at an early stage. Most clinicians have experienced this situation at least once.

A positive diagnosis for HIB is often difficult in a patient with cellulitis, for clinicians are often reluctant to aspirate from the inflamed tissue. If blood cultures are positive for HIB or if the clinical picture is compatible and the urinary latex test is positive, the diagnosis can be assumed to be correct. With no positive results, it is prudent to treat the patient with an antibiotic that would also treat *S. aureus* infections.

If an aspirate is obtained from a patient with septic arthritis, it often will confirm the bacterial cause of the infection; but if it is not obtained, positive blood cultures and/or positive urinary latex tests must provide the answers. If the child is already receiving an oral antibiotic, all the same difficulties with negative cultures mentioned previously prevail. If there is doubt about the cause of the arthritis, the patient must be treated with antibiotics (and surgical drainage, if indicated) that would be suitable for both *S. aureus* infections and for HIB.

Pericarditis always requires drainage. If the drainage is performed early in the course of disease, a positive culture for HIB from the fluid or blood is likely. If, however, the child has been on antibiotics and cultures are negative, a positive latex agglutination test result for HIB from the pericardial fluid or urine would be useful.

Pneumonia remains the most difficult of all the infections to document, for there is question about the meaning of positive latex agglutination tests in these patients (see previous discussion). A positive blood culture or positive latex agglutination test from pleural fluid may be confirmatory, but these tests may not be positive even if they are performed.

Laboratory tests

Gram stain and culture are the tests of choice to document infection. However, prior antibiotic treatment often makes blood cultures sterile. CSF cultures are less critically affected, particularly by the prior use of oral antibiotics, and thus may still be positive. Additionally, diseases with localized infection (arthritis and epiglottitis) have a lower level of bacteremia, and positive cultures may be missed if an inadequate volume of blood is taken for culture.

Several methods of antigen detection are useful even when the organisms have been made nonviable by antibiotics. The most popular and sensitive is the latex particle agglutination test that uses anti-PRP antibody on latex particules that agglutinate in the presence of PRP antigen. This test may be negative, however, if there is an overabundance of PRP antigen or, alternately, too little antigen. It is also occasionally falsely positive because of cross-reactivity with some *Escherichia coli*, *Streptococcus pneumoniae*, *S. aureus*, or *Neisseria meningitidis* strains. Nevertheless, a positive latex test result in the presence of a strongly suggestive clinical course is useful.

DIFFERENTIAL DIAGNOSIS

Meningitis. The most common cause of meningitis in the developed world in children 3 months to 3 years of age has been HIB. The disease is indistinguishable from other causes of meningitis by clinical signs and symptoms alone. The chapters in this book on bacterial and aseptic meningitis deal with clinical symptoms, so they are not discussed here. With the advent of HIB immunization in children as young as 2 months of age in the United States, HIB as a cause of meningitis in this age group should diminish. *N. meningitidis* and *S. pneumoniae* would then be the leading causes of meningitis in this age group (Wenger et al., 1990). HIB meningitis can be differentiated from the previously mentioned causes of bacterial meningitis, by the results of CSF culture or by a positive blood culture with a compatible CSF picture. A positive urinary latex test for HIB with a compatible clinical course and CSF analysis would also be acceptable. Other possible diagnoses would include *Streptococcus agalactiae* (group B streptococcus) or *Listeria monocytogenes* in infants and tubercular meningitis or aseptic meningitis in a child of any age. A patient with tubercular meningitis typically has CSF lymphocytosis, increased protein, and decreased glucose. One with aseptic meningitis may have CSF pleocytosis and slightly elevated protein, but the glucose level is usually within normal limits.

Epiglottitis. The initial symptoms for a patient with epiglottitis include upper airway obstruction and a toxic appearance. Symptoms often appear rapidly, frequently in just a few hours. In areas where epiglottitis is common, it is customary to visualize the epiglottis with an anesthesiologist or intensivist present so that the child can be immediately intubated if necessary. The epiglottis is cherry red and swollen. It is useful to swab the epiglottis for bacterial culture at the time of intubation. If the epiglottis is not typical in appearance (for epiglottitis) but the child requires intubation, sending the swab for viral culture is useful. Most viruses causing a similar clinical syndrome have other symptoms of a respiratory infection (e.g., cough, coryza, conjunctivitis) and have a longer period of recovery. Children presenting with drooling and their head placed forward to facilitate air entry occasionally will have other pharyngeal structures (uvula or posterior pharynx) red and swollen, and often HIB will grow from their blood or mucosal surface culture.

There is evidence that virtually all cases of epiglottitis in young children, as determined by inspection of the epiglottis during intubation, are caused by HIB. HIB was isolated from 114 of 123 (93%) blood cultures collected from epiglottitis patients in a study in Melbourne, Australia, and no other pathogens were isolated (Gilbert, 1990). When the diagnosis is not bacteriologically confirmed, it is usually because appropriate specimens were not taken.

Pneumonia. The diagnosis of HIB pneumonia is difficult because blood cultures may not be positive, due to prior antibiotic therapy or an associated low level of bacteremia. If there is a pleural effusion, aspiration of fluid for culture or latex agglutination may provide a positive re-

sult. However, the value of only a urinary latex agglutination result positive for HIB is debatable. The presence of a significant effusion is suggestive that the pneumonia may be due to HIB, for up to 90% of HIB pneumonias in some reports have effusions (compared to only 10% for *S. pneumoniae*). Drainage of a large effusion may not be required for recovery unless there is empyema, but it usually will speed the healing process.

Septic arthritis. Septic arthritis apparently occurs secondarily to seeding synovial surfaces subsequent to bacteremia. Large joints, particularly the hip, are most commonly affected and should be surgically drained to avoid permanent damage. If the child was febrile and/or irritable before diagnosis, he may already be taking an antibiotic; thus blood cultures may be negative. If a small amount of antigen is in the blood or if the urine is dilute, the urinary latex agglutination test may be negative as well. In this case only an aspirate of the joint for culture and latex agglutination testing may provide a diagnosis. In the absence of a positive culture it is prudent to treat for possible *S. aureus* septic arthritis also, for it is common in the same age group, and the symptoms are identical. If the child is very young, it is important to determine whether contiguous osteomyelitis is present.

Cellulitis. Cellulitis of the face or around the orbit (periorbital) often develops rapidly. There is some suggestion that facial cellulitis may be associated with maxillary sinusitis or bottle feeding. These superficial skin infections are markedly different from the deep orbital tissue infection, orbital cellulitis, that commonly has associated ipsilateral ethmoid sinusitis. Computed tomographic (CT) imaging may be required to distinguish the difference, for the eyelid is often too swollen to allow inspection of eye movement. The inability to move the eye suggests orbital infection, and decompression of the orbit is often required to avoid permanent sequelae. A positive microbiological diagnosis can be made in these infections only if there is a positive blood culture or aspirate from the infected tissue. A positive urinary latex agglutination test result alone is suggestive, and some would believe it sufficient. However, if the diagnosis is uncertain, treatment to include *S. pneumoniae* and *Streptococcus pyogenes* would be prudent.

COMPLICATIONS

Most of the complications of HIB disease occur in the youngest patients who have meningitis. This is not unexpected. The youngest children often have the most fulminant disease and have the fewest focal symptoms to alert parents and physicians of their diagnosis before the disease progresses to meningitis, the consequences of which necessarily affect the brain.

Subdural fluid. Subdural effusions are frequently associated with HIB meningitis. Some of these effusions probably represent subdural empyemas, and there is debate about which of them require surgical drainage. Treating the child with antibiotics and performing serial CT scans or other appropriate imaging procedures to document whether the effusion or empyemas resolve are appropriate measures. Children with these fluid collections often have persistent fever, which is compatible with the presence of persistent HIB antigen (particularly LOS) in the subdural space causing the febrile reaction. Subdural fluid HIB antigen tests in some patients are positive for as long as 1 month after initial treatment, although cultures of the fluid are sterile.

Hearing loss. The most common sequela of HIB disease is hearing loss, which has been reported in 5% to 15% of cases. Prior treatment of the child with oral antibiotics may actually increase the incidence of hearing loss, probably by decreasing bacteremia and hence symptoms but masking smoldering central nervous system (CNS) infection. The available evidence indicates that treatment of meningitis with steroids in addition to antibiotics decreases the incidence of hearing loss (see p. 256).

Intellectual functioning. A sizeable minority of children (5% to 20%) will have significant intellectual impairment after HIB meningitis. In the United States, as compared to other developed nations, there are sequelae after HIB disease, but the median and mean ages of patients with meningitis are younger in the United States, which may predispose the patients to more complications. In addition, studies have examined more subtle measurements of intellectual functioning in the United States. A disturbingly high percentage (up to 40%) of patients have "soft" intellectual problems such as the inability to concentrate or specific learning disabilities when compared to their siblings or peers (Sell, 1987). With the advent of preventive immunization, the incidence of all of these sequelae should decrease.

PROGNOSIS

In the United States the death rate due to HIB disease is approximately 3% of those known infected (Wenger et al., 1990). Meningitis results in the highest death rate, for it occurs in the youngest children and affects the brain. Mental retardation, hearing loss, and mild neurological abnormalities have also been described, with the rates of each dependent on the population examined and the intensity of investigation.

IMMUNITY

The protective role of polyribosyl-ribitol phosphate (PRP) antibodies was first demonstrated by Fothergill and Wright in 1933. They noted an increased incidence of HIB disease when maternal antibody began to wane at 4 to 6 months of age. In common with other polysaccharide antigens, PRP alone is T-cell independent and thus does not induce immunological memory; the ability to respond to PRP with production of antibody (particularly IgG2) is not acquired until approximately 18 to 24 months of age. Thus the greatest period of susceptibility to disease is from 4 to 24 months of age, which is the peak incidence of HIB disease in the United States. This lack of response to polysaccharide antigen is also responsible for the susceptibility of these children to *N. meningitidis* and *S. pneumoniae* infections. Immunization for the prevention of these diseases has necessitated the conjugation of the polysaccharide to a protein moiety to induce the infant immune system to make antibody to the polysaccharide, induce memory, and thus protect itself. This is discussed in "Recommendations for Vaccine Use" at the end of this chapter.

Thus children who acquire HIB infection at an early age may not mount an immunological response. They may be susceptible to the disease if infected again before acquiring the ability to mount this response. Therefore even children who have had HIB disease should be immunized as recommended with the new conjugate vaccines designed for use in children as young as 2 months of age.

EPIDEMIOLOGICAL FACTORS

The HIB nasopharyngeal carriage rate is generally less than 5%, but most children have acquired antibody to PRP by the age of 5 years without becoming ill, suggesting that they have been exposed to HIB or cross-reacting polysaccharides of other organisms. Disease is more common in children from crowded conditions such as day-care centers or crowded social conditions, and although there is seasonal variation in disease, clear-cut epidemics do not occur.

Worldwide, the yearly incidence and type of HIB disease vary by country, but approximately 90% to 95% of disease occurs before the age of 5, regardless of location. The case attack rate per 100,000 children less than 5 years of age is 50 to 60 in Australia and Scandinavia and 60 to 130 in the United States. In certain ethnic groups such as Alaskan Eskimos, American Indians, and Australian aboriginals, the case attack rate can be as high as 400 per 100,000 children less than 5 years of age (1% to 2% of all children). When the incidence is high (e.g., as in Alaskan Eskimos), the median age of disease is low (6 months), and epiglottitis is rare. In Australia and Finland where the incidence of disease is lower, the median age is higher (27 months), and 30% to 40% of the disease type is epiglottitis.

The differences in incidence of disease in different locations may be due in part to both genetic and environmental factors. Alaskan Eskimos in the same environment as non-Eskimos have a higher incidence of HIB disease, despite apparently adequate antibody levels. In addition, black Americans without the Km1 allotype have a higher incidence of disease than do black Americans with this allotype.

Population-based epidemiological studies in Australia, Finland, and the United States have demonstrated differences in the case attack rate for all invasive HIB disease and, in particular, in the relative frequency of the major clinical manifestations, namely, meningitis and epiglottitis (Table 8-1). A recent comprehensive study from Australia showed that the annual case attack rate of invasive HIB infections was 58.5 per 100,000 in children less than 5 years of age, and almost two thirds (64%) of cases occurred in children more than 18 months of age (Gilbert et al., 1990). Meningitis (mean age, 20 months) and epiglottitis (mean age, 36 months) each accounted for approximately 40% of infections (attack rates of 23 per 100,000 each).

Population-based studies from Finland show that the HIB case attack rate (52 per 100,000) and the proportion of cases of meningitis (46%) and epiglottitis (29%) are similar to those in Australia (Takala et al., 1989).

The attack rate for HIB disease is higher in the United States, even in populations that are primarily Caucasian. Studies from the United States estimate that the overall HIB disease rate

Table 8-1. Estimated incidence of invasive *Haemophilus influenzae* type b disease

Population/place	Annual rate per 100,000 children <5 years of age		
	Meningitis	*Epiglottitis*	*Mean age (mos)*
Alaskan natives	601	5	10
Australia (aboriginal)	450	0	7
Navajo Indians	152	0	8
United States (average)	19-69	5-15	8-15
Sweden	27	28*	30
Finland	26	13	28
Australia	25	23*	27
England	18	9	24

Modified from Clements DA, Gilbert GL: Aust N Z J Med 1990; 20:828-834, and Broome CV: Pediatr Infect Dis 1987; 6:779-782.
*Includes patients with clinically but not bacteriologically confirmed epiglottitis (of which more than 95% are probably caused by HIB).

is 60 to 100 per 100,000, of which approximately 60% are meningitis and 5% to 15% are epiglottitis.

In general, meningitis occurs at an earlier age than epiglottitis so that populations with a higher proportion of cases of meningitis have a lower mean age overall for HIB disease. In addition, populations with higher HIB attack rates also have a lower mean age of meningitis relative to those populations with lower attack rates. Thus overall a lower mean age of disease is relative to HIB disease incidence and disease manifestations (Fig. 8-3). A hypothesis could be that there is a pool of susceptible young children that gradually diminishes over time, coincident with the maturation of the immune system; if the environment provides for early exposure to the HIB organism, the frequency of meningitis is increased, and if exposed later, the children are less likely to become diseased even if infected, and their diseases more likely will be localized. This hypothesis is, however, still unproven.

Sex distribution. Generally, the sex distribution for HIB disease manifestations, except pneumonia and epiglottitis, is equal. There is perhaps a small predominance of males when all studies are considered together, but it is small.

The distribution for epiglottitis, however, is unequivocally dominated by males. Most studies show a 1.5 to 2.0:1 male:female ratio. In studies of HIB pneumonia there is a predominance of males (2:1), but as previously mentioned, complete case ascertainment for pneumonia is questionable, which may (or may not) bias this finding.

Age distribution. HIB disease is primarily a disease of children 3 months to 5 years of age. Most disease manifestations, except epiglottitis, are concentrated in the younger ages. Epiglottitis, although varying in incidence in different populations, has a median age of disease of 2 to 3 years (compared to 12 to 18 months for most other disease manifestations). The reason for this difference in age distribution is not known. Except for epiglottitis, the incidence of HIB disease is inversely proportional to the level of anti-PRP antibody measured in children's serum.

The age distribution of HIB disease is best demonstrated by data from Australia where the incidence of epiglottitis is common. Data from the United States give similar age distributions except that the meningitis cases tend to occur even earlier in life. The overall distribution of disease is dependent on the predominant dis-

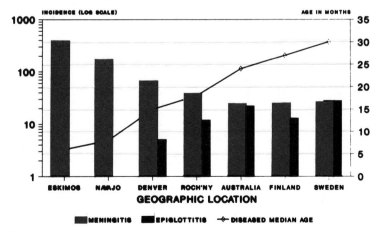

Fig. 8-3. Median age by country by disease type. (Modified from Clements DA, Gilbert GL: Aust N Z J Med 1990; 20:828-834.)

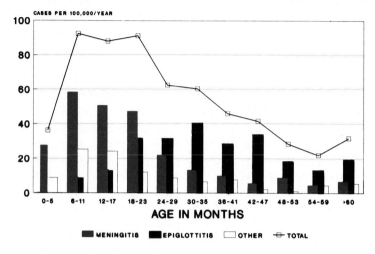

Fig. 8-4. Australian age distribution of disease. (Modified from Ward JI, Cochi S: In Plotkin SA, Mortimer EA, editors: Vaccines, ed 1. Philadelphia: WB Saunders Co, 1988, p 303.)

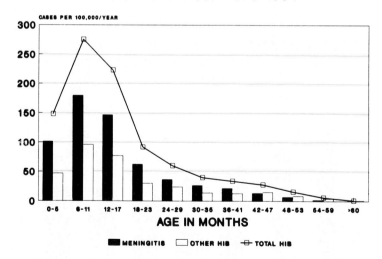

Fig. 8-5. United States' age distribution of disease. (Modified from Gilbert GL et al. Pediatr Infect Dis 1990; 9:252-257.

ease manifestations. Most other causes of HIB disease have an age distribution similar to that of meningitis (Figs. 8-4 and 8-5).

Seasonal incidence and year-to-year variation. Apparently there is very little year-to-year variation in HIB disease incidence in countries in which HIB disease has been systematically followed (Finland and Australia). There is, however, a seasonal variation. HIB is least common in the summer months, and disease clusters around the winter months, although some investigators have shown a bimodal fall-spring distribution.

RISK FACTORS

Infection rates depend on host susceptibility and exposure to the infectious agent. Protection from HIB disease in the first few months of life is provided by maternal antibody; thereafter the risk is relatively high until the child can mount an antibody response to HIB polysaccharide antigen, which develops gradually over the first few years of life.

Two studies from the United States have reported that crowded conditions increase the risk of HIB disease (Cochi et al., 1986; Istre et al., 1985). Crowding can result from smaller or fewer rooms per family unit or an increased number of persons per family. Attendance at day-care centers also appears to increase the risk of HIB disease, and children with HIB infection are more likely to have siblings who attend day-care centers or school. Breast-feeding apparently provides protection, but children who breast-feed may be less likely to be exposed to environments in which there is a large number of other children. After controlling for the number of siblings and residence size, family income is not an apparent risk factor for disease.

Family members of children with HIB disease, particularly siblings 3 to 6 years of age, are often HIB carriers. In an Australian study in which day-care exposure and siblings were risk factors for HIB disease, the risk of disease by attending day care centers was modified by whether the child had siblings, suggesting that day care has an effect similar to an increased number of siblings. Both of these measures probably are related to crowding and/or the potential for organism transmission.

Some unknown genetic factors may increase the risk of HIB disease. Australian Aboriginals, Eskimos, and native American Indians have a particularly high incidence of HIB disease. The environmental exposure may be the predominant determinant in the setting of a homogeneous genetic background. Black Americans who lack the Km1 immunoglobulin allotype have an increased incidence of HIB disease, but the reasons for this increase in disease rate are unknown.

TREATMENT

Until 1974 HIB was universally susceptible to ampicillin. Beginning in that year, sporadic reports of resistance to ampicillin began to appear. Chloramphenicol, used routinely before the development of ampicillin, became commonly used again. The advent of second-generation cephalosporins provided another possible treatment for HIB disease in subsequent years, but variable CNS penetration and treatment failures precluded their use. At present, with 15% to 50% of HIBs producing β-lactamase, the antibiotics of choice are the third-generation cephalosporins, cefotaxime and ceftriaxone. These two antibiotics have very low minimal inhibitory concentrations (MICs) against all HIB, regardless of whether they produce β-lactamase. Some clinicians have concluded that ampicillin can be used if the HIB organism isolated does not produce β-lactamase, but HIB isolates both sensitive and resistant to ampicillin have been recovered from the same patient on occasion.

Although chloramphenicol is infrequently used at present, there are recent reports of resistance to this antibiotic resulting from the ability of some HIB organisms to produce chloramphenicol acetyltransferase.

PREVENTIVE MEASURES
Immunization

PRP alone. In 1974 100,000 Finnish children were immunized with unconjugated PRP or with meningococcal group A vaccine in a trial to prevent an outbreak of meningococcal A disease. In the 4 years after vaccination there were 20 cases of HIB disease in children more than 18 months of age in the group that received meningococcal vaccine and only two cases in the PRP vaccine group—90% vaccine efficacy (Peltola et al., 1984). Protective efficacy for the polysaccharide antigen was not demonstrated in children less than 18 months of age. In an attempt to overcome the inability of the polysaccharide antigen alone to protect the youngest children, PRP was subsequently conjugated to one of several proteins to stimulate antibody production better and to convert the immunogen to a T-cell dependent antigen.

In spite of the limitations of the use of PRP alone as an immunogen to children more than 2 years of age, it was judged cost-effective and was licensed for use in the United States in 1985. Because PRP is at least partially effective in children 18 to 24 months old, it was also recommended at that time that high-risk children (those attending day-care centers and close contacts of cases) in the 18- to 24-month age group be vaccinated with the proviso that they be vaccinated again at 24 months of age.

Replacement immunoglobulin therapy and the 1974 vaccine trials suggested that an anti-PRP antibody level greater than 0.15 $\mu g/ml$ would be protective. However, because antibody levels fall over time, a higher level (>1.0 $\mu g/ml$) after immunization was postulated to be required for sustained protection.

In Finnish children more than 18 months of age PRP immunization was 90% protective against HIB disease in 1974. However, when licensed in the United States for children more than 2 years of age, vaccine efficacy averaged only 60% as estimated by several retrospective case-control studies (Ward et al, 1988). This may have been due to differences in populations or possibly the differences in use of vaccine under controlled vs. uncontrolled conditions. Nevertheless, it gives reasons for caution when extrapolating results of vaccine trials from one population to another.

PRP conjugate vaccines. After unsuccessful attempts to enhance PRP immunogenicity by changing the PRP polymer length and mixing PRP with diphtheria and tetanus toxoids and pertussis vaccine (DTP) or with pertussis vaccine, PRP was conjugated (covalently linked) to one of several protein carriers, including a mutant diphtheria toxin (PRP-OC), a diphtheria toxoid (PRP-D), an outer membrane protein of *N. meningitidis* (PRP-OMP), and a tetanus toxoid (PRP-T). The amount of specific antibody produced after immunization depends on the method of conjugation and the age of the child. It is not clear whether a level of 1.0 $\mu g/ml$ of anti-PRP antibody is required in response to T-cell dependent vaccines to maintain protection. A lower antibody level may be protective if there is a prompt anamnestic response to a second PRP exposure as a result of receiving the vaccine or of natural infection.

PRP-D. PRP-D contains PRP conjugated to diphtheria toxoid with a six-carbon spacer. In children more than 14 months of age one 20 μg (PRP) dose gives antibody levels greater than 1 $\mu g/ml$ in 67% of children. For children 9 to 15 months old two doses are required to give the same levels. In younger children the antibody produced is primarily IgM and thus relatively short-lived, whereas proportionately higher levels of IgG are produced in older children. The antibody levels achieved are considerably higher than those with PRP alone in children less than 7 months of age. In children less than 6 months of age three injections fail to achieve levels greater than 1 $\mu g/ml$, and levels decline rapidly in the subsequent year. A booster dose of the conjugate or PRP vaccine alone at 18 months produces a good response. These data encouraged the use of this vaccine in two efficacy trials, one in Alaska and the other in Finland.

In 1985 the PRP-D vaccine was given to Finnish children in a three-dose schedule at 3, 5, and 7 months of age. The protective efficacy was 83% for one injection, 90% for two injections, and 100% for three injections. However, the antibody response was relatively poor in children less than 7 months of age, and invasive disease occurred less often in this age group. The same vaccine was also used in a trial in Alaskan children but was not protective. A genetic or environmental factor may contribute to the early mean age of disease in Alaskan children and, because of the poor antibody response in the youngest children, may have been responsible for the difference in vaccine efficacy reported. PRP-D is presently licensed for use in children at 18 to 24 months of age in the United States, several countries in Europe, and Australia.

PRP-OC. Low-molecular-weight oligosaccharides of PRP are coupled to a mutant version of diphtheria toxin in this vaccine. It was the first conjugate vaccine licensed for use in children at 2 months of age in the United States. There is little antibody response to the initial dose of vaccine at 2 months of age, but there is a brisk and sustained antibody response to subsequent doses of vaccine. Like all conjugate vaccines, there are almost no side effects to vaccination. The present recommendation for vaccination includes three doses of vaccine by 6 months of age, preferably 2 months apart, with a booster at 15 months of age.

PRP-OMP. PRP was conjugated to a protein from group B *N. meningitidis*. This vaccine, PRP-OMP, is very immunogenic with the first dose given. Its demonstrated efficacy in the Navajo population (even after one dose) in which there is a very early median age of HIB disease was particularly impressive. The only case of disease (arthritis) in the immunized group was in a child who was more than 1 year of age and who had failed to receive her booster immunization. PRP-OMP subsequently was licensed for use in children as young as 2 months of age. It requires two immunizations in the first 6 months of life, preferably 2 months apart, with a booster at 12 months of age.

Response to subsequent doses of vaccine is less than that to PRP-CRM, and although it apparently is T-cell dependent, PRP-OMP does not boost to the same level as the other licensed product. However, there is an extremely good antibody response to the first dose of vaccine. There are no significant side effects to receiving this vaccine.

PRP-T. This conjugate vaccine is very immunogenic in young children. It has been approved for use by the FDA on the basis of immunogenicity information alone.

Others

There has been considerable controversy about the use of rifampin to prevent secondary cases of HIB. The evidence is sufficient that rifampin, taken orally, will markedly decrease the carrier rate of HIB in the pharynx (estimates are as high as 95%). What is not clear is the advantage this has in stopping the spread of disease. Several studies show that family members or close contacts often carry the organism in the throat, which is presumably where the diseased child obtained his infection. But unless there is another susceptible child in the environment, rifampin treatment may be of little use. At pres-

ent, the recommendations are to treat all members of a family, including the patient, with rifampin (20 mg/kg/day, maximum, 600 mg) once daily for 4 days if there is another child less than 48 months of age in the home. Treatment of contacts at day-care centers should be individualized, but in general, prophylaxis at day-care centers is no longer recommended routinely.

Two approaches other than immunization have been taken to decrease disease incidence in populations in which the median age of patients with HIB disease is very young. In the Navajo Indians maternal immunization with HIB before delivery, boosting the mother's anti-PRP IgG levels, has been performed. In addition, newborns of Navajo mothers have received repeated doses of intramuscular immunoglobulin to boost IgG levels. Both of these strategies have had some effect on increasing anti-PRP antibody in the newborn, but the advent of conjugated HIB vaccines that can be given at 2 months of age may have obviated the need for these therapies.

It is expected that in populations in which the conjugated HIB vaccines are used there will be significant decreases in HIB disease and therefore in sequelae. The health benefit in decreased morbidity and mortality rates for the children and in decreased suffering by the families will be most welcome. Because these vaccines were licensed for use in children less than 6 months of age at the end of 1990 in the United States, it will be a few years before efficacy can be proven.

• • •

The recommendations of the Advisory Committee on Immunization Practices (ACIP) for the use of HIB vaccines are as follows (MMWR 1991;40:Jan 11).

RECOMMENDATIONS FOR VACCINE USE

1. **On the basis of the above considerations, the ACIP recommends that all children receive one of the conjugate vaccines licensed for infant use (HbOC or PRP-OMP), beginning routinely at 2 months of age** (Table 8-2). Administration of the vaccine series may be initiated as early as age 6 weeks.

2. **If HbOC is to be used, previously unvaccinated infants 2-6 months of age should receive three doses**

Table 8-2. ACIP-recommended *Haemophilus influenzae* type b (Hib) routine vaccination schedule

Vaccine	2 months	4 months	6 months	12 months	15 months
HbOC	Dose 1	Dose 2	Dose 3		Booster
PRP-OMP	Dose 1	Dose 2		Booster	

Table 8-3. Detailed vaccination schedule for *Haemophilus* b conjugate vaccines

Vaccine	Age at 1st dose (months)	Primary series	Booster
HbOC	2-6	3 doses, 2 mo apart	15 mo*
(Lederle-Praxis)	7-11	2 doses, 2 mo apart	15 mo*
	12-14	1 dose	15 mo*
	15-59	1 dose	—
PRP-OMP	2-6	2 doses, 2 mo apart	12 mo*
(Merck, Sharp and	7-11	2 doses, 2 mo apart	15 mo*
Dohme)	12-14	1 dose	15 mo*
	15-59	1 dose	—
PRP-D	15-59	1 dose	—
(Connaught)			

*At least 2 months after previous dose.

given at least 2 months apart. Unvaccinated infants 7-11 months of age should receive two doses of HbOC, given at least 2 months apart, before they are 15 months old (Table 8-3). Unvaccinated children 12-14 months of age should receive a single dose of vaccine before they are 15 months of age. **An additional dose of HbOC should be given to all children at 15 months of age, or as soon as possible thereafter, at an interval not less than 2 months after the previous dose.** The other two conjugate vaccines licensed for use at 15 months of age may be used for this dose, but there are no data demonstrating that a booster response will occur. An interval as short as 1 month between doses is acceptable but not optimal.

3. **If PRP-OMP is to be used, previously unvaccinated infants 2-6 months of age should receive two doses 2 months apart and a booster dose at 12 months of age.** Children 7-11 months of age not previously vaccinated should receive two doses 2 months apart and a booster dose at 15 months of age (or as soon as possible thereafter), not less than 2 months after the previous dose. Children 12-14 months of age not previously vaccinated should receive a single dose and a booster dose at 15 months of age (or as soon as possible thereafter), not less than 2 months after the previous dose. The other two conjugate vaccines licensed for use at 15 months of age may be used for this dose,

but there are no data demonstrating that a booster response will occur. An interval as short as 1 month between doses is acceptable but not optimal.

4. **Unvaccinated children 15-59 months of age may be given any one of the three conjugate vaccines licensed for this age group.**

5. **Ideally, the same conjugate vaccine should be used throughout the entire vaccination series (according to the schedule outlined in Table 8-3).** No data exist regarding the interchangeability of different conjugate vaccines with respect to safety, immunogenicity, or efficacy. However, situations will arise in which the vaccine provider does not know which type of Hib conjugate vaccine the child to be vaccinated had previously received. Under these circumstances, it is prudent for vaccine providers to ensure that as a minimum an infant 2-6 months of age receives a primary series of three doses of conjugate vaccine. These recommendations may change as data become available regarding the response to different conjugate vaccines in a primary series.

6. **Children <24 months of age who have had invasive Hib disease should still receive vaccine, since many children of that age fail to develop adequate immunity following natural disease.** The vaccine series can be initiated (or continued) at the time of hospital discharge.

7. **Chemoprophylaxis of household or day-care classroom contacts of children with Hib disease should be directed at both vaccinated and unvaccinated contacts because immune individuals may asymptomatically carry and transmit the organism.** Because of the time required to generate an immunologic response, vaccination following exposure should not be used to prevent secondary cases. However, the ACIP strongly supports extensive use of the Hib vaccine for infants attending day-care facilities; that action should substantially decrease the occurrence of primary cases of Hib disease in day-care facilities. If every child in a household or day-care classroom has been fully vaccinated, chemoprophylaxis is unnecessary.

8. **Conjugate vaccine may be given simultaneously with diphtheria and tetanus toxoids and pertussis vaccine adsorbed (DTP); combined measles, mumps, rubella vaccine (MMR); oral poliovirus vaccine (OPV); or inactivated poliovirus vaccine (IPV).** Any of the vaccines may be injected in the thigh, and two injections may be given in the same deltoid. All licensed conjugate vaccines should be administered by the intramuscular route. There are no known contraindications to simultaneous administration of any Hib conjugate vaccine with either pneumococcal or meningococcal vaccine.

9. No efficacy data are available on which to base a recommendation concerning use of the vaccine for older children and adults with the chronic conditions associated with an increased risk of Hib disease. Studies suggest, however, good immunogenicity in patients with sickle cell disease, leukemia, patients who have had splenectomies, or who have HIV infection, and administering vaccine to these patients is not contraindicated.

Side effects and adverse reactions

Reported reactions to the three conjugate vaccines have been mild among both infants and children. In one study, approximately 300 1- to 6-month-old infants who received HbOC vaccine (without simultaneous administration of DTP) were evaluated; within 24 hours of injection, no serious side effects were noted. Following the third dose, 2.2% were noted to have a temperature >38.3 C, 2.2% had localized redness, 1.1% had swelling, and <1% had warmth. Adverse events following the first and second doses were less frequent.

Serious adverse reactions to PRP-OMP also have been rare. Among 4,459 healthy Navajo infants 6-12 weeks of age, no differences were reported in the type and frequency of serious adverse events among those who received PRP-OMP and those who received placebo. Of the infants in the group who were

2-14 months of age, 3%-4.3% had a temperature >38.3 C within 48 hours of receiving a second dose of vaccine, 0.7%-1.2% had erythema of >2.5 cm in diameter, and 0.9%-3.7% had swelling and induration of >2.5 cm in diameter. Adverse events following the first dose were less frequent.

Precautions and contraindications

Conjugate vaccines that contain either diphtheria toxoid or protein should not be considered as an immunizing agent against diphtheria; no changes in the schedule for administering DTP are recommended. A conjugate vaccine that contains meningococcal protein should not be considered as an immunizing agent against meningococcal disease.

REFERENCES

Barenkamp SJ, Granoff DM, Pittman M. Outer membrane protein subtypes and biotypes of *Haemophilus influenzae* type b: relation between strains isolated in 1934-1954 and 1977-1980. J Infect Dis 1983;148:1127.

Broome CV. Epidemiology of *Haemophilus influenzae* type b infections in the United States. Pediatr Infect Dis 1987;6:779-782.

Clements DA, Gilbert GL. Immunisation for the prevention of *Haemophilus influenzae* type b infections: a review. Aust NZ J Med 1990;20:828-834.

Cochi SL, Fleming DW, Hightower AW, et al. Primary invasive *Haemophilus influenzae* type b disease: a population-based assessment of risk factors. J Pediatr 1986;108:887-896.

Cochi SL, O'Mara D, Preblud SR. Progress in *Haemophilus* type b polysaccharide vaccine use in the United States. Pediatrics 1988;81:166-168.

Gilbert GL, Clements DA, Broughton S. *Haemophilus influenzae* type b infections in Victoria, Australia 1985-87. A population based study to determine the need for immunization. Pediatr Infect Dis 1990;9:252-257.

Goldberg F, Berne AS, Oski FA. Differentiation of orbital cellulitis from preseptal cellulitis by computed tomography. Pediatrics 1978;62:1000-5.

Isaacs D. Problems in determining the etiology of community-acquired childhood pneumonia. Pediatr Infect Dis 1989;8:143-8.

Istre CR, Conner JS, Broome CV, et al. Risk factors for primary invasive *Haemophilus influenzae* disease: increased risk from day care attendance and school age household members. J Pediatr 1985;106:190-185.

Kilian M. A taxonomic study of the genus *Haemophilus* with the proposal of a new species. J Clin Microbiol 1976;93:9-62.

Michaels RH, Stonebraker FE, Robbins JB. Use of antiserum agar for detection of *Haemophilus influenzae* type b in the pharynx. Pediatr Res 1975;9:513-6.

Moxon ER. Virulence genes and prevention of *Haemophilus influenzae* infections. Arch Dis Child 1985;60:1193-6.

Musser JM, Granoff DM, Pattison PE, Selander RK. A population genetic framework for the study of invasive diseases caused by serotype b strains of *Haemophilus influenzae*. Proc Natl Acad Sci 1985;82:5078-82.

Musser JM, Kroll JS, Moxon ER, Selander RK. Clonal populations structure of encapsulated *Haemophilus influenzae*. Infect Immun 1988;56:1837-1845.

Peltola H, Kayhty H, Virtanen M, Makela PH. Prevention of *Haemophilus influenzae* type b bacteremic infections with the capsular polysaccharide vaccine. N Engl J Med 1984;310:1566-1569.

Sell SH. Haemophilus influenzae type b meningitis: manifestations and long term sequelae. Pediatr Infect Dis 1987;6:775-778.

Takala AK, Eskola J, Peltola H, Mäkelä PH. Epidemiology of invasive *Haemophilus influenzae* type b disease among children in Finland before vaccination with *Haemophilus influenzae* type b conjugate vaccine. Pediatr Infect Dis 1989;8:297-302.

Takala AK, van Alphen L, Eskola J, Palmgren J, et al. *Haemophilus influenzae* type b strains of outer membrane subtypes 1 and 1c cause different types of invasive disease. Lancet 1987;2:647-650.

van Alphen L, Geelen L, Jonsdottir K, et al. Distinct geographical distribution of HIB subtypes in Western Europe. J Infect Dis 1987;156:216-218.

Ward JI, Broome CV, Harrison LJ, et al. *Haemophilus influenzae* type b vaccines: lessons for the future. Pediatrics 1988a;81:886-892.

Ward JI, Cochi S. *Haemophilus influenzae* Vaccines. In Plotkin SA, Mortimer EA eds. Vaccines. Philadelphia: WB Saunders, 1988, p 303.

Wenger JD, Hightower AW, Facklam RR, et al. Bacterial meningitis in the United States, 1986: report of a multistate surveillance study. J Infect Dis 1990;162:1316-1323.

9

VIRAL HEPATITIS: A, B, C, D, AND E

The term *viral hepatitis* refers to a primary infection of the liver caused by at least five etiologically and immunologically distinct viruses: hepatitis A (HAV), hepatitis B (HBV), hepatitis C (HCV), hepatitis D (HDV), and hepatitis E (HEV). Hepatitis may occur also during the course of disease caused by the following viruses: cytomegalovirus (CMV), Epstein-Barr virus (EBV), herpes simplex virus (HSV), and varicella-zoster virus (VZV).

Hepatitis A is synonymous with *infectious hepatitis*, an ancient disease described by Hippocrates and formerly known as *epidemic jaundice*, acute *catarrhal jaundice*, and other designations. The fulminant form of the disease was called *acute yellow atrophy of the liver*.

Hepatitis B is synonymous with *serum hepatitis*, a disease with a more recent history. The first known outbreak occurred in 1883 among a group of shipyard workers who were vaccinated against smallpox with glycerinated lymph of human origin (Lürman, 1885). Later, an increased incidence of the disease was observed among patients attending venereal disease clinics, diabetic clinics, and other facilities in which multiple injections were given with inadequately sterilized syringes and needles contaminated with the blood of a carrier. The most extensive outbreak occurred in 1942 when yellow fever vaccine containing human serum caused 28,585 cases of hepatitis B infection with jaundice among U.S. military personnel. It was unknown at the time of vaccination that the human serum component of the vaccine was contaminated

with HBV. The additional aliases of hepatitis B recorded in the literature include *homologous serum jaundice, transfusion jaundice, syringe jaundice,* and *postvaccinal jaundice*.

Hepatitis C was formerly designated *parenterally transmitted non-A, non-B hepatitis* (PT-NANB). Non-A, non-B (NANB) hepatitis was recognized as a clinical entity in the 1970s when specific tests for the identification of HAV and HBV infections became available. The identification of HCV as the most common cause of PT-NANB hepatitis was reported in 1989 (Choo et al., Kuo et al.).

Hepatitis delta virus (HDV) is a "defective" RNA virus that can replicate only in the presence of acute or chronic HBV infection. The genome of HDV codes for an internal antigen (HDAg), but the virus is encapsulated by hepatitis B surface antigen (HBsAg) of the helper HBV. The delta antigen was discovered by Rizzetto et al. in 1977.

Hepatitis E was previously called *enterically transmitted NANB* (ET-NANB). Serological studies of various outbreaks of ET-NANB hepatitis revealed no evidence of HAV or HBV infection (Khuroo, 1980). In retrospect, it is clear that these outbreaks were caused by HEV, an agent that was cloned by Reyes et al. in 1990.

ETIOLOGY
Hepatitis A

Before the mid-1960s knowledge of the properties of HAV was derived from human volunteer studies. The agent survived a temperature of 56° C for 30 minutes (Havens et al., 1944) and was inactivated by heating at 98° C for 1 minute (Krugman et al., 1970). It retained its infectivity after storage at −18° C to −70° C for several years. HAV was more resistant to chlorine than many bacteria found in drinking water.

Oral or parenteral administration of the virus caused hepatitis after an incubation period ranging from 15 to 40 days, averaging approximately 30 days. Extensive studies with the MS-1 strain of HAV and the MS-2 strain of HBV confirmed observations by Havens et al. (1944) and Neefe et al. (1946) that hepatitis A and B viruses were immunologically distinct (Krugman et al., 1967).

In 1966 Deinhardt et al. reported the successful transmission of hepatitis A to marmoset monkeys. Later, additional studies by his group (Holmes et al., 1969) and by Lorenz et al. (1970), Mascoli et al. (1973), Provost et al. (1973), and

Maynard (1974) confirmed the successful transmission of human HAV to marmosets. In addition, Dienstag et al. (1975b) successfully transmitted HAV to susceptible chimpanzees.

In 1973 Feinstone et al. reported the identification of 27 nm viruslike particles in the stools of adults who had been infected with the MS-1 strain of HAV. These particles were identified by immune electron microscopy (IEM). These findings were confirmed by Maynard (1974), who induced hepatitis in marmosets by inoculating them with stool filtrates containing the 27 nm particles.

Human HAV was further characterized by Provost et al. (1975b), who reported that the 27 nm particles appeared to have the physical, chemical, and biological characteristics of an enterovirus. It has been designated enterovirus type 27 (Melnick, 1982). Electron micrographs comparing HAV with HBV are shown in Fig. 9-

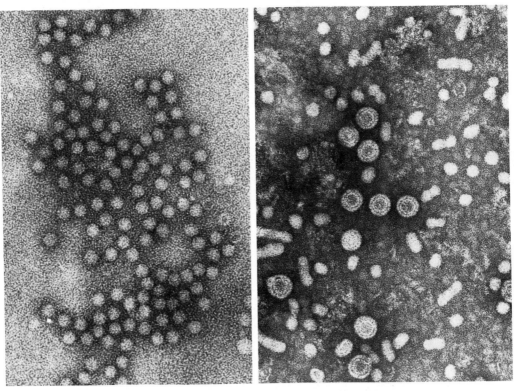

Type A   Type B

Fig. 9-1. Electron micrographs of type A and type B hepatitis viruses. Type A: Note 27 nm particles, uniform in size. Type B: Note 43 nm Dane particles (hepatitis B virus) and spherical and filamentous particles 20 nm in diameter (hepatitis B surface antigen). (From Provost PJ et al: Am J Med Sci 1975; 270:87.)

1. Unlike HBV, HAV is a simple, nonenveloped virus with a nucleocapsid that has been designated hepatitis A antigen (HA Ag). The HAV capsid consists of 32 capsomeres arranged in icosahedral conformation; it is composed of four virion polypeptides (VP1, VP2, VP3, and VP4). A single-stranded molecule of RNA is present inside the capsid.

Purified HAV is inactivated by formalin, ultraviolet irradiation, heating at 100° C for 5 minutes, or treatment with chlorine (Provost et al., 1975b; Peterson et al., 1982). The purified virus was shown by IEM as specifically aggregated by hepatitis A antibody (anti-HAV).

Miller et al. (1975) prepared HA Ag from infected marmoset liver for use in an immune adherence hemagglutination antibody (IAHA) test. Both HA Ag and anti-HAV can be detected by various established serological methods, including IEM (Feinstone et al., 1973), radio-immunoassay (RIA) (Hollinger et al., 1975), enzyme immunoassay (EIA) (Duermeyer et al., 1978), and immunofluorescence (IF) (Murphy et al., 1978). The RIA and EIA tests are the most practical for serodiagnosis of acute hepatitis A.

In 1979 Provost and Hilleman reported the propagation of human HAV in primary explant cell cultures of marmoset livers and in the normal fetal rhesus kidney cell line (FRhK6). Provost et al. (1981) subsequently isolated HAV directly from acute-phase human stool specimens by in vitro propagation in an FRhK6 line. Other workers demonstrated that HAV could be cultivated in human diploid fibroblasts (Gauss-Muller et al., 1981), in human amniotic (FL) and Vero cells (Kojima et al., 1981), and in African green monkey kidney (AGMK) cell cultures (Daemer et al., 1981). HAV propagates in the cytoplasm and is noncytopathic.

The HAV genome has been cloned by various investigators (Ticehurst et al., 1983; Baroudy et al., 1985). Modern molecular biological techniques have provided insight into the structure and organization of the virus, thereby revealing similarities to and differences from other enteroviruses.

Hepatitis B

The human volunteer studies of the 1940s indicated that hepatitis B was highly infectious by inoculation. These studies suggested that HBV caused a parenteral infection characterized by a long incubation period of 50 to 180 days and, unlike HAV, was not infectious by mouth.

Studies in the 1960s provided evidence for the existence of two types of viral hepatitis with distinctive clinical, epidemiological, and immunological features (Krugman et al., 1967). One type, MS-1, resembled hepatitis A; it was characterized by an incubation period of 30 to 38 days and a high degree of contagion by contact. The other type, MS-2, resembled hepatitis B; it had a longer incubation period of 41 to 108 days. Contrary to the prevailing concept, the MS-2 strain of HBV was infectious both by mouth and parenterally.

The successful transmission of HBV to chimpanzees was achieved in the early 1970s (Maynard et al., 1972; Barker et al., 1973). The chimpanzee has proved to be a highly sensitive animal model for the study of hepatitis B infection.

The discovery of Australia antigen by Blumberg et al. (1965) and its subsequent association with hepatitis B had a major impact on the understanding of the etiology and natural history of the disease.

By the early 1970s the agent responsible for hepatitis B had been identified and characterized. Electron microscopic examination of serum obtained from patients with acute or chronic type B hepatitis revealed the following types of viruslike particles: (1) spherical particles, 20 nm in diameter (Bayer et al., 1968); (2) filamentous particles, 100 nm or more in length and 20 nm in diameter (Hirschman et al., 1969); and (3) "Dane particles," approximately 42 nm in diameter (Dane et al., 1970) (see Fig. 9-1). The available evidence indicates that the Dane particle is the complete hepatitis B virion and that the 20 nm spherical particles represent excess virus-coat (HBsAg) material. The HBsAg and Dane particles occur free in serum.

Hepatitis B virus (Dane particle). The HBV, a complex 42 nm virion, is a member of a new class of viruses designated *hepadna*. The precise nomenclature of HBV is hepadna virus type 1 (Melnick, 1982). Unlike HAV, it has not been propagated successfully in cell culture. Nevertheless, its biophysical and biochemical properties have been well characterized, and the HBV genome has been cloned and sequenced.

A schematic illustration of the structure of

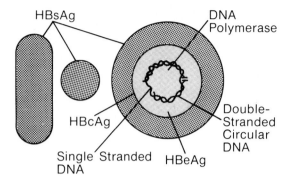

Fig. 9-2. Schematic illustration of the hepatitis B virus and its antigens: hepatitis B surface antigen *(HBsAg)*, hepatitis B core antigen *(HBcAg)*, and hepatitis B e antigen *(HBeAg)*.

HBV and its antigens is shown in Fig. 9-2. The virus is a double-shelled particle; its outer surface component, the hepatitis B surface antigen (HBsAg), is immunologically distinct from the inner core component, the hepatitis B core antigen (HBcAg). The core contains the genome of HBV, a single molecule of partially double-stranded DNA. One of the strands is incomplete, leaving a single-stranded or gap region. Additional components of the core include DNA-dependent DNA polymerase and hepatitis B e antigen (HBeAg).

A simple, direct molecular hybridization test has been developed to detect HBV DNA in serum. Studies by various investigators have revealed that most HBeAg-positive sera have detectable HBV DNA (Lieberman et al., 1983; Scotto et al., 1983).

Hepatitis B surface antigen. The HBsAg particle contains approximately seven polypeptides. Multiple antigenic specificities of HBsAg are associated with these polypeptides. Serological analysis of HBsAg particles indicates that (1) they share a common group-specific determinant *a* and (2) they usually carry at least two mutually exclusive subdeterminants, *d* or *y* and *w* or *r* (LeBouvier, 1972). The subtypes are the phenotypic expressions of distinct genotype variants of HBV. Four principal phenotypes have been recognized: *adw, adr, ayw,* and *ayr.* Other complex permutations of these subdeterminants and new variants are listed in Table 9-1. The subtypes are valuable epidemiological markers of infection. Protection against infection apparently is conferred by antibody against the *a* specificity.

Table 9-1. Nomenclature of hepatitis B antigens and antibodies

HBV	Hepatitis B virus; a 42 nm double-shelled virus, originally known as the Dane particle
HBsAg	Hepatitis B surface antigen; the hepatitis B antigen found on the surface of the virus and on the accompanying unattached spherical (22 nm) and tubular particles
HBcAg	Hepatitis B core antigen; the hepatitis B antigen found within the core of the virus
HBeAg	The e antigen, which is closely associated with hepatitis B infection
anti-HBs	Antibody to hepatitis B surface antigen
anti-HBc	Antibody to hepatitis B core antigen
anti-HBc	Antibody to the e antigen

Subdeterminants of hepatitis B surface antigen:

ayw1	(a_1y2)	*adw₂*	(a_2^1dw)
ayw2	(a_2^1yw)	*adw₄*	(a_3dw)
ayw3	(a_2^3yw)	*adr*	
ayw4	(a_3yw)	*adyw*	
ayr			

From World Health Organization Expert Committee on Viral Hepatitis: Advances in viral hepatitis, WHO Tech Rep Ser No. 602, 1977.

Various tests for the detection of HBsAg and anti-HBs have been developed. These techniques have proved very useful for various studies involving (1) the testing of blood donors and blood products, (2) the diagnosis of acute and chronic hepatitis and the hepatitis B carrier state, (3) the epidemiology of hepatitis B infections, (4) various investigations designed to enhance knowledge of the pathogenesis and immunological aspects of the disease, and (5) the evaluation of active and passive immunization procedures for the prevention of HBV infections.

Hepatitis C

Studies in chimpanzees by Bradley et al. (1987) revealed the presence of a transmissible agent in blood products that caused NANB hepatitis. The agent was sensitive to organic solvents, and it was less than 80 nm in diameter as assessed by filtration. Using large quantities of Bradley's well-characterized highly infectious plasma as a source of virus, Choo et al. (1989)

cloned the genome of this NANB agent, HCV. The physical characteristics of HCV indicate that it is a flavivirus-like agent; it contains a positive single-stranded RNA molecule.

Hepatitis D

The 35 nm HDV double-shelled particle resembles HBV on electron microscopy. It has an external coat antigen of HBsAg provided by the genome of HBV (the helper virus) and an internal delta antigen (HDAg) provided by the HDV genome. A small circular RNA molecule is associated with the HDAg; it is single stranded. HDV RNA isolated from infected liver is present in linear or circular forms. The structure and replicative cycle of HDV place it outside of any known family of animal viruses.

Hepatitis E

Viruslike particles, 27 to 30 nm in diameter, were detected by Balayan et al. (1981) in fecal samples from a volunteer who ingested an aqueous extract of feces obtained from patients with enterically transmitted NANB hepatitis. A similar agent was transmitted to marmosets and chimpanzees by Bradley et al. (1987). This cause of ET-NANB hepatitis is the HEV. The virus apparently is very labile. Its biophysical properties indicate that it is a calcivirus-like agent.

PATHOLOGY
Acute viral hepatitis

The histological features of acute viral hepatitis caused by various hepatitis viruses (A, B, C, D, and E) may be indistinguishable. The characteristic findings on biopsy include necrosis and inflammation of the lobule, architectural consequences of the necrosis, and proliferation of the mesenchymal and bile duct elements. Anicteric hepatitis shows the same histological appearance as icteric but usually with less severity.

During the fully developed stage of hepatitis there are degeneration and death of liver cells, proliferation of the Kupffer cells, mononuclear cell infiltration, and bile duct proliferation. The hepatic cell changes involve the entire lobule, with a concentration of lesions in the centrolobular areas. The cells are usually swollen, but occasionally they are shrunken. As the lesions progress, there may be a variable degree of collapse, condensation of reticulin fibers, and accumulation of ceroid pigment and large phagocytic cells, first within the lobules and later in the portal tracts. In HEV infection the typical changes are focal necrosis with little infiltration and no lobular predilection. The focal lesions resemble those seen in drug-associated toxic hepatitis.

During the recovery period the following residual changes may be seen: pleomorphic liver cells around central veins, focal inflammatory infiltration of portal tracts, and a mild degree of fibrosis extending from the portal tracts. Liver cell necrosis is slight or absent, but ceroid pigment may be found in the portal tracts.

Complete resolution is the usual course of all types of viral hepatitis. In most cases complete regeneration of the liver cells is observed after 2 or 3 months. However, other possible consequences include chronic persistent or chronic active hepatitis, resolution of hepatitis with postnecrotic scarring, cirrhosis, or fatal massive necrosis.

Chronic active hepatitis

Chronic active hepatitis caused by HBV, HCV, and HDV is characterized histologically by accumulations of lymphocytes and plasma cells that are located in the portal tracts and in foci of necrosis scattered throughout the hepatic lobules. Other findings include disruption of the limiting plate of the hepatic lobule adjacent to the portal tract and extension of the inflammatory reaction out of the portal tract into the hepatic parenchyma. The hepatocytes undergoing necrosis in these areas apparently are entrapped by the inflammatory infiltrate (so-called "piecemeal necrosis"). Small clusters of hepatocytes may be surrounded by the inflammatory process, thereby creating a "rosette" appearance.

The inflammation may vary in severity and distribution. A predominance of plasma cells may be found in patients with lupoid hepatitis.

The pattern of lobular collapse and necrosis bridging portal areas and central veins has been termed *submassive necrosis* or *bridging necrosis* (Boyer and Klatskin, 1970). These findings during a biopsy indicate a poor prognosis.

The presence of portal fibrosis is variable. In more severe cases there is a marked deposition of fibrous tissue in the portal areas accompanied by collapse of the hepatic lobular architecture and formation of fibrous tissue "bridges" between adjacent portal areas and central veins. In advanced stages the extensive cirrhosis may mask the chronic inflammatory process, resulting in histological evidence of cryptogenic or macronodular cirrhosis.

Chronic persistent hepatitis

In patients with chronic persistent hepatitis the lymphocytic inflammatory infiltration is confined chiefly to the portal tracts. The lobular architecture of the liver is preserved, evidence of hepatocellular damage is minimal or absent, and fibrosis is only slight or absent. Piecemeal necrosis, very typical with chronic active hepatitis, is lacking in chronic persistent hepatitis.

Fulminant hepatitis

In patients with fulminant hepatitis with death occurring within 10 days, the size of the liver is reduced, and its color is yellow or mottled (acute yellow atrophy). Histological findings include extensive, diffuse necrosis and loss of hepatocytes, which are replaced by an inflammatory infiltrate composed of both polymorphonuclear and monocytic cells. The lobular structure of the liver may be collapsed. Occasionally, however, the architecture of the liver may be well preserved. Kupffer cells and histiocytes contain phagocytized material from disintegrated liver cells. Bile thrombi may be seen in the canaliculi. Portal triads that usually are retained are filled with monocytes, lymphocytes, and polymorphonuclear cells. Occasionally, surviving liver tissue may be seen in the periphery of the lobules.

Regeneration of liver tissue may begin if patients survive for several days. The regeneration appears as clusters of cells scattered randomly throughout the liver. As regeneration advances, these "pseudolobules" of liver parenchyma appear to form adenoma-like groups of liver cells unrelated to the normal lobular architecture and lacking central veins.

Patients who survive fulminant hepatitis usually have a remarkable recovery of liver function. Little or no residual liver damage is seen in biopsy specimens, although occasionally a coarse lobular type of cirrhosis is noted (Karvountzis et al., 1974).

IMMUNOPATHOLOGY
Hepatitis A

Hepatitis A antigen is detected in the cytoplasm of hepatocytes shortly before onset of acute hepatitis. Viral expression decreases rapidly after the appearance of clinical and histological manifestations and IgM-specific anti-HAV. These findings indicate that hepatocellular damage is caused chiefly by immunological rather than cytotoxic factors. Propagation of HAV in tissue culture is not associated with a cytopathic effect.

Hepatitis B and C

The pathological and clinical consequences of hepatitis B and C infections are related to at least two factors: (1) HBV and HCV are not cytopathogenic, and (2) liver cell necrosis is in great part the result of host defenses.

Cell necrosis may be the result of a cellular and immune response to HBV and HCV infection. Acute hepatitis with recovery may be associated with an efficient immune response that eliminates virus-infected cells by means of spotty necrosis. Viral antigens (HBsAg and HBcAg) that may be present in the liver before elicitation of the immune response are eliminated at the height of the acute disease. In contrast, chronic forms of hepatitis B and C may be the result of a quantitatively and/or qualitatively ineffective immune response.

Under the conditions of high-grade immunosuppression such as occurs in kidney transplant recipients, HBV may persist in the liver without any substantial liver cell damage. On the other hand, in patients with chronic active hepatitis the occurrence of piecemeal necrosis may be a consequence of a partially deficient immune state. The available evidence indicates that an immune defect resulting in the incomplete elimination of infected hepatocytes is a cause of chronic HBV infection.

CLINICAL MANIFESTATIONS

The similarities and differences between the clinical manifestations of viral hepatitis types A, B, C, D, and E are listed in Table 9-2. The incubation period of hepatitis A ranges between 15 and 40 days, and the onset of symptoms is usually acute. In contrast, the incubation period of hepatitis B is longer (50 to 180 days), and the onset more commonly is insidious. The incubation period of hepatitis C may be the same as that of both type A and type B hepatitis; it may range between 1 and 5 months. In general, the clinical features of hepatitis C resemble type B infection more than type A.

The clinical picture shows great variation.

Table 9-2. Viral hepatitis types A, B, D, C, and E: comparison of clinical, epidemiological, and immunological features

Features	A	B	D	C	E
Virus	HAV	HBV	HDV	HCV	HEV
Family	Picornavirus	Hepadnavirus	Satellite	Flavivirus	Calicivirus
Genome	RNA	DNA	RNA	RNA	RNA
Incubation period	15-40 days	50-180 days	21-90 days	1-5 months	2-9 weeks
Type of onset	Usually acute	Usually insidious	Usually acute	Usually insidious	Usually acute
Prodrome: arthritis and rash	Not present	May be present	Unknown	May be present	Not present
Mode of transmission					
Oral (fecal)	Usual	No	No	No	Usual
Parenteral	Rare	Usual	Usual	Usual	No
Other	Food or water-borne	Intimate (sexual) contact, perinatal	Intimate (sexual) contact less common	Intimate (sexual) contact less common	Waterborne transmission in developing countries
Sequelae					
Carrier	No	Yes	Yes	Yes	No
Chronic hepatitis	No cases reported	Yes	Yes	Yes	No cases reported
Mortality	0.1%-0.2%	0.5%-2.0% in uncomplicated cases; may be higher in complicated cases	2%-20%	1%-2% in uncomplicated cases; may be higher in complicated cases	20% in pregnant women; 1%-2% in general population
Immunity					
Homologous	Yes	Yes	Yes	Yes	Yes
Heterologous	No	No	No	No	No

In children the acute disease is generally milder, and its course is shorter than in adults. In children or adults jaundice may be inapparent or evanescent, or it may persist for many weeks. The course of the disease often may be separated into two phases: preicteric and icteric. However, occasionally jaundice may be the initial symptom.

Preicteric phase

Fever, when present, appears during the preicteric phase of the disease; often it is absent or fleeting in young children, but in adolescents and adults it may last for 5 days. The temperature ranges from 37.8° to 40° C (100° to 104° F) and generally is accompanied by headache, las-

situde, anorexia, nausea, vomiting, and abdominal pain. Urticaria and arthralgia or arthritis occurring during the preicteric phase usually are manifestations of hepatitis B. The liver may be enlarged and tender, and splenomegaly and lymphadenopathy may be present in some patients.

Icteric phase

Jaundice begins to emerge as the fever subsides; it usually is preceded by the appearance of dark urine (biliuria). In young children the transition to the icteric phase is most often marked by disappearance of symptoms. On the other hand, in adults and older children the icteric phase may be accompanied by an exacer-

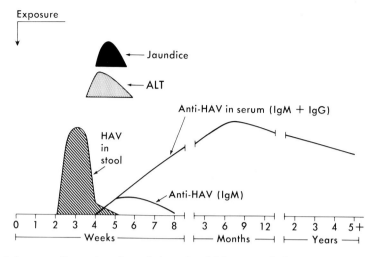

Fig. 9-3. Schematic illustration of serial clinical and laboratory findings in a patient with type A hepatitis. Hepatitis A virus *(HAV)* is detected in stool during the latter part of the incubation period before onset of the disease. Appearance of hepatitis A antibody *(anti-HAV)* coincides with disappearance of HAV in stool. IgM-specific anti-HAV is detected at the time of onset of disease; IgG-specific anti-HAV appears approximately 1 week later. (Modified from Frösner GG: Munch Med Wochenschr 1977; 119:825.)

bation of some of the original symptoms such as anorexia, nausea, vomiting, and abdominal pain. Mental depression, bradycardia, and pruritus, all frequently occurring in adults, are uncommon in children. The stools may be clay colored, but this is an inconstant finding. The icteric phase persists from a few days to as long as a month, with an average duration of 8 to 11 days in children in contrast to 3 to 4 weeks in adults. As jaundice fades, the patient's symptoms subside. As a rule, convalescence is rapid and uneventful. Excessive weight loss is more common in adults than in children. In small infants and children less than 3 years of age hepatitis is usually anicteric.

Jaundice is a very rare manifestation of neonatal hepatitis B infection. Most HBV-infected infants born to mothers who are HBV carriers have a chronic asymptomatic infection.

Hepatitis A

The course of hepatitis A is shown in Fig. 9-3. After an incubation period of approximately 30 days, there is a spiking rise in serum alanine aminotransferase (ALT) levels. The duration of abnormal ALT levels in children is brief, rarely exceeding 2 to 3 weeks.

The serum bilirubin value usually becomes abnormal when ALT reaches peak levels. The increased level of serum bilirubin may be tran-

sient, and the duration may be as short as 1 day or may persist for more than 1 month. In general, jaundice is transient in children and more prolonged in adults.

The following tests are available for the detection of hepatitis A antibody: IAHA, RIA, and EIA. As indicated in Fig. 9-3, RIA anti-HAV is detected very early—at the time of onset of disease. Initially, RIA anti-HAV is predominantly IgM; later it is exclusively IgG. The time of appearance of EIA anti-HAV is the same for RIA, and the test apparently is equally sensitive.

The duration of illness caused by HAV is variable, ranging from several weeks to several months. The degree of morbidity and the duration of jaundice correlate directly with the patient's age. Even with prolonged acute illness lasting several months, complete resolution of hepatitis usually occurs. Unlike hepatitis B, C, and D, HAV infection does not cause chronic liver disease. Viremia is transient; it is not characterized by a chronic carrier state. Although the outcome of HAV infection is usually favorable, fulminant hepatitis may occur. McNeil et al. (1984) reported three deaths (0.14%) in a series of 2,174 consecutive virologically or serologically confirmed *hospitalized* cases. Thus the death rate among all hepatitis A cases must be negligible.

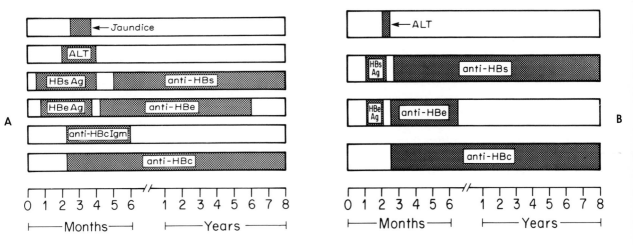

Fig. 9-4. A, Acute hepatitis B followed by recovery, showing results of serial tests for serum alanine aminotransferase *(ALT)*, hepatitis B surface antigen *(HBsAg)* and its antibody *(anti-HBs)*, hepatitis B e antigen *(HBeAg)* and its antibody *(anti-HBe)*, hepatitis B core antibody *(anti-HBc)*, and anti-HBc IgM. **B,** Subclinical hepatitis B infection followed by an immune response. Shaded areas denote "abnormal" or "detectable," and white areas denote "normal" or "not detectable." (From Krugman S: Pediatr Rev 1985; 7:3-11.)

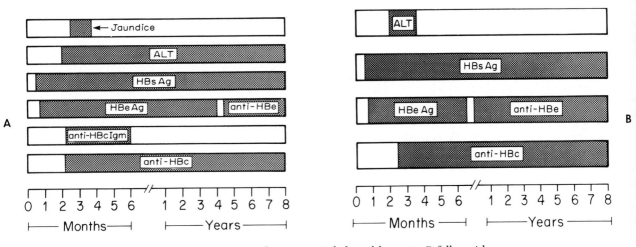

Fig. 9-5. A, Chronic hepatitis B infection. **B,** Subclinical hepatitis B followed by an asymptomatic chronic carrier state. See Fig. 9-4 for key. (From Krugman S: Pediatr Rev 1985; 7:3-11.)

Hepatitis B

The course of hepatitis B infection is shown in Figs. 9-4 and 9-5. The incubation period may range from 2 to 6 months. The detection of HBsAg in the blood of a patient with acute hepatitis is indicative of HBV infection. The characteristic laboratory findings and the profile of abnormal liver function are shown in Table 9-3 and Fig. 9-4.

HBsAg may be detected by RIA 6 to 30 days after a parenteral exposure and 56 to 60 days after an oral exposure (Krugman, 1979; Krugman et al., 1979). The antigen may be detected approximately 1 week to 2 months before the appearance of abnormal levels of ALT and jaundice. In most patients with acute hepatitis B, HBsAg is consistently present during the latter part of the incubation period and during the preicteric phase of the disease. The antigen may become undetectable shortly after onset of jaundice.

The pattern of serum ALT activity is illus-

Table 9-3. Detection of hepatitis B surface antigen (HBsAg), antibody to HBsAg (anti-HBs), antibody to hepatitis B core antigen (anti-HBc), hepatitis B e antigen (HBeAg), and antibody to HBeAg (anti-HBe) during the course of type B hepatitis infection

Time of hepatitis B infection	HBsAg	anti-HBs	anti-HBc	HBeAg	anti-HBe
Late incubation period	+	0	0	+	0
Early in course of acute hepatitis (<1 week)	+	0	+	+	0
Late in course of acute hepatitis (1 to 4 weeks)	+ or 0	+ or 0	+	+ or 0	0 or +
Convalescence from acute hepatitis					
Early (4 to 8 weeks)	0	+ or 0	+	0	+ or 0
Late (>8 weeks)	0	+	+	0	+ or 0

+, present; 0, not present.

trated in Fig. 9-4, *A*. After an incubation period of approximately 50 days, the serum ALT values become abnormal, rising gradually over a period of several weeks. The duration of abnormal ALT activity may be prolonged, usually exceeding 30 to 60 days.

As indicated in Fig. 9-4, *A*, the first antibody that is detectable is anti-HBc. It appears approximately 1 week or more after the onset of hepatitis. The anti-HBc titers, predominantly IgM, are usually high for several months. Thereafter IgM values decline to low or undetectable levels, but anti-HBc persists for many years (Chau et al., 1983). The commercially available test for anti-HBc IgM is a solid-phase immunoassay; its cut-off assay value was established to differentiate high levels of antibody (positive) from low or undetectable levels (negative). The test is negative in healthy HBsAg carriers and in patients with cirrhosis. It may be positive in those with chronic hepatitis characterized by marked inflammatory changes without cirrhosis.

The anti-HBc IgM assay should be useful for differentiating recent from past HBV infections and identifying acute hepatitis B in patients whose HBsAg has declined to undetectable levels before the appearance of anti-HBs (window phase). Antibody to the HBsAg usually appears late, approximately 2 weeks to 2 months after HBsAg is no longer detectable. Anti-HBs is detected in approximately 80% of patients with hepatitis B who eventually become HBsAg negative. In the remainder the antibody levels are too low for detection. Anti-HBs may be detected in approximately 5% to 10% of HBsAg carriers.

The results of tests for HBsAg, HBeAg, anti-HBs, and anti-HBc during the course of hepatitis B are shown in Table 9-3 and in Figs. 9-4 and 9-5.

Most patients with hepatitis B infection recover completely. However, progression to chronic hepatitis with persistence of HBsAg has been reported in 3% of Taiwanese university students (Beasley et al., 1983), in 8% of homosexual men (Szmuness et al., 1981), and in 13% of Eskimos (McMahon et al., 1985). The risk of chronic hepatitis B infection in infants born to mothers who are HBsAg- and HBeAg-positive carriers may exceed 60% (see p. 154). Other serious consequences of acute HBV infection include fulminant hepatitis (see p. 155), cirrhosis, and hepatocellular carcinoma (see p. 156).

Hepatitis C

Most patients with HCV infection are anicteric, especially those who have the contact-acquired sporadic form. The incubation period ranges from 1 to 5 months. The clinical signs and symptoms of the acute illness are milder than those with HAV and HBV infections. However, biochemical evidence of chronic liver disease develops in approximately 50% of patients with posttransfusion hepatitis C (Alter, 1985). As indicated in Fig. 9-6, the ALT elevations fluctuate over prolonged periods of time.

The interval between exposure to HCV or onset of illness and detection of anti-HCV may be prolonged. In recipients of transfusions the mean interval from onset of hepatitis to anti-HCV detection may be 15 weeks (range, 4 to 32

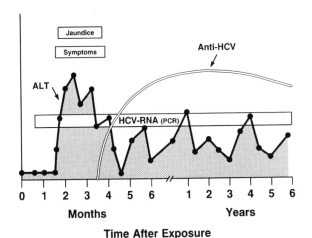

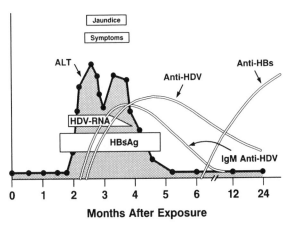

Fig. 9-6. Typical course of a case of acute hepatitis C that progresses to chronic infection and disease. *ALT,* alanine aminotransferase; *HCV-RNA,* hepatitis C virus ribonucleic acid; *PCR,* polymerase chain reaction; *anti-HCV,* antibody to hepatitis C virus. (From Hoofnagle JH, DiBisceglie AM: Semin Liver Dis 1991; 11:78.)

Fig. 9-7. Typical course of a case of acute delta hepatitis coinfection. *ALT,* alanine aminotransferase; *HBsAg,* hepatitis B surface antigen; *HDV-RNA,* hepatitis delta virus ribonucleic acid; *anti-HDV,* antibody to HDV; *anti-HBs,* antibody to HBsAg. (From Hoofnagle JH, DiBisceglie AM: Semin Liver Dis 1991; 11:79.)

weeks). In general, anti-HCV persists in patients with chronic disease; it may disappear in those with acute resolving hepatitis C (Alter et al., 1989; Farci et al., 1991).

The course of a typical case of posttransfusion hepatitis C is shown in Fig. 9-6. Evidence of viremia was detected by the use of polymerase chain reaction (PCR) technology 2 weeks after a transfusion of HCV-contaminated blood. (Unfortunately, PCR, a research tool, is not available in clinical practice.) The first increase in ALT values was detected at 8 weeks, and anti-HCV was detectable at 11 weeks. A 6-year follow-up revealed persistence of positive PCR, detectable anti-HCV, and biopsy evidence of chronic active hepatitis. Long-term prospective studies of patients with posttransfusion (NANB) hepatitis (HCV disease) have revealed evidence of progression to cirrhosis and to hepatocellular carcinoma.

Hepatitis D

The clinical manifestations and course of type D hepatitis resemble those of acute or chronic hepatitis B. In general, however, hepatitis D is a more severe disease. The mortality rate of acute HDV hepatitis has ranged from 2% to 20%, as compared with less than 1% for acute

hepatitis B. In addition, cirrhosis and complications of portal hypertension occur more often and progress more rapidly in patients with hepatitis D.

Acute delta hepatitis occurs as either a coinfection or superinfection of hepatitis B (see Table 9-2). In coinfection there is a simultaneous onset of acute HBV and HDV infection. In superinfection a chronic HBV carrier is infected with HDV.

The course of acute delta coinfection is shown in Fig. 9-7. During the latter part of the incubation period HBsAg, followed by HDV RNA, appears. Thereafter serum ALT levels begin to rise, followed by the development of clinical symptoms and jaundice. Serum ALT activity is often biphasic. Resolution of acute liver disease follows clearance of HBsAg and cessation of HDV replication. The antibody to HDV (anti-HDV) that appears shortly after onset of clinical disease is transient.

The course of acute delta superinfection followed by the development of chronic delta hepatitis is shown in Fig. 9-8. At the time of exposure to HDV this patient was an asymptomatic chronic HBsAg carrier with normal ALT values. At the end of the incubation period there are (1) a rise in serum ALT values, (2) appearance and persistence of HDV RNA, followed by (3) appearance of IgM anti-HDV, which is transient,

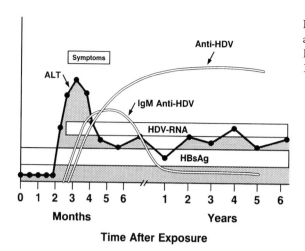

Fig. 9-8. Typical course of a case of acute delta hepatitis superinfection. See Fig. 9-7 for key. (From Hoofnagle JH, DiBisceglie AM: Semin Liver Dis 1991; 11:80.)

and (4) a rise of IgG anti-HDV to high levels that persist.

Hepatitis E

The clinical manifestations and course of hepatitis E are essentially the same as those for hepatitis A. However, there are several striking differences. During various epidemics the disease has been rare in children and common in adolescents and young adults.

HEV, like HAV, does not cause chronic liver disease. In most patients the illness is self-limiting, and there is no evidence of a chronic carrier state. However, unlike hepatitis A, hepatitis E can be a devastating disease in pregnant women. Whereas the mortality rate from hepatitis A in pregnant women is less than 1%, it has ranged from 10% to 20% in outbreaks of hepatitis E. The deaths are caused by fulminant hepatitis. Mortality is highest during the third trimester and lowest during the first trimester. The mortality rate in nonpregnant women is the same as that among men, less than 1%.

At the present time a practical serological test to confirm a diagnosis of hepatitis E is not available. Immune electron microscopy was the first-generation test used by investigators. Second-generation tests such as RIA and EIA are being evaluated for their sensitivity and specificity.

NEONATAL HEPATITIS B INFECTION

HBV is the most common and most important cause of neonatal hepatitis infection. To date, perinatal transmission of HAV, HCV, HDV, and HEV has not been well documented. It is unlikely that HAV and HEV will prove to be problems because these infections are not characterized by a carrier state. The risk of perinatal transmission of HCV is unknown at the present time.

Perinatal transmission of HBV from mother to infant during the course of pregnancy or at the time of birth was first reported by Stokes et al. (1954). They observed an infant born by cesarean section to a mother who was a hepatitis B carrier. The infant, who developed hepatitis with jaundice at 2 months of age, later died at age 18 months with advanced fibrosis of the liver.

The availability of tests to detect HBsAg has enabled various investigators to study infants whose mothers had acute hepatitis B or an asymptomatic chronic carrier state during pregnancy (Schweitzer et al., 1972; Stevens et al., 1975). Signs of neonatal hepatitis B infection (antigenemia) are usually not present at the time of birth but may be detected between 2 weeks and 5 months of age. Approximately 5% of infants are infected in utero and approximately 95% at the time of birth. Certain infants escape infection completely; others develop only persistent antigenemia with no liver disease; others may develop severe chronic active hepatitis; and still others may develop fulminant hepatitis (Fawaz et al., 1975).

Perinatal transmission of hepatitis B infection from mother to infant depends in great part on the presence of HBeAg. Infection is most likely to occur if the mother is HBeAg-positive (Stevens et al., 1975). Infants born to HBeAg-positive carrier mothers have a 60% to 90% chance of contracting chronic hepatitis B infection and possible subsequent progression to cirrhosis and hepatocellular carcinoma. In contrast, the attack rate of hepatitis B in infants whose HBsAg-positive mothers are anti-HBe positive is less than 20%. These infants usually recover completely, and chronic hepatitis is rare, but occasionally the infection may be fulminant with a fatal outcome (Delaplane et al., 1983).

Possible routes of transmission from mother to baby include (1) leakage of virus across the placenta late in pregnancy or during labor, (2) ingestion of amniotic fluid or maternal blood, and (3) breast-feeding, especially if the mother has cracked nipples. Studies by Alter (1980) with HBsAg-positive and HBeAg-positive pregnant chimpanzees revealed that cesarean section and postdelivery isolation did not prevent infection of newborn chimpanzees. They became HBsAg-positive in spite of these precautions.

Infants who inadvertently receive contaminated blood or blood products during the neonatal period may subsequently develop severe hepatitis B. Dupuy et al. (1975) described their experience with 14 infants 2 to 5 months of age, admitted to the hospital with severe or fulminant hepatitis. Of the 14 infants, 11 had serological evidence of hepatitis B infection. Of the 11 infants with hepatitis B, seven received blood derivatives during the neonatal period, and four were exposed to their mothers who were chronic HBsAg carriers. The case fatality rate was very high; eight of the 14 infants died.

COURSE AND COMPLICATIONS

Various factors can affect the course of hepatitis infection: age, type of virus, and immunocompetence. In general, hepatitis A and E are mild or inapparent infections in infants and children. However, they are generally more severe in adults. In contrast, infants infected with HBV are more likely to develop chronic hepatitis B than older children and adults. Unlike hepatitis A, hepatitis B, C, and D infections are more likely to progress to chronic liver disease.

Acute hepatitis

The duration of illness caused by HAV is variable, ranging from several weeks to several months. The degree of morbidity and duration of jaundice correlate directly with age. Even with prolonged acute illness lasting several months, complete resolution of hepatitis usually occurs. Most patients with hepatitis A recover completely. Hepatitis B, C, and D, on the other hand, are associated with more debility and a substantial risk of chronic liver disease. In rare instances acute hepatitis may progress to a fulminant fatal outcome.

Chronic persistent hepatitis

Chronic persistent hepatitis is a pathological diagnosis based on a liver biopsy. It is an inflammatory process involving only the portal areas. This form of hepatitis usually lasts longer than 6 months, and it is more common and less severe than chronic active hepatitis. In general, the patient is asymptomatic and usually has mild hepatomegaly and moderate elevation of serum aminotransferases without jaundice. Chronic persistent hepatitis may resolve after several years or may progress to chronic active hepatitis. These patients may be HBsAg carriers.

Chronic active hepatitis

Chronic active hepatitis, also referred to as *chronic aggressive hepatitis*, is more likely to progress to cirrhosis. The disease is characterized by chronic and recurrent episodes of jaundice, abnormal levels of serum aspartate aminotransferase (AST) and ALT, and evidence of portal hypertension with ascites if the disease progresses to cirrhosis. Severe episodes of hepatic necrosis may terminate in hepatic failure.

Most patients with chronic hepatitis (persistent and/or active) have not had a past history of acute illness with jaundice. The disease usually follows mild, anicteric forms of hepatitis.

Fulminant hepatitis

The occurrence of hepatic failure within the first few days or within 4 weeks after onset of acute hepatitis indicates a fulminant course. When the course is more prolonged and hepatic failure occurs after 1 to 3 months of illness, the term *subacute hepatitis* is used; it is associated with portal hypertension, ascites, and submassive hepatic necrosis.

Fulminant hepatitis usually is characterized by mental confusion, emotional instability, restlessness, bleeding manifestations, and coma.

during the course of the disease. The presence of IgM-specific anti-HAV indicates hepatitis A infection. The interpretation of various serological tests for the diagnosis of hepatitis B infection is shown in Table 9-3. Identification of the five types of hepatitis requires knowledge of their epidemiological features and interpretation of the specific serological tests.

DIFFERENTIAL DIAGNOSIS

Before jaundice emerges, the following diseases may be considered in the differential diagnosis: infectious mononucleosis, acute appendicitis, gastroenteritis, influenza, and, in some parts of the world, malaria, dengue, and sandfly fever. The diagnosis of these diseases may be established by the detection of specific etiological agents, by serological tests, or by the subsequent course.

In the presence of jaundice the diseases that may be confused with viral hepatitis are congenital or acquired hemolytic jaundice or obstructive jaundice caused by blockage of the bile ducts by stone or tumor or, in infants, congenital atresia; hepatocellular jaundice resulting from chemical poisons, cirrhosis, or neoplasm of the liver (primary or metastatic); spirochetal jaundice (Weil's disease); yellow fever; acute cholangitis; and jaundice associated with various other infections such as infectious mononucleosis, brucellosis, amebiasis, malaria, and syphilis. Before considering these diseases in the differential diagnosis, it would be important to rule out a diagnosis of hepatitis A (absence of IgM anti-HAV) and hepatitis B (absence of HBsAg and IgM anti-HBc). At the present time the test for anti-HVC is not useful for the diagnosis of acute HCV infection. A negative test does not rule out HCV infection; it may not be detectable for several months after onset of disease. A positive test may be indicative of a past unrelated infection.

Hemolytic jaundice

Hemolytic jaundice can be differentiated from obstructive jaundice by the history, the presence of anemia, positive Coombs' test, presence of urobilin in the stools, and absence of bilirubinuria.

Extrahepatic obstructive jaundice

Calculi and neoplasms are rare in children. In infancy congenital obliteration of the bile ducts

may present difficulties at first. The distinction should be clear in the course of the illness as the jaundice progressively deepens and the stools remain chalky or gray. Serum aminotransferase levels are lower than those found with viral hepatitis.

Hepatocellular jaundice

Hepatocellular jaundice or parenchymal jaundice caused by chemical poisons may be difficult to diagnose in the absence of a history of ingestion of toxic agents. The history is also important in the recognition of cirrhosis or neoplasm, both of which are uncommon in children in the United States.

Drug-associated hepatitis

Hepatitis induced by the following drugs may be clinically, biochemically, and morphologically indistinguishable from viral hepatitis: pyrazinamide, isoniazid, zoxazolamine, gold, and cinchophen. A clinical picture similar to the cholestatic form of the disease may be produced by the phenothiazine derivatives (e.g., chlorpromazine), methyltestosterone, and contraceptive drugs. Fatal toxic hepatitis has been described in a child receiving indomethacin for rheumatoid arthritis.

Jaundice associated with infection

In patients with jaundice associated with infection the diagnosis is established by demonstrating the specific etiological agent or a rise in the specific antibody in convalescence. Jaundice in the neonatal period should suggest bacterial sepsis, syphilis, CMV infection, toxoplasmosis, congenital rubella, HSV, or Coxsackie B infections. Neonatal hepatitis associated with these infections is present at the time of birth or several days thereafter. In contrast, hepatitis B is usually detected several weeks to as long as 5 months after birth. The diagnosis is established by detection of HBsAg in the blood.

TREATMENT
Acute viral hepatitis

The management of patients with acute hepatitis involves decisions about (1) the duration of bed rest, (2) the choice of a diet, and (3) the value of various nonspecific drugs. At the present time there is no antiviral agent that has been shown to alter the course of either type A or type B hepatitis consistently.

Bed rest is recommended for patients who are symptomatic during the acute stage of the disease. Studies by Chalmers et al. (1955) provided the basis for a more liberal attitude toward bed rest during the convalescent period. They observed that ad-lib activity was preferable to rigidly enforced bed rest for prolonged periods of time.

The liberal attitude toward bed rest described by Chalmers et al. in the 1950s is just as pertinent in the 1990s. Resumption of normal activity is usually gradual. Progressively decreasing serum aminotransferase and bilirubin levels are helpful guides to increasing activity. It is not necessary to restrict the activity of an asymptomatic patient for the many weeks and months that the transaminase levels may be elevated. Generally, children return to normal activity much sooner than adults.

Diet is best regulated by the patient's appetite. While anorexia exists, liquids such as chicken soup and fruit juices should be given. It is recommended that with the return of appetite, a normal diet be given that is nutritious, properly balanced, and palatable. There is no contraindication to ingesting fats in moderate amounts.

Corticosteroids and antiviral agents are not recommended for the treatment of acute hepatitis infections caused by HAV, HBV, HCV, HDV, and HEV.

Chronic persistent hepatitis

Since chronic persistent hepatitis is usually a benign, self-limited disorder, normal activity is advised, and dietary restrictions are unnecessary. Corticosteroid or other immunosuppressive forms of therapy are not indicated.

Chronic active hepatitis

Patients with chronic active hepatitis may be permitted to carry out normal activities on an ad-lib basis. There is no evidence that bed rest and limitation of activity are of benefit. Alcohol should be avoided. A normal, well-balanced diet is recommended. The effect of various antiviral and immunomodulatory agents has been evaluated for the treatment of chronic hepatitis B, C, and D infections.

Chronic hepatitis B. Several studies have revealed that the use of corticosteroids may be detrimental in treating chronic hepatitis B (Hoofnagle, 1987). Adenine arabinoside (Ara-A)

and its monophosphate derivative have not been shown effective. To date the most promising agent has been α or (leukocyte)-interferon.

Various controlled studies in adults have revealed that it is possible to eliminate HBV replication and to ameliorate liver disease in approximately 40% of patients treated with α-interferon (Hoofnagle et al., 1988). However, it should be noted that (1) the therapy involved a 3- to 6-month course of daily or three times per week subcutaneous inoculations; (2) relapses occurred in approximately 50% of responders after therapy was discontinued; and (3) potential side effects included fever, chills, myalgia, anorexia, irritability, weight loss, and hair loss. In one small trial in Hong Kong the effect of α-interferon on chronic hepatitis B in Asian children was not encouraging (Lai et al., 1987).

Chronic hepatitis C. Corticosteroid therapy has not been effective against chronic hepatitis C. Recombinant α-interferon therapy was evaluated in a double-blind, placebo-controlled trial (DiBisceglie et al., 1989). Approximately 50% of patients treated with 2 million units of α-interferon three times weekly for 6 months responded with a fall of ALT values to normal and an improvement in liver histology. However, in most patients relapses occurred after cessation of interferon therapy. This treatment is experimental at the present time.

Chronic hepatitis D. Corticosteroid therapy has not been beneficial in treating chronic hepatitis D; it is not recommended. A controlled trial with α-interferon revealed transient improvement. Cessation of interferon therapy was followed by a return of viral replication and liver disease (Rizzetto et al., 1986).

Fulminant hepatitis

Sudden onset of mental confusion, emotional instability, restlessness, coma, and hemorrhagic manifestations in a patient with hepatitis requires prompt therapy. The rationale for the treatment is to combat the deleterious systemic effects of liver failure. The major objective of treatment of fulminant hepatitis is to reduce the load of nitrogenous products entering the portal circulation. Failure of the compromised liver to remove and detoxify these products is probably responsible for the cerebral dysfunction. The following measures are used: (1) restriction of protein intake, (2) removal of protein already in the gastrointestinal tract (use of a laxative and high colonic irrigations), and (3) suppression of the bacterial population of the bowel (use of neomycin sulfate by mouth or nasogastric tube).

The following therapeutic procedures of unproved benefit have been used: (1) corticosteroids, (2) exchange transfusion, (3) cross-perfusion with human, baboon, or pig liver, and (4) total body perfusion. Studies by the Acute Hepatic Failure Study Group (1977) failed to show any difference in survival rates between groups treated with hepatitis B immune serum globulin (HBIG) as compared with those treated with standard immune globulin (IG). There have been isolated reports of dramatic improvement after liver transplantation.

PROGNOSIS

The prognosis of various types of viral hepatitis has been discussed in the sections devoted to clinical manifestations and to course and complications.

Hepatitis A is a relatively benign disease. Occasionally the illness may be prolonged, but eventually there is complete recovery with no evidence of chronic liver disease. Fatal fulminant hepatitis A may occur, but it is an extraordinarily rare phenomenon.

Most patients with hepatitis B recover completely. However, the risk of chronic infection is extremely variable; it may be low in young healthy adults (approximately 3%) or very high in infants born to HBsAg- and HBeAg-carrier mothers (60% to 90%). The overall risk is near 10%. Chronic hepatitis B infection may progress to cirrhosis of the liver and primary hepatocellular carcinoma. The risk of fatal fulminant hepatitis B is low (<2%) except when there is superinfection with HDV. Under these circumstances the mortality rate may be as high as 30% (Hadler et al., 1984).

Observations of patients with posttransfusion and community-acquired hepatitis C have revealed a relatively high incidence of chronic liver disease—approximately 50% (Alter, 1985; Sampliner et al., 1984). Fulminant hepatitis is an occasional outcome. The overall mortality rate is 1% to 2%. Studies in Japan have revealed that HCV infection is associated with the development of hepatocellular carcinoma (Saito et al., 1990).

Hepatitis E is a relatively benign disease that does not progress to chronic hepatitis. However,

it is a highly fatal disease in pregnant women (Kane et al., 1984).

EPIDEMIOLOGICAL FACTORS
Hepatitis A

The geographical distribution of hepatitis A is worldwide. It is endemic in parts of the world such as the Mediterranean littoral and parts of Africa, South America, Central America, and the Orient, where its presence creates a danger to susceptible military and civilian persons working or traveling in such areas.

Although no age group is immune, the highest incidence in civilian populations occurs among persons less than 15 years of age. In military groups the youngest persons are the ones chiefly affected. Persons of either sex are equally susceptible to infection.

The well-defined autumn-winter seasonal incidence has changed; no consistent seasonal patterns have been observed. In general, at the present time the incidence of hepatitis is fairly constant throughout the year.

Abundant evidence favors transmission through intestinal-oral pathways. HAV is found in the stools of both naturally and experimentally infected persons. Various studies have revealed that HAV is detectable in blood and stools during the latter part of the incubation period. Viremia is no longer detectable after onset of jaundice when anti-HAV appears. Fecal shedding of HAV persists for approximately 1 week after onset of jaundice (Krugman et al., 1962; Dienstag et al., 1975a). These findings indicate that the infection is usually spread during the preicteric phase of the disease and that it is generally not communicable after the first week of jaundice.

Epidemics long have been known to occur in association with poor sanitation in military camps. Explosive waterborne, milkborne, and foodborne epidemics have been reported. Ingestion of raw shellfish from polluted waters has caused many epidemics. For example, an epidemic of hepatitis A in Shanghai, China, in 1988 involved more than 300,000 persons who had eaten raw hairy clams. HAV was isolated from the gills and digestive tracts of the contaminated clams.

There is evidence also for human association as the principal mode of spread. HAV may be transmitted through the use of blood, blood products, or contaminated needles, syringes,

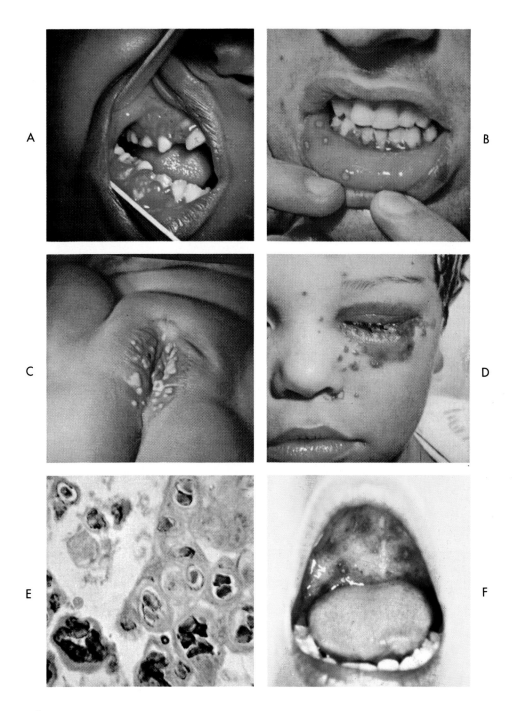

Plate 2

Herpes simplex infections. **A,** Primary herpetic gingivostomatitis in a child. **B,** Same disease in a young adult. **C,** Primary HSVI vulvovaginitis in an infant. **D,** Primary herpetic kerato-conjunctivitis. **E,** Biopsy of herpetic vesicle. Eosinophilic intranuclear inclusions and giant cells. (×800.) **F,** Ulcerative lesions on palate and tongue in hand-foot-and-mouth syndrome caused by Coxsackie A-16 virus. (**A** to **E** from Blank H, Rake G. Viral and rickettsial diseases of the skin, eye, and mucous membranes of man. Boston: Little, Brown & Co., 1955; **F** courtesy James D Cherry, MD)

and stylets. However, this potential mode of transmission is very rare, chiefly because viremia is transient in hepatitis A infection, and a carrier state does not exist.

When hepatitis A occurs in circumscribed situations such as households, day-care centers, orphanages, institutions for mentally handicapped children, military installations, and children's camps, it may smolder for months or years, or it may strike in explosive outbreaks. In families secondary cases may occur in approximately 20 to 30 days.

Seroepidemiological surveys by various investigators have provided valuable information about the distribution of anti-HAV in various population groups (Miller et al., 1975; Szmuness et al., 1976; Villarejos et al., 1976). The investigators observed a striking correlation between the presence of anti-HAV and socioeconomic status. Persons from lower socioeconomic groups were more likely to have detectable anti-HAV (past hepatitis A infection) than those from middle and upper socioeconomic groups. The detection of anti-HAV was strongly correlated with age. In New York City the prevalence increased gradually in adults, reaching peak levels in persons 50 years of age or older. In Costa Rica, however, peak levels were reached by 10 years of age. It is clear that the prevalence of anti-HAV (1) varies among different population groups, (2) increases with age, and (3) is independent of sex and race.

It is likely that the continued improvement of environmental and socioeconomic conditions will decrease the probability of exposure to hepatitis A, thereby changing a predominantly childhood infection to one that is more apt to occur in adults. This changing epidemiological pattern was typical for poliomyelitis during the first half of the twentieth century in the United States. Poliomyelitis, like hepatitis A, is currently a more severe and more disabling disease in adults than in children.

Hepatitis B

Early epidemiological concepts indicated that HBV was transmitted exclusively by the parenteral route. It is now clear, however, that other modes of transmission play an important role in the dissemination of the HBV. The experimental demonstration of oral transmission and the demonstration that contact-associated transmission is common have altered previous epidemiological concepts. The term *contact-associated hepatitis* includes one or more of the following possible modes of transmission: (1) oral-oral, (2) sexual, (3) perinatal, and (4) intimate physical contact of any type. Hepatitis B antigen has been detected in saliva (Ward et al., 1972), in semen (Heathcote et al., 1974), and in many other body fluids.

The major reservoirs of HBV are healthy chronic carriers and patients with acute hepatitis. The infection is transmitted to susceptible persons by transfusion of blood, plasma, or other blood products or by the use of inadequately sterilized needles and syringes. Medical and paramedical personnel may be infected by accidental inoculation or ingestion of contaminated materials. Outbreaks have occurred among drug addicts using unsterilized equipment. Tattooing and acupuncture have been responsible for transmitting the infection. Patients and personnel in the following areas are at high risk: renal dialysis, intensive care, and oncology units and various laboratories in which potentially contaminated blood and tissues are examined.

Seroepidemiological surveys to detect the presence of HBsAg and anti-HBs have confirmed the worldwide distribution of the disease. The antigen has been detected in all populations, even in those living in the most remote areas devoid of parenteral modes of transmission. The antigen is most prevalent among persons living under crowded conditions and with poor hygienic standards, thus accounting for the endemicity of the disease in institutions for mentally retarded persons and in certain developing countries of the world.

The HBsAg carrier rate may range from 0.1% to more than 10%; it is dependent on such factors as geographical location, age, and sex. The carrier rate is higher in tropical, underdeveloped areas than in temperate, developed countries; it is higher in urban than in rural communities and higher among males than among females. As indicated in Table 9-4, the prevalence of anti-HBs in various populations ranges from 3.1% in Switzerland to 78% in Taiwan.

The period of infectivity of patients with hepatitis B is dependent on the presence or absence of a carrier state. HBsAg is detectable in the blood during the latter part of the incubation period and for a variable period after onset of

Table 9-4. Prevalence of antibody to hepatitis B surface antigen (anti-HBs) in the populations surveyed for HAV infections

Country	Number tested	Number anti-HBs positive	Percent positive
United States	1000	108	10.8
Switzerland	98	3	3.1
Belgium	133	7	5.3
Yugoslavia	97	33	34.0
Israel	112	17	15.2
Taiwan	123	96	78.0
Senegal	96	60	62.5

From Szmuness W et al: Am J Epidemiol 1977; 106:392.

jaundice. Infectivity has also been associated with the presence of HBeAg and a high titer of HBsAg. For example, perinatal transmission of hepatitis B infection from HBsAg-positive mothers to their infants is highly likely if they are HBeAg-positive. On the other hand, HBsAg-positive and anti–HBe-positive mothers are much less likely to transmit infection.

Hepatitis C

The availability of a specific serological test to detect anti-HCV has clarified the epidemiology of parenterally transmitted and sporadic HCV infection. The distribution of the disease is worldwide, with an estimated 100 million HCV carriers. In the United States hepatitis C may be the cause of 20% to 40% of all acute hepatitis cases. Persons at high risk of contracting HCV infection include transfusion recipients, intravenous drug users, hemodialysis patients, and health care workers with frequent blood contact. Promiscuous homosexual and heterosexual persons have a low risk of contracting HCV infection, which is not true for HBV. Perinatal transmission of HCV has not been well documented.

Hepatitis D

The epidemiology of hepatitis D is characterized by striking similarities to and certain differences from hepatitis B (see Table 9-2). The modes of transmission are the same except that HDV perinatal infection is rare. In general, the prevalence of HDV correlates with the prevalence of HBV in the following high-risk groups: intravenous drug users, hemophiliacs, and institutionalized mentally retarded patients. In contrast, HDV has not been reported as prevalent in the following HBV high-risk groups: homosexual men and chronic carriers in such highly endemic areas as Southeast Asia, Southern Africa, and Alaska.

Superinfection of chronic HBV carriers has been responsible for epidemics of HDV-associated fulminant hepatitis in Venezuela, Colombia, and Brazil (Hadler et al., 1984; Buitrago et al., 1986). In the United States and in Northern Europe HDV is most common in drug abusers.

Hepatitis E

The epidemiology of hepatitis E is characterized by certain similarities to and many differences from hepatitis A (see Table 9-2). Both hepatitis E and hepatitis A are enterically transmitted diseases that are spread through the fecal-oral route.

Hepatitis A is worldwide in distribution; it is predominantly an infection of children, and the secondary attack rate in household contacts is approximately 10% to 20%. In contrast, hepatitis E has occurred predominantly in certain developing areas of the world during the course of waterborne outbreaks. Hepatitis E is most common in adults but rare in children, and the secondary attack rate in household contacts has been relatively low, less than 3% (Kane et al., 1984).

Hepatitis E epidemics have occurred in China, Southeast and Central Asia, Northern and Western Africa, Mexico, and Central America. The epidemics have either been extensive, involving thousands of persons, or smaller focal outbreaks. With the exception of a few imported cases, hepatitis E has not occurred in the United States (DeCock et al., 1987). Hepatitis E, unlike hepatitis A, is a highly fatal disease in infected pregnant women in whom the mortality rate may be 10% to 20%.

• • •

A detailed discussion of recommendations for prevention of viral hepatitis follows. These recommendations of the Immunization Practices Advisory Committee (ACIP) were reported in the February 9, 1990, issue of the Public Health Service, Centers for Disease Control *Morbidity and Mortality Weekly Report*.

IMMUNE GLOBULINS

Immune globulins are important tools for preventing infection and disease before or after exposure to hepatitis viruses. Immune globulins used in medical practice are sterile solutions of antibodies (immunoglobulins) from human plasma. They are prepared by cold ethanol fractionation of large plasma pools and contain 10%-18% protein. In the United States, plasma is primarily obtained from paid donors. Only plasma shown to be free of hepatitis B surface antigen (HBsAg) and antibody to human immunodeficiency virus (HIV) is used to prepare immune globulins.

Immune globulin (IG) (formerly called immune serum globulin, ISG, or gamma globulin) produced in the United States contains antibodies against the hepatitis A virus (anti-HAV) and the HBsAg (anti-HBs). Hepatitis B immune globulin (HBIG) is an IG prepared from plasma containing high titers of anti-HBs.

There is no evidence that hepatitis B virus (HBV), HIV (the causative agent of acquired immunodeficiency syndrome [AIDS]), or other viruses have ever been transmitted by IG or HBIG commercially available in the United States. Since late April 1985, all plasma units for preparation of IGs have been screened for antibody to HIV, and reactive units are discarded. No instances of HIV infection or clinical illness have occurred that can be attributed to receiving IG or HBIG, including lots prepared before April 1985. Laboratory studies have shown that the margin of safety based on the removal of HIV infectivity by the fractionation process is extremely high. Some HBIG lots prepared before April 1985 have detectable HIV antibody. Shortly after being given HBIG, recipients have occasionally been noted to have low levels of passively acquired HIV antibody, but this reactivity does not persist.

Serious adverse effects from IGs administered as recommended have been rare. IGs prepared for intramuscular administration should be used for hepatitis prophylaxis. IGs prepared for intravenous administration to immunodeficient and other selected patients are not intended for hepatitis prophylaxis. IG and HBIG are not contraindicated for pregnant or lactating women.

HEPATITIS A
Recommendations for IG prophylaxis for hepatitis A

Numerous field studies conducted in the past 4 decades confirm that IG given before exposure or during the incubation period of hepatitis A is protective against clinical illness. Its prophylactic value is greatest (80%-90%) when given early in the incubation period and declines thereafter. Recent tests have shown slightly decreased titers of anti-HAV in current IG lots compared with lots tested 8 years previously; however, no differences in IG efficacy have been noted.

Preexposure prophylaxis

The major group for whom preexposure prophylaxis is recommended is international travelers. The risk of hepatitis A for U.S. citizens traveling abroad varies with living conditions, length of stay, and the incidence of hepatitis A infection in areas visited. In general, travelers to developed areas of North America, western Europe, Japan, Australia, and New Zealand are at no greater risk of infection than they would be in the United States. For travelers to developing countries, risk of infection increases with duration of travel and is highest for those who live in or visit rural areas, trek in back country, or frequently eat or drink in settings of poor sanitation. Nevertheless, recent studies have shown that many cases of travel-related hepatitis A occur in travelers with "standard" tourist itineraries, accommodations, and food and beverage consumption behaviors. In developing countries, travelers should minimize their exposure to hepatitis A and other enteric diseases by avoiding potentially contaminated water or food. Travelers should avoid drinking water (or beverages with ice) of unknown purity and eating uncooked shellfish or uncooked fruits or vegetables that they did not prepare.

IG is recommended for all susceptible travelers to developing countries. IG is especially important for persons who will be living in or visiting rural areas, eating or drinking in settings of poor or uncertain sanitation, or who will have close contact with local persons (especially young children) in settings with poor sanitary conditions. Persons who plan to reside in developing areas for long periods should receive IG regularly.

For travelers, a single dose of IG of 0.02 ml/kg of body weight is recommended if travel is for <3 months. For prolonged travel or residence in developing countries, 0.06 ml/kg should be given every 5 months. For persons who require repeated IG prophylaxis, screening for total anti-HAV before travel is useful to define susceptibility and eliminate unnecessary doses of IG for those who are immune. IG produced in developing countries may not meet the standards for purity required in most developed countries. Persons needing repeat doses overseas should use products that meet U.S. license requirements.

However, studies with inactivated hepatitis A vaccine have confirmed their safety, immunogenicity and efficacy. Hepatitis A vaccines will be licensed for use in 1993. In the future it is likely that inactivated HAV vaccine will replace IG for preexposure prophylaxis.

Postexposure prophylaxis

Hepatitis A cannot be reliably diagnosed on clinical presentation alone, and serologic confirmation of index patients is recommended before contacts are treated. Serologic screening of contacts for anti-HAV before they are given IG is not recommended because screening is more costly than IG and would delay its administration.

For postexposure IG prophylaxis, a single intramuscular dose of 0.02 ml/kg is recommended. IG should be given as soon as possible after last exposure; giving IG more than 2 weeks after exposure is not indicated.

Specific recommendations for IG prophylaxis for hepatitis A depend on the nature of the HAV exposure.

1. Close personal contact. IG is recommended for all household and sexual contacts of persons with hepatitis A.

2. Day-care centers. Day-care facilities attended by children in diapers can be important settings for HAV transmission. IG should be administered to all staff and attendees of day-care centers or homes if a) one or more children or employees are diagnosed as having hepatitis A, or b) cases are recognized in two or more households of center attendees. When an outbreak (hepatitis cases in three or more families) occurs, IG should also be considered for members of households that have children (center attendees) in diapers. In centers not enrolling children in diapers, IG need only be given to classroom contacts of an index patient.

3. Schools. Contact at elementary and secondary schools is usually not an important means of transmitting hepatitis A. Routine administration of IG is not indicated for pupils and teachers in contact with a patient. However, when an epidemiologic investigation clearly shows the existence of a school- or classroom-centered outbreak, IG may be given to persons who have close contact with patients.

4. Institutions for custodial care. Living conditions in some institutions, such as prisons and facilities for the developmentally disabled, favor transmission of hepatitis A. When outbreaks occur, giving IG to residents and staff who have close contact with patients with hepatitis A may

reduce the spread of disease. Depending on the epidemiologic circumstances, prophylaxis can be limited or can involve the entire institution.

5. Hospitals. Routine IG prophylaxis for hospital personnel is not indicated. Rather, sound hygienic practices should be emphasized. Staff education should point out the risk of exposure to hepatitis A and should emphasize precautions regarding direct contact with potentially infective materials.

   Outbreaks of hepatitis A occur occasionally among hospital staff, usually in association with an unsuspected index patient who is fecally incontinent. Large outbreaks have occurred from contact with infected infants in neonatal intensive care units. In outbreaks, prophylaxis of persons exposed to feces of infected patients may be indicated.

6. Offices and factories. Routine IG administration is not indicated under the usual office or factory conditions for persons exposed to a fellow worker with hepatitis A. Experience shows that casual contact in the work setting does not result in virus transmission.

7. Common-source exposure. IG use might be effective in preventing foodborne or waterborne hepatitis A if exposure is recognized in time. However, IG is not recommended for persons exposed to a common source of hepatitis infection after cases have begun to occur, since the 2-week period during which IG is effective will have been exceeded.

   If a food handler is diagnosed as having hepatitis A, common-source transmission is possible but uncommon. IG should be administered to other food handlers but is usually not recommended for patrons. However, IG administration to patrons may be considered if all of the following conditions exist: a) the infected person is directly involved in handling, without gloves, foods that will not be cooked before they are eaten, and b) the hygienic practices of the food handler are deficient or the food handler has had diarrhea, and c) patrons can be identified and treated within 2 weeks of exposure. Situations in which repeated exposures may have occurred, such as in institutional cafeterias, may warrant stronger consideration of IG use.

Hepatitis B prevention strategies in the United States

The incidence of reported acute hepatitis B cases increased steadily over the past decade and reached a peak in 1985 (11.50 cases/10^5/year), despite the introduction of hepatitis B vaccine 3 years previously. Incidence decreased modestly (18%) by 1988, but still remains higher than a decade ago. This minimal impact of hepatitis B vaccine on disease incidence is attributable to several factors. The sources of infection for most cases include intravenous drug abuse (28%), heterosexual contact with infected persons or multiple partners (22%), and homosexual activity (9%). In addition, 30% of patients with hepatitis B deny any of the recognized risk factors for infection.

The present strategy for hepatitis B prevention is to vaccinate those individuals at high risk of infection. Most persons receiving vaccine as a result of this strategy have been persons at risk of acquiring HBV infection through occupational exposure, a group that accounts for approximately 4% of cases. The major deterrents to vaccinating the other high-risk groups include their lack of knowledge about the risk of disease and its consequences, the lack of public-sector programs, the cost of vaccine, and the inability to access most of the high-risk populations.

For vaccine to have an impact on the incidence of hepatitis B, a comprehensive strategy must be developed that will provide hepatitis B vaccination to persons before they engage in behaviors or occupations that place them at risk of infection. Universal HBsAg screening of pregnant women was recently recommended to prevent perinatal HBV transmission. The previous recommendations for selective screening failed to identify most HBsAg-positive pregnant women. As an alternative to high-risk-group vaccination, universal vaccination of infants and adolescents needs to be examined as a possible strategy to control the transmission of disease (see p. 171).

Hepatitis B prophylaxis

Two types of products are available for prophylaxis against hepatitis B. Hepatitis B vaccines, first licensed in 1981, provide active immunization against HBV infection, and their use is recommended for both preexposure and postexposure prophylaxis. HBIG provides temporary, passive protection and is indicated only in certain postexposure settings.

HBIG

HBIG is prepared from plasma preselected to contain a high titer of anti-HBs. In the United States, HBIG has an anti-HBs titer of >100,000 by radioimmunoassay (RIA). Human plasma from which HBIG is prepared is screened for antibodies to HIV; in addition, the Cohn fractionation process used to prepare this product inactivates and eliminates HIV from the final product. There is no evidence that the causative agent of AIDS (HIV) has been transmitted by HBIG.

Hepatitis B vaccine

Two types of hepatitis B vaccines are currently licensed in the United States. Plasma-derived vaccine consists of a suspension of inactivated, alum-adsorbed, 22-nm, HBsAg particles that have been purified from human plasma by a combination of biophysical (ultracentrifugation) and biochemical procedures. Inactivation is a threefold process using 8M urea, pepsin at pH 2, and 1:4,000 formalin. These treatment steps have been shown to inactivate representatives of all classes of viruses found in human blood, including HIV. Plasma-derived vaccine is no longer being produced in the United States, and use is now limited to hemodialysis patients, other immunocompromised hosts, and persons with known allergy to yeast.

Currently licensed recombinant hepatitis B vaccines are produced by *Saccharomyces cerevisiae* (common baker's yeast), into which a plasmid containing the gene for the HBsAg has been inserted. Purified HBsAg is obtained by lysing the yeast cells and separating HBsAg from yeast components by biochemical and biophysical techniques. These vaccines contain more than 95% HBsAg protein. Yeast-derived protein constitutes no more than 5% of the final product.

Hepatitis B vaccines are packaged to contain 10-40 μg HBsAg protein/ml and are absorbed with aluminum hydroxide (0.5 mg/ml). Thimerosal (1:20,000 concentration) is added as a preservative.

The recommended series of three intramuscular doses of hepatitis B vaccine induces an adequate antibody response* in >90% of healthy adults and in >95% of infants, children, and adolescents from birth through 19 years of age. The deltoid (arm) is the recommended site for hepatitis B vaccination of adults and children; immunogenicity of vaccine for adults is substantially lower when injections are given in the buttock. Larger vaccine doses (two or four times normal adult dose) or an increased number of doses (four doses) are required to induce protective antibody in a high proportion of hemodialysis patients and may also be necessary for other immunocompromised persons (such as those on immunosuppressive drugs or with HIV infection).

Field trials of the vaccines licensed in the United States have shown 80%-95% efficacy in preventing infection or clinical hepatitis among susceptible persons. Protection against illness is virtually complete for persons who develop an adequate antibody response after vaccination. The duration of protection and need for booster doses are not yet fully defined. Between 30% and 50% of persons who develop adequate antibody after three doses of vaccine will lose

---

*An adequate antibody response is ≥10 milliInternational Units (mIU)/ml, approximately equivalent to 10 sample ratio units (SRU) by RIA or positive by enzyme immunoassay (EIA), measured 1-6 months after completion of the vaccine series.

Table 9-5. Recommended doses and schedules of currently licensed HB vaccines

Group	Vaccine					
	Heptavax-B*,†		Recombivax HB*		Engerix-B*,§	
	Dose (µg)	(ml)	Dose (µg)	(ml)	Dose (µg)	(ml)
Infants of HBV-carrier mothers	10	(0.5)	5	(0.5)	10	(0.5)
Other infants and children <11 years	10	(0.5)	2.5	(0.25)	10	(0.5)
Children and adolescents 11-19 years	20	(1.0)	5	(0.5)	20	(1.0)
Adults >19 years	20	(1.0)	10	(1.0)	20	(1.0)
Dialysis patients and other immunocompromised persons	40	(2.0)¶	40	(1.0)**	40	(2.0)¶,††

* Usual schedule: three doses at 0, 1, 6 months.
† Available only for hemodialysis and other immunocompromised patients and for persons with known allergy to yeast.
§ Alternative schedule: four doses at 0, 1, 2, 12 months.
¶ Two 1.0-ml doses given at different sites.
** Special formulation for dialysis patients.
†† Four-dose schedule recommended at 0, 1, 2, 6 months.

detectable antibody within 7 years, but protection against viremic infection and clinical disease appears to persist. Immunogenicity and efficacy of the licensed vaccines for hemodialysis patients are much lower than in normal adults. Protection in this group may last only as long as adequate antibody levels persist.

Vaccine usage

Primary vaccination comprises three intramuscular doses of vaccine, with the second and third doses given 1 and 6 months, respectively, after the first. Adults and older children should be given a full 1.0 ml/dose, while children <11 years of age should usually receive half (0.5 ml) this dose. See Table 9-5 for complete information on age-specific dosages of currently available vaccines. An alternative schedule of four doses of vaccine given at 0, 1, 2, and 12 months has been approved for one vaccine for postexposure prophylaxis or for more rapid induction of immunity. However, there is no clear evidence that this regimen provides greater protection than the standard three-dose series. Hepatitis B vaccine should be given only in the deltoid muscle for adults and children or in the anterolateral thigh muscle for infants and neonates.

For patients undergoing hemodialysis and for other immunosuppressed patients, higher vaccine doses or increased numbers of doses are required. A special formulation of one vaccine is now available for such persons (Table 9-5). Persons with HIV infection have an impaired response to hepatitis B vaccine. The immunogenicity of higher doses of vaccine is unknown

for this group, and firm recommendations on dosage cannot be made at this time.

Vaccine doses administered at longer intervals provide equally satisfactory protection, but optimal protection is not conferred until after the third dose. If the vaccine series is interrupted after the first dose, the second and third doses should be given separated by an interval of 3-5 months. Persons who are late for the third dose should be given this dose when convenient. Postvaccination testing is not considered necessary in either situation.

In one study, the response to vaccination by the standard schedule using one or two doses of one vaccine, followed by the remaining doses of a different vaccine, was comparable to the response to vaccination with a single vaccine. Moreover, because the immunogenicities of the available vaccines are similar, it is likely that responses in such situations will be comparable to those induced by any of the vaccines alone.

The immunogenicity of a series of three low doses (0.1 standard dose) of plasma-derived hepatitis B vaccine administered by the intradermal route has been assessed in several studies. The largest studies of adults show lower rates of developing adequate antibody (80%-90%) and twofold to fourfold lower antibody titers than with intramuscular vaccination with recommended doses. Data on immunogenicity of low doses of recombinant vaccines given intradermally are limited. At this time, intradermal vaccination of adults using low doses of vaccine should be done only under research protocol, with appropriate informed consent and with postvaccination testing to identify persons with inadequate response who would be eligible for revaccination. Intradermal vaccination is not recommended for infants or children.

All hepatitis B vaccines are inactivated (noninfective) products, and there is no evidence of interference with other simultaneously administered vaccines.

Data are not available on the safety of hepatitis B vaccines for the developing fetus. Because the vaccines contain only noninfectious HBsAg particles, there should be no risk to the fetus. In contrast, HBV infection of a pregnant woman may result in severe disease for the mother and chronic infection of the newborn. Therefore, pregnancy or lactation should not be considered a contraindication to the use of this vaccine for persons who are otherwise eligible.

Vaccine storage and shipment

Vaccine should be shipped and stored at 2° C-8° C but not frozen. *Freezing destroys the potency of the vaccine.*

Side effects and adverse reactions

The most common side effect observed following vaccination with each of the available vaccines has been soreness at the injection site. Postvaccination surveillance for 3 years after licensure of the plasma-derived vaccine showed an association of borderline significance between Guillain-Barré syndrome and receipt of the first vaccine dose. The rate of this occurrence was very low (0.5/100,000 vaccinees) and was more than compensated by disease prevented by the vaccine even if Guillain-Barré syndrome is a true side effect. Such postvaccination surveillance information is not available for the recombinant hepatitis B vaccines. Early concerns about safety of plasma-derived vaccine have proven to be unfounded, particularly the concern that infectious agents such as HIV present in the donor plasma pools might contaminate the final product.

Effect of vaccination on carriers and immune persons

Hepatitis B vaccine produces neither therapeutic nor adverse effects for HBV carriers. Vaccination of individuals who possess antibodies against HBV from a previous infection is not necessary but will not cause adverse effects. Such individuals will have a postvaccination increase in their anti-HBs levels. Passively acquired antibody, whether acquired from HBIG or IG administration or from the transplacental route, will not interfere with active immunization.

Prevaccination serologic testing for susceptibility. The decision to test potential vaccine recipients for prior infection is primarily a cost-effectiveness issue and should be based on whether the costs of testing

balance the costs of vaccine saved by not vaccinating individuals who have already been infected. Estimation of cost-effectiveness of testing depends on three variables: the cost of vaccination, the cost of testing for susceptibility, and the expected prevalence of immune individuals in the group.

Testing in groups with the highest risk of HBV infection (HBV marker prevalence >20%) is usually cost-effective unless testing costs are extremely high. Cost-effectiveness of screening may be marginal for groups at intermediate risk. For groups with a low expected prevalence of HBV serologic markers, such as health professionals in their training years, prevaccination testing is not cost-effective.

For routine testing, only one antibody test is necessary (either anti-HBc or anti-HBs). Anti-HBc identifies all previously infected persons, both carriers and those who are not carriers, but does not differentiate members of the two groups. Anti-HBs identifies persons previously infected, except for carriers. Neither test has a particular advantage for groups expected to have carrier rates of <2%, such as health-care workers. Anti-HBc may be preferred to avoid unnecessary vaccination of carriers for groups with higher carrier rates. If RIA is used to test for anti-HBs, a minimum of 10 sample ratio units should be used to designate immunity (2.1 is the usual designation of a positive test). If EIA is used, the positive level recommended by manufacturers is appropriate.

Postvaccination testing for serologic response and revaccination of nonresponders

Hepatitis B vaccine, when given in the deltoid, produces protective antibody (anti-HBs) in >90% of healthy persons. Testing for immunity after vaccination is not recommended routinely but is advised for persons whose subsequent management depends on knowing their immune status (such as dialysis patients and staff). Testing for immunity is also advised for persons for whom a suboptimal response may be anticipated, such as those who have received vaccine in the buttock, persons ≥50 years of age, and persons known to have HIV infection. Postvaccination testing should also be considered for persons at occupational risk who may have needle-stick exposures necessitating postexposure prophylaxis. When necessary, postvaccination testing should be done between 1 and 6 months after completion of the vaccine series to provide definitive information on response to the vaccine.

Revaccination of persons who do not respond to the primary series (nonresponders) produces adequate antibody in 15%-25% after one additional dose and in 30%-50% after three additional doses when the primary vaccination has been given in the deltoid. For persons who did not respond to a primary vaccine series given in the buttock, data suggest that revaccination in the arm induces adequate antibody in >75%. Revaccination with one or more additional doses should be considered for persons who fail to respond to vaccination in the deltoid and is recommended for those who have failed to respond to vaccination in the buttock.

Need for vaccine booster doses

Available data show that vaccine-induced antibody levels decline steadily with time and that up to 50% of adult vaccinees who respond adequately to vaccine may have low or undetectable antibody levels by 7 years after vaccination. Nevertheless, both adults and children with declining antibody levels are still protected against hepatitis B disease. Current data also suggest excellent protection against disease for 5 years after vaccination among infants born to hepatitis B-carrier mothers. For adults and children with normal immune status, booster doses are not routinely recommended within 7 years after vaccination, nor is routine serologic testing to assess antibody levels necessary for vaccine recipients during this period. For infants born to hepatitis B-carrier mothers, booster doses are not necessary within 5 years after vaccination. The possible need for booster doses after longer intervals will be assessed as additional information becomes available.

For hemodialysis patients, for whom vaccine-induced protection is less complete and may persist only as long as antibody levels remain above 10 mIU/ml, the need for booster doses should be assessed by annual antibody testing, and booster doses should be given when antibody levels decline to <10 mIU/ml.

Groups recommended for preexposure vaccination

Persons at substantial risk of HBV infection who are demonstrated or judged likely to be susceptible should be vaccinated. They include the following:

1. Persons with occupational risk. HBV infection is a major infectious occupational hazard for health-care and public-safety workers. The risk of acquiring HBV infection from occupational exposures is dependent on the frequency of percutaneous and permucosal exposures to blood or blood products. Any health-care or public-safety worker may be at risk for HBV exposure depending on the tasks that he or she performs. If those tasks involve contact with blood or blood-contaminated body fluids, such workers should be vaccinated. Vaccination should be considered for other workers depending on the nature of the task.

   Risks among health-care professionals vary during the training and working career of each individual but are often highest during the professional training period. For this reason, when possible, vaccination should be com-

pleted during training in schools of medicine, dentistry, nursing, laboratory technology, and other allied health professions before workers have their first contact with blood.

2. Clients and staff of institutions for the developmentally disabled. Susceptible clients in institutions for the developmentally disabled should be vaccinated. Staff who work closely with clients should also be vaccinated. The risk in institutional environments is associated not only with blood exposure but may also be consequent to bites and contact with skin lesions and other infective secretions. Susceptible clients and staff who live or work in smaller (group) residential settings with known HBV carriers should also receive hepatitis B vaccine. Clients discharged from residential institutions into community settings should be screened for HBsAg so that the community programs may take appropriate measures to prevent HBV transmission. These measures should include both environmental controls and appropriate use of vaccine.

   Staff of nonresidential day-care programs (e.g., schools, sheltered workshops for the developmentally disabled) attended by known HBV carriers have a risk of HBV infection comparable to that among health-care workers and therefore should be vaccinated. The risk of HBV infection for clients appears to be lower than the risk for staff. Vaccination of clients in day-care programs may be considered. Vaccination of classroom contacts is strongly encouraged if a classmate who is an HBV carrier behaves aggressively or has special medical problems that increase the risk of exposure to his/her blood or serous secretions.

3. Hemodialysis patients. Hepatitis B vaccination is recommended for susceptible hemodialysis patients. Although seroconversion rates and anti-HBs titers are lower than those for healthy persons, for those patients who do respond, hepatitis B vaccine will protect them from HBV infection and reduce the necessity for frequent serologic screening. Some studies have shown higher seroconversion rates and antibody titers for patients with uremia who were vaccinated before they required dialysis. Identification of patients for vaccination early in the course of their renal disease is encouraged.

4. Sexually active homosexual men. Susceptible sexually active homosexual men should be vaccinated regardless of their age or the duration of their homosexual practices. Persons should be vaccinated as soon as possible after their homosexual activity begins. Homosexual and bisexual men known to have HIV infection

should be tested for anti-HBs response after completion of the vaccine series and should be counseled accordingly.

5. Users of illicit injectable drugs. All users of illicit injectable drugs who are susceptible to HBV should be vaccinated as early as possible after their drug abuse begins.

6. Recipients of certain blood products. Patients with clotting disorders who receive clotting-factor concentrates have an increased risk of HBV infection. Vaccination is recommended for these persons, and it should be initiated at the time their specific clotting disorder is identified. Prevaccination testing is recommended for patients who have already received multiple infusions of these products.

7. Household and sexual contacts of HBV carriers. Household contacts of HBV carriers are at high risk of HBV infection. Sexual contacts appear to be at greatest risk. When HBV carriers are identified through routine screening of donated blood, diagnostic testing in hospitals, prenatal screening, screening of refugees from certain areas, or other screening programs, they should be notified of their status. All household and sexual contacts should be tested and susceptible contacts vaccinated.

8. Adoptees from countries of high HBV endemicity. Families accepting orphans or unaccompanied minors from countries of high or intermediate HBV endemicity should have the children screened for HBsAg. If the children are HBsAg-positive, family members should be vaccinated.

9. Other contacts of HBV carriers. Persons in casual contact with carriers in settings such as schools and offices are at minimal risk of HBV infection, and vaccine is not routinely recommended for them. At child-care centers, HBV transmission between children or between children and staff has rarely been documented. Unless special circumstances exist, such as behavior problems (biting or scratching) or medical conditions (severe skin disease) that might facilitate transmission, vaccination of contacts of carriers in child care is not indicated.

10. Populations with high endemicity of HBV infection. In certain U.S. populations, including Alaskan Natives, Pacific Islanders, and refugees from HBV-endemic areas, HBV infection is highly endemic, and transmission occurs primarily during childhood. In such groups, universal hepatitis B vaccination of infants is recommended to prevent disease transmission during childhood. In addition, more extensive programs of "catch-up" childhood vaccination should be considered if resources are available.

Immigrants and refugees from areas with highly endemic HBV disease (particularly Africa and eastern Asia) should be screened for HBV markers upon resettlement in the United States. If an HBV carrier is identified, all susceptible household contacts should be vaccinated. Even if no HBV carriers are found within a family, vaccination should be considered for susceptible children <7 years of age because of the high rate of interfamilial HBV infection that occurs among these children. Vaccination is recommended for all infants of women who were born in areas in which infection is highly endemic.

11. Inmates of long-term correctional facilities. The prison environment may provide a favorable setting for the transmission of HBV because of the use of illicit injectable drugs and because of male homosexual practices. Moreover, it provides an access point for vaccination of percutaneous drug abusers. Prison officials should consider undertaking screening and vaccination programs directed at inmates with histories of high-risk behaviors.

12. Sexually active heterosexual persons. Sexually active heterosexual persons with multiple sexual partners are at increased risk of HBV infection. Risk increases with increasing numbers of sexual partners. Vaccination is recommended for persons who are diagnosed as having recently acquired other sexually transmitted diseases, for prostitutes, and for persons who have a history of sexual activity with multiple partners in the previous 6 months.

13. International travelers. Vaccination should be considered for persons who plan to reside for more than 6 months in areas with high levels of endemic HBV and who will have close contact with the local population. Vaccination should also be considered for short-term travelers who are likely to have contact with blood from or sexual contact with residents of areas with high levels of endemic disease. Ideally, hepatitis B vaccination of travelers should begin at least 6 months before travel to allow for completion of the full vaccine series. Nevertheless, a partial series will offer some protection from HBV infection. The alternative four-dose schedule may provide better protection during travel if the first three doses can be delivered before travel (second and third doses given 1 and 2 months, respectively, after first).

Postexposure prophylaxis for hepatitis B

Prophylactic treatment to prevent hepatitis B infection after exposure to HBV should be considered in the following situations: perinatal exposure of an infant born to an HBsAg-positive mother, accidental percutaneous or permucosal exposure to HBsAg-positive blood, sexual exposure to an HBsAg-positive person, and household exposure of an infant <12 months of age to a primary care giver who has acute hepatitis B.

Various studies have established the relative efficacies of HBIG and/or hepatitis B vaccine in different exposure situations. For an infant with perinatal exposure to an HBsAg-positive and HBeAg-positive mother, a regimen combining one dose of HBIG at birth with the hepatitis B vaccine series started soon after birth is 85%-95% effective in preventing development of the HBV carrier state. Regimens involving either multiple doses of HBIG alone, or the vaccine series alone, have 70%-85% efficacy.

For accidental percutaneous exposure, only regimens including HBIG and/or IG have been studied. A regimen of two doses of HBIG, one given after exposure and one a month later, is about 75% effective in preventing hepatitis B in this setting. For sexual exposure, a single dose of HBIG is 75% effective if given within 2 weeks of last sexual exposure. The efficacy of IG for postexposure prophylaxis is uncertain. IG no longer has a role in postexposure prophylaxis of hepatitis B because of the availability of HBIG and the wider use of hepatitis B vaccine.

Recommendations on postexposure prophylaxis are based on available efficacy data and on the likelihood of future HBV exposure of the person requiring treatment. In all exposures, a regimen combining HBIG with hepatitis B vaccine will provide both short- and long-term protection, will be less costly than the two-dose HBIG treatment alone, and is the treatment of choice.

Perinatal exposure and recommendations

Transmission of HBV from mother to infant during the perinatal period represents one of the most efficient modes of HBV infection and often leads to severe long-term sequelae. Infants born to HBsAg-positive and HBeAg-positive mothers have a 70%-90% chance of acquiring perinatal HBV infection, and 85%-90% of infected infants will become chronic HBV carriers. Estimates are that >25% of these carriers will die from primary hepatocellular carcinoma (PHC) or cirrhosis of the liver. Infants born to HBsAg-positive and HBeAg-negative mothers have a lower risk of acquiring perinatal infection; however, such infants have had acute disease, and fatal fulminant hepatitis has been reported. Based on 1987 data in the United States, an estimated 18,000 births occur to HBsAg-positive women each year, resulting in approximately 4,000 infants who become chronic HBV carriers. Prenatal screening of all pregnant women identifies those who are HBsAg-positive and allows treatment of their newborns with HBIG and hepatitis B vaccine, a reg-

imen that is 85%-95% effective in preventing the development of the HBV chronic carrier state. The following are perinatal recommendations:

1. All pregnant women should be routinely tested for HBsAg during an early prenatal visit in each pregnancy. This testing should be done at the same time that other routine prenatal screening tests are ordered. In special situations (e.g., when acute hepatitis is suspected, when a history of exposure to hepatitis has been reported, or when the mother has a particularly high-risk behavior, such as intravenous drug abuse), an additional HBsAg test can be ordered later in the pregnancy. No other HBV marker tests are necessary for the purpose of maternal screening, although HBsAg-positive mothers identified during screening may have HBV-related acute or chronic liver disease and should be evaluated by their physicians.

2. If a woman has not been screened prenatally or if test results are not available at the time of admission for delivery, HBsAg testing should be done at the time of admission, or as soon as possible thereafter. If the mother is identified as HBsAg-positive >1 month after giving birth, the infant should be tested for HBsAg. If the results are negative, the infant should be given HBIG and hepatitis B vaccine.

3. Following all initial positive tests for HBsAg, a repeat test for HBsAg should be performed on the same specimen, followed by a confirmatory test using a neutralization assay. For women in labor who did not have HBsAg testing during pregnancy and who are found to be HBsAg-positive on first testing, initiation of treatment of their infants should not be delayed by more than 24 hours for repeat or confirmatory testing.

4. Infants born to HBsAg-positive mothers should receive HBIG (0.5 ml) intramuscularly once they are physiologically stable, preferably within 12 hours of birth (Table 9-6). Hepatitis B vaccine should be administered intramuscularly at the appropriate infant dose. The first dose should be given concurrently with HBIG but at a different site. If vaccine is not immediately available, the first dose should be given as soon as possible. Subsequent doses should be given as recommended for the specific vaccine. Testing infants for HBsAg and anti-HBs is recommended when they are 12-15 months of age to monitor the success or failure of therapy. If HBsAg is not detectable and anti-HBs is present, children can be considered protected. Testing for anti-HBc is not useful, since maternal anti-HBc can persist for >1 year. HBIG and hepatitis B vaccination do not interfere with routine childhood vaccinations. Breast-feeding

Table 9-6. Hepatitis B virus postexposure recommendations

	HBIG		Vaccine	
Exposure	Dose	Recommended timing	Dose	Recommended timing
Perinatal	0.5 ml IM	Within 12 hours of birth	0.5 ml IM*	Within 12 hours of birth†
Sexual	0.06 ml/kg IM	Single dose within 14 days of last sexual contact	1.0 ml IM*	First dose at time of HBIG treatment†

* For appropriate age-specific doses of each vaccine, see Table 9-5.
† The first dose can be given the same time as the HBIG dose but in a different site; subsequent doses should be given as recommended for specific vaccine.

poses no risk of HBV infection for infants who have begun prophylaxis.

5. Household members and sexual partners of HBV carriers identified through prenatal screening should be tested to determine susceptibility to HBV infection, and, if susceptible, should receive hepatitis B vaccine.

6. Obstetric and pediatric staff should be notified directly about HBsAg-positive mothers so that neonates can receive therapy without delay after birth and follow-up doses of vaccine can be given. Programs to coordinate the activities of persons providing prenatal care, hospital-based obstetrical services, and pediatric well-baby care must be established to assure proper follow-up and treatment both of infants born to HBsAg-positive mothers and of other susceptible household and sexual contacts.

7. In those populations under U.S. jurisdiction in which hepatitis B infection is highly endemic (including certain Alaskan natives, Pacific Island groups, and refugees from highly endemic areas accepted for resettlement in the United States), universal vaccination of newborns with hepatitis B vaccine is the recommended strategy for hepatitis B control. HBsAg screening of mothers and use of HBIG for infants born to HBV-carrier mothers may be added to routine hepatitis B vaccination when practical, but screening and HBIG alone will not adequately protect children from HBV infection in endemic areas. In such areas, hepatitis B vaccine doses should be integrated into the childhood vaccination schedule. More extensive programs of childhood hepatitis B vaccination should be considered if resources are available.

On February 26, 1991, the ACIP recommended that universal vaccination of infants be incorporated in the routine immunization sched-

ule for infants and children in the United States. The two options proposed by the ACIP committee and the Committee on Infectious Diseases of the American Academy of Pediatrics are as follows: Option 1—first dose at birth, second dose at 1 to 2 months, and third dose at 6 to 18 months; option 2—first dose at 1 to 2 months, second dose at 4 months, and third dose at 6 to 18 months. The ACIP recommendations describing a comprehensive strategy for eliminating transmission of HBV in the United States through universal childhood vaccination is described in detail in the following CDC *Morbidity and Mortality Weekly Report* (MMWR 1991; 40[No. RR-13]:1-25).

REFERENCES

Acute Hepatic Failure Study Group. Failure of specific immunotherapy in fulminant type B hepatitis. Ann Intern Med 1977;86:272.

Alpert E, Isselbacher KJ, Schur PH: The pathogenesis of arthritis associated with viral hepatitis. N Engl J Med 1971;285:185.

Alter HJ: The infectivity of the healthy hepatitis B surface antigen carrier. In Bianchi L, Gerok W, Sickinger K, Stalder GA, eds: Virus and the liver. Lancaster, England: M.T.P. Press, Ltd., 1980, p 261.

Alter HJ. Posttransfusion hepatitis: Clinical features, risk, and donor testing. In Dodd RY, Barker LF, eds: Infection, immunity and blood transfusion. New York; Alan R Liss, 1985, pp 47-69.

Alter JH, Purcell RH, Shih JW, et al. Detection of antibody to hepatitis C virus in prospectively followed transfusion recipients with acute and chronic non-A, non-B hepatitis. N Engl J Med 1989;321:1494-1500.

Bacon PA, Doherty SM, Zuckerman AJ: Hepatitis B antibody in polymyalgia rheumatics. Lancet 1975;2:476.

Balayan MS, Anlzhaparidze AG, Savinskaya SS, et al. Evidence for a virus in non-A, non-B hepatitis transmitted via the fecal-oral route. Intervirology 1981;20:23.

Barker LF et al: Transmission of type B viral hepatitis to chimpanzees. J Infect Dis 1973;127:648.

Baroudy BM, Ticehurst JR, Miele TA, et al. Sequence analysis of hepatitis A virus cDNA coding for capsed proteins and RNA polymerase. Proc Natl Acad Sci USA 1985; 82:2143-2147.

Bayer ME, Blumberg BS, Werner B: Particles associated with Australia antigen in the sera of patients with leukemia, Down's syndrome and hepatitis. Nature 1968; 218:1057.

Beasley RP, Hwang L-Y, Lin C-C, et al. Incidence of hepatitis among students at a university in Taiwan. Am J Epidemiol 1983;117:213-222.

Blumberg BS, Alter HJ, Visnich S. A "new" antigen in leukemia sera. JAMA 1965;191:541.

Boyer JL, Klatskin G. Pattern of necrosis in acute viral hepatitis. Prognostic value of bridging (subacute hepatic necrosis). N Engl J Med 1970;283:1063.

Bradley DW, Krawczynski K, Cook EH, et al. Enterically transmitted non-A, non B hepatitis: Serial passage of disease in cynomologous macaques and tumorous and recovery of disease-associated 27-34 nm viruslike particles. Proc Natl Acad Sci 1987;84:6277-6281.

Brzosko WJ et al. Glomerulonephritis associated with hepatitis B surface antigen immune complexes in children. Lancet 1974;2:477.

Buitrago B, Popper H, Hadler SC, et al. Specific histologic features of Santa Marta hepatitis. A severe form of hepatitis D virus infection in northern South America. Hepatology 1986;6:1285-1291.

CDC. Protection against viral hepatitis. MMWR 1990; 39/ 52:1-26.

Chalmers TG et al. Treatment of acute infectious hepatitis. Controlled studies of the effects of diet, rest, and physical reconditioning on the acute course of the disease and on the incidence of relapses and residual abnormalities. J Clin Invest 1955;34:1163.

Chau KH, Hargie MP, Decker RH, et al. Serodiagnosis of recent hepatitis B infection by IgM class anti-HBc. Hepatology 1983;3:141.

Choo QL, Kuo G, Weiner AJ, et al. Isolation of a cDNA derived from blood-borne non-A, non-B viral hepatitis genome. Science 1989;244:359-361.

Combes B et al. Glomerulonephritis with deposition of Australia antigen-antibody complexes in glomerular basement membrane. Lancet 1971;2:234.

Daemer RJ, Feinstone SM, Gust ID, et al. Propagation of human hepatitis A virus in African Green Monkey Kidney cell culture: primary isolation and serial passage. Infect Immunol 1981;32:388.

Dane DS, Cameron CH, Briggs M. Virus-like particles in serum of patients with Austrialia-antigen-associated hepatitis. Lancet 1970;1:695.

DeCock, KMD, Bradley DW, Sanford NL, et al. Epidemic non-A, non-B hepatitis in patients from Pakistan. Ann Intern Med 1987;106:227.

Deinhardt, F et al. Studies on the transmission of human viral hepatitis to marmoset monkeys. I. Transmission of disease, serial passages, and description of liver lesions. J Exp Med 1966;125:673.

Delaplane D, Yogev R, Crussi G, Schulman ST. Fatal hepatitis in early infancy. Pediatrics 1983;72:176.

Desmyter J et al. Administration of human fibroblast interferon in chronic hepatitis-B infection. Lancet 1976;2:645.

DiBisceglie AM, Hoofnagle JH. Antiviral therapy of chronic viral hepatitis. Am J Gastroenterol 1990;85:650-654.

DiBisceglie AM, Martin P, Kassianides C, et al. Recombinant interferon alpha therapy for chronic hepatitis C. A randomized, double-blind, placebo-controlled trial. N Engl J Med 1989;321:1506-1510.

Dienstag JL, Feinstone SM, Kapikian AZ, Purcell RH. Fecal shedding of hepatitis-A antigen. Lancet 1975a;1:765.

Dienstag JL et al. Experimental infection of chimpanzees with hepatitis A virus. J Infect Dis 1975b;132:532.

Duermeyer W, van der Veen J, Koster B. ELISA in hepatitis A. Lancet 1978;1:823.

Dupuy JW, Frommel D, Alagille D. Severe viral hepatitis type B in infants. Lancet 1975;1:191.

Edmondson HA. Needle biopsy in differential diagnosis of acute liver disease. JAMA 1965;191:136.

Farci P, Alter HJ, Wong D, et al. A long term study of hepatitis C virus replication in non-A, non-B hepatitis. N Engl J Med 1991;325:98-104.

Fawaz KA, Grady GF, Kaplan MM, Gellis SS. Repetitive maternal-fetal transmission of fatal hepatitis B. N Engl J Med 1975;293:1357.

Feinstone SM, Kapikian AZ, Purcell RH. Hepatitis A: detection by immune electron microscopy of a virus-like antigen associated with acute illness. Science 1973; 182:1026.

Gauss-Muller V, Frosner GG, Deinhardt F. Propagation of hepatitis A virus in human embryo fibroblasts. J Med Virol 1981;7:233.

Gerber MA, Thung SN. The diagnostic value of immunohistochemical demonstration of hepatitis viral antigens in the liver. Hum Pathol 1987;18:771-774.

Gianotti F. Papular acrodermatitis of childhood: an Australia antigen disease. Arch Dis Child 1973;48:794.

Gimson AE, Tedder RS, White YS, et al. Serological markers in fulminant hepatitis B Gut 1983;24:615-617.

Gocke DJ. Extrahepatic manifestations of viral hepatitis. Am J Med Sci 1975;270:49.

Gocke DJ et al. Association between polyarteritis and Australia antigen. Lancet 1970;3:1149.

Gocke DJ et al. Vasculitis in association with Australia antigen. J Exp Med 1971;134:330.

Govindarajan S, Chin KP, Redeker AG, et al. Fulminant B viral hepatitis: role of delta agent. Gastroenterology 1984;86:1417-1420.

Hadler SC, DeMonzon M, Ponzetto A, et al. Delta virus infection and severe hepatitis: an epidemic in Yuepa Indians of Venezuela. Ann Intern Med 1984;100:339-344.

Havens WP Jr, Ward R, Drill VA, Paul JR. Experimental production of hepatitis by feeding icterogenic materials. Proc Soc Exp Biol Med 1944;53:206.

Heathcote J, Cameron CH, Dane DS. Hepatitis-B antigen in saliva and semen. Lancet 1974;1:71.

Hirschman RJ et al. Virus-like particles in sera of patients with infectious and serum hepatitis. JAMA 1969;208:1667.

Hollinger FB, Bradley DW, Dreesman GR et al. Detection of hepatitis A viral antigen by radioimmunoassay. J Immunol 1975;115:1464.

Holmes ZW et al. Hepatitis in marmosets: induction of disease with coded specimens from a human volunteer study. Science 1969;165:816.

Hoofnagle JH. Antiviral treatment of chronic type B hepatitis. Ann Intern Med 1987; 107:413-415.

Hoofnagle JH, DiBisceglie AM. Serologic diagnosis of acute and chronic viral hepatitis. Sem Liver Dis 1991.

Hoofnagle JH, Peters M, Mullen KD, et al. Randomized, controlled trial of recombinant human alpha interferon in patients with chronic hepatitis B. Gastroenterology 1988;95:1318-1325.

Ishimaru Y et al. An epidemic of infantile papular acrodermatitic (Gianotti's disease) in Japan associated with hepatitis B surface antigen subtype *ayw*. Lancet 1976;1:707.

Kane MA, Bradley DW, Shrestha SM, et al. Epidemic non-A, non-B hepatitis in Nepal. JAMA 1984;252:3140-3145.

Karvountzis GD, Redeker AG, Peters RL. Long term followup studies of patients surviving fulminant viral hepatitis. Gastroenterology 1974;67:870.

Khuroo MS. Study of an epidemic of non-A, non-B hepatitis. Am J Med 1980;68:818-824.

Kohler PF et al. Chronic membranous glomerulonephritis caused by hepatitis B antigen-antibody immune complexes. Ann Intern Med 1974;81:488.

Kojima S, Shibayoma T, Sato A et al. Propagation of human hepatitis A virus in conventional cell lines. J Med Virol 1981;7:273.

Krugman S. Viral hepatitis, type B: prospects for active immunization. Am J Med Sci 1975;270:391.

Krugman S. Incubation period of type B hepatitis. N Engl J Med 1979;300:625.

Krugman S, Friedman H, Lattimer C. Viral hepatitis, type A: identification by specific complement fixation and immune adherence tests. N Engl J Med 1975;292:1141.

Krugman S, Giles JP. Viral hepatitis: new light on an old disease. JAMA 1970;212:1019.

Krugman S, Giles JP. Viral hepatitis type B (MS-2 strain): further observations on natural history and prevention. N Engl J Med 1973;288:755.

Krugman S, Giles JP, Hammond J. Infectious hepatitis: evidence for two distinctive clinical, epidemiological and immunological types of infection. JAMA 1967;200:365.

Krugman S, Giles JP, Hammond J. Hepatitis virus: effect of heat on the infectivity and antigenicity of the MS-1 and MS-2 strains. J Infect Dis 1970;122:432.

Krugman S, Giles JP, Hammond J. Viral hepatitis, type B (MS-2 strain): prevention with specific hepatitis B immune serum globulin. JAMA 1971a;218:1665.

Krugman S, Giles JP, Hammond J. Viral hepatitis, type B (MS-2 strain): studies on active immunization. JAMA 1971b;217:41.

Krugman S, Ward R. Infectious hepatitis: current status of prevention with gamma globulin. Yale J Biol Med 1962;34:329.

Krugman S, Ward R, Giles JP. The natural history of infectious hepatitis. Am J Med 1962;32:717.

Krugman S, Ward R, Giles JP, Jacobs AM. Infectious hepatitis: studies on the effect of gamma globulin and on the incidence of inapparent infection. JAMA 1960;174:825.

Krugman S et al: Viral hepatitis, type B: DNA polymerase activity and antibody to hepatitis B core antigen. N Engl J Med 1974;290:1331.

Krugman S et al. Viral hepatitis, type B: studies on natural history and prevention re-examined. N Engl J Med 1979;300:101.

Kuo G, Choo QL, Alter HJ, et al. An assay for circulating antibodies to a major ecologic virus of human non-A, non-B hepatitis. Science 1989;244:362-364.

Lai CL, Lok ASF, Lin HJ, et al. Placebo-controlled trial of recombinant alpha-2 interferon in Chinese patients with chronic hepatitis B infection. Lancet 1987;2:877-880.

LeBouvier GL. Subspecificities of the Australia antigen complex. Am J Dis Child 1972;123:420.

Levo Y et al. Association between hepatitis B virus and essential mixed cryoglobulinemia. N Engl J Med 1977;296:1501.

Lieberman HM, La Breeque DR, Kew MC, et al. Detection of hepatitis B virus DNA directly in human serum by a simplified molecular hydribization tests: comparison to HBeAg/anti-HBe status in BHsAg carriers. Hepatology 1983;3:285.

Lorenz D et al. Hepatitis in the marmoset. *Saguinus mystax*, Proc Soc Exp Biol Med 1970;135:348.

Lürman A. Eine Icterusepidemie. Berl Klin Wochenschr 1885;22:20.

MacNab GM, Alexander JJ. Lecatsas G, et al. Hepatitis B surface antigen produced by a human hepatoma cell line. Br J Cancer 1976;34:509.

Mascoli CC et al. Recovery of hepatitis agents in the marmoset from human cases occuring in Costa Rica. Proc Soc Exp Biol Med 1973;143:276.

Maynard JE. Infectivity studies of hepatitis A and B in non human primates. Proc Int Assoc Biol Stand Symposium on Viral Hepatitis. Milan, Italy: December 16-19, 1974.

Maynard JE, Berquist KR, Krushak DH, Purcell RH. Experimental infection of chimpanzees with the virus of hepatitis B. Nature 1972;237:514.

McMahon BJ, Alward WLM, Hall DB, et al. Acute hepatitis B virus infection: relation of age to the clinical expression of disease and subsequent development of the carrier state. J Infect Dis 151:1985;599-603.

McNeil M, Hoy JF, Richards MJ, et al. Etiology of fatal hepatitis in Melbourne. Med J Aust 1984;2:637-640.

Melnick JL. Classification of hepatitis A virus as enterovirus type 72 and of hepatitis B virus as hepadna virus, type 1. Intervirology 1982;18:105.

Meltzer M et al. Cryoglobulinemia—a clinical and laboratory study. II. Cryoglobulins with rheumatoid factor activity. Am J Med 1966;40:837.

Mill WJ et al. Specific immune adherence assay for human hepatitis A antibody. Application of diagnostic and epidemiologic investigations. Proc Sec Exp Biol Med 1975;149:254.

Miller WJ et al. Specific immune adherence assay for human hepatitis A antibody. Application of diagnostic and epidemiologic investigations. Proc Soc Exp Biol Med 1975;149:254.

Morrow RH Jr, Smetana HF, Sai FT, et al. Unusual features of viral hepatitis in Accra, Ghana. Ann Intern Med 1968;68:1250-1264.

Murphy BL, Maynard JE, Bradley DW, et al. Immunofluorescence of hepatitis A virus antigen in chimpanzees. Infect Immunol 1978;21:663.

Neefe JR, Gellis SS, Stokes J Jr. Homologous serum hepatitis and infectious (epidemic) hepatitis. Studies in volunteers bearing on immunological and other characteristics of the etiological agents. Am J Med 1946;1:3.

Perillo RP, Schiff ER, Davis GL, et al. A randomized controlled trial of interferon alpha-2b alone and after prednisone withdrawal for the treatment of chronic hepatitis B. N Engl J Med 1990;323:295-301.

Peterson DA, Hurley TR, Hoff JC et al. Hepatitis A virus infectivity and chlorine treatment. In Szmuness W, Alter HJ, Maynard JE, eds. Proceedings, 1981 International Symposium on Viral Hepatitis. Philadelphia: Franklin Institute Press, 1982, p 624.

Plouvier B, Wattre P, Devulder B. HBsAg in superficial artery of a patient with polymyalgia rheumatica. Lancet 1978;2:932.

Popper H, Shih JW-K, Gerin JL, et al. Woodchuck hepatitis and hepatocellular carcinoma: correlation of histologic with virologic observations. Hepatology 1981;1:91.

Provost PJ, Giesa PA, McAleer WJ, et al. Isolation of hepatitis A virus in vitro in cell culture directly from human specimens. Proc Soc Exp Biol Med 1981;167:201.

Provost PJ, Hilleman MR. Propagation of human hepatitis A virus in cell culture in vitro. Proc Soc Exp Biol Med 1979;160:213.

Provost PJ. Ittensohn OL, Villarejos VM, Hilleman MR. A specific complement fixation test for human hepatitis A employing CR326 virus antigen. Diagnosis and epidemiology. Proc Soc Exp Biol Med 1975;148:961.

Provost PJ, Wolanski BS, Miller WJ, Ittensohn OL. Biophysical and biochemical properties of CR326 human hepatitis virus. Am J Med Sci 1975;270:87.

Provost PF et al. Recovery of hepatitis agents in the marmoset from human cases occurring in Costa Rica. Proc Soc Exp Biol Med 1973;142:1257.

Reyes GR, Purdy MA, Kim JP. Isolation of cDNA from virus responsible for enterically transmitted non-A, non-B hepatitis. Science 1990;247:1335-1339.

Rizzetto M, Canese MG, Arico S, et al. Immunofluorescence detection of new antigen–antibody system associated to hepatitis B virus in liver and serum of HBsAg carriers. Gut 1977;18:997-1003.

Rizzetto M, Ponzetto A, Borino A. Hepatitis delta virus infection: clinical and epidemiological aspects. In Viral hepatitis and liver disease. New York; Alan R Liss, 1988, pp 389-394.

Rizzetto M, Rosina F, Saracco G, et al. Treatment of chronic delta hepatitis with alpha 2 recombinant interferon. J Hepatol 1986;3:S229-233.

Saito I, Miyamura T, Ohbayashi A, et al. Hepatitis C virus infection is associated with the development of hepatocellular carcinoma. Proc Natl Acad Sci USA 1990;87:6547-6549.

Sampliner RE, Woronow DI, Alter HJ, et al: Community-acquired non-A, non-B hepatitis. J Med Virol 1984;13:125-130.

Schweitzer IL, Wing A, McPeak C, Spears RL. Hepatitis and hepatitis-associated antigen in 56 mother-infant pairs. JAMA 1972;220:1092.

Scotto J, Hadchouel M, Herej C et al. Detection of hepatitis B virus DNA in serum by a simple spot hybridization technique. Comparison with results for other viral markers. Hepatology 1983;3:279.

Sergent I et al. Vasculitis with hepatis B antigenemia. Long term observations in nine patients. Medicine 1976;55:1.

Shafritz DA, Kew MC. Identification of integrated hepatitis B virus DNA sequences in human hepatocellular carcinoma. Hepatology 1981;1:1.

Shrestha SM, Kane MA. Preliminary report of non-A, non-B hepatitis in Kathmandu Valley. J Inst Med 1983;5:1-10.

Smedile A, Farci P, Verme G, et al. Influence of delta infection on severity of hepatitis B. Lancet 1982;2:945.

Stevens CE et al. Vertical transmission of hepatitis B antigen in Taiwan. N Engl J Med 1975;292:771.

Stokes J Jr, et al. The carrier-state in viral hepatitis. JAMA 1954;154:1059.

Szmuness W. Hepatocellular carcinoma and hepatitis B virus: evidence for a causal association. Prog Med Virol 1978;24:40.

Szmuness W, Stevens CE, Zang EA, et al. A controlled clinical trial of the efficacy of the hepatitis B vaccine (Heptavax B): a final report. Hepatology 1981;1:377-385.

Szmuness W et al. Distribution of antibody to hepatitis A antigen in urban adult population. N Engl J Med 1976;295:755.

Szmuness W et al. The prevalence of antibody to hepatitis A antigen in various parts of the world. A pilot study. Am J Epidemiol 1977;106:392.

Tabor E, Krugman S, Weiss EC, et al. Disappearance of hepatitis B surface antigen during an unusual case of fulminant hepatitis B. J Med Virol 1981;8:277-282.

Ticehurst JR, Recaniello VR, Baroudy BM, et al. Molecular cloning and characterization of hepatitis A virus with DNA. Proc Natl Acad Sci USA 1983;80:5885.

Toda G, Ishimaru Y, Mayumi M, Oda T. Infantile papular acrodermatitis (Gianotti's disease) and intrafamilial occurrence of acute hepatitis B with jaundice: age dependency of clinical manifestations of hepatitis B virus infection. J Infect Dis 1978;138:211.

Trepo CH, Thiyolet J. Hepatitis associated antigen and periarteritis nodosa (PAN). Vox Sang 1970;19:410.

Trey C. The fulminant hepatic surveillance study. CMA J 1972;106:525.

Villarejos VM et al. Seroepidemiologic investigations of human hepatitis caused by A, B, and a possible third virus. Proc Soc Exp Biol Med 1976;152:524.

Wands JR et al. The pathogenesis of arthritis associated with acute HB, Ag-positive hepatitis: complement activation and characterization of circulating immune complexes. Gastroenterology 1974;67:813.

Ward R, Borchert B, Wright A, Kline E. Hepatitis B antigen in saliva and mouth washing. Lancet 1972;2:726.

World Health Organization Expert Committee on Viral Hepatitis. Advances in viral hepatitis. WHO Tech Rep Ser No 602, 1977.

10

HERPES SIMPLEX VIRUS INFECTIONS

Herpes simplex viruses (HSV) are among the most widely disseminated infectious agents of humans. The ubiquity of these viruses is not generally appreciated because they often do not produce overt disease. The various clinical syndromes caused by HSV in infants and children, particularly neonatal infections, gingivostomatitis, encephalitis, and infections in the immunocompromised, however, are clinically significant problems.

ETIOLOGY

HSV, a member of the herpesvirus group, is composed of an inner core containing linear double-stranded DNA, surrounded concentrically by an icosahedral capsid of approximately 100 nm, an amorphous material termed the tegument, and an outer envelope composed of lipids and glycoproteins. Enveloped HSV particles range in size from 150 to 200 nm. HSV usually is considered the prototype of the human herpesviruses, and cytomegalovirus (CMV), varicella-zoster virus (VZV), and Epstein-Barr virus (EBV) resemble it in morphological appearance. The two antigenic types of HSV, designated types 1 (HSV-1) and 2 (HSV-2), show 50% homology of their DNA (Nahmias and Dowdle, 1968). The two types can be distinguished by the following means: (1) restriction enzyme analysis of the DNA (Buchman et al., 1978; Buchman et al., 1979), (2) antigenic structure determined by Western blotting (Growdon et al., 1987), and (3) certain antibody determinations (see below). Subtypes of HSV-1 and HSV-2 can be further distinguished by analysis of viral DNA with restriction enzymes (Buchman et al., 1978; Buchman et al., 1979; Corey, 1982). Subtypes differ in less than 10% of their DNA, and they do not show significant antigenic variation, so they can only be distinguished from one another by DNA analysis.

HSV DNA encodes for a number of structural and nonstructural viral proteins and glycoproteins. As with all of the herpesviruses, replication occurs in a regulated cascading sequence, with immediate early (α) genes controlling subsequent transcription and translation of early (β) and late (γ) gene products (Whitley, 1990). Certain α genes initiate viral transcription, β genes control synthesis of proteins and enzymes such as thymidine kinase necessary for viral replication, and γ genes encode structural proteins of HSV, including the glycoproteins (g). There are at least nine envelope glycoproteins of HSV, designated gB through gJ. These glycoproteins are antigenic and therefore play an important role in generating immune responses by the infected host. They also play important roles in viral infectivity. Some glycoproteins (gB, gC, gD, and gH) mediate viral attachment to and penetration of host cells; gC binds to the C3b component of complement, and gE binds to the Fc portion of IgG.

The relative importance of immune responses to each of the glycoproteins and to nonstructural proteins (α gene products) for protection of the host is the subject of much investigation. Infection with one HSV does not result in immunity to the other type, but there is some indication that partial protection is induced against HSV-2 infection when there is preexisting immunity to type 1 (Boucher et al., 1990; Breinig et al., 1990).

Antibody responses to each type of HSV cannot be distinguished by routine antibody assays, but they may be detected by Western blot, using known strains of HSV-1 and HSV-2 as antigens. Antibodies to types 1 and 2 can also be distinguished by using gG as the antigen in an immunological antibody assay such as enzyme-linked immunosorbent assay (ELISA) since gG is distinct for each type of HSV (Whitley, 1990).

HSV is readily transmitted to a variety of animals, but only in rabbits does the virus reactivate in vivo. Animal models are useful for studying viral latency and the effects of antiviral drugs.

Tissue cultures infected with HSV show characteristic cytopathic effects characterized by degeneration and clumping of the cells and the presence of typical intranuclear inclusion bodies and giant cells. Infection in tissue cultures is at first focal, reflecting cell-to-cell viral spread, and then generalized throughout a culture, reflecting release of infectious virus into supernatant media.

HSV-1 has been associated chiefly with non-genital infections of the mucous membranes of the mouth, lips, and eyes and of the central nervous system (CNS). HSV-2 most commonly has been associated with genital and neonatal infections. There are no strict anatomical barriers, however; therefore HSV-1 can cause genital and neonatal infection, and HSV-2 can infect the oral mucosa.

Latency

All of the herpesviruses share the characteristic of becoming latent after primary infection; the virus may subsequently reactivate periodically and produce clinical symptoms in certain individuals. The phenomenon of latent infection permits long-term persistence of the virus within the host and potential future transmissibility to others. Presumably, HSV reaches the ganglia during primary infection when the sensory nerve endings, as well as the skin or mucous membranes, are invaded by the virus. Based on studies in animals, HSV is thought to reach the ganglia by retrograde axonal transport. Various factors such as fever, sunlight, stress, and trauma may trigger a recurrent infection, but at times no stimulus is apparent. Sites and, possibly, mechanisms of latent infection vary for different herpesviruses; for both HSV-1 and HSV-2, however, the site of latency is the sensory ganglia. Surgical transection of the trigeminal nerve frequently results in the appearance of herpetic vesicles in the facial skin. In studies of ganglia obtained at autopsy from patients with no clinical evidence of HSV infection at death, it was found that HSV-1 or HSV-2 can be isolated in tissue culture by cocultivation techniques from approximately 50% of trigeminal ganglia and 15% of sacral ganglia (Baringer, 1974; Baringer and Swoveland, 1973).

There is no morphological or antigenic evidence of the presence of HSV in latently infected ganglia; however, limited amounts of viral RNA are detectable. During latent infection there is consistent expression of RNA that is transcribed in the opposite orientation to and overlapping the part of the α gene encoding a viral protein termed the infected cell protein 0 (ICP0). This RNA is referred to as the latency-associated transcript (LAT); it is hypothesized to play a major role in regulating whether an infection will produce a virus or remain latent (Stevens et al., 1988; Croen et al., 1987, 1991). The presence of LAT markedly reduces ICP0 expression (Farrell et al., 1991). The role of this transcript in latency, however, has been seriously questioned since latent HSV infection in animals can be established in its absence; therefore the HSV LAT cannot be essential, and its role in latency remains unknown (Steiner et al., 1989).

Immunological factors have long been hypothesized to control reactivation of HSV since immunocompromised patients are at high risk to develop reactivation syndromes, but no specific abnormal or absent immunological reactions have been consistently implicated. In general, HSV can reactivate despite specific humoral and cell-mediated immunity. The following cells or cell-mediated immune reactions may play roles in host defense against HSV: macrophages, cytotoxic T cells, natural killer (NK) cells, antibody-dependent cellular cytotoxicity (ADCC), and cytokines released as a result of antigenic stimulation of lymphocytes and macrophages (Corey and Spear, 1986). Antibody may play a role by neutralization of virus and participation in ADCC. It seems most likely that specific immune reactions in the host determine the extent to which reactivated HSV is able to multiply and cause disease. The phenomena of viral latency and reactivation, however, probably are regulated by the latently infected cell rather than controlled by the immune system.

PATHOLOGY

The characteristic lesion caused by HSV on the skin is a vesicle and on the mucous membranes is an ulcer. The epidermis but not the dermis is usually involved so that healing followed by scarring is uncommon. Invaded epithelial cells are destroyed by the virus and the associated inflammatory response of the host except for an intact superficial cornified layer that covers the vesicle; in the ulcer this upper layer is not present. Cells invaded by HSV demonstrate the following characteristics: coalescence to form multinucleated giant cells, nuclear de-

generation, ballooning, and intranuclear inclusions. Cells in deeper tissues characteristically exhibit hemorrhagic necrosis. A biopsy specimen of a herpetic vesicle showing eosinophilic intranuclear inclusions and giant cells is shown in Plate 2, *E*.

CLINICAL MANIFESTATIONS OF PRIMARY INFECTIONS

The clinical manifestations of primary herpetic infections are determined by a variety of factors including (1) the portal of entry of the virus and (2) host factors such as age, immune competence, and integrity of the cutaneous barrier. The various clinical entities that may be encountered are listed in Fig. 10-1. The most common type of HSV infection in children is acute gingivostomatitis. The other diseases are relatively uncommon or rare. The incubation period for primary infection is approximately 6 days, with a range of 2 to 20 days.

The host-parasite relationship for HSV is

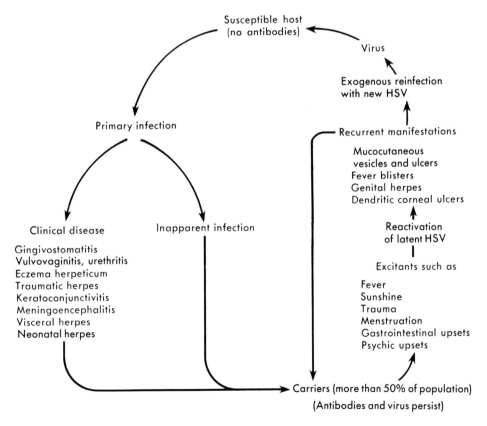

Fig. 10-1. The host-parasite relationship of herpes simplex virus in man. (Modified from Blank H, Rake G: Viral and rickettsial diseases of the skin, eye, and mucous membranes of man, Boston: Little, Brown & Co, 1955.)

shown in Fig. 10-1. Primary infection of a susceptible host is frequently inapparent for both HSV-1 and HSV-2 (Boucher et al., 1990; Breinig et al., 1990; Brock et al., 1990; Langenberg et al., 1989; Strand et al., 1986). Clinically apparent primary infections may be characterized by a vesicular eruption, fever, and other constitutional symptoms. Recurrent clinical infections usually are characterized by a localized vesicular eruption and absence of constitutional symptoms. The primary infection can be asymptomatic, and recurrent infections can be symptomatic. The primary infection, however, may be symptomatic with asymptomatic recurrences, or there may be any other combination of symptomatic and asymptomatic infections (Corey and Spear, 1986; Langenberg et al., 1989; Strand et al., 1986). Because of this phenomenon, it is impossible to differentiate between primary and recurrent HSV infections on clinical grounds alone. Primary infections are defined as those that occur in individuals with no preexisting type-specific antibody to HSV.

Acute herpetic gingivostomatitis

Acute herpetic gingivostomatitis almost always is caused by HSV-1. Most children have no symptoms during their primary infection with the virus; an estimated 5% will develop clinically apparent gingivostomatitis.

Primary infection of the mucous membranes of the mouth occurs most often in the 1- to 4-year age group and occasionally in adolescents and adults. The illness begins with the abrupt onset of fever (39.4° to 40.6° C; 103° to 105° F), irritability, anorexia, and sore mouth. Along with these constitutional symptoms, striking lesions appear on the mucous membranes of the oropharynx. The gums are swollen, reddened, friable, and bleed very easily (Plate 2, A and B). White 2 to 3 mm plaques or shallow ulcers with red areolae develop on the buccal mucosa, tongue, palate, and fauces. The lesions usually appear in the mouth first. Occasionally, however, they may develop first on the tonsils and subsequently progress forward. The regional anterior cervical lymph nodes become enlarged and tender.

Satellite vesicular lesions around the mouth are not uncommon. Infants with gingivostomatitis who are thumbsuckers can also infect the thumb (or other fingers) by self-inoculation.

The disease varies considerably in severity and duration. It may be extremely mild, with a paucity of lesions, low-grade fever, and minimal constitutional symptoms. Under these circumstances, the patient improves within 5 to 7 days. On the other hand, an occasional infant will be desperately ill with high fever, extensive hemorrhagic mouth lesions, evidence of dehydration and acidosis, and a course that does not abate until the tenth to fourteenth day.

Acute herpetic vulvovaginitis

Acute herpetic vulvovaginitis is usually a sexually transmitted infection. An exception is vulvovaginitis that is an unusual manifestation of HSV-1 infection in children secondary to autoinoculation from gingivostomatitis (Krugman, 1952). Vulvovaginitis caused by HSV-2 is not uncommon in sexually active adolescents and adults. The counterpart of this disease in sexually active males is development of penile ulcers and vesicles caused by HSV. The spectrum of disease is similar to that of herpetic gingivostomatitis, with a high percentage of subclinical infections (Brock et al., 1990; Corey and Spear, 1986; Johnson et al., 1989; Strand et al., 1986). In infants and children who develop isolated vulvovaginitis caused by HSV, the virus should be typed since the possibility of child abuse must be considered if HSV-2 is implicated.

Symptomatic patients often complain of dysuria, and children may refuse to void. The perineal area is usually reddened, edematous, and studded with painful shallow white ulcers 2 to 4 mm in diameter. Many of these lesions coalesce to form larger ulcers (Plate 2, C). The regional inguinal lymph nodes are enlarged and tender. Fever and constitutional symptoms subside within 5 to 7 days, and nonmucosal lesions become crusted by the tenth to fourteenth day. Healing is complete without scarring by the end of the third week.

Eczema herpeticum (Kaposi's varicelliform eruption)

Eczema herpeticum, a manifestation of herpetic infection of the skin, was first described by Kaposi in 1887. It is characterized by vesicular and crusting eruptions superimposed on atopic eczema or chronic dermatitis (Lynch et al., 1945). Primary infection usually is more severe than secondary infection. This disease starts abruptly with high fever (40° to 40.6° C; 104° to 105° F), irritability, and restlessness followed by the appearance of crops of vesicles concentrated chiefly on the eczematous skin. In areas of broken skin there may be ulcers and weeping, with a hemorrhagic component. A smaller number of lesions may involve the normal skin. The lesions may appear in crops over a period of 7 to 9 days, then rupture and become crusted within a few days. Thus as the disease progresses in some children, it may resemble varicella.

Like other herpetic infections, this disease varies considerably in severity from extremely mild to potentially rapidly fatal, especially if it is primary. Severe cases have been related to deficient cell-mediated immunity to HSV (Vestey et al., 1990). Extensive areas of weeping, oozing skin may be associated with severe fluid loss and with bacterial superinfection.

Traumatic herpetic infections

Traumatic herpetic infections of the skin are similar to eczema herpeticum except that they are localized rather than generalized. The site of an abrasion, burn, or break in the skin may be infected with HSV. The source of the virus may be a sympathetic parent or caretaker who "kissed to make well" the injured site for reassurance. HSV also may be transmitted during athletic activities such as wrestling, in which there are both skin trauma and close physical contact with others. Vesicular lesions that develop at the site of inoculation may be associated with fever, constitutional symptoms, and regional lymphadenopathy. Another form is due to trauma to a nerve that is latently infected with HSV with resultant reactivation of the virus. These syndromes may be difficult to differentiate clinically.

Acute herpetic keratoconjunctivitis

Primary herpetic infections of the eye are relatively rare. Fever and constitutional symptoms are associated with keratoconjunctivitis and preauricular adenopathy. Usually the infection is unilateral. The cornea has a hazy appearance, and the patient may be unable to close the eyelid (Plate 2, *D*). A purulent and membranelike exudate is present. The skin around the eye may exhibit discrete vesicles. The eye usually clears completely in 2 weeks if the infection is confined chiefly to the conjunctiva. Superficial corneal

involvement is characterized by the formation of typical dendritic ulcers. These infections may cause a serious impairment of sight. Deep infections such as keratitis disciformis, hypopyon keratitis, and iridocyclitis are almost always accompanied by significant scarring.

Acute herpetic encephalitis and meningoencephalitis

Primary infection of the CNS is an unusual manifestation of HSV infection in children. Infection of the CNS with HSV-2 beyond the neonatal period (often in conjunction with genital HSV) in an otherwise healthy individual is almost always associated with a self-limited form of meningitis rather than encephalitis, although occasionally it may cause a serious illness (Boucquey et al., 1990). An estimated 15% of patients with primary genital HSV infection will have mild concomitant meningitis (Kohl, 1988).

In contrast, HSV-1 causes a rapidly progressive, fatal type of encephalitis, with death after 1 to 2 weeks in approximately 70% of patients who are untreated. The clinical manifestations of 113 biopsy-proved cases of HSV encephalitis are listed in Table 10-1. The encephalitis frequently may be localized in the frontotemporal area, simulating a mass lesion, or it may be wide-

Table 10-1. Historical findings and signs at presentation of 113 patients with biopsy-proved herpes simplex encephalitis

Characteristics	Number/total	Percent
Historical findings		
Altered consciousness	109/112	97
Fever	101/112	90
Personality change	62/87	71
Headache	89/110	81
Vomiting	51/111	46
Recurrent herpes labialis	24/108	22
Memory loss	14/59	24
Signs and presentation		
Dysphasia	58/76	76
Autonomic nervous system dysfunction	53/88	60
Ataxia	22/55	40
Seizures	43/112	38
Hemiparesis	41/107	38

Modified from Whitley RJ et al: JAMA 1982; 247:318.

spread, involving both cerebral hemispheres. The cerebrospinal fluid (CSF) usually shows pleocytosis with a predominance of lymphocytes. Computerized tomography (CT) and magnetic resonance imaging (MRI) often can be used to localize the area of affected brain (Kohl, 1988; Schroth et al., 1987).

Approximately 25% of patients with herpes encephalitis are experiencing a primary infection, but there is no known clinical difference between primary and secondary HSV infection in this instance. The virus is believed to reach the brain either by the hematogenous route, from olfactory neurons of the respiratory mucosa, or from infected ganglia. No immunological component has been identified, and immunocompromised patients are not at increased risk to develop this form of HSV infection (Kohl, 1988).

Neonatal HSV infections

HSV infections in premature and newborn infants are usually caused by HSV-2, most often the consequence of primary maternal genital HSV-2 infection at term. Characteristically, the mother's genital infection is asymptomatic, she is delivered vaginally, and the infant is unwittingly exposed to the virus during delivery. Less commonly, the infant is infected by HSV-1 secondary to primary maternal gingivostomatitis at term (Amortegui et al., 1984) or exposure to someone else with HSV infection, such as a father or grandparent. The reported incidence of neonatal herpes is 1 in 8,000 live births (Sullivan-Bolyai et al., 1983b).

Until recently, the inability to dintinguish accurately between type-specific antibodies of HSV led to confusion and controversy about whether antibodies could protect an infant from the virus (Nahmias et al., 1971; Yeager et al., 1980). It is now becoming apparent, based on a small number of reported cases, that the presence of specific antibodies in an infant is likely to play at least some role in protection after exposure (Sullender et al., 1988). To a large extent, this may account for the observation in prospective studies that the rate of infection during primary maternal HSV-2 infection is approximately 50%, whereas during recurrent infection it is less than 8% (Prober et al., 1987). In a report by Prober et al. none of 34 infants born vaginally to women with recurrent HSV at delivery later

were found infected; all had detectable neutralizing antibodies to HSV-2 (Prober et al., 1987). Similarly, high titers of ADCC antibodies at presentation in HSV-infected neonates have not been associated with disseminated infections, but high titers are seen in babies who have been exposed to HSV but have not been infected or have had only localized infections (Kohl, 1991; Kohl et al., 1989).

Rarely, infants may be infected in utero with either HSV-1 or HSV-2 during an episode of maternal viremia that may or may not have been clinically apparent (Florman et al., 1973; Hutto et al., 1987; Rabalais et al., 1990). The spectrum of congenital disease varies from chronic to fulminant; some infants have died within days of birth, and others have survived with severe neurological sequelae. Most have evidence of acute, chronic, or recurrent skin infections with HSV. Infants with zosteriform rashes present at birth have had HSV infection (Music et al., 1971; Rabalais et al., 1990).

The clinical picture of full-blown neonatal herpes is well recognized. At the end of the first week of life, the infant develops fever or hypothermia, progressively increasing icterus, hepatosplenomegaly, and vesicular skin lesions. Anorexia, vomiting, lethargy, respiratory distress, cyanosis, and circulatory collapse may follow. Untreated, the outcome is frequently fatal. The presence of skin vesicles is helpful in distinguishing neonatal herpes from other infections; however, they may be absent in approximately 20% of affected babies. In infants without rash, neonatal HSV infection should be considered when there are signs and symptoms of bacterial meningitis but no bacterial cause can be identified (Arvin et al., 1982), and if there is an interstitial pneumonic process beginning at approximately 4 days of age. Infected infants are usually also febrile and thrombocytopenic and have evidence of liver involvement (Anderson, 1987; Hubbell et al., 1988). Fulminant hepatitis has also been described as the initial symptom of neonatal HSV (Benador et al., 1990). An infant with HSV infection of the CNS has been reported who did not develop symptoms until he was 2 months old, when he developed a skin lesion caused by HSV-2 (Thomas et al., 1989).

Whitley et al. (1980) have classified neonatal

HSV into three presenting groups on the basis of their experience with 95 proven cases. These groups include (1) disseminated disease (hepatitis, pneumonia, and/or disseminated intravascular coagulation, with or without CNS involvement) in 51%, (2) isolated CNS involvement in 32%, and (3) disease localized to the eye, skin, or mouth in 17%. Untreated, the mortality rates were 85%, 50%, and 0%, respectively (Whitley et al., 1980).

HSV in immunocompromised hosts

In the immunocompromised host HSV infections may show two unusual courses: (1) disseminated disease may occur with widespread dermal, mucosal, and visceral involvement; or (2) disease may remain localized but with a greatly prolonged course, persisting for periods as long as 9 months with indolent, often painful ulcerative lesions (Schneidman et al., 1979). These two forms of the infection appear more likely in patients whose T-lymphocyte function is depressed. In immunocompromised patients both primary and recurrent HSV infections may be severe.

Other illnesses associated with HSV

Other illnesses associated with HSV include infection of the fingers (herpetic whitlow) (Gill et al., 1988), respiratory infection, including epiglottitis (Bogger-Goren, 1987; Schwenzfeier and Fechner, 1976); lymphadenitis with lymphangitis (Sands and Brown, 1988; Tamaru et al., 1990); parotitis (Arditi et al., 1988); and erythema multiforme (Arditi et al., 1988; Brown et al., 1987a), which may result from hypersensitivity of the host to HSV. All are either unusual or rare in children. Although it once was thought that HSV played at least some causal role in cervical cancer, based on available current evidence, this is now considered unlikely (Meigner et al., 1986).

RECURRENT INFECTIONS

Recurrent herpetic infections are more common than clinically apparent primary infections. The most common type is herpes labialis, the well-known fever sore that is manifested by vesicular lesions at the corner of the mouth. Other recurrent lesions may appear on any part of the skin or mucous membranes. As indicated before, these are generally mild and not associated with constitutional symptoms. Two exceptions to this general rule are HSV encephalitis, which may be a primary or secondary infection, and severe HSV in the immunocompromised patient, which may be recurrent and yet severe (Corey and Spear, 1986).

DIAGNOSIS

Infection with HSV should be suspected in a patient who develops fever, constitutional symptoms, and a vesicular exanthem or enanthem. The diagnosis can be confirmed by (1) isolation of virus from, or demonstration of viral antigens in, the local lesions, (2) serological tests showing a significant rise in the level of antibodies during convalescence from a primary infection, and (3) histological evidence of type A intranuclear inclusion bodies and multinucleated giant cells in infected tissue.

Isolation of virus and viral antigen tests

HSV can be cultivated in a variety of cell cultures; inoculation of these cultures produces cytopathic changes that are usually evident within 24 to 48 hours. Cultures with suspected infection can be stained with fluorescein-labeled monoclonal antibodies so that identification and simultaneous typing of HSV can be performed rapidly and the results made available to the clinician. Cultures are now available in many hospital laboratories since HSV is rather easy to propagate and grows rapidly. Culture is superior to Papanicolaou and Tzanck smears since these tests are nonspecific and may yield false-positive and false-negative reactions.

Newer diagnostic tests may be available in some hospital laboratories. Smears from skin or mucous membrane lesions for direct staining with fluorescein-tagged monoclonal antibodies are very useful for rapid diagnosis. For preparing smears, vigorous swabbing of an open ulcer or ruptured vesicle should be performed to include epithelial cells that harbor the virus in the specimen. An ELISA that identifies HSV antigens in samples from lesions with sensitivity equal to that of culture may be used for rapid identification of HSV, although it will not distinguish between types 1 and 2 (Baker et al., 1989; Dascal et al., 1989).

Diagnosis is often difficult when HSV encephalitis or pneumonia is suspected. In the latter case smears of tracheal or bronchial secretions may be submitted to the diagnostic laboratory, but positive results may reflect asymptomatic shedding of virus from the respiratory tract rather than true infection. When CNS infection is suspected, skin lesions may or may not be present; in any case they offer no specific diagnostic clues. To make a certain diagnosis of herpes encephalitis, a brain biopsy may be required. At present, performing a brain biopsy for diagnosis of HSV encephalitis is controversial. Proponents cite its diagnostic sensitivity and specificity, low rate of complications, and ability to limit the use of the antiviral acyclovir (ACV) to patients with proven disease (Hanley et al., 1987; Whitley et al., 1986). Opponents cite the risk of complications of the procedure, delay in ACV therapy, potential for false-negative results, and lack of serious toxicity of ACV (Fishman, 1987; Wasiewski and Fishman, 1988). When a brain biopsy can be performed readily and safely in the care of an experienced neurosurgeon, it is probably worth the small risk of complications (approximately 2%). In hospitals in which there is little or no experience with this procedure, however, it may be more acceptable to treat expectantly with ACV. The reported incidence of false-negative results for biopsied brain specimens is approximately 4% (Kohl, 1988). CT and/or MRI can be used to localize the affected area of the brain, and an electroencephalogram (EEG) may provide nonspecific clues such as periodic slow and sharp waves that suggest HSV encephalitis. The abnormalities of the CT scan in neonates with HSV probably will not be localized to the temporal and/or frontal lobes of the brain as in herpes encephalitis in an older child but more likely will be generalized. At times in patients with neonatal HSV of the CNS the CT scan is normal (Noorbehesht et al., 1987). Brain biopsy material can be examined by culture for virus or viral antigens and/or by electron microscopy. Demonstration of HSV by in situ hybridization in brain biopsy specimens has been reported (Bamborschke et al., 1990).

It is rare to isolate HSV from CSF in patients with either neonatal or postnatal HSV encephalitis, although it is more common to isolate the virus from the CSF of neonates. The presence of antibodies to HSV in CSF, if significantly greater in titer than the serum titer, is considered diagnostic of HSV encephalitis (Kahlon et al., 1987). These antibodies are not always detected early enough in the illness, however, to make this test useful in providing guidance about whether or not to institute antiviral therapy (Van Loon et al., 1989). HSV antigens have also been detected in the CSF of patients with proven HSV encephalitis by an immunoblot assay using monoclonal antibodies. This test is highly sensitive and specific, but it has not become widely available on a clinical basis, perhaps because it too may be negative early in the illness when it is desirable to initiate therapy (Lakeman et al., 1987). An especially promising technique for diagnosis of HSV encephalitis is polymerase chain reaction (PCR) (Rowley et al., 1990; Aurelius et al., 1991). In PCR DNA is amplified and detected with a molecular probe; this technique has been successful diagnostically in a number of patients early in the illness. It is specific, accurate, and rapidly performed, although it is currently available only on a research basis.

The interest in diagnosing maternal HSV in pregnant women at term, especially in those with asymptomatic infections, has been great. It is now recognized, based on studies of over 6,000 pregnant women cultured before and at delivery, that performing maternal genital cultures from those women who have a history of genital HSV is not only expensive but yields little useful information. Women who had positive cultures during pregnancy were not likely to have positive cultures at delivery, and only a minority of infants at risk are identified if asymptomatic viral shedding is looked for only in women with a past history of genital herpes (Arvin et al., 1986; Prober et al., 1988). The ELISA assay for HSV (Baker et al., 1989; Dascal et al., 1989) has not yet been evaluated with regard to identification of women with active genital HSV at delivery. This assay will identify patients shedding HSV antigen who may or may not be infectious to their infants. Furthermore, this method may not be sensitive enough to identify asymptomatic women who are shedding tenfold less virus than women with symptoms (Hardy et al., 1990). Diagnosis using PCR has been evaluated in a small group of women at term. PCR was positive in eight of eight women with genital lesions from which HSV-2 was also isolated in tissue culture and in 11 of 11 women with asymptomatic genital HSV infections at delivery

(Hardy et al., 1990). Diagnosis of HSV by PCR remains a research procedure, but it is expected to become clinically useful in the future.

Serological tests

Although neither as rapid or specific as demonstration of virus in lesions, paired samples of sera from the acute and convalescent phases of an illness may be tested for HSV antibodies for diagnostic purposes in a variety of suspected herpetic infections. The levels of these antibodies begin to rise by the end of the first week of illness after a primary infection. Often, however, there is no rise in antibody titer with recurrent HSV infection, and these tests may yield false-positive results since rising levels of antibodies to HSV may also be seen with VZV infections.

An ELISA method in which gG of HSV-1 and HSV-2 is used for the antigen is an important newly developed antibody test. With this assay, antibodies specific to either type of HSV can be measured; therefore it is possible to determine if an individual has been infected with either or both types of HSV (Corey and Spear, 1986; Johnson et al., 1989). This test is not yet available commercially.

Histological studies

The demonstration of acidophilic intranuclear inclusion bodies, multinucleated giant cells, and ballooning degeneration of the epithelial cells of a lesion from biopsy material reinforces the diagnosis of HSV. Immunofluorescence with specific antiserum or monoclonal antibodies is important to confirm a tissue diagnosis.

DIFFERENTIAL DIAGNOSIS
Acute herpetic gingivostomatitis

Acute herpetic gingivostomatitis usually can be recognized clinically and requires no laboratory confirmation. The following diseases may be confused with it.

Herpangina. The lesions of herpangina, caused by group A Coxsackie virus, are clinically indistinguishable in appearance from those of HSV (p. 73). However, the distribution of the lesions makes it possible to separate these two conditions. With herpangina they usually are confined to the anterior fauces and soft palate, and gingivitis does not occur; whereas with her-

petic infection, gingivitis is a typical manifestation.

Acute membranous tonsillitis. Acute membranous tonsillitis secondary to streptococcal infection, EBV infection, diphtheria, and other infectious agents may simulate herpetic involvement of the tonsillar area. Invariably, herpetic lesions appear on the tongue, buccal mucosa, palate, and gingival tissues. Cultures and blood smears are the most helpful diagnostic laboratory procedures.

Thrush. Thrush generally is not associated with fever and constitutional symptoms. Lesions are polymorphous elevated white plaques without ulceration.

Acute herpetic vulvovaginitis

Acute involvement of the skin of the perineal area may simulate herpetic vulvovaginitis. The following conditions are most commonly confused.

Ammoniacal dermatitis with secondary infection. Fever and systemic symptoms are absent as a rule with this condition. The lesions extend onto the thighs and diaper area.

Gonorrheal and monilial vulvovaginitis. Lesions can be identified by appropriate cultures.

Impetigo. Lesions are usually present elsewhere, particularly on the nares and other sites readily scratched. Viral diagnostic procedures (see "Diagnosis") and bacterial cultures may provide helpful diagnostic information.

Eczema herpeticum

Herpetic infection of eczematous skin lesions must be differentiated from the following conditions.

Eczema with secondary bacterial infection. These lesions may resemble eczema herpeticum, but fever and constitutional symptoms are usually not present.

Varicella. Varicella is not an unusually severe infection in children with eczema, and the rash does not become disseminated or confluent.

Eczema vaccinatum. This disease may be almost impossible to distinguish clinically from eczema herpeticum, and the diagnosis requires the performance of laboratory procedures. Fortunately, however, eczema vaccinatum has become a disease of the past since routine vaccination of children for eczema is no longer performed.

Traumatic herpes infections

Traumatic herpetic infections may be confused with herpes zoster or with secondary bacterial infection of the site that has been traumatized. Performing methods of viral diagnosis of HSV may be necessary to make a certain diagnosis.

Acute herpetic keratoconjunctivitis

A variety of bacteria, including *Haemophilus*, pneumococci, and staphylococci, and viruses such as picornaviruses, influenza viruses, rubeola, and adenoviruses may cause conjunctivitis. Adenovirus infection with enlargement of the preauricular lymph nodes may be an isolated phenomenon or may be accompanied by respiratory symptoms. Differentiation requires assessment of the history and accompanying symptoms and physical findings of the patient. Cultures and scrapings are often required to make the correct diagnosis.

Neonatal HSV

In infants with vesicular skin lesions HSV may be confused with varicella. Historical information concerning exposure to varicella or VZV is helpful. It may be necessary either to identify the viral antigen in the vesicular lesion or to perform a culture. In infants without skin lesions neonatal HSV infection may be confused with bacterial sepsis, enteroviral infections, pneumonia, or meningitis. The average length of time until onset of pneumonia caused by group B β-hemolytic streptococcus is 20 hours of age, whereas HSV pneumonia begins on average at 5 days of age (Hubbell et al., 1988). Rapid diagnosis is important because early treatment with either appropriate antimicrobials or antivirals improves the outcome. If skin lesions are not present, the diagnosis may be made by isolation of HSV from the mouth or conjunctiva or, more rarely, from the urine or CSF (Hammerberg et al., 1983). Occasionally, it may be possible to isolate HSV from buffy coat cells if the infant has viremia (Golden, 1988). On rare occasions it is necessary to obtain a biopsy of the brain to diagnose infants with obvious CNS involvement and no skin lesions (Arvin et al., 1982; Koskiniemi et al., 1989). Infants with positive throat cultures only in the first 24 hours of life born vaginally to women with genital herpes have been reported (Arvin et al., 1986). These infants appear to "carry" HSV briefly but are not actually infected.

HSV encephalitis

Many other conditions mimic HSV encephalitis. They include vascular disease, brain abscess, other forms of viral encephalitis (enterovirus, mumps, EBV, measles, influenza, arbovirus), cryptococcal infection, tumor, toxic encephalopathy, Reye's syndrome, toxoplasmosis, tuberculosis, and lymphocytic choriomeningitis. Although it remains a controversial procedure, a brain biopsy may be necessary to distinguish HSV encephalitis from the conditions that mimic it (Whitley et al., 1981).

COMPLICATIONS

Bacterial complications rarely occur in a patient with acute gingivostomatitis. Dehydration and acidosis may result from the patient's refusal of fluids because of extensive and painful lesions in the mouth. Eczema herpeticum occasionally may become secondarily infected with bacteria, which may be a potential focus for the development of septicemia.

PROGNOSIS

The prognosis of patients with acute herpetic gingivostomatitis is excellent. Extensive eczema herpeticum, neonatal HSV, and herpes simplex encephalitis are highly fatal if not treated with an antiviral drug. Early therapy of eczema herpeticum is associated with a good prognosis. The prognosis of neonatal HSV and herpes encephalitis has greatly improved since the development of antiviral drugs, particularly ACV.

As is true for many HSV infections, the prognosis for patients with neonatal herpes depends on the extent of the infection at the time antiviral therapy is begun. Early therapy improves the outcome, but progression of the disease (e.g., development of chorioretinitis) has been reported despite antiviral treatment. Poor prognosis has been associated with acute primary maternal disease at delivery, prematurity, visceral involvement, and EEG abnormalities (Koskiniemi et al., 1989). Collaborative studies of Whitley et al. (1991) on 202 infants infected with HSV-1 or HSV-2 have revealed the following information. The death rate for patients who have been treated for disseminated HSV infection is approximately 60%, and for those treated for encephalitis it is approximately 15%. Approximately 60% of survivors of disseminated disease and 30% to 40% of those surviving encephalitis are developing normally at 1 year of age (Whitley et al., 1991a and b; Whitley and Hutto, 1985). The mortality after neonatal HSV infection limited to the skin, eye, and/or mouth is essentially nil, with approximately 10% having sequelae. There is no difference in prognosis for babies treated with vidarabine or ACV (Whitley et al., 1991a and b). The prognosis has been reported as better after HSV-1 than after HSV-2 neonatal encephalitis (Corey et al., 1988; Whitley et al., 1991b). For example, of 15 infants with HSV-2 encephalitis, only 23% were normal at 18 months of age, whereas of nine who had encephalitis caused by HSV-1, all were normal at the same age. These infants had all been treated appropriately with vidarabine or ACV (Corey et al., 1988).

Treatment with ACV has also decreased the mortality and morbidity of herpes encephalitis beyond the neonatal period, and ACV therapy has proved to offer a better prognosis than vidarabine (Whitley et al., 1986). The mortality rate for 32 patients treated with ACV was approximately 30%, as compared to 54% in 37 who received vidarabine. Roughly 40% of ACV-treated patients were free of sequelae 6 months later, compared to only 14% of vidarabine-treated patients. The better the condition of the patient before initiation of therapy, particularly with regard to neurological status, the better will be the outcome (Whitley et al., 1986).

IMMUNITY

Many infants are born with HSV antibodies passively acquired from the mother. This passive immunity is somewhat protective, but it disappears by approximately 6 months of age. Active immunity in the form of long-lasting humoral and cellular immune responses develops after an apparent or inapparent primary infection with HSV. This immunity to HSV, however, is incomplete and does not necessarily protect against future exogenous herpetic infections or against recurrent endogenous herpetic infections, although the infection may be modified (Buchman et al., 1979). The virus may reactivate after latent infection, and reinfection may also occur. In addition, patients may have latent infection with more than 1 type of HSV (Whitley

et al., 1982a). A prior infection with HSV-1 appears to attenuate the severity of subsequent infection with HSV-2 (Corey and Spear, 1986; Johnson et al., 1989).

Host factors important in defense have been analyzed best in infants. Although the presence of neutralizing antibodies in infants does not necessarily prevent disseminated infection, they may attenuate the illness considerably (Arvin et al., 1986; Sullender et al., 1987; Yeager et al., 1980). The functions of NK cells and T lymphocytes, including production of cytokines such as interleukin-2 and interferon, are all immature in infants, which appears to predispose infants to serious infection with HSV (Kohl, 1989; Kohl et al., 1988; Sullender et al., 1987). In all probability, in the healthy child and adult antibodies and cellular immunity act in concert in host defense against HSV.

EPIDEMIOLOGICAL FACTORS

In lower socioeconomic groups most individuals have been infected with HSV-1 before 6 years of age. In contrast, in upper socioeconomic groups much of the population may escape primary HSV-1 infection in the first decade of life; in these groups therefore young adults are more likely to experience primary HSV-1 gingivostomatitis. For HSV-2 infections, as with other sexually transmitted diseases, the highest rate of infection is during the second and third decades. Herpetic infections are worldwide in distribution.

Not all of the details about the spread of HSV are known, but it appears that one means of transmission is by intimate contact. Infectious virus may be recovered from saliva, skin and mucosal lesions, and urine, all of which are potential sources. Patients with recurrent lesions are infectious to others for a shorter period of time than those with primary infections.

An extensive study of the natural history of herpetic infection in 4,191 Yugoslavian children has been reported (Juretic, 1966). The incidence of clinically apparent infection, primary herpetic gingivostomatitis, was 12%. The peak incidence according to age was in the second year of life, and there was no seasonal variation. Adults with herpetic lesions were the chief source of infection. Nine minor epidemics were observed. The incubation period was 2 to 12 days, with a mean of 6 days.

A seroepidemiological study of HSV-2 infection in 4,201 participants in which a type-specific (gG) antibody assay was used revealed the following. Between 1976 and 1980, 16.4% of the U.S. population between 15 and 74 years of age had detectable antibodies to HSV-2. The prevalence of antibodies increased from less than 1% positive in children less than 15 years old to 20.2% in young adults. The highest prevalence of positive titers in elderly individuals was 19.7% in whites and 64.7% in blacks (Johnson et al., 1989).

Neonatal HSV is usually acquired from a maternal genital source. Maternally transmitted HSV infections in the perinatal period apparently are increasing in incidence (Sullivan-Bolyai et al., 1983b). Intrauterine infection has been reported but seems rare (Florman et al., 1973; Hutto et al., 1987; Stone et al., 1989). Delivery of an infant by cesarean section usually will prevent neonatal infection if the fetal membranes remain intact or have been ruptured for less than 4 hours before delivery. Most infants who develop neonatal HSV are born vaginally to mothers with no history or knowledge of genital HSV infection. Although an infant may be infected with HSV after exposure to a woman with recurrent HSV (Growdon et al., 1987), the high-risk situation for transmission is not in women with a history of recurrent genital HSV but in those with no history of this disease. Transmission to an infant is far greater after maternal primary infection than after maternal recurrent genital HSV.

The effects of a first episode of genital herpes during pregnancy on the fetus have been analyzed prospectively in a report of 29 women infected in various trimesters and their offspring (Brown et al., 1987b). This study confirmed the serious nature of primary in contrast to secondary infection during pregnancy since there were 3 of 15 infected offspring in the first group and 0 of 14 infected in the second. In addition, the incidence of premature birth and intrauterine growth retardation increased in the babies whose mothers had a primary infection during pregnancy, especially if the infection occurred in the third trimester.

Infants may on occasion be inadvertently infected through scalp monitors during delivery (Parvey and Ch'ien, 1980), during breast-feeding (Sullivan-Bolyai et al., 1983a), in intensive care nurseries (Hammerberg et al., 1983), and from family members besides the mother (Yeager et al., 1983). The availability of molecular biological techniques for viral "fingerprinting," using restriction endonucleases to evaluate the DNA of HSV isolates, has been invaluable in proving many of these transmissions.

TREATMENT

The treatment of mucocutaneous HSV is chiefly supportive. Infants require careful observation for possible dehydration. Fluids should be given intravenously if necessary. Citrus fruit juices and other irritating liquids should be avoided. Cold drinks such as apple, pear, and peach juices often seem well tolerated. Only those children with extensive oral involvement should be treated with specific antiviral chemotherapy; intravenous ACV (10 mg/kg every 8 hours) should usually be given. Some pediatricians may first try administration of oral ACV since the medication is now available in a suspension formulation (200 mg/5 ml). Unfortunately, however, the dosage for infants with primary HSV gingivostomatitis is not known (Arvin, 1987). In a study of 174 nonimmunocompromised adults with oral herpes, many of whom probably had secondary HSV, a dose of 400 mg five times a day by mouth for 5 days hastened the healing if therapy was begun in the very early stages of the illness (Spruance et al., 1990). ACV is relatively nontoxic; the main associated adverse effects include rash, gastrointestinal discomfort, and mild azotemia, which can be avoided by maintenance of good hydration.

ACV is both an inhibitor of and a faulty substrate for viral DNA polymerase; because ACV requires phosphorylation by a viral enzyme to exert its antiviral effects, it is relatively nontoxic to uninfected cells that lack the enzyme. This tolerability, plus its proven efficacy against many herpesviruses, makes ACV a very significant antiviral drug. Approximately 20% of the oral formulation is absorbed by the gastrointestinal tract. ACV is marketed in topical, oral, and intravenous formulations. Topical ACV has very little use, except possibly for its placebo effect in patients with recurrent nasolabial herpes. Topical ACV shortens the course of primary genital HSV from an average of 14 to 11 days. This interval is shortened significantly further by administration of oral ACV (200 mg five times a day for an adult), which is the treatment of choice for primary genital herpes. Frequently, recurring genital HSV can be suppressed by long-term oral administration of ACV (400 to 800 mg per day [two to four 200 mg capsules in divided doses]) (Gold and Corey, 1987; Guinan, 1986; Merz et al., 1988; Straus et al., 1989). Therapy with ACV must be considered carefully for any child with an infection that is not life threatening since, although short-term toxicity is minimal, data on possible long-term toxicity are not yet available and will not be for a number of years. The drug first was used in the late 1970s and early 1980s. No long-term adverse effects have been described.

Children with herpetic keratoconjunctivitis should be treated with topical trifluridine; topical ophthalmic ACV ointment is not a licensed product in the United States. Children with conjunctivitis and mucosal and/or cutaneous lesions should also be treated with oral ACV. The care of children with this disease should be supervised by an ophthalmologist. However, some infants with neonatal HSV present with conjunctivitis; special consideration should be taken with infants less than 1 month old. They should receive intravenous ACV and topical ophthalmic ointment (Liesegang, 1988) and should be evaluated for systemic HSV infection.

Serious HSV infections such as encephalitis and neonatal HSV should be treated with intravenous ACV (10 mg/kg every 8 hours) for 2 to 3 weeks. Immunocompromised children with severe mucocutaneous involvement should be given 5 to 10 mg/kg every 8 hours, usually for 5 to 7 days. Lower dosages should be used for children with renal compromise (Balfour and Englund, 1989).

For both neonatal HSV and HSV encephalitis, it is often necessary to begin therapy before a proven diagnosis since the earlier treatment is begun, the better the outcome (Sullivan-Bolyai et al., 1986; Whitley et al., 1986; Whitley and Hutto, 1985). Treatment with ACV for 1 to 2 days before obtaining a diagnostic culture usually will not interfere with obtaining a positive result (Balfour and Englund, 1989). All babies under 1 month of age who have HSV infection must be treated intravenously, even if their symptoms are mild, since the incidence of progression to CNS or disseminated disease is more than 50% in babies presenting with infection localized to the skin, mouth, or eye.

The increased awareness of neonatal HSV and the use of antiviral therapy appear to have made a significant impact on the presentation of the disease. For example, during the 1970s approximately 50% of infants presented with disseminated disease, but now the rate has been reduced to less than 25%. Moreover, the frequency of skin, eye, and mouth infections has increased recently to approximately 40% from approximately 20% (Whitley et al., 1988).

Close follow-up of patients after treatment of neonatal HSV and HSV encephalitis is also critical since rare relapses in both diseases have been reported (Brown et al., 1987a; Gutman et al., 1986; Kohl, 1988). In most instances of relapse retreatment with ACV for several weeks is believed helpful, but it is not known whether additional therapy with orally administered ACV on a long-term basis will add any additional benefit. Relapse of HSV encephalitis caused by hypersensitivity to HSV, a form of postinfectious encephalitis, has been reported (Koenig et al., 1979), as has relapse after treatment for only 10 days (VanLandingham et al., 1988).

Resistance of HSV to ACV is an emerging problem (Hirsch and Schooley, 1989). HSV may become resistant in three ways. Most commonly, it may cease producing thymidine kinase, the enzyme that phosphorylates ACV into an active antiviral compound. It may also induce either an altered form of thymidine kinase or an altered form of DNA polymerase (Balfour and Englund, 1989). Strains of HSV resistant to ACV have been found in acquired immunodeficiency syndrome (AIDS) patients. These strains have limited ability to spread to others since they are also less invasive than ACV-sensitive strains of HSV. Resistance to ACV may arise rapidly in immunocompromised patients, and although the ability to detect these strains remains a research tool, clinically useful methods to detect them are being developed (Englund et al., 1990). Since the ACV-resistance of HSV is increasing, the wisdom of using prophylactic therapy in patients with non-life-threatening herpetic illnesses must be carefully considered in every instance.

Vidarabine currently is rarely used to treat severe HSV infections since it is more toxic and, in general, less effective than ACV (Skoldenberg et al., 1984; Whitley et al., 1986). A case has been described in which an infant exposed to HSV at birth was treated prophylactically with vidarabine and developed a disseminated HSV illness while still on this therapy (Feder, 1988).

Certain forms of therapy for HSV infections that were once proposed but have now been discarded include systemic iododeoxyuridine (IDUR), topical neutral red dye and light, and topical vidarabine.

Drugs in the developmental stage for future use against HSV include foscarnet (phosphonoformate) and BVdU (E-5-[2-bromovinyl]-2'-deoxyuridine) (McKinlay and Otto, 1987).

PREVENTIVE MEASURES

Most herpetic infections are difficult to prevent. Children with eczema should avoid contact with others with HSV infections if possible. Infants whose mothers have active genital HSV during labor should be delivered by cesarean section, particularly if the membranes are intact or have been ruptured for less than 4 hours. Newborn infants should not have contact with persons with active herpes labialis. The advantages of a successful herpes simplex vaccine are apparent; attempts to develop one are in progress, including efforts with subunit vaccines and with a live attenuated vaccine (Whitley, 1990).

The risk-benefit ratio of administration of ACV to pregnant women who develop primary HSV to prevent infection of the infant or to prevent infection of an infant delivered vaginally to a woman with known genital HSV is unknown. Therefore neither of these possible preventive strategies is encouraged at this time.

REFERENCES

Amortegui AJ, Macpherson TA, Harger JH. A cluster of neonatal herpes simplex infections without mucocutaneous manifestations. Pediatrics 1984;73:194-198.

Anderson RD. Herpes simplex virus infection of the neonatal respiratory tract. Am J Dis Child 1987;141:274-276.

Arditi M, Shulman S, Langman CB, et al. Probable herpes simplex type 1-related acute parotitis, nephritis, and erythema multiforme. Pediatr Infect Dis 1988;7:427-428.

Arvin AM. Oral therapy with acyclovir in infants and children. Pediatr Infect Dis 1987;6:56-58.

Arvin AM, Hensleigh PA, Prober C, et al. Failure of antepartum maternal cultures to predict the infant's risk of exposure to herpes simplex virus at delivery. N Engl J Med 1986;315:796-800.

Arvin AM, Yeager AS, Bruhn FW, Grossman M. Neonatal herpes simplex infection in the absence of mucocutaneous lesions. J Pediatr 1982;100:715-721.

Aurelius E, Johansson B, Skoldenberg B, et al. Rapid diagnosis of herpes simplex encephalitis by nested polymerase chain reaction assay of cerebrospinal fluid. Lancet 1991;1:189-192.

Baker DA, Gonik B, Milch PO, et al. Clinical evaluation of a new virus ELISA: a rapid diagnostic test for herpes simplex virus. Obstet Gynecol 1989;73:322-325.

Balfour HH, Englund JA. Antiviral drugs in pediatrics. Am J Dis Child 1989;143:1307-1316.

Bamborschke S, Porr A, Huber M, Heiss W-D. Demonstration of herpes simplex virus DNA in CSF cells by in situ hybridization for early diagnosis of herpes encephalitis. J Neurol 1990;237:73-76.

Baringer JR. Recovery of herpes simplex virus from human sacral ganglions. N Engl J Med 1974;291:828.

Baringer JR, Swoveland R. Recovery of herpes simplex virus from human trigeminal ganglions. N Engl J Med 1973;288:648-650.

Benador N, Mannhardt W, Schranz D, et al. Three cases of neonatal herpes simplex virus infection presenting as fulminant hepatitis. Eur J Pediatr 1990;149:555-559.

Bogger-Goren S. Acute epiglottis caused by herpes simplex virus. Pediatr Infect Dis 1987;6:1133-1134.

Boucher FD, Yasukawa LL, Bronzan RN, et al. A prospective evaluation of primary genital herpes simplex virus type 2 infections acquired during pregnancy. Pediatr Infect Dis 1990;9:499-504.

Boucquey D, Chalon M-P, Sindic CJM, et al. Herpes simplex virus type 2 meningitis without genital lesions: an immunoblot study. J Neurol 1990;237:285-289.

Breinig MK, Kingsley LA, Armstrong JA, et al. Epidemiology of genital herpes in Pittsburgh: serologic, sexual, and racial correlates of apparent and inapparent herpes simplex infections. J Infect Dis 1990;162:299-305.

Brock BV, Selke MA, Benedetti J, et al. Frequency of asymptomatic shedding of herpes simplex virus in women with genital herpes. JAMA 1990;263:418-420.

Brown ZA, Ashley R, Douglas J, et al. Neonatal herpes simplex virus infection: relapse after initial therapy and transmission from a mother with an asymptomatic genital herpes infection and erythema multiforme. Pediatr Infect Dis 1987a;6:1057-1061.

Brown ZA, Vontver LA, Benedetti J, Critchlow CW, et al. Effects on infants of a first episode of genital herpes during pregnancy. N Engl J Med 1987b;317:1246-1251.

Buchman TG, Roizman B, Adams G, Stover BH. Restriction endonuclease fingerprinting of herpes simplex virus DNA: a novel epidemiologic tool applied to a nosocomial outbreak. J Infect Dis 1978;138:488-498.

Buchman TG, Roizman B, Nahmias AJ. Demonstration of exogenous genital reinfection with herpes simplex virus type 2 by restriction endonuclease fingerprinting of viral DNA. J Infect Dis 1979;140:295-304.

Corey L. The diagnosis and treatment of genital herpes. JAMA 1982;248:1041-1049.

Corey L, Spear P. Infections with herpes simplex viruses. N Engl J Med 1986;314:686-691, 749-757.

Corey L, Stone EF, Whitley RJ, Mohan K. Difference between herpes simplex virus type 1 and type 2 neonatal encephalitis in neurological outcome. Lancet 1988;1:1-4.

Croen KD, Ostrove JM, Dragovic LJ, et al. Latent herpes simplex virus in human trigeminal ganglia. N Engl J Med 1987;317:1427-1432.

Croen KD, Ostrove JM, Dragovic LJ, et al. Characterization of herpes simplex virus type 2 latency-associated transcription in human sacral ganglia and in cell culture. J Infect Dis 1991;163:23-28.

Dascal A, Chan-Thim J, Morahan M, et al. Diagnosis of herpes simplex virus infection in a clinical setting by a direct antigen detection enzyme immunoassay. J Clin Microbiol 1989;27:700-704.

Englund JA, Zimmerman ME, Swierkosz EM, et al. Herpes simplex virus resistant to acyclovir: a study in a tertiary care center. Ann Intern Med 1990;112:416-422.

Farrell MJ, Dobson AT, Feldman L. Herpes simplex virus latency-associated transcript is a stable intron. Proc Natl Acad Sci USA 1991;88:790-794.

Feder HM. Disseminated herpes simplex infection in a neonate during prophylaxis with vidarabine. JAMA 1988; 259:1054-1055.

Fishman RA. No, brain biopsy need not be done in every patient suspected of having herpes simplex encephalitis. Arch Neurol 1987;44:1291-1292.

Florman AL, Gershon AA, Blackett PR, Nahmias AJ. Intrauterine infection with herpes simplex virus: resultant congenital malformations. JAMA 1973;225:129-132.

Gill MJ, Arlett J, Buchan K. Herpes simplex virus infection of the hand. Am J Med 1988;84:89-93.

Gold D, Corey L. Acyclovir prophylaxis for herpes simplex infection. Antimicrob Ag Chemo 1987;31:361-367.

Golden SE. Neonatal herpes simplex viremia. Pediatr Infect Dis 1988;7:425-426.

Growdon WA, Apodaca L, Cragun J, et al. Neonatal herpes simplex virus infection occurring in second twin of an asymptomatic mother. JAMA 1987;257:508-511.

Guinan ME. Oral acyclovir for treatment and suppression of genital herpes simplex virus infection. JAMA 1986; 255:1747-1749.

Gutman LT, Wilfert CM, Eppes S. Herpes simplex virus encephalitis in children: analysis of cerebrospinal fluid and progressive neurodevelopmental deterioration. J Infect Dis 1986;154:415-421.

Hammerberg O, Watts J, Chernesky M, et al. An outbreak of herpes simplex virus type 1 in an intensive care nursery. Pediatr Infect Dis 1983;2:290-294.

Hanley DF, Johnson RT, Whitley RJ. Yes, brain biopsy should be a pre-requisite for herpes simplex encephalitis treatment. Arch Neurol 1987;44:1289-1290.

Hardy DA, Arvin AM, Yasukawa LL, et al. Use of polymerase chain reaction for successful identification of asymptomatic genital infection with herpes simplex virus in pregnant women at delivery. J Infect Dis 1990; 162:1031-1035.

Hirsch MS, Schooley RT. Resistance to antiviral drugs: the end of innocence. N Engl J Med 1989;320:313-314.

Hubbell C, Dominguez R, Kohl S. Neonatal herpes simplex pneumonitis. Rev Infect Dis 1988;10:431-438.

Hutto C, Arvin AM, Jacobs R, et al. Intrauterine herpes simplex infections. Ann Intern Med 1987;110:97-101.

Johnson RE, Nahmias AJ, Magder LS, Lee F, et al. A seroepidemiologic survey of the prevalence of herpes simplex virus type 2 infection in the United States. N Engl J Med 1989;321:7-12.

Juretic M. Natural history of herpetic infection. Helv Pediatr Acta 1966;21:356.

Kahlon J, Chatterjee S, Lakeman F, et al. Detection of antibody to herpes simplex virus in the cerebrospinal fluid of patients with herpes simplex encephalitis. J Infect Dis 1987;155:38-44.

Koenig H, Rabinowitz SG, Day E, Miller V. Post-infectious encephalomyelitis after successful treatment of herpes simplex encephalitis with adenine arabinoside. N Engl J Med 1979;300:1089-1093.

Kohl S. Herpes simplex virus encephalitis in children. Pediatr Clin N Am 1988;35:465-483.

Kohl S. The neonatal human's immune response to herpes simplex virus infection: a critical review. Pediatr Infect Dis 1989;8:67-74.

Kohl S. Role of antibody-dependent cellular cytotoxicity in defense against herpes simplex virus infections. J Infect Dis 1991;13:108-114.

Kohl S, West MS, Loo LS. Defects in interleukin-2 stimulation of neonatal natural killer cytotoxicity to herpes simplex virus-infected cells. J Pediatr 1988;112:976-981.

Kohl S, West MS, Prober CG, et al. Neonatal antibody dependent cellular cytotoxicity antibody levels are associated with the clinical presentation of neonatal herpes simplex virus infection. J Infect Dis 1989;160:770-776.

Koskiniemi M, Happonen M-M, Jarvenpaa A-L, et al. Neonatal herpes simplex virus infection: a report of 43 patients. Pediatr Infect Dis 1989;8:30-35.

Krugman S. Primary herpetic vulvovaginitis: report of a case; isolation and identification of herpes simplex virus. Pediatrics 1952;9:585.

Lakeman FD, Koga J, Whitley RJ. Detection of antigen to herpes simplex virus in cerebrospinal fluid from patients with herpes simplex encephalitis. J Infect Dis 1987; 155:1172-1178.

Langenberg A, Benedetti J, Jenkins J, et al. Development of clinically recognizable genital lesions among women previously identified as having "asymptomatic" herpes simplex virus type 2 infection. Ann Intern Med 1989; 110:882-887.

Liesegang TJ. Ocular herpes simplex infection: pathogenesis and current therapy. Mayo Clin Proc 1988;63:1092-1105.

Lynch FW, Evans CA, Bolin VS, Steves RJ. Kaposi's varicelliform eruption: extensive herpes simplex as a complication of eczema. Arch Dermatol Syph 1945;51:129.

McKinlay M, Otto MJ. Recent developments in antiviral chemotherapy. Infect Dis Clin North Am 1987;1:479-493.

Meigner B, Norrild B, Thunning C, et al. Failure to induce cervical cancer in mice by long-term frequent vaginal exposure to live or inactivated herpes simplex virus. Int J Cancer 1986;38:387-394.

Merz GJ, Jones CC, Mills J, et al. Long-term acyclovir suppression of frequently recurring genital herpes simplex virus infection. JAMA 1988;260:201-206.

Music SI, Fine EM, Togo Y. Zoster-like disease in the newborn caused by herpes simplex virus. N Engl J Med 1971;284:24-26.

Nahmias AJ, Dowdle WR. Antigenic and biologic differences in herpesvirus hominis. Prog Med Virol 1968;10:110.

Nahmias AJ et al. Perinatal risk associated with maternal genital herpes simplex virus infection. Am J Obstet Gynecol 1971;110:825.

Noorbehesht B, Enzmann DR, Sullender W, et al. Neonatal herpes simplex encephalitis: correlation of clinical and CT findings. Radiology 1987;162:813-819.

Parvey LS, Ch'ien LT. Neonatal herpes simplex virus infection introduced by fetal-monitor scalp electrodes. Pediatrics 1980;65:1150-1153.

Prober G, Hensleigh PA, Boucher FD, et al. Use of routine viral cultures at delivery to identify neonates exposed to herpes simplex virus. N Engl J Med 1988;318:887-891.

Prober CG, Sullender WM, Yasukawa LL, et al. Low risk of herpes simplex virus infections in neonates exposed to the virus at the time of vaginal delivery to mothers with recurrent genital herpes simplex virus infections. N Engl J Med 1987;316:240-244.

Rabalais GP, Yusk JW, Wilkerson SA. Zosteriform denuded skin caused by intrauterine herpes simplex virus infection. Pediatr Infect Dis 1990;10:79-81.

Rowley AH, Whitley RJ, Lakeman FD, Wolinsky SM. Rapid detection of herpes-simplex-virus DNA in cerebrospinal fluid of patients with herpes simplex encephalitis. Lancet 1990;1:440-441.

Sands M, Brown R. Herpes simplex lymphangitis. Arch Intern Med 1988;148:2066-2067.

Schneidman DW, Barr RJ, Graham JH. Chronic cutaneous herpes simplex. JAMA 1979;241:592.

Schroth G, Gawehn J, Thron A, et al. Early diagnosis of herpes simplex encephalitis by MRI. Neurology 1987;37:179-183.

Schwenzfeier CW, Fechner RE. Herpes simplex of the epiglottis. Arch Otolaryngol 1976;102:374-375.

Skoldenberg B, Forsgren M, Alestig K, et al. Acyclovir versus vidarabine in herpes simplex encephalitis: randomized multicentre study in consecutive Swedish patients. Lancet 1984;2:707-711.

Spruance SL, Stewart JCB, Rowe N, et al. Treatment of recurrent herpes simplex labialis with oral acyclovir. J Infect Dis 1990;161:185-190.

Steiner I, Spivack JG, Lirette R, et al. Herpes simplex virus type 1 latency-associated transcripts are evidently not essential for latent infection. EMBO J 1989;8:505-511.

Stevens JG, Haarr L, Porter DD, et al. Prominence of the herpes simplex virus latency-associated transcript in trigeminal ganglia from seropositive humans. J Infect Dis 1988;158:117-123.

Stone KM, Brooks CA, Guinan ME, Alexander ER. National surveillance for neonatal herpes simplex virus infections. Sex Trans Dis 1989;16:152-156.

Strand A, Vahlne A, Svennerholm B, et al. Asymptomatic virus shedding in men with genital herpes infection. Scand J Infect Dis 1986;18:195-197.

Straus S, Seidlin M, Takiff H, et al. Effect of oral acyclovir treatment on symptomatic and asymptomatic virus shedding in recurrent genital herpes. Sex Trans Dis 1989;16:107-113.

Sullender WM, Miller JL, Yasukawa LL, et al. Humoral and cell-mediated immunity in neonates with herpes simplex virus infection. J Infect Dis 1987;155:28-37.

Sullender WM, Yasukawa LL, Schwartz M, et al. Type-specific antibodies to herpes simplex virus type 2 (HSV-2) glycoprotein G in pregnant women, infants exposed to maternal HSV-2 infection at delivery, and infants with neonatal herpes. J Infect Dis 1988;157:164-171.

Sullivan-Bolyai J, Fife KH, Jacobs RF, et al. Disseminated neonatal herpes simplex type 1 from a maternal breast lesion. Pediatrics 1983a;71:455-457.

Sullivan-Bolyai J, Hull HF, Wilson C, et al. Herpes simplex virus infection in King County, Washington. JAMA 1983b;250:3059-3062.

Sullivan-Bolyai JZ, Hull HF, Wilson C, et al. Presentation of neonatal herpes simplex virus infections: implications for a change in therapeutic strategy. Pediatr Infect Dis 1986;5:309-314.

Tamaru J, Mikata A, Horie H, et al. Herpes simplex lymphadenitis. Am J Surg Pathol 1990;14:571-577.

Thomas EE, Scheifele DW, MacLean BS, Ashley R. Herpes simplex type 2 aseptic meningitis in a two-month-old infant. Pediatr Infect Dis 1989;8:184-186.

Van Loon AM, Van der Logt JTM, Heessen FWA, et al. Diagnosis of herpes simplex virus encephalitis by detection of virus-specific immunoglobulins A and G in serum and cerebrospinal fluid by using an antibody-capture enzyme-linked immunosorbent assay. J Clin Microbiol 1989;27:1983-1987.

VanLandingham KE, Marsteller HB, Ross GW, Hayden FG. Relapse of herpes simplex encephalitis after conventional acyclovir therapy. JAMA 1988;259:1051-1053.

Vestey JP, Howie SEM, Norval M, et al. Severe eczema herpeticum is associated with prolonged depression of cell-mediated immunity to herpes simplex virus. In Current problems in dermatology, Basel, Switzerland: S. Karger, 1990, pp 158-161.

Wasiewski WW, Fishman MA. Herpes simplex encephalitis: the brain biopsy controversy. J Pediatr 1988;113:575-578.

Whitley R. Herpes simplex viruses. In B Fields ed. Virology, ed 2. New York: Raven Press, 1990, pp 1843-1887.

Whitley RJ, Alford CA, Hirsch MS, et al. Vidarabine versus acyclovir therapy in herpes simplex encephalitis. N Engl J Med 1986;314:144-149.

Whitley R, Arvin A, Prober C, et al. Predictors of morbidity and mortality in neonates with herpes simplex virus infections. N Engl J Med 1991a;324:450-454.

Whitley R, Arvin A, Prober C, et al. A controlled trial comparing vidarabine with acyclovir in neonatal herpes simplex virus infection. N Engl J Med 1991b;324:444-454.

Whitley RJ, Corey L, Arvin AM, et al. Changing presentation of herpes simplex viral infection in neonates. J Infect Dis 1988;158:109-116.

Whitley RJ, Hutto C. Neonatal herpes simplex virus infections. Pediatr Rev 1985;7:119-126.

Whitley RJ, Lakeman FD, Nahmias AJ, Roizman B. DNA restriction-enzyme analysis of herpes simplex virus isolates obtained from patients with encephalitis. N Engl J Med 1982a;307:1060-1062.

Whitley RJ, Nahmias AJ, Visintine AM, et al. The natural history of herpes simplex virus infection of mother and child. Pediatrics 1980;66:489-494.

Whitley RJ, Soong S, Hirsch MS, et al. Herpes simplex encephalitis: vidarabine therapy and diagnostic problems. N Engl J Med 1981;304:313-318.

Whitley RJ, Soong S, Linneman C Jr, et al. Herpes simplex encephalitis. JAMA 1982b;247:317-320.

Yeager A, Arvin AM, Urbani LJ, Kemp JA. Relationship of antibody to outcome in neonatal herpes simplex virus infections. Infect Immunol 1980;29:532-538.

Yeager A, Ashley R, Corey L. Transmission of herpes simplex virus from father to neonate. J Pediatr 1983;103:905-907.

11

INFECTIONS IN THE IMMUNOCOMPROMISED CHILD

LINDA L. LEWIS
PHILIP A. PIZZO

The risk for infections in children undergoing intensive cytotoxic therapy for cancer has been investigated extensively over the last 20 years, resulting in advances in the diagnosis and treatment of serious infections. In this chapter the alterations of host defense that heighten the risk for infection, the current diagnostic considerations, and the principles of treatment and prevention of these complications are reviewed.

HOST-DEFENSE DISTURBANCES ASSOCIATED WITH INCREASED RISK OF INFECTION

Alterations in host defense mechanisms increase the risk for viral, bacterial, fungal, and protozoan pathogens (Table 11-1). Although specific defects in host defense can increase susceptibility to particular types of organisms (e.g., with splenectomy and the increased risk for bacteremia with encapsulated bacteria), most commonly the immunocompromised child has deficiencies of multiple components of the immune network, rendering him at risk for a wide variety of potential infectious complications.

Anatomical abnormalities resulting in breaks in skin or mucosal integrity or mechanical obstruction of a usually patent body cavity or lumen provide an environment conducive to the rapid multiplication of potential pathogens. Oral and gastrointestinal (GI) mucosal surfaces may be disrupted by chemotherapeutic regimens, allowing normal or hospital-acquired flora access to the bloodstream. Enlarged lymph nodes, tumor mass, or scar tissue from previous surgical procedures or radiation therapy may obstruct body passages allowing overgrowth of microorganisms in usually sterile sites, transmigration of bacteria across mucosal surfaces, or proximal perforation.

Bacteremias with organisms such as fastidious streptococci, *Peptococcus*, or *Capnocytophaga* also can implicate certain body sites (e.g., the oral cavity) as the potential source of infection. Similarly, bacteremia with gram-negative aerobes, anaerobes, enterococcus, or other enteric pathogens (e.g., *Streptococcus bovis*) should prompt investigation of the GI tract as the source of infection. Frequent hospitalization and frequent use of antibiotics or chemotherapeutic agents can alter the "normal" flora of many patients with chronic illnesses and produce an endogenous microflora more likely to result in infectious complications.

Asplenia, whether surgical, congenital, or functional, predisposes to serious infections with encapsulated bacteria such as *Streptococcus pneumoniae, Haemophilus influenzae, Klebsiella* spp., and *Neisseria meningiditis*. The increased risk of salmonella infections in patients with sickle cell disease has been attributed to both splenic dysfunction and humoral immune deficits. Of note, patients who underwent splenectomy after trauma apparently are less likely to develop overwhelming infections than those asplenic for other reasons, presumably because of the presence of residual splenic rests that provide functional activity (Rubin et al., 1991).

Table 11-1. Predominant pathogens in compromised patients: Association with selected defects in host defenses

Host-defense impairment	Bacteria	Fungi	Viruses	Other
Neutropenia	Gram-negative Enteric organisms (*E. coli, K. pneumoniae, Enterobacter* and *Citrobacter* spp.) *Pseudomonas aeruginosa* Gram-positive Staphylococci (coagulase-negative and positive) Streptococci (group D, α-hemolytic) Anaerobes (anaerobic streptococci, *Clostridium* spp., *Bacteroides* spp.)	*Candida* spp. (*C. albicans, C. tropicalis,* other species) *Aspergillus* spp. (*A. fumigatus, A. flavus*)		
Abnormal cell-mediated immunity	*Legionella* *Nocardia asteroides* *Salmonella* spp. Mycobacteria (*M. tuberculosis* and atypical mycobacteria) Disseminated infection from live mycobacterial vaccine (BCG)	*Cryptococcus neoformans* *Histoplasma capsulatum* *Coccidioides immitis* *Candida*	Varicella-zoster virus Herpes simplex virus Cytomegalovirus Epstein-Barr virus Hepatitis B Disseminated infection from live virus vaccines (vaccinia, measles, rubella mumps, yellow fever, polio)	*Pneumocystis carinii* *Toxoplasma gondii* *Cryptosporidium* *Strongyloides stercoralis*
Immunoglobulin abnormalities	Gram-positive *S. pneumoniae* *S. aureus* Gram-negative *Haemophilus influenzae* *Neisseria* spp. enteric organisms		Enteroviruses (including polio)	*Giardia lamblia*
Complement abnormalities C3, C5	Gram-positive *S. pneumoniae* Staphylococci Gram-negative *H. influenzae, Neisseria* spp. enteric organisms			

	Bacteria	Fungi	Viruses	Parasites
C5-C9	*Neisseria* spp. (*N. gonorrhoeae, N. meningitidis*)			
Anatomical disruption				
Oral cavity	α-Hemolytic streptococci, oral anaerobes (*Peptococcus, Peptostreptococcus*)	*Candida*	Herpes simplex virus	
Esophagus	Staphylococci, other colonizing organisms	*Candida*	Herpes simplex virus	
Lower gastrointestinal tract	Gram-positive Group D streptococci Gram-negative Enteric organisms Anaerobes (*B. fragilus, C. perfringens*)	*Candida*	Cytomegalovirus	*S. stercoralis*
Skin (intravenous catheter)	Gram-positive Staphylococci, streptococci Corynebacteria *Bacillus* spp. Gram-negative *P. aeruginosa* enteric organisms Mycobacteria *M. fortuitum, M. chelonei*	*Candida Aspergillus Malassezia furfur*		
Urinary tract	Gram-positive Group D streptococci Gram-negative Enteric organisms *P. aeruginosa*	*Candida*		
Splenectomy	Gram-positive *S. pneumoniae* DF2 bacillus Gram-negative *S. pneumoniae H. influenzae Salmonella*			*Babesia*

The ability of granulocytes to respond appropriately to infection requires migration of the cells to the site of infection (chemotaxis), phagocytosis, and killing of the organism. Defects in all of these steps have been described with hereditary disorders and with hematological malignancies and as the result of certain medications. Chronic granulomatous disease (CGD) of childhood, perhaps the best understood inherited leukocyte disorder, most commonly is due to an X-linked recessive disorder. Because of faulty metabolism of hydrogen peroxide, superoxide, and oxygen radicals, intracellular killing of bacteria by neutrophils is deficient. Patients with this disease are most susceptible to recurrent infections with catalase-producing bacteria such as *Staphylococcus aureus*, *Serratia*, *Escherichia coli*, *Pseudomonas*, and *Candida*. Recent advances in understanding the disease have led to therapy for some patients with interferon-γ resulting in a significant decrease in infections and in the need for hospitalization (Esekowitz et al., 1988; Sechler et al., 1988; The International Chronic Granulomatous Disease Cooperative Study Group, 1991). Myeloperoxidase deficiency; deficiency of the synthesis of β-2 integrin chain, CD18; Chédiak-Higashi syndrome; and glucose-6-phosphate dehydrogenase (G6PD) deficiency all affect granulocytic microbicidal functions, predisposing patients to bacterial infections, particularly soft-tissue abscesses, dermatitis, adenitis, and sinopulmonary infections.

Abnormal neutrophil function also has been documented in a number of hematological diseases, including acute myelogenous leukemia, preleukemia, and myelodysplastic syndromes. Neutrophils from some of these patients have decreased myeloperoxidase, elastase, and other granule constituents (Davey et al., 1988). Cytotoxic agents and radiation therapy may also result in abnormalities of granulocyte functioning. These deficits may relate to increased risk of infectious complications.

Defects in cell-mediated immunity can result from congenital disorders or acquired deficits secondary to lymphoid malignancies, certain immunosuppressive drugs, some chronic illnesses, and viral infections, including human immunodeficiency virus (HIV) infection. Abnormal cellular immunity arises when the normal T-lymphocyte–macrophage interactions fail, predisposing the patient to infections with intracellular organisms such as *Salmonella*, *Listeria*, mycobacteria, cytomegalovirus (CMV), herpes simplex virus (HSV), varicella-zoster virus (VZV), Epstein-Barr virus (EBV), *Histoplasma*, *Cryptococcus*, *Coccidioides*, *Toxoplasma*, and *Pneumocystis carinii* (Van Der Meer, 1988). Several congenital disorders affect cellular immunity either as isolated T-lymphocyte dysfunction (as in Nezelof's syndrome) or in combination with defects of humoral immunity (as in severe combined immune deficiency).

For many years the use of corticosteroids also has been implicated in increased risk of infection. Although steroids adversely affect several host-defense mechanisms such as wound healing, lymphocyte function, and lymphokine production, they are also notorious as agents that decrease granulocyte chemotaxis to sites of infection, thus "masking" the usual signs and symptoms of inflammation (Cupps and Fauci, 1982).

Immunosuppressive drugs may interfere with cellular immunity by different mechanisms. The cytotoxic agents have profound effects on cell proliferation. Corticosteroids decrease production of and response to cytokines by macrophages and induce lymphopenia through a redistribution of these cells (Cupps and Fauci, 1982). Cyclosporin A, a potent immunosuppressive agent used to prevent rejection in solid-organ transplant patients, is associated with disturbances of T-helper cell population, inhibits production of interleukin-2 (IL-2) and interferon-γ, and can alter the risk for infectious complications.

The most rapidly increasing group of immunocompromised children at risk for serious infectious complications are those with HIV infection. A detailed discussion of HIV-related risks of infection and immunosuppression is presented in Chapter 1.

Nevertheless, the most frequent reason for host compromise in children remains cancer and its treatment. Indeed, infection is a major cause of morbidity in children with cancer, especially in association with neutropenia. The relationship between falling neutrophil numbers, absolute neutrophil count, and risk of infection was first reported in 1966 by investigators at the National Cancer Institute. This group followed 52 leukemia patients through the course of their illness and treatment, charting white blood cell counts, absolute numbers of neutrophils and lymphocytes, clinically and microbiologically diagnosed infections, fevers without proven infections, and relapses and remissions of the underlying malignancy. These investigators concluded the following: (1) the risk of infection related directly to the number of circulating neutrophils, with an increased incidence of infection when the absolute neutrophil count fell below 1000 cells/mm^3 and especially when the absolute neutrophil count reached levels below 100/mm^3; (2) the risk of infection was greater for all absolute neutrophil count levels during relapse; (3) the most important factor in predicting risk of infection was the duration of neutropenia, with episodes longer than 3 weeks leading to the highest rates of infection and highest mortality; and (4) the degree of fall in the absolute neutrophil count was not as important as the final level that resulted (Bodey et al., 1966). Since the time of this report, the relationship between cancer, neutropenia, and infection has been clearly established, and advances in management have focused attention on this high-risk group of patients. Studies performed during the last two decades confirm that patients with an absolute neutrophil count less than 500 cells/mm^3 comprise a population who require urgent empiric therapy when they become febrile. The considerations that surround the diagnosis, treatment, and prevention of infections in these neutropenic patients offer a paradigm for the management of any immunocompromised child and are the focus of this chapter.

INFECTIONS ENCOUNTERED IN IMMUNOCOMPROMISED PATIENTS
Bacterial infections

By far, the majority of organisms infecting compromised children arise from endogenous flora of the respiratory or GI tracts or the skin. With hospitalizations and treatment there is a shift in the endogenous flora, manifested by colonization with gram-negative organisms and, at some institutions, more resistant bacteria.

During the past 30 years there has been an evolving shift in the cause of the bacterial infections in neutropenic patients. In the 1950s and early 1960s gram-positive organisms (especially S. aureus) predominated. With the use of more intensive chemotherapy in the late 1960s

and 1970s, gram-negative bacteria, especially Enterobacteriaceae species (Van der Waaij et al., 1977) and *Pseudomonas aeruginosa*, emerged as the predominant pathogens. Because infections with gram-negative bacilli, especially *Pseudomonas*, were associated with the rapid onset of overwhelming sepsis and a high mortality rate (Bodey et al., 1985), guidelines for empirical therapy emerged as the standard of practice. Although gram-negative organisms still were important, certain of these organisms, *P. aeruginosa* in particular, inexplicably declined as pathogens during the 1980s. Currently, gram-positive organisms, including the staphylococci (both coagulase positive and negative), α-hemolytic streptococci, and enterococci, predominate at most large medical centers (Pizzo et al., 1978; Wade et al., 1982). Such shifts have an impact on the management and outcome of patients with neutropenia.

In spite of their numerical preponderance, anaerobic bacteria are less commonly associated with bacteremia in immunocompromised hosts, accounting for only approximately 5% of episodes. Anaerobes have, however, been associated with specific clinical syndromes, including intra-abdominal abscesses, peritonitis, mucositis, or perianal cellulitis. Most anaerobes isolated under these circumstances are *Bacteroides* or *Clostridium* spp. (Fainstein et al., 1989). *C. difficile* toxin-mediated GI disease may also cause a variety of symptoms from mild gastroenteritis to severe pseudomembranous colitis but rarely results in bacteremia.

Fungal infections

During recent years the increased use of intensive chemotherapy for almost all varieties of pediatric cancers has resulted in more regimens that result in prolonged neutropenia. Under these circumstances fungi have emerged as a major cause of infectious complications. The duration of neutropenia after initiation of antibiotics apparently was the significant risk factor for an invasive mycosis in a recent multivariate analysis (Wiley et al., 1990). Moreover, invasive mycoses are most likely to occur as secondary infections during periods of prolonged neutropenia. The majority of fungal infections in children with cancer are caused by *Candida* spp., with *Aspergillus* spp. the second most frequent cause of invasive mycoses. Depending on the patients' underlying cancer, treatment regimen, and geographical location, a variety of other fungal organisms, including *Cryptococcus*, *Histoplasma*, *Coccidioides*, the Zygomycetes, *Fusarium*, *Trichosporon*, and the dematiaceous molds, may also result in serious infection. Although some of these fungi, particularly *Candida albicans*, comprise part of the normal GI or skin flora, most invasive mycoses in immunocompromised hosts represent nosocomial infections. Alterations of mucosal surfaces by chemotherapy, surgery, or tumor invasion may increase the risk of invasive disease, and certain species such as *Candida tropicalis* or *Torulopsis glabrata* may be intrinsically more invasive (Wingard et al., 1979; Aisner et al., 1976). Other fungi such as *Aspergillus* and *Mucor* are not part of the normal microbial flora and are most often acquired from environmental sources. Yeasts such as *Cryptococcus neoformans* and *Histoplasma capsulatum* more commonly produce infection in patients with impaired cell-mediated immunity, and although rarely considered nosocomial processes, they can result from either primary or secondary infection.

Virus infections

Viruses also have emerged as important pathogens in neutropenic or otherwise immunocompromised children. Early epidemiological studies probably underestimated the importance of viruses as pathogens since techniques for viral detection or isolation were less reliable in the 1960s and 1970s. It has been well-documented that the herpes group viruses may cause severe and even life-threatening infections in this population. HSV and VZV were clearly identified as the most common viral pathogens in a comprehensive, prospective study of 150 pediatric leukemia patients, but significant morbidity was associated with isolation of a wide variety of other viruses, including the influenza viruses, parainfluenza viruses, CMV, measles, adenovirus, enteroviruses, respiratory syncytial virus, and rhinoviruses. Because of difficulties in obtaining specimens from some sites (e.g., lower respiratory tract, central nervous system [CNS], or liver), this study was unable to make conclusions about the cause-and-effect relationship of virus detection and most clinical syndromes. The investigators were able to document an increased incidence of virus infections in patients during induction or relapse compared to patients who were in remission. Furthermore, there was an increased rate of virus isolation from patients with acute myeloblastic leukemia compared to those with acute lymphoblastic leukemia (Wood and Corbitt, 1985).

Similar to fungus infections, virus infections may represent either primary or secondary processes. HSV, VZV, and CMV commonly affect large numbers of children early in life and may become latent for long periods, only to recur as reactivation disease when the immune system fails during cancer, chemotherapy, organ transplantation, or HIV infection. Primary VZV in leukemic children carries with it the potential for serious pneumonitis, encephalitis, hepatitis, Reye's syndrome, purpura fulminans, and a mortality rate of 7% to 14% (Feldman et al., 1975). Zoster, which represents recrudescent VZV, contributes little to the virus-associated mortality when it occurs as localized cutaneous disease, but it can disseminate cutaneously and potentially viscerally in up to 26% of compromised patients (Strauss et al., 1988). CMV infection in compromised patients may be manifest as a spectrum of involvement ranging from asymptomatic viral shedding to life-threatening pneumonitis. Among bone marrow transplant patients the incidence of CMV infection is greater in patients already seropositive (Meyers et al., 1986), but there is some evidence that, although it occurs more frequently, reactivation CMV disease results in less morbidity than primary infection (Chou, 1986). Those at highest risk for serious morbidity and mortality are seronegative individuals who receive seropositive organs or leukocyte-containing blood products (Rubin, 1990).

Infections caused by common respiratory viruses were documented in 25% of the febrile episodes encountered in one series of neutropenic patients followed at the National Cancer Institute (Cotton et al., 1984). Unfortunately, the role of these viruses in illness could not be predicted on the basis of presenting symptoms, chest radiograph, degree of fever, or the duration of neutropenia, so this information did not have much impact on patient management. Improvement in rapid diagnostic assays and increased treatment options for viral infections make this one of the most rapidly changing areas in the care of febrile, immunosuppressed patients.

Parasites

P. carinii has been the major pathogenic protozoan organism, although there have always been arguments about its exact taxonomic position (Bartlett and Smith, 1991), in immunocompromised children. In children with cancer *P. carinii* is most often a reactivation infection, in contrast to its presumptive role as a primary infection in young infants with HIV infection. In cancer patients *P. carinii* causes a more rapidly progressive, severe infection characterized by lower numbers of cysts than in HIV patients, although there is no difference in the overall mortality (Kovacs et al., 1984). A variety of other protozoan pathogens are seen in HIV-infected adults, but since they frequently occur as reactivations of latent infections, organisms such as *Toxoplasma gondii* and *Cryptosporidium* are relatively unusual in children. Infections with *Strongyloides stercoralis*, frequently seen in patients with adult T-cell leukemia and human T lymphotropic virus I (HTLV-I) infection, are rare complications in children.

DIAGNOSTIC EVALUATION

In nonneutropenic cancer patients infection is the presumed cause of fever in less than 20% of the episodes. More often, fever is a consequence of the use of chemotherapeutic agents or of the underlying malignancy. Although "tumor fever" occurs in less than 5% of children with leukemia or lymphoma, it may be present in up to 25% of children with solid tumors associated with necrosis. Unless these children are neutropenic or have rapidly falling neutrophil counts after receiving chemotherapy, empiric therapy is unnecessary, and treatment can be based on whether an infectious cause can be demonstrated. An exception to this approach pertains to nonneutropenic children who have central venous catheters. Because these patients are at increased risk of bacteremia (Hiemenz et al., 1986), the authors' current practice is to admit these children for administration of intravenous antibiotics while blood cultures are in progress (see "Central Venous Catheter–Associated Infection").

In a neutropenic patient the occurrence of a single oral temperature greater than 38.5° C or three episodes of temperature greater than 38.0° C within a 24-hour period mandates hospital admission for evaluation and empiric antibiotic therapy. The importance of empiric therapy is underscored by the fact that among the 1,001 febrile episodes that occurred in 324 pediatric and young adult patients followed at the National Cancer Institute, there were no clearly definable signs, symptoms, treatment modalities, or invasive procedures that were predictive of bacteremia (Pizzo et al., 1982b). In fact, the classic signs of inflammation may be notably absent in neutropenic patients. At the same time, the patient's clinical status may change over time, making serial (at least daily) examinations of critical importance. Each patient should have at least two sets of blood cultures obtained before the institution of antibiotics, and if a central venous catheter is present, blood cultures should be obtained both from peripheral venipuncture and from all lumens of the indwelling device. Urinalysis and urine culture should also be done before antibiotics are given. Cultures of any other potentially infected sites revealed by the history or initial examination should be pursued aggressively for the source of fever. A chest radiograph obtained at the onset of illness not only provides information about infiltrates that may be present at the time of presentation but also provides a baseline by which to monitor the evolution of infiltrates as neutrophils recover or as secondary infections arise. Routine serum electrolyte profiles, including liver and kidney function tests, allow monitoring of organ system dysfunction or antibiotic toxicities and should be part of the initial evaluation. Special diagnostic procedures such as thoracentesis, paracentesis, lumbar puncture, sinus radiography, other imaging studies, or surgical biopsy should be pursued as indicated by the patient's presentation and clinical course.

Although colonization with a particular organism usually precedes infection, the use of routine surveillance cultures has not proved useful. In a series of 652 episodes of neutropenia with fever, serial surveillance cultures of nose, throat, urine, and stool were evaluated. The clinical value of this information was limited, however, because no single body site was predictive of bacteremia, multiple organisms were frequently isolated from the same site, the organisms responsible for sepsis were often known before the results of the surveillance cultures, and the results of the cultures rarely influenced initial patient management. The cost of such surveillance is tremendous and is not justified on the basis of available data (Kramer et al., 1982).

PRINCIPLES OF EMPIRIC THERAPY

The morbidity and mortality associated with fever in neutropenic children have been greatly reduced by the rapid initiation of empiric antibiotics. This policy evolved during the 1960s and 1970s when it became clear that a delay in starting antibiotics of even 24 to 48 hours while waiting for results of cultures could have disastrous consequences, particularly when gram-negative organisms ultimately were identified. Not surprisingly, the earliest empiric regimens were directed against gram-negative pathogens, particularly *P. aeruginosa*. To optimize the benefits of empiric antibiotic therapy, the regimen should have a broad spectrum of activity that includes *Pseudomonas*, effectiveness in the absence of neutrophils, ability to achieve high serum bactericidal concentrations quickly, an acceptable incidence of adverse side effects, and a low potential for the emergence of resistant pathogens (Rubin et al., 1991).

Monotherapy vs. combination antibiotics

Numerous antibiotic regimens have been proposed and used for the initial management of the febrile neutropenic child over the last 25 years. To provide broad coverage against the many potential pathogens, the use of combinations of antibiotics has been the standard practice at most institutions. Although both the carboxypenicillins (carbenicillin and ticarcillin) and the more recent ureido- and piperazyl penicillins (azlocillin and piperacillin) have excellent activity against gram-negative bacteria, including *P. aeruginosa*, when used alone, resistant organisms can emerge. Thus an aminoglycoside or another β-lactam antibiotic must be combined with an extended-spectrum penicillin. Similarly, in the neutropenic patient aminoglycosides cannot be used alone since clinical and microbiological failures frequently occur. Nonetheless, combinations of a penicillin plus an aminoglycoside have proved highly effective, although the use of aminoglycosides requires careful monitoring of serum levels to ensure adequate therapy and reduce the likelihood of toxicity. The selection of a particular aminoglycoside should be based on local antibiotic resistance patterns.

During the late 1970s and early 1980s two major developments have raised the possibility that single agent therapy may be an effective empiric regimen: (1) the availability of new β-lactam antibiotics with extended gram-negative activity and (2) the gradual decrease in the prevalence of gram-negative organisms, especially *Pseudomonas*, at many centers. The third-generation cephalosporins such as ceftazidime and cefoperazone and the carbapenem imipenem-cilastatin represent significant advances in activity that make them attractive for use in febrile, immunocompromised patients. The newer cephalosporins have been studied as monotherapy in at least 13 separate trials, and although a variety of combination regimens were used, in comparison the investigators concluded that monotherapy was equivalent to combination therapy in nine of these studies (Pizzo et al., 1985). A comparison of ceftazidime alone vs. "standard" combination therapy (in this case, cephalothin, gentamicin, and carbenicillin) conducted at the National Cancer Institute encompassed 550 consecutive admissions for fever and neutropenia. For both initial regimens the outcome was successful in 98% of the patients who presented with unexplained fever. Success was also similar for the two regimens in patients who had documented infections (89% and 91%), but many of these patients required modification of their initial antibiotic therapy. Patients requiring more frequent modifications in therapy usually were those with documented infections and those who remained neutropenic for longer than 1 week. This study also confirmed a shift toward a higher percentage of unexplained febrile episodes (72%) than documented infections and assumed that this phenomenon was related to the early initiation of antibiotics with any defined fever (Pizzo et al., 1986).

More recently, a new trial at the National Cancer Institute has explored the use of imipenem-cilastatin, the first in the carbapenem class of antibiotics, as monotherapy for initial empiric antibiotic therapy. In this study patients were randomized to receive either imipenem or ceftazidime as initial therapy for neutropenia-associated fever. Although analysis of the data collected in this trial has not been completed, it appears that in at least 500 episodes studied to date there is no clear difference in overall outcome in the two treatment groups (Pizzo, unpublished data). A higher number of patients in the imipenem group required modification of antibiotics secondary to nausea than was expected, but fewer modifications were made in order to provide coverage for anaerobic infections.

A number of studies have also investigated the use of intravenous ciprofloxacin, a fluoroquinolone antibiotic with broad-spectrum activity, as initial treatment in febrile neutropenic adults. Although the studies have included relatively small numbers of patients, this agent achieved a successful outcome in a majority of patients (Rolston et al., 1989), although there was some indication that a higher incidence of secondary streptococcal infections occurred (Bayston et al., 1989). At present, the quinolone antibiotics are not approved for use in children because of concern for potential age-related arthropathy; however, emerging data are beginning to suggest that ciprofloxacin may be safe for use in pediatric patients.

Although the third-generation cephalosporins and the carbapenems have excellent gram-negative activity and coverage of a number of grampositive organisms, none are active against the methicillin-resistant staphylococci. This factor, together with the increased frequency of grampositive infections (particularly caused by coagulase-negative staphylococci and α-streptococci), has led several investigators to evaluate the inclusion of vancomycin as part of initial empiric therapy. Although these studies have suggested that the early use of vancomycin reduces the incidence of secondary infections or even the need for empiric amphotericin B, there was no difference in mortality in patients randomized to receive initial vancomycin or not (Karp et al., 1986). The experience at the National Cancer Institute has suggested that patients could be treated successfully with pathogen-directed vancomycin and that there was no adverse effect on outcome when vancomycin was not included as part of the initial empiric regimen. Importantly, this pathogen-directed use of vancomycin is much more cost-effective than if vancomycin were simply given to every patient with fever and neutropenia (Rubin et al., 1988).

At present, recommendations for the addition of vancomycin to empiric regimens for the treatment of fever during neutropenia should be based on local experience and institutional antibiotic resistance patterns. Recently, the Working Committee of the Infectious Diseases Society of America established guidelines for the use of antimicrobial agents in neutropenic patients that outline all acceptable regimens (Hughes et al., 1990).

Modifications and length of therapy

The question of how long to continue therapy or when to modify the empiric treatment regimen frequently arises in the management of the febrile neutropenic patient. Indeed, empiric therapy really relates to the management of patients until the results of the pretreatment cultures become available. Even when a pathogen is isolated in a febrile, neutropenic child, the evidence suggests that during the period of neutropenia broad-spectrum antibiotic coverage should be continued (Pizzo et al., 1980). Specific clinical settings that develop during an episode may also warrant a change in therapy. Table 11-2 lists some common events for which modifications of the empiric regimen are warranted.

The appropriate length of antibiotic therapy in a febrile neutropenic patient depends on the clinical setting and the length of neutropenia. Minimal data exist to support specific recommendations about length of therapy, especially in those patients with no defined site of infection. In patients with fever of unexplained origin who become afebrile and have resolution of neutropenia in less than 7 days, it is probably reasonable to discontinue antibiotics and observe them carefully. Those who become afebrile but remain neutropenic may benefit from continuing antibiotic therapy for a full 14 days or until the resolution of neutropenia (Pizzo et al., 1984). Limited evidence supports either of these positions, but it has been demonstrated that discontinuing antibiotics after 7 days of empiric therapy in patients who remain neutropenic may result in recurrent fever and hypotensive events (Pizzo et al., 1979). Any neutropenic patient in whom antibiotics are discontinued must be observed closely since evidence of recurrent fever mandates reinstitution of antibiotic therapy.

In patients with a defined site of infection who have resolution of both fever and neutropenia and show a good response to antibiotics, the length of therapy can be based on usual standards of treatment. For those patients who remain neutropenic antibiotics should be continued until there is microbiological and clinical

resolution of the infection and the patient has been afebrile for at least 7 days. Under those circumstances the patient should also be free of mucosal or skin lesions and must, again, be observed closely for evidence of recurrent infection at the same or another site (Hughes et al., 1990).

Empiric antifungal therapy

Standard practice is to begin empiric antifungal therapy if a patient remains febrile and neutropenic without an obvious source after 4 to 7 days of receiving broad-spectrum antibiotics. This policy has been based on an accumulating body of knowledge and experience in caring for both pediatric and adult cancer patients. Studies from different groups have documented the rate of serious fungal infection in this patient population as 9% to 31% (Pizzo et al., 1982a; EORTC International Antimicrobial Therapy Cooperative Group, 1989; Wiley et al., 1990). These rates include cases diagnosed at autopsy, emphasizing the difficulty in making a diagnosis of fungal infection even in some cases of disseminated disease. Empiric amphotericin B (usually 0.5 mg/kg/day) has appeared to decrease the rates of documented fungal infection. However, doses of amphotericin B used in empiric therapy may be less effective with some fungi (e.g., *Aspergillus* and *C. tropicalis*), and infection with these organisms may benefit from higher doses of antifungals.

In spite of its potential benefit, amphotericin B has considerable toxicity, making the search for newer and less toxic antifungal agents an important priority. Among the most promising are the imidazoles such as ketoconazole and thiazoles such as fluconazole and itraconazole. Ketoconazole has been compared to amphotericin B in two trials of neutropenic patients already receiving antibiotic therapy with reported equivalent efficacy (Hathorn et al., 1985; Fainstein et al., 1987). Unfortunately, because of its lack of activity against *Aspergillus* spp. and *C. tropicalis* and the lack of a parenteral form, ketoconazole cannot be recommended for routine use in this setting (Walsh, 1990). Fluconazole will be investigated as a potential agent for empiric antifungal therapy and prophylaxis at the National Cancer Institute in the near future. In addition, liposomal formulations of amphotericin B are also being investigated at a number of

Table 11-2. Modifications of therapy during fever and neutropenia

Clinical event	Possible modifications in therapy
Breakthrough bacteremia	If gram-positive isolate, add vancomycin If gram-negative isolate (presumably resistant), change regimen
Catheter-associated soft-tissue infections	Add vancomycin (and gram-negative coverage if not already being given)
Severe oral mucositis or necrotizing gingivitis	Add specific anaerobic agent (clindamycin, metronidazole); may need trial of acyclovir
Esophagitis	Trial of clotrimazole, ketoconazole, fluconazole, or amphotericin B; may need trial of acyclovir
Diffuse or interstitial pneumonitis	Trial of trimethoprim-sulfamethoxazole and erythromycin in addition to broad-spectrum antibiotics if the patient remains neutropenic
New infiltrate in neutropenic patient receiving antibiotics	If neutrophil count rising, may observe If neutrophil count not recovering, pursue biopsy; if biopsy not possible, add amphotericin B
Perianal cellulitis	If patient already on broad-spectrum antibiotics, add a specific anaerobic agent If not on antibiotics, begin broad-spectrum regimen with anaerobic coverage
Prolonged fever and neutropenia	After 1 week of antibiotics, add amphotericin B

centers and appear to have greatly decreased toxicity over the currently available preparation.

CLINICAL SYNDROMES OF INFECTION IN COMPROMISED CHILDREN

More than half of children with fever and neutropenia have no definable site of infection. Of those with clinically or microbiologically documented infections, 10% to 15% may have bacteremia with any of a wide variety of organisms, and a small percentage may have fungemia. The range of infections seen in two different large series of febrile, neutropenic patients at the National Cancer Institute are compiled in Table 11-3. Some of these clinical syndromes and their management in neutropenic or immunocompromised children are discussed in more detail.

Pulmonary infiltrates

Pulmonary infections are the most common localized infection seen in neutropenic hosts and initially can have a wide range of symptoms and radiographic appearances. In children who are severely neutropenic there may be no obvious infiltrate at the time of the initial evaluation. Use of invasive diagnostic procedures such as bronchoalveolar lavage must be considered for a child with respiratory symptoms and a "normal" chest x-ray result if the initial evaluation provides no cause for the clinical manifestations.

A localized pulmonary infiltrate at the onset of fever in a neutropenic child should be considered bacterial and should be treated with broad-spectrum antibiotics while the initial as-

sessment proceeds. Routine childhood pathogens such as *S. pneumoniae, H. influenzae,* and *Mycoplasma* must be considered in addition to the pathogens associated with immunocompromised hosts such as the gram-negative enteric bacteria (including *E. coli, Klebsiella pneumoniae,* and *Pseudomonas* spp.). *Legionella* pneumonia should be considered, especially if the patient also has diarrhea and headache. Localized infiltrates that fail to improve with broad-spectrum antibiotic therapy usually represent infection with mycobacteria, fungi (especially *Aspergillus* spp.), *Nocardia,* or multiply resistant bacteria.

Interstitial infiltrates in immunocompromised patients are more likely to represent a nonbacterial process. *P. carinii* is the entity most frequently diagnosed in interstitial pneumonitis in children not receiving prophylactic trimethoprim-sulfamethoxazole. A high index of suspicion should be maintained for any compromised patient but especially for those receiving steroid therapy or those with significant defects in cellular immunity. Common symptoms include fever, dry cough, and significant hypoxemia. An arterial blood gas study and an induced sputum examination to look for cysts should be performed when *P. carinii* is being considered. The incidence of *P. carinii* in this patient population has been decreased dramatically by the routine use of trimethoprim-sulfamethoxazole for prophylaxis in high-risk patients (Hughes et al., 1987). In nonneutropenic hosts with diffuse infiltrates who are unable to undergo biopsy an empiric trial of trimethoprim-sulfamethoxazole and erythromycin is reasonable (Browne et al., 1990). *Legionella, Mycoplasma,* and viral infections may also cause diffuse or interstitial infiltrates. Of the viral pathogens, CMV has been linked most frequently to serious pneumonias, especially in allogeneic bone marrow transplant patients (Meyers, 1986). CMV pneumonitis is suspected when CMV is found by culture or hybridization in bronchoalveolar lavage fluid, but confirmation requires lung or transbronchial biopsy. Therapeutic options for CMV pneumonitis are limited, although a regimen of ganciclovir and intravenous immune globulin appears successful in some patients (Emmanuel et al., 1988).

Whether localized or diffuse, infiltrates that

Table 11-3. Documented sites of infection in febrile, neutropenic cancer patients

Site of infection	Source A*	Source B†	Total
Sepsis	81	109	190
Lungs	28	88	116
Skin	42	43	85
HEENT	11	69	80
Gastrointestinal tract	4	35	39
Urinary tract	22	29	51
Other	2	38	40

*Pizzo PA, et al.: Medicine 1982; 61:153.
†Pizzo PA, et al.: N Engl J Med 1986; 315:552.

of candidemia in children whose central catheters were removed or retained. Pediatr Infect Dis 1989;8:99.

Esekowitz RAB, Dinaur MC, Jaffe HS, et al. Partial correction of the phagocytic defect in patients with x-linked chronic granulomatous disease by subcutaneous interferon gamma. N Engl J Med 1988;319:146.

Fainstein V, Bodey GP, Elfing L, et al. Amphotericin B or ketoconazole therapy of fungal infections in neutropenic cancer patients. Antimicrob Agents Chemother 1987; 31:11.

Fainstein V, Elting LS, Bodey GP. Bacteremia caused by nonsporulating anaerobes in cancer patients: a 12-year experience. Medicine 1989;68:151.

Feldman S, Hughes WT, Daniel CB. Varicella in children with cancer: seventy-seven cases. Pediatrics 1975;56:388.

Gabrilove JL, Jakubowski A, Scher H, et al. Effect of granulocyte colony-stimulating factor on neutropenia and associated morbidity due to chemotherapy for transitional-cell carcinoma of urothelium. N Engl J Med 1988; 318:1414.

Gershon AA, Steinberg SP, and the Varicella Vaccine Collaborative Study Group of the National Institute of Allergy and Infectious Diseases. Persistence of immunity to varicella in children with leukemia immunized with live attenuated varicella vaccine. N Engl J Med 1989;320:892.

Glenn J, Cotton D, Wesley R, Pizzo P. Anorectal infections in patients with malignant diseases. Rev Infect Dis 1988;10:42.

Groopman JE, Molina J-M, Scadden DT. Hematopoietic growth factors: biology and clinical applications. N Engl J Med 1989;321:1449.

Hathorn J, Thaler M, Skelton J, et al. Empiric amphotericin B versus ketoconazole in febrile granulocytopenic cancer patients (Abstract 248). Proceedings of the 25th Interscience Conference on Antimicrobial Agents and Chemotherapy, 1985.

Hiemenz J, Skelton J, Pizzo PA. Perspective on the management of catheter related infections in cancer patients. Pediatr Infect Dis 1986;5:6.

Hill H. Infections complicating congenital immunodeficiency syndromes. In Rubin RH, Young LS ed. Clinical approach to infection in the compromised host, New York: Plenum Medical Book Co, 1988, pp. 407-438.

Hughes WT, Armstrong D, Bodey GP, et al. Guidelines for the use of antimicrobial agents in neutropenic patients with unexplained fever. J Infect Dis 1990;161:381.

Hughes WT, Kuhn S, Chaudhary S, et al. Successful chemoprophylaxis for Pneumocystis carinii pneumonitis. N Engl J Med 1977;297:1419.

Hughes WT, Rivera GK, Schell MJ, et al. Successful intermittent chemoprophylaxis for Pneumocystis carinii pneumonitis. N Engl J Med 1987;316:1627.

International Chronic Granulomatous Disease Cooperative Study Group: a controlled trial of interferon gamma to prevent infection in chronic granulomatous disease. N Engl J Med 1991;324:509.

Karp JE, Dick JD, Angelopulos C, et al. Empiric use of vancomycin during prolonged treatment-induced granulocytopenia: randomized, double-blind, placebo-controlled clinical trial in patients with acute leukemia. Am J Med 1986;81:237.

Karp JE, Merz WG, Hendricksen C, et al. Oral norfloxacin for prevention of gram-negative bacterial infections in patients with acute leukemia and granulocytopenia: a randomized, double-blind, placebo-controlled trial. Ann Intern Med 1987;106:1.

Kovacs JA, Hiemenz JW, Macher AM, et al. Pneumocystis carinii pneumonia: a comparison between patients with the acquired immunodeficiency syndrome and patients with other immunodeficiencies. Ann Intern Med 1984;100:663.

Kramer BK, Pizzo PA, Robichaud DJ et al. Role of serial microbiological surveillance and clinical evaluation in the management of cancer patients with fever and granulocytopenia. Am J Med 1982;72:561.

Laver J, Moore MAS. Clinical use of recombinant human hematopoietic growth factors. J Natl Cancer Inst 1989; 81:1370.

Masar H. The management of pneumonias in immunocompromised patients. JAMA 1985;253:1769.

McFarland LV, Mulligan ME, Kwok RYY, Stamm WE. Nosocomial acquisition of Clostridium difficile infection. N Engl J Med 1989;320:204.

Meyers JD. Infection in bone marrow transplant recipients. Am J Med 1986;81(suppl 1A):27.

Meyers JD, Flournoy N, Thomas ED. Risk factors for cytomegalovirus infection after human marrow transplantation. J Infect Dis 1986;153:478.

Meyers JD, Reed EC, Shepp DH, et al. Acyclovir for prevention of cytomegalovirus infection and disease after allogeneic marrow transplantation. N Engl J Med 1988; 318:70.

Ohno R, Tomonaga I, Kobayashi T, et al. Effect of granulocyte colony-stimulating factor after intensive induction therapy in relapsed or refractory acute leukemia. N Engl J Med 1990;323:871.

Pizzo PA. Considerations for the prevention of infectious complications in patients with cancer. Rev Infect Dis 1989;11(suppl 7):S1551.

Pizzo PA, Commers J, Cotton D, et al. Approaching the controversies in the antibacterial management of cancer patients. Am J Med 1984;76:436.

Pizzo PA, Hathorn JW, Hiemenz J, et al. A randomized trial comparing ceftazidime alone with combination antibiotic therapy in cancer patients with fever and neutropenia. N Engl J Med 1986;315:552.

Pizzo PA, Ladisch S, Robichaud K. Treatment of gram-positive septicemia in cancer patients. Cancer 1980;45:206.

Pizzo PA, Ladisch S, Simon RM, et al. Increasing incidence of gram-positive sepsis in cancer patients. Med Pediatr Oncol 1978;5:241.

Pizzo PA, Robichaud KJ, Gill FA, Witebsky FG. Empiric antibiotic and antifungal therapy of cancer patients with prolonged fever and granulocytopenia. Am J Med 1982;72:101.

Pizzo PA, Robichaud KJ, Gill FA, et al. Duration of empiric antibiotic therapy in granulocytopenic cancer patients. Am J Med 1979;67;194.

Pizzo PA, Robichaud KJ, Wesley R, Commers JR. Fever in the pediatric and young adult patient with cancer: a prospective study of 1001 episodes. Medicine 1982b;61:153.

Pizzo PA, Thaler M, Hathorn J, et al. New beta-lactam antibiotics in granulocytopenic patients: new options and new questions. Am J Med 1985;79(suppl 2A):75.

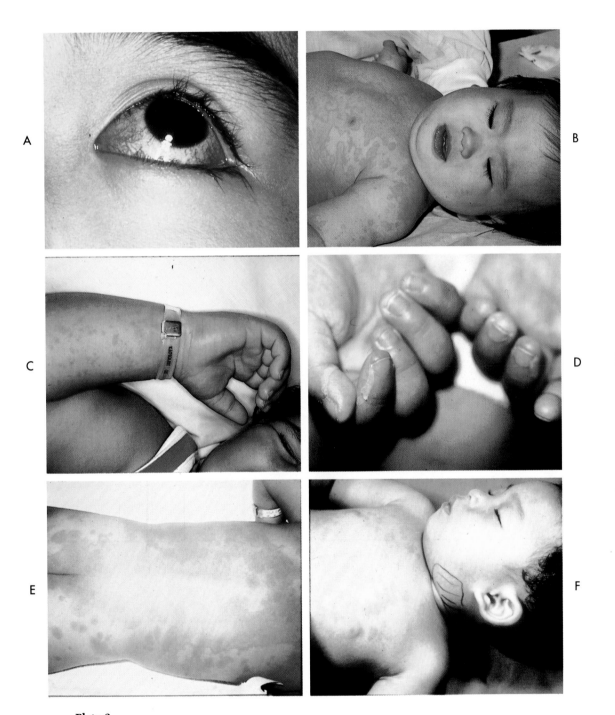

Plate 3

Some clinical signs of Kawasaki syndrome. **A,** Discrete vascular injection of the bulbar conjunctiva. **B,** Generalized lip erythema with mild edema, cracking, and bleeding fissures. **C,** Diffuse red-purple discoloration of the palm(s). **D,** Desquamation beginning at the fingertips just below the nailbeds. **E,** Diffuse erythematous, nonvesicular and nonbullous, polymorphic rash. **F,** Unilaterally enlarged cervical lymph node.

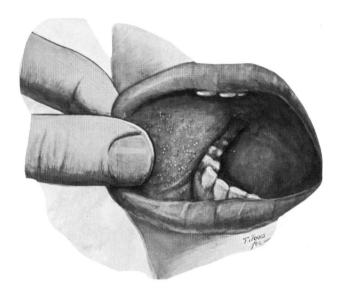

Plate 4
Koplik's spots. (From Zahorsky J, Zahorsky TS. Synopsis of pediatrics. St. Louis. The C.V. Mosby Co., 1953.)

Roilides E, Walsh TJ, Pizzo PA, Rubin M. Granulocyte colony-stimulating factor enhances the phagocytic and bactericidal activity of normal and defective human neutrophils. J Infect Dis 1991;163:579.

Rolston KVI, Haron E, Cunningham C, Bodey GP. Intravenous ciprofloxacin for infections in cancer patients. Am J Med 1989;87(suppl 5A):261.

Rubin RH. Impact of cytomegalovirus infection on organ transplant recipients. Rev Infect Dis 1990;12(suppl 7):S754.

Rubin M, Hathorn JW, Marshall D, et al. Gram-positive infections and the use of vancomycin in 550 episodes of fever and neutropenia. Ann Intern Med 1988;108:30.

Rubin M, Walsh TJ, Pizzo PA. Clinical approach to infections in the compromised host. In Benz E, Cohen H, Furip B, et al (eds). Hematology: Basic Principles and Practice, 1991, pp. 1063-1114.

Saral R, Burns WH, Laskin OL, et al. Acyclovir prophylaxis of herpes simplex virus infections: a randomized, double-blind, controlled trial in bone-marrow-transplant recipients. N Engl J Med 1981;305:63.

Schmidt GM, Horak DA, Niland JC, et al. A randomized, controlled trial of prophylactic ganciclovir for cytomegalovirus pulmonary infection in recipients of allogeneic bone marrow transplants. N Engl J Med 1991;324:1005.

Sechler JMF, Malech HL, White CJ, Ballin JI. Recombinant human interferon-gamma reconstitutes defective phagocyte function in patients with chronic granulomatous disease of childhood. Proc Natl Acad Sci USA 1988;85:4874.

Shamberger RC, Weinstein HJ, Delorey MJ, Levey RH. The medical and surgical management of typhlitis in children with acute nonlymphocytic (myelogenous) leukemia. Cancer 1986;57:603.

Skibber JM, Matter GJ, Pizzo PA, Lotze MT. Right lower quadrant pain in young patients with leukemia: a surgical perspective. Ann Surg 1987;206:711.

Straus SE, Ostrove JM, Inchauspe G, et al. Varicella-zoster virus infectious: biology, natural history, treatment and prevention. Ann Intern Med 1988;108:221.

Van Der Meer JWM. Defects in host-defense mechanisms. In Rubin RH, Young LS (ed). Clinical approach to infection in the compromised host. New York: Plenum Medical Book Co, 1988, pp 439-466.

Van der Waaij D, Tielemans-Speltie TM, Roeck-Houben AMJ. Infection by and distribution of biotyped of Enterobacteriaceae species in leukaemic patients treated under ward conditions and in units for protective isolation in seven hospitals in Europe. Infection 1977;5:188.

Wade JC, Schimpff SC, Newman KA, Wiernik PH. *Staphylococcus epidermidis:* an increasing cause of infection in patients with granulocytopenia. Ann Intern Med, 1982; 97:503.

Wagner ML, Rosenberg HS, Fernbach DJ, Singleton EB. Typhlitis: a complication of leukemia in childhood. Am J Roentgenol 1970;109:341.

Walsh TJ. Invasive pulmonary aspergillosis in patients with neoplastic diseases. Sem Resp Infect 1990;5:111.

Wiley JM, Smith N, Leventhal BG, et al. Invasive fungal disease in pediatric acute leukemia patients with fever and neutropenia during induction chemotherapy: a multivariate analysis of risk factors. J Clin Oncol 1990;8:280.

Wingard JR, Merz WG, Saral RR. *Candida tropicalis:* a major pathogen in immunocompromised patients. Ann Intern Med 1979;91:539.

Wood DJ, Corbitt G. Viral infections in childhood leukemia. J Infect Dis 1985;152:266.

Yu VL, Muder RR, Poorsattar A. Significance of isolation of aspergillus from the respiratory tract in diagnosis of invasive pulmonary aspergillosis: results from a three-year prosective study. Am J Med 1986;81:249.

Ziegler EJ, Fisher CJ, Spring CL, et al. Treatment of gram-negative bacteremia and septic shock with HA-1A human monoclonal antibody against endotoxin. N Engl J Med 1991;324:429.

Ziegler EJ, McCutchan JA, Fierer J, et al. Treatment of gram-negative bacteremia and shock with human antiserum to a mutant *Escherichia coli*. N Engl J Med 1982;307:1225.

12

KAWASAKI SYNDROME

MARIAN E. MELISH

Kawasaki syndrome, or mucocutaneous lymph node syndrome, is an acute febrile multisystem vasculitis affecting children. It was first described by Dr. Tomisaku Kawasaki in Japan in 1967 (Kawasaki, 1967; Kawasaki et al., 1974). Dr. Kawasaki's particular genius was the clear description of the disease and the identification of six clinical criteria, which remain the foundation of diagnosis 25 years later. Originally termed "benign" mucocutaneous lymph node syndrome, it is no longer considered necessarily benign. It was recognized in the early 1970s that death caused by myocardial infarction occurred in approximately 2% of cases; subsequently, it has been appreciated that approximately 30% of patients develop clinical evidence of cardiac disease, 20% develop coronary artery abnormalities large enough for detection by echocardiogram, and 30% develop inflammatory arthritis. In North America Kawasaki syndrome currently is a more common cause of acquired heart disease and inflammatory arthritis than acute poststreptococcal rheumatic fever. No longer confined to the Orient, Kawasaki syndrome has been recognized on all continents in children of all racial groups. Although the cause of this disorder remains unexplained, therapy is available. Intravenous gamma globulin given during the first week of illness has a dramatic effect on the clinical illness and reduces the likelihood of coronary abnormalities from greater than 20% to less than 5% (Furusho et al., 1984; Newburger et al., 1986; Newburger, 1991).

ETIOLOGY

Because of its febrile, exanthematous, and self-limited clinical characteristics, Kawasaki syndrome is widely believed to have a microbial cause. Despite intensive investigation, the causative agent had not been discovered by 1992. Recent studies (Shulman and Rowley, 1986; Burns et al., 1987) reporting the detection of reverse transcriptase, possibly indicating a retroviral cause, have not been confirmed by others (Melish et al., 1989; Marchette et al., 1990) or in subsequent experiments in one of the original laboratories (Shulman and Rowley, 1986). Although the human herpesvirus family, especially Epstein-Barr virus, has come under suspicion, all, including the newest member (human herpes virus 6), have been exonerated (Marchette et al., 1990).

PATHOLOGY AND PATHOGENESIS

By the mid-1970s it became evident that approximately 2% of children affected with Kawasaki syndrome, originally considered a benign condition, died suddenly, generally between 10 and 40 days from onset in the subacute or convalescent stage of illness (Kawasaki et al., 1974).

At autopsy, the major findings are multisystem vasculitis with special predilection for the coronary arteries (Fujiwara and Hamashima, 1978; Landing and Larson, 1977). The immediate cause of death is acute thrombosis of inflamed coronary arteries in more than 80% of fatal cases. In some deaths occurring early (within the first 2 weeks after onset), pancarditis with inflammation in the atrioventricular conduction system is thought to result in death from fatal arrhythmias or intractable congestive heart failure, whereas some late deaths (months to years after acute disease) apparently are secondary to coronary stenosis with chronic myocardial ischemia. Rupture of a coronary aneurysm is rare. Involvement of other arteries, particularly large and medium-sized muscular arteries, is variable and scattered. The history of the vascular lesion is directly related to the stage of illness at the time of death, demonstrating that the insult in Kawasaki syndrome is episodic and has a self-limited relationship to the acute illness rather than being chronic or progressive.

Early lesions (<10 days from onset of fever) are characterized by acute inflammation involving the intima of the coronary arteries. There is also an intense perivascular infiltration in the adventitia, with evidence of acute inflammation in the microvessels or vasa vasorum supplying the arterial wall. The media is spared, and aneurysmal dilation is absent. The clinical correlation is that the first evidence of coronary dilation by serial echocardiography appears at a mean of 10 days in those children ultimately developing coronary aneurysms. At this early stage carditis with an acute polymorphonuclear infiltrate in the pericardium, in the perivascular spaces of the myocardium, and in the endothelium, especially the mitral, tricuspid, and aortic valves, is present. Polymorphonuclear leukocyte infiltration is notable in the atrioventricular conduction system.

By the second week of illness through the sixth week, the intensity and nature of the inflammatory infiltrate progressively change, maturing from a dominant polymorphonuclear cell infiltrate to a less intense infiltrate composed predominantly of plasma cells and lymphocytes. The inflammation of the pericardium, myocardium, and endocardium gradually subsides. In the blood vessel wall destruction of the media appears, with multiple fractures of the internal elastic lamina and the development of aneurysmal dilation. The cause of death at this stage almost invariably involves coronary thrombosis close to the origin of the vessel, with massive myocardial infarction. Deaths occurring during this stage represent the most commonly encountered cardiac pathology of Kawasaki syndrome and are indistinguishable from a previously described pathological entity, infantile periarteritis nodosa. Infantile periarteritis nodosa was encountered rarely from the late nineteenth century to 1975; it was characterized by a fatal 2- to 6-week illness compatible with what is now recognized as Kawasaki syndrome. Both Kawasaki syndrome and infantile periarteritis nodosa have major differences from classic periarteritis nodosa, which is generally a chronic progressive illness of older children and adults, resulting in hypertension and renal and pulmonary disease and involving most often small and medium-sized muscular arteries, especially in the lung, kidney, and intestines.

Patients whose deaths occur more than 2 months from onset generally show little or no evidence of inflammation in the vessel walls or the heart. There is evidence of stenosis and myocardial infarction, both recent and remote, and the cause of death is generally acute infarction or chronic myocardial ischemia.

Although changes in multiple arteries, especially axillary, iliac, and femoral arteries and extraparenchymal portions of arteries supplying the stomach, spleen, and intestines, are seen, the intensity of involvement of other vessels in fatal cases is nearly always less than that found in the heart. Nonspecific changes in the lymph nodes, including focal necrosis with microthrombi, T-zone hyperplasia, macrophage infiltration of B zones, immunoblast proliferation, and mononuclear cell infiltration, have been described.

Recently, considerable progress has been made in elucidating aspects of the immunopathogenesis of vasculitis in Kawasaki syndrome. An acute rise and a convalescent fall of all classes of immunoglobulins occur during the illness so that 50% of IgE values and 80% of IgM values exceed 2 standard deviations for age-matched norms (Eluthesen et al., 1985). Immunoregulatory abnormalities resulting in a dramatic increase in the numbers of circulatory B cells spontaneously secreting immunoglobulin have been reported. The increase in immunoglobulin is polyclonal, with a very high proportion of activated B cells, apparently the result of a relative and absolute depression of suppressor T cells, which results in an elevated T-helper–T-suppressor ratio in the acute stage. T cells from patients with early Kawasaki syndrome stimulate normal, control B cells to produce immunoglobulins. The relative and absolute T-suppressor deficiency resolves rapidly with time, with normalization at 2 to 3 weeks of illness (Leung et al., 1983; Mason et al., 1985).

Immune complexes can be detected in more than 50% of patients by either C1q or Raji cell assays. These immune complexes are present very early in the illness, tend to peak approximately 4 weeks after onset, and become undetectable in late convalescence. The quantity of immune complexes in patients with Kawasaki syndrome is lower than that found in those with systemic lupus erythematosus but higher than that found in normal, afebrile children (Levin et al., 1985; Ono et al., 1985). Concentrations of complement are of special interest because of the increased levels of immune complexes in Kawasaki syndrome. C3 is universally elevated in weeks 1 through 3 of illness and then becomes normal, whereas C4 remains normal throughout the illness (Eluthesen et al., 1985). The coexistence of immune complexes with normal or high complement values in Kawasaki syndrome is markedly different from the classic immune complex disorders in which there is complement consumption, generally with renal involvement. Renal involvement is extremely unusual in Kawasaki syndrome. With Kawasaki syndrome, immune complexes may aggregate platelets, resulting in release of vasoactive factors. It is possible that the immune complexes bind directly to the vascular endothelium and induce an inflammatory reaction.

Increased elaboration of cytokines from peripheral blood mononuclear cells and high levels of serum interleukin-1 (IL-1), tumor necrosis factor (TNF), and interferon-gamma (IFN-γ) have been documented (Maury et al., 1989; Leung et al., 1989; Leung, 1989). Serum-soluble interleukin-2 (IL-2) receptor levels are increased in the acute phase and early subacute phase (up to 14 days), becoming normal thereafter (Lang et al., 1990). This provides another marker of lymphocyte activation that is associated with increased production of the cytokine IL-2.

Endothelial injury with Kawasaki syndrome may be related both to increased cytokine production, which may induce novel endothelial cell antigens, and to the generation of harmful autoantibodies to these new antigens. IgG and IgM antibodies, which are cytotoxic to cultured human umbilical vein endothelial cells that have been exposed to IFN-γ, IL-1, or TNF, can be detected in early illness. These novel cytokine-induced antigens might also make the endothelial cell surface more thrombogenic and induce adhesion antigens that could attract inflammatory cells (Leung et al., 1986).

In all of these studies the period of most intense cytokine elaboration and immune activation occurs during the acute and early subacute phase, coinciding with the period of most intense vascular inflammation through aneurysm formation. Leukotriene B_4 production by polymorphonuclear cells is increased in the subacute phase 13 to 29 days from onset. This powerful endogenous chemoattractant released from polymorphonuclear cells at an inflammatory site may play a role in attracting more inflammatory cells to the site, thus prolonging the period of intense inflammation (Hamasaki et al., 1989).

The strongest evidence of the importance of immunological factors in the pathogenesis of vasculitis in Kawasaki syndrome is provided by the remarkable beneficial effect of large-dose intravenous gamma globulin (IVIG) on both the acute febrile illness and the prevalence of coronary aneurysms. After IVIG therapy, B-cell activation and cytokine secretion are reduced, and T-suppressor cells return more rapidly to normal. Endothelial cell activation antigens disappeared after treatment in four of six patients in whom skin biopsies were performed before and while being given IVIG (Leung, 1989). The possible importance of endothelial cell antigens is demonstrated by a necropsy study that showed that endothelial cells of coronary arteries from Kawasaki syndrome patients, but not from normal individuals, expressed the major histocompatibility class II activation antigen (Terai et al., 1990). Prompt reversal of cytokine elaboration and other aspects of immune activation affecting endothelial cell function and antigen expression provide an attractive explanation of the still unknown mechanism of action of high-dose IVIG. Other theories attempting to explain the beneficial action of IVIG in this disease include down regulation of immunoglobulin production by a negative-feedback mechanism, specific immunoglobulin neutralization of the elusive causative agent or toxin, and nonspecific blockade of attachment sites for immune complexes or harmful autoantibodies on the vascular endothelium.

EPIDEMIOLOGY

The epidemiology of Kawasaki syndrome demonstrates that the disease virtually is restricted to young children: 50% are less than 2 years of age, 80% are less than 4 years, and cases are rare in individuals over the age of 12 years. Males outnumber females by a ratio of 1.4 to 1.6:1. Race-specific incidence rates developed from active surveillance in diverse locations such as Japan, Hawaii, Los Angeles, Chicago, and Heilbronn, Germany, demonstrate that Japanese and Korean children have an annual incidence of 40 to 150 cases per 100,000 children less than 5 years old, whereas Caucasian children in the diverse areas outside of Japan have rates of 6 to 10 cases per 100,000 children less than 5 years old. Intermediate rates have been recorded for children of black, Hispanic, Chinese, Filipino, and Polynesian ancestry. These rates are higher than that obtained from a nationwide passive surveillance in the United States and Britain (1.1 and 1.5 per 100,000 children <5 years old) but undoubtedly more accurately represent the true incidence. Projecting these figures to the United States as a whole, an estimated 3,000 to 5,000 cases occur per year, a figure close to that reported for Lyme disease. Community-wide epidemics generally occurring in the winter and spring with a 2- to 4-year interepidemic frequency have been recorded in several well-studied communities in Japan and North America. In these outbreaks no point-source exposure or direct person-to-person spread is apparent. In Japan two national pandemics have occurred with temporal-geographical spread from region to region, but such spread has not been reported in North America where outbreaks to date have been limited to single communities. Epidemiological and case-control investigations have demonstrated no striking climatic or urban-rural differences, no evidence of association with drugs or immunizations, no evidence to suggest insect vector or animal contact transmission, and no evidence of parenteral spread, contact with specific environmental toxins, or diets unusual for age. Two intriguing associations—exposure to freshly shampooed carpets and residence near a body of standing water—have been found in some investigations but not in others (Patriarca et al., 1982; Rauch, 1987; Klein et al., 1986; Rogers, 1986; Burns et al., 1991).

The clinical and epidemiological features of sudden onset, the febrile exanthematous and self-limited character of the disease, and the regular occurrence of epidemics at 2- to 4-year intervals suggest a microbial cause. The widespread nature of the community-wide outbreaks with little evidence of direct person-to-person spread, the epidemic periodicity, and the restriction to young children further suggest that the elusive causative agent probably is highly transmissible and human associated, spreading widely through the community, producing infection and immunity in nearly all individuals by the age of 12 years, but resulting in clinically apparent disease in only a few, particularly those with a race-related genetic predisposition to disease. The 2- to 4-year interepidemic frequency, superimposed on endemic occurrence, coincides with the age of greatest occurrence and suggests that outbreaks can be generated when a sufficient number of new susceptibles have been added to the population by birth. No evidence has yet been found supporting a bacterial cause, for no bacterial agent has been isolated regularly from a normally sterile site. The possibility that an agent constituting the normal flora of the respiratory tract or the gut might have pathological potential, perhaps through elaboration of a toxin, has been suggested. A novel, difficult to cultivate virus would be equally likely.

CLINICAL MANIFESTATIONS

In its fully developed form Kawasaki syndrome is a distinctive clinical entity with a predictable clinical course. Because no single pathognomonic laboratory test or clinical sign has yet emerged, the diagnosis must be made by careful adherence to clinical criteria (see box and Plate 3). These criteria were described by Dr. Kawasaki and are discussed in detail below.

Fever

The fever usually begins abruptly and is of a remittent, high-spiking nature, with two to four peaks per day. The temperature usually ranges from 38.5° to more than 40° C. Unless the patient is treated with a combination of aspirin and

PRINCIPAL DIAGNOSTIC CRITERIA FOR KAWASAKI SYNDROME

Five of the six criteria are necessary to make a secure diagnosis.
- Fever
- Conjunctival injection
- Changes in the mouth
    Erythema, fissuring, and crusting of the lips
    Diffuse oropharyngeal erythema
    Strawberry tongue
- Changes in the peripheral extremities
    Induration of hands and feet
    Erythema of palms and soles
    Desquamation of fingertips and toetips approximately 2 weeks after onset
    Transverse grooves across fingernails 2 to 3 months after onset
- Erythematous rash
- Enlarged lymph node mass measuring more than 1.5 cm in diameter

IVIG, the mean duration of fever exceeds 10 days but ranges from 5 to 35 days. The fever drops dramatically to the normal range in more than 80% of patients within 24 hours of single-dose IVIG treatment.

Conjunctival changes

In patients with Kawasaki syndrome there is discrete vascular injection of the bulbar conjunctiva, which is more severe than injection in the tarsal or palpebral conjunctiva. Finding a zone of decreased infection around the iris (limbal sparing) is characteristic. Some patients also have follicular palpebral conjunctivitis. These findings develop in the first week of illness. There is no associated exudate, and edema of the conjunctiva and corneal ulceration do not occur, thus distinguishing the conjunctivitis of Kawasaki syndrome from the purulent conjunctivitis of Stevens-Johnson syndrome. Mild acute iridocyclitis or anterior uveitis also occurs early in the acute phase and is diagnosed by visualization of cells or "flare" during office slit-lamp examination. The finding rapidly resolves and rarely is associated with photophobia or eye pain.

Mouth changes

Any or all of the following mouth changes can occur in patients with Kawasaki syndrome: lip involvement, strawberry tongue, and oropharyngeal erythema. Lip changes first appear 2 to 5 days after onset of fever, starting as generalized erythema with mild edema. Erythema and edema progressively increase over the next several days, with cracking and bleeding. The development of fissures coincides with lip changes. A strawberry tongue develops with prominent hypertrophied papillae. The tongue is usually reddened; the white strawberry tongue characteristic of early scarlet fever is encountered less often. Patients may have diffuse oropharyngeal erythema, but exudates on the tonsils and vesicles and ulcers within the mouth are rarely encountered; therefore their appearance should prompt consideration of an alternate diagnosis.

Hand and foot lesions

Changes in the hands and feet are among the most distinctive features of Kawasaki syndrome. The first and most constant finding is the development of diffuse red-purple discoloration of the palms and soles 2 to 5 days after onset of fever. This erythema may wrap partially around the fingers and soles and extend a few centimeters up the wrists. Discrete macules on the palms and soles as seen in measles and other viral illnesses are not part of Kawasaki syndrome and constitute strong evidence against the diagnosis. The hands and feet may be edematous or firmly indurated. Patients often refuse to stand or walk because of discomfort from edema, and older children find the edema of their hands prevents using crayons and scissors. In the subacute phase of illness, days 10 to 20 from onset of fever, a characteristic desquamation begins at the fingertips just under the nailbed. It is followed by toe desquamation a few days later. Extensive desquamation of the entire palm and sole, with the shedding of large, thick sheets of skin, usually is present. This desquamation differs considerably from the fine, branny flakes that begin at the sides of the fingernails as a characteristic of the convalescent stage of scarlet fever. A transverse groove across the fingernails and toenails (Beau's lines) becomes apparent 6 to 8 weeks after onset and grows out with the nail.

Rash

The rash of Kawasaki syndrome is deeply erythematous, nonvesicular, and nonbullous, but it is polymorphic in both its nature and distribution. The most common type of rash consists of raised, deeply erythematous pruritic plaques of varying sizes ranging from 2 to more than 10 mm in diameter. These lesions resemble intensely erythematous urticaria or incompletely developed target lesions of the erythema multiforme type. The second most frequently encountered type of rash is maculopapular. It may be widely scattered or coalescent. This type of rash strongly resembles that of measles, but it rarely has the same distribution and does not progress from the face and trunk to the extremities in a centripetal fashion. A generalized or blotchy scarlatiniform erythroderma occurs in approximately 10% of cases. Rarely have the authors encountered a flat erythema marginatum rash in small infants. The distribution of rash is very variable; in some patients it is truly generalized, and in others it is more prominent on the trunk or on the extremities. Occasionally, the rash is most prominent on or even limited to the lower abdomen and perineal area.

Lymph nodes

An enlarged lymph node mass is seen in approximately 50% of cases. When present, it is virtually always unilateral and cervical, with considerable firm induration measuring from 1.5 to 7 cm in diameter. It may be extremely tender and have overlying erythema. At times it may result in acute torticollis or swallowing difficulty.

Once present, rash, hand and foot erythema, edema, and lymph node swelling persist throughout the febrile phase and disappear dramatically when the fever resolves. Conjunctival infection and mouth changes resolve more gradually.

Associated features

The associated features of Kawasaki syndrome attest to its multisystemic nature (see box). Sterile pyuria reflecting urethritis is found in three quarters of patients. Arthritis developing in the first week of illness tends to involve multiple joints, including the small interphalangeal joints and large weight-bearing joints. Arthrocentesis during this phase reveals copious, thick purulent fluid, with a mean white blood cell count (WBC)

ASSOCIATED FEATURES (IN ORDER OF FREQUENCY)
Pyuria and urethritis
Arthralgia and arthritis
Aseptic meningitis
Diarrhea
Abdominal pain
Myocardiopathy
Pericardial effusion
Obstructive jaundice
Hydrops of gallbladder
Acute mitral insufficiency
Myocardial infarction

---

of $125,000/mm^3$ up to $300,000$ WBC/mm^3. Glucose determinations are within normal limits; gram stain results and cultures are invariably negative. Approximately one third of patients with arthritis have the onset in the first 10 days of illness. Arthritis developing after 10 days has a predilection for large weight-bearing joints, especially the knees and ankles. It is associated with slightly less intense inflammation as measured by the WBC count of the joint fluid. Gastrointestinal complaints, including abdominal pain, severe diarrhea, and nausea, occur in approximately one third of children during the early stages of the disease. Central nervous system (CNS) involvement, with severe lethargy, semicoma, and aseptic meningitis, occurs in one quarter of the patients. Obstructive jaundice and acute gallbladder hydrops are seen in approximately 5% of patients.

The most important associated feature of Kawasaki syndrome is involvement of the heart. Clinical cardiac disease occurs in approximately 20% of patients and most often is manifested as pericardial effusion, transient myocardiopathy with congestive heart failure, and/or arrhythmias. Angiographic and two-dimensional echocardiographic studies performed on a routine basis 4 to 8 weeks after onset demonstrate coronary artery aneurysms in approximately 20% of patients.

Clinical course

The clinical course of Kawasaki syndrome is triphasic. The acute febrile phase of the disease is marked by rash, conjunctival injection, strawberry tongue, edema and erythema of the hands and feet, lymphadenitis, aseptic meningitis, and hepatic dysfunction. Without aspirin or IVIG treatment, this phase generally lasts 8 to 15 days (mean, 11). After defervescence, the physical findings disappear rapidly, but the child remains irritable and anorectic. Arthritis and cardiac disease may develop in the subacute phase of the illness, which is marked also by desquamation and thrombocytosis. The subacute phase persists until the child's behavior returns to normal, approximately 3 weeks after onset. The subacute and early convalescent periods (3 to 4 weeks from onset) constitute the time of greatest risk of sudden death from acute coronary artery thrombosis.

Laboratory abnormalities with Kawasaki syndrome are quite nonspecific. In the acute phase most patients have leukocytosis with abundant band-form neutrophils. Increased acute phase reactants, with elevated sedimentation rate, C-reactive protein, or alpha$_1$-antitrypsin, are universally found during the acute and subacute stages; they return to normal 8 to 12 weeks after onset. The platelet count shows a gradual rise from normal levels, becoming elevated above 450,000 between days 7 and 10 and peaking between days 15 and 25. Virtually all patients ultimately have elevated platelet counts, which may persist for 3 months after onset.

DIAGNOSIS

Management of Kawasaki syndrome starts with diagnosis. Kawasaki syndrome should be considered in the differential diagnosis of patients with fever and any of the following: generalized polymorphous erythematous rash, conjunctival injection, characteristic changes in the mouth, characteristic changes in the hands and feet, or unilateral cervical lymph node swelling measuring greater than 1.5 cm. A secure diagnosis of Kawasaki syndrome is made in patients who fulfill five of the six criteria and for whom other illnesses that may mimic Kawasaki syndrome have been excluded. The most commonly encountered diseases to exclude are (1) nonspecific exanthems, presumably viral, (2) measles, (3) streptococcal and staphylococcal infections with scarlatiniform eruptions, (4) infectious mononucleosis, and (5) hypersensitivity reactions. If all clinical features of Kawasaki syndrome are present, it is not necessary to wait until the fifth day from onset before making the diagnosis and beginning therapy (Levy and Koren, 1990).

Some "incomplete" cases of Kawasaki syndrome do not fulfill the diagnostic criteria but are at risk for the development of coronary artery aneurysms. Children under the age of 6 months are particularly likely to develop coronary abnormalities while not expressing complete diagnostic criteria (Burns et al., 1986). Most young infants with Kawasaki syndrome fulfill diagnostic criteria, but many of the manifestations are milder or more subtle than those usually seen in older children. Therefore Kawasaki syndrome should be considered even if the diagnostic criteria are not fulfilled; in some cases patients with incomplete forms should receive care just as patients who fulfill all the clinical criteria.

The laboratory tests provide modest diagnostic support. An elevated C-reactive protein result or elevated sedimentation rate is almost universal in patients with Kawasaki syndrome and is not commonly found in patients with viral exanthems, hypersensitivity reactions, or measles. Platelet count elevation greater than 450,000/mm^3 is usually seen in patients presenting after the seventh day of illness, but the platelet count is usually normal for the first week. An analysis of reported cases of atypical Kawasaki syndrome with coronary abnormalities demonstrated that platelet elevation and elevated sedimentation rate were universal in these cases. The authors' experience in Hawaii and with the 900 patients in the U.S. Multicenter Study Group experience corroborates that finding to the point that a diagnosis of Kawasaki syndrome is extremely unlikely if the platelet count and a full panel of acute phase inflammatory reactants (sedimentation rate, C-reactive protein, alpha$_1$-antitrypsin) are normal after day 7.

TREATMENT
Intravenous immune globulin

As soon as the disease can be diagnosed, patients should have a baseline echocardiogram and receive IVIG, 2 g/kg given in a 10- to 12-hour infusion (Fig. 12-1). This dosage has recently been demonstrated as equally efficacious in reducing the risk of coronary disease as a schedule of 400 mg/kg/day given for 4 consecutive days. The single-dose schedule is superior

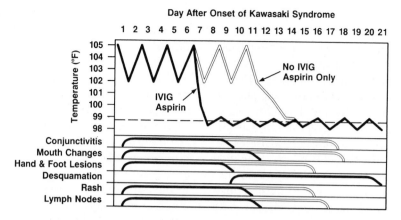

Fig. 12-1. Effect of IVIG and aspirin on the course of Kawasaki syndrome.

to the four-dose schedule in rapidity of return of fever and acute phase reactants to normal (Newburger, 1990; Newburger et al., 1991). Single-dose infusion is safe, having been given to 273 children in a controlled trial with no significant adverse effects. Pulse, heart rate, and blood pressure should be monitored at the beginning of infusion, at 30 minutes, at 1 hour, and then at 2 hours during infusion. Although this dose does provide a substantial fluid and protein load, it does not increase the risk of congestive heart failure, even in patients with decreased myocardial function.

No large clinical experience is available demonstrating efficacy of lower-dose single-infusion therapy. Multiple studies in Japan have also demonstrated efficacy for multiple-dose regimens of more than 1 g/kg. Total doses at or below 1 g/kg have been ineffective in reducing the incidence of coronary abnormalities.

No data are available to guide therapy of patients encountered later than 10 days from onset. If patients are still febrile or have other signs of active disease, including progressive coronary dilation, IVIG therapy should be instituted, for it may result in prompt clinical improvement. Patients who have become afebrile and have normal coronary arteries by day 21 of illness are unlikely to benefit from receiving IVIG but should receive aspirin 3 to 5 mg/kg once daily. Currently, no evidence suggests any beneficial effect of IVIG in patients who have already developed coronary aneurysms once active inflammation has subsided.

Aspirin

On the same day that IVIG is administered, the patient should start to receive aspirin. The dose of aspirin best studied in the United States is 100 mg/kg/day until the fever is controlled or until day 14 of illness, followed by a dose of 5 to 10 mg/kg/day (40 to 80 mg by mouth once daily) until the sedimentation rate and platelet count are normal, approximately 3 months from onset of illness. The appropriate dose of aspirin in Kawasaki syndrome has been controversial. Theoretically, high-dose aspirin (>80 mg/kg/day) adjusted to produce a serum total salicylate level of 18 to 28 mg/dl might decrease the intensity of the vasculitis, whereas much lower doses (3 to 10 mg/kg/day) would provide optimal inhibition of platelet aggregation. Both regimens have supporters in North America. Japanese clinicians generally have received an intermediate antipyretic dose of 30 to 50 mg/kg/day. To date there is no conclusive evidence favoring any of these dosages.

Difficulty in obtaining therapeutic anti-inflammatory serum salicylate levels during the acute phase of illness has been reported. Koren et al. (1985) associates found this difficulty related to both impaired bioavailability and enhanced clearance of salicylate. Because IVIG appears to have potent anti-inflammatory effects, a lower dose of aspirin throughout the illness may be more appropriate. A study to answer this important question is currently underway. Salicylate levels should be obtained if symptoms of vomiting, hyperpnea, lethargy, or liver function abnormalities develop while the patient is receiving high-dose aspirin. To decrease the risk of Reye's syndrome, aspirin administration can be interrupted for a few days if patients develop varicella or influenza during the follow-up phase.

Monitoring

All patients with Kawasaki syndrome should be admitted to the hospital for administration of IVIG and for observation until the fever is controlled. Cardiovascular function should be monitored carefully. Once a child's fever has subsided, it is unlikely that significant congestive heart failure or myocardial dysfunction will occur. The patient should be evaluated within a week after discharge and should have an echocardiogram between 21 and 28 days after onset of fever. If baseline and 3- to 4-week echocardiograms reveal normal results with no evidence of coronary abnormality, further echocardiograms are unnecessary. The peak period to demonstrate coronary abnormalities detectable by echocardiogram is 3 to 4 weeks after onset. In a recent study of more than 800 patients, the authors found no new abnormalities at 8 weeks if the 3- to 4-week echocardiogram was normal. Patients with no evidence of coronary abnormalities should receive 80 mg of aspirin per day for approximately 3 months, the period required for both the platelet count and the sedimentation rate to return to normal.

Myocardial infarction

Myocardial infarction occurs most commonly in patients with giant coronary aneurysms, 8 mm or greater, in the first year after onset of Kawasaki syndrome. Patients with a history of giant aneurysms are also at higher risk for later coronary thrombosis than those with smaller lesions. Parents of all children with coronary abnormalities should be instructed to contact a physician and alert the emergency medical system if chest pain, dyspnea, extreme lethargy, or syncope develop. Prompt fibrinolytic therapy with streptokinase, urokinase, or tissue plasminogen activator should be attempted at a tertiary care center if acute coronary thrombosis is diagnosed.

Noncardiac complications

Kawasaki syndrome is a multi-system disease, but, except for cardiac complications, other systemic involvement is generally self-limited. In most patients with arthritis, joint inflammation occurs in the acute stage and is intense and painful but self-limited, usually lasting less than 2 weeks. Although the authors have treated patients with both high-dose aspirin (100 mg/kg/day) and other nonsteroidal anti-inflammatory drugs, particularly tolmetin sodium (20 mg/kg/day in three divided doses), they have not been impressed with prompt temporal response to anti-inflammatory therapy. Many patients with large effusions appear to benefit most from arthrocentesis, which usually must be done only once. Abdominal pain-diarrhea complex, also a feature of the early acute stage, usually responds to intravenous hydration and supportive care. Gallbladder hydrops, presenting clinically as a right upper-quadrant mass, sometimes in association with obstructive jaundice, can be confirmed by diagnostic ultrasonography and can be monitored until resolution occurs. Surgical removal of the dilated gallbladder is not necessary, for this complication is self-limited. A rare complication seen in the acute febrile stage is peripheral vasoconstriction threatening distal extremities. It is usually seen only in patients with severe systemic illness and widespread vascular involvement. This complication has been managed either with prostaglandin E_1 infusion (0.007 to 0.03 mg/kg/minute), maintained over several days in an intensive care unit with constant hemodynamic monitoring (Westphalen et al., 1988), or with systemic heparinization and corticosteroid pulse therapy (methylprednisolone, 25 mg/kg intravenous push). There are anecdotal reports of success with both approaches but no controlled experience. Telephone consultation with a center treating large numbers of Kawasaki syndrome patients should be sought by the physician faced with rare or serious complications.

LONG-TERM MANAGEMENT

Patients with no history of coronary artery abnormalities. There is no need for administration of aspirin or other antiplatelet medications beyond 3 months or for restriction of physical activities. Cardiac evaluation and electrocardiograms obtained every 2 to 3 years may be warranted.

Patients with transient or small coronary aneurysms. These patients should receive long-term antiplatelet therapy with aspirin (3 to 5 mg/kg/day) at least until resolution of abnormalities, preferably indefinitely. Restricting physical activities is not necessary unless there are cardiac stress test abnormalities. Patients should be followed with yearly cardiac evaluations and have periodic stress testing when they are over the age of 5 years. Echocardiograms should be performed yearly or more often until stable regression has been demonstrated. Angiography is indicated if electrocardiographic or stress test abnormalities develop.

Patients with giant aneurysms, 8 mm or greater. Indefinite therapy with aspirin (3 to 5 mg/kg once daily, with or without dipyridamole, 3 to 4 mg/kg/day in three doses) is advised. Anticoagulant therapy with warfarin (Coumadin) and/or subcutaneous heparin may be added, especially during the first 2 years after onset. Cardiac evaluation should be performed every 6 months along with periodic stress testing, and yearly or more frequent echocardiograms should be performed to monitor aneurysm size. Angiography should be performed to define the extent of disease at least once and whenever symptoms or stress tests indicate myocardial ischemia. Physical activity is regulated on the basis of stress test results and the level of anticoagulation. Patients with obstructive lesions or signs of ischemia may need evaluation for possible surgical intervention. These patients require consultation with a pediatric cardiologist with extensive experience managing Kawasaki syndrome patients.

PROGNOSIS

Kawasaki syndrome is primarily an acute and self-limited disease; however, cardiac damage sustained when the disease is active may be permanent and progressive. This damage may manifest soon after onset or may not become apparent until years later. From multiple studies it is clear that approximately 20% of all patients untreated with IVIG develop coronary artery aneurysms that are detectable by angiography or two-dimensional echocardiography. These abnormalities may appear as early as 7 days and as late as 4 weeks after onset of the syndrome. The risk of coronary aneurysms is lowered to 4% by 8 weeks overall if IVIG is given in the first 10 days of illness. For infants less than 1 year of age, even with IVIG treatment, the risk of coronary abnormalities at 8 weeks is 12% (Newburger et al., 1991). Patients with coronary artery abnormalities are at risk for myocardial infarction, sudden death, and myocardial ischemia for a period of at least 5 years after onset of illness (Kato et al., 1986). Regression of aneurysms is known to occur. Approximately two thirds of patients with coronary aneurysms at 8 weeks after onset have regression within 1 year to apparently normal vessels by angiography or echocardiography. Approximately one third continue to have coronary dilation. Among patients whose aneurysms regress, stenosis, tortuosity, and thrombosis of coronary vessels may occur (Kato, Inoue, and Akagi, 1988). Patients with giant aneurysms (coronary lumen >8 mm in diameter) are at risk for the development of significant stenosis with resultant myocardial ischemia (Tatara and Kusakawa, 1987). The risk of giant aneurysm, originally found in 3% to 7% of all patients, has also been dramatically lowered by the use of IVIG (Rowley et al., 1988). Chung and the United States Multicenter Kawasaki Disease Study Group (1989) administered IVIG to more than 800 patients. Six of these patients developed giant aneurysms; three had coronary dilation at the time IVIG was begun.

A mortality rate of approximately 2% was reported in the mid-1970s. Currently, in Japan the mortality rate is approximately 0.1% (Kawasaki, 1989). This improvement in mortality came during a decade in which there was (1) widespread use of aspirin; (2) awareness of the possibility of cardiac disease, with more intensive follow-up and supportive care; and (3) increased recognition of Kawasaki syndrome, possibly leading to the inclusion of milder cases in the total. The true long-term prognosis for patients with Kawasaki syndrome is not well understood, for long-term follow-up studies into the second and third decade after disease have not been performed. Inoue et al. (1989) have surveyed cardiologists in Japan and found adults with newly detected coronary aneurysms discovered by angiography performed to evaluate myocardial infarction or ischemia. One quarter of these patients had a history of Kawasaki syndrome or compatible childhood illness 19 to 60 years before discovery of coronary aneurysms.

Other complications of Kawasaki syndrome such as arthritis and hepatic disease apparently are entirely self-limited, last for less than 3 months, and are not associated with chronic or progressive disability or recurrent attacks.

Recurrence of Kawasaki syndrome is uncommon, with approximately 3% of patients suffering one or more episodes. Recurrences may occur as long as 8 years after the first attack.

PREVENTION

Without knowledge about its cause, no effective preventive strategies for Kawasaki syndrome have been determined.

ISOLATION AND QUARANTINE

To date there has been no evidence of point-source exposure or direct person-to-person spread. Therefore isolation and quarantine are not indicated.

REFERENCES

Burns JC, Geha RS, Schneeberger EE, et al. Polymerase activity in lymphocyte culture supernatants from patients with Kawasaki disease. Nature 1987;323:814-816.

Burns JC, Wiggins JW, Toews WH, Glode M. Clinical spectrum of Kawasaki syndrome in infants younger than 6 months of age. J Pediatr 1986;109:759-763.

Burns JC, Wilbert MH, Mary GP, et al. Clinical and epidemiologic characteristics of patients referred for evaluation of possible Kawasaki disease. J Pediatr 1991;118:680-686.

Chung KJ, U.S. Multicenter Kawasaki Study Group. Incidence and prognosis of giant coronary artery aneurysms in Kawasaki disease (Abstract 1123). Circulation 1989;80:II-282.

Eluthesen K, Marchette N, Melish ME. Immunoglobulins, complimental circulating immune complexes in Kawasaki syndrome. Presented at the 21st Interscience Conference on Antimicrobial Agents and Chemotherapeutics, November 1985.

Fujiwara H, Hamashima Y. Pathology of the heart in Kawasaki disease. J Pediatr 1978;61:100-107.

Furusho K, Kamiya T, Nakano H, et al. High-dose intravenous gamma globulin for Kawasaki disease. Lancet 1984;2:1055-1058.

Hamasaki Y, Ichimaru T, Koga H, et al. Increased in-vitro leukotriene B4 production by stimulated polymorphonuclear cells in Kawasaki disease. Acta Pediatr Jpn Overseas Ed 1989;31:346-348.

Inoue O, Akagi T, Kato H. Fate of giant coronary artery aneurysms in Kawasaki disease: long term follow-up study (Abstract 1046). Circulation 1989;80:II-262.

Kato H, Ichinose E, Kawasaki T. Myocardial infarction in Kawasaki disease. J Pediatr 1986;108:923-928.

Kato H, Inoue O, Akagi T. Kawasaki disease: cardiac problems and management. Pediatr Rev 1988;9:209-217.

Kawasaki T. Acute febrile mucocutaneous syndrome with lymphoid involvement with specific desquamation of the fingers and toes in children [Japanese]. Jpn J Allerg 1967;16:178-222.

Kawasaki T, Kosaki F, Okawa S, et al. A new infantile acute febrile mucocutaneous lymph node syndrome (MLNS) prevailing in Japan. Pediatrics 1974;54:271-276.

Kawasaki T. Kawasaki disease. Asian Med J 1989;32:497-506.

Klein BS, Rogers MF, Patrican LA, et al. Kawasaki syndrome: a controlled study of an outbreak in Wisconsin. Am J Epidemiol 1986;124:306-316.

Koren G, Rose V, Levi S. Probable efficacy of high dose salicylates in reducing coronary involvement in Kawasaki disease. JAMA 1985;254:767.

Landing BH, Larson EJ. Are infantile periarteritis nodosa with coronary artery involvement and fatal mucocutaneous lymph node syndrome the same? Comparison of 20 patients from North America with patients from Hawaii and Japan. J Pediatr 1977;59:651-662.

Lang BA, Silverman ED, Laxer RM, et al. Serum soluble interleukin-2 receptor levels in Kawasaki disease. J Pediatr 1990;116:592-596.

Leung DYM. Immunomodulation by intravenous immune globulin in Kawasaki disease. J Allergy Clin Immunol 1989;84:588-894.

Leung DYM, Chu ET, Wood N, et al. Immunoregulatory T cell abnormalities in mucocutaneous lymph node syndrome. J Immunol 1983;130:2002-2004.

Leung DYM, Collins T, LaPierre LA, et al. IgM antibodies present in the acute phase of Kawasaki syndrome lyse cultured vascular endothelial cells stimulated by gamma interferon. J Clin Invest 1986;77:1428-1435.

Leung DYM, Kurt-Jones E, Newberger JW, et al. Endothelial cell activation and high interleukin-1 secretion in the pathogenesis of acute Kawasaki disease. Lancet 1989;2:1298-1302.

Levin M, Holland PC, Nokes TJC, et al. Platelet immune complex interaction in pathogenesis of Kawasaki disease and childhood polyarteritis. Br Med J 1985;290:1456-1460.

Levy M, Koren G. Atypical Kawasaki disease: analysis of clinical presentation and diagnostic clues. Pediatr Infect Dis 1990;9:122-126.

Marchette NJ, Melish ME, Hicks R, et al. Epstein-Barr virus and other herpes virus infections in Kawasaki syndrome. J Infect Dis 1990;161:680-684.

Mason WH, Jordan SC, Sakai R, et al. Circulating immune complexes in Kawasaki syndrome. Pediatr Infect Dis 1985;4:48-51.

Maury CPJ, Sal E, Pelkemen P. Elevated circulating tumor necrosis factor in patients with Kawasaki disease. J Lab Clin Med 1989;113:651.

Melish ME, Marchette NJ, Kaplan JC, et al. Absence of significant RNA-dependent DNA polymerase activity in lymphocytes from patients with Kawasaki syndrome. Nature 1989;337:288-290.

Newberger JW, Takahashi M, Beiser AS, et al. A single infusion of intravenous gamma globulin compared to four daily doses in the treatment of acute Kawasaki syndrome. N Engl J Med 1991;324:1633-1637.

Newburger JW, Takahashi M, Burns JC, et al. The treatment of Kawasaki syndrome with intravenous gamma globulin. N Engl J Med 1986;315:341-347.

completely within several days, or it may be a rapidly progressive and fulminating disease, terminating fatally within 24 hours. Between these two extremes are many variations. In general, approximately 60% of patients recover completely; 15% die; and 25% subsequently show manifestations of brain damage such as mental retardation, recurrent convulsive seizures, severe behavior disorders, nerve deafness, hemiplegia, and paraplegia. The course is unpredictable. It is not unusual for a child to be in a coma for several weeks and subsequently to recover completely without sequelae.

Other CNS complications of measles include cerebellar ataxia, retrobulbar neuritis, and hemiplegia caused by infarctions in the distribution of major arteries (Tyler, 1957). Although the pathogenesis of measles encephalomyelitis remains obscure, it does not seem to involve viral replication in the CNS but more closely resembles the neuropathological findings of experimental allergic encephalomyelitis, suggesting an autoimmune-mediated process (Johnson et al., 1984).

Infants with dehydration and hyperelectrolytemia may present a neurological picture that closely resembles that of measles encephalomyelitis. Correction of the water and electrolyte disturbance is usually followed by rapid improvement.

Subacute sclerosing panencephalitis

The rare condition of subacute sclerosing panencephalitis (SSPE) can be considered a late complication of measles, with an incidence of approximately one per 100,000 cases. It has clinical and pathological features that are characteristic of a slowly progressing viral infection. The syndrome, first described by Dawson in 1934 and by van Bogaert in 1945, has also been called *subacute inclusion-body encephalitis*.

The early clinical manifestations are characterized by insidious and progressive behavioral and intellectual deterioration, possibly initially manifested by declining school performance. These symptoms are associated with awkwardness, stumbling, and falling. Later, the course may be characterized by involuntary myoclonic seizures and increasing mental deterioration that frequently are followed by death within a 6-month period. The confirmatory laboratory findings include (1) an electroencephalogram

with paroxysmal spiking at regular intervals and depressed activity between spikes; (2) elevation of the CSF globulin, predominantly the IgG fraction; (3) an exceptionally high serum measles antibody titer; and (4) detectable oligoclonal measles antibody in the CSF.

Pathological and clinical differences have been observed between SSPE and acute encephalomyelitis. The early neuropathological features of SSPE include perivascular round cell infiltration, neuronal degeneration, and intranuclear and intracytoplasmic inclusion bodies. Later, extensive gliosis and demyelination occur. The demonstration of measles-virus antigen in the brain and the serological findings incriminate the virus itself as the causative agent or, more probably, a defective variant of the virus. Further confirmation of the role of measles virus in SSPE has been provided by electron microscopic demonstration of paramyxovirus nucleocapsids in the inclusion bodies, immunofluorescence with specific measles antiserum of affected cells, and recovery in the laboratory by cocultivation techniques of infectious measleslike virus from brain biopsy or autopsy specimens.

Using immunoprecipitation methods, Hall and Choppin (1981) found a relative lack of antibodies to M protein in serum and CSF of patients with SSPE. However, there were high levels of antibody to other viral proteins. The onset of SSPE occurs many months or many years after an attack of measles. Epidemiologic studies have shown a possible relationship to age of the person. It is usually the youngest male child in the family who develops SSPE, even though older siblings had measles at the same time. Moreover, the initial measles infection is usually very mild. It has been postulated that during the course of a relatively mild or inapparent infection, the virus may survive and persist as a defective virion. The defects are apparently in expression of the M, H, and F genes of the measles virus. The following case report describes a child who had measles at 6 months of age and developed SSPE at 8 years of age.

CASE REPORT. M.R., an 8-year-old girl, was admitted to Bellevue Hospital on November 12, 1966, with a 3-month history of myoclonic seizures and progressive deterioration of behavior manifested by confusion, regression, frequent falls, and bizarre speech. Her growth and development were normal before the onset of present illness. She had a history of measles at 6 months of age. During a 9-month period of observation at the hospital, the course of the disease was characterized by gradual mental and motor deterioration. The electroencephalogram was abnormal and characteristic of hypsarrhythmia. CSF examination revealed no cells, normal concentration of glucose, and a protein concentration of 90 mg/dl. The results of measles HI antibody tests in serum were as follows: December 1966—1:16,384; March 1967—1:8192; April 1967—1:4096; May 1967—1:2048; August 1967—1:512; and January 1968—1:512. Measles HI antibody was not detected in the CSF.

A follow-up study of 46 children with natural measles revealed a geometric mean HI antibody titer of approximately 1:128 1 to 7 years after onset of disease; the titers ranged from a low of 1:4 to a high of 1:2048. In view of this experience, the observation of a measles virus HI antibody titer of 1:16,384 is highly significant in a child who had measles 7 years previously; it suggests a causative association (Berman et al., 1968).

Other complications

Purpura, thrombocytopenic and nonthrombocytopenic, rarely may complicate measles. The deleterious effect of measles on pregnancy and on tuberculosis was clearly demonstrated in the southern Greenland epidemic. Of 26 pregnant women with measles, half either aborted or gave birth to premature infants; there were no congenital malformations. There apparently were a reactivation of previously arrested cases, a striking increase of new cases of tuberculosis, and an increased mortality rate with this disease.

A positive tuberculin test may temporarily revert to negative during the course of measles. This anergy may persist for as long as 6 weeks. In the majority of cases the tuberculin test becomes positive again within 2 weeks.

Pneumomediastinum and subcutaneous emphysema may occur in rare instances. Bloch and Vardy (1968) described four cases that occurred during an epidemic in a small town in the northern Negev in Israel.

Corneal ulceration is a potentially serious complication that fortunately is very rare. However, nearly all patients have a mild superficial keratoconjunctivitis.

Appendicitis may develop, perhaps as a result of lymphoid hyperplasia in the appendix, and

may be so extensive it obliterates the lumen. In most instances perforation occurs before the complication is recognized.

In certain areas of the world (Africa, India, and Central and South America) where measles is a severe and often fatal disease, the following complications are frequently observed: severe diarrhea and dehydration, kwashiorkor, pyogenic infections of the skin, cancrum oris, and septicemia.

Among children with human immunodeficiency virus (HIV) infection, measles has an enhanced severity, with a higher incidence of pneumonia, hospitalization, and death (Krasinski and Borkowsky, 1989) (see also Chapter 1). Of four measles deaths in New Jersey in early 1991, two were in HIV-infected patients; of nine in New York City, two were in HIV-infected patients.

PROGNOSIS

The prognosis of measles has improved significantly during the past three decades. Many of the serious bacterial complications are easily controlled by antimicrobial therapy. In general, the prognosis is better in older children than in infants. A preexisting tuberculous infection may be aggravated. The majority of deaths are the result of severe bronchopneumonia or encephalitis. In 1989 and 1990 in outbreaks in the United States the reported case fatality rates were from three to four per 1,000 (Centers for Disease Control, 1991).

Modified measles, which is rarely complicated, has an excellent prognosis.

IMMUNITY
Active immunity

One attack of measles is generally followed by permanent immunity. Most so-called recurrent attacks reflect errors in diagnosis. The available evidence suggests that in most cases lasting immunity follows an attack of modified measles also. Contemporary studies indicate that comparable lasting immunity will follow immunization with live attenuated measles virus vaccine. Markowitz et al. (1990a) reviewed extensively the literature on duration and quality of measles vaccine–induced immunity in the 27 years since licensure of vaccine. Although a number of issues remain unresolved, waning immunity has been demonstrated in only a very

Serial determinations of hemagglutination-inhibition (HI) antibody

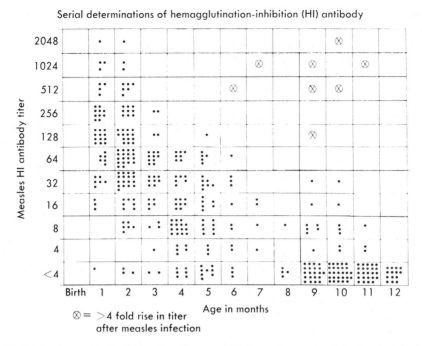

⊗ = >4 fold rise in titer after measles infection

Fig. 13-5. Measles antibody during the first year of life—a longitudinal study of 107 infants. Note the disappearance of passive antibody by 12 months of age and the occurrence of eight cases of measles from 6 to 11 months of age. ⊗, Greater than fourfold rise in titer after measles infection. (From Krugman S, Giles JP, and Friedman H: PAHO/WHO Scientific Publication No 147, May 1967, pp 353-360.)

small proportion of vaccinees (Edmonson et al., 1990).

Passive immunity

Neutralizing antibodies for measles virus are present in convalescent serum and in pooled adult serum. These antibodies are contained in the immune globulin (IG) fraction that has been used for passive immunization. Passively acquired measles antibody is detected in cord blood and is usually not measurable after the infant reaches 12 months of age. The results of a longitudinal study of measles immunity during the first year of life are shown in Fig. 13-5.

Studies by Albrecht et al. (1977) revealed the presence of passively acquired measles-neutralizing antibody in serum specimens obtained from 12-month-old infants who had no detectable HI antibody.

EPIDEMIOLOGICAL FACTORS

Patients with measles harbor the virus in their nasopharyngeal secretions during the acute stage of the disease. Epidemiological evidence suggests that the patients are contagious for at least 7 days after the onset of the first symptom. Contacts may acquire the infection (1) *directly*, by being sprayed with droplets emanating from a cough or sneeze, (2) *indirectly*, by a third person, or (3) by airborne spread. The most common mode of spread is by direct contact. Indirect contact within a house or a hospital ward is also possible, but is an unlikely mode of transmission. In crowded settings such as classrooms, residential institutions, day-care centers, and homes, the spread of large respiratory droplets accounts for the major amount of communicability. Airborne spread by viruses persisting in fine droplets for several hours has also been demonstrated in physicians' waiting rooms.

An extraordinary study of an epidemic in Greenland in 1962 may contribute to a better understanding of the *communicability* of measles (Littauer and Sørenson, 1965). A correlation between time of exposure and communicability was observed during this epidemic. It was obvious that the available health facilities would be inadequate to cope with the problems associated with a major outbreak. Accordingly, it was decided that a "guided epidemic" would be the best solution for a potentially critical situation. The area was divided into three quarantinable units: the 800 inhabitants of the town of Umanak, the 500 inhabitants of the four most remote settlements, and the 700 inhabitants of the five nearest settlements. The plan involved the deliberate exposure of large groups of susceptible individuals to a person or persons with measles; half the adults and half the children in each household were asked to volunteer for "artificial infection."

The results of this unique plan were very interesting. Approximately 400 persons visited a patient named Josef on the first day of his measles rash. Josef coughed twice in the face of each person. In spite of this exposure, not a single contact acquired measles! Consequently, 3½ weeks later the procedure was repeated, but this time patients in the catarrhal, prerash stage of measles were chosen as the source of infection. Under these circumstances the disease was successfully transmitted to the susceptible contacts.

Measles virus is present in the nasopharynx during the first day of rash and during the catarrhal period of the disease. The failure to transmit the infection on the first day of the rash was due to the minimal quantity of virus present at that time. The larger quantities of virus present during the catarrhal period are undoubtedly responsible for the communicability of the disease.

During the prevaccine era (before 1963) the *age incidence* varied with the particular environment. In general, measles was a disease of childhood. In congested urban areas the highest incidence occurred in the infant and preschool age groups. In rural and less crowded urban areas the highest incidence was in children 5 to 10 years of age. In epidemics that occurred in isolated communities children of all ages were equally affected. In developing countries measles is most common in infants 1 to 2 years of age and is frequently seen in those less than 12 months old. Because of this early occurrence among small infants for whom morbidity and mortality are often very marked, a number of programs have been initiated to evaluate the immunogenicity, safety, and efficacy of several higher-titered live virus measles vaccines (Pre-

blud and Katz, 1988) administered as early as age 4 to 6 months (Aaby et al., 1988; Markowitz et al., 1990c; Tidjani et al., 1989; Whittle et al., 1988a,b). The disease is extremely rare in infants less than 3 to 4 months of age because of passively acquired maternal antibodies. If the mother, however, has never had measles, the newborn infant will be susceptible.

Seasonal incidence in the temperate zones is fairly consistent. Measles is essentially a winter-spring disease, with the peak of the outbreak occurring during March and April. In heavily populated areas epidemics usually occurred at intervals of 2 to 3 years during the prevaccine era. This periodicity was in part caused by the accumulation of a new crop of susceptible children during this interval. The extensive use of live attenuated measles virus vaccine since licensure in 1963 has had a profound effect on the incidence of measles (Fig. 13-6).

Following the initiation in 1966 of major federal funding for measles vaccine programs, a precipitous drop in the reported cases of disease resulted so that by 1981 a reduction of greater than 99% from prevaccine years had occurred. In 1983 an all-time low was reached, with fewer than 1,500 cases in contrast to the half million or more reported annually before 1963. In 1989 and 1990 a striking increase in measles cases was observed, especially among inner-city, poor, unimmunized, preschool children (see inset of Fig. 13-6). This resulted in great part from a failure to reach these infants and children with recommended health care measures, including basic immunizations (Katz, 1991).

Geographical distribution is worldwide. Modern air transportation can carry an infected individual to all parts of the world within the incubation period.

Measles is one of the most highly contagious diseases. The secondary attack rate after an intimate household exposure is greater than 90%. The reduced intimacy and duration of exposure in a school, bus, or hospital ward are followed by a lower attack rate in susceptible persons— less than 25%.

TREATMENT

Measles is a self-limited disease. The course of uncomplicated infection is not altered by antimicrobial therapy. Treatment is chiefly supportive.

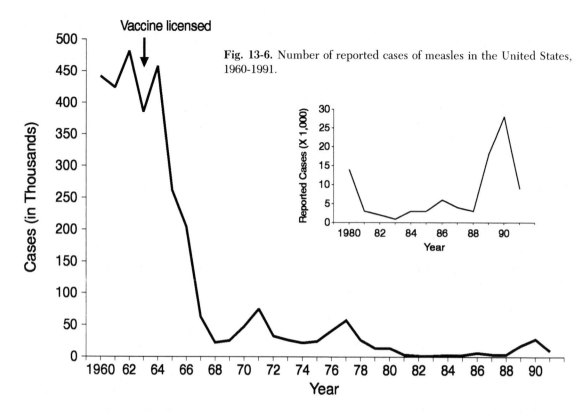

Fig. 13-6. Number of reported cases of measles in the United States, 1960-1991.

Studies in Africa by Barclay et al. (1987) and by Hussey and Klein (1990) have demonstrated the striking beneficial effects of giving vitamin A to children with severe measles. Hussey and Klein, in a randomized, double-blind trial of hospitalized children (median age, 10 months), found that those who received 400,000 IU of vitamin A within 5 days of onset of rash had less croup, recovered more rapidly from pneumonia and diarrhea, spent fewer days in the hospital, and had a much lower mortality rate than those given a placebo. Only 2 of 92 patients died among the vitamin A recipients; 10 of 97 placebo patients died. The World Health Organization has recommended vitamin A supplementation for all children in regions where vitamin A deficiency exists or where the measles mortality rate is 1% or higher.

Supportive therapy

Bed rest is advisable and not difficult to enforce during the febrile period. The diet should be either liquid or soft as tolerated. When the child becomes afebrile and the anorexia subsides, regular indoor activity and diet may be resumed.

The measles *cough* is difficult to control. Most cough medicines are not very effective.

The *coryza*, too, is unaffected by treatment and runs a self-limited course. Generally, nose drops are ineffective and unnecessary. The skin around the nares, however, should be protected with petrolatum.

The *conjunctivitis* usually requires no medication. The eyelids should be cleansed with warm water to remove any secretions or crusts. The cornea should be examined for possible ulceration. Corneal complications should be treated by an ophthalmologist. If photophobia is present, bright lights should be avoided; it is depressing and unnecessary to darken the room completely.

Infants with very high fever and children with headache should be treated with appropriate doses of antipyretic drugs.

Prevention of bacterial complications

Antibacterial drugs should not be routinely administered to children with measles for the purpose of preventing bacterial complications. These agents not only may fail to achieve this goal but also may have the adverse effect of encouraging overgrowth by antibiotic-resistant bacteria or fungi that later may be responsible for complicating secondary infections (pneumonia, otitis, mastoiditis, sinusitis). This was demonstrated clearly by Weinstein (1955) in his studies of measles and its complications in the prevaccine era. Consequently, each case of measles should be carefully evaluated before antimicrobial agents are prescribed. The following factors pertaining to the host, the environment, and the disease may influence the decision to administer or withhold these drugs.

Host factors. Age and past experience influence the development of complications. Infants are more prone to develop complications than are older children. Children with a past history of recurrent otitis media are particularly susceptible.

Environmental factors. Patients at home are less likely to acquire a secondary infection than those in hospital wards.

Disease factors. A mild case of measles is usually uncomplicated and need not be treated. A severe case, however, more likely will be complicated by otitis media or pneumonia.

Treatment of complications

The complications of measles may be treated as follows.

Otitis media. The pathogenesis and the treatment of otitis media complicating measles are no different than those following other respiratory virus infections. For a complete discussion, see Chapter 17.

Pneumonia. Bacterial pneumonia may be caused by *Streptococcus pneumoniae*, hemolytic streptococci, *Staphylococcus* species, or *Haemophilus influenzae*. These infections are discussed in Chapters 8, 27, and 28.

Bronchiolitis. The treatment of infants who develop complicating bronchiolitis is difficult. The details are discussed in Chapter 21.

Obstructive laryngitis and laryngotracheitis. The development of a severe measles croup requires emergency treatment. The child should be hospitalized and placed in an intensive care unit. Treatment of this complication is discussed in detail in Chapter 21.

Encephalitis. Treatment is primarily symptomatic. Convulsive seizures may be controlled by barbiturates. If bulbar involvement is present, the management would be similar to that of bulbar poliomyelitis (p. 79).

The use of large doses of IG was recommended for treatment, but the value of this procedure was never demonstrated. A careful statistical study was carried out by Greenberg et al. in 1955 comparing 51 children with measles encephalitis treated with IG and 108 children who received no IG. The course of the encephalitis in the IG-treated group did not appear to differ from that of the untreated group.

The use of corticosteroids remains controversial. The very favorable clinical experience reported by Applebaum and Abler in 1956 with 17 treated cases and by Allen in 1957 with 10 treated cases appeared impressive. Although the number of cases was small (27), the reported incidence of 26 complete recoveries was striking. On the other hand, in 1959 Meade reported comparable results without corticosteroid therapy. He cited a personal observation of more than 50 patients, many with respiratory paralysis and status epilepticus, who recovered without sequelae. The evidence for the efficacy of corticosteroids in the treatment of measles encephalitis is not convincing.

An important aspect of the treatment of encephalitis is the supportive medical and nursing care necessary to tide over a comatose child for a period of days and sometimes weeks. This includes careful attention to hydration and nutrition and the prevention and treatment of intercurrent infections.

PREVENTIVE MEASURES
Immune globulin

Measles can be modified or prevented by human IG, which induces passive immunity of approximately 4 weeks' duration. Consequently, it may have to be repeated if reexposure occurs more than 1 month after inoculation. IG is given intramuscularly. The dose for modification of the disease is 0.04 ml per kilogram of body weight and for prevention, 0.2 ml per kilogram of body weight.

Measles virus vaccines

The following guidelines for the use of the currently licensed measles vaccine are extracted from the recommendations of the Immunization Practices Advisory Committee (ACIP), as published in *MMWR* (1989;38:1-2).

MEASLES VIRUS VACCINE

Live measles virus vaccine* used in the United States is prepared in chick-embryo-cell culture. It is available in monovalent (measles only) form and in

---

*Official name: Measles Virus Vaccine, Live Attenuated.

two combinations: measles-rubella (MR) and measles-mumps-rubella (MMR) vaccines.*

Measles vaccine produces an inapparent or mild, noncommunicable infection. Measles antibodies develop in at least 95% of susceptible children vaccinated at ≥15 months of age. Although the titers of vaccine-induced antibodies are lower than those following natural disease, both serologic and epidemiologic evidence indicate that vaccine-induced protection appears to be long-lasting in most individuals.

Vaccine shipment and storage

The administration of improperly stored vaccine may fail to provide protection against measles. Although the current measles vaccine may be more thermostable than vaccine produced in the past, it should be stored at 2-8 C (35.6-46.4 F) or colder during storage. Vaccine must be shipped at 10 C (50 F) or colder and may be shipped on dry ice. It must be protected from light, which may inactivate the virus. Reconstituted vaccine must be stored in a refrigerator (not frozen) and discarded if not used within 8 hours.

VACCINE USAGE
General recommendations (Tables 13-1 and 13-2)

All vaccines containing measles virus are recommended for routine use for children 15 months of age. Persons born in or after 1957 who lack documentation of measles immunity (see "Measles Immunity") are considered susceptible and should be vaccinated if there are no contraindications (see "Precautions and Contraindications"). All vaccinations should be documented in the patient's permanent medical record. A parental history of vaccination, by itself, is not considered adequate documentation. A physician should not provide an immunization record for a patient unless s/he has administered the vaccine or has seen a record that documents vaccination. Most persons born before 1957 are likely to have been naturally infected with measles virus and generally need not be considered susceptible; however, vaccination may be offered to these persons if there is reason to believe they may be susceptible.

Both doses of measles vaccine should be given as combined MMR vaccine when given on or after the first birthday. The combined vaccine is preferred to assure immunity to all three viruses. Mumps revaccination is particularly important. Recent studies have shown that mumps can occur in highly vaccinated populations, resulting in substantial numbers of cases among persons with histories of prior mumps vacci-

nation. Although rubella vaccine failure has not been a major problem, the potential consequences of rubella vaccine failure are substantial (i.e., congenital rubella syndrome), and the use of MMR should provide an additional safeguard against such failures.

The most commonly used laboratory test for assessing immunity to measles has been the hemagglutination-inhibition (HI) test. Other more sensitive assays, such as the enzyme immuno-assay (EIA), are now being used by many laboratories. Persons with measles-specific antibody, detectable by any test, are considered immune. Routine serologic screening to determine measles immunity is not generally recommended, although it may be cost-effective in some situations (e.g., large prepaid medical programs). However, the test may not be widely available, and screening requires that tracking systems be established to assure that identified susceptibles return for vaccination. In addition, screening for antibodies for mumps and rubella would further decrease the cost-effectiveness of this strategy.

Dosage

Two doses of measles vaccine, generally given as MMR, are recommended for all children after the first birthday. The dose is 0.5 ml and should be given subcutaneously.

Age at vaccination
Routine childhood immunization schedule for most areas of the United States

The first dose of measles vaccine should be given when children are ≥15 months of age. The second dose should routinely be given when children enter kindergarten or first grade (4-6 years of age).

The recommended time for the second dose is based primarily on administrative considerations. The current childhood immunization schedule recommends other vaccines (diphtheria and tetanus toxoids, and pertussis vaccine [DTP] and oral poliovirus vaccine [OPV]) when children enter school; therefore, an additional provider visit for the second dose of measles vaccine is not necessary. In addition, most school authorities have systems at this grade level for identifying and tracking children with incomplete immunizations.

Because many of the vaccine failures in recent outbreaks of measles have occurred among 10 to 19-year-old children and adolescents, administering the second dose at the time of school entry may not achieve full impact on the incidence of measles for 5 to 15 years. For the impact to occur more rapidly, some localities may choose to give students the second dose at an older age (e.g., when they enter middle school or junior high school). In deciding when to administer the second dose, health officials should consider how

---

*Available in the United States as Attenuvax® (single antigen), M-R-Vax® (measles-rubella) and M-M-R (measles-mumps-rubella), from the Merck, Sharp and Dohme Co.

Table 13-1. 1989 Recommendations for measles vaccination

Routine childhood schedule, United States	
Most areas	Two doses*†
	• First dose at 15 months
	• Second dose at 4-6 years (entry to kindergarten or first grade)‡
High-risk areas§	Two doses*†
	• First dose at 12 months
	• Second dose at 4-6 years (entry to kindergarten or first grade)‡
Colleges and other educational institutions post–high school	Documentation of receipt of two doses of measles vaccine after the first birthday† or other evidence of measles immunity.‖
Medical personnel beginning employment	Documentation of receipt of two doses of measles vaccine after the first birthday† or other evidence of measles immunity.‖

*Both doses should preferably be given as combined measles, mumps, rubella vaccine (MMR).
†No less than 1 month apart. If no documentation of any dose of vaccine, vaccine should be given at the time of school entry or employment and no less than 1 month later.
‡Some areas may elect to administer the second dose at an older age or to multiple age groups (see "Age at Vaccination").
§A county with more than five cases among preschool-aged children during each of the last 5 years, a county with a recent outbreak among unvaccinated preschool-aged children, or a county with a larger inner-city urban population. These recommendations may be applied to an entire county or to identified risk areas within a county.
‖Prior physician-diagnosed measles disease, laboratory evidence of measles immunity, or birth before 1957.

Table 13-2. Recommendations for measles outbreak control*

Outbreaks in preschool-aged children	Lower age for vaccination to as low as 6 months of age in outbreak area if cases are occurring in children <1 year of age.†
Outbreaks in institutions: day-care centers, K-12th grades, colleges, and other institutions	Revaccination of all students and their siblings and of school personnel born in or after 1957 who do not have documentation of immunity to measles.‡
Outbreaks in medical facilities	Revaccination of all medical workers born in or after 1957 who have direct patient contact and who do not have proof of immunity to measles.‡ Vaccination may also be considered for workers born before 1957.
	Susceptible personnel who have been exposed should be relieved from direct patient contact from the 5th to the 21st day after exposure (regardless of whether they received measles vaccine or IG) or—if they become ill—for 7 days after they develop rash.

*Mass revaccination of entire populations is not necessary. Revaccination should be limited to populations at risk, such as students attending institutions where cases occur.
†Children initially vaccinated before the first birthday should be revaccinated at 15 months of age. A second dose should be administered at the time of school entry or according to local policy.
‡Documentation of physician-diagnosed measles disease, serologic evidence of immunity to measles, or documentation of receipt of two doses of measles vaccine on or after the first birthday.

they can best achieve a high vaccination rate since this is essential to assure maximum impact of a two-dose schedule. Some localities may want to provide a second dose to multiple age groups from kindergarten through 12th grade to achieve complete immunization of all school-aged children more rapidly.

Children who have received two doses of live measles vaccine on or after the first birthday (at least 1 month apart) do not need an additional dose when they enter school. Children who have no documentation of live measles vaccination when they enter school should be admitted after the first dose. A second dose should be given according to local policy, but no less than 1 month later.

Routine childhood immunization schedule for areas with recurrent measles transmission

Initial vaccination with MMR at 12 months of age is recommended for children living in high-risk areas. This strategy assumes that the benefit of preventing measles cases between 12 and 15 months of age outweighs the slightly lower efficacy of the vaccine when given at this age. A high-risk area is defined as: (1) a county with more than five cases among preschool-aged children during each of the last 5 years, (2) a county with a recent outbreak among unvaccinated preschool-aged children, or (3) a county with a large inner-city urban population. These recommendations may be implemented for an entire county or only in defined high-risk areas.

Revaccination of persons vaccinated according to earlier recommendations
Previous vaccination with live vaccine

Persons vaccinated with live measles vaccine before their first birthday should be considered unvaccinated. If they are entering kindergarten or first grade, college or other post-high school educational institutions (see "Special Situations"), or beginning employment in a medical facility (see "Special Situations") and cannot provide documentation of immunity to measles (see "Measles Immunity"), they should receive two doses of vaccine no less than 1 month apart.

Live attenuated Edmonston B vaccine (distributed from 1963-1975) was usually administered with immune globulin (IG) or high-titer measles immune globulin (MIG; no longer available in the United States). This vaccine, administered on or after the first birthday, is acceptable as an effective first dose of vaccine. A second dose should be administered as recommended above. However, if a further attenuated measles vaccine (i.e., Schwarz or Moraten) was given simultaneously with IG or MIG, the IG or MIG may have impaired the immune response to vaccination. Persons who received measles vaccine of un-

known type or further attenuated measles vaccine accompanied by IG or MIG should be considered unvaccinated and should be given two doses of vaccine as outlined above.

Previous vaccination with inactivated vaccine or vaccine of unknown type

Inactivated (killed) measles vaccine was available in the United States only from 1963 to 1967 but was available through the early 1970s in some other countries. It was frequently given as a series of two or three injections. Some persons who received inactivated vaccine are at risk of developing severe atypical measles syndrome when exposed to the natural virus. Consequently, such persons should receive two doses of live vaccine separated by no less than 1 month. Persons vaccinated with inactivated vaccine followed within 3 months by live vaccine should be revaccinated with two doses of live vaccine. Revaccination is particularly important when the risk of exposure to natural measles virus is increased, as may occur during international travel.

A wide range (4%-55%) of recipients of inactivated measles vaccine who were later revaccinated with live measles vaccine have had reactions to the live vaccine. Most of these reactions have been mild, consisting of local swelling and erythema, with or without low-grade fever lasting 1-2 days. Rarely, more severe reactions, including prolonged high fevers and extensive local reactions, have been reported. However, recipients of inactivated measles vaccine are more likely to have serious illness when exposed to natural measles than when given live measles virus vaccine.

These same recommendations for revaccination apply to persons vaccinated between 1963 and 1967 with vaccine of unknown type, since they may have received inactivated vaccine. Since inactivated measles vaccine was not distributed in the United States after 1967, persons vaccinated after 1967 with a vaccine of unknown type need not be revaccinated routinely unless the original vaccination occurred before the first birthday or was accompanied by IG or MIG. However, such persons should receive a second dose if they are entering college, beginning employment in medical facilities, or planning international travel.

Measles immunity

Persons are considered immune to measles if they (1) were born before 1957, (2) have documentation of physician-diagnosed measles, (3) have laboratory evidence of immunity to measles, or (4) have documentation of adequate vaccination. Eventually, adequate vaccination will be defined as receipt of one dose of live measles vaccine on or after the first birthday for children before they enter school and two doses of measles vaccine on or after the first birthday for children who are entering or have entered school.

For localities implementing the second dose for students at ages beyond school entry (e.g., entry to middle school or junior high school), acceptable evidence of immunity will be one dose at school entry and two doses for students older than the routine age of the second dose (see "Age at Vaccination").

Since most areas will implement the two-dose schedule one age group at a time, criteria for adequate vaccination will vary in the interim. For example, if the two-dose schedule is implemented in 1990, children in kindergarten or first grade will need to have documentation of two doses of measles vaccine after the first birthday to be considered adequately vaccinated. However, a single dose of vaccine will be acceptable evidence of adequate vaccination for children in higher grades. Two years later, children in kindergarten through second or third grade will need two doses of measles vaccine for acceptable evidence of adequate vaccination. Similar criteria would apply if the second-dose strategy is implemented at an older age (see "Age at Vaccination").

The interim vaccination criteria for adequate measles vaccination noted above apply to routine settings only. During outbreaks, all persons at risk and born in or after 1957 who are in kindergarten, first grade, or beyond will need two doses on or after the first birthday as evidence of adequate vaccination (see "Outbreak Control").

Individuals exposed to disease
Use of vaccine

Exposure to measles is not a contraindication to vaccination. If live measles vaccine is given within 72 hours of measles exposure, it may provide some protection. This approach is preferable to using IG for persons ≥12 months of age. If the exposure does not result in infection, vaccination should induce protection against subsequent measles infection.

Use of IG

IG can prevent or modify measles in a susceptible person if given within 6 days of exposure. The recommended dose of IG is 0.25 ml/kg (0.11 ml/lb) of body weight (maximum dose = 15 ml). IG may be especially indicated for susceptible household contacts of measles patients, particularly contacts <1 year of age, pregnant women, or immunocompromised persons, for whom the risk of complications is increased. The recommended dose of IG for immunocompromised persons is 0.5 ml/kg of body weight (maximum dose = 15 ml). Live measles vaccine should be given 3 months later (when passively acquired measles antibodies should have disappeared) if the individual is then at least 15 months old. IG should not be used to control measles outbreaks.

Special situations
Recommendations for colleges and other institutions

Colleges, technical schools, and other institutions for post-high school education should require documentation of two doses of live measles–containing vaccines, documentation of prior physician-diagnosed measles disease, or laboratory evidence of measles immunity before entry for all students born in or after 1957. Students who have no documentation of live measles vaccination or other evidence of measles immunity at the time of school entry should be admitted after receiving the first dose. A second dose should be given no less than 1 month later. Institutions may wish to extend this requirement to all classes.

Recommendations for medical facilities

Medical personnel are at higher risk for acquiring measles than the general population. Hospitals should require evidence of two live measles vaccinations, documentation of physician-diagnosed measles disease, or laboratory evidence of measles immunity for medical staff beginning employment who will have direct patient contact. Persons born in or after 1957 who have no documentation of vaccination or other evidence of measles immunity should be vaccinated at the time of employment and revaccinated no less than 1 month later. If resources are available, institutions may wish to extend this recommendation to all medical personnel, not just those beginning employment. Since some medical personnel who have acquired measles in medical facilities were born before 1957, institutions may consider requiring at least one dose of measles vaccine for older employees who are at risk of occupational exposure to measles.

Recommendations for international travel

Persons traveling abroad should be immune to measles. The protection of young adults who have escaped measles disease and have not been vaccinated is especially important. Consideration should be given to providing a dose of measles vaccine to persons born in or after 1957 who travel abroad, who have not previously received two doses of measles vaccine, and who do not have other evidence of measles immunity (see "Measles Immunity").

The age for measles vaccination should be lowered for children traveling to areas in which measles is endemic or epidemic. Children 12-14 months of age should receive MMR vaccine before their departure. Children 6-11 months of age should receive a dose of monovalent measles vaccine before departure, although there is no specific contraindication to the use of MMR for this age group if monovalent measles vaccine is not available. Seroconversion rates observed for measles, mumps, and rubella antigens are significantly less among children vaccinated before the first birthday then among older children. Children who receive monovalent measles vaccine or MMR before their first birthday should be considered unvaccinated and should receive two doses of MMR at later ages. Whereas the optimal age for the first revaccination dose is 15 months, the age for revaccination may be as low as 12 months if the child remains in a high-risk area (see "Routine childhood immunization schedule for areas with recurrent measles transmission"). The second revaccination dose would normally be given when a child enters school or according to local policy.

Since virtually all infants <6 months of age will be protected by maternally derived antibodies, no additional protection against measles is necessary in this age group.

SIDE EFFECTS AND ADVERSE REACTIONS

More than 170 million doses of measles vaccine were distributed in the United States from 1963 through 1988. The vaccine has an excellent record of safety. From 5%-15% of vaccinees may develop a temperature of ≥103 F (≥39.4 C) beginning 5-12 days after vaccination and usually lasting several days. Most persons with fever are otherwise asymptomatic. Transient rashes have been reported for approximately 5% of vaccinees. Central nervous system conditions, including encephalitis and encephalopathy, have been reported with a frequency of less than one per million doses administered. The incidence of encephalitis or encephalopathy after measles vaccination of healthy children is lower than the observed incidence of encephalitis of unknown etiology. This finding suggests that the reported severe neurologic disorders temporally associated with measles vaccination were not caused by the vaccine. These adverse events should be anticipated only in susceptible vaccinees and do not appear to be age-related. After revaccination, reactions should be expected to occur only among the small proportion of persons who failed to respond to the first dose.

Personal and family history of convulsions

As with the administration of any agent that can produce fever, some children may have a febrile seizure. Although children with a personal or family history of seizures are at increased risk for developing idiopathic epilepsy, febrile seizures following vaccinations do not in themselves increase the probability of subsequent epilepsy or other neurologic disorders. Most convulsions following measles vaccination are simple febrile seizures, and they affect children without known risk factors.

An increased risk of these convulsions may occur among children with a prior history of convulsions or those with a history of convulsions in first-degree family members (i.e., siblings or parents). Although the precise risk cannot be determined, it appears to be low.

In developing vaccination recommendations for these children, the Committee considered a number of factors, including risks from measles disease, the large proportion (5%-7%) of children with a personal or family history of convulsions, and the fact that convulsions following measles vaccine are uncommon and have not been associated with permanent brain damage. The Committee concluded that the benefits of vaccinating these children greatly outweigh the risks. They should be vaccinated just as children without such histories.

Because the period for developing vaccine-induced fever occurs approximately 5-12 days after vaccination, prevention of febrile seizures is difficult. Prophylaxis with antipyretics is one alternative, but these agents may not be effective if given after the onset of fever. They would have to be initiated before the expected onset of fever and continued for 5-7 days. However, parents should be alert to the occurrence of fever after vaccination and should treat their children appropriately.

Children who are being treated with anticonvulsants should continue to take them after measles vaccination. Because protective levels of most currently available anticonvulsant drugs (e.g., phenobarbitol) are not achieved for some time after therapy is initiated, prophylactic use of these drugs does not seem feasible.

The parents of children who have either a personal or family history of seizures should be advised of the small increased risk of seizures following measles vaccination. In particular, they should be told in advance what to do in the unlikely event that a seizure occurs. The permanent medical record should document that the small risk of postimmunization seizures and the benefits of vaccination have been discussed.

Revaccination risks

There is no evidence of increased risk from live measles vaccination in persons who are already immune to measles, as a result of either previous vaccination or natural disease.

PRECAUTIONS AND CONTRAINDICATIONS
Pregnancy

Live measles vaccine, when given as a component of MR or MMR, should not be given to women known to be pregnant or who are considering becoming pregnant within the next 3 months. Women who are given monovalent measles vaccine should not become pregnant for at least 30 days after vaccination. This precaution is based on the theoretical risk of fetal infection, although no evidence substantiates this theoretical risk. Considering the importance of protecting adolescents and young adults against measles, asking women if they are pregnant, excluding those who are, and explaining the theoretical risks to the others before vaccination are sufficient precautions.

Febrile illness

The decision to administer or delay vaccination because of a current or recent febrile illness depends largely on the cause of the illness and the severity of symptoms. Minor illnesses, such as a mild upper-respiratory infection with or without low-grade fever, are not contraindications for vaccination. For persons whose compliance with medical care cannot be assured, every opportunity should be taken to provide appropriate vaccinations.

Children with moderate or severe febrile illnesses can be vaccinated as soon as they have recovered. This wait avoids superimposing adverse effects of vaccination on the underlying illness or mistakenly attributing a manifestation of the underlying illness to the vaccine. Performing routine physical examinations or measuring temperatures are not prerequisites for vaccinating infants and children who appear to be in good health. Asking the parent or guardian if the child is ill, postponing vaccination for children with moderate or severe febrile illnesses, and vaccinating those without contraindications are appropriate procedures in childhood immunization programs.

Allergies

Hypersensitivity reactions following the administration of live measles vaccine are rare. Most of these reactions are minor and consist of a wheal and flare or urticaria at the injection site. More than 170 million doses of measles vaccine have been distributed in the United States, but only five reported cases of immediate allergic reactions have occurred among children who had histories of anaphylactic reactions to egg ingestion. These reactions could potentially have been life threatening. Four children experienced difficulty in breathing, and one of these four had hypotension. Persons with a history of anaphylactic reactions (hives, swelling of the mouth and throat, difficulty in breathing, hypotension, and shock) following egg ingestion should be vaccinated only with extreme caution. Protocols have been developed for vaccinating such persons. However, persons are not at increased risk if they have egg allergies that are not anaphylactic in nature; they can be vaccinated in the usual manner. Persons with allergies only to chickens or feathers are not at increased risk of reaction to measles vaccination.

MMR vaccine and its component vaccines contain trace amounts of neomycin. Although the amount present is less than that usually used for a skin test to determine hypersensitivity, persons who have experienced anaphylactic reactions to neomycin should not be given these vaccines. Most often, neomycin allergy is manifested by contact dermatitis rather than anaphylaxis. A history of contact dermatitis to neomycin is not a contraindication to receiving measles vaccine. Live measles virus vaccine does not contain penicillin.

Recent administration of IG

Vaccine virus replication and stimulation of immunity usually occurs 1-2 weeks after vaccination. When the live measles vaccine is given after IG or specific IG preparations, the vaccine virus might not replicate successfully, and the antibody response could be diminished. Measles vaccine should not be given for at least 6 weeks, and preferably for 3 months, after a person has been given IG, whole blood, or other antibody-containing blood products. If vaccine is given to a person who has received such products within the preceding 3 months, the dose should not be counted and the person should be revaccinated approximately 3 months later unless serologic testing indicates that measles-specific antibodies have been produced. For international travelers, measles vaccination should precede the administration of IG by at least 2 weeks to preclude interference with replication of the vaccine virus. If the interval between measles vaccination and subsequent administration of an IG preparation is <14 days, vaccination should be repeated 3 months later, unless serologic testing indicates that antibodies were produced.

Tuberculosis

Tuberculosis may be exacerbated by natural measles infection. Live measles virus vaccine has not been shown to have such an effect. Tuberculin skin testing is not a prerequisite for measles vaccination. If tuberculin testing is needed for other reasons, it can be done the day of vaccination. Otherwise, the test should be postponed for 4-6 weeks, since measles vaccination may temporarily suppress tuberculin reactivity.

Altered immunocompetence

Replication of vaccine viruses can be enhanced in persons with immune-deficiency diseases and in persons with immunosuppression, as occurs with leukemia, lymphoma, generalized malignancy, or therapy with alkylating agents, antimetabolites, radiation, or large doses of corticosteroids. For this reason, patients with such conditions or therapies (except patients with symptomatic infection with human immunodeficiency virus [HIV]; see below) should not be given live measles virus vaccine.

Patients with leukemia in remission who have not received chemotherapy for at least 3 months may receive live-virus vaccines. Short-term (<2 weeks), low- to moderate-dose systemic corticosteroid therapy, topical steroid therapy (e.g., nasal, skin), long-term alternate-day treatment with low to moderate doses of short-acting systemic steroids, and intra-articular, bursal, or tendon injection of corticosteroids are not immunosuppressive in their usual doses and do not contraindicate the administration of measles vaccine.

The growing number of infants and preschoolers with HIV infection has directed special attention to the appropriate immunization of such children. Asymptomatic children do not need to be evaluated and tested for HIV infection before decisions concerning vaccination are made. Asymptomatic HIV-infected persons in need of MMR should receive it. MMR should be considered for all symptomatic HIV-infected children, including children with acquired immunodeficiency syndrome (AIDS), since measles disease in these children can be severe. Limited data on MMR vaccination among both asymptomatic and symptomatic HIV-infected children indicate that MMR has not been associated with severe or unusual adverse events, although antibody responses have been unpredictable.

The administration of high-dose intravenous immune globulin (IVIG) at regular intervals to HIV-infected children is being studied to determine whether it will prevent a variety of infections. MMR vaccine may be ineffective if it is administered to a child who has received IVIG during the preceding 3 months.

Management of patients with contraindications to measles vaccine

If immediate protection against measles is required for persons with contraindications to measles vaccination, passive immunization with IG, 0.25 ml/kg (0.11 ml/lb) of body weight (maximum dose = 15 ml), should be given as soon as possible after known exposure. Exposed symptomatic HIV-infected and other immunocompromised persons should receive IG regardless of their previous vaccination status; however, IG in usual doses may not be effective in such patients. For immunocompromised persons, the recommended dose is 0.5 ml/kg of body weight if IG is administered intramuscularly (maximum dose = 15 ml). This corresponds to a dose of protein of approximately 82.5 mg/kg (maximum dose = 2,475 mg). Intramuscular IG may not be needed if a patient with HIV infection is receiving 100-400 mg/kg IGIV at regular intervals and the last dose was given within 3 weeks of exposure to measles. Because the amounts of protein administered are similar, high-dose IGIV may be as effective as IG given intramuscularly. However, no data are available concerning the effectiveness of IGIV in preventing measles.

Simultaneous administration of vaccines

In general, simultaneous administration of the most widely used live and inactivated vaccines does not impair antibody responses or increase rates of adverse reactions. The administration of MMR vaccine yields results similar to the administration of individual measles, mumps, and rubella vaccines at different sites or at different times.

There are equivalent antibody responses and no clinically significant increases in the frequency of adverse events when DTP, MMR, and OPV or inactivated poliovirus vaccine (IPV) are administered either simultaneously at different sites or at separate times. Routine simultaneous administration of MMR, DTP, and OPV (or IPV) is recommended for all children ≥15 months of age who are eligible to receive these vaccines. Vaccination with MMR at 15 months followed by DTP, OPV (or IPV), and *Haemophilus influenzae* b conjugate vaccine (HbCV) at 18 months remains an acceptable alternative for children with caregivers known to be generally compliant with other health-care recommendations. No data are available on the concomitant administration of HbCV or *H. influenzae* b polysaccharide vaccine (HbPV) and OPV and MMR vaccine. If the child might not be brought back for future vaccinations, the simultaneous administration of all vaccines (including DTP, OPV, MMR, and HbCV or HbPV) is recommended, as appropriate to the recipient's age and previous vaccination status.

OUTBREAK CONTROL

All reports of suspected measles cases should be investigated promptly. A measles outbreak exists in a community whenever one case of measles is confirmed. Once this occurs, preventing the dissemination of measles depends on the prompt vaccination of susceptible persons. Control activities should not be delayed for laboratory results on suspected cases. Persons who cannot readily provide documentation of measles immunity (see "Measles Immunity") should be vaccinated or excluded from the setting (e.g., school). Documentation of vaccination is adequate only if the date of vaccination is provided. Almost all persons who are excluded from an outbreak area because they lack documentation of immunity quickly comply with vaccination requirements. Persons who have been exempted from measles vaccination for medical, religious, or other reasons should be excluded from the outbreak area until at least 2 weeks after the onset of rash in the last case of measles.

School-based outbreaks

During outbreaks in day-care centers; elementary, middle, junior, and senior high schools; and colleges and other institutions of higher education, a program of revaccination with MMR vaccine is recommended in the affected schools. Consideration should be given to revaccination in unaffected schools that may be at risk of measles transmission. Revaccination should include all students and their siblings and all school personnel born in or after 1957 who cannot provide documentation that they received two doses of measles-containing vaccine on or after their first birthday or other evidence of measles immunity (see "Measles Immunity"). Persons revaccinated, as well as unvaccinated persons receiving their first dose as part of the outbreak control program, may be immediately readmitted to school. Mass revaccination of entire communities is not necessary.

Quarantine

Imposing quarantine measures for outbreak control is both difficult and disruptive to schools and other organizations. Under special circumstances restriction of an event might be warranted; however, such action is not recommended as a routine measure for outbreak control.

Outbreaks among preschool-aged children

The risk of complications from measles is high among infants <1 year of age. Therefore, considering the benefits and risks, vaccination with monovalent measles vaccine is recommended for infants as young as 6 months of age when exposure to natural measles is considered likely. MMR may be administered to children before the first birthday if monovalent measles vaccine is not readily available. Children vaccinated before the first birthday should be revaccinated when they are 15 months old and when they enter school to ensure adequate protection (see "General Recommendations").

Medical settings

If an outbreak occurs in the areas served by a hospital or within a hospital, all employees with direct patient contact who were born in or after 1957 who cannot provide documentation they received two doses of measles vaccine on or after their first birthday or other evidence of immunity to measles (see "Measles Immunity") should receive a dose of measles vaccine. Since some medical personnel who have acquired measles in medical facilities were born before 1957, vaccination of older employees who may have occupational exposure to measles should also be considered during outbreaks. Susceptible personnel who have been exposed should be relieved from direct patient contact from the fifth to the 21st day after exposure regardless of whether they received vaccine or IG after the exposure. Personnel who become ill should be relieved from patient contact for 7 days after they develop rash.

DISEASE SURVEILLANCE AND REPORTING OF ADVERSE EVENTS
Disease surveillance

As the incidence of measles declines in the United States, aggressive surveillance becomes increasingly important. Effective surveillance can delineate inadequate levels of protection, define groups needing special attention, and assess the effectiveness of control activities.

Known or suspected measles cases should be reported immediately to local health departments. Serologic confirmation should be attempted for every suspected case of measles that cannot be linked to a confirmed case. Reporting of suspected cases and implementation of outbreak-control activities should not be delayed pending laboratory results.

The traditional serologic diagnosis of measles requires a significant rise in antibody titer between acute- and convalescent-phase sera. However, the diagnosis can also be made by demonstrating the presence of IgM antibody in a single specimen. Correct interpretation of serologic data depends upon the proper timing of specimen collection in relation to rash onset. This timing is especially important for interpreting negative IgM results, since IgM antibody peaks approximately 10 days after rash onset and is usually undetectable 30 days after rash onset.

Asymptomatic reinfection can occur in persons who have previously developed antibodies, whether from vaccination or from natural disease. Symptomatic reinfections are rare. These reinfections have been accompanied by rises in measles antibody titers.

Reporting of adverse events

The National Childhood Vaccine Injury Act of 1986 requires physicians and other health care providers who administer vaccines to maintain permanent immunization records and to report occurrences of adverse events specific in the Act. These adverse events, as well as other adverse events that require medical attention, must be reported to the U.S. Department of Health and Human Services. Although there eventually will be one system for reporting adverse events following immunizations, two separate systems currently exist. The appropriate reporting method depends on the source of funding used to purchase the vaccine. If a vaccine was purchased with public funds, adverse events should be reported to the appropriate local, county, or state health department. The state health department submits its report to CDC. If vaccine was purchased with private money, adverse events should be reported directly to the Food and Drug Administration.

ISOLATION AND QUARANTINE

In general, isolation and quarantine procedures are of limited value in the prophylaxis of measles. Exposure usually occurs before the diagnosis is obvious. Attempts to isolate siblings from each other are useless. The availability of IG and live attenuated measles virus vaccine for household and other susceptible contacts has obviated the need for quarantine.

the fifth day or later. Gram-stained smear and culture may be negative in pretreated patients, but antigen detection tests are usually still useful. The CSF glucose and protein concentrations generally will remain abnormal for several days despite effective treatment.

DIFFERENTIAL DIAGNOSIS

Acute bacterial meningitis can simulate other inflammatory diseases that involve the meninges either directly or indirectly. Typical cases do not usually pose a diagnostic dilemma. In some instances, however, the spinal fluid findings in patients with bacterial disease do not conform to the typical picture, and confusion can occur in distinguishing viral or mycobacterial meningitis from meningitis caused by the usual bacterial agents.

Aseptic meningitis. In children with aseptic or proved viral meningitis the spinal fluid commonly shows an increase in lymphocytes and a normal or only slightly decreased glucose concentration, with a slightly elevated protein concentration. Early in the disease the CSF can reveal a large number of polymorphonuclear cells, but a repeat lumbar tap 12 to 24 hours later will demonstrate the typical lymphocyte predominance in CSF (see Chapter 35).

Tuberculous meningitis. This condition may be clinically indistinguishable from acute bacterial meningitis. The diagnosis is established by (1) an increase in number of CSF leukocytes, usually from 50 to 500 cells/mm³, with a predominance of lymphocytes, a low glucose, elevated protein concentrations, and a culture negative for the usual pathogenic organisms but subsequently positive for tubercle bacilli; (2) a positive tuberculin skin test; (3) chest roentgenograms showing evidence of a tuberculous lesion; and (4) a positive history of contact with an active case of tuberculosis.

Brain abscess. Brain abscess can result from head trauma, chronic otitis media and sinusitis, or septic embolization in children with cyanotic congenital heart disease. The symptoms are usually not as acute as those of meningitis, and focal neurological signs can be present. Results of the spinal fluid examination are highly variable and can either be normal or show an increase in leukocytes, a normal glucose value, and a slightly elevated protein concentration. The cul-

ture of the CSF specimen is usually sterile. Rupture of the abscess into the subarachnoid space or ventricles will result in purulent meningitis with a positive CSF culture.

Brain tumor. The findings with a brain tumor are similar to those with brain abscess except that the course is more insidious, fever is usually absent, and the patient is usually not acutely ill.

Meningismus. Meningismus is characterized by symptoms and signs of meningeal irritation and normal results from spinal fluid examination and culture. It is usually associated with pneumonia, acute otitis media, acute tonsillitis, or other infectious diseases.

Lead encephalopathy. Lead encephalopathy in infants and children can simulate meningitis. The spinal fluid has a normal glucose concentration, an increased protein concentration, and normal or slightly elevated lymphocyte count. Helpful diagnostic aids include (1) a blood smear showing basophilic stippling, (2) roentgenographic evidence of a line of increased density at the metaphyseal ends of the long bones in growing children, (3) coproporphyrinuria, and (4) an increased blood lead value.

COMPLICATIONS

Complications of acute bacterial meningitis can develop early in the course of illness, either before diagnosis or after several days of the start of treatment.

Systemic circulatory manifestations. Systemic circulatory manifestations usually occur during the first hospital day of acute bacterial meningitis. Peripheral circulatory collapse is one of the most dramatic and most serious complications of meningitis. It most frequently is associated with meningococcemia but can accompany other types of infection. Profound shock usually develops early in the course of the illness and, if untreated, progresses rapidly to a fatal outcome. Disseminated intravascular coagulation (DIC) can be an associated finding. Gangrene of the distal extremities can occur in patients with fulminating hemorrhagic meningococcal meningitis. It commonly has been recognized that antibiotic therapy can initially aggravate these systemic phenomena, probably as a result of release of cell wall or membrane active components such as endotoxin from rapidly lysed microorganisms. Many patients also develop the syndrome of inappropriate antidiuretic hormone (SIADH) secretion, and fluid restriction is usually recommended in the initial management of patients with meningitis. However, systemic blood pressure must be monitored frequently to avoid hypovolemic episodes that may compromise cerebral perfusion.

Neurological complications. Focal neurological findings such as hemiparesis, quadriparesis, facial palsy, and visual field defects occur early or late in approximately one fifth of patients with meningitis and may correlate with persistent abnormal neurological examinations on long-term follow-up assessments. Presence of focal signs can be associated with cortical necrosis, occlusive vasculitis, or thrombosis of the cortical veins. Extension of the meningeal inflammatory process can involve the second, third, sixth, seventh, and eighth cranial nerves that course through the subarachnoid space. Damage of the auditory nerve and cochlear aqueduct can lead to reversible or permanent deafness in 5% to 20% of cases. Hydrocephalus of either the communicating or obstructive type is occasionally seen in patients in whom treatment has been either suboptimal or delayed, occurring more often in younger infants. Brain abscesses can rarely complicate the course of meningitis, particularly in newborn infants infected with *Citrobacter diversus* or *Proteus* species.

Seizures. Seizure disorders occur before or in the first 2 days after admission to the hospital in up to one third of patients with meningitis. Although most of these episodes are generalized, focal seizures are more likely to presage an adverse neurological outcome. In addition, seizures that are difficult to control or that persist beyond the fourth hospital day and seizures that occur for the first time late in the patient's hospital course have a greater likelihood of being associated with neurological sequelae.

Subdural collections of fluid. Subdural effusions are not generally associated with signs and symptoms, usually resolve spontaneously, are present in more than one third of patients with meningitis, and usually are not associated with permanent neurological abnormalities (Snedeker et al., 1990). These collections are less commonly present with meningococcal than with *H. influenzae* or pneumococcal meningitis. Subdural effusions occur principally in infants

less than 2 years of age. Indications for performing needle puncture of a subdural effusion include a clinical suspicion that empyema is present, a rapidly enlarging head circumference in a child without hydrocephalus, focal neurological findings, and/or evidence of increased intracranial pressure.

Arthritis. Joint involvement may be present initially or develop during the course of bacterial meningitis. Early occurrence suggests direct invasion of the joint by the microorganism, usually *H. influenzae* type b, whereas arthritis that develops after the fourth day of therapy is believed an immune complex–mediated event that usually involves several joints and is most frequently seen with meningococcal infections.

Other complications. Buccal or preseptal cellulitis, pneumonia, and pericarditis can also be present in patients with bacterial meningitis, particularly complicating invasive *H. influenzae* infections in infants.

PROGNOSIS

The prognosis in individual patients with bacterial meningitis is correlated with many factors, including (1) age of patient, (2) duration of illness before effective antibiotic therapy is instituted, (3) microorganism, (4) number of bacteria or the quantity of active bacterial products in CSF at the time of diagnosis, (5) intensity of the host's inflammatory response, and (6) time needed to sterilize CSF cultures.

As a rule, the younger the patient, the poorer the prognosis. The highest mortality and morbidity rates occur in the neonatal period. Infections caused by group B streptococci, gram-negative enteric bacilli, and pneumococci are associated with poorer outcome from disease. Delay in starting antimicrobial therapy or in sterilizing CSF cultures has been recognized to increase the rate of adverse outcome. The amount of bacteria or their products correlates with an increased host production of inflammatory mediators such as TNF, IL-1, and prostaglandins. The greater the host's inflammatory response in the subarachnoid space to the microorganism and its products, the greater the likelihood of permanent sequelae.

With adequate antimicrobial and appropriate supportive therapy, the chances for survival today are excellent, especially in infants and chil-

Table 14-2. Daily dosages of recommended antimicrobial agents for treatment of bacterial meningitis in pediatric age groups*

| Drugs | Neonates† | | Infants and children |
	0-7 days	8-28 days	
Amikacin‡	15-20 div q 12	20-30 div q 8	20-30 div q 8
Ampicillin	100-150 div q 12	150-200 div q 8 or 6	200-300 div q 6
Cefotaxime	100 div q 12	150-200 div q 8 or 6	200-225 div q 6 or 8
Ceftazidime	60 div q 12	90 div q 8	125-150 div q 8
Ceftriaxone	—	—	80-100 div q 12 or once daily
Chloramphenicol‡	25 once daily	50 div q 12	75-100 div q 6
Gentamicin‡	5 div q 12	7.5 div q 8	7.5 div q 8
Nafcillin or oxacillin	100-150 q 12	150-200 q 8 or 6	200 q 6
Penicillin G	100,000-150,000 div q 12	150,000-200,000 div q 8 or 6	250,000 div q 6 or 4
Tobramycin‡	5 div q 12	6 div q 8	6 div q 8
Vancomycin‡	30 div q 12	45 div q 8	40-60 div q 6

*Dosages are expressed in milligrams per kilogram of body weight per day and divided (div) for administration every (q) 12, 8, or 6 hours. Penicillin is expressed in units per kilogram.
†Daily dosages may be different for very low-birth-weight infants (Prober, et al: Pediatr Infect Dis J 1990;9:111).
‡Serum concentrations should be monitored and dosages adjusted accordingly.

dren for whom case fatality rates have been reduced to less than 10%. Long-term sequelae, however, have not changed dramatically, despite the advent of extraordinarily active β-lactam antibiotics and highly sophisticated intensive care management. The incidence rate of residual abnormalities in postmeningitic children is approximately 15% (range, 10% to 30%). Infants and children who survive bacterial meningitis are more apt to have seizures, hearing deficits, learning and/or behavioral problems, and lower intelligence compared with their siblings who did not have meningitis.

TREATMENT

Optimal management of infants and children with bacterial meningitis requires appropriate antimicrobial therapy, fluid and electrolyte adjustments, control of cardiovascular stability and intracranial pressure, and anticonvulsant therapy. The role of corticosteroids has been studied in animal models of meningitis and in patients with bacterial meningitis, and continuing emerging experimental and clinical evidence suggests that dexamethasone therapy is beneficial in rapidly modulating the meningeal inflammatory response and in improving long-term outcome in infants and children (Lebel et al., 1988).

Antimicrobial therapy

Optimal antibiotic therapy entails the selection of appropriate agents that are effective against the likely pathogens and are able to attain adequate bactericidal activity in CSF. The initial empiric regimen chosen for treatment should be broad enough to cover the potential organisms for the age group involved. Recommended dosages are listed in Table 14-2.

Newborn infants. In the neonatal period the organisms most often responsible for meningitis are group B *Streptococcus, E. coli* and other gram-negative enteric bacilli, and *L. monocytogenes*. The initial empiric regimen used conventionally has been ampicillin (or penicillin G) and an aminoglycoside. Because of the emergence of aminoglycoside-resistant gram-negative enteric bacilli in some neonatal units, the concern about possible adverse auditory and renal effects, and the relatively low bactericidal activity of aminoglycosides in the CSF, approximately 30% of centers in the United States are now using ampicillin and cefotaxime for initial, empiric treatment of neonatal meningitis. Although ampicillin and cefotaxime are effective for treatment of bacterial meningitis, there is concern that the routine use of a cephalosporin in neonatal intensive care units will lead to rapid emergence of resistant organisms, especially among *Enterobacter cloacae, Proteus* species, and *Serratia* species. By contrast, the use of cefotaxime is advantageous from the standpoint of achieving high CSF bactericidal activity against most coliforms and of avoiding the necessity to monitor serum concentrations of the aminoglycoside to attain safe and therapeutic concentrations. Ceftriaxone, although equivalent in efficacy to cefotaxime, is not recommended for use in the neonatal period because of the potential displacement of bilirubin from albumin-binding sites and its inhibitory effect on growth of the bacterial flora of the intestinal tract. We continue to recommend ampicillin and an aminoglycoside for initial empiric treatment of suspected neonatal meningitis; when the specific pathogen is identified and results of susceptibilities are known, antimicrobial therapy can be modified. In newborns with meningitis caused by susceptible gram-negative enteric organisms cefotaxime can be used safely and effectively, either alone or combined with an aminoglycoside. For meningitis caused by group B streptococci or *L. monocytogenes* ampicillin alone is usually satisfactory after an initial 48 to 72 hours of combined therapy with an aminoglycoside. The possible exception is for disease caused by a tolerant strain (inhibited but not killed by achievable CSF concentrations of ampicillin) of group B *Streptococcus*, in which case combination therapy is continued for the entire course.

The duration of therapy for neonatal meningitis depends on the clinical response and duration of positive CSF cultures after therapy is initiated. Ten to 14 days is usually satisfactory for disease caused by group B *Streptococcus* and *L. monocytogenes*, and a minimum of 2 weeks of treatment after sterilization of CSF cultures is required for gram-negative enteric meningitis. Because of the unpredictable clinical course of illness and the unreliability of the clinical examination in assessing response to therapy in neonates, the authors believe that the CSF should be examined and cultured at completion of therapy to determine whether additional treatment is required. Additionally, they recommend a cranial computed tomographic (CT) scan or magnetic resonance imaging (MRI) be performed to be certain that intracranial complications have not occurred.

One- to 3-month-old infants. Infants 1 to 3 months old are considered as a special category because of the broad array of possible causative agents implicated in causing meningitis. These agents include the pathogens encountered in neonates and those that usually cause disease in older infants, namely, *H. influenzae* type b, *S. pneumoniae*, and *N. meningitidis*. Ampicillin and cefotaxime or ampicillin and ceftriaxone constitutes a suitable initial empiric regimen since in some patients *Listeria* or enterococci (resistant to the cephalosporin) can be the causative agent.

Infants and children. Conventional therapy with ampicillin and chloramphenicol has been effective for many years. Attention has recently focused, however, on cefotaxime and ceftriaxone for treatment of meningitis in infants and children because of their extraordinary in vitro activity against the common meningeal pathogens, their excellent safety record, and their ability to sterilize promptly CSF cultures. Moreover, because of the unpredictable metabolism of chloramphenicol in young infants and of the pharmacological interactions of this agent when administered concomitantly with phenobarbital, phenytoin, rifampin, or acetaminophen, serum concentrations should be monitored to avoid toxic or subtherapeutic values. In a recent survey of directors of pediatric infectious disease training programs in the United States only one third of responding centers were using ampicillin and chloramphenicol as initial empiric therapy, whereas the remaining two thirds used cefotaxime or ceftriaxone (Word and Klein, 1989).

Cefuroxime, a second-generation cephalosporin, has also been used for treatment of bacterial meningitis. However, several recent reports have documented delayed sterilization of CSF cultures in 10% to 15% of patients with *Haemophilus* meningitis treated with this agent compared with those treated with ceftriaxone. In this regard delayed sterilization resulting from cefuroxime therapy has been associated with a greater likelihood of hearing impairment.

Another reason for using third-generation cephalosporins in the management of meningitis is the fact that currently 5% to 15% of *S. pneumoniae* strains in the United States are relatively resistant to penicillin (minimum inhibitory concentration [MIC], 0.1 to 1.0 µg/ml) and a few are truly resistant (MIC, >1.0 µg/ml) (Istre et al., 1987). Some of these strains are also resistant to chloramphenicol. *N. meningitidis* strains in the United States remain susceptible to penicillin.

Seven days of treatment is satisfactory for most infants and children with uncomplicated meningococcal meningitis, 7 to 10 days for *Haemophilus* disease, and 10 days or longer for pneumococcal meningitis. Performing a lumbar puncture at completion of therapy in a child with uncomplicated meningitis is not recommended because the information obtained is not useful in predicting which patient will develop bacteriological relapse (Schaad et al., 1981).

Steroid therapy

Three prospective, double-blind, placebo-controlled studies evaluating 260 infants and children have been published recently. Dexamethasone was given intravenously 30 minutes or more after the first parenterally administered dose of either cefuroxime or ceftriaxone in a regimen of 0.6 mg/kg/day in four divided doses for 4 days. At approximately 24 hours after onset of therapy, dexamethasone-treated patients had a significantly higher CSF concentration of glucose and lower concentrations of lactate and protein compared with that in patients receiving placebo. In addition, IL-1β and TNF α concentrations in CSF were lower in patients given dexamethasone. Children receiving dexamethasone had significantly fewer neurological and audiological sequelae compared with those in placebo recipients. Dexamethasone treatment was not associated with delayed sterilization of CSF cultures or with a higher incidence of relapse. Two children (1.5%) developed gastrointestinal bleeding while receiving the steroid.

A prospective, double-blind, placebo-controlled study was performed in 104 Costa Rican infants and children to evaluate the efficacy of dexamethasone when given 15 minutes before the initial cefotaxime dose for treatment of meningitis. Patients who received the steroid had significant improvement in the indices of meningeal inflammation, greater reduction in intracranial pressure, and better estimated cerebral perfusion pressures 12 to 24 hours after treatment was initiated than did children who received placebo (Odio et al., 1991). Clinical follow-up assessments for an average of 15 months revealed significantly fewer patients with neurological and audiological sequelae in the dexamethasone-treated group.

Based on this information, the authors believe that the advantages of dexamethasone treatment, especially when given before the first parenterally administered antibiotic dose, clearly outweigh the possible disadvantages and that its use should be strongly considered for therapy of bacterial meningitis in infants and children, regardless of the severity of illness. Its usefulness in infants younger than 6 weeks must await a currently conducted multicenter collaborative neonatal meningitis study.

SUPPORTIVE THERAPY

Adequate oxygenation, prevention of hypoglycemia and hyponatremia, anticonvulsant therapy, and measures oriented to decrease intracranial hypertension and to avoid fluctuation in cerebral blood flow are a crucial part of the management of patients with bacterial meningitis.

Infants and children with alteration of consciousness, pupillary changes, and/or cardiovascular instability should have intracranial pressure monitored. Among measures to reduce abnormal pressures are elevation of the head of the bed to approximately 30 degrees, avoidance of vigorous suctioning and chest physiotherapy, maintenance of normal serum osmolarity, fluid restriction to treat inappropriate secretion of antidiuretic hormone (dehydration and hypotension should be avoided), and use of mannitol to decrease cerebral edema.

Optimal cerebral perfusion can be maintained by controlling fever to reduce the brain's metabolic demands, by hyperventilation to reduce arterial carbon dioxide tension ($PaCO_2$) to a range of 25 to 30 mm Hg, and by maintaining arterial blood pressures within normal limits (Ross and Scheld, 1989).

PREVENTION
Vaccination

Immunization is potentially the most effective means of preventing bacterial meningitis in children. Sixty to seventy percent of all *H. influenzae* meningitis cases occur in infants younger than 18 months old. The new conjugated *Haemophilus* vaccines are considerably more immunogenic than the initial polysaccharide vaccine, and studies in Finland and in the United States have demonstrated immunogenicity and protection after initiation of a two to three-dose vaccine regimen at 2 to 3 months of age (Black et al., 1991; Madore et al., 1990; Mäkelä et al., 1990; Santosham et al., 1991). Vaccination beginning at this age was approved for routine use in the United States in late 1990; a three- or four-dose regimen is recommended (see Chapter 8).

A polyvalent meningococcal vaccine, containing the purified polysaccharide capsules of group A, C, Y, and W135 organisms, is available but is not recommended for general use in infants and young children. The vaccine is recommended for children older than 2 years of age who are at high risk of infection such as those with asplenia or with terminal complement component deficiencies.

The currently manufactured pneumococcal vaccine is composed of purified capsular polysaccharide antigen from 23 pneumococcal serotypes. It is recommended for children older than 2 years of age who are at increased risk of developing pneumococcal disease, including those with asplenia, especially patients with sickle cell hemoglobinopathies, with nephrotic syndrome, and with recurrent meningitis after head trauma.

Chemoprophylaxis

Administration of ampicillin during labor to mothers with prenatal vaginal or rectal group B streptococcal colonization and presence of an obstetrical risk factor of premature labor, prolonged rupture of membranes, or intrapartum fever has been associated with reduced rates of neonatal colonization and of early-onset streptococcal sepsis (Gotoff, 1984). For logistical and cost-effective reasons, however, chemoprophylaxis presently is routinely recommended only for pregnant women who have previously delivered an infant with invasive group B streptococcal infection and for the asymptomatic twin of an infant with infection caused by this organism (see Chapter 24).

In infants and children rifampin prophylaxis for *Haemophilus* disease is recommended for all household contacts of an index case and for the index case when at least one contact is younger than 4 years of age, regardless of the immunization status of the contacts. The dose is 20 mg/kg daily given for 4 days. The index case should receive rifampin at or near completion of therapy for the *H. influenzae* infection. Management

of day-care and extended home-care groups must be individualized. The efficacy of rifampin prophylaxis in day-care attendees is unproved, and the difficulties in delivering prophylaxis to many individuals in such centers can be considerable. Accordingly, prophylaxis is recommended only after two cases of disease have occurred among attendees within 2 months in a day-care or home-care setting. Contacts who have received *Haemophilus* vaccine should also receive rifampin prophylaxis to eradicate the organism from the nasopharynx (see Chapter 8).

Household and day-care or nursery school contacts of an index case of meningococcal disease should be given rifampin prophylaxis in a dosage of 10 mg/kg given every 12 hours for five doses or in the same regimen as recommended for *Haemophilus* prophylaxis. One intramuscular dose of ceftriaxone has been reported in one study (Schwartz et al., 1988) as more effective than oral rifampin in eliminating meningococcal group A nasopharyngeal carriage, thereby allowing its use when oral rifampin cannot be taken (e.g., during pregnancy) or when compliance with the oral regimen is unlikely.

REFERENCES

Appelbaum PC, Scragg JN, Bowen AJ, et al. *Streptococcus pneumoniae* resistant to penicillin and chloramphenicol. Lancet 1977;2:995.

Arditi M, Ables L, Yogev R. Cerebrospinal fluid endotoxin levels in children with *H. influenzae* meningitis before and after administration of intravenous ceftriaxone. J Infect Dis 1989;160:1005.

Auslander MC, Meskan ME. The pattern and stability of post meningitic hearing loss in children. Laryngoscope 1988;98:940.

Baker CJ. Prevention of neonatal group B streptococcal disease. Pediatr Infect Dis 1983;2:1.

Black SB, Shinefield H, Fireman B, et al. Efficacy in infancy of oligosaccharide conjugate *Haemophilus influenzae* type b (HbOC) vaccine in a United States population of 61,080 children. Pediatr Infect Dis 1991;10:97-104.

Burnes LE, Hodgman JE, Cass AB. Fatal circulatory collapse in premature infants receiving chloramphenicol. N Engl J Med 1959;261:1318.

Converse GM, Gwaltney JM Jr, Strassburg DA, et al. Alteration of cerebrospinal fluid findings by partial treatment of bacterial meningitis. J Pediatr 1973;83:220.

Dajani AS, Asmar BI, Thirumoorthi MC. Systemic *Haemophilus influenzae* disease: an overview. J Pediatr 1979;94:355.

Del Rio M, Chrane D, Shelton S, et al. Ceftriaxone versus ampicillin and chloramphenicol for treatment of bacterial meningitis in children. Lancet 1983;1:1241.

Dodge PR, Swartz MN. Bacterial meningitis. A review of selected aspects. N Engl J Med 1965;272:725 + .

Feldman HA. Meningococcal disease. JAMA 1966;196:105.

Feldman WE. Concentrations of bacteria in cerebrospinal fluid of patients with bacterial meningitis. J Pediatr 1976;88:549.

Feldman WE. Relation of concentrations of bacteria and bacterial antigen in cerebrospinal fluid to prognosis in patients with bacterial meningitis. N Engl J Med 1977;296:433.

Fishman RA. Brain edema. N Engl J Med 1975;193:706.

Fraser DW, Darby CP, Koehler RE, et al. Risk factors in bacterial meningitis. J Infect Dis 1973;127:271.

Galaid EI, Cherubin CE, Marr JS, et al. Meningococcal disease in New York City, 1973 to 1978. Recognition of groups Y and W-135 as frequent pathogens. JAMA 1980;244:2167.

Gartner JC, Michaels RM. Meningitis from a pneumococcus moderately resistant to penicillin. JAMA 1979;241:1707.

Ginsburg CM, McCracken GH Jr, Rae S, et al. *Haemophilus influenzae* type b disease: incidence in a day care center. JAMA 1977;128:604.

Girgis NI, Farid Z, Makhail IA, et al. Dexamethasone treatment for bacterial meningitis in children and adults. Pediatr Infect Dis J 1989;8:848.

Gotoff SP. Chemoprophylaxis of early onset group B streptococcal disease. Pediatr Infect Dis J 1984;3:401.

Graham DR, Band JD. *Citrobacter diversus* brain abscess and meningitis in neonates. JAMA 1981;245:1923.

Istre GR, Tarpay M, Anderson M, et al. Invasive disease due to *Streptococcus pneumoniae* in an area with a high rate of relative penicillin resistance. J Infect Dis 1987;156:732.

Jacobs MR, Koornhof HJ, Robins-Browne RM, et al. Emergence of multiply resistant pneumococci. N Engl J Med 1978;299:735.

Jacobs RF, His S, Wilson CB, et al. Apparent meningococcemia: clinical features of disease due to *Haemophilus influenzae* and *Neisseria meningitidis*. Pediatrics 1983; 72:469.

Kaplan SL, Feigin RD. Treatment of meningitis in children. Pediatr Clin North Am 1983;30:259.

Kaplan SL, Goddard J, Van Kleeck M, et al. Ataxia and deafness in children due to bacterial meningitis. Pediatrics 1981;68:8.

Kessler SL, Dajani AS. *Listeria* meningitis in infants and children. Pediatr Infect Dis 1990;9:61.

Klein JO, Feigin RD, McCracken GH Jr. Report of the Task Force on diagnosis and management of meningitis. Pediatrics 1986;78:959.

Lebel MH, Freij BJ, Syrogiannopoulos GA, et al. Dexamethasone therapy for bacterial meningitis; results of two double-blind, placebo-controlled trials. N Engl J Med 1988;319:964.

Lebel MH, Hoyt MJ, McCracken GH Jr. Comparative efficacy of ceftriaxone and cefuroxime for treatment of bacterial meningitis. J Pediatr 1989;114:1049.

Leedom MJ, Inler D, Matties AW, et al. The problems of sulfadiazine-resistant meningococci. Antimicrob Agents Chemother 1966;6:281.

Linnan MJ, Mascola L, Lou XD, et al. Epidemic listeriosis associated with Mexican-style cheese. N Engl J Med 1988:319:823.

Madore DV, Johnson CL, Phipps DC, et al. Safety and immunologic response to *Haemophilus influenzae* type b oligosaccharide-CRM 197 conjugate vaccine in 1- to 6-month-old infants. Pediatrics 1990;85:331.

Mäkelä PH, Eskola J, Peltola H, et al. Clinical experience with *Haemophilus influenzae* type b conjugate vaccines. Pediatrics 1990;85(4S):651.

McCracken GH Jr. Neonatal septicemia and meningitis. Hosp Pract 1976;11:89.

McCracken GH Jr. New developments in the management of children with bacterial meningitis. Pediatr Infect Dis 1984;3:532.

McCracken GH Jr, Lebel MH. Dexamethasone therapy for bacterial meningitis in infants and children. Am J Dis Child 1989;143:287.

Mertsola J, Ramilo O, Mustafa MM, et al. Release of endotoxin after antibiotic treatment of gram negative bacterial meningitis. Pediatr Infect Dis 1989;8:904.

Minns RA, Engleman HM, Stirling H. Cerebrospinal fluid pressure in pyogenic meningitis. Arch Dis Child 1989;64:814.

Mustafa MM, Ramilo O, Sáez-Llorens X, et al. Cerebrospinal fluid prostaglandins, interleukin-1β and tumor necrosis factor in bacterial meningitis: clinical and laboratory correlations in placebo and dexamethasone-treated patients. Am J Dis Child 1990;144:883.

Nelson JD. How preventable is bacterial meningitis? N Engl J Med 1982;307:1265.

Nelson JD. Cerebrospinal fluid shunt infections. Pediatr Infect Dis 1984;3:530.

Odio CM, Faingezicht I, Paris M, et al. The beneficial effects of early dexamethasone administration on infants and children with bacterial meningitis. N Engl J Med 1991; 324:1525-1531.

Paredes A, Taber LH, Yow MD, et al. Prolonged pneumococcal meningitis due to an organism with increased resistance to penicillin. Pediatrics 1976;58:378.

Portnoy JM, Olsen LC. Normal cerebrospinal fluid values in children: Another Look. Pediatrics 1985;75:484.

Prober CG, Stevenson DK, Benitz WE. The use of antibiotics in neonates weighing less than 1200 grams. Pediatr Infect Dis 1990;9:111.

Ramilo O, Sáez-Llorens X, Mertsola J, et al. Tumor necrosis factor α/cachectin and interleukin-1β initiate meningeal inflammation. J Exp Med 1990;172:497.

Rapkin RH. Repeat lumbar punctures in the diagnosis of meningitis. Pediatrics 1974;54:34.

Rodriguez AF, Kaplan SL, Mason EO Jr. Cerebrospinal fluid values in the very low birth weight infant. J Pediatr 1990;116:971.

Ross KL, Scheld WM. The management of fulminant meningitis in the intensive care unit. Infect Dis Clin North Am 1989;3:137.

Sáez-Llorens X, Ramilo O, Mustafa MM, et al. Molecular pathophysiology of bacterial meningitis: current concepts and therapeutic implications. J Pediatr 1990;116:671.

Sáez-Llorens X, Umana MA, Odio CM, et al. Brain abscess in infants and children. Pediatr Infect Dis 1989;8:449.

Sande MA, Tauber MG, Scheld M, McCracken GH Jr. Pathophysiology of bacterial meningitis: summary of the workshop. Pediatr Infect Dis 1989;8:929.

Santosham M. Wolff M, Reid R, et al. The efficacy in Navajo infants of a conjugate vaccine consisting of *Haemophilus influenzae* type b polysaccharide and *Neisseria meningitidis* outer-membrane protein complex. N Engl J Med 1991;324:1767-1772.

Schaad MB, Nelson JD, McCracken GH Jr. Recrudescence and relapse in bacterial meningitis of childhood. Pediatrics 1981;67:188.

Scheld WM, Fletcher DD, Fink FN, et al. Response to therapy in an experimental rabbit model of meningitis due to *Listeria monocytogenes*. J Infect Dis 1979;140:287.

Schwartz B, Al-Ruwais A, As'Ashi J, et al. Comparative efficacy of ceftriaxone and rifampicin in eradicating pharyngeal carriage of group A *Neisseria meningitidis*. Lancet 1988;1:1239.

Sell SH. Long term sequelae of bacterial meningitis in children. Pediatr Infect Dis 1983;2:90.

Shapiro ED. Prophylaxis for contacts of patients with meningococcal or *Haemophilus influenzae* type b disease. Pediatr Infect Dis 1982;1:132.

Siegel JD, Shannon KM, DePasse BM. Recurrent infection associated with penicillin-tolerant group B streptococci: a report of two cases. J Pediatr 1981;99:920.

Snedeker JD, Kaplan SL, Dodge PR, et al. Subdural effusion and its relationship with neurologic sequelae of bacterial meningitis in infancy: a prospective study. Pediatrics 1990;86:163.

Syrogiannopoulos GA, Hansen EJ, Erwin AL, et al. *Haemophilus influenzae* type b lipooligosaccharide induces meningeal inflammation. J Infect Dis 1988;157:237.

Tauber MG. Brain edema, intracranial pressure, and cerebral blood flow in bacterial meningitis. Pediatr Infect Dis 1989;8:915.

Tauber MG, Schibl AM, Hackbarth CJ, et al. Antibiotic therapy, endotoxin concentration in cerebrospinal fluid, and brain edema in experimental *Escherichia coli* meningitis in rabbits. J Infect Dis 1987;156:456.

Tikhomirov E. Meningococcal meningitis: global situation and control measures. World Health Stat Quartan 1987;40:98.

Toews WH, Bass JW. Skin manifestations of meningococcal infection. Am J Dis Child 1974;127:173.

Tuomanen E. Molecular mechanisms of inflammation in experimental pneumococcal meningitis. Pediatr Infect Dis 1987;6:1146.

Toumanen E, Liu H, Hengstler B, et al. The induction of meningeal inflammation by components of the pneumococcal cell wall. J Infect Dis 1985;151:859.

Tureen JH, Dworkin RJ, Kennedy SL, et al. Loss of cerebrovascular autoregulation in experimental meningitis in rabbits. J Clin Invest 1990;85:577.

Umaña MA, Odio CM, Castro E, et al. Evaluation of aztreonam and ampicillin vs. amikacin and ampicillin for treatment of neonatal bacterial infections. Pediatr Infect Dis 1990;9:175.

Waage A, Halstensen A, Espevik T. Association between tumor necrosis factor in serum and fatal outcome in patients with meningococcal disease. Lancet 1987;1:355.

Ward JI, Fraser DW, Baroff LJ, et al. *Haemophilus influenzae* meningitis a national study of secondary spread in household contacts. N Engl J Med 1979;301:122.

Word BM, Klein JO. Therapy of bacterial sepsis and meningitis in infants and children: 1989 poll of directors of programs in pediatric infectious diseases. Pediatr Infect Dis 1989;3:635.

15

MUMPS (EPIDEMIC PAROTITIS)

Mumps is an acute contagious disease caused by a paramyxovirus that has a predilection for glandular and nervous tissue. Mumps is characterized most commonly by enlargement of the salivary glands, particularly the parotid glands. One or more of the following manifestations of mumps may be associated with or may occur without parotitis: meningoencephalitis, orchitis, pancreatitis, and other glandular involvement. Inapparent infection occurs in a significant percentage of persons (30% to 40%).

ETIOLOGY

Mumps is caused by a specific virus belonging to the parainfluenza subgroup of the paramyxoviruses. It ranges in size from 90 to 135 nm. It is infective for monkeys and chick embryos and produces cytopathic effects in a variety of tissue cultures of primary monkey kidney, human embryonic kidney, and human diploid fibroblasts. Infectivity is lost as a result of heating at 55° to 60° C for 20 minutes and after exposure to formalin or to ultraviolet light. Infectivity is maintained for years at temperatures of −20° to −70° C.

Mumps virus has an antigenic relationship to other members of the myxovirus group, including Newcastle disease virus and parainfluenza viruses.

PATHOLOGY

The mumps-infected parotid gland is rarely available for pathological examination. The interstitial tissue shows edema and infiltration with lymphocytes. The cells of the ducts degenerate, with accumulation of necrotic debris and polymorphonuclear leukocytes in the lumina. Inclusion bodies are not seen.

Mumps orchitis is characterized by edema and a perivascular lymphocytic infiltrate that progresses to involve the interstitial tissue. There are focal hemorrhage and destruction of germinal epithelium, producing plugging of the tubules by epithelial debris, fibrin, and polymorphonuclear leukocytes.

PATHOGENESIS

The current concept of the pathogenesis of mumps stems from experience gained from a variety of epidemiological, immunological, clinical, and experimental studies. The virus probably enters through the nose or mouth. Proliferation takes place in either the parotid gland or the superficial epithelium of the respiratory tract. This is followed by viremia, with subsequent localization of virus in glandular or nervous tissue. The parotid gland is most often involved. Mumps virus has been isolated from human saliva, blood, urine, and cerebrospinal fluid (CSF) during the acute phase of the illness. The salivary glands, brain, and spinal cord of experimentally infected monkeys also have yielded virus. The concept of mumps as a generalized infection has been well documented.

CLINICAL MANIFESTATIONS

For a long time the terms *mumps* and *epidemic parotitis* were used interchangeably.

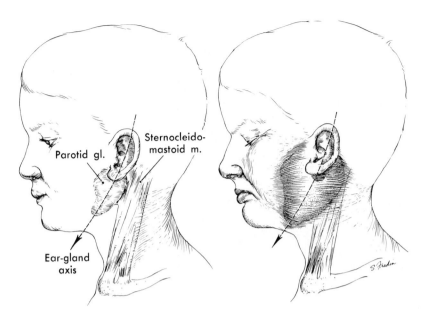

Fig. 15-1. Schematic drawing of parotid gland infected with mumps, *right*, compared with normal gland, *left*. An enlarged cervical lymph node is usually posterior to the imaginary line.

Mumps was recognized as primarily an infection of the salivary glands. The isolation of the virus and the development of serological specific tests, however, have contributed to a better understanding of the pathogenesis and a clarification of the clinical picture of the disease.

Infection with mumps virus usually develops after an incubation period of 16 to 18 days. In approximately 30% to 40% of the patients the resulting infection is inapparent. The remaining 60% to 70% of the patients develop an illness of variable severity, with symptoms that depend on the site or sites of infection. In the majority of instances clinical mumps is characterized only by parotitis, either unilateral or bilateral. Additional relatively common manifestations include submaxillary and sublingual gland infection, orchitis, and meningoencephalitis. Pancreatitis, oophoritis, thyroiditis, and other glandular infections are relatively rare. These various manifestations of mumps may precede, accompany, follow, or occur without parotitis.

Salivary gland involvement

The classic illness is ushered in by fever, headache, anorexia, and malaise. Within 24 hours the child complains of an "earache" localized near the lobe of the ear and aggravated by chewing movements of the jaw. The following day the enlarged parotid is noticeable and rapidly progresses to its maximum size within 1 to 3 days. The fever usually subsides after a variable period of 1 to 6 days, with the temperature returning to normal before the glandular swelling disappears.

The normal parotid gland is not palpable. It is horseshoe in shape, with the concave portion adjacent to the lobe of the ear (Fig. 15-1). An imaginary line bisecting the long axis of the ear and passing through the ear lobe divides the gland into two relatively equal parts. These anatomical relationships are not altered by the enlarging parotid gland. As the swelling progresses, the lobe of the ear is displaced upward and outward. During the phase of rapid parotid enlargement, the pain and tenderness may be very severe. These symptoms subside after the swelling has reached its peak. The enlarged parotid gradually decreases in size over a period of 3 to 7 days. Thus the swelling may be present for possibly 6 to 10 days. Usually one parotid gland enlarges first, and within a few days the other enlarges. Occasionally, both sides swell simultaneously. Approximately 25% of all patients have unilateral parotitis.

The submaxillary swelling, when present, may be seen and palpated beneath the mandible

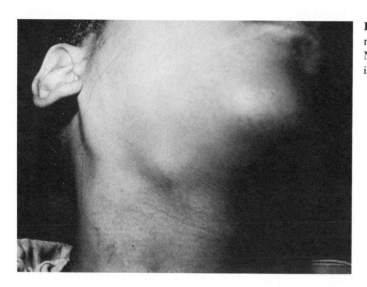

Fig. 15-2. Patient with mumps showing right parotid and submaxillary swelling. Note displacement of ear and characteristic location of both glands.

just anterior to the angle of the jaw and directly beneath the anterior portion of the masseter muscle (Fig. 15-2). During the early stages the edema surrounding the submaxillary gland may spread over the mandible onto the cheek and downward toward the neck. When submaxillary mumps occurs without parotitis, it is clinically indistinguishable from cervical adenitis.

Sublingual mumps is usually bilateral and begins as a swelling in the submental region and on the floor of the mouth. Of the three salivary glands, the sublinguals are the least commonly involved.

The clinical picture of mumps just described is the classic one. The disease, however, is extremely variable. Occasionally, the appearance of local glandular swelling and tenderness may be the only manifestation of infection. Fever and constitutional symptoms may be absent.

Frequently, the orifices of the ducts show inflammatory changes. The openings of Stensen's (parotid) and Wharton's (submaxillary) ducts may be reddened and edematous.

Patients with extensive salivary gland involvement may develop edema in the presternal area. It has been postulated that this is caused by an obstruction of the lymphatic vessels by the enlarged salivary glands.

Epididymo-orchitis

Epididymo-orchitis is the second most common manifestation of mumps infection in the adult male. It usually follows parotitis, but it may precede it or occur as an isolated manifestation of mumps. Epididymitis invariably is associated with the orchitis. Unilateral involvement occurs in 20% to 30% of males who develop the disease after puberty. The incidence of bilateral orchitis is low—approximately 2%. Under epidemic conditions the incidence of orchitis may be higher. In 1959 Philip et al. described an epidemic of 363 cases of mumps in a "virgin" population on St. Lawrence Island in the Bering Sea. The incidence of orchitis in males more than 10 years of age was approximately 35%; bilateral orchitis occurred in approximately 12%. Orchitis develops within the first 2 weeks of infection, most commonly during the first week. In rare instances it may be delayed to the third week. As indicated in the following case report, mumps orchitis may occur in the absence of salivary gland involvement.

CASE 1. M.R., a 33-year-old man, was admitted to the Bellevue Hospital Infectious Disease Unit on December 5, 1958. He had a history of fever, chills, and right testicular swelling of 4 days' duration. Physical examination revealed a temperature of 102° F and an enlarged, tender right testicle. The salivary glands were not palpable. The diagnosis of mumps orchitis was confirmed by a significant rise in the level of mumps complement-fixing antibody during convalescence; the antibody titer was 1:32 on December 10 and ≥1:128 on December 22, 1958.

Orchitis begins abruptly with fever, chills, headache, nausea, vomiting, and lower abdominal pain. The systemic reaction usually parallels the extent of gonadal involvement. The temperature may vary from normal to 41.1° C (106°

F). The duration of fever rarely exceeds 1 week. It persists for 3 days or less in approximately 20% of cases, 4 days or less in 50%, and 5 days or less in 80%. The temperature falls by crisis in approximately half the cases and by lysis in the remainder.

With the appearance of the fever, the testis begins to swell rapidly and becomes very painful and tender. It may increase in size very slightly or to as much as four times that of the normal gland. As the fever subsides, the pain and swelling disappear. The tenderness, however, persists for a longer period. As the testis decreases in size, a change of consistency is noted—loss of turgor. In approximately half of the cases this is subsequently followed by atrophy. However, at least half of the involved glands do return to normal.

One of the most important concerns of men with mumps orchitis is the fear that sexual impotence and sterility will follow. Most orchitis is unilateral. Even with bilateral involvement, it would be rare to have complete atrophy of both glands. The extensive experience with mumps orchitis in World Wars I and II failed to demonstrate that impotence and sterility are frequent consequences of this infection.

Meningoencephalitis

Central nervous system (CNS) involvement is another common manifestation of mumps. Symptomatic disease has been estimated to occur in approximately 10% of all cases. In a study by Bang and Bang (1944) 62% of 371 patients with mumps parotitis had cells in the CSF. Of this group 106 (28%) had CNS symptoms. Mumps meningoencephalitis usually follows the parotitis by 3 to 10 days. However, it may precede or even occur in the absence of salivary gland involvement (Fig. 15-3).

The illness is characterized by fever, headache, nausea, vomiting, nuchal rigidity, change in sensorium, and, only rarely, convulsions. Brudzinski's and Kernig's signs can be elicited. The CSF shows pleocytosis, with a predominance of lymphocytes, normal glucose content, and elevated protein level. Although the glucose content is usually normal, cases with hypoglycorrhachia have been reported (Wilfert, 1969). The temperature usually falls by lysis over a pe-

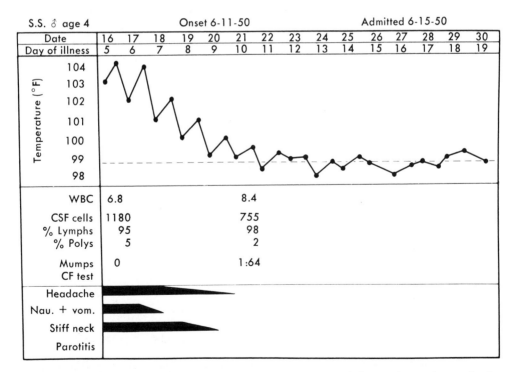

Fig. 15-3. Diagram of clinical course of mumps meningoencephalitis without salivary gland involvement. Pleocytosis with predominance of lymphocytes was found. The diagnosis was established by the development of complement-fixing antibody between the fifth and tenth days of illness.

riod of 3 to 10 days. As the fever subsides, the symptoms clear, and recovery is usually uneventful. The infection follows the course of benign aseptic meningitis (Chapter 35) and usually has no sequelae.

Pancreatitis

Pancreatitis is a severe but uncommon manifestation of mumps infection. There is a sudden onset of severe epigastric pain and tenderness associated with fever, chills, extreme weakness, prostration, nausea, and repeated bouts of vomiting. The symptoms gradually subside over a period of 3 to 7 days, and the patient usually recovers completely.

Other clinical manifestations

The development of fever, nausea, vomiting, and lower abdominal pain in the female with mumps points to *oophoritis*. When the right ovary is involved, the signs and symptoms may be indistinguishable from those of acute appendicitis.

Many other glands may be involved in the infection. *Thyroiditis*, *mastitis*, *dacryoadenitis*, and *bartholinitis* are rare manifestations of mumps. In general, except for the symptoms caused by the local swelling, the course is essentially the same as for any other mumps infection.

DIAGNOSIS
Confirmatory clinical factors

The following factors should point to mumps as a diagnostic possibility: (1) a history of exposure to mumps 2 to 3 weeks before onset of illness, (2) a compatible clinical picture of parotitis or other glandular involvement, and (3) signs of aseptic meningitis.

In the classic case of so-called epidemic parotitis, confirmatory laboratory procedures are usually unnecessary. In the absence of parotitis or in the presence of recurrent parotitis, however, use of the following specific diagnostic aids may be necessary.

Isolation of causative agent

Mumps virus can be recovered from the saliva, mouth washings, or urine during the acute phase of parotitis and from the CSF early in the course of meningoencephalitis. The isolation may be made by inoculating the amniotic cavities of 8-day chick embryos or susceptible cell cultures. The isolation of mumps virus is not a routine laboratory procedure.

Serological tests

There are at least four serological tests used to demonstrate the development of specific mumps antibody: complement fixation (CF), hemagglutination-inhibition (HI), enzyme-

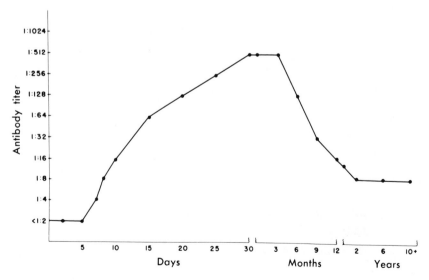

Fig. 15-4. Schematic curve illustrating development of mumps complement-fixing antibody. A significant rise in the level of antibody can be demonstrated in the serum by the end of the second week of illness. The acute and convalescent serum specimens should be tested simultaneously.

linked immunosorbent assay (ELISA), and virus neutralization. The CF and ELISA tests are the most practical and most reliable of these diagnostic procedures.

The formation of mumps CF antibody after infection is shown in Fig. 15-4. The antibody becomes detectable in the blood by the end of the first week, and by the end of the second week a fourfold or greater rise in antibody titer can be demonstrated. When a diagnosis of mumps is suspected, acute and convalescent sera should be tested simultaneously. A fourfold or greater rise in the level of antibody confirms the diagnosis. This test is particularly useful for the diagnosis of mumps meningoencephalitis without parotitis, as is illustrated in Fig. 15-3.

Ancillary laboratory findings

The serum amylase level is elevated in both mumps parotitis and pancreatitis. The levels seem to parallel the parotid swelling. The values reach a peak during the first week, gradually returning to normal by the second and third weeks. Serum amylase determinations are abnormal in approximately 70% of cases of mumps parotitis. The finding of normal serum amylase levels may aid in the identification of obscure swellings about the jaw that resemble parotid involvement.

The white blood cell count may be normal or slightly elevated. Usually there is a slight predominance of lymphocytes, but at times the reverse is true.

DIFFERENTIAL DIAGNOSIS
Parotitis

Mumps parotitis may be simulated by various conditions affecting the parotid glands or neighboring lymph nodes.

Anterior cervical or preauricular adenitis. Involvement of the lymph nodes, with surrounding edema, may simulate mumps parotitis. The parotid gland can usually be identified by its characteristic location, consistency, and outline. Its anatomical relationship to the ear is illustrated in Fig. 15-1. A line bisecting the long axis and lobe of the ear passes through the center of the gland. It has a brawny consistency with a well-defined posterior border and ill-defined anterior and inferior borders. In contrast, an enlarged lymph node has a well-defined, discrete border, is firm, and does not have the charac-

teristic anatomical relationship to the ear. The appearance of the opening of Stensen's duct does not help very much. An elevated serum amylase level would point to parotid involvement. A mumps antibody test will clarify the diagnosis.

Suppurative parotitis. In suppurative parotitis the skin over the gland is usually red and hot, and the gland is exquisitely tender. Pus may be expressed from Stensen's duct by massaging the gland. An increase in the number of polymorphonuclear leukocytes is usually present. Although aerobic bacteria such as *Staphylococcus aureus* are the most common cause of acute suppurative parotitis, occasionally anaerobic bacteria *(Bacteroides, Fusobacterium,* and *Peptostreptococcus)* may be responsible (Brook and Finegold, 1978).

Recurrent parotitis. Recurrent parotitis, a condition of unknown and probably varied causes, is characterized by frequent recurrent swellings of the parotid gland. Infection and hypersensitivity to certain drugs such as iodides and phenothiazines may have a role in the causation of this disease. Roentgenographic studies of the duct system reveal evidence of sialectasia in some cases. The individual attack may be clinically indistinguishable from mumps parotitis. The submaxillary and sublingual glands, which are frequently associated with mumps parotitis, are not involved in recurrent parotitis. The history of previous attacks and a negative or unchanging CF test will clarify the diagnosis.

Calculus. A calculus that obstructs Stensen's duct causes a swelling of the parotid gland that is usually intermittent.

Coxsackie virus infection. In 1957 Howlett et al. described a syndrome of parotitis and herpangina caused by Coxsackie virus.

Parainfluenza 3 virus infection. In 1970 Zollar and Mufson reported on two children in whom acute parotitis was associated with detection of parainfluenza 3 virus and a significant rise in the level of homologous antibody.

Mixed tumors, hemangiomas, and lymphangiomas of the parotid. Mixed tumors, hemangiomas, and lymphangiomas of the parotid are responsible for chronic enlargement of the gland and are confused with mumps only during the early stages.

Mikulicz's syndrome. In Mikulicz's syndrome there is chronic bilateral parotid and lacrimal

16

OSTEOMYELITIS AND SUPPURATIVE ARTHRITIS

JOHN D. NELSON

Suppurative skeletal infections are relatively uncommon in childhood, but when they occur, they are most likely to afflict young children. More than half of all cases occur in children younger than 5 years of age. This is a time of rapid skeletal growth, so damage to the growth plate or to joints has the potential for lifelong consequences. Skeletal infections are often difficult to recognize or localize early in the course of illness, and many are difficult to manage medically and surgically. Because prompt medical and surgical intervention probably decreases the likelihood of permanent sequelae, physicians who care for children should be aware of the earliest signs and symptoms of suppurative skeletal infections and be aggressive about establishing the diagnosis.

PATHOGENESIS AND EPIDEMIOLOGY

The majority of bone and joint infections are hematogenous in origin. However, infection less commonly can follow penetrating injuries or various medical and surgical maneuvers (e.g., arthroscopy, prosthetic joint surgery, intraarticular steroid injection, and various orthopedic surgeries on bones). Impaired host defenses also can increase the risk of skeletal infection.

Significant blunt trauma is a preceding event in approximately one third of cases of osteomyelitis. Animal models of experimental osteomyelitis involve inflicting trauma to a bone of an animal that is bacteremic. The unique anatomy of the ends of long bones explains the predilection for localization of blood-borne bacteria.

In the metaphysis are tiny vascular loops in which blood flow is sluggish. Rupture of some of these vessels as a result of trauma provides a favorable environment for multiplication of bacteria.

In the newborn and young infant there are blood vessels connecting the metaphysis and epiphysis, so it is common for pus from the metaphysis to rupture into the joint space. However, in the latter part of the first year of life the physis (growth plate) forms, there are no transphyseal blood vessels, and purulent infection of the joint occurs only rarely when the synovial attachment allows perforation of the periosteum to occur within the joint space. Bone is not distensible, so pus under pressure, prevented from decompressing into the joint, moves laterally through cortical vascular channels and accumulates under the loosely attached periosteum. After growth ceases, once again blood vessels connect the metaphysis and epiphysis.

Preceding trauma is less common in patients with suppurative arthritis, and the pathogenesis of hematogenous arthritis is poorly understood. The synovium is rich in blood vessels, and insignificant, unremembered trauma may play a role in pathogenesis. Possibly synovial membrane receptors for bacteria play a role in localization. For example, *Haemophilus influenzae* type b accounts for only approximately 10% of cases of osteomyelitis in children in the first 2 years of life (Lebel and Nelson, 1988), but it is the pathogen in 45% of cases of arthritis in that age group (Fink and Nelson, 1986).

Table 16-1. Frequency of disease by age group*

| | | Age groups (yr) | | | |
Disease	Number of cases	<2	2-5	6-10	11-15
Osteomyelitis					
Number	399	127	101	108	63
Percent	100	32	25	27	16
Arthritis					
Number	682	362	172	102	46
Percent	100	53	25	15	7

*Based on J Nelson's series of cases.

Both conditions are most common in young children (Table 16-1); this is particularly true of arthritis, in which one half of all cases occurs in the first 2 years of life and three fourths of all cases by 5 years of age. The figures for osteomyelitis in those two age groups are approximately one third and one half, respectively.

Skeletal infections consistently occur more commonly in boys than in girls in all reported series. The male:female ratio is approximately 2:1 in most series. If trauma is truly an important risk factor, it may be that the life-style of boys predisposes to traumatic events.

Apparently there is no particular predilection for arthritis or osteomyelitis based on race. In most series the racial distribution of cases reflects that of the local population.

CLINICAL FINDINGS

The earliest signs and symptoms of skeletal infection are often subtle. This is particularly true of the neonate, who characteristically is not ill. In a report summarizing 83 cases of neonatal osteomyelitis from the literature, 52% had no fever, and only 8% were described as appearing septic or toxic (Nelson, 1983). In infants only pseudoparalysis of an extremity or apparent pain on movement of the affected extremity may be present.

In older infants and children the majority has fever and localized signs. Redness and swelling of skin and soft tissue overlying the site of infection usually are seen earlier in patients with arthritis than in those with osteomyelitis. The exception is with hip involvement in which these signs are usually absent because of the deep location of that joint. In other joints the bulging,

Table 16-2. Infected bones in 372 patients with monosteal disease and 27 patients with polyosteal disease*

Bone	Monosteal	Polyosteal
Femur	93	12
Tibia	89	18
Humerus	50	8
Fibula	16	10
Phalanx	18	5
Calcaneus	18	0
Radius	13	4
Ischium	14	1
Metatarsus	8	0
Ulna	7	3
Ilium	7	0
Vertebra	7	2
Sacrum	3	0
Skull	3	0
Talus	3	1
Clavicle	2	2
Rib	2	1
Scapula	2	1
Carpal bone	2	0
Cuneiform	2	0
Pubis	3	1
Sternum	3	0
Metacarpus	2	0
One case each: maxilla, mandible, cuboid, bone of pyriform aperture, acetabulum	6	0

*Based on J Nelson's series of cases.

infected synovium is relatively near the surface, whereas the metaphyses are located deeper under the soft tissues. Local swelling and redness in a patient with osteomyelitis mean that the infection has spread out of the metaphysis into the subperiosteal space and that there is a secondary soft-tissue inflammatory response.

Nonspecific systemic signs of infection such as nausea, vomiting, diarrhea, and headache are not prominent features of skeletal infections even though many of the patients are bacteremic. If those signs are present, disseminated infection syndrome with multiple foci of disease should be suspected; this is most likely to occur with *Staphylococcus aureus* or *H. influenzae* type b infection.

Long bones are principally involved in osteo-

Table 16-3. Distribution of affected joints in patients with septic arthritis

Joint	Dallas series (646 joints, 591 patients)		Five other series (377 joints, 357 patients)	
	Total joints	Percentage	Total joints	Percentage
Knee	258	40	144	38
Hip	146	23	121	32
Elbow	89	14	21	6
Ankle	85	13	52	14
Wrist	27	4	3	1
Shoulder	28	4	11	3
Hand/foot	8	1	15	4
Other	5	1	10	2

Modified from Fink CW, Nelson JD: Clin Rheum Dis 1986;12:423-435.

Table 16-4. Monarticular and polyarticular involvement in septic arthritis

Joints	Dallas series (591 joints)		Other series (307 joints)	
	Number of patients	Percentage	Number of patients	Percentage
Monarticular	552	93.4	295	96
Two joints	26	4.4	8	2.6
Three joints	10	1.7	3	1
Four joints	3	0.5	1	0.3

Modified from Fink CW, Nelson JD: Clin Rheum Dis 1986;12:423-435.

myelitis (Table 16-2). The femur and tibia are equally affected and together constitute almost half of all cases. The bones of the upper extremities account for one fourth of all cases. Flat bones are less commonly affected.

Joints of the lower extremity constitute three quarters of all cases of arthritis. The elbow, wrist, and shoulder joints are involved in approximately 20% of cases, and small joints uncommonly are infected.

A single locus usually is involved in bone or joint infection. Multifocal osteomyelitis and polyarticular arthritis occur in fewer than 10% of cases (Tables 16-3 and 16-4). An exception is gonococcal infection, which is polyarticular in more than half of the cases.

DIAGNOSIS

The differential diagnosis of bone and joint infection includes trauma, cellulitis, pyomyositis, malignancy, and collagen vascular diseases. It is not unusual for patients with leukemia or neuroblastoma to present with fever and focal signs suggesting bone or joint infection. A biopsy establishes the diagnosis. History and roentgenographic findings help in distinguishing trauma from infection. Pyomyositis is rare outside central Africa and parts of southeast Asia. Sonography and magnetic resonance imaging (MRI) are very helpful in identifying pyomyositis. In most cases the differential diagnosis between cellulitis and similar soft-tissue findings secondary to bone and joint infection becomes obvious during physical examination. When there is doubt, three-phase radionuclide scanning can be helpful. Various collagen vascular diseases may mimic arthritis if the patient has a single joint involved. In most cases multiple joint involvement, disease in other organ systems, failure to respond to antibiotic therapy, and the chronic or remittent nature of the process lead to the correct diagnosis.

Results from routine laboratory tests such as the white blood count and differential count, erythrocyte sedimentation rate, and C-reactive protein are nonspecific and not helpful in dif-

oral antibiotic regimen have been published (Nelson, 1983).

The oral regimen decreases the risk of nosocomial infections related to prolonged intravenous therapy, is more comfortable for the patient, and permits treatment outside the hospital if compliance with taking the medicine can be assured.

Surgical therapy

No randomized, prospective study has compared two or more surgical procedures in patients with skeletal infections. The measures used derive from training and experience. For example, after arthrotomy some surgeons leave drains and some do not. Of those who use drains, some use collapsible drains and some use rigid ones. Of those who use rigid drains, some use suction and some do not. None of these things has been evaluated in a controlled manner.

Hip joint infection is a surgical emergency because of the vulnerability of the blood supply to the head of the femur. When a penetrating injury has occurred and the presence of a foreign body is likely, surgical intervention is indicated. In other situations the need for surgery is individualized.

For joints other than the hip daily percutaneous needle aspirations of synovial fluid are done. Generally one or two subsequent aspirations suffice. If fluid is still accumulating after 4 to 5 days, arthrotomy is performed. At the time of surgery the joint is flushed with sterile saline solution. Antibiotics are not instilled because they are irritating to synovial tissue, and adequate amounts of antibiotic are achieved in joint fluid with systemic administration (Nelson, 1971).

If frank pus is obtained from subperiosteal or metaphyseal aspiration, the patient is taken to surgery for drainage through a cortical window. In one series incision and drainage were done in 36% of cases of arthritis and in 69% of cases of osteomyelitis (Syrogiannopoulos and Nelson, 1988).

Physical medicine

The major role of physical medicine is a preventive one. If a child is allowed to lie in bed with an extremity in flexion, limitation of extension can develop in a few days. The affected extremity should be kept in extension with sand

bags, splints or, if necessary, casts. Casts are indicated when there is a potential for pathological fracture.

After 2 or 3 days when pain is easing, passive range of motion exercises are started and then continued until the child resumes normal activity.

In neglected cases with flexion contractures prolonged physical therapy is required.

Duration of antibiotic therapy

Prolonged courses of antibiotic therapy have traditionally been recommended, but there has been a trend toward shorter courses.

The Centers for Disease Control guidelines recommend 7 days of therapy for gonococcal tenosynovitis (Centers for Disease Control, 1989). As mentioned previously, 7 postoperative days of treatment is adequate for *Pseudomonas* osteochondritis or arthritis. Immunocompromised patients generally require prolonged courses of therapy as do patients with fungal or tuberculous disease.

For the usual case of staphylococcal, streptococcal, or *Haemophilus* infection, treatment is continued for a minimum of 3 weeks provided that the signs of inflammation have disappeared. Duration of antibiotic therapy should be individualized, and if clinical response has been slow, a course of 4 to 6 weeks commonly is used.

PROGNOSIS

Because children are in a dynamic state of growth, sequelae of skeletal infections may not become apparent for months or years, so long-term follow-up is important.

In a series of 40 neonates with osteomyelitis treated during 1970 to 1979 10 had severe sequelae, and six had moderate sequelae (Bergdahl et al., 1985). Major problems relate to retarded growth of an affected bone. Growth disturbance was evident in 20 of 36 nonoperated foci and in 4 of 19 operated foci.

Relapses and chronic infections are uncommon. A group of 50 infants and children with osteomyelitis was followed for an average of 36 months (range, 12 to 56 months) after treatment (Dunkle and Brock, 1982). At diagnosis 32 were classified as acute, 15 as subacute (symptoms for longer than 7 days), and 3 as chronic. Relapses occurred in only two patients, one of whom was originally classified as acute and the other as chronic. In another series (Vaughan et al., 1987) eight of 60 patients did not respond to antibiotics within 48 hours and required surgical drainage. Of the remaining 52 patients, 35 patients were treated with parenteral antibiotics for an average of 21 days, and 17 were treated parenterally for 8 days, followed by 4 weeks of oral antibiotics. Chronic infection ensued in one of the operatively treated patients and in two of the remaining 52.

In 49 patients with suppurative arthritis of weight-bearing joints followed an average of 4.3 years (range, 18 months to 12 years) after treatment 13 patients (27%) had sequelae, and in eight (16%) ambulation was impaired (Howard et al., 1976). Residual damage was more common with hip (40% of cases) and ankle (33%) involvement than with knee joint (10%) disease. Sequelae were equally common after *H. influenzae* and *S. aureus* infection. Evaluation at the time of hospital discharge correctly identified only four of the 13 children with sequelae, and four others who were normal at follow-up had been thought to have permanent damage at discharge. Children with sequelae tended to have been sick longer before diagnosis, and in them drainage of pus was delayed.

Thirty-seven children with hip joint infection treated at the Mayo Clinic from 1943 through 1973 had long-term (mean, 8.3 years) follow-up evaluation (Morrey et al., 1976). Nineteen had satisfactory results, and 18 had unsatisfactory results. "Unsatisfactory" was defined as more than 2.5 cm limb length discrepancy (7 patients), persisting pain (5 patients), limitation of motion (7 patients), or need for secondary surgical procedures (9 patients). Duration of symptoms was the most important prognostic factor. There were no sequelae among the nine patients treated within 4 days of onset of symptoms. Of 11 patients with symptoms for more than 1 week, only two had satisfactory results. Associated metaphyseal osteomyelitis was another bad prognostic sign: only two of 14 had a satisfactory result.

Even with appropriate medical and surgical therapy, there is a potential for permanent disabling sequelae in patients with skeletal infections. Prompt recognition and vigorous medical, surgical, and physical therapy offer the best hope for a satisfactory outcome.

REFERENCES

Adeyokunnu AA, Hendrickse RG: Salmonella osteomyelitis in childhood. Arch Dis Child 1980;55:175-184.

Ash JM, Gilday DL: The futility of bone scanning in neonatal osteomyelitis in children, J Nucl Med 1980;21:417-420.

Bergdahl S, Ekengren K, Eriksson M: Neonatal hematogenous osteomyelitis: risk factors for long-term sequelae. J Pediatr Orthop 1985;5:564-568.

Björkstén B, Gustavson KH, Eriksson B, et al: Chronic recurrent multifocal osteomyelitis and pustulosis palmoplantaris. J Pediatr 1978;93:227-231.

Broderick A, Perlman S, Dietz F: *Pseudomonas* bursitis: Inoculation from a catfish. Pediatr Infect Dis 1985;4:693-694.

Capitanio MA, Kirkpatrick JA: Early roentgen observations in acute osteomyelitis. Am J Roentgenol 1970;108:488-496.

Centers for Disease Control. 1989 sexually transmitted diseases treatment guidelines, MMWR 1989; 38(No. S-8):24-25.

Dan M: Septic arthritis in young infants: Clinical and microbiologic correlations and therapeutic implications. Rev Infect Dis 1984;6:147-155.

Demopulos GA, Bleck EE, McDougall IR: Role of radionuclide imaging in the diagnosis of acute osteomyelitis. J Pediatr Orthop 1988;8:558-565.

Dorr U, Zieger M, Hauke H: Ultrasonography of the painful hip. Prospective studies in 204 patients. Pediatr Radiol 1988;19:36-40.

Dubey L, Krasinski K, Hernanz-Schulman M: Osteomyelitis secondary to trauma or infected contiguous soft tissue. Pediatr Infect Dis J 1988;7:26-34.

Dunkle LM, Brock N: Long-term follow-up ambulatory management of osteomyelitis. Clin Pediatr 1982;21:650-655.

Edwards MS, Baker CJ, Wagner ML, et al: An etiologic shift in infantile osteomyelitis: the emergence of group B streptococcus. J Pediatr 1978;93:578-583.

Eisenberg JM, Kitz DS: Savings from outpatient antibiotic therapy for osteomyelitis. Economic analysis of a therapeutic strategy. JAMA 1986;255:1584-1588.

Fajardo JE, Mickunas VH, deTriquet JM: Suppurative arthritis and hemophilia. Pediatr Infect Dis 1986;5:593-594.

Fink CW: Reactive arthritis. Pediatr Infect Dis J 1988; 7:58-65.

Fink CW, Nelson JD: Septic arthritis and osteomyelitis in children. Clin Rheum Dis 1986;12:423-435.

Fisher MC, Goldsmith JF, Gilligan PH: Sneakers as a source of *Pseudomonas aeruginosa* in children with osteomyelitis following puncture wounds. J Pediatr 1985;106:607.

Giedion A, Holthusen W, Masel LF, et al: Subacute and chronic "symmetrical" osteomyelitis. Ann Radiol (Paris) 1972;15:329-342.

Goldenberg DL, Reed JI: Bacterial arthritis. N Engl J Med 1985;312:764-771.

Green NE, Beauchamp RD, Griffin PP: Primary subacute epiphyseal osteomyelitis. J Bone Joint Surg (Am) 1981;63:107-114.

Haueisen DC, Weiner DS, Weiner SD: The characterization of "transient synovitis of the hip" in children. J Pediatr Orthop 1986;6:11-17.

Herndon WA, Alexieva BT, Schwindt ML, et al: Nuclear imaging for musculoskeletal infections in children. J Pediatr Orthop 1985;5:343-347.

Howard JB, Highgenboten CL, Nelson JD: Residual effects of septic arthritis in infancy and childhood. JAMA 1976;236:932-935.

Hummell DS, Anderson SJ, Wright PF, et al: Chronic recurrent multifocal osteomyelitis: are mycoplasmas involved? N Engl J Med 1987;317:510-511.

Jacobs RF, McCarthy RE, Elser JM: *Pseudomonas* osteochondritis complicating puncture wounds of the foot in children: a 10-year evaluation. J Infect Dis 1989;160:657.

Jacobs RF, Adelman L, Sack CM, et al: Management of *Pseudomonas* osteochondritis complicating puncture wounds of the foot. Pediatrics 1982;69:432-435.

Jacobson HG: Musculoskeletal applications of magnetic resonance imaging. JAMA 1989;262:2420-2427.

Jurik AG, Helmig O, Ternowitz T, et al: Chronic recurrent multifocal osteomyelitis: a follow-up study. J Pediatr Orthop 1988;8:49-58.

King SM, Laxer RM, Manson D, et al: Chronic recurrent multifocal osteomyelitis: a noninfectious inflammatory process. Pediatr Infect Dis 1987;6:907-911.

Lebel MH, Nelson JD: *Haemophilus influenzae* type b osteomyelitis in infants and children. Pediatr Infect Dis J 1988;7:250-254.

Likitnukul S, McCracken GH Jr, Nelson JD: Arthritis in children with bacterial meningitis. Am J Dis Child 1986;140:424-426.

Lilien LD, Harris VJ, Ramamurthy RS, et al: Neonatal osteomyelitis of the calcaneus: complications of heel puncture. J Pediatr 1976;88:478-480.

Majeed HA, Kalaawi M, Mohanty D, et al: Congenital dyserythropoietic anemia and chronic recurrent multifocal osteomyelitis in three related children and the association with Sweet syndrome in two siblings. J Pediatr 1989;115:730-734.

Meyers S, Lonon W, Shannon K: Suppurative bursitis in early childhood. Pediatr Infect Dis 1984;3:156-158.

Mok PM, Reilly BJ, Ash JM: Osteomyelitis in the neonate. Radiology 1982;145:677-682.

Morrey BF, Bianco AJ, Rhodes KH: Suppurative arthritis of the hip in children. J Bone Joint Surg (Am) 1976;58:388-392.

Morrissy RT, Haynes DW: Acute hematogenous osteomyelitis: A model with trauma as an etiology. J Pediatr Orthop 1989;9:447-456.

Mustafa MM, Sáez-Llorens X, et al: Acute hematogenous pelvic osteomyelitis in infants and children. Pediatr Infect Dis 1990;9:416-421.

Nelson JD: Acute osteomyelitis in children. Infect Dis Clin North Am 1990;4:513-522.

Nelson JD: A critical review of the role of oral antibiotics in the management of hematogenous osteomyelitis, in Remington JS, Swartz MN (ed): Current clinical topics in infectious diseases. New York: McGraw-Hill, 1983, pp 64-74.

Nelson JD: Antibiotic concentrations in septic joint effusions. N Engl J Med 1971;284:349-353.

Nelson JD: Bone and joint infections. Pediatr Infect Dis 1983;2:S45-S50.

Ogden JA, Lister G: The pathology of neonatal osteomyelitis. Pediatrics 1975;55:474-478.

Paisley JW: Septic bursitis in childhood. J Pediatr Orthop 1982;2:57-61.

Pappo AS, Buchanan GR, Johnson A: Septic arthritis in children with hemophilia. Am J Dis Child 1989;143:1226-1227.

Peltola H, Vahvanen V, Aalto K: Fever, C-reactive protein, and erythrocyte sedimentation rate in monitoring recovery from septic arthritis: a preliminary study. J Pediatr Orthop 1984;4:170-174.

Rao S, Solomon N, Miller S, et al: Scintigraphic differentiation of bone infarction from osteomyelitis in children with sickle cell disease. J Pediatr 1985;107:685-688.

Rodgriquez W, Ross S, Khan W, et al: Clindamycin in the treatment of osteomyelitis in children. Am J Dis Child 1977;131:1088-1093.

Rosenbaum DM, Blumhagen JD: Acute epiphyseal osteomyelitis in children. Radiology 1985;156:89-92.

Rubin RH, Fischman AJ, Callahan JR, et al: In-labeled nonspecific immunoglobulin scanning in the detection of focal infection. N Engl J Med 1989;321:935-940.

Rush PJ, Shore A, Inman R, et al: Arthritis associated with *Haemophilus influenzae* meningitis: septic or reactive? J Pediatr 1986;109:412-414.

Sadat-Ali M, Sankaran-Kutty, Kannan Kutty: Recent observations on osteomyelitis in sickle-cell disease. Int Orthop 1985;9:97-99.

Sáez-Llorens X, Mustafa M, Ramilo O, et al: Tumor necrosis factor alpha and interleukin-1 beta in synovial fluid of infants and children with suppurative arthritis, Am J Dis Child 1990;144:353-356.

Sundberg SB, Savage JP, Foster BK: Technetium phosphate bone scan in the diagnosis of septic arthritis in childhood. J Pediatr Orthop 1989;9:579-585.

Syrogiannopoulos GA, McCracken GH Jr, Nelson JD: Osteoarticular infections in children with sickle cell disease. Pediatrics 1986;78:1090-1096.

Syrogiannopoulos GA, Nelson JD: Duration of antimicrobial therapy for acute suppurative osteoarticular infections. Lancet 1988;1:37-40.

Vaughan PA, Newman NM, Rosman MA: Acute hematogenous osteomyelitis in children. J Pediatr Ortho 1987;7:652-655.

Waldvogel FA, Vasey H: Osteomyelitis: The past decade. N Engl J Med 1980;303:360-370.

Yousefzadeh DK, Jackson JH: Neonatal and infantile candidal arthritis with or without osteomyelitis: a clinical and radiographical review of 21 cases, Skeletal Radiol 1980;5:77-90.

17

OTITIS MEDIA

JEROME O. KLEIN

Acute otitis media and middle ear effusion are among the most common illnesses of childhood. After every episode of acute otitis media, fluid persists in the middle ear for varying periods of time, usually weeks to months. The signs of acute infection resolve with appropriate antibiotic therapy, but the middle ear effusion, now sterile (in episodes of bacterial infection), persists. Conductive hearing loss usually accompanies middle ear effusion, although the extent of the loss varies from child to child. Because of the frequency of acute otitis media and accompanying hearing loss, pediatricians have been concerned that children who suffer from persistent or recurrent middle ear disease might also suffer from delay or impairment of speech, language, or cognitive abilities.

EPIDEMIOLOGY

Otitis media is a disease of infants and young children. By 3 years of age, most children have had at least one episode of acute otitis media, and up to one half have had recurrent acute otitis media (three or more episodes). The peak age-specific attack rate occurs during the second half of the first year of life. Few children have first episodes of acute otitis media after 3 years of age (Teele et al., 1989). Among the variables associated with acute otitis media are sex (males have more middle ear disease than females); race (there is an extraordinary incidence of infection in some racial groups such as American Indians, Alaskan and Canadian Eskimos, and African and Australian aboriginal children); age at first epi-

sode (the earlier in life the first episode occurs, the more likely the child is to have recurrent disease); sibling history of acute otitis media and recurrent acute otitis media (suggesting a genetic basis for the disease); breast-feeding (infants who are breast-fed for as little as 3 months have less disease in the first year of life than children who are not breast-fed); and frequent exposure to infectious agents such as occurs in day-care centers (Teele et al., 1989; Wald et al., 1988).

ETIOLOGY

The microbiology of otitis media has been documented by appropriate culture of middle ear fluids obtained by needle aspiration (Bluestone and Klein, 1990) (Table 17-1). The findings of bacteriological studies performed in the United States and Scandinavia are remarkably consistent: *Streptococcus pneumoniae* is the most frequent agent in all age groups; *Haemophilus influenzae* is an important pathogen in all age groups; *Moraxella catarrhalis* is isolated from middle ear fluids with increasing frequency; *Streptococcus pyogenes* has been a significant pathogen in some studies from Scandinavia but not in studies done in the United States; and *Staphylococcus aureus*, gram-negative enteric bacilli, and anaerobic bacteria are infrequent causes of otitis media (Table 17-1).

Because *S. pneumoniae* is the most important cause of otitis media, investigators have carefully studied the types responsible for infection of the middle ear. The results indicate that relatively

Table 17-1. Bacterial pathogens isolated from middle ear fluids in children with acute otitis media*

Pathogen	Mean (%)	Range (%)
Streptococcus pneumoniae	39	27-52
Haemophilus influenzae	27	16-52
Moraxella catarrhalis	10	2-27
Streptococcus pyogenes	3	0-11
Staphylococcus aureus	2	0-16
None or nonpathogens	28	12-35

*Data from nine reports from United States and Canada, 1980-1987.

Table 17-2. Bacterial pathogens isolated from 169 infants with otitis media during the first 6 weeks of life*

Microorganism	Percent of infants with pathogen
Respiratory bacteria	
Streptococcus pneumoniae	18.3
Haemophilus influenzae	12.4
S. pneumoniae and H. influenzae	3.0
Staphylococcus aureus	7.7
Streptococci, groups A and B	3.0
Moraxella catarrhalis	5.3
Enteric bacteria	
Escherichia coli	5.9
Klebsiella-Enterobacter	5.3
Pseudomonas aeruginosa	1.8
Miscellaneous	5.3
None or nonpathogens	32.0

*Reports from Honolulu, Hawaii (Bland, 1972); Dallas, Texas (Tetzlaff et al., 1977); Denver, CO (Berman et al., 1978); and Huntsville, AL, and Boston, MA (Shurin et al., 1978).

few types are responsible for most disease. The eight most common types in order of decreasing frequency are types 19, 3, 6, 23, 14, 1, 18, and 7. All are included in the pneumococcal vaccine.

Otitis media caused by *H. influenzae* is associated with nontypeable strains in the vast majority of patients. In approximately 10% the otitis is due to type b; some of these children are toxic and may have bacteremia and meningitis. At one time *H. influenzae* was believed of limited importance to otitis media in school-age children and adolescents, but several studies indicate that this organism is a significant cause of otitis media in all age groups (Grönroos et al., 1964; Howie et al., 1970; Herberts et al., 1971; Schwartz et al., 1977).

Gram-negative enteric bacilli are responsible for approximately 20% of cases of otitis media in young infants (to 6 weeks of age), but these organisms are rarely present in the middle ear effusion of older children. Other than the greater prevalence of otitis media caused by gram-negative bacilli and the presence of other organisms responsible for neonatal sepsis such as group B streptococci and *S. aureus*, the bacteriology of otitis in the infant up to 6 weeks of age is similar to that in older children (Table 17-2) (Bland, 1972; Tetzlaff et al., 1977; Berman et al., 1978; Shurin et al., 1978).

Studies in Cleveland (Shurin et al., 1983) and Pittsburgh (Kovatch et al., 1983) indicate a significant increase in isolation of *M. catarrhalis*.

During the period 1980 to 1981, *M. catarrhalis* was isolated from 27% and 19% of children with acute otitis media, respectively. Approximately three fourths of the isolates produced β-lactamase and were therefore resistant to ampicillin.

Epidemiological data suggest that viral infection is associated with acute otitis media (Henderson et al., 1982). Respiratory syncytial virus, influenza virus, rhinoviruses, and enteroviruses without concurrent bacterial pathogens (Chonmaitre et al., 1986; Arola et al., 1990) have been isolated from middle ear fluids from some children. In addition, there is evidence of viral infection obtained by enzyme-linked immunosorbent assay techniques (ELISA) that identify viral antigens in middle ear fluids in children with acute otitis media (Klein et al., 1982).

Only one report of isolation of a mycoplasma (*Mycoplasma pneumoniae*) from middle ear fluid of a child with acute otitis media has been published (Sobeslavsky et al., 1965).

Chlamydia trachomatis infection results in a mild but prolonged pneumonitis in infants that may be accompanied by otitis media. *C. trachomatis* has been isolated from middle ear fluids of such infants (Tipple et al., 1979).

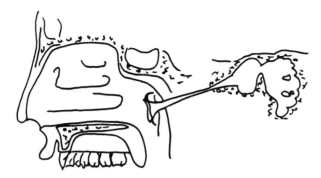

Fig. 17-1. Position of the eustachian tube relative to the nasopharynx and the middle ear. The eustachian tube is a double-horned organ with the proximal two thirds lying in cartilage and the distal one third in bone. The segments are connected by the narrow isthmus, the site most vulnerable to obstruction. Thus the system consists of the nares, nasopharynx, eustachian tube, middle ear, and mastoid air cells.

PATHOGENESIS

The pathogenesis of otitis media must be approached with the understanding that the disease involves a system having contiguous parts, including the nares, nasopharynx, eustachian tube, middle ear, and mastoid antrum and air cells (Fig. 17-1). The middle ear resembles a flattened box, which is approximately 15 mm from top to bottom, 10 mm wide, and only 2 to 6 mm deep. The lateral wall includes the tympanic membrane and the medial wall the oval and round windows. The mastoid air cells lie behind, and the orifice of the eustachian tube is in the superior portion of the front wall.

The eustachian tube connects the middle ear with the posterior nasopharynx, and its lateral one third lies in bone and is open. The medial two thirds are in cartilage, and the walls are in apposition except during swallowing or yawning. In the young infant the eustachian tube is both shorter and proportionately wider than in the older child; the cartilaginous and osseous portions of the tube form a relatively straight line. In an older child the angle of the tube is more acute. These anatomical differences may predispose some infants to early and repeated illness.

The eustachian tube has at least three important physiological functions with respect to the middle ear: protection of the ear from nasopharyngeal secretions, drainage into the nasopharynx of secretions produced within the middle ear, and ventilation of the middle ear to equalize air pressure within the box with pressure in the external ear canal. When one or more of these functions is compromised, the result may be obstruction of the tube, accumulation of secretions in the middle ear, and, if pyogenic organisms are present, development of suppurative otitis media. Dysfunction of the eustachian tube because of anatomical or physiological factors apparently is the most important feature of the pathogenesis of infection of the middle ear.

CLINICAL MANIFESTATIONS

Otalgia (ear pain), otorrhea (ear drainage), hearing impairment affecting one or both ears, and fever suggest infection of the middle ear. However, many children with otitis media do not have these signs. Infants may manifest only general signs of distress, including irritability, bouts of crying, diarrhea, and feeding problems. Acute otitis media is usually defined by the presence of middle ear effusion accompanied by a sign or symptom of acute illness.

Hyperemia of the tympanic membrane caused by injection of blood vessels is an early sign of otitis media. But redness of the tympanic membrane may be caused by inflammation elsewhere in the system since the mucous membrane is continuous from the nares and eustachian tube and lines the walls of the middle ear cleft. Thus a "red ear" alone does not establish the diagnosis of otitis media.

Fluid in the middle ear persists for variable periods of time after onset of the acute episode.

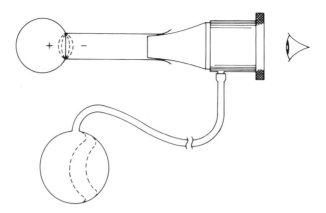

Fig. 17-2. Use of the pneumatic otoscope. The normal tympanic membrane moves inward with positive pressure in the ear canal and outward with negative pressure. The presence of effusion or negative pressure dampens movement of the tympanic membrane.

At the conclusion of a 10- to 14-day course of antimicrobial therapy, approximately two thirds of children still have fluid in the middle ear. The fluid in the middle ear persists in approximately 40% of children at 1 month, 20% at 2 months, and 10% at 3 months after onset of acute otitis. Children should be observed until fluid has cleared.

DIAGNOSIS
Clinical

Pneumatic otoscopy provides an assessment of mobility of the tympanic membrane. The normal tympanic membrane moves inward with positive pressure and outward with negative pressure (Fig. 17-2). The motion observed is proportional to the pressure applied by gently squeezing and then releasing the rubber bulb attachment on the head of the otoscope. Normal mobility of the tympanic membrane is indicated when positive, then negative pressure is applied and the membrane moves rapidly inward and outward like a sail in a brisk wind. Either presence of fluid in the middle ear or high negative middle ear pressure dampens tympanic membrane mobility.

Tympanometry uses an electroacoustic impedance bridge to record compliance of the tympanic membrane and middle ear pressure. After a small probe is inserted into the external canal by means of a snug-fitting cuff, a tone of fixed characteristics is delivered by an oscillator-amplifier through the probe. The compliance of the tympanic membrane is measured by a microphone while the external canal pressure is varied by a pump manometer. The tone is delivered at a given intensity as the air pressure in the canal is varied over a positive and negative range. The recording that results—the tympanogram—reflects the dynamics of the middle ear system, including the tympanic membrane, middle ear, mastoid air cells, and eustachian tube. The technique is reliable, simple, and readily carried out by nonprofessional personnel. However, there are technical problems in applications of presently available instruments to young children, particularly those less than 7 months of age. Tympanometry is of particular value in diagnosis of ambiguous cases of otitis media, in screening for ear disease, and in training of students and young physicians.

The acoustic otoscope is a hand-held instrument that uses principles of reflected energy from the middle ear space to provide information about the presence or absence of middle ear effusion. A microphone located in the probe tip measures the level of transmitted and reflected sound. Acoustic energy is reflected back toward the probe tip from the ear canal and ear drum. The more sound reflected, the greater is the likelihood of the presence of an effusion.

Microbiology

The results of bacterial cultures of the nasopharynx and oropharynx correlate poorly with those of middle ear fluids. Thus cultures of the upper respiratory tract are of limited value in specific bacteriological diagnosis of otitis media. If the child is toxic or has localized infection elsewhere, culture of blood and/or the focus of infection should be performed.

Needle aspiration of a middle ear effusion provides immediate and specific information about the bacteriology of the infection. Although the consistent results of investigations of the bacteriology of acute otitis media provide a guide to the most likely pathogens, S. *pneumoniae* and H. *influenzae*, needle aspiration should be considered in selected children. These children include those who are critically ill at first visit and those who fail to respond adequately to initial therapy and remain toxic and febrile 48 to 72 hours after onset of therapy. Also included are patients with altered host defenses who may be infected with an unusual agent such as those with malignancy or immunosuppressive disease, newborn infants, and those with chronic otitis media.

When spontaneous perforation occurs, the exudate in the ear canal is contaminated with flora from the canal. Culture should be obtained, after cleansing the canal with alcohol, by needle aspiration of fluid emerging from the area of perforation or preferably from within the middle ear.

COMPLICATIONS AND SEQUELAE

Suppurative complications of acute infection of the middle ear are uncommon. Contiguous spread of infection, however, may be responsible for mastoiditis, petrositis, labyrinthitis, brain abscess, and meningitis.

Of more concern, at present, is impairment of hearing associated with fluid in the middle ear. Audiograms of children with middle ear effusion usually indicate a mild to moderate conductive hearing loss. The median loss is approximately 25 dB (Fria et al., 1985), which is the equivalent of putting plugs in the ears. The hearing loss is conductive and due to the presence of fluid in the middle ear and is less influenced by the quality of fluid (serous, mucoid, or purulent) than by its volume (partially or completely filling the middle ear space). The conductive hearing impairment is usually reversed with resolution of the middle ear effusion. High negative pressure in the middle ear or atelectasis, both in the absence of middle ear effusion, may also result in conductive hearing loss.

Sensorineural hearing loss is uncommonly associated with otitis media. Permanent sensorineural loss has been described, presumably as a result of the spread of microorganisms or products of inflammation through the round window membrane or because of a suppurative complication of acute otitis media such as labyrinthitis. Permanent hearing loss also may result from irreversible inflammatory changes, including adhesive otitis media and ossicular discontinuity.

The significance of hearing loss associated with acute infection or persistent middle ear effusion is uncertain. Retrospective studies suggest that chronic middle ear disease with effusion occurring during the first few years of life has adverse effects on development of speech and language, hearing, intelligence, and performance in school (Holm and Kunze, 1969; Kaplan et al., 1973; Lewis, 1976; Needleman, 1977; Zinkus et al., 1978).

Recent longitudinal studies indicate that children who had recurrent episodes of otitis media or persistent middle ear effusion perform less well on tests of speech, language, and cognitive abilities than do their disease-free peers. These data suggest that delay or impairment of development may be an important sequela of otitis media. Boston children observed for ear disease from birth were evaluated at age 7 years by Teele et al. (1990). Estimated time with middle ear effusion during the first 3 years of life was associated significantly with lower scores on tests of cognitive abilities (full-scale, performance, and verbal intelligence quotients), speech and language (articulation and use of morphological markers), and school performance (lower scores in mathematics and reading).

TREATMENT
Acute otitis media

The preferred antimicrobial agent for the patient with otitis media must be active against S. *pneumoniae*, H. *influenzae*, and M. *catarrhalis*. Group A streptococci and S. *aureus* are infrequent causes of acute otitis media and need not be considered in initial therapeutic decisions. Gram-negative enteric bacilli must be considered when otitis media occurs in the newborn infant, in the patient with a depressed immune

Table 17-3. Antimicrobial agents for acute otitis media

Drug (trade name)	Dosage (kg/day)	Issues about usage
Amoxicillin (Amoxil)	40 mg in three doses	β-Lactamase susceptible
Amoxicillin-clavulanate (Augmentin)	40 mg in three doses	Diarrhea
Cefaclor (Ceclor)	40 mg in two to three doses	Serum-sickness–like reactions
Cefixime (Suprax)	8 mg in one dose	Diarrhea
Cefprozil (Cefzil)	30 mg in two doses	
Cefuroxime axetil (Ceftin)	250-500 mg (total/day) in two doses	Available only as tablets
Erythromycin-sulfisoxazole (Pediazole)	40 mg in four doses	Rare hematological effects of sulfa; gastric distress of erythromycin
Trimethoprim-sulfamethoxazole (Bactrim, Septra)	8 mg* in three doses	Rare hematological effects; not recommended for group A streptococcal infections

*Trimethoprim component.

response, and in the patient with suppurative complications of chronic otitis media. Amoxicillin is the current drug of choice for initial treatment since it is effective against the major pathogens and less expensive than alternative regimens.

The increasing proportion of β-lactamase–producing non-typeable *H. influenzae* and *M. catarrhalis* raises concerns about continued usage of amoxicillin for initial therapy of acute otitis media. The vast majority of *M. catarrhalis* strains are β-lactamase producers. The proportion of β-lactamase–producing strains of *H. influenzae* isolated from middle ear fluids varies from 21% in a multicenter study (Doern et al., 1988) to 60% in a recent report from Northern Virginia and Washington, D.C. (Schwartz and Rodriguez, 1989). Nevertheless, amoxicillin is still the drug of choice for treating acute otitis media in most communities. The physician should safeguard the child against possible treatment failure by instructing the parent to call if signs and symptoms have not resolved significantly within 48 hours. At that time the illness can be reassessed, and an alternative antimicrobial agent may be considered if no other disease is present. Alternative agents include amoxicillin-clavulanate, four cephalosporins (cefaclor, cefixime, cefprozil, and cefuroxime axetil), and

two sulfa-containing combinations (erythromycin-sulfisoxazole and trimethoprim-sulfamethoxazole). Clinical and microbiological data indicate that all are of approximately equivalent efficacy. The choice should be made on the basis of cost (trimethoprim-sulfamethoxazole is the least expensive), side effects (concern about the hematological effects of the sulfonamides, diarrhea associated with amoxicillin-clavulanate, serum-sickness–like disease associated with cefaclor), and convenience of administration (once-a-day dosage and stability at room temperature of cefixime) (Table 17-3).

Nasal and oral decongestants, administered either alone or in combination with an antihistamine, are currently among the most popular medications for the treatment of acute otitis media with effusion. The common concept is that these drugs reduce congestion of the respiratory mucosa and relieve the obstruction of the eustachian tube that results from inflammation caused by respiratory infection. The results of clinical trials, however, indicate no significant evidence of efficacy of any of these preparations used alone or in combination for relief of signs of disease or decrease in time spent with fluid in the middle ear after acute infection (Collip, 1961; Fraser et al., 1977; Olson et al., 1978).

Chronic otitis media with effusion

Appropriate management of the child with chronic otitis media remains controversial. The major goal is to establish and to maintain an aerated middle ear that is free of fluid and has a normal mucosa and thus to achieve normal hearing. Current therapies include prolonged courses of antimicrobial agents, myringotomy, adenoidectomy, and use of tympanostomy (ventilating) tubes. Before the introduction of antimicrobial agents, myringotomy was the major method of managing suppurative otitis media. Currently, the use of myringotomy is limited to the relief of intractable ear pain, hastening resolution of mastoid infection, and drainage of persistent middle ear effusion that is unresponsive to medical therapy.

Enlarged adenoids may obstruct the orifice of the eustachian tube in the posterior portion of the nasopharynx and interfere with adequate ventilation and drainage of the middle ear. Recent studies of the use of adenoidectomy in children with prolonged effusions in the middle ear identify a beneficial effect in reducing time spent with effusion in selected children (Gates et al., 1987; Paradise et al., 1990).

Tympanostomy tubes, resembling small collar buttons placed in the tympanic membrane, provide drainage of middle ear fluid and ventilate the middle ear. The effect in children who have impaired hearing because of the presence of fluid is restoration of normal hearing. Placement of the tube treats the effect and not the cause of the persistent effusion. The criteria for placement of ventilating tubes, management of tubes once they are placed, and long-term benefits, if any, are uncertain. The indications for placement of tympanostomy tubes include persistent middle ear effusions that are unresponsive to adequate medical treatment, persistent tympanic membrane retraction pockets with impending cholesteatoma, and persistent negative pressure with significant hearing loss (Bluestone and Shurin, 1974).

PREVENTION

A study in Rochester, New York, suggested that chemoprophylaxis may be of value in the prevention of signs of acute infection in children with recurrent otitis media (Perrin et al., 1974). A significant decrease in new episodes of otitis occurred in children receiving sulfisoxazole compared with children receiving a placebo. Other studies (Maynard et al., 1972; Biedel, 1978; Schwartz et al., 1982; Liston et al., 1983; Schuller, 1983; Principi et al., 1989) corroborate the results of the Rochester study. The data are persuasive that children who are prone to recurrent episodes of acute infection of the middle ear are benefited by the following program:

1. Enrollment criteria—children who have had three documented episodes of acute otitis media in 6 months or four episodes in 12 months

2. Drugs and dosage—amoxicillin or sulfisoxazole offers the advantages of demonstrated efficacy, safety, and low cost; the drugs can be administered once a day in one half the therapeutic dosage (sulfisoxazole, 50 mg/kg of body weight; amoxicillin, 20 mg/kg)

3. Duration—approximately 6 months, usually during the winter and spring seasons when respiratory tract infections are most frequent

4. Observation—children should be examined at approximately 1-month intervals when free of acute signs to determine if middle ear effusion is present; management of prolonged middle ear effusion should be considered separately from prevention of recurrences of acute infection

Prevention of disease by use of bacterial vaccines has been considered because of the limited number of pathogens responsible for acute otitis media. Since the vast majority of *H. influenzae* strains responsible for otitis media are nontypeable and current vaccines are prepared from type b capsular polysaccharide, prospects for a vaccine against this organism lie in the future. A polyvalent pneumococcal vaccine is effective in prevention of bacteremia and pneumonia due to types of *S. pneumoniae* present in the vaccine.

Use of pneumococcal vaccine for prevention of recurrences of otitis media in Finnish and American children under 2 years of age resulted in fewer episodes of type-specific infection, but the experience of immunized children with acute otitis media was not significantly different than that of children who received only control materials (Makela et al., 1981; Sloyer et al., 1981; Teele et al., 1981). Although some episodes of acute otitis media may be prevented (particularly in children 2 years of age and older, who respond more uniformly to the polysaccharide antigens), the reduction may not be sufficient to alter the experience of children with infections of the middle ear significantly.

REFERENCES

Arola M, Ruuskanen O, Ziegler T, et al. Clinical role of respiratory virus infection in acute otitis media. Pediatrics 1990;86:848-855.

Berman SA, Balkany TJ, Simmons MA. Otitis media in infants less than 12 weeks of age: differing bacteriology among inpatients and outpatients. J Pediatr 1978;93:453.

Biedel CW. Modification of recurrent otitis media by short-term sulfonamide therapy. Am J Dis Child 1978;132:681-683.

Bland RD. Otitis media in the first six weeks of life: diagnosis, bacteriology, and management. Pediatrics 1972;49:187.

Bluestone CD, Klein JO. Otitis media, atelectasis, and eustachian tube dysfunction. In Bluestone CD, Stool S, (eds). Philadelphia: WB Saunders, 1990, pp 372-379.

Bluestone CD, Shurin PA. Middle ear disease in children. Pathogenesis, diagnosis, and management. Pediatr Clin North Am 1974;21:379.

Chonmaitree T, Howie VM, Truant AL. Presence of respiratory viruses in middle ear fluids and nasal wash specimens from children with acute otitis media. Pediatrics 1986;77:698.

Collip PJ. Evaluation of nose drops for otitis media in children. Northwest Med 1961;60:999.

Doern GV, Jorgensen JH, Thornsberry C, et al. National collaborative study of the prevalence of antimicrobial resistance among clinical isolates of Haemophilus influenzae. Antimicrob Agents Chemother 1988;32:180-185.

Fraser JG, Mehta M, Fraser PM. The medical treatment of secretory otitis media: a clinical trial of three commonly used regimens. J Laryngol Otol 1977;91:757.

Fria TJ, Cantekin EI, Eichler JA. Hearing acuity of children with otitis media with effusion. Arch Otolaryngol 1985;111:10-16.

Gates GA, Avery CA, Prihoda TJ, Cooper JC. Effectiveness of adenoidectomy and tympanostomy tubes in the treatment of chronic otitis media with effusion, N Engl J Med 1987;317:1444-1451.

Grönroos JA, et al. The etiology of acute middle ear infection. Acta Otolaryngol 1964;58:149.

Henderson FW, Collier AM, Sanyal MA, et al. A longitudinal study of respiratory viruses and bacteria in the etiology of acute otitis media with effusion. N Engl J Med 1982;306:1377-1383.

Herberts G, Jeppsson PH, Nylen O. Acute otitis media. Pract Otorhinolaryngol 1971;33:191.

Holm VA, Kunze LH. Effect of chronic otitis media on language and speech development. Pediatrics 1969;43:833.

Howie V, Ploussard J, Lester R. Otitis media: a clinical and bacteriologic correlation. Pediatrics 1970;45:29.

Kaplan GJ, et al. Long-term effects of otitis media. A ten-year cohort study of Alaskan Eskimo children. Pediatrics 1973;52:577.

Klein BS, Dollette FR, Yolken RH. The role of respiratory syncytial virus and other viral pathogens in acute otitis media. J Pediatr 1982;101:16-20.

Kovatch AJ, Wald ER, Michaels RH. β-Lactamase-producing Branhamella catarrhalis causing otitis media in children. J Pediatr 1983;102:261-264.

Lewis N. Otitis media and linguistic incompetence. Arch Otolaryngol 1976;102:387.

Liston TE, Foshee WS, Pierson WD. Sulfisoxazole chemoprophylaxis for frequent otitis media. Pediatrics 1983;71:524-530.

Makela PH, Leinonen M, Pukander J, et al. A study of the pneumococcal vaccine in prevention of clinically acute attacks of recurrent otitis media. Rev Infect Dis 1981;3(suppl):124.

Maynard JE, Fleshman JK, Tschopp CF. Otitis media in Alaskan Eskimo children. JAMA 1972;219:597-599.

Needleman H. Effects of hearing loss from early recurrent otitis media on speech and language development. In Jaffee B (ed). Hearing loss in children. Baltimore: University Park Press, 1977.

Olson AL, Klein SW, Charney E, et al. Prevention and therapy of serous otitis media by oral decongestant: a double-blind study in pediatric practice. Pediatrics 1978;61:679.

Paradise JL, Bluestone CD, Rogers KD, et al. Efficacy of adenoidectomy for recurrent otitis media in children previously treated with tympanostomy-tube placement: results of parallel randomized and non-randomized trials. JAMA 1990;263:2066-2073.

Perrin JM, et al. Sulfisoxazole as chemoprophylaxis for recurrent otitis media. A double-blind crossover study in pediatric practice. N Engl J Med 1974;291:664.

Principi N, Marchisio P, Massironi E, et al. Prophylaxis of recurrent acute otitis media and middle-ear effusion: comparison of amoxicillin with sulfamethoxazole and trimethoprim. Am J Dis Child 1989;143:1414-1418.

Schuller DE. Prophylaxis of otitis media in asthmatic children. Pediatr Infect Dis 1983;2:280-283.

Schwartz RH, Puglise J, Rodriguez WJ. Sulfamethoxazole prophylaxis in the otitis media-prone child, Arch Dis Child 1982;57:590-593.

Schwartz RH, Rodriquez WJ. Amoxicillin as the drug of choice for acute otitis media: isn't it time for its reassessment in some areas of the country? Pediatr Infect Dis 1989;8:806-807.

Schwartz R, Rodriguez J, Khan WN, Ross S. Acute purulent otitis media in children older than 5 years: incidence of Haemophilus as a causative organism. JAMA 1977;238:1032.

Shurin PA, Marchant CD, Kim CH, et al. Emergence of beta-lactamase-producing strains of Branhamella catarrhalis as important agents of acute otitis media. Pediatr Infect Dis 1983;2:34-38.

Shurin PA, et al. Bacterial etiology of otitis media during the first six weeks of life. J Pediatr 1978;92:893.

Sloyer JL Jr, Ploussard JH, Howie VM. Efficacy of pneumococcal polysaccharide vaccine in preventing acute otitis media in infants in Huntsville, Alabama. Rev Infect Dis 1981;3(suppl):119.

Sobeslavsky O, et al. The etiological role of *Mycoplasma pneumoniae* in otitis media in children. Pediatrics 1965;35:652.

Teele DW, Klein JO, Greater Boston Collaborative Study Group. Use of pneumococcal vaccine for prevention of recurrent acute otitis media in infants in Boston, Rev Infect Dis 1981;3(suppl):113.

Teele DW, Klein JO, Chase C, et al. Otitis media in infancy and intellectual ability, school achievement, speech, and language at age 7 years. J Infect Dis 1990;162:685-694.

Teele DW, Klein JO, Rosner B. Greater Boston Otitis Media Study Group. Epidemiology of otitis media during the first seven years of life in children in greater Boston: a prospective, cohort study. J Infect Dis 1989;160:83-94.

Tetzlaff TR, Ashworth C, Nelson JD. Otitis media in children less than 12 weeks of age. Pediatrics 1977;59:827.

Tipple MA, Beem MO, Saxon EM: Clinical characteristics of afebrile pneumonia associated with *Chlamydia trachomatis* infections in infants less than 6 months of age. Pediatrics 1979;63:192.

Wald ER, Dashefshy B, Byers et al. Frequency and severity of infections in day care. J Pediatr 1988;112:540-544.

Zinkus PW, Gottlieb MI, Schapiro M. Developmental and psycho-educational sequelae of chronic otitis media. Am J Dis Child 1978;132:1100.

18

PARVOVIRUS INFECTIONS

RUSSELL E. WARE

Viruses within the Parvoviridae family are among the smallest known DNA-containing viruses. Within this family is the genus *Parvovirus*, members of which replicate autonomously (i.e., without assistance from a helper virus) and have a broad vertebrate host range. Parvoviruses have long been recognized as causing illness in small mammals, but only recently have they been identified as causing disease in humans. Parvovirus B19, hereafter referred to as *B19*, is currently the only known human pathogen within the Parvoviridae family of viruses. Over the past 15 years B19 has been implicated in a wide spectrum of both acute and chronic diseases.

Cossart et al. (1975) first reported the presence of the parvovirus in human sera. While screening serum samples for the presence of hepatitis B surface antigen, these investigators found that several specimens (one of which was encoded B19) had small spherical viral particles with many disrupted fragments and empty shells. Serological testing demonstrated that the agent was distinct from hepatitis B virus and that up to 40% of adults had preexisting IgG antibody to the new antigen (Cossart et al., 1975; Paver and Clarke, 1976). The virus subsequently was categorized by genetic and biochemical analysis as belonging within the genus *Parvovirus* (Summers et al., 1983).

As a new viral agent not associated with any particular disease, B19 initially was a mysterious human pathogen. However, the availability of serological tests for B19 infection allowed screening of sera from patients and soon led to the identification of several categories of human disease caused by this agent.

CLINICAL MANIFESTATIONS OF PARVOVIRUS B19

The clinical manifestations of B19 infection are protean and are discussed as separate entities. However, infection may cause more than one disease manifestation in a given patient. Experimental infection in normal volunteers (Anderson et al., 1985) has demonstrated that illness can occur during both the acute viremic phase and the convalescent phase when immune mechanisms contribute to the pathogenesis of disease. It is currently believed that as many as 20% of infected persons have subclinical illness.

Erythrocyte aplasia

The clinical illness known as the *transient aplastic crisis* is a temporary cessation of erythrocyte production that is usually diagnosed in patients with hemolytic anemia. In this condition the patient has mild respiratory symptoms followed by the onset of fatigue, pallor, and worsening anemia. The peripheral hemoglobin concentration may fall below 4 g/dl, with no compensatory increase in reticulocytes, but the white blood cell and platelet counts remain normal. The patient typically recovers within a week and does not have a recurrence.

In the early 1980s two teams of investigators (Pattison et al., 1981; Serjeant et al., 1981) discovered that the majority of patients with sickle cell disease and transient aplastic crisis had acute B19 infection (i.e., detectable B19 viremia but no specific B19 antibody). Transient erythrocyte aplasia was also reported in patients with a variety of other hemolytic anemias, suggesting that B19 might have a tropism for actively dividing erythroid bone marrow precursors. Mortimer et al. (1983a) demonstrated that B19 inhibited in vitro erythroid colony formation and was directly cytotoxic to the progenitor erythroid cell. The successful propagation of B19 with the erythroid fraction of human bone marrow was reported by Ozawa et al. (1986, 1987).

The proposed pathophysiology of the aplastic crisis involves the infection of erythroid progenitor cells by B19, with subsequent reticulocytopenia and anemia; presumably only patients with accelerated rates of erythropoiesis would develop signs and symptoms of anemia. The production of specific B19 antibody leads to clearance of the virus and resolution of the illness. Patients with immunodeficiency, either primary (Kurtzman et al., 1987) or secondary to suppressive chemotherapy (Van Horn et al., 1986), can develop chronic hypoplastic anemia as a result of prolonged viremia associated with an inability to form specific IgG antibody to B19.

Erythema infectiosum (fifth disease)

Erythema infectiosum is a mildly contagious childhood illness associated with a characteristic rash and mild constitutional symptoms. The illness typically begins with the sudden onset of an erythematous face (so-called "slapped-cheek" appearance), followed by a generalized lacy maculopapular rash on the extremities and trunk. The rash remains evanescent over several weeks, particularly if the skin is irritated or exposed to sunlight. Erythema infectiosum occurs in outbreaks, particularly within families or schools, and is believed contagious upon close contact with affected individuals.

Several investigators (Anderson et al., 1984; Plummer et al., 1985; Nunoue et al., 1985) clearly established an epidemiological link between erythema infectiosum and parvovirus B19 infection. In most cases of erythema infectiosum, however, B19 viremia could not be demonstrated, although IgM antibodies to B19 routinely were detected. Erythema infectiosum therefore can be considered an immune-mediated illness, probably in part as a result of circulating immune complexes of B19 virus and antibody.

Arthropathy

Whereas erythema infectiosum is the common clinical presentation of parvovirus B19 infection in otherwise healthy children, acute arthritis is the more typical presentation in affected adults. Two large studies (White et al., 1985; Reid et al., 1985) demonstrated that the joint manifestations mainly affect women and consist of a symmetrical polyarthritis of the wrists, hands, knees, and ankles. The pathophysiology presumably is immune mediated because it temporally occurs 2 to 4 weeks after infection, with the development of IgG antibodies against B19. The prognosis for patients with B19 arthropathy is generally good, although chronic cases have been described.

Fetal infection

The issues surrounding transplacental infection with parvovirus B19 are not completely resolved at this time. B19 can infect the developing fetus and cause fatal nonimmune hydrops (Knott et al., 1984; Brown et al., 1984). The demonstration of B19 DNA in a variety of fetal tissues (Bond et al., 1986; Porter et al., 1988) suggests a complex pathophysiology, but severe erythroid aplasia and perhaps direct myocardial infection contribute to the hydropic fetal demise.

Important and controversial issues concerning B19 infection relate to the risk of transplacental infection of the fetus (Anand et al., 1987; Woernle et al., 1987; Kinney et al., 1988; Ware, 1989; Anderson, 1990). Reports of fetal demise clearly have documented that B19 infection can have a fatal outcome but have not allowed an estimate of the true fetal risks of B19 infection. In 1989 the Centers for Disease Control offered the following guidelines and risk estimates: approximately 50% of adults are already seropositive to B19, and parvovirus B19 is not highly contagious; therefore the chance of maternal infection during an outbreak of B19 infection is 15% to 25%, depending on the nature of the exposure. After maternal infection the fetus has only a 10% chance of acquiring the virus transplacentally, for a maximal risk of fetal death after maternal exposure of 1.5% to 2.5%.

A recent study from Great Britain (Hall et al., 1990) has refined this estimate by documenting that most B19-infected pregnant women do not suffer fetal loss and that fetal infection is not necessarily fatal. This study indicated that after maternal B19 infection, the rate of transplacental transmission is 33% and the risk of fetal death caused by B19 in an infected pregnancy is 9%.

At this time it is recommended that an exposed pregnant woman be tested for IgG antibodies to document previous infection. If the woman is at risk, serial ultrasonography and maternal serum α-fetoprotein measurements should be performed (Carrington et al., 1987; Bernstein and Capeless, 1989). Intrauterine blood transfusions have been used successfully in affected hydropic fetuses (Schwartz et al., 1988), but the benefits of this clinical approach have not been proved. The use of intravenous immunoglobulin to provide specific B19 antibodies has not been reported for this setting.

Immunocompromised hosts

Chronic and/or severe anemia from parvovirus B19 infection has been documented in patients with altered immune function. Prolonged infection has been reported in patients with congenital immunodeficiency (Kurtzman et al., 1987; Kurtzman et al., 1989) and also in patients with immune defects acquired after antineoplastic therapy (Van Horn et al., 1986; Kurtzman et al., 1988), bone marrow transplantation (Weiland et al., 1989), or infection with the human immunodeficiency virus (Frickhofen et al., 1990; Griffin et al., 1991). Typical findings include chronic erythroid hypoplasia with prolonged viremia and IgM antibodies, with no specific IgG antibodies present. Therapy with intravenous immunoglobulin has been tried in this clinical setting with some success (Kurtzman et al., 1989), probably by providing B19 antibody titers sufficient for temporary clearance of the viremia.

Experimental infection

Much of the clinical information about pathogenesis and mechanisms of B19 infection has been derived from studies involving healthy human volunteers. A study by Anderson et al. (1985) demonstrated that 1 week after intranasal inoculation of parvovirus B19, constitutional symptoms (e.g., fever, malaise, and pruritus) developed coincident with the presence of high titers of B19 virus in the blood and nasopharynx. At this same time erythroid progenitors in the bone marrow were becoming depleted as a result of direct viral infection and cytolysis (Potter et al., 1987). Two weeks after exposure, specific IgM could be detected in all previously seronegative volunteers, and effects on the peripheral blood counts were noted. Reticulocytopenia and slight leukopenia and thrombocytopenia typically occurred but resolved within 1 week. By the third week after exposure specific IgG could be detected, and patients developed the arthritis and rash typical of immune-complex disease (Anderson et al., 1985).

ROUTES OF TRANSMISSION

Previous epidemiological studies of erythema infectiosum suggested that parvovirus B19 is spread from person to person by droplet infection, as a result of the occurrence of outbreaks among people in close physical contact such as schoolmates or family members. The study on healthy volunteers by Anderson et al. (1985) documented viral isolation in blood and nasopharyngeal secretions, with no detectable virus in urine or stool. A recent study (Bell et al., 1989) documented that hospital workers are at risk of contracting nosocomial B19 infection from patients with erythrocyte aplasia and suggested that respiratory and contact isolation be used for these hospitalized patients.

Transmission of parvovirus B19 has also been documented to occur following coagulation factor replacement therapy (Mortimer et al., 1983b), although heat treatment may reduce the incidence of infection. Viral transmission has not been reported but is theoretically possible after routine erythrocyte transfusions or organ transplantation.

DIAGNOSIS

Identification of parvovirus B19 infection initially depended on the visualization of viral particles in the serum by electron microscopy (Cossart et al., 1975). Subsequent tests used parvovirus B19 antisera for the detection of B19 viral antigens (Cohen et al., 1983; Anderson et al., 1986). The construction of a cloned molecular B19 nucleotide probe (Clewley, 1985) allowed the detection of B19 DNA in blood cells and specific tissues. The highly sensitive polymerase chain reaction test has been used for the detection of B19 DNA in clinical specimens (Clewley, 1989).

The determination of antibody response to B19 infection has been another important tool in the diagnosis of disease and in the identification of patients with either acute or chronic B19 infection. Assays are available for both IgM and IgG responses to B19 (Anderson et al., 1986). In acute infection the patient typically will develop specific IgM antibody to B19 during the second week after inoculation, then develop IgG antibody by the third week (Anderson et al., 1985).

Antibody titers may be obtained through state health departments and the Centers for Disease Control in Atlanta, Georgia.

DIFFERENTIAL DIAGNOSIS

Erythema infectiosum may be confused with rubella on occasion, but ordinarily the facial appearance and reticular rash on the extremities is so characteristic it is diagnostic.

COMPLICATIONS

Complications of erythema infectiosum are extremely unusual in children. Adults, especially females, may develop arthritis that may last for months and rarely may become chronic. Immunocompromised patients, who may develop prolonged viremia, may develop a protracted, severe anemia.

THERAPY

The only specific therapy currently available is intravenous immunoglobulin. Since most B19 infections are self-limited, therapy mainly has been used in immunocompromised patients with prolonged anemia for whom red blood cell transfusions may also be necessary. Intrauterine transfusion in the setting of fetal hydrops has been described but is of unknown utility.

PREVENTION

Preventive measures have not yet become available.

REFERENCES

Anand A, Gray ES, Brown T, et al. Human parvovirus infection in pregnancy and hydrops fetalis. N Engl J Med 1987;316:183.

Anderson LJ. Human parvoviruses. J Infect Dis 1990;161:603.

Anderson LJ, Tsou C, Parker RA, et al. Detection of antibodies and antigens of human parvovirus B19 by enzyme-linked immunosorbent assay. J Clin Microbiol 1986;24:522.

Anderson MJ, Higgins PG, Davis LR, et al. Experimental parvoviral infection in humans. J Infect Dis 1985;152:257.

Anderson MJ, Lewis E, Kidd IM, et al. An outbreak of erythema infectiosum associated with human parvovirus infection. Epidemiol Infect 1984;93:83.

Bell LM, Naides SJ, Stoffman P, et al. Human parvovirus B19 infection among hospital staff members after contact with infected patients. N Engl J Med 1989;321:485.

Bernstein IM, Capeless EL. Elevated maternal serum alpha-fetoprotein and hydrops fetalis in association with fetal parvovirus B-19 infection. Obstet Gynecol 1989;74:456.

Bond PR, Caul EO, Usher J, et al. Intrauterine infection with human parvovirus (letter). Lancet 1986;1:448.

Brown T, Anand A, Ritchie LD, et al. Intrauterine parvovirus infection associated with hydrops fetalis (letter). Lancet 1984;2:1033.

Carrington D, Gilmore DH, Whittle MJ, et al. Maternal serum α-fetoprotein—a marker of fetal aplastic crisis during intrauterine human parvovirus infection. Lancet 1987;1:433.

Centers for Disease Control. Risks associated with human parvovirus B19 infection. MMWR 1989;38:81.

Clewley JP. Detection of human parvovirus using a molecularly cloned probe. J Med Virol 1985;15:173.

Clewley JP. Polymerase chain reaction assay of parvovirus B19 DNA in clinical specimens. J Clin Microbiol 1989;27:2647.

Cohen BJ, Mortimer PP, Pereira MS. Diagnostic assays with monoclonal antibodies for the human serum parvovirus-like virus (SPLV). J Hyg 1983;91:113.

Cossart YE, Cant B, Field AM, et al. Parvovirus-like particles in human sera. Lancet 1975;1:72.

Frickhofen N, Abkowitz JL, Safford M, et al. Persistent B19 parvovirus infection in patients infected with human immunodeficiency virus Type 1 (HIV-1): a treatable cause of anemia in AIDS. Ann Intern Med 1990;113:926.

Griffin TC, Squires JE, Timmons CF, et al. Chronic human parvovirus B19-induced erythrocyte hypoplasia as the initial manifestation of human immunodeficiency virus infection. J Pediatr 1991;118:899.

Hall SM and Public Health Laboratory Service Working Party on Fifth Disease. Prospective study of human parvovirus (B19) infection in pregnancy. Br Med J 1990;300:1166.

Kinney JS, Anderson JL, Farrar J, et al. Risk of adverse outcomes of pregnancy after human parvovirus B19 infection. J Infect Dis 1988;157:663.

Knott PD, Welply GAC, Anderson MJ. Serologically proved intrauterine infection with parvovirus (letter). Br Med J 1984;289:1660.

Antigens

Among the many bacteria that affect humans, *B. pertussis* has been one of the most difficult to study in terms of its biological anatomy. Indeed, only in the last 15 years or so has it been possible to dissect the organism and relate its various components to disease pathogenesis and immunity in man, although as yet imperfectly. Previously, various physiological effects and attributes of the organism, recognized in the laboratory and to some extent in man, could not be assigned to identifiable components. Therefore from the clinical standpoint the development of an effective subcellular pertussis vaccine, free of potentially toxic components irrelevant to immunity, could not be pursued on any logical scientific basis until recently. A brief review of the constituents of the organism and their probable or possible roles in disease pathogenesis and immunity follows.

A component of *B. pertussis* assigned considerable importance in the pathogenesis and immunology of pertussis has been variously designated *lymphocytosis promoting factor (LPF)*, *pertussis toxin*, or *pertussigen*, with the first term used most commonly. The existence of this component has long been recognized because of its physiological actions, identified in man and in laboratory animals; however, only in the last 15 years has it become evident that these actions are produced by a single molecule. LPF is associated with the production of lymphocytosis in man and experimental animals. It is also the histamine sensitizing factor (HSF), the effect of which has been long recognized in experimental animals, although this effect is of no apparent consequence in man. LPF also stimulates the release of insulin in man and animals; in animals, but not in man, significant hypoglycemia results. LPF has a variety of other actions, including mitogenicity in the laboratory and hemagglutination (Wardlaw and Parton, 1988).

It is likely that LPF plays an important role in the pathogenesis of pertussis. Although sometimes designated as a toxin, it exerts its major effects locally on the host. It appears to facilitate attachment of the organism to respiratory cilia and is an important contributor to respiratory mucosal damage. LPF is immunogenic and is a major factor in the induction of immunity in the mouse protection test, which is used as the standard measure of potency for whole-cell pertussis vaccines. Antibodies to LPF develop in humans after infection or immunization, and it is highly probable that antibodies to LPF are important in clinical immunity to pertussis.

Filamentous hemagglutinin (FHA) is an antigen that apparently plays a single role, that of facilitating attachment of the organism to respiratory cilia, in disease pathogenesis and clinical immunity. It is nontoxic for cells. FHA is vigorously immunogenic, producing measurable antibodies (as does LPF), and there is evidence that these antibodies contribute to clinical protection against pertussis.

Strains of the genus *Bordetella* produce a number of agglutinating capsular antigens. Agglutinogens 1 through 6 are found only in strains of *B. pertussis;* agglutinogen 7 is found in all three members of the genus; and factors 14 and 12 occur in *B. parapertussis* and *B. bronchiseptica*, respectively. These agglutinogens apparently are not active in the pathogenesis of pertussis. However, they are immunogenic, and there is seroepidemiological evidence that they (or some component closely associated with them) play a role in inducing clinical immunity to pertussis. This evidence derives from studies in the United Kingdom that suggested that efficacy of whole-cell pertussis vaccines depends on a match between the agglutinogens present in the vaccine strain and those in strains circulating in the community (Public Health Laboratory Service, 1973).

Another component of the organism that has attracted recent attention, particularly in relation to its potential role as a protective antigen, is the 69K outer membrane protein, so named because of its molecular weight. The 69K protein is closely associated with, or may be identical to, agglutinogen 1. It is of interest because serum antibodies to it are found after disease or immunization with the whole-cell vaccine, and these antibodies are protective against respiratory infection with *B. pertussis* in mice (Shahin et al., 1990).

Adenylate cyclase is a cellular enzyme that disrupts host cell metabolism and very likely participates in ciliary destruction. It is also immunogenic, but there is no evidence to date that antibodies to this enzyme play a role in clinical immunity.

Another identified component of the organism is tracheal toxin, which very likely plays a role in cell damage. A relatively small molecule, tracheal toxin is not immunogenic. A heat-labile toxin, also known as dermonecrotic toxin, is also produced. It is lethal when given systemically and produces dermonecrosis. It appears to play no role in clinical immunity, and whether or how it participates in the pathogenesis of the disease is unknown.

In common with other gram-negative bacteria, B. pertussis produces an endotoxin. Compared to the endotoxins of enteric bacilli, the toxicity of this lipopolysaccharide is weak, being one tenth to one one-hundredth as potent. It is not immunogenic, and there is no evidence that it participates in the pathogenesis of the disease.

EPIDEMIOLOGY

Pertussis is highly contagious, transmitted primarily by intimate respiratory contact. Nearly all nonimmune, exposed household contacts acquire the disease, and approximately 50% of susceptible individuals exposed in school settings develop pertussis. Because there is no effective transplacental immunity, young infants, in whom the disease is most dangerous, are fully susceptible.

In the absence of immunization it is likely that no person escapes pertussis. Curiously, the disease is more often reported in girls than in boys, and mortality rates are higher in girls. An explanation for this phenomenon is not evident; it may be, given that almost every unimmunized child acquires pertussis, that the disease is inexplicably more severe and therefore more recognizable, and thus reported, in females. In the past pertussis was both endemic and epidemic; major increases in incidence occurred every 3 or 4 years (usually 3). Widespread immunization has not altered this cyclic pattern, although incidence rates, both endemic and peak, are strikingly lower (Cherry, 1984).

Seasonal influences on the incidence of pertussis in the United States are difficult to interpret. National data for the prevaccine era do not exist, and there is no unanimity among descriptions of the seasonal epidemiology of pertussis before widespread use of the vaccine. Some reports indicated higher incidence in the summer when young infants probably were in more contact with each other. Others stated that the peak incidence was in late winter and early spring, and some alleged no seasonal variation. However, examination of tabulated deaths from pertussis by month for the 5 years 1936 through 1940, allowing a 4- to 8-week lag between onset and date of death, provides support for the assertion that the incidence of pertussis was highest during the first half of the calendar year, at least in younger children, the group most likely to succumb from the disease. Closer examination of these mortality data shows that this seasonal variation was accounted for by the 2 years (1937 and 1938) when deaths were the highest (70% greater than the other 3 years). Recorded deaths for the 3 years with fewer deaths show no month-to-month variation. This suggests that in colder, temperate zones such as the United States pertussis was endemic year-round before the advent of widespread immunization and that epidemic whooping cough was more apt to occur in the winter and spring. Remarkably, the seasonal epidemiology of pertussis is presently very different. Examination of the annual summaries published by the Centers for Disease Control for the years 1979 through 1989 shows that the disease is reported two to five times as frequently in the latter 6 months of the year as in the first half. Although these data comprise the dates that cases are reported, this observation remains valid when cases are tabulated by dates of onset (Cochi, 1991). No explanation is available for the past and current seasonality of pertussis or for the apparent shift.

There have also been remarkable changes in the age distribution of pertussis from the prevaccine era to the present, but these changes very likely are explained by widespread immunization beginning in the 1950s. Before World War II approximately half of all reported cases occurred in elementary school-age children, who served as the major reservoir of the disease. Less than 20% of cases occurred in infants under 1 year of age, but 50% to 70% of all deaths occurred in this age group. Preschool children, age 1 to 4 years, accounted for another 40% of cases, but the mortality rate was lower than in infants. With some state-to-state variation, 40% to 55% of reported cases were in children 5 to 14 years. Fewer than 1% of reported cases occurred in individuals older than 14 years (Dauer, 1943).

The present age distribution of whooping cough in the United States has changed markedly, very likely as a consequence of several in-

Table 19-1. Age distribution of reported pertussis cases in the United States, 1979-1981 and 1987-1989

		Percent by age group in years				
Year	Total cases	<1	1-4	5-14	15-19	>19
1979-1981	4,601	56	26	12	2	4
1987-1989	10,430	46	26	12	7	9

Data from Centers for Disease Control from annual summaries published in the *Morbidity and Mortality Weekly Report* for the respective years.

terrelated factors. The first is widespread immunization against the disease. A second factor is the requirement for immunization before school entry in the United States. In some states this requirement includes day-care and preschool classes, but in most states immunization requirements are initiated on entry into elementary school. A factor of indeterminable impact is possible enhanced recognition and reporting of pertussis as a result of augmented interest in the disease and better diagnostic methods. Finally, it is increasingly recognized that pertussis occurs in adolescents and young adults, ranging from mild atypical cases to the full-blown syndrome (Mortimer, 1990). Whether this phenomenon has always existed and has only come to attention because of decreased rates of pertussis in other age groups, is a consequence of waning of vaccine-induced immunity resulting from the comparative decline of the incidence of pertussis and the consequent lack of reinforcement of immunity caused by casual exposure to the disease, and/ or results from better laboratory methods for diagnosis is uncertain. It is logical to assume, but not proven, that these adult infections, whether mild or severe, represent important sources of continuing transmission of *B. pertussis*. Table 19-1 compares the age distributions of pertussis for 1979 through 1981 and 1987 through 1989 in the United States. Because there is firm evidence that partially immune adolescents and young adults with pertussis often exhibit mild symptoms, these data probably underestimate the true incidence of infection in older persons. Whatever the reasons, the striking reductions in pertussis morbidity and mortality in the United States have been associated with clear-cut changes in the age distribution of reported cases.

Determining the effects of race on pertussis epidemiology is complicated by a number of factors. In the late 1930s overall pertussis mortality rates for blacks strikingly exceeded those for whites (Dauer, 1943). This was in part due to the fact that disease incidence rates for blacks were considerably higher in infants and very young children, who are at highest risk of death, than for whites. Additionally, age-specific mortality rates for blacks were higher in all age groups. These differences in morbidity and mortality are undoubtedly explained in large part by socioeconomic status. Curiously, the overall mortality rate from pertussis was always higher in rural areas in the United States; it is likely that this is in part explained by very high mortality rates in blacks in the rural South. These differences persisted through the first decade or two of the pertussis vaccine era, probably for similar reasons and because of lower rates of immunization in blacks, related to socioeconomic status. It is therefore unlikely that any differences in morbidity and mortality by race are related to race per se (Dauer, 1943).

PATHOLOGY

The pathological findings in patients with pertussis are primarily bronchopulmonary; changes in other organs are of anoxic origin stemming from bronchopulmonary damage. The key changes are bronchial and bronchiolar, with ciliary damage and destruction, edema, the accumulation of mucoid secretions, and relatively little inflammatory infiltration. Secondary findings are bronchiolar obstruction, atelectasis, areas of bronchopneumonia, and, occasionally, spotty emphysematous changes. Pneumothorax is uncommon, and secondary bacterial pneumonia such as lobar pneumonia is extremely rare. Mortality from pertussis relates directly to the severity of pulmonary involvement (Lapin, 1943).

Secondary findings occur mainly in the brain and are of two varieties. The first comprises edema and other findings characteristic of anoxia. Hemorrhages constitute the other cerebral changes. They may be moderately extensive but more often are small, including petechiae.

PATHOGENESIS

Knowledge of the actions of the various components of B. pertussis permits the development of an hypothesis about the series of pathological events that occur in the course of whooping cough. Because the likelihood of infection varies directly with the intimacy and duration of contact, it is probable that large numbers of organisms are required to infect the respiratory tract. Attachment of organisms to respiratory cilia is facilitated by LPF and FHA. After attachment it is necessary for the organism to evade host defenses; major roles in this process are presumably played by LPF and adenylate cyclase. It is logical that tracheal toxin and dermonecrotic toxin participate. Cell damage is a consequence of the actions of LPF and adenylate cyclase. It is probable that tracheal and dermonecrotic toxins also contribute (Wardlaw and Parton, 1988).

The role of the 69K protein is uncertain; it may relate to cell adherence. There is no evidence that agglutinogens play a role in pathogenesis. Similarly, there is no evidence that the rather weak endotoxin of B. pertussis contributes to disease manifestations (Wardlaw and Parton, 1988).

An obvious contribution of LPF is induction of the characteristic lymphocytosis of pertussis. There is no evidence that LPF induces histamine stimulation of clinical consequence during the illness, nor does the insulin-stimulating activity exert any clinically recognizable effect in man. B. pertussis is noninvasive; accordingly, all the manifestations of pertussis except lymphocytosis may be explained by the unique effects on respiratory endothelium with disruption of function or cell death (Wardlaw and Parton, 1988).

As a consequence of ciliary destruction or dysfunction, the normal toilet of the pulmonary tree is compromised. The processes that remove foreign material, cell debris, and secretions are im-

paired, resulting in the accumulation of more difficult-to-expel mucoid secretions, thus compounding the problem. Retained secretions obstruct smaller bronchi and bronchioles, with consequent atelectasis and occasional emphysema. Nonspecific bronchopneumonia occurs frequently.

The thick ropy secretions that accumulate are very difficult to expel, resulting in episodes of repetitious, continuous coughing, often followed by vomiting. The mechanism of vomiting is probably the accumulation of this viscid material in the pharynx. The characteristic whoop follows a protracted spasm that has nearly emptied the bronchopulmonary tree of air and represents an attempt to inspire through vocal cords that may be partially narrowed because of secretions and consequent spasm. Indeed, it may well be that in some instances inspiration is possible only when some relaxation of vocal chords occurs as a result of severe anoxia.

The mechanism of the encephalopathy, often with permanent brain damage or death, that sometimes occurs in the course of pertussis was the subject of considerable debate in the past. A hypothesis often voiced was that one or another toxic product of B. pertussis was responsible. No such toxin has been identified; currently, there is general consensus that encephalopathy during the course of pertussis is explained by anoxia engendered by the episodes of paroxysmal coughing and, in some instances, by cerebral hemorrhages of varying extent that result from the combination of increased intracranial pressure during paroxysms and the vascular effects of anoxia.

In those children who die of pertussis there are three apparent mechanisms of death that often act in concert. Severe bronchopulmonary disease with bronchopneumonia is of major importance. Often associated with it is the above-described central nervous system damage. In the past, and perhaps in the developing world today, inanition secondary to repeated emesis following spasms of coughing was undoubtedly a major factor in mortality from whooping cough in infants and children. Additionally, in the past in the United States and presently in the developing world, other underlying disorders such as low birth rate, malnutrition, gastrointestinal infections, and other debilitating conditions, including measles and severe respiratory illnesses, strongly compromise survival of infants and children with whooping cough.

CLINICAL MANIFESTATIONS

The incubation period of pertussis is between 7 and 13 days. In some partially immune individuals it may be a few days longer. The initial symptoms are nonspecific. Throughout the course of the disease fever is absent or low. There may be mild coryza-like symptoms, plus a mild, dry cough. The cough progresses in frequency and severity, and approximately 2 weeks after onset, spells of paroxysmal coughing are recognized. The paroxysms progress in severity and frequency; ultimately, dozens of such spells may occur daily. As the paroxysms increase, the characteristic whoop occurs, often followed by vomiting. With severe paroxysms cyanosis often occurs, the eyes roll back, and the child may appear semiconscious. When a paroxysm terminates, it appears that the respiratory tract has been nearly emptied of air; the characteristic whoop is produced by the initial attempt to inspire through the glottis, which may be narrowed by spasm caused by the irritative effects of the secretions and the cough. The vomiting apparently is a consequence of thick mucoid secretions in the pharynx. Frequently, a series of paroxysms may occur in immediate succession. Severe paroxysms are very frightening to the child and to all observers. After a severe episode the child appears exhausted. In full-blown pertussis paroxysms with whooping usually persist at least 2 weeks and may continue for 6 weeks. The paroxysms frequently are precipitated by a variety of events such as feeding, crying, or even hearing another person cough; in the past when several children with pertussis were in the same hospital room, a paroxysm in one child would precipitate episodes in others. In convalescence the cough gradually disappears over a month or more, although minor exacerbations may occur with exertion or in the course of an intercurrent respiratory infection.

The two major and potentially lethal complications of pertussis, bronchopneumonia and encephalopathy, are most apt to occur at the height of the paroxysmal stage. In patients with severe whooping cough it may be difficult to maintain adequate intake of fluid and nourishment be-cause of the vicious cycle of feeding inducing paroxysms and vomiting. In the past when the incidence of whooping cough was high, particularly in infants, some nurses in contagious disease hospitals were highly valued for their skill and patience in feeding and refeeding infants with severe whooping cough.

DIAGNOSIS

The clinical picture of full-blown pertussis is so characteristic that the disease is readily suspected and recognized by physicians, other health-care personnel, and grandmothers who have had prior experience with its manifestations, particularly if a paroxysm is observed. The presence of pertussis in the community or a history of exposure provides strongly supportive evidence; however, the source of infection may be an individual with a mild, atypical illness, particularly a household member with waning immunity. Also strongly supportive of the diagnosis is absolute lymphocytosis, which is usually present at the beginning of the paroxysmal stage and persists for 3 or 4 weeks (Fig. 19-1).

Proof of the diagnosis of pertussis is achieved by recovery of the organism on culture (Onorato and Wassilak, 1987). The organism is most readily recovered during the catarrhal stage but disappears within 2 or 3 weeks after the onset of paroxysms (Fig. 19-1). The best source of material for culture is nasopharyngeal mucus obtained by the use of a transnasal swab. Use of cough plates, often the practice in the past, is less frequently successful.

Isolation of *B. pertussis* depends on careful transport and efficient processing of the materials obtained for culture and is particularly enhanced if the clinical microbiologist is experienced with the organism. If the specimen will not be planted for 1 to 2 hours, the swab should be placed in 0.25 to 0.50 ml of casamino acids solution with a pH of 7.2 to prevent drying of the swab. When the specimen will be shipped to another laboratory or when holding time exceeds 2 hours, other organisms may overgrow *B. pertussis*. Therefore swabs should be placed in modified Stuart's medium or Mishulow's charcoal agar. These media are better able to maintain the viability of organisms and to support the growth under the conditions of transport, but there is a decreased recovery rate of *B. pertussis*

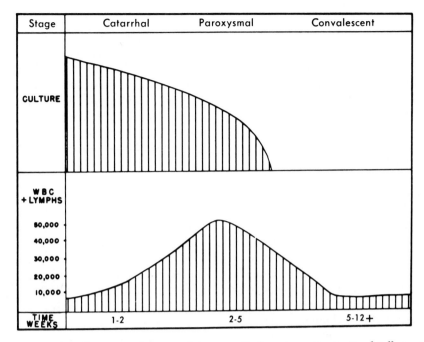

Fig. 19-1. Diagram illustrating diagnostic laboratory findings in pertussis. *Bordetella pertussis* may be recovered, usually during catarrhal and early paroxysmal stages (first 4 weeks of illness). The white blood cell count usually is elevated during the paroxysmal stage (second to fifth weeks). Lymphocytes predominate.

from transport media as compared to direct inoculation. Modified Bordet-Gengou agar is recommended for primary isolation of the organism. The addition of 0.25 to 0.5 unit/ml of penicillin to a second plate is useful in inhibiting the growth of the gram-positive flora of the respiratory tract without affecting growth of *B. pertussis* organisms.

In addition to a specific pattern of biochemical reactions, serological identification of *B. pertussis* will confirm the isolation. A slide agglutination test can be performed with a standard inoculum of organisms and specific antiserum, which is available commercially (Onorato and Wassilak, 1987).

Fluorescent antibody (FA) staining has been used to identify *B. pertussis* from direct smears of nasopharyngeal swabs and for identification of organisms growing on Bordet-Gengou plates. The FA examination of nasopharyngeal swab material is often unreliable even in experienced hands. The FA procedure cannot substitute for cultural isolation of the organism, but it can offer the advantage of more rapid laboratory identification of organisms after isolation. The Ana-

lytical Bacteriology Section of the Centers for Disease Control and many of the state bacteriology laboratories are prepared to culture and/or examine secretions by FA techniques for *B. pertussis*.

At present, assessment of antibodies in the serum is usually accomplished by measuring agglutinins. Few laboratories in the United States are prepared to perform tests for *B. pertussis* agglutinin titers. The current microagglutination tests give titers that have not been correlated with protection against disease. Since these agglutinins are not the protective antibodies, they give only an indirect assessment of immunity, although they do assess experience with *B. pertussis* as an infection or as a vaccine. After infection, there may be only a slight rise in agglutinins, and it tends to occur weeks into the illness. An acute and convalescent pair of sera is needed to define an antibody rise that is indicative of recent contact with antigen.

Other generally available, specific, and reliable serological measures of infection with *B. pertussis* are needed. Specific tests for antibodies to LPF and FHA have been developed, and enzyme-linked immunosorbent assays (ELISAs) for IgG, IgM, and IgA antibodies correlate well with infection and are of considerable use in recognizing culture-negative pertussis, including mild or asymptomatic infections (Granstrom et al., 1988; Steketee et al., 1988). As yet, however, these tests are not available for routine use.

Most instances of the whooping cough syndrome in infants and children represents true pertussis, particularly during outbreaks, although on rare occasions other disorders may mimic whooping cough and result in confusion. Parapertussis, caused by a somewhat similar organism, is usually a milder illness but with many of the same symptoms. Certain viral infections, notably those caused by adenoviruses and *Chlamydia*, may mimic the disease. Confusion occasionally arises in some children with bronchiolitis or protracted bronchopneumonia. Previously unrecognized cystic fibrosis may cause confusion as may respiratory foreign bodies. In the past tuberculosis with hilar nodes pressing on the trachea or bronchi occasionally resulted in similar symptoms. Ordinarily, however, there is little confusion, but other conditions should be suspected when confirmatory or supportive evidence such as a positive culture, lymphocytosis, and epidemiological linkage to another case or to an outbreak is lacking.

More important than misclassifying other conditions as pertussis at the present time is the problem of failure to diagnose pertussis in cases that are mild or atypical as a consequence of waning immunity. Such mild illnesses may display no characteristics that distinguish them from a wide variety of other, more common respiratory disorders, and pertussis is not suspected. Mild cases in older siblings or parents in a household are often recognized retrospectively when an infant, as yet unimmunized, develops full-blown whooping cough. In individuals with mild disease the diagnosis, even if suspected early, may be difficult to make. The organism may be more difficult to recover on culture, either because of the lack of copious respiratory secretions or because the number of organisms is small. Additionally, lymphocytosis may be inhibited by residual antibody to LPF. Nonetheless, such individuals appear to constitute a major reservoir for pertussis and a source of infection for others.

COMPLICATIONS

There are three major complications of pertussis: respiratory problems, effects on the central nervous system, and malnutrition. Respiratory complications usually comprise varying degrees of atelectasis and nonspecific bronchopneumonia. Localized emphysema may occur, but pneumothorax is rare. True lobar pneumonia is uncommon. In the past 90% of deaths caused by pertussis resulted from pulmonary complications; this proportion is no doubt reduced considerably at present by modern measures of intensive care, including mechanical ventilation and, perhaps, antimicrobial therapy.

Central nervous system complications occur rarely in the course of pertussis, particularly during the paroxysmal stage, and they may be severe (Litvak et al., 1948). They apparently are secondary to anoxia and/or cerebral hemorrhages that are usually petechial but may be larger. The clinical findings are those of nonspecific encephalopathy, usually including repeated convulsions and obtundation. Visual disturbances and paralyses may occur. Central nervous system complications are most frequent in young infants. Estimates of the precise risk of encephalopathy associated with whooping cough are quite imprecise because they are based on hospitalized cases and do not include in the denominator the much larger numbers of children with pertussis who do not require hospitalization. However, from two populations in which it was possible to estimate the total number of cases of pertussis, the apparent risks of severe encephalopathy were 1:11,000 and 1:12,500 (Litvak et al., 1948; Miller et al., 1985). Undoubtedly the risk is markedly age dependent; it is probably negligible in older children and much higher in young infants. Permanent sequelae, with seizure disorders, developmental retardation, and pareses, frequently ensue. There is also evidence, mostly but not all anecdotal, that milder forms of encephalopathy, insufficiently severe to warrant hospitalization, exist and may be associated with more subtle neurological disturbances, including developmental disorders.

In the past in the United States malnutrition secondary to repeated vomiting and sometimes progressing to inanition was a major problem, particularly in infants. It remains as a serious complication in developing countries where it is often superimposed on or concomitant with other debilitating factors. The combination of large populations of unimmunized children with consequently high rates of pertussis and high case-fatality rates explains the excessive mortality from whooping cough in these countries.

Minor complications of pertussis include otitis media and hemorrhagic phenomena such as epistaxis, petechiae, and subconjunctival bleeding. In infants and children young enough to have lower incisors, ulceration of the frenum may occur because of protrusion of the tongue during coughing spells. Occasionally, a hernia may become manifest because of increased abdominal pressure during coughing spells, and rarely, prolapse of the rectum occurs.

PROGNOSIS

In the United States the mortality rate has declined remarkably since the turn of the century. At that time approximately one of every 200 children born alive died of pertussis before the fifth birthday; in the last decade this risk has been reduced to no more than one in 500,000. This decline cannot be attributed solely to the advent of pertussis vaccines; indeed, by the late 1930s, before pertussis vaccine was available, the mortality rate from pertussis in young children had declined approximately 80% from 1900. This remarkable decline by 1940 must be attributed to a decrease in the case-fatality rate because nearly every child experienced pertussis, a highly contagious disease. Undoubtedly, many factors contributed to this decline in the case-fatality rates. Probable or possible factors include the diminished frequency of diarrheal diseases of infancy as a result of pasteurization of milk, better nutrition, improved socioeconomic status, and diminished family size, resulting both in diminished likelihood of high-risk young infants and in better supportive care of ill infants. With the advent of increasingly widespread immunization against pertussis beginning in the late 1940s, there was a striking acceleration in the decline of mortality from pertussis. A similar decrease was observed in Britain a few years later when pertussis immunization was instituted. Although vaccine-induced near elimination of pertussis is clearly the major factor in this accelerated decline, undoubtedly case-fatality rates have also decreased as a result of better supportive care, including respiratory

assistance, better nutrition, and, perhaps, the availability of antibiotics (Mortimer and Jones, 1979).

TREATMENT

The treatment of pertussis is largely supportive. In most instances the disease, although fatiguing or exhausting, protracted, and very unpleasant, can be managed at home. Most patients who require hospitalization are young infants. For children managed at home maintenance of adequate nutrition and hydration is ordinarily easily achieved. Providing high humidity is probably of no value. Cough suppressants, if used at all, should be used in low doses to avoid interference with expulsion of secretions (Bass, 1985).

For those children who must be hospitalized, usually infants, symptomatic management depends on disease manifestations and their severity. The infant or child with severe pertussis must be constantly monitored so that immediate help can be provided for severe paroxysms. A means of suction should be at hand. In patients unable to handle their own secretions, removal of mucoid material is facilitated by placing the child in a head-down position (45 to 60 degrees) to take advantage of gravity. Suction of the oropharynx with a catheter large enough to permit flow of tenacious secretions is required during paroxysms. In a severely ill child oxygen may be needed. The child's state of hydration must be monitored and maintained at an adequate level. Caloric intake also requires observation, although during the most severe phase of the disease optimal intake may not be possible.

Specific therapy is less than satisfactory. Serum immune globulin and hyperimmune antipertussis globulin, no longer available, are of no value, although a recent study of a high-dose experimental preparation suggests the contrary and the need for further study (Granstrom, 1991). *B. pertussis* is susceptible to a number of antibiotics in vitro, but the only agent with useful clinical efficacy is erythromycin. Erythromycin may be expected to eradicate *B. pertussis* from the upper respiratory tract; for this reason all persons with pertussis should receive 14 days of treatment to minimize transmission. Unfortunately, erythromycin has not been shown to exert any effect on the clinical course of full-blown pertussis. There is evidence that it will prevent or modify the course of the disease when given during the incubation period before the onset of symptoms. There is also some evidence that, when given early in the catarrhal stage, it will ameliorate symptoms and/or shorten the course of the disease. Unfortunately, the potential use of erythromycin is sorely compromised because exposure usually is not recognized and because the symptoms of those with early pertussis in the catarrhal stage are indistinguishable from the symptoms of those with a common respiratory infection. Nonetheless, in a household with a case of recognized pertussis, all family members, with or without symptoms, promptly should receive a full course of erythromycin in an effort to prevent further disease and subsequent spread.

IMMUNITY

After an attack of pertussis, immunity to the disease has been considered lifelong (Mortimer, 1990). Old anecdotes exist about grandmothers who acquired whooping cough from their grandchildren, but these episodes are very rare and poorly documented. In some instances these second attacks may have been parapertussis, an immunologically distinct disorder, or other infections caused by viruses or chlamydia.

The proportion of individuals protected against clinical pertussis by full immunization with the whole-cell vaccine is high but not as high as the proportion protected by the natural disease. Vaccine failures are approximately 10%, with some variation perhaps caused by the intensity of exposure. The likelihood of children acquiring pertussis increases with years elapsed since the last dose. Also, many individuals with waning immunity after immunization may be infected, as measured by serological studies. They experience symptoms ranging from few or none to the full clinical syndrome. This phenomenon has been observed most often following vaccine-induced immunity but appears to occur in those who experienced the natural disease many years previously as well. This apparent loss of immunity has become particularly evident in recent years because of an increase in the incidence of reported cases of pertussis in adolescents and young adults; the increase is both relative and absolute. This increase has strong implications for future pertussis control for the reason that older individuals with the disease,

whether full-blown or unrecognized, undoubtedly constitute an important reservoir for disease transmission, particularly to young infants who are as yet unprotected. Therefore one of the reasons for efforts to develop a less reactive, acellular pertussis vaccine is the anticipation that it might be acceptable for use in adults.

PREVENTION

Because treatment of pertussis is far from satisfactory, transmission occurs from early or unrecognized infections, and passive immunization is ineffective, active immunization is the mainstay of pertussis control worldwide (Cherry, 1984; Mortimer and Jones, 1979). Beginning approximately in 1910, a few years after identification and isolation of the organism, various attempts were made to develop vaccines for primary immunization. For many years these hit-or-miss efforts were largely unsuccessful. Most preparations comprised killed, whole organisms, although around 1940 futile attempts were made to immunize with cell-free filtrates of cultures of the organism. By the early 1940s clinically effective whole-cell preparations were produced, and by 1945 they were licensed and marketed. Pertussis vaccine was standardized by federal regulation in 1954, and current whole-cell pertussis vaccines are relatively unchanged since that time except for technical refinements such as better control of the number of organisms required for an immunizing dose.

Early attempts to produce an effective pertussis vaccine were hampered by the lack of a surrogate measure for estimation of clinical efficacy; accordingly, clinical trials were required. This situation was ameliorated to a large extent in the mid-1940s by the development of the mouse protection test, in which mice, immunized with the vaccine in question, are challenged by injecting live pertussis organisms intracerebrally. Quantitation of the immunogenicity of the test vaccine is accomplished by comparing survival rates with those achieved by a standard vaccine of known potency, expressed in so-called mouse protection units. Each dose contains approximately 4 mouse protection units; a total of 8 or more units in the first three primary immunization doses is considered satisfactory. For whole-cell vaccines the mouse protection test correlates with clinical efficacy in man. This test, bizarre as it may seem, has served well over the years in assessing the efficacy of whole-cell pertussis vaccines, thus avoiding the necessity for clinical trials in children.

Current killed, whole-cell pertussis vaccines are combined with diphtheria and tetanus toxoids and adsorbed onto an aluminum salt, comprising the familiar diphtheria and tetanus toxoids and pertussis vaccine (DTP). Three doses of DTP are recommended in infancy, with a reinforcing dose approximately 1 year later and another at entry to elementary school. Because of the alleged reactivity of whole-cell pertussis vaccine in older children and adults, it is not recommended for individuals 7 years and older.

Whole-cell pertussis vaccines, widely used in the industrialized world during the past three or four decades, have achieved a remarkable record of success. For the 10 years 1978 through 1987, an average of less than six deaths from pertussis was reported annually in the United States. Additionally, in 1981 a low of only 1,248 cases was reported, compared to more than 220,000 40 years previously. Acknowledging that the disease is vastly underreported, even if recognized, this is a remarkable achievement (Sutter and Cochi, 1992).

For many years it has been recognized that DTP is undesirably reactive (Mortimer and Jones, 1979). Most of the reactivity is attributable to the pertussis component (Cody et al., 1981). Local reactions include pain at the site of injection in approximately half of all recipients; redness and swelling are observed in approximately 40%. Systemic reactions include fever of 38° C or more in nearly half of recipients; more than half display irritability. Drowsiness is noted in approximately one third and anorexia in approximately 20%. These systemic symptoms are largely limited to the first 48 hours after injection; fever is most apt to occur between 6 and 12 hours after receipt of the vaccine.

Rare but disturbing events that occur after DTP injection include so-called hypotensive-hyporesponsive episodes. These episodes usually occur within a few hours of the injection and always within 12 hours. Duration is usually a matter of minutes or 1 or 2 hours but rarely episodes have lasted longer (up to 36 hours). The best estimate of their frequency is 1 per 1,750 doses but with a wide confidence interval. These episodes are frightening to observe because the

child appears cold, clammy, and bluish and responds poorly. Nonetheless, spontaneous recovery occurs, and death has not been observed. The mechanism is unclear; similar episodes have been observed following administration of diphtheria and tetanus toxoids (DT) (Pollock and Morris, 1983).

As would be expected, febrile convulsions occur occasionally after DTP injection but appear to be without sequelae (Baraff et al, 1988; Cody et al., 1981; Shields et al., 1988). The best estimate of their frequency is 1 per 1,750 doses, with a wide confidence interval and variation with age. Occasionally, convulsions after DTP injection occur in the absence of fever; rarely, more complex or protracted seizures may occur with or without fever. It is likely that most, if not all, of these more worrisome convulsive episodes represent the precipitation of overt manifestations of preexisting central nervous system disorders by the systemic effects of DTP. Persistent, inconsolable crying has also been observed after the child was given DTP or, less often, DT. These episodes are without sequelae and probably are caused by pain at the site of injection (Cody et al., 1981).

For nearly 60 years, beginning with the original hit-or-miss experimental vaccines, there have been dozens of anecdotal reports suggesting that, on occasion, within 1 or 2 days after injection pertussis vaccine produces acute, severe encephalopathy, sometimes with permanent brain damage or death (Cherry et al., 1988). Because the disease itself was known to produce encephalopathy and because other vaccines such as those for rabies and smallpox were recognized to cause severe neurological sequelae, these rare events were accepted as an unfortunate price to pay for the control of a serious disease. As widespread use of the vaccine reduced the threat of the disease markedly, these events became magnified in importance, not only in the United States but also in other industrialized nations, including the United Kingdom, Japan, and Sweden. Widespread publicity about these occurrences caused near boycotts of pertussis vaccine in the United Kingdom and Japan, with reappearance of major outbreaks of the disease (Cherry, 1984; Kanai, 1980; Noble, 1987). In the United States similar publicity about these alleged injuries exerted only a minor effect on vaccine use, but widespread litigation ensued, resulting in major price increases because of insurance costs. These problems prompted systematic efforts to assess the causative role of pertussis vaccine in severe neurological disease, both in the United States and in the United Kingdom, with the latter nation being particularly suited to such studies because of the organization of its health care system.

In the British National Childhood Encephalopathy Study (NCES) over a 3-year period, during which time approximately 2,100,000 doses of DTP were administered, 1,182 children age 3 months to 3 years with acute encephalopathic disorders without obvious causes were studied (Miller et al., 1981, 1985). For each of these children two age-matched controls were selected, and for all case and control children it was determined whether a vaccine had been administered in the prior 28 days and, if so, when. After elimination from the analysis of children with infantile spasms, a disorder shown to bear no causative relationship to DTP in another part of the study, it was estimated that the relative risk for acute encephalopathy with permanent brain damage, based on seven cases, was 4.7, with a wide confidence interval. Because the approximate number of doses of DTP distributed in the United Kingdom during the period of the study was known, it could be estimated that the risk of acute encephalopathy with permanent brain damage was 1 per 330,000 doses, again with a wide confidence interval (Pollock and Morris, 1983).

The NCES, superbly designed and executed, has been subjected to exhaustive (and exhausting) analysis and re-analysis, not only by the investigators themselves but also by others. A 10-year follow-up of subjects and controls has been performed and on preliminary analysis continues to show an increased risk of serious neurological disease after administration of DTP, although the numbers are small (Madge et al., 1990).

Unfortunately, this study has failed to resolve the question of whether pertussis vaccine produces acute encephalopathy with permanent brain damage on rare occasions, and it is unlikely that further analyses will be of help because of the small number of affected subjects who received DTP within 7 days before onset. Further, several of these children showed evidence of other, unrelated disorders. It is also possible that

one or more of these children, all apparently normal before administration of DTP, did have some preexisting but unrecognized neurological impairment, the manifestations of which were brought out by the known systemic effects of DTP. Whether the analysis is limited to the 3-day interval following DTP injection or the 7-day interval is used also influences the results. Differing approaches and assumptions have resulted in analyses of the data with quite disparate results, including some that indicate no risk at all (Bowie, 1990; Miller et al., 1988; Stephenson, 1988).

Four other studies, none of which in itself is of sufficient size to provide a definitive answer, in toto provide support for the lack of an association between pertussis vaccine and acute encephalopathy with permanent brain damage (Cherry, 1990). As a result of these various studies, the most conservative statement that can be made is either that pertussis vaccine does not cause acute neurological disease with permanent sequelae or if it does, the rate is too low for measurement and never will be known. It is impossible to prove an absolute negative. Nonetheless, it is very clear that most, if not all, of the various neurological ills that have been attributed anecdotally to pertussis vaccine represent either coincidence or the precipitation of inevitable events in children with underlying neurological disorders by the well-known systemic effects of pertussis vaccine, including fever. The estimate of one instance of permanent neurological damage per 330,000 doses of DTP has no validity.

Temporal association between DTP administration and the onset of infantile spasms or the occurrence of sudden infant death syndrome (SIDS) (or an excess of deaths from any other cause) is pure coincidence (Howson and Fineberg, 1992). There is no causative relationship between DTP and other disorders such as hyperactivity, learning problems, infantile autism, behavior problems, transverse myelitis, or other overt, subtle, or slowly progressive neurological conditions (Bellman et al., 1983; Butler et al., 1982; Cherry, 1990; Golden, 1990). A detailed review and analysis of the evidence related to reactions to pertussis vaccine has been published (Howson and Fineberg, 1992). This special committee report indicates that the evidence is insufficient to conclude that DTP causes chronic neurological damage, although it may cause acute encephalopathic symptoms. The report also concludes that DTP does not cause SIDS or infantile spasms on the basis of the available data. This report is an authoritative resource for information regarding these and other alleged reactions to DTP.

Unfortunately, the differentiation between association and causation in relation to pertussis vaccine and neurological injury is not understood by the vast majority of the general public and, indeed, by some physicians. Accordingly, inaccurate portrayals of the risks of pertussis vaccine continue to appear in the media, and litigation over alleged pertussis vaccine injuries continues to soar. The advent of the federally sponsored vaccine injury compensation program has resulted in an enormous increase in legal claims for alleged injuries. However, this increase appears to involve the compensation program and not civil litigation. Unfortunately, the compensation program is endangered because the costs are far greater than expected because both the congressional act that established the program and those who adjudicate the claims appear to assume that temporal association and causation are synonymous and that the expected benign minor symptoms following DTP injection such as irritability, sleepiness, or decreased appetite indicate encephalopathy, shock-collapse, or imminent SIDS as alleged by plaintiff lawyers.

ACELLULAR PERTUSSIS VACCINE

The identification and isolation of many of the components of *B. pertussis* responsible for the organism's physiological and immunogenic characteristics beginning in the late 1970s have provided the basis for the development of acellular pertussis vaccines extracted from the supernatant fluid of both cultures of *B. pertussis*. These extracted vaccines are free of components irrelevant to clinical immunity, presumably reducing reactivity (Martin, 1990).

The first of these vaccines for clinical use was produced in Japan and consists of adsorbed preparations in combination with diphtheria and tetanus toxoids. All of the six products produced by different manufacturers in Japan contain LPF and FHA in varying amounts. Five contain agglutinogens as well, and the 69K protein is present in at least one of these five. LPF is detoxified

by formalin, and most of the endotoxin is removed. These vaccines were not subjected to field trials for clinical efficacy before licensure but instead were licensed on the basis of serological responses and passage of the mouse protection test, even though this test was originally standardized with whole-cell vaccines and it is not clear whether protection of mice is mediated similarly to protection in man (British Medical Research Council, 1956).

Beginning in late 1981 acellular vaccines replaced whole-cell preparations for immunization of Japanese children, and vaccination was initiated at 2 years of age because of concern that the more immature nervous system of the infant was more susceptible to injury and the assumption that herd-immunity plus prevention of home exposure to older siblings would protect younger children. Because this strategy was less than satisfactory for the protection of infants, the age of initiation of immunization with DTP in Japan was lowered to 3 months in 1989. It is, however, clear that these six vaccines as a group effectively controlled pertussis in children 2 years and older in Japan (Kimura and Kuno-Sakai, 1990).

In part because of the Japanese experience, acellular pertussis vaccines of varying antigen content and produced by a variety of techniques have been developed by at least a dozen manufacturers in the United States and Europe and are in various stages of evaluation. Replacement of current pertussis vaccines by less reactive acellular preparations is highly desirable, even though whole-cell pertussis vaccines have been largely exonerated as a cause of brain damage. Because a less reactive vaccine would minimize unpleasantness for the child and the family, would offer the prospect of providing reinforcing doses for older children and adults, and would increase the likelihood of completion of the immunization series, which is particularly important in the developing world in which pain-relief medications are not readily available, these preparations are being pursued.

Several Japanese acellular pertussis vaccines have been studied in the United States and Japan. These vaccines apparently are satisfactorily immunogenic and of low reactivity (Anderson et al., 1988; Blumberg et al., 1990; Edwards et al., 1986). There are, however, only limited data regarding efficacy of individual products. One study has attempted to assess the clinical efficacy of two Japanese acellular preparations of pertussis vaccine but without diphtheria and tetanus toxoids in Swedish infants (Ad Hoc Group, 1988). In this placebo-controlled trial a specially prepared preparation containing only detoxified LPF and another containing detoxified LPF and FHA were used. Point estimates of efficacy for culture-proven pertussis were 54% and 69%, respectively, for the single and double antigen preparations. Both vaccines were 80% efficacious in preventing severe whooping cough. Continuing follow-up after the study was unblinded has indicated persistence of efficacy for at least an additional year (Storsaeter et al., 1990). The study has also suggested that the addition of FHA to LPF offers better protection against infection and colonization than does LPF alone.

A household contact study in Japan of a Japanese absorbed DTP that contained LPF, FHA, agglutinogens, and the 69K protein indicated that this vaccine was 98% protective against severe pertussis in children 2 years and older; including mild or suspected cases indistinguishable from viral respiratory infections, efficacy was 81% (Mortimer et al., 1990). Because the results of the Swedish trial in infants are considered unsatisfactory by many and because the household contact study of the four-antigen preparation in Japanese children was limited to those 2 years and older, at least two field trials of Japanese acellular pertussis vaccines as the primary immunogen in infants are currently in progress.

Nonetheless, the low reactivity of these acellular vaccines, their immunogenicity, and the results of controlled and uncontrolled clinical observations suggest that current whole-cell vaccines will be replaced as primary immunogens by acellular preparations within a few years. Indeed, in late 1991 the FDA licensed one adsorbed, acellular DTP product containing LPF, FHA, agglutinogens, and the 69K protein for use as the fourth and fifth doses (15 months and 5 to 7 years). Additionally, it is likely that future acellular pertussis vaccines will be produced by genetic engineering rather than by extraction from broth cultures.

Several problems remain. First, the protective antigens of *B. pertussis* are not defined precisely, although it is probable that there are at least two. Accordingly, the components necessary for optimal vaccine efficacy are not yet defined. Related to the lack of definition of the protective antigens is a second problem—the lack of a satisfactory serological surrogate for clinical protection in man. Until such is available, difficult and costly clinical field trials are required for demonstration of efficacy. Third, an important question is whether the goal of pertussis immunization is simply to prevent overt disease in recipients or whether it is desirable to prevent infection, with or without mild symptoms, as well as severe disease. It is at least arguable that prevention of severe disease but not infection would permit continuing circulation of *B. pertussis* in populations, with consequent reinforcement of clinical immunity. However, because a satisfactory method for protecting infants too young to have been immunized is not currently foreseeable, the more desirable goal probably is the prevention of infection and disease to minimize exposure of infants.

Guidelines extracted from the Advisory Committee on Immunization Practices (ACIP) concerning use of DTP vaccine are given on p. 54 (Chapter 4).

REFERENCES

Ad Hoc Group for the Study of Pertussis Vaccines. Placebo-controlled trial of two acellular pertussis vaccines in Sweden—protective efficacy and adverse events. Lancet 1988;1:955-960.

Anderson EL, Belshe RB, Bartram J. Differences in reactogenicity and antigenicity of acellular and standard pertussis vaccines combined with diphtheria and tetanus in infants. J Infect Dis 1988;157:731-737.

Baraff LJ, Shields WD, Beckwith L, et al. Infants and children with convulsions and hypotonic-hyporesponsive episodes follwoing diptheria-tetanus-pertussis immunization: follow-up evaluation. Pediatrics 1988;81:789-794.

Bass JW. Pertussis: current status of prevention and treatment. Pediatr Infect Dis 1985;4:614-619.

Bellman MH, Ross EM, Miller DL. Infantile spasms and pertussis immunisation. Lancet 1983;1:1031-1034.

Blumberg D, Mink CM, Cherry JD, et al. Comparison of an acellular pertussis-component diphtheria-tetanus-pertussis (DTP) vaccine with a whole-cell pertussis-component DTP vaccine in 17- to 24-month-old children, with measurement of 69-kilodalton outer membrane protein antibody. J Pediatr 1990;117:46-51.

Bowie C. Viewpoint. Lessons from the pertussis vaccine court trial. Lancet 1990;335:397-399.

British Medical Research Council. Vaccination against whooping-cough. Relation between protection in children and results of laboratory tests. Br Med J 1956;2:454-462.

Butler NR, Haslum M, Golding J, Stewart-Brown S. Recent findings from the 1970 child health and education study: preliminary communication. J R Soc Med 1982;75:781-784.

Centers for Disease Control. Summary of notifiable diseases, United States 1989. MMWR 1989(38);54:55-59.

Cherry JD. The epidemiology of pertussis and pertussis vaccine in the United Kingdom and the United States: a comparative study. In Lockhart JD (ed). Current problems in pediatrics, Chicago: Year Book Medical Publishers, 1984, p 78.

Cherry JD. "Pertussis vaccine encephalopathy": it is time to recognize it as the myth it is. JAMA 1990;263:1679-1680.

Cherry JD, Brunell PA, Golden GS, Karzon DT. Report of the Task Force on Pertussis and Pertussis Immunization— 1988. Pediatrics 1988;81(suppl):939-984.

Cochi SL. Personal communication, 1991.

Cody CL, Baraff LJ, Cherry JD, et al. Nature and rates of adverse reactions associated with DTP and DT immunizations in infants and children. Pediatrics 1981;68:650-660.

Dauer CC. Reported whooping cough morbidity and mortality in the United States. Public Health Rep 1943;58:661-676.

Edwards KM, Lawrence E, Wright PF. Diphtheria, tetanus, and pertussis vaccine. A comparison of the immune response and adverse reactions to conventional and acellular pertussis components. Am J Dis Child 1986;140:867-871.

Golden GS. Pertussis vaccine and injury to the brain. J Pediatr 1990;116:854-861.

Granstrom G, Wretlind B, Salenstedt C-R, Granstrom M. Evaluation of serologic assays for diagnosis of whooping cough. J Clin Microbiol 1988;26:1818-1823.

Granstrom M, Olinder-Neilsen AM, Holmblad P, et al. Specific immunoglobulin for treatment of whooping cough. Lancet 1991;338:1230-1233.

Howson CP, Fineberg HV. Adverse events following pertussis and rubella vaccines. Summary of a report of the Institute of Medicine. JAMA 1992;267:392-396.

Institute of Medicine. CP Howson, CJ Howe, HV Fineberg (eds). Committee report: adverse effects of pertussis and rubella vaccines. Washington: National Academy Press, 1991.

Kanai K. Japan's experience in pertussis epidemiology and vaccination in the past thirty years. Jpn J Sci Biol 1980;33:107-143.

Kimura M, Kuno-Sakai J. Developments in pertussis immunisation in Japan. Lancet 1990;336:30-32.

Lapin LH. Whooping cough. Springfield, Ill: Charles C Thomas, Publisher, 1943.

Litvak AM, Gibel H, Rosenthal SE, Rosenblatt P. Cerebral complications in pertussis. J Pediatr 1948;32:357-379.

Madge N, Miller D, Ross E, Wadsworth J. The National Childhood Encephalopathy Study: a 10-year followup. In Manclark CR (ed). Sixth international symposium on pertussis (abstracts). DHHS Publication No. (FDA) 90-1162.

Bethesda, MD: Public Health Service, US Department of Health and Human Services, 1990.

Miller D, Wadsworth J, Diamond J, Ross E. Pertussis vaccine and whooping cough as risk factors for acute neurological illness and death in young children. Dev Biol Stand 1985;61:389-394.

Miller D, Wadsworth J, Ross E. Severe neurological illness: further analyses of the British National Childhood Encephalopathy study. Tokai J Exp Clin Med 1988; 13(suppl):145-155.

Miller DL, Ross EM, Alderslade R, et al. Pertussis immunisation and serious acute neurological illness in children. Br Med J 1981;282:1595-1599.

Mortimer EA Jr. Perspective. Pertussis and its prevention: a family affair. J Infect Dis 1990;161:473-479.

Mortimer EA Jr, Jones PK. An evaluation of pertussis vaccine. Rev Infect Dis 1979;1:927-932.

Mortimer EA Jr, Kimura M, Cherry JD, et al. Protective efficacy of the Takeda acellular pertussis vaccine combined with diphtheria and tetanus toxoids following household exposure of Japanese children. Am J Dis Child 1990;144:899-904.

Noble GR, Bernier RH, Esber EC, et al. Acellular and whole-cell pertussis vaccine in Japan: report of a visit by U.S. scientists. JAMA 1987;257:1351-1356.

Onorato IM, Wassilak SGF. Laboratory diagnosis of pertussis: the state of the art. Pediatr Infect Dis 1987;6:145-151.

Pollock TM, Morris J. A 7-year survey of disorders attributed to vaccination in North West Thames region. Lancet 1983;1:753-757.

Public Health Laboratory Service. Efficacy of whooping-cough vaccines used in the United Kingdom before 1968. Br Med J 1973;1:259-262.

Shahin RD, Brennan MJ, Li ZM, et al. Characterization of the protective capacity and immunogenicity of the 69-kD outer membrane protein of Bordetella pertussis. J Exp Med 1990;171:63-73.

Shields WD, Nielsen C, Buch D, et al. Relationship of pertussis immunization to the onset of neurologic disorders: a retrospective epidemiologic study. J Pediatr 1988;113:801-805.

Steketee RW, Burstyn DG, Wassilak SGF, et al. A comparison of laboratory and clinical methods for diagnosing pertussis in an outbreak in a facility for the developmentally disabled. J Infect Dis 1988;157:441-449.

Stephenson JBP. A neurologist looks at neurological disease temporally related to DTP immunization. Tokai J Exp Clin Med 1988;13:157-164.

Storsaeter J, Hallander H, Farrington CP, et al. Secondary analyses of the efficacy of two acellular pertussis vaccines evaluated in a Swedish phase III trial. Vaccine 1990;6:457-461.

Sutter RW, Cochi SL. Pertussis hospitalizations and mortality, 1985-1988. Evaluation of the completeness of national reporting. JAMA 1992;267:386-391.

Wardlaw AC, Parton R, eds. Pathogenesis and immunity in pertussis. New York: John Wiley & Sons, 1988.

20

RABIES (HYDROPHOBIA, RAGE, LYSSA)

Human rabies is a rare, fatal encephalomyelitis caused by a rhabdovirus that is usually transmitted to man by the bite of a rabid animal. In the United States the average annual incidence of human rabies declined from 40 cases during the 1940s to zero to two cases per year since 1980. Monoclonal serotyping of rabies isolates from four human cases of rabies occurring in the United States in the 1980s revealed viruses similar to those in the country of origin of the patient. The important feature was an incubation period of 11 months to 6 years, with probable acquisition of infection before entry into the United States (Smith et al., 1991). Rabies in *domestic* animals has shown a similar decrease. In 1946 there were more than 8,000 cases of rabies in dogs, compared with 550 cases in all domestic animals in 1988. Rabid domestic animals comprise 12% of all rabid animals but are responsible for 64% of exposures requiring treatment. Rabid cats are the most commonly reported rabid domestic species in the United States.

There were 4,724 confirmed cases of wildlife rabies in 47 states in 1988 (Centers for Disease Control, 1989) (Fig. 20-1). These data originate in state and federal laboratories of the United States but reflect the worldwide epizootic in wildlife hosts, extending from the Arctic Circle to the tropics in both hemispheres. Wild animals currently constitute the most important source of infection for domestic animals in the United States. Transmission from one domestic species to another rarely occurs in the United States.

The general treatment of the bite and the question of whether or not to immunize those persons bitten or scratched by animals suspected of being rabid is a difficult decision. Skunks and raccoons are the main sources of rabies for domestic animals. The decision must be made immediately after exposure because the likelihood that any prophylactic measure will contribute to the prevention of rabies diminishes rapidly as the interval between exposure and treatment increases.

Although occasionally a case of rabies may develop in persons who receive antirabies treatment, evidence from laboratory and field experience in many parts of the world indicates that postexposure prophylaxis can be highly effective when appropriately used.

ETIOLOGY

Rabies virus was the first virus transmitted experimentally to a laboratory animal.

Physical and chemical properties

Rabies virus is bullet shaped and has a symmetrical structure like a beehive. The virus measures 80 to 180 nm in diameter. The negative single-stranded genome is nonsegmented RNA approximately 1,000 nucleotides long. The genome has been cloned and several genes sequenced. The glycoprotein of the spikes on the surface of the virus is encoded by the G gene, which has been sequenced. This is the attachment protein and is the antigen eliciting neutralizing antibodies. The virulence of virus is

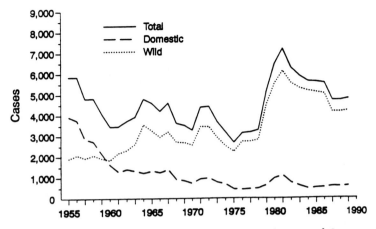

Fig. 20-1. Rabies in wild and domestic animals, by year, in the United States and Puerto Rico, 1955 to 1989. (From MMWR 1990; 38:36.)

dramatically altered by single amino acid substitutions in the glycoprotein. Monoclonal antibodies against the glycoprotein distinguish strains of virus and are clarifying the epidemiology of rabies.

Rabies virus survives storage at 4° C for weeks and in the frozen state for much longer periods in the absence of carbon dioxide; therefore in dry-ice cabinets it must be stored in sealed glass ampules. It keeps for years in the dried state at 4° C. Rabies virus is killed by temperatures of 56° C in 1 hour and of 60° C in 5 minutes. It is quickly inactivated by sunlight and ultraviolet light. The virus is resistant to phenol and thimerosol (Merthiolate). It is inactivated by β-propiolactone, ether, formalin, mercury bichloride, and nitric acid.

Host range

Rabies virus has an extensive host range; all warm-blooded animals are susceptible. Introduction of virus by virtually any route usually gives rise to infection, but the intracerebral inoculation with virus from canines almost invariably produces fatal encephalomyelitis. Widely distributed in infected animals, virus is found in the central nervous system (CNS), saliva, urine, lymph, milk, and blood. The salivary glands of infected dogs have yielded high titers of virus; lesser quantities have been detected in the lacrimal glands, pancreas, kidney, adrenal glands, and breast tissue. In humans, rabies virus has been recovered from various parts of the CNS, including the olfactory bulbs, horn of Ammon,

frontal and occipital cortices, and medulla. It has also been recovered from both cervical and abdominal sympathetic ganglia, salivary glands, adrenal glands, myocardium, walls of both small and large intestines, mesenteric lymph nodes, tonsillar and pharyngeal tissues, and lungs.

The term *street virus* is used to designate strains freshly isolated in the laboratory. Such strains are characterized by incubation periods that usually vary from 10 days to several months. Current evidence suggests incubation periods may be several years. These viruses produce either prolonged excitation and viciousness (furious type) or depression and paralysis with early onset (dumb type) or, as occurs in most infected dogs, some manifestations of both types. Street virus rabies is almost always associated with the presence of Negri bodies.

The term *fixed virus* refers to strains transferred in series from brain to brain, usually in the rabbit, characterized by a short and constant incubation period of 4 to 6 days, absence of Negri bodies, and diminished ability to spread centrifugally. The Pasteur strain of fixed virus has been maintained in rabbits since its original isolation in 1882 and is the strain generally used for human vaccination (Semple type).

Rabies virus has also been propagated in both chick and duck embryos, in tissue cultures of mouse and chick embryos and hamster kidney, and in a human diploid cell line (WI-38). After many serial transfers were made in the chick embryo, the Flury strain became attenuated, that is, lost its pathogenicity for animals injected intramuscularly but retained its immunogenic capacity. This modified living virus is used for immunization of dogs. A killed virus vaccine prepared from duck embryos has been used in humans since 1957; its main advantages are the absence of CNS tissue in the vaccine and decreased incidence of the neuromyelitic accidents that may follow injections of Semple vaccine. The duck embryo vaccine has beeen replaced by an inactivated human diploid cell rabies vaccine (see p. 320).

Immunological properties

Both neutralizing and complement-fixing antibodies are formed in the course of rabies infection, and they may develop as a result of vaccination. The level of neutralizing antibody to glycoprotein is associated with protection against illness. Cell-to-cell spread of virus is prevented by neutralizing antibody in vitro. Postexposure administration of antibody may prevent virus from reaching the CNS.

A measurable cytotoxic T-cell response is generated, but the role in pathogenesis or protection is unknown. In vitro the cellular response contributes to clearance of virus from cells, and this can be enhanced by antibody.

PATHOLOGY

The principal changes produced by rabies virus are found throughout the CNS, consisting mainly of neuronal necrosis, which is most pronounced in the thalamus, hypothalamus, substantia nigra, pons, and medulla. The cranial nerve nuclei are severely damaged, and mononuclear cell infiltration is likely to be greater there than elsewhere. The spinal cord shows neuronal changes, especially in the posterior horns.

The most distinctive feature of the pathological changes is the presence of Negri bodies, which are pathognomonic of rabies. These specific inclusion bodies are found in the cytoplasm of nerve cells. They consist of acidophilic structures approximately 2 to 10 μm in diameter, are sharply demarcated, and are usually round or oval; they occur most abundantly in the hippocampus (horn of Ammon), basal ganglia, pons, and medulla.

Changes similar to those in the brain may be found in the sympathetic ganglia and dorsal root ganglia of the spinal cord. The salivary glands may show degenerative changes of the acinar cells and neurons; Negri bodies may be found in the latter.

PATHOGENESIS

In general, the *attack rate* in persons bitten by rabid animals is hard to estimate; it depends on the extent and location of the bites and the dose of virus entering the wound. Lacerations of the head and neck are followed by higher attack rates than those of the feet and ankles. The amount of virus reaching the nerves is influenced by several additional factors: (1) lack of virus in saliva of 50% of rabid dogs; (2) protection afforded by clothing so that little or no virus enters the wound; and (3) removal or inactivation of virus by soap and water, benzalkonium (Zephiran), and other agents.

Rabies virus in saliva is inoculated into tissue by a bite. Available evidence indicates that rabies virus multiplies initially in the muscle at the inoculation site, reaches neuromuscular junctions, and travels through the axoplasm of peripheral nerves to dorsal root ganglia and the CNS. After multiplication in neurons centrally, the virus travels peripherally along nerve pathways to invade many distal tissues and organs. Host response is limited, perhaps because virus is sequestered from the immune system during the long incubation period, and little inflammatory response or measurable host response can be demonstrated.

CLINICAL MANIFESTATIONS

The incubation period is usually 1 to 2 months, but wide ranges from 10 days to 6 years have been observed. It probably will be short after multiple severe lacerations and the introduction of large doses of virus.

The illness may begin, as do other kinds of encephalitis, with prodromal symptoms of malaise, fever, headache, anorexia, nausea, sore throat, drowsiness, irritability, and restlessness. The patient may complain of hyperesthesia, paresthesia, or anesthesia in the area of the bite and along the course of the involved peripheral nerves.

Progress of the infection is associated with increased anxiety and hyperexcitability accompanied by mounting fever. Delirium, involuntary twitching movements, and generalized convulsions are often seen. Maniacal behavior may alternate with periods of lethargy. Violent spasmodic contractions of the muscles of the patient's mouth, pharynx, or larynx when he attempts to drink or when he merely sees water are the striking characteristics that gave rabies its common name—*hydrophobia*. These painful spasms may be set off by relatively mild stimuli such as noise or light touch. The patient may drool profusely from the mouth to avoid swallowing, which is associated with painful spasm.

Within a few days the patient's condition worsens, the pulse rate increases, respirations become more labored or irregular, and the temperature rises steadily. Periods of responsiveness become less frequent, and muscular spasms may give way to paralysis. Peripheral vascular collapse, coma, and death quickly follow. The disease runs its entire course usually in no more than 5 to 6 days and ends fatally.

In 5% to 20% of patients the clinical picture of rabies may be that of an ascending, symmetrical, flaccid paralysis without hyperexcitability or spasmodic muscle contractions. This picture resembles that of Guillain-Barré syndrome so that, in the absence of known history of rabies virus exposure, such patients may go through the entire course of illness with no suspicion of the diagnosis of rabies until the characteristic findings are observed at autopsy (Baer, 1975).

The cerebrospinal fluid (CSF) is usually normal: the pressure is normal or slightly increased; the fluid is clear; and in most cases the number of cells is not increased. In patients with pleocytosis the CSF cell count rarely exceeds 100, and the cells are mostly mononuclear leukocytes. There may be a slight increase in the level of protein.

The peripheral white blood cell count shows a slight increase in number of leukocytes that may reach 20,000 to 30,000, with a predominance of polymorphonuclear leukocytes. Abnormal urinary findings may include albumin, casts, reducing substances, and acetone.

CASE 1. An 11-year-old boy was bitten on the forehead by a dog 32 days before onset of the disease; the wound was cauterized, but no antirabies vaccine was given. The patient's illness began with headache, drowsiness, anorexia, and malaise that progressed in 2 days to delirium accompanied by fever and vomiting. Delirium associated with visual hallucinations and delusions of persecution were the outstanding and persistently recurring features. He was often manic and struck and bit attendants. Except for transient difficulty in swallowing and slurring of speech on the fourth and fifth days, there was a striking ab-

sence of localizing neurological signs. The CSF was normal. The temperature was sustained between 38.9° and 40.3° C (102° and 104.5° F) for 1 week. On the tenth day, irregular respirations were observed with periods of apnea lasting as long as 45 seconds. He died on the twelfth day from respiratory and circulatory failure. Postmortem touch preparations of the hippocampus showed typical Negri bodies, and rabies virus was isolated from various parts of the brain and other tissues.

DIAGNOSIS

In a typical case rabies is easily recognized. The characteristic history is that of an animal bite followed in several weeks or months by the onset of overwhelming encephalitis; the CNS signs include excitement, anxiety, maniacal behavior, and delirium associated with spasmodic concentrations of muscles concerned with swallowing and speech. Clinical laboratory findings are generally of little help.

In humans the diagnosis is made best by demonstration of antigen in a skin biopsy. Corneal impressions have been difficult to obtain and unreliable for detection of antigen. During the first week of illness, virus can be isolated occasionally from saliva, CSF, and urine and consistently from brain. Virus can be demonstrated by immunofluorescence, by identification of Negri bodies, or by inoculation of brain tissue into mice. Primary isolation of virus is accomplished in mice, although cell culture can be used. The presence of IgM antibody in blood and CSF indicates acute infection. Polymerase chain reaction (PCR) may improve sensitivity and specificity of diagnosis.

Tetanus may be confused with rabies. Excitement accompanied by spasms of the laryngeal and pharyngeal muscles is not so common in patients with tetanus and is virtually constant in patients with rabies. Tetanus is characterized by trismus and spasmodic contractions of the muscles of the body.

PROGNOSIS

Rabies was considered 100% lethal until recent years.

CASE 2. *Probable human rabies with survival.* On October 10, 1970, in Lima, Ohio, a 6-year-old boy was bitten on his left thumb by a bat while he was asleep. The bat was captured by the boy's father and was submitted to the Ohio Health Department, where rabies was confirmed on examination of the brain by fluorescent antibody (FA) technique. On October 14 a 14-day course of treatment with duck-embryo vaccine (DEV) was begun on the boy.

The boy showed no symptoms until October 30 when he complained of neck pain, and during the next several days he became lethargic and showed malaise and anorexia. His condition worsened, and on November 4 he entered a local hospital with a temperature of 40° C (104° F). During the next 10 days, the boy's temperature dropped, but he became more lethargic. On November 13 stiffness of the neck developed, and the CSF yielded 125 white blood cells. During the next several days, the boy's condition deteriorated; he showed total aphasia, weakness of left arm, bilateral Babinski's signs, and coma. A tracheostomy was done because of respiratory difficulty, tachypnea, and increased pharyngeal secretions. The patient was in and out of coma for a week and then gradually began to improve. In December his condition continued to improve, and he was able to walk with assistance and speak in short sentences. As of October 1971, the patient was reported as normal.

Efforts to establish the diagnosis included biopsy of the brain, which was negative for rabies virus by culture, and FA tests. There were no detectable serum antibodies to St. Louis encephalitis, eastern or western equine encephalomyelitis, or leptospirosis. Serum complement-fixing antibody titer to California virus was 1:8 on October 13, and biweekly determinations through December 3 remained the same. Serum neutralizing antibody titers against rabies were 1:300 on November 13, rose to 1:37,000 on November 27, and remained between 1:39,000 and 1:47,000 during December and January. The question arose, could the 14-day course of treatment with DEV be responsible for these high antibody titers? In answer, it can be said after a 14-day course of treatment with DEV, rabies antibody titers rarely exceed 1:500 and therefore that illness of the magnitude seen in this patient strongly support the diagnosis of rabies. Indeed, the only aspect of this patient's course not compatible with rabies infection is recovery. The clinical management of this patient included the continuous monitoring of cardiac and pulmonary functions, the prevention of hypoxia by prophylactic tracheostomy, and intensive pulmonary assistance. These measures may have contributed to the arrest of clinical illness and eventual recovery.

EPIDEMIOLOGICAL FACTORS

Geographical distribution of rabies includes most of the world. The mammalian host range is so large that areas free of rabies are primarily island nations. The British Isles, Switzerland, Australia, New Zealand, and the Hawaiian Islands are rabies free through eradication efforts and quarantine to eliminate enzootic cycles. It is common in Africa and Southwest Asia and is particularly prevalent in India.

Rabies occurs in any climate and in any season.

Rabies is no respecter of age. The incidence is high in children, probably because of their increased chance of exposure resulting from their friendliness toward animals and their inability to defend themselves against attack.

The *natural reservoirs* of rabies are wild and domestic animals. From the ecological viewpoint, two types of rabies can be distinguished: (1) the natural form of the disease, occurring in wild animals such as foxes, skunks, and raccoons, and (2) the domestic form, occurring in dogs, cats, and cattle.

In the United States the importance of dogs as vectors of rabies has declined greatly. Currently, the most important source of infection for domestic animals is wild animals, especially skunks, foxes, bats, and raccoons. However, in geographical proximity, Mexico continues to have human exposure to rabid dogs.

Mexico recognized 74 cases of rabies in 1988; 92% had been bitten by rabid dogs. More than 8,000 clinically identified cases of rabies in animals and almost 5,000 cases of laboratory diagnosed disease were recorded; 93% of the rabid animals were dogs, 2% cats, 2% bats, and 2% other.

On the other border, Canada reported 2,284 laboratory confirmed and 129 clinically diagnosed cases of animal rabies in 1988. Foxes (45%), skunks (28%), cattle (14%), cats (4%), and dogs (3%) were the rabid animals; 76% were from Ontario.

Winkler (1968) has pointed out the possibility of airborne respiratory infection acquired in caves inhabited by large numbers of infected bats. Although transmission by inhalation is probably very rare, it must be considered in patients with compatible clinical illnesses who have a history of visits to bat-infested caves. Spelunkers may be listed among those with "high-risk" vocations or avocations for whom preexposure prophylaxis is justified.

A highly unusual case was reported of human-to-human transmission or rabies (Houff et al., 1979). This resulted from a corneal transplant to a healthy recipient from a donor who had died of a CNS illness with progressive ascending paralysis similar to Guillain-Barré syndrome. One month after the transplant procedure, the recipient developed an acute fatal meningoencephalitis, which only at autopsy was recognized as rabies. Studies of the donor's and the recipient's eyes then demonstrated the presence of rabies virus in both.

PREVENTIVE MEASURES

Attack rates in persons bitten by rabid animals and the effect of specific prophylactic measures are shown in Table 20-1. Sabeti et al. (1964) described the results of treatment of individuals bitten in Iran by wolves proved rabid. The evidence is clear that use of the combination of hyperimmune serum and vaccine was superior to vaccine alone, especially in cases of head bites, which are associated with shorter incubation periods and higher attack rates than are those in which the head and neck are not involved.

In 1964 Veeraraghaven et al. (cited by Johnson, 1965) compared the attack rates in persons bitten by proved rabid animals in India during 1946 to 1962 when a total of 581 persons exposed in this manner were given a complete course of antirabies vaccine; of them, 49 (8.4%) died. By contrast, of 153 persons who were not vaccinated, 77 (50%) died (Table 20-1).

With use of the new human diploid cell strain rabies vaccines (Wiktor et al., 1977), there now have been several convincing studies of efficacy in postexposure rabies prophylaxis. Bahmanyar et al. (1976) described the successful protection of eight groups, totaling 45 persons, who were severely bitten in Iran by six dogs and two wolves that were proved rabid. A total of only six doses of vaccine was administered to each patient plus an initial injection of antirabies serum prepared in mules. None developed rabies despite deep wounds of the extremities and in some cases the face and head. In Germany all of 31 persons bitten by animals that were proved rabid were protected from rabies by a similar vaccine schedule (Kuwert et al., 1976).

Vaccines

The most recent development in the evolution of rabies vaccines, which began with Pasteur in 1885, has been the preparation of a new antigen from virus grown in human diploid cell cultures (WI-38), inactivated and concentrated. This material is highly immunogenic, free of serious reactions, and effective in postexposure prophylaxis as described previously. It has also been reliable in stimulating high antibody titers when administered in a three-dose schedule to high-risk individuals before exposure (Plotkin and Wiktor, 1979).

The following guidelines for the use of currently licensed vaccine(s) are extracted from the recommendations of the Immunization Practices

Table 20-1. Attack rates in human beings bitten by animals proved to be rabid—effect of specific preventive measures

Authors	Persons bitten		Number of rabies deaths	Mortality (%)	Type of prophylaxis
	Number	*On head*			
Sabeti et al., 1964*	96	Yes	38	40	Vaccine alone
	71	No	6	8.4	
TOTAL	167		44	26	
	50	Yes	3	6	Serum and
	24	No	0	0	vaccine
TOTAL	74		3	4	
Veeraraghaven et al., 1964*	153	†	77	50	No vaccine
	581	†	49	8.4	Vaccine

*Cited by Johnson HN: Rabies virus. In Horsfall FL Jr, Tamm I (eds). Viral and rickettsial diseases of man, ed 4. Philadelphia: JB Lippincott, 1965, pp 826 and 832.
†No data.

Advisory Committee (ACIP) (MMWR 1991; 40:1-19).

RABIES PREVENTION—UNITED STATES, 1991*

Data on the efficacy of active and passive rabies immunization have come from both human and animal studies. Evidence from laboratory and field experience in many areas of the world indicates that postexposure prophylaxis combining local wound treatment, passive immunization, and vaccination is uniformly effective when appropriately applied. However, rabies has occasionally developed among humans when key elements of the rabies postexposure prophylaxis treatment regimens were omitted or incorrectly administered (see "Postexposure Treatment Outside the United States").

RABIES IMMUNIZING PRODUCTS

There are two types of rabies immunizing products.

1. Rabies vaccines induce an active immune response that includes the production of neutralizing antibodies. This antibody response requires approximately 7-10 days to develop and usually persists for ≥2 years.
2. Rabies immune globulins (RIG) provide rapid, passive immune protection that persists for only a short time (half-life of approximately 21 days).

In almost all postexposure prophylaxis regimens, both products should be used concurrently.

---

*For assistance with problems or questions about rabies prophylaxis, contact your local or state health department. If local or state health department personnel are unavailable, call the Division of Viral and Rickettsial Diseases, Center for Infectious Diseases, CDC ([404] 639-1075 during working hours or [404] 639-2888 nights, weekends, and holidays).

Vaccines licensed for use in the United States

Two inactivated rabies vaccines are currently licensed for preexposure and postexposure prophylaxis in the United States.

Rabies vaccine, human diploid cell (HDCV)

HDCV is prepared from the Pitman-Moore strain of rabies virus grown in MRC-5 human diploid cell culture and concentrated by ultrafiltration. The vaccine is inactivated with betapropiolactone and is supplied in forms for:

1. Intramuscular (IM) administration, a single-dose vial containing lyophilized vaccine (Pasteur-Merieux Sérum et Vaccins, Imovax® Rabies, distributed by Connaught Laboratories, Inc., Phone: 800-VACCINE) that is reconstituted in the vial with the accompanying diluent to a final volume of 1.0 ml just before administration.
2. Intradermal (ID) administration, a single-dose syringe containing lyophilized vaccine (Pasteur-Merieux Sérum et Vaccins, Imovax® Rabies I.D., distributed by Connaught Laboratories, Inc.) that is reconstituted in the syringe to a volume of 0.1 ml just before administration.

A human diploid cell-derived rabies vaccine developed in the United States (Wyeth Laboratories, Wyvac®) was recalled by the manufacturer from the market in 1985 and is no longer available.

Rabies vaccine, adsorbed (RVA)

RVA (Michigan Department of Public Health) was licensed on March 19, 1988; it was developed and is currently distributed by the Biologics Products Program, Michigan Department of Public Health. The vaccine is prepared from the Kissling strain of Challenge Virus Standard (CVS) rabies virus adapted to fetal rhesus lung diploid cell culture. The vaccine virus is inactivated with betapropiolactone and con-

---

RABIES IMMUNIZING PRODUCTS, UNITED STATES, 1991

Human rabies vaccine
Rabies Vaccine, Human Diploid Cell (HDCV)
    Intramuscular .... Imovax® Rabies
    Intradermal .... Imovax® Rabies I.D.
Rabies Vaccine Adsorbed (RVA)

Rabies immune globulin (RIG)
Rabies Immune Globulin, Human (HRIG):   Hyperab®
                                           Imogam® Rabies

centrated by adsorption to aluminum phosphate. Because RVA is adsorbed to aluminum phosphate, it is liquid rather than lyophilized. RVA is currently available only from the Biologics Products Program, Michigan Department of Public Health. Phone: (517) 335-8050.

Both types of rabies vaccines are considered equally efficacious and safe when used as indicated. The full 1.0-ml dose of either product can be used for both preexposure and postexposure prophylaxis. Only the Imovax® Rabies I.D. vaccine (HDCV) has been evaluated by the ID dose/route for preexposure vaccination; the antibody response and side effects after ID administration of RVA have not been studied. *Therefore, RVA should not be used intradermally.*

Rabies immune globulins licensed for use in the United States

HRIG (Cutter Biological [a division of Miles Inc.], Hyperab®; and Pasteur-Merieux Sérum et Vaccins, Imogam® Rabies, distributed by Connaught Laboratories, Inc.) is an antirabies gamma globulin concentrated by cold ethanol fractionation from plasma of hyperimmunized human donors. Rabies neutralizing antibody content, standardized to contain 150 international units (IU) per ml, is supplied in 2-ml (300 IU) and 10-ml (1,500 IU) vials for pediatric and adult use, respectively.

Both HRIG preparations are considered equally efficacious and safe when used as described in this document.

POSTEXPOSURE PROPHYLAXIS: RATIONALE FOR TREATMENT

Physicians should evaluate each possible exposure to rabies and if necessary consult with local or state public health officials regarding the need for rabies prophylaxis (Table 20-2). In the United States, the following factors should be considered before specific antirabies treatment is initiated.

Type of exposure

Rabies is transmitted only when the virus is introduced into open cuts or wounds in skin or mucous membranes. If there has been no exposure (as described in this section), postexposure treatment is not necessary. The likelihood of rabies infection varies with the nature and extent of exposure. Two categories of exposure (bite and nonbite) should be considered.

Bite

Any penetration of the skin by teeth constitutes a bite exposure. Bites to the face and hands carry the highest risk, but the site of the bite should not influence the decision to begin treatment.

Nonbite

Scratches, abrasions, open wounds, or mucous membranes contaminated with saliva or other potentially infectious material (such as brain tissue) from a rabid animal constitute nonbite exposures. If the material containing the virus is dry, the virus can be considered noninfectious.

Table 20-2. Rabies postexposure prophylaxis guide, United States, 1991

Animal type	Evaluation and disposition of animal	Postexposure prophylaxis recommendations
Dogs and cats	Healthy and available for 10 days observation	Should not begin prophylaxis unless animal develops symptoms of rabies*
	Rabid or suspected rabid	Immediate vaccination
	Unknown (escaped)	Consult public health officials
Skunks, raccoons, bats, foxes, and most other carnivores; woodchucks	Regarded as rabid unless geographic area is known to be free of rabies or until animal proven negative by laboratory tests†	Immediate vaccination
Livestock, rodents, and lagomorphs (rabbits and hares)	Consider individually	Consult public health officials. Bites of squirrels, hamsters, guinea pigs, gerbils, chipmunks, rats, mice, other rodents, rabbits, and hares almost never require antirabies treatment

*During the 10-day holding period, begin treatment with HRIG and HDCV or RVA at first sign of rabies in a dog or cat that has bitten someone. The symptomatic animal should be killed immediately and tested.

†The animal should be killed and tested as soon as possible. Holding for observation is not recommended. Discontinue vaccine if immunofluorescence test results of the animal are negative.

Other contact by itself, such as petting a rabid animal and contact with the blood, urine, or feces (e.g., guano) of a rabid animal, does not constitute an exposure and is not an indication for prophylaxis.

Although occasional reports of transmission by non-bite exposure suggest that such exposures constitute sufficient reason to initiate postexposure prophylaxis under some circumstances, nonbite exposures rarely cause rabies. The nonbite exposures of highest risk appear to be exposures to large amounts of aerosolized rabies virus, organs (i.e., corneas) transplanted from patients who died of rabies, and scratches by rabid animals. Two cases of rabies have been attributed to airborne exposures in laboratories, and two cases of rabies have been attributed to probable airborne exposures in a bat-infested cave in Texas.

The only documented cases of rabies caused by human-to-human transmission occurred among six recipients of transplanted corneas. Investigations revealed each of the donors had died of an illness compatible with or proven to be rabies. The six cases occurred in four countries: Thailand (two cases), India (two cases), United States (one case), and France (one case). Stringent guidelines for acceptance of donor corneas have reduced this risk.

Apart from corneal transplants, bite and nonbite exposures inflicted by infected humans could theoretically transmit rabies, but no such cases have been documented. Adherence to respiratory precautions will minimize the risk of airborne exposure.

Animal rabies epidemiology and evaluation of involved species

Wild animals

All bites by wild carnivores and bats must be considered possible exposures to the disease. Postexposure prophylaxis should be initiated when patients are exposed to wild carnivores unless (1) the exposure occurred in a part of the continental United States known to be free of terrestrial rabies and the results of immunofluorescence antibody testing will be available within 48 hours or (2) the animal has already been tested and shown not to be rabid. If treatment has been initiated and subsequent immunofluorescence testing shows that the exposing animal was not rabid, treatment can be discontinued.

Signs of rabies among carnivorous wild animals cannot be interpreted reliably; therefore, any such animal that bites or scratches a person should be killed at once (without unnecessary damage to the head) and the brain submitted for rabies testing. If the results of testing are negative by immunofluorescence, the saliva can be assumed to contain no virus, and the person bitten does not require treatment.

If the biting animal is a particularly rare or valuable specimen and the risk of rabies small, public health authorities may choose to administer postexposure treatment to the bite victim in lieu of killing the animal for rabies testing. Such animals should be quarantined for 30 days.

Rodents (such as squirrels, hamsters, guinea pigs, gerbils, chipmunks, rats, and mice) and lagomorphs (including rabbits and hares) are almost never found to be infected with rabies and have not been known to cause rabies among humans in the United States. However, from 1971 through 1988, woodchucks accounted for 70% of the 179 cases of rabies among rodents reported to CDC. In all cases involving rodents, the state or local health department should be consulted before a decision is made to initiate postexposure antirabies prophylaxis.

Exotic pets (including ferrets) and domestic animals crossbred with wild animals are considered wild animals by the National Association of State Public Health Veterinarians (NASPHV) and the Conference of State and Territorial Epidemiologists (CSTE) because they may be highly susceptible to rabies and could transmit the disease. These animals should be killed and tested rather than confined and observed when they bite humans.

Domestic animals

In areas where canine rabies is not enzootic (including virtually all of the United States and its territories), a healthy domestic dog or cat that bites a person should be confined and observed for 10 days. Any illness in the animal during confinement or before release should be evaluated by a veterinarian and reported immediately to the local health department. If signs suggestive of rabies develop, the animal should be humanely killed and its head removed and shipped, under refrigeration, for examination by a qualified laboratory. Any stray or unwanted dog or cat that bites a person should be killed immediately and the head submitted as described for rabies examination.

In most developing countries of Asia, Africa, and Central and South America, dogs are the major vector of rabies; exposures to dogs in such countries represent a special threat. Travelers to these countries should be aware that >50% of the rabies cases among humans in the United States result from exposure to dogs outside the United States. Although dogs are the main reservoir of rabies in these countries, the epizootiology of the disease among animals differs sufficiently by region or country to warrant the evaluation of all animal bites.

Exposures to dogs in canine rabies-enzootic areas outside the United States carry a high risk; some authorities therefore recommend that postexposure rabies treatment be initiated immediately after such exposures. Treatment can be discontinued if the dog or cat remains healthy during the 10-day observation period.

Circumstances of biting incident and vaccination status of exposing animal

An unprovoked attack by a domestic animal is more likely than a provoked attack to indicate that the animal is rabid. Bites inflicted on a person attempting to feed or handle an apparently healthy animal should generally be regarded as provoked.

A fully vaccinated dog or cat is unlikely to become infected with rabies, although rare cases have been reported. In a nationwide study of rabies among dogs and cats in 1988, only one dog and two cats that were vaccinated contracted rabies. All three of these animals had received only single doses of vaccine; no documented vaccine failures occurred among dogs or cats that had received two vaccinations.

POSTEXPOSURE PROPHYLAXIS: LOCAL TREATMENT OF WOUNDS AND VACCINATION

The essential components of rabies postexposure prophylaxis are local wound treatment and the administration, in most instances, of both HRIG and vaccine (Table 20-3). Persons who have been bitten by animals suspected or proven rabid should begin treatment within 24 hours. However, there have been instances when the decision to begin treatment was not made until many months after the exposure because of a delay in recognition that an exposure had

occurred and awareness that incubation periods of >1 year have been reported.

In 1977, the World Health Organization (WHO) recommended a regimen of RIG and six doses of HDCV over a 90-day period. This recommendation was based on studies in Germany and Iran. When used this way, the vaccine was found to be safe and effective in protecting persons bitten by proven rabid animals and induced an excellent antibody response in all recipients. Studies conducted in the United States by CDC have shown that a regimen of one dose of HRIG and five doses of HDCV over a 28-day period was safe and induced an excellent antibody response in all recipients.

Local treatment of wounds

Immediate and thorough washing of all bite wounds and scratches with soap and water is an important measure for preventing rabies.

Immunization
Vaccine usage

Two rabies vaccines are currently available in the United States; either is administered in conjunction with HRIG at the beginning of postexposure therapy. A regimen of five 1-ml doses of HDCV or RVA should be given intramuscularly. The first dose of the five-dose course should be given as soon as possible after

Table 20-3. Rabies postexposure prophylaxis schedule, United States, 1991

Vaccination status	Treatment	Regimen*
Not previously vaccinated	Local wound cleansing	All postexposure treatment should begin with immediate thorough cleansing of all wounds with soap and water.
	HRIG	20 IU/kg body weight. If anatomically feasible, up to one-half the dose should be infiltrated around the wound(s) and the rest should be administered IM in the gluteal area. HRIG should not be administered in the same syringe or into the same anatomical site as vaccine. Because HRIG may partially suppress active production of antibody, no more than the recommended dose should be given.
	Vaccine	HDCV or RVA, 1.0 ml, IM (deltoid area†), one each on days 0, 3, 7, 14 and 28.
Previously vaccinated‡	Local wound cleansing	All postexposure treatment should begin with immediate thorough cleansing of all wounds with soap and water.
	HRIG	HRIG should not be administered.
	Vaccine	HDCV or RVA, 1.0 ml, IM (deltoid area†), one each on days 0 and 3.

*These regimens are applicable for all age groups, including children.

†The deltoid area is the only acceptable site of vaccination for adults and older children. For younger children, the outer aspect of the thigh may be used. Vaccine should never be administered in the gluteal area.

‡Any person with a history of preexposure vaccination with HDCV or RVA; prior postexposure prophylaxis with HDCV or RVA; or previous vaccination with any other type of rabies vaccine and a documented history of antibody response to the prior vaccination.

exposure. Additional doses should be given on days 3, 7, 14, and 28 after the first vaccination. For adults, the vaccine should always be administered IM in the deltoid area. For children, the anterolateral aspect of the thigh is also acceptable. The gluteal area should never be used for HDCV or RVA injections, since administration in this area results in lower neutralizing antibody titers.

Postexposure antirabies vaccination should always include administration of both passive antibody and vaccine, with the exception of persons who have previously received complete vaccination regimens (preexposure or postexposure) with a cell culture vaccine, or persons who have been vaccinated with other types of vaccines and have had documented rabies antibody titers.

Because the antibody response after the recommended postexposure vaccination regimen with HDCV or RVA has been satisfactory, routine postvaccination serologic testing is not recommended.

HRIG usage

HRIG is administered only once (i.e., at the beginning of antirabies prophylaxis) to provide immediate antibodies until the patient responds to HDCV or RVA by actively producing antibodies. If HRIG was not given when vaccination was begun, it can be given through the seventh day after administration of the first dose of vaccine. Beyond the seventh day, HRIG is not indicated since an antibody response to cell culture vaccine is presumed to have occurred. The recommended dose of HRIG is 20 IU/kg. This formula is applicable for all age groups, including children. If anatomically feasible, up to one-half the dose of HRIG should be thoroughly infiltrated in the area around the wound and the rest should be administered intramuscularly in the gluteal area. *HRIG should never be administered in the same syringe or into the same anatomical site as vaccine.* Because HRIG may partially suppress active production of antibody, no more than the recommended dose should be given.

VACCINATION AND SEROLOGIC TESTING

The effectiveness of rabies vaccines is primarily measured by their ability to protect persons exposed to rabies. An estimated one million people worldwide have received rabies postexposure prophylaxis with HDCV since its introduction 12 years ago.

In studies of animals, antibody titers have been shown to be markers of protection. Antibody titers will vary with time since the last vaccination.

Serologic response shortly after vaccination

All persons tested at CDC 2-4 weeks after completion of preexposure and postexposure rabies prophylaxis according to ACIP guidelines have demonstrated an antibody response to rabies. Therefore, it is not necessary to test serum samples from patients completing preexposure or postexposure prophylaxis to document seroconversion unless the person is immunosuppressed. If titers are obtained, specimens collected 2-4 weeks after preexposure or postexposure prophylaxis should completely neutralize challenge virus at a 1:25 serum dilution by the rapid fluorescent focus inhibition test (RFFIT). (This dilution is approximately equivalent to the minimum titer of 0.5 IU recommended by the WHO.)

Serologic response and preexposure booster doses of vaccine

Two years after primary preexposure vaccination, a 1:5 serum dilution will fail to neutralize challenge virus completely (by RFFIT) among 2%-7% of persons who received the three-dose preexposure series intramuscularly and 5%-17% of persons who received the three-dose series intradermally. If the titer falls below 1:5, a preexposure booster dose of vaccine is recommended for a person at continuous or frequent risk (Table 20-4) of exposure to rabies. The following guidelines are recommended for determining when serum testing should be performed after primary preexposure vaccination:

1. A person in the continuous risk category (Table 20-4) should have a serum sample tested for rabies antibody every 6 months.
2. A person in the frequent risk category (Table 20-4) should have a serum sample tested for rabies antibody every 2 years.

POSTEXPOSURE TREATMENT OUTSIDE THE UNITED STATES

U.S. citizens and residents who are exposed to rabies while traveling outside the United States in countries where rabies is endemic may sometimes receive postexposure therapy with regimens or biologics that are not used in the United States. The following information is provided to familiarize physicians with some of the regimens used more widely abroad. These schedules have not been submitted for approval by the Food and Drug Administration (FDA) for use in the United States. If postexposure treatment is begun outside the United States using one of these regimens or biologics of nerve tissue origin, it may be necessary to provide additional treatment when the patient reaches the United States. State or local health departments should be contacted for specific advice in such cases.

Costs are reduced primarily by substituting various schedules of ID injections (0.1 ml each) of HDCV (or newer tissue culture-derived rabies vaccines for humans) for IM injection of HDCV. Two such regimens are efficacious among persons bitten by rabid animals.

Table 20-4. Rabies preexposure prophylaxis guide, United States, 1991

Risk category	Nature of risk	Typical populations	Preexposure recommendations
Continuous	Virus present continuously, often in high concentrations. Aerosol, mucous membrane, bite, or nonbite exposure. Specific exposures may go unrecognized.	Rabies research lab worker*; rabies biologics production workers.	Primary course. Serologic testing every 6 months; booster vaccination when antibody level falls below acceptable level.†
Frequent	Exposure usually episodic, with source recognized, but exposure may also be unrecognized. Aerosol, mucous membrane, bite, or nonbite exposure.	Rabies diagnostic lab workers,* spelunkers, veterinarians and staff, and animal-control and wildlife workers in rabies enzootic areas. Travelers visiting foreign areas of enzootic rabies for more than 30 days.	Primary course. Serologic testing or booster vaccination every 2 years.†
Infrequent (greater than population at large)	Exposure nearly always episodic with source recognized. Mucous membrane, bite, or nonbite exposure.	Veterinarians and animal-control and wildlife workers in areas of low rabies enzooticity. Veterinary students.	Primary course; no serologic testing or booster vaccination.
Rare (population at large)	Exposures always episodic. Mucous membrane, or bite with source unrecognized.	U.S. population at large, including persons in rabies epizootic areas.	No vaccination necessary.

*Judgment of relative risk and extra monitoring of vaccination status of laboratory workers is the responsibility of the laboratory supervisor.

†Minimum acceptable antibody level is complete virus neutralization at a 1:5 serum dilution by RFFIT. Booster dose should be administered if the titer falls below this level.

One of these regimens consists of 0.1-ml ID doses of HDCV given at eight different sites (deltoid, suprascapular, thigh, and abdominal wall) on day 0; four ID 0.1-ml doses given at four sites on day 7 (deltoid, thigh); and one ID 0.1-ml dose given in the deltoid on both day 28 and 91. Another ID regimen shown to be efficacious and now widely used in Thailand employs Purified VERO Cell Rabies Vaccine (Pasteur-Merieux), with 0.1-ml doses given at two different sites on days 0, 3, and 7, followed by one 0.1-ml booster on days 30 and 90.

Strategies designed to hasten the development of active immunity have concentrated on administering more IM or ID doses at the time postexposure prophylaxis is initiated with fewer doses thereafter. The most extensively evaluated regimen in this category,

developed in Yugoslavia, has been the 2-1-1 regimen (two 1.0-ml IM doses on day 0, and one each on days 7 and 21). However, when using HRIG in conjunction with this schedule, there may be some suppression of the neutralizing antibody response.

Purified antirabies sera of equine origin (Sclavo; Pasteur-Merieux; Swiss Serum and Vaccine Institute, Bern) have been used effectively in developing countries where HRIG may not be available. The incidence of adverse reactions has been low (0.8%-6.0%) and most of those that occurred were minor.

Although no postexposure vaccine failures have occurred in the United States during the 10 years that HDCV has been licensed, seven persons have contracted rabies after receiving postexposure treatment with both HRIG and HDCV outside the United

Table 20-5. Rabies preexposure prophylaxis schedule, United States, 1991

Type of vaccination	Route	Regimen
Primary	IM	HDCV or RVA, 1.0 ml (deltoid area), one each on days 0, 7, and 21 or 28
	ID	HDCV, 0.1 ml, one each on days 0, 7, and 21 or 28
Booster*	IM	HDCV or RVA, 1.0 ml (deltoid area), day 0 only
	ID	HDCV, 0.1 ml, day 0 only

*Administration of routine booster dose of vaccine depends on exposure risk category as noted in Table 20-4.

States. An additional six persons have contracted the disease after receiving postexposure prophylaxis with other cell culture-derived vaccines and HRIG or ARS. However, in each of these cases, there was some deviation from the recommended postexposure treatment protocol. Specifically, patients who contracted rabies after postexposure prophylaxis did not have their wounds cleansed with soap and water or other antiviral agents, did not receive their rabies vaccine injections in the deltoid area (i.e., vaccine was administered in the gluteal area), or did not receive passive vaccination around the wound site.

PREEXPOSURE VACCINATION AND POSTEXPOSURE THERAPY OF PREVIOUSLY VACCINATED PERSONS

Preexposure vaccination should be offered to persons among high-risk groups, such as veterinarians, animal handlers, certain laboratory workers, and persons spending time in foreign countries where canine rabies is endemic. Other persons whose activities bring them into frequent contact with rabies virus or potentially rabid dogs, cats, skunks, raccoons, bats, or other species at risk of having rabies should also be considered for preexposure prophylaxis.

Preexposure prophylaxis is given for several reasons. First, it may provide protection to persons with inapparent exposures to rabies. Second, it may protect persons whose postexposure therapy might be delayed. Finally, preexposure vaccination does not eliminate the need for HRIG and decreasing the number of doses of vaccine needed—a point of particular importance for persons at high risk of being exposed to rabies in areas where immunizing products may not be available or where they may carry a high risk of adverse reactions.

Primary preexposure vaccination
Intramuscular primary vaccination

Three 1.0-ml injections of HDCV or RVA should be given intramuscularly (deltoid area), one each on days 0, 7, and 21 or 28 (Table 20-5). In a study in the United States, >1,000 persons received HDCV according to this regimen. Antibody was demonstrated in serum samples of all subjects when tested by the RFFIT. Other studies have produced comparable results.

Intradermal primary vaccination

A regimen of three 0.1-ml doses of HDCV, one each on days 0, 7, and 21 or 28, is also used for preexposure vaccination (Table 20-5).

Pasteur-Merieux developed a syringe containing a single dose of lyophilized HDCV (Imovax® Rabies I.D.) that is reconstituted in the syringe just before administration. The syringe is designed to deliver 0.1 ml of HDCV reliably and was approved by the FDA in 1986. The 0.1-ml ID doses, given in the area over the deltoid (lateral aspect of the upper arm) on days 0, 7, and 21 or 28, are used for primary preexposure vaccination. One 0.1-ml ID dose is used for booster vaccination (see Table 20-4). The 1.0-ml vial is not approved for multi-dose ID use. *RVA should not be given by the ID dose/route.*

Chloroquine phosphate (administered for malaria chemoprophylaxis) interferes with the antibody response to HDCV. Accordingly, HDCV should not be administered by the ID dose/route to persons traveling to malaria-endemic countries while the person is receiving chloroquine. The IM dose/route of preexposure prophylaxis provides a sufficient margin of safety in this situation. For persons who will be receiving both rabies preexposure prophylaxis and chloroquine in preparation for travel to a rabies-enzootic area, the ID dose/route should be initiated at least 1 month before travel to allow for completion of the full three-dose vaccine series before antimalarial prophylaxis begins. If this schedule is not possible, the IM dose/route should be used.

Booster vaccination
Preexposure booster doses of vaccine

Persons who work with live rabies virus in research laboratories or vaccine production facilities (continuous risk category; see Table 20-4) are at the highest risk of inapparent exposures. Such persons should have a serum sample tested for rabies antibody every 6 months (Table 20-5). Booster doses (IM or ID) of vaccine should be given to maintain a serum titer corresponding to at least complete neutralization at a 1:5 serum dilution by the RFFIT. The frequent risk category includes other laboratory workers, such as those doing rabies diagnostic testing, spelunkers, veterinarians and staff, animal-control and wildlife officers in areas where animal rabies is epizootic, and international travelers living or visiting (for >30 days) in areas where canine rabies is endemic. Persons among this group should have a serum sample tested for rabies antibody every 2 years and, if the titer is less than complete neutralization at a 1:5 serum dilution by the RFFIT, should have a booster dose of vaccine. Alternatively, a booster can be administered in lieu of a titer determination. Veterinarians and animal control and wildlife officers working in areas of low rabies enzooticity (infrequent exposure group) do not require routine preexposure booster doses of HDCV or RVA after completion of primary preexposure vaccination (Table 21-4).

Postexposure therapy of previously vaccinated persons

If exposed to rabies, persons previously vaccinated should receive two IM doses (1.0 ml each) of vaccine, one immediately and one 3 days later. Previously vaccinated refers to persons who have received one of the recommended preexposure or postexposure regimens of HDCV or RVA, or those who received another vaccine and had a documented rabies antibody titer. HRIG is unnecessary and should not be given in these cases.

Preexposure vaccination and serologic testing

Because the antibody response after these recommended preexposure prophylaxis vaccine regimens has been satisfactory, serologic testing is not necessary except for persons suspected of being immunosuppressed.

UNINTENTIONAL INOCULATION WITH MODIFIED LIVE RABIES VIRUS

Veterinary personnel may be inadvertently exposed to attenuated rabies virus while administering modified live rabies virus (MLV) vaccines to animals. Although there have been no reported rabies cases among humans resulting from exposure to needle sticks or sprays with licensed MLV vaccines, vaccine-induced rabies has occurred among animals given these vaccines. Absolute assurance of a lack of risk for humans, therefore, cannot be given. The best evidence for low risk is the absence of recognized cases of vaccine-associated disease among humans despite frequent inadvertent exposures.

MLV animal vaccines that are currently available are made with one attenuated strain of rabies virus: high egg passage (HEP) Flury strain. The HEP Flury strain has been used in animal vaccines for more than 25 years without evidence of associated disease among humans; therefore, postexposure treatment is not recommended following exposure to this type of vaccine by needle sticks or sprays.

Because the data are insufficient to assess the true risk associated with any of the MLV vaccines, preexposure vaccination and periodic boosters are recommended for all persons whose activities either bring them into contact with potentially rabid animals or who frequently handle attenuated animal rabies vaccine.

ADVERSE REACTIONS
Human diploid cell rabies vaccine and rabies vaccine adsorbed

Reactions after vaccination with HDCV and RVA are less serious and common than with previously available vaccines. In studies using a three-dose postexposure regimen of HDCV, local reactions, such as pain, erythema, and swelling or itching at the injection site, have been reported among 30%-74% of recipients. Systemic reactions, such as headache, nausea, abdominal pain, muscle aches, and dizziness, have been reported among 5%-40% of recipients. Three cases of neurologic illness resembling Guillain-Barré syndrome that resolved without sequelae in 12 weeks have been reported. In addition, a few other subacute central and peripheral nervous system disorders have been temporally associated with HDCV vaccine, but a causal relationship has not been established.

An immune complex-like reaction occurs among approximately 6% of persons receiving booster doses of HDCV 2-21 days after administration of the booster dose. In no cases have the illnesses been life-threatening.

The reaction has been associated with the presence of betapropiolactone-altered human serum albumin in the HDCV and the development of immunoglobulin E (IgE) antibodies to this allergen. Among persons who have received their primary vaccination series with HDCV, administration of boosters with a purified HDCV produced in Canada (Connaught Laboratories Ltd., Rabies Vaccine Inactivated [Diploid Cell Origin]-Dried) does not appear to be associated with this reaction. This vaccine is not yet licensed in the United States.

Vaccines and immune globulins used in other countries

Many developing countries use inactivated nerve tissue vaccines made from the brains of adult animals or suckling mice. Nerve tissue vaccine (NTV) is reported to induce neuroparalytic reactions among approximately 1 per 200 to 1 per 2,000 vaccines; suckling mouse brain vaccine (SMBV) causes reactions in among approximately 1 per 8,000.

Human rabies immune globulins

Local pain and low-grade fever may follow receipt of HRIG. Although not reported specifically for HRIG, angioneurotic edema, nephrotic syndrome, and anaphylaxis have been reported after injection of

clinical syndromes; for example, rhinoviruses most often are associated with the common cold, respiratory syncytial virus (RSV) with pneumonia and bronchiolitis of infants, parainfluenza viruses with croup, and *Mycoplasma pneumoniae* with atypical pneumonia.

More than 200 nonbacterial agents etiologically related to acute respiratory infections have been identified, and more than 90% of acute respiratory tract infections probably are caused by nonbacterial agents. Since relatively few causative agents are susceptible to antimicrobial treatment, precise diagnostic criteria are needed. Without the availability of a laboratory capable of performing accurate rapid viral diagnosis, it is often difficult to confirm a viral cause during the acute phase of illness when precision is most needed. By the same token, successful culture of bacteria from the nasopharynx does not establish those bacteria as causative agents.

This chapter initially describes various causative agents—viruses, bacteria, chlamydiae, and fungi—associated with acute respiratory tract illness and estimates the contribution made by each agent to the various clinical syndromes. A following section is concerned with clinical manifestations and treatment of acute respiratory tract infections.

VIRUSES

In 1940 only a few viruses had been established as causative agents of respiratory tract diseases of humans; the current total number is well over 200. In Table 21-1 the viruses most frequently associated with respiratory tract infections are presented in tabular form with the clinical syndromes they cause.

Orthomyxoviruses and paramyxoviruses

The orthomyxoviruses implicated in human respiratory infections include influenza virus types A, B, and C. The paramyxoviruses include parainfluenza virus types 1, 2, 3, and 4; measles virus; and RSV. In general, infants are more likely than adults to experience life-threatening infection and lower tract involvement with influenza, parainfluenza, and RSV infection. In infants the clinical spectrum of lower respiratory tract disease associated with these agents is diverse and overlaps.

In the Northern Hemisphere the influenza viruses, RSV, and the parainfluenza viruses cause outbreaks of respiratory illness during the winter months. During a single winter season epidemics of illness caused by particular respiratory pathogens tend not to coincide.

These viruses have the following biophysical characteristics: medium size, ranging from 100 to 300 nm; generally pleomorphic; a nucleic acid core consisting of RNA; enveloped; possession of essential lipids; and inactivated by ether and acids.

These respiratory viruses generally are transmitted via aerosolized droplets shed by infected individuals. These droplets are deposited on surface respiratory tract mucosal cells to which the virus may attach and then penetrate the lining

Table 21-1. Viruses in acute respiratory tract disease

| Group of agents | Serotypes | | Clinical syndromes |
	Number	Number associated with respiratory illness	
Respiratory syncytial virus	2	2	Bronchiolitis; pneumonia; bronchitis; upper respiratory tract infection
Parainfluenza virus	4	4	Croup; bronchitis; bronchiolitis; pneumonia
Influenza virus	3	3	Influenza; croup; upper respiratory tract infection; pneumonia
Coronavirus	3 or more	3+	Common colds in adults
Nonpolio enteroviruses	65	Variable	Febrile pharyngitis (pediatric age group); colds in military recruits; herpangina; pleurodynia
Rhinovirus	100+	100+	Common colds
Adenovirus	42	Many	Both upper and lower respiratory tract disease in children, infants, and military recruits; bronchiolitis obliterans; pertussis syndrome

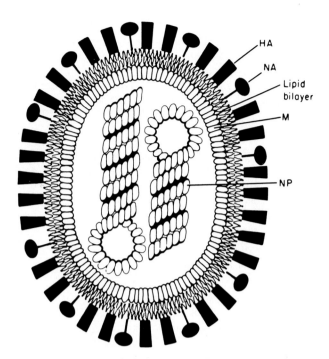

HA
NA
Lipid biloyer
M
NP

Fig. 21-1. Schematic diagram of the arrangement suggested for the structural components in the influenza virion. The two types of surface projections, hemagglutinin subunits consisting of HA polypeptides and neuraminidase subunits consisting of NA polypeptides, are on the external surface of a lipid bilayer; the mode of their attachment to the bilayer is unknown. On the internal surface of the bilayer is a layer of the membrane polypeptide M, and within it are the ribonucleoprotein composed of NP polypeptides and the viral RNA. The location of the P polypeptides is uncertain. (From Compano RW, Choppin PW: Compr Virol 1975; 4:198.)

cells of a susceptible host. Hand contact with contaminated materials followed by direct digital inoculation of the conjunctiva or nasal mucosa is the route for rhinovirus infections and RSV (Hendley, et al., 1973; Hall and Douglas, 1981). For most viruses, however, inhalation of infected aerosols is the apparent route of major importance.

Influenza viruses. Influenza viruses A, B, and C were first described in 1933, 1940, and 1949, respectively. The single-stranded RNA genome is found in eight segments. The viruses are pleomorphic and usually spherical particles, 80 to 100 nm in diameter (Fig. 21-1). The surface of the virus (types A and B) is covered by two types of projections 10 nm long, one possessing hemagglutinin activity (HA) and the other neuraminidase activity (NA). The HA spike is responsible for adsorption of the virus to the host cell. In addition, the HA spike is responsible for the characteristic agglutination of erythrocytes by the influenza virus. The NA spike is respon-

sible for the receptor-destroying activity of type A and B viruses. Neuraminidase cleaves neuraminic acid residues on host cell receptors, allowing elution of the virus from the receptors, and thereby facilitates the cell-to-cell spread of the virus.

The hemagglutinin is the specific envelope antigen, and the differences in this antigen among various strains of virus can be identified by hemagglutination-inhibition (HI) tests. The virus is neutralized by antibody to the hemagglutinin. In contrast, neuraminidase antibody does not neutralize the virus, but it does modify infection, probably by its effect on the release of virus from the cells. Three types of hemagglutinin (H1, H2, H3) and two types of neuraminidase (N1, N2) are recognized.

Influenza viruses vary in their antigenic stability. Antigenic changes occur mainly in the hemagglutinin and neuraminidase proteins. Type A virus is least stable and is characterized by frequent minor antigenic changes and occasional major antigenic changes. Type C virus is most stable, and type B is intermediate between A and C, undergoing only minor antigenic changes. The classification of influenza viruses before 1972 was based on the type of ribonucleoprotein antigen, and the subtype was dependent on the hemagglutinin antigen (e.g., A2). However, when it became obvious that neuraminidase undergoes antigenic variation independent of hemagglutinin variation, it was proposed that the influenza virus strain be designated by the antigenic type of its hemagglutinin and neuraminidase—for example, A/Hong Kong/68 (H3N2) (Table 21-2). This designation indicates that the virus was isolated from a person in Hong Kong in 1968 and that it contains HA type 3 and NA type 2 antigens.

The term *antigenic drift* describes relatively frequent minor changes in H or N that result in the occurrence of annual localized epidemics of influenza type A or B. The term *antigenic shift* refers to the periodic change in the dominant antigenic composition of influenza type A virus. Antigenic shift occurs when there is a major change in the antigenic type of either the hemagglutinin or neuraminidase (e.g., in 1968 the surface antigen shifted from H2N2 to H3N2). In each of the four decades between the 1940s and the 1970s major variants emerged with dominant antigens relatively new to most people. When the population at large has no immunity, antigenic shift heralds a pandemic so that localized epidemics of influenza spread worldwide. The last major antigenic shift resulting in pandemic influenza occurred in 1977. Since that time H1N1 and H3N2 strains of influenza type A have cocirculated.

Since the breadth of antibody is dependent on experience with strains of varied composition, inexperienced children exhibit the highest incidence of infection by any and all strains and also have the most limited antibody reflection of viral antigens. With the passage of time, antibody to succeeding dominants is acquired, but large gaps exist in the immunity of the community to viral antigens that prevailed when the older segments of the population were young. Such gaps in acquired immunity permit epidemic spread of influenza strains with newly rearranged antigenic composition.[*]

---

[*] Francis T Jr: Problems of acute respiratory disease. Yale J Biol Med 1961-1962; 34:191.

Table 21-2. Designation of influenza type A strains prevalent in the United States

Prototype strain designation	Surface antigens		Years of prevalence
	H	*N*	
A/PR/34	HO	N1	1934-1946
A/FM/47	H1	N1	1947-1956
A/Japan/57	H2	N2	1957-1968
A/Hong Kong/69	H3	N2	1968-1972
A/England/72	H3	N2	1972-1974
A/Port Chalmers/73	H3	N2	1974-1975
A/Victoria/75	H3	N2	1975-1978
A/New Jersey/76	Hsw1	N1	1976-1977
A/Texas/77	H3	N2	1977-1978
A/USSR/77	H1	N1	1977-1979
A/Brazil/78	H1	N1	1978-1979
A/Bangkok/79	H3	N2	1979-1981
A/Philippines/82	H3	N2	1982-1986
A/Chile/83	H1	N1	1983-1984
A/Taiwan/86	H1	N1	1986-1991
A/Sichuan/87	H3	N2	1987-1988
A/Shanghai/87	H3	N2	1989-1990

Antigenic drift results from mutations affecting the RNA segments coding for hemagglutinin or neuraminidase, whereas antigenic shift results from a new segment of RNA, probably resulting from genetic reassortment. Because influenza A viruses have been isolated from horses, pigs, and many species of birds, the prevailing theory of the constantly shifting antigens suggests that genetic reassortants occur with strains of influenza in these animal reservoirs.

Clinical manifestations of disease caused by both influenza A and B. Disease caused by type B probably is generally milder than that caused by type A. The clinical illness is characterized by a sudden rise in temperature, rigors, myalgia, headache, lassitude, and anorexia. Respiratory symptoms include a sore throat, nasal congestion, conjunctivitis, and a nonproductive cough. The illness generally lasts several days and may be followed by a period of asthenia. Children are more likely to present with croup, bronchiolitis, gastrointestinal complaints, conjunctivitis, and otitis media.

Influenza A and B may be complicated by the development of pneumonia. The pneumonia may be due to the virus itself or to bacterial superinfection. Other complications of influenza include myositis, myocarditis, Reye syndrome, Guillain-Barré syndrome, and aseptic meningitis. Both myositis and Reye syndrome have been associated more frequently with influenza B, whereas Guillain-Barré has been associated more frequently with influenza A.

Comparatively little is known about influenza virus C; outbreaks of disease from it are usually limited to young children and to persons in military installations. In contrast to influenza viruses A and B, influenza virus C seems to have a single stable antigen. Antibody appears early in life and persists in persons in older age groups, in whom the disease is seldom seen.

Influenza virus reaches the respiratory tract via droplet infection. After a short incubation period of 1 to 2 days, it is possible to detect virus in the nasopharynx. Viremia is probably a very rare occurrence. The neuraminidase of the virus decreases the viscosity of the mucus covering of the respiratory tract, thereby exposing the cellular receptors and facilitating the spread of virus-containing fluid to the lower respiratory tract. If specific antibody is present at the portal of entry, the infection may be aborted. This can be achieved by high levels of serum antibody and/or the presence of local secretory antibody (IgA).

Pathological changes include evidence of inflammation of the upper respiratory tract with destruction of ciliated epithelial cells. If the infection has progressed to involve the lungs, the findings include interstitial inflammation, necrosis of the bronchiolar and alveolar epithelium, and alveoli filled with red blood cells (RBCs), white blood cells (WBCs), and hyaline membranes. Secondary bacterial infection may be caused by staphylococci, pneumococci, or *Haemophilus influenzae*.

Parainfluenza viruses. Parainfluenza viruses comprise four antigenic types: 1, 2, 3, and 4, which apparently are very stable and have not exhibited the continuing antigenic variation so characteristic of influenza A viruses. Parainfluenza viruses have certain biophysical characteristics in common with the influenza viruses, but they also have some unique characteristics, including the ability to hemolyze certain kinds of RBCs and to fuse cell membranes. They are pleomorphic with diameters of 150 to 200 nm; the genome is nonsegmented negative-stranded RNA coding for six structural proteins.

Unlike the influenza viruses, the parainfluenza viruses possess a single surface spike (HN) for both HA and NA. The HN glycoprotein attaches to host cell moieties and initiates infection. A second surface glycoprotein, the fusion (F) glycoprotein, mediates viral envelope fusion to the target cell and viral penetration into the host cell. Proteolytic cleavage of the F glycoprotein by host cell enzymes is required for viral infectivity. The anatomical location of host cell enzymes capable of cleaving the F glycoprotein may help determine the particular tissue tropism of the parainfluenza viruses.

Most parainfluenza viruses are readily detected and grown in primary or continuous tissue cultures of monkey and human kidney. Cytopathogenic effects may be scant or lacking in first passage, but the presence of virus can be recognized by adding guinea pig RBCs to the culture and observing adsorption of the red cells to the kidney monolayer (hemadsorption technique).

Clinical syndromes and epidemiology of parainfluenza viruses. Parainfluenza virus types 1, 2, and 3 were recovered from 40% of 2,359 infants and children with croup, bronchitis, bronchiolitis, or pneumonia and from 6% of 3,377 children with mild rhinitis, pharyngitis, or bronchitis or a combination of the three (Parrott et al., 1962). Altogether, types 1, 2, and 3 constitute the agents most commonly associated with croup. Each of the three types also most frequently manifests as croup. More specifically, parainfluenza virus type 1 has been found chiefly in association with croup and is a major cause of severe croup in young children. Parainfluenza virus type 3 is second only to RSV as the cause of bronchiolitis in young infants. Parainfluenza virus type 4 is isolated infrequently and tends to cause only a mild upper respiratory illness.

Epidemic outbreaks of croup associated with parainfluenza virus types 1 and 2 generally occur in the autumn of the year. Parainfluenza virus type 3–related respiratory infections tend to occur endemically throughout the year. Springtime outbreaks of illness secondary to parainfluenza virus type 3 have also been noted.

Serological studies indicate that primary infection with the parainfluenza virus usually takes place in the first 3 to 5 years of life. Illness associated with primary infection caused by parainfluenza virus types 1 and 2 is most likely to occur in the child older than 2 years of age. The relatively older age at which primary infection occurs with types 1 and 2 suggests a protective role for passively acquired maternal antibody. Illness with primary parainfluenza virus type 3 infection generally occurs in the first year of life. Studies also suggest that infants born with high levels of maternal neutralizing antibody to parainfluenza virus type 3 are at lower risk of having serious illness with type 3 infection.

Most adults have circulating antibodies to parainfluenza virus. The presence of antibody, however, does not preclude reinfection. Severity of illness is related to previous experience with the virus and, accordingly, to age. Thus primary infection is usually expressed as febrile respiratory illness, and approximately one third of the patients have involvement of the lower respiratory tract. Reinfection results in either mild upper respiratory tract disease or no disease. Mild afebrile coldlike illness was observed in adult human volunteers given parainfluenza virus types 1 and 3 experimentally through the nose and throat. Most of the volunteers had specific neutralizing antibody before they were given virus, and there was no difference in serum antibody levels between those in whom illness developed and those who escaped illness. The presence of serum antibody did not prevent illness, but the illness was mild and confined to the upper respiratory tract.

In later studies conducted with human volunteers Smith et al. (1966) showed that the presence or absence of IgA neutralizing antibody in the nasal secretions was critical in determining whether or not the volunteer would be reinfected after challenge with parainfluenza virus type 1 (Table 21-3). Although an inactivated type 1 parainfluenza virus vaccine stimulated the production of neutralizing antibody in the serum of adult volunteers, the response in their nasal secretions was minimal. The implications of these important studies are (1) that the presence of secretory IgA antibodies in the nasal secretions is a better index of resistance to infection of the upper respiratory tract than the level of serum antibody and (2) that a live attenuated virus vaccine offers a better chance than inactivated virus vaccine to stimulate the production of neutralizing antibodies in nasal secretions.

Respiratory syncytial virus. RSV is the most

Table 21-3. Response of volunteers to inoculation with parainfluenza virus type 1*

	Presence or absence of virus neutralizing activity in nasal secretions at time of challenge	
	Present	*Absent*
Number of men inoculated	29	51
Virus recovery	2†	33
Upper respiratory tract illness associated with type 1 virus	4†	29
Upper respiratory tract illness not associated with type 1 virus	7	2

*Data from Smith CB, et al: N Engl J Med 1966; 275:1145.
†P <0.01.

important single agent responsible for respiratory disease in early life. RSV was first isolated in 1956 from a chimpanzee with coryza by Morris et al., who named it chimpanzee coryza agent (CCA). The next year Chanock and Finberg (1957) recovered the first strains in human beings from children with pneumonia, described the characteristic syncytial cytopathic changes, and suggested the term *respiratory syncytial virus*.

Properties of RSV. RSV is a highly pleomorphic, enveloped, negative-stranded RNA virus that matures at the limiting membrane of the infected cell. It measures 90 to 300 nm in diameter. The nonsegmented RNA genome encodes for 10 viral proteins. The outer viral envelope is studded with spikelike glycoprotein projections of which there are two major types. The G glycoprotein mediates attachment of the virus to host cells, and the F glycoprotein facilitates the spread of infection in the host by inducing cell-to-cell fusion. RSV has no hemagglutinin or neuraminidase activities.

RSV is the only human pathogen in the genus *Pneumovirus*. It has been suggested that RSV and pneumonia virus of mice may comprise a third subgroup of myxoviruses distinct from the orthomyxoviruses and the paramyxoviruses (Joncas et al., 1969).

RSV is relatively unstable at temperatures of 37° C and above, and approximately 90% of its infectivity is lost after slow freezing. However, when frozen rapidly and stored at $-70°$ C, the virus remains stable. RSV is rapidly destroyed at pH 3 and also by exposure to a 20% solution of ether for 18 hours at 4° C. In contrast to myxoviruses, hemagglutination or hemadsorption has not been demonstrated with RSV.

On the other hand RSV experimentally has been shown capable of infecting a number of animals, including the chimpanzee, baboon, monkey, ferret, mink, chinchilla, guinea pig, hamster, and mouse. Signs of illness developed only in the chimpanzee and cebus monkey. RSV can be recovered in high titer from the nasal turbinates of infected ferrets.

Tissue culture. RSV multiplies in cultures of several primary, diploid, and heteroploid human cells, including HeLa and HEp-2 cells. The virus also grows in primary simian and bovine kidney cell cultures. In addition to causing the characteristic formation of syncytial areas in the cell cultures, the virus causes some of the cells to become rounded and to degenerate independently without fusing with other cells in the monolayer.

Antigenic composition. There are two major antigenic groups of RSV strains (designated 1 or 2 or A and B) resulting from the variability in the G protein. These strain differences have been determined through the use of monoclonal antibodies. A and B groups co-circulate in the same community during the same season. Primary infection with group A provides a broader neutralizing antibody response than does primary infection with group B. However, after multiple infections, broadly reactive neutralizing antibody is demonstrable.

Within the A and B groups apparently are subgroups based on antigenic differences. Variations among group and subgroup isolates have been noted among laboratories throughout the United States and Canada in the same year and between years for the same laboratory. These differences suggest that RSV outbreaks are community based (Anderson et al., 1991).

Role of immunological factors in pulmonary disease in infants. Early untoward experiences with inactivated RSV vaccines led some investigators to postulate an immune reaction in the pathogenesis of bronchiolitis and pneumonia (Chanock et al., 1969). Suggested mechanisms of pathogenicity include an IgE-mediated re-action, an immune complex reaction, an antibody-dependent cell-mediated cytotoxicity reaction, or an imbalance of various responses. The production of local respiratory tract secretory antibody in the lung, humoral antibody, and cell-mediated immune responses may all be important (Chanock et al., 1970).

Full protection against RSV infection is not conferred by transplacental IgG antibodies; nonetheless, infants with higher levels of maternal antibody are infected less often or are less severely ill if infected than are those with low serum antibody titers (Glezen et al., 1981). It has been suggested that serum antibody reaches the lung and confers protection if adequate titers are present. Reinfections are less severe than primary infections and may represent a combination of acquired immunity and an increase with age in the diameters of affected air passages (Henderson et al., 1979a).

Clinical syndromes associated with RSV. Approximately 50% of children are infected with RSV during the first year of life, and virtually all infants have experienced infection by 2 years of age. RSV has been etiologically linked with five clinical syndromes: mild upper respiratory tract illness, croup, bronchitis, bronchiolitis, and pneumonia. As many as 40% of infants infected in the first 6 months of life will present with lower respiratory tract involvement, with bronchiolitis and pneumonia the most important manifestations. Estimates of the morbidity attributable to RSV in the first year of life are hospitalization rates of 10 per 1,000 infants and clinic or emergency room visits of 110 per 1,000. Parrott et al. (1973), who collected data over an 8-year period at the Children's Hospital in Washington, D.C., isolated RSV from 29.6% of patients with pneumonia. Studies confirming these results have been reported from other parts of the United States and from Australia. Since immunity to infection with RSV is short lived, reinfection is common throughout life. Primary infection with RSV, like infection with parainfluenza virus, usually is more severe than reinfection, which in adults takes the form of mild upper respiratory tract illness. Serum antibody may protect against the development of pulmonary disease, whereas the waning of local antibody in the upper respiratory tract allows infection to occur.

Nonobstructive apnea may occur as a complication of RSV infection. Children born prematurely and who are chronologically young at the time of primary infection are most at risk of developing apnea, which may be the presenting manifestation of infection.

Infection with RSV can also predispose the young child to otitis media. Both bacteria and RSV have been isolated from the middle ear fluid of children with otitis media and RSV infection. Bacterial pneumonia may also complicate the course of RSV infection.

Beyond the prevalence of acute disease in infancy is the question of the role these earlier episodes play in the development of chronic obstructive airway disease later in childhood. In a prospective follow-up study 25% to 50% of infants with bronchiolitis had recurrent wheezing episodes (Rooney and Williams, 1971). Pullan and Hey (1982) demonstrated continuing abnormalities of pulmonary function 10 years after acute illness. A sequential follow-up study of 29 children for 8 years after RSV infection in infancy revealed that half the group had abnormally low oxyhemoglobin levels for 3 to 4 years and 21% for the full 8 years. Spirometry measurements confirmed the presence of peripheral airway obstruction (Hall et al., 1984).

Outbreaks of illness caused by RSV among infants and children tend to occur annually for sharply defined periods in either mid-winter or spring. This annual epidemic pattern is unlike that of influenza virus A, which tends to recur at intervals of 2 or 3 years, that of influenza virus B, with its 4- to 6-year cycle, or that of parainfluenza virus type 3, which is virtually endemic, being easily detectable in the community almost every month of the year.

RSV is transmitted by direct inoculation of respiratory droplets, requiring close person-to-person contact, or through fomites, with subsequent self-inoculation. It does not appear to occur after more distant contact with small-particle aerosols. Excreted virus may persist on environmental surfaces for hours. Nosocomial spread of RSV among hospitalized infants and the personnel caring for them is a major problem.

Adenoviruses

The adenoviruses were first discovered in 1953 by Rowe et al., who unmasked several agents from adenoids removed from healthy children and grown in tissue culture. Currently, adenoviruses form a clearly defined group of viruses represented by over 42 antigenic types isolated from human beings and a number of other types recovered from primates, dogs, cows, mice, and avian species. Adenoviruses are 80 nm in diameter; possess double-stranded linear DNA; have an icosahedral structure with 252 capsomeres; are resistant to the action of ether and acid but are heat labile, being destroyed at 56° C for 30 minutes; and share a common, but not identical, soluble complement-fixing antigen. Neutralizing antibody responses are type specific. The viruses carry many antigenic determinants, including those associated with the hexons, pentons, and fibers of the virion. They can be divided into six subgroups on the basis of the molecular characterization of their DNA. They contain at least 12 structural polypeptides and replicate and produce inclusions within the nuclei of infected cells. The most favorable cultures in vitro have been human lines of epithelial origin (HeLa, KB, HEp-2), primary human embryonic kidney, and fetal diploid lines.

Primary infection with adenoviruses usually occurs in early life, either as an asymptomatic infection or as acute upper respiratory tract disease. Surveillance studies suggest that approximately 5% of acute respiratory tract disease in children less than 5 years of age is due to adenoviruses. Adenovirus is most frequently isolated from children with coryza, otitis media, and pharyngitis (Edwards et al., 1985). Adenovirus-associated pharyngitis is typically exudative and may be difficult to distinguish from streptococcal tonsillitis. Adenovirus type 1 through 7, 14, and 21 may be implicated in cases of upper respiratory tract disease with associated pharyngitis or conjunctivitis.

The adenoviruses also can cause diseases of the lower respiratory tract, including croup, bronchiolitis, and pneumonia. Lower respiratory tract illness caused by adenoviruses may be difficult to distinguish from illness caused by other viral respiratory pathogens. Occasionally, fatal pneumonia in very young infants has been described associated with types 3, 4, 7, and 21. The authors saw a fatal case in an infant 9 months old whose lungs revealed necrotizing bronchitis and pneumonia and intranuclear inclusions characteristic of adenoviral infection. Adenovirus type 3 was detected in the lung suspension and was also isolated from the patient's lung tissue.

Infection caused by adenovirus is generally endemic, with infection occurring throughout the year. Like the other respiratory viruses, the virus is more commonly isolated from October through May. Sporadic outbreaks of respiratory illness caused by adenoviruses have occurred in school-age children living closely together in institutions such as boarding schools and camps.

Although they usually are considered primarily as respiratory tract pathogens, adenoviruses may produce viremia, and disease may arise in distant sites. It has also been suggested that the penton protein of the virus may act as an exotoxin, producing systemic effects. Table 21-4 lists some of the clinical syndromes attributed to adenovirus infections. Outbreaks of keratoconjunctivitis caused by adenovirus types 8, 11, 19, or 37 have been associated with nosocomial infections caused by ophthalmic instruments and solutions. Acute paroxysmal cough with lymphocytosis indistinguishable from *Bordetella pertussis* infection has been attributed to adenovirus. Mufson and Belshe (1976) have reviewed the association of adenoviruses, especially types 11 and 21, with a syndrome of dysuria, frequency, hematuria, and viruria. The enteric adenoviruses, in particular types 40 and 41, have been significantly associated with community-acquired diarrhea (Kotloff et al., 1989) (see Chapter 7).

Among college students and other adult civilians the incidence of adenoviral infection has been low. Young military recruits, on the other hand, were especially prone in the past to epidemics of acute respiratory disease and atypical pneumonia, often with rubella-like rash caused chiefly by adenovirus type 4 and, to a lesser extent, types 3 and 7. Adenoviruses cause between 5% and 10% of respiratory illnesses in civilians and between 8% and 50% of respiratory illnesses in military recruits.

Picornaviruses

A family of viruses consisting of the rhinoviruses and the enteroviruses (poliovirus, Coxsackie virus, and ECHO virus subgroups), has been designated *picornaviruses* (*pico*, very small RNA). They measure 20 to 30 nm and are characterized by a nucleic acid core of single-stranded RNA, absence of essential lipid as shown by resistance to the action of ether, and cationic stabilization of thermal inactivation (see Chapter 5).

Rhinoviruses. Rhinoviruses can be isolated from the upper respiratory tract and are the principal cause of mild upper respiratory illness in adults.

Rhinoviruses share many of the properties of enteroviruses, including particle diameter of 20 to 30 nm, RNA core, resistance to ether, and in general, cytopathic effects in tissue culture. In primary cultures of monkey or human embryonic kidney cells or in human embryonic lung cell lines, rhinoviruses grow best at slightly lower temperatures (33° C) and more acidic pH than enteroviruses. Rhinoviruses differ sharply from the enteroviruses in their sensitivity to acid; all strains of rhinovirus are completely or almost completely inactivated at pH 3 to 5, and enteroviruses are not. From studies published so far, there apparently are at least 100 different serological types of rhinoviruses.

Rhinovirus colds are one of the most common infections in humans worldwide. Epidemiological investigations indicate that rhinoviruses cause common colds and upper respiratory tract infections in adults and children and occasionally lower respiratory tract illnesses in children. Rhinovirus illness rates are highest for young children and infants and decrease with advancing age. Peaks of infection tend to occur in the spring and fall of the year. British scientists, using volunteers, have shown that a number of strains will produce colds. Virus can be isolated from nasopharyngeal washings in the first 3 to 5 days of illness.

Table 21-4. Adenovirus infections

Respiratory tract	Other
Upper respiratory infection (URI)	Keratoconjunctivitis
	Hepatitis
Exudative pharyngotonsillitis	Intussusception
	Diarrhea
Adenoidal-pharyngeal-conjunctival (APC) fever	Interstitial nephritis
	Hemorrhagic cystitis
Bronchitis	Rash disease
Pertussis syndrome	Meningoencephalitis
Bronchiolitis	Myocarditis
Pneumonia	
Bronchiolitis obliterans	

Enteroviruses. The properties of enteroviruses and their role in causing diverse clinical syndromes, including aseptic meningitis, paralysis, pleurodynia, febrile exanthem, and myocarditis in newborn infants, are described in Chapter 5. The contribution of enteroviruses to the cause of respiratory illness is less clear.

Group A Coxsackie viruses, notably types 2 through 6, 8, and 10, have been etiologically linked with herpangina, an acute illness characterized by fever, vomiting, sore throat, and the appearance of small vesicles or punched-out ulcers in and around the throat (Chapter 5). Steigman et al. (1962) reported the isolation of group A Coxsackie virus type 10 from patients with a summer febrile disease that they called *acute lymphonodular pharyngitis*, characterized by the appearance of discrete raised nonulcerative lesions on the anterior pillars, soft palate, and uvula. Another clinical syndrome associated with group A Coxsackie virus type 16 was observed in Toronto in 1957 and in California in 1961. The illness was characterized by a vesicular enanthem on the buccal mucosa, tongue, gums, and palate; another feature, which does not appear with herpangina, was a papulovesicular exanthem involving the hands, feet, legs, and buttocks in approximately 25% of the patients; the name *hand-foot-and-mouth disease* is often used to designate this syndrome.

A number of group A and B Coxsackie viruses have been associated with other respiratory illnesses. Coxsackie A21 and A24 have been associated with mild upper respiratory illness. Pharyngitis caused by Coxsackie A21 has occurred in outbreaks in military populations. In addition to causing epidemic pleurodynia, which has certain characteristics of a respiratory disease such as cough and chest pain, group B Coxsackie viruses types 4 and 5 have been implicated in febrile respiratory tract illness accompanied by cough and nasal discharge. These agents have also been associated with influenza-like illness (see Chapter 5).

ECHO viruses may also cause human infections characterized by upper respiratory tract and enteric tract diseases and common cold–like illnesses. ECHO virus types 1 to 4, 6 to 9, 11, 16, 19, 20, 22, and 25 are known causes of a mild upper respiratory tract illness.

Suggestive evidence linking enteroviruses with cases of pneumonia, bronchiolitis, bronchitis, and croup in infants under 2 years of age has been reported. Serious and sometimes fatal cases of enteroviral-associated pneumonia have been described as well. It may be difficult clinically to distinguish lower respiratory tract disease caused by enteroviruses from other viral lower respiratory tract infections. However, infection caused by enteroviruses typically occurs in the summer and early fall, whereas infection caused by the majority of respiratory pathogens occurs during the winter.

Coronaviruses

The coronaviruses are enveloped, single-stranded RNA viruses. They are large viruses measuring 60 to 220 nm in diameter. There are four recognized antigenic groups of coronaviruses. It remains unclear how many strains are capable of causing human infection, which usually results in either respiratory or gastrointestinal illness since the virus apparently is tropic for either respiratory tract or gastrointestinal tract epithelial cells. The virus has been associated with a cold syndrome in adults. More serious lower respiratory tract infection possibly may occur. Although rhinoviruses tend to circulate in the fall and spring of the year, coronaviruses tend to cause illness during the winter months.

Herpesviruses

Herpes simplex virus types 1 and 2, varicella-zoster virus, cytomegalovirus, and Epstein-Barr virus (EBV) are five of the members of the herpesvirus group for which humans serve as the usual hosts and reservoirs (Chapters 3, 6, 10, and 34). The herpesvirus group is included in this discussion of respiratory viruses because (1) herpes simplex virus is one of the common causes of acute pharyngitis with vesicles or ulcers, (2) varicella-zoster virus may cause pneumonia, complicating chickenpox, particularly in adults and immunocompromised patients of all ages, (3) involvement of the lungs with pneumonia occurs in cytomegalovirus infection, and (4) EBV is a cause of acute tonsillopharyngitis in infectious mononucleosis. Andiman et al. (1981) reported a study of 15 children with pulmonary infiltrates in whose sera they detected antibody to EBV, indicative of current or recent infection with that virus. Eight of the 15 had evidence of coexistent infection with a second pathogen—either viral, bacterial, or mycoplasmal. They speculated that EBV might be a primary or coprimary causative agent or that it was reactivated in the presence of infection with the other pathogen.

Lymphocytic choriomeningitis virus

Lymphocytic choriomeningitis (LCM) virus, a member of the arenavirus group, may cause human infection characterized by onset with respiratory manifestations such as cough and sore throat, by an influenza-like syndrome, or occasionally, by severe systemic involvement, including pneumonia.

LCM virus is one of 14 arenaviruses, only four of which are known as pathogenic for man (Junin, Machupo, Lassa, and LCM). They are ether-sensitive, enveloped viruses containing single-stranded, segmented, linear RNA. The membranous envelope shows surface spikes, and the agent is pleomorphic with diameters of 60 nm to 280 nm. All the arenaviruses are characterized by persistent tolerant infections in their natural hosts, which are a variety of rodents. LCM virus is enzootic in mice, guinea pigs, and hamsters.

Infected gray house mice excrete virus in the saliva and urine, thus providing the most likely source of human infection. There is no evidence of person-to-person spread. The virus is preserved in the frozen state at $-70°$ C and by lyophilization. LCM virus may be isolated from the spinal fluid, blood, and urine by injecting these materials into mice, newborn hamsters, guinea pigs, or tissue culture. Complement-fixing, neutralizing, and indirect fluorescent antibodies (FA) are detected in convalescent sera within 30 days.

RICKETTSIAE

Coxiella burnetii (formerly *Rickettsia burnetii*) is the cause of Q fever, an acute illness characterized by sudden onset of fever, chills, headache, malaise, and weakness that progresses to cough, chest pain, and the picture of atypical pneumonia. The properties of *C. burnetii* and the clinical manifestations of Q fever are described in Chapter 30.

CHLAMYDIAE

A number of investigators have studied the role of *Chlamydia trachomatis* in the etiology of pneumonia among infants during the first months of life (Schachter et al., 1975; Beem and Saxon, 1977). The organism had previously been considered mainly an oculogenital pathogen responsible for neonatal conjunctivitis and for nongonococcal urethritis of adult males. Infants born of mothers with positive uterine cervical cultures have a great likelihood of chlamydial colonization and subsequent development of inclusion conjunctivitis and pneumonia. The full spectrum and epidemiology of this lower respiratory tract infection remain the object of current research. *C. psittaci* is another species of the genus, long recognized for its association with human respiratory disease contracted from a variety of avian sources. Pneumonia or milder respiratory illness has been reported among owners of or dealers in pet birds.

The chlamydiae are small, intracellular, obligate parasites considered a group of bacteria. They possess a cell wall, contain both RNA and DNA, replicate by binary fission, and are inactivated by some antibiotics (erythromycin, chloramphenicol, tetracyclines, and sulfonamides). *Chlamydia* species pathogenic for humans are *C. trachomatis*, *C. psittaci*, and *C. pneumoniae*. The species differ in morphology, staining qualities with iodine, antigenic structure, and their usual hosts. *C. psittaci* infects animals and birds with occasional spillover to man. Human infections are characterized by a febrile interstitial pneumonia, ornithosis, acquired by inhalation of dried excreta or secretions from infected birds. Originally only psittacine birds (parrots and parakeets) were considered the reservoir, but many other species of domestic and wild birds actually can harbor the organisms. In sheep and cattle *C. psittaci* is a major cause of abortions.

C. trachomatis is further subdivided into those agents associated with lymphogranuloma venereum (LGV) and the trachoma-inclusion conjunctivitis (TRIC) group. This latter group received increasing attention as a cause of pneumonia in infants (Beem and Saxon, 1977). Other clinical syndromes caused by TRIC infections include trachoma, neonatal inclusion conjunctivitis, and genital tract infections (nongonococcal urethritis, cervicitis, salpingitis, and epididymitis). (See Chapter 25.)

C. pneumoniae (previously called the TWAR agent) recently has been identified as an important agent of pneumonia and other respiratory syndromes in older children and adults. Infections of children who are less than school age is infrequent in most areas, as documented by antibody prevalence surveys. Infection in younger children, however, has been found in the Philippines. Disease caused by *C. pneumoniae* typically is mild and protracted, similar to other types of atypical pneumonia. Symptoms of pharyngitis (sore throat, hoarseness) or sinusitis may accompany the lower respiratory tract involvement of *C. pneumoniae* infection and, when present, may suggest this diagnosis. Systemic complications of *C. pneumoniae* infection have not been documented. A recent report discusses *C. pneumoniae* infection in children with sickle cell disease and the "acute chest syndrome" of fever and new pulmonary infiltrates (Miller et al., 1991). Thus both mycoplasmal and chlamydial pneumonias may be unusually severe in children with sickle cell disease.

Chlamydiae grow in the yolk sac of the embryonated chicken's egg but more conveniently in cell culture systems. A variety of cells will successfully propagate *C. psittaci*, but the conditions for in vitro growth of *C. trachomatis* are more fastidious. A favorite technique uses the McCoy mouse fibroblast cell line pretreated with 5-iodo-2'-deoxyuridine (idoxuridine). Serological assays for specific chlamydial antibodies are done by immunofluorescent methods with monoclonal antibody. Giemsa stains of infected conjunctival epithelial cells show the inclusion bodies of *C. trachomatis* under the oil immersion lens. *C. trachomatis* may be responsible for 30% of pneumonias necessitating hospitalization in the first 6 months of life (Harrison et al., 1978). In a prospective study of 244 infants, 25% of whose mothers had cervical cultures positive for *C. trachomatis* antenatally, the exposed infants subsequently had twice the rate of pneumonia and recurrent otitis media in the first 6 months of life (Schaefer et al., 1985). Ancillary laboratory findings from infants with pneumonia include a peripheral eosinophilia and an elevation of IgG and IgM.

Diagnosis of *C. pneumoniae* infection is accomplished by culture of respiratory secretions on HeLa 229 cells or by detection of specific antibody with a microimmunofluorescence test. The identity of organisms seen in tissue culture is confirmed with FA staining using a specific monoclonal antibody. The organism is sensitive to erythromycin and therapy seems to give a satisfactory clinical response. Treatment should continue for 10 to 14 days. However, relapse may occur after such a course, and further therapy may be needed.

BACTERIA

It is not easy to assess the present-day quantitative role of bacteria in acute respiratory tract disease. The estimate that the primary cause is nonbacterial in more than 90% of acute respiratory tract infections does not negate the importance of bacteria as both primary and secondary invaders. Patients with lower respiratory tract infections of severity sufficient to require hospitalization are more apt to have bacterial disease than those whose illnesses permit ambulatory care. At the extremes of life, in the newborn and geriatric patient, bacterial pneumonia may be more common, with higher morbidity and mortality. Group A β-hemolytic streptococcus is the most common bacterial cause of acute tonsillopharyngitis with exudate or membrane (Chapter 28).

Acute epiglottitis is the most important respiratory syndrome caused by *H. influenzae* type b (HIB). This disorder generally occurs in the absence of meningitis or other manifestations of infection with *H. influenzae* type b. In addition, epiglottitis occurs at a somewhat later age; the mean age for epiglottitis patients is 40 months as compared to approximately 9 months for patients with meningitis, septic arthritis, and cellulitis caused by the same organism. Pneumonia and empyema caused by HIB have been identified with increased frequency in recent years (Ginsberg et al., 1979). Identification of the *H. influenzae* type b capsular polysaccharide in serum, exudates, or urine may be of great value in making this diagnosis. It may be anticipated that since the introduction in 1990 of a conjugated *H. influenzae* type b vaccine that is immunogenic in young infants, the incidence of these infections will decline sharply in coming years.

With the multiplicity of different agents, especially viruses, capable of causing any one respiratory syndrome, it is difficult to measure the present-day role of bacteria as the cause of acute respiratory tract disease. To make a precise etiological diagnosis, the physician must have access to clinical diagnostic laboratories capable of isolating and identifying nonbacterial and bacterial agents. Of available laboratory tests, the quantitative assay for C-reactive protein may be the most closely correlated with bacterial infection. C-reactive protein rises sharply early in the course of pneumonia and other systemic bacterial infections but remains in the normal range during the course of comparable viral infection.

The differential diagnosis between viral and nonviral illness is often made on clinical grounds that are imprecise, even though they may include a WBC count and differential, an examination of the polymorphonuclear cells for toxic granulations, an erythrocyte sedimentation rate (ESR), and occasionally the clinical response to a "therapeutic trial" of antibiotic therapy. In addition, it may be necessary to use invasive procedures to obtain cultures from such normally sterile locations as lung, pleural fluid, or sinus or middle ear cavities. Potential bacterial pathogens such as pneumococci, H. influenzae, and staphylococci frequently are present in the upper respiratory tract as colonizers; such bacteria generally can be identified even in healthy children.

Thus isolation of a potential bacterial pathogen in the upper respiratory tract generally does not prove its etiological involvement in infections such as pneumonia or sinusitis. Respiratory viruses do not cause prolonged carriage but may themselves lead to secondary bacterial infection.

Early in the course of some lower respiratory tract infections a specific bacteriological diagnosis may be made when appropriate specimens (sputum, pleural fluid, blood) are available for Gram stain and culture or antigenic analysis by techniques such as countercurrent immunoelectrophoresis (CIE).

Despite these obstacles to precise definition of etiology, it is clear that bacteria continue to figure prominently in both primary and secondary roles in acute upper and lower respiratory tract illnesses. For example, an inestimable number of cases of streptococcal infections occur annually in the United States; pneumonias complicating epidemic influenza are mostly bacterial and are chiefly responsible for the deaths that follow influenza; and staphylococcal pneumonia with its various complications continues to present a formidable problem, especially in early life.

Hemolytic streptococci (Streptococcus pyogenes)

Group A hemolytic streptococci are the main *bacterial* cause of upper respiratory tract infections, including tonsillopharyngitis with exudate or membrane and febrile nasopharyngitis in infants. S. pyogenes is also an occasional cause of otitis media and sinusitis. These organisms are seldom responsible for laryngitis (croup) or pneumonia. The characteristics of hemolytic streptococci and the epidemiological, immunological, and pathological aspects and clinical manifestations of streptococcal infections are discussed in Chapter 28.

Staphylococci

The chief contribution of staphylococci to respiratory tract illness is as the cause of severe pneumonia. Pneumonia caused by *Staphylococcus aureus* is a particularly severe and fulminant bacterial pneumonia that frequently is seen during influenza epidemics or at times when S. aureus infections are prevalent in the community. Nosocomial infection was a particular problem in nurseries in the 1950s and 1960s; however, bacterial tracheitis attributed to staphylococcal infection has reemerged as a recognized clinical entity (Nelson, 1984). In addition to the local infection, S. aureus involvement of the respiratory tract can produce various toxigenic complications. Toxic shock syndrome, for example, has been reported as a complication of staphylococcal sinusitis in children. The properties of staphylococci and the pathogenesis, pathological and immunological aspects, and clinical manifestations of staphylococcal infections are presented in detail in Chapter 27.

Pneumococci

Pneumococci are important agents of pneumonia, sinusitis, otitis media, a syndrome of occult bacteremia, and pyogenic meningitis in children. Control of these infections has been difficult because of their extremely wide distribution, the presence of multiple capsular serotypes without cross-reactivity of the protective antibodies that are produced after infection or colonization, and the relatively poor immunogenicity of the currently available pneumococcal vaccines in infants.

Streptococcus pneumoniae is a gram-positive, lancet-shaped cell surrounded by a polysaccharide capsule, an M protein specific for each serological type, and a carbohydrate (C substance) common to all. The capsule, acting as a protective shell against phagocytes, provides a significant factor in the virulence of the organism; pneumococci without capsules are avirulent. The presence of type-specific, anti-capsular antibody is a critical determinant of immunity to pneumococcal infections. In the immune state type-specific antibody combines with capsular polysaccharide, thereby promoting phagocytosis, and it is also responsible for the Neufeld (quellung) reaction.

Pneumococci are grown on various bacteriological media, including blood agar and beef infusion broth with 0.5% dextrose and 5% to 10% blood or serum. Pneumococcal cultures are differentiated from other streptococcal species by their bile solubility and their inhibition by optochin (ethylhydrocupreine hydrochloride). On blood agar the colonies are smooth, glistening, 0.5 to 1.5 cm in diameter and α-hemolytic. Encapsulated pneumococci give a mucoid appearance to their colonies.

At least 83 specific antigenic types of pneumococci have been described. The most frequent types encountered in adults with pneumonia are types 8, 4, 1, 14, 3, 7, 12, 6, 18, 9, 19, and 23, in descending order of frequency, as reported by Austrian et al. (1976) in their collaborative study of more than 3,600 patients in the United States. Among children, the serotypes most commonly identified with disease are 19, 23, 14, 3, 6, and 1. Gray et al.(1980) noted similar distributions of pneumococcal types in children with bacteremia, meningitis, and otitis media with one addition, type 18.

Pneumococci are common inhabitants of the normal upper respiratory tract. Factors that may predispose to invasive pneumococcal infection include (1) preceding viral infections, (2) bronchial obstruction and atelectasis, (3) alteration of mucociliary function by allergy, irritants, and other agents, (4) pulmonary congestion with cardiovascular problems, (5) splenectomy, agammaglobulinemia, lymphocytic leukemia, and sickle cell disease, (6) antibody deficiency states, (7) human immunodeficiency virus (HIV) infection, and (8) the absence of acquired immunity, which is present in infants.

Among infants and children pneumococci cause pneumonia, otitis media, mastoiditis, and sinusitis as a direct result of colonization in the respiratory tract. More distant foci of pneumococcal illness include meningitis and, infrequently, cellulitis, peritonitis, arthritis, osteomyelitis, endocarditis, and pericarditis. Occult bacteremia is relatively common in febrile children under 2 years, whereas fulminant, overwhelming septicemia may occur in patients with functional or anatomical absence of the spleen.

Most pneumococci remain highly sensitive to penicillin with minimum inhibitory concentrations (MIC) of 0.05 μg/ml or less. In 1977 resistant strains of S. pneumoniae were recovered from South African children with pneumonia, meningitis, and/or bacteremia. These organisms were resistant to penicillin, ampicillin, methicillin, erythromycin, cephalothin, tetracycline, aminoglycosides, and chloramphenicol. The only antibiotics to which these virulent organisms were sensitive were rifampin, vancomycin, and bacitracin (Jacobs et al. 1978). A high nasopharyngeal carrier rate was detected among contacts of the patients. MICs to penicillin were from 1 to 8 μg/ml. Cates et al. (1978) isolated a penicillin-resistant pneumococcus type 14 (MIC 4 μg/ml) from an immune-deficient girl in Minnesota, but this organism fortunately was sensitive to erythromycin, chloramphenicol, trimethoprim-sulfamethoxazole, and clindamycin. Other resistant S. pneumoniae organisms have been recovered from ill children in California and Texas.

At present, highly resistant pneumococci are uncommon in the United States. However, these resistant organisms are extremely widespread in other areas, including Europe, and so may at any time be carried into new areas by individual patients or may appear after importation by unknown routes. Examples from recent surveys include the presence of penicillin resistance in 70% of pneumococci isolated from children in Hungary compared with 1% and 7% obtained in surveys in Belgium and Japan, respectively (Marton et al., 1991). Resistance to co-trimoxazole, erythromycin, chloramphenicol, and tetracycline also was identified in these surveys, either alone or as part of a pattern of multiple drug resistance. Drugs useful in treating infections caused by resistant pneumococci include vancomycin, cefotaxime, ceftriaxone, and rifampin. Chloramphenicol may be used if the strain is known as susceptible. Several investigational agents also appear promising.

In addition to the highly resistant pneumococci described above, a second pattern of resistance to penicillin, termed *relative resistance*, is more commonly seen in the United States. Relatively resistant strains have MIC values greater than 0.1 and less than 1.0 μg/ml. These organisms have undergone mutations in the penicillin-binding proteins, enzymes involved in cell wall synthesis. Diminished binding results in the diminished effect of the drug on the growing cells.

Routine screening for resistance should be done with agar-disk diffusion and a 1.0 μg oxacillin disk. Oxacillin is used because the activity of penicillin against relatively resistant cells is sufficient to cause difficulty in interpreting the zones of inhibition.

Prevention of pneumococcal infection is an important goal, particularly for high-risk patients. Prophylactic daily administration of low-dose penicillin (125 mg of penicillin V twice daily) has been used successfully in children with sickle cell disease (Gaston et al., 1986) and could reasonably be used in others with predisposing disorders such as asplenia or in those receiving intensive chemotherapy. Clearly, this approach might prove ineffective with any significant increase in drug resistance in a particular location. Children taking such prophylaxis may thus remain susceptible to pneumococcal disease and should be monitored closely for signs of acute infection. Immune globulins of human origin contain those antibodies present in the plasma of the adult donors from which they are prepared. Thus gamma globulin preparations contain a wide variety of antipneumococcal antibody. For prevention, however, frequent administration and high doses may be needed. Thus in a recent trial of an intravenous immune globulin (IVIG), doses of 400 mg/kg were given monthly to children with HIV infection. As compared with results in placebo recipients, a reduction of approximately 50% was seen in the incidence of serious pneumococcal infection (Mofenson et al., 1991).

Vaccine-induced prevention of pneumococcal infection has been difficult to achieve, both for healthy children and for those more susceptible because of underlying disorders. The current vaccine is composed of 25 μg of the purified capsular polysaccharides of 23 different pneumococcal serotypes. Adequate antibody responses do not develop in the first 2 years of life, the period, unfortunately, during which risk of infection is greatest. The vaccine is recommended for use in children 2 years old or older who are at increased risk of acquiring pneumococcal infection or of being severely affected by such infection. Children in this category include those with (1) sickle cell anemia, (2) asplenia, whether functional or anatomical, (3) HIV infection, or (4) nephrotic syndrome and those about to undergo cytoreduction therapy for Hodgkin's disease. Detailed recommendations for managing the above circumstances are cited in the Report of the Committee on Infectious Diseases (1991).

Moraxella (Branhamella) catarrhalis

This organism recently has achieved new recognition as an important respiratory pathogen, being a frequent agent of acute otitis media, sinusitis, and, in adults, of acute bronchopulmonary infection. *M. catarrhalis* is a respiratory tract colonizer with no other known reservoir. Carriage of the organism is most common in very young children, is most frequent in the presence of respiratory tract symptoms, although *M. catarrhalis* is not thought to cause such symptoms, and is highly seasonal, with prevalence greatest in the fall and winter. It is remarkable that β-lactamase production by this species was first recognized in the late 1970s and that at about the same time its frequency as an agent of otitis media increased at least threefold.

M. catarrhalis occurs slightly less frequently than *H. influenzae* in sinus and middle ear aspirates, being found singly or in combination with other agents in 10% to 25% of cases. At present, approximately 75% of *B. catarrhalis* isolates produce β-lactamase and thus are resistant to penicillin and ampicillin. No other resistance factors are found with any frequency. Clinical isolates of *M. catarrhalis* are highly susceptible to erythromycin, to trimethoprim-sulfamethoxazole, and to one orally administered cephalosporin, cefixime. In addition, the β-lactamase produced by this agent may be inhibited by the β-lactamase inhibitors clavulanate and sulbactam; combinations containing these drugs would also be effective in treating infections caused by *Moraxella*.

Clinical features of otitis media and sinusitis caused by *M. catarrhalis* have not differed from those associated with other agents. Disseminated infection and pyogenic complications have not been described, even when drugs such as ampicillin with limited in vitro activity against the resistant strains are widely used. *M. catarrhalis* is rarely an agent of other infections such as bacteremia, meningitis, endocarditis, and ophthalmia neonatorum.

Haemophilus influenzae

H. influenzae is a small, gram-negative, pleomorphic bacillus found in encapsulated or nonencapsulated forms. Virulent *H. influenzae* possess a type-specific capsular polysaccharide. Six distinct antigenic types, a through f, have been identified by capsular swelling (Neufeld [quellung] reaction) and precipitin or agglutination tests. More than 90% of serious *H. influenzae* infections in infants and children are caused by type b. Nonencapsulated strains are nontypeable and have been associated with otitis media, sinusitis, and chronic bronchitis. Nonencapsulated *H. influenzae* in found frequently in nasopharyngeal cultures of normal children and adults. Respiratory tract disease caused by *H. influenzae* type b takes the form of epiglottitis, pneumonia (often with empyema), mastoiditis, sinusitis, and otitis media (Chapters 8 and 17). Nonrespiratory illness includes meningitis (Chapters 8 and 14), orbital cellulitis, buccal cellulitis, arthritis and osteomyelitis (Chapter 16), pericarditis, and, rarely, endocarditis. Immunity to the organism is associated with the development of type-specific bactericidal anticapsular antibodies that can be detected and quantitated in the serum.

Culture of *H. influenzae* in the laboratory requires enriched media containing a heat-stable (X) factor and heat-labile (V) factor. Antigen detection with antiserum against the capsular polysaccharide (polyribosyl-phosphate, or PRP, of type b) has been helpful in detecting organisms rapidly in infected body fluids such as sputum, blood, pleural fluid, urine, and cerebrospinal fluid (CSF).

As with the pneumococci, changes in antibiotic sensitivity have altered the considerations of chemotherapy for *H. influenzae* infections. Since 1974 strains of ampicillin-resistant *H. influenzae* have been recovered from patients throughout the United States and other nations. From 5% to 25% of isolates from children with invasive disease produce β-lactamase (penicillinase) and are therefore resistant to ampicillin therapy. Thus cefotaxime, ceftriaxone, or cefuroxime is currently the initial drug of choice for infants and children with systemic *H. influenzae* infection. (Cefuroxime should not be used to treat meningitis.) To complicate matters further, a few strains of chloramphenicol-resistant *H. influenzae* have been detected in Europe and the United States, but they are still rare. It is important to test clinical isolates from blood, CSF, joint fluid, and other sources associated with invasive infections for sensitivity to these drugs. At present, clinical outcomes reported with chloramphenicol, cefotaxime, ceftriaxone, and, with susceptible strains, ampicillin apparently are identical (Chapter 8).

Some of the cephalosporins have been subjected to clinical study, with favorable results reported with cefotaxime in invasive *H. influenzae* infections (see Chapter 14 and Appendix A).

Bordetella pertussis

B. pertussis, a common respiratory tract pathogen, is mentioned here because the manifestations in the catarrhal stage of pertussis are those of an upper respiratory tract infection, and often the true cause is unsuspected. Moreover, the severity of pertussis and the mortality in infancy, usually from complicating pneumonia, are not generally appreciated. The characteristics of *B. pertussis* and the clinical manifestations of pertussis are discussed in Chapter 19.

Corynebacterium diphtheriae

Despite widespread immunization practices, *C. diphtheriae* may occur as the pathogen responsible for membranous tonsillitis and laryngitis. It is mentioned here to emphasize the importance of early recognition of diphtheria because delay in treatment with antitoxin may jeopardize the patient's life. The cause and other aspects of diphtheria are discussed in Chapter 4.

Legionella pneumophila

As the result of an outbreak of pneumonia in 1976 following a national convention of the American Legion in Philadelphia, a new disease was identified, studied retrospectively and prospectively, associated etiologically with a previously unrecognized bacterium, and correlated with a wide spectrum of clinical manifestations. Legionnaires' disease has occurred both in outbreaks and sporadically since initial recognition and examination of sera dating back to 1973. The clinical manifestations range from mild febrile pneumonia to the adult respiratory distress syndrome and may be accompanied by extrapulmonary involvement, including encephalopathy, rhabdomyolysis, and gastrointestinal and renal dysfunction. Cases have been reported throughout the United States and also from England and Spain.

The organism responsible for legionnaires' disease is a gram-negative bacillus, *L. pneumophila*, that is exceedingly fastidious and difficult to grow in vitro. As a result, most diagnostic studies rely on serological techniques for antibody increases and/or on direct demonstration of the organism in infected tissues, using special stains. Sputum, pleural fluid, bronchial washings, and lung biopsies or aspirates can all be examined by immunofluorescence and by a modification of the Dieterle spirochete stain (Lattimer et al., 1978). Both in vitro and in vivo the organism may be sensitive to erythromycin, which has been used with some success among patients.

Only a few cases have been described among children (Ryan et al., 1979). Because the illness occurs with enhanced morbidity and mortality in the aged and in the immunocompromised, more cases may be recognized in pediatric populations with underlying disorders such as cancer, immunodeficiency, and hematologic malignancies (Sturm et al., 1981; Kovatch et al., 1984).

Mycoplasma pneumoniae

Although it is now classified as a bacterium, for many years the agent of cold agglutinin-positive primary atypical pneumonia was thought to be a virus. There is evidence that this bacterium, in addition to causing primary atypical pneumonia (both cold agglutinin positive and occasionally cold agglutinin negative) in adults, is an important pathogen for pneumonia and wheezing associated with respiratory infections in children (Henderson et al., 1979b).

The mycoplasmas are ubiquitous, free-living bacteria found in many insects, animals, and plants. They are unable to synthesize a cell wall.

Characteristically, they grow down into nutrient agar and produce a "fried egg" appearance with dark centers and a light periphery. Only one species, *M. pneumoniae*, has been proved to cause significant disease in humans. There is evidence that other related family members (*Ureaplasma urealyticum* and *M. hominis*) play a role in human urogenital tract disease and occasionally in systemic or neonatal infections. *M. pneumoniae* is a filamentous, pleomorphic, 10×200 nm, moderately motile bacterium. It has an electron-dense core at one end with a terminal differentiated structure for attachment to host cell membranes by neuraminic acid receptors. On human ciliated respiratory tract mucosal cells, the bacterium remains extracellular but exerts a toxic effect that interferes with ciliary function and mucosal cell metabolism. *M. pneumoniae* is resistant to cell wall–active antibiotics such as penicillin but is sensitive to the tetracyclines and erythromycin.

Much of the knowledge of human respiratory infections with *Mycoplasma* emanates from studies begun during World War II of atypical pneumonia among military recruits. Eaton et al. (1944) reported the recovery of an agent from filtered sputum or lung suspensions obtained from patients with cold agglutinin-positive primary atypical pneumonia. Material passed to hamsters and cotton rats induced pneumonia that could be prevented by using convalescent patients' serum. In 1957 Liu confirmed Eaton's work by providing unequivocal evidence of infection of human beings with the Eaton agent.

In 1962 Chanock et al. grew the agent on artificial medium. The morphological and staining properties of colonies on agar plates identified the organism as belonging to the genus *Mycoplasma* (Fig. 21-2). With the use of paired serum specimens from patients with *M. pneumoniae* pneumonia, it was observed that acute-phase serum failed to stain the colonies, whereas convalescent-phase serum diluted 1:40 gave rise to intense fluorescence of the colonies (Fig. 21-3).

To complete the etiological postulates, Chanock et al. (1963) infected human volunteers experimentally. Of 27 volunteers with no detectable antibody, three developed pneumonia; four, febrile respiratory tract illness without pneumonia; nine, myringitis with or without bullae and hemorrhage; and four, afebrile res-

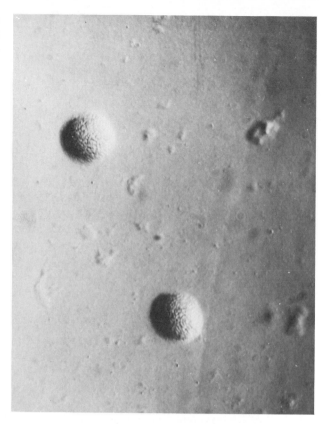

Fig. 21-2. Typical colonies of *Mycoplasma pneumoniae* on agar plate. (×600.) (From Chanock RM, et al. In Pollard M [ed]. Perspectives in virology, vol 3. New York: Harper & Row, 1963.)

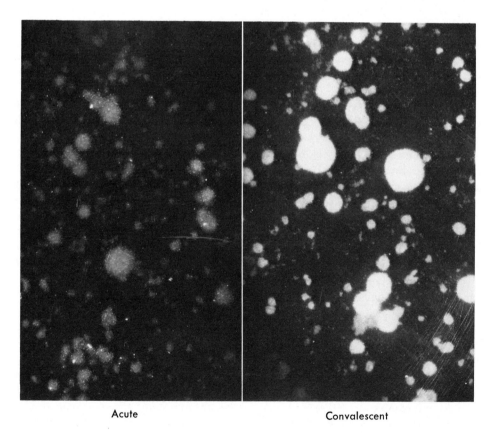

Acute   Convalescent

Fig. 21-3. Agar colonies stained with acute- and convalescent-phase sera from patient with *Mycoplasma pneumoniae* pneumonia. Acute-phase serum fails to stain colonies of *M. pneumoniae*, which indicates absence of antibody; convalescent-phase serum produces intense fluorescence of colonies, indicating presence of antibody. (From Chanock RM, et al. In Pollard M [ed]. Perspectives in virology, vol 3. New York: Harper & Row, 1963.)

piratory tract illness. All 27 volunteers acquired antibody. Febrile respiratory tract illness without pneumonia developed in other groups of volunteers after administration of *M. pneumoniae* artificially propagated on agar. Of 30 volunteers given these materials, 27 showed development of antibody.

Associated clinical syndromes. Community spread of *M. pneumoniae* occurs in protracted outbreaks that may extend through the entire respiratory disease season. The incubation period averages 14 days but is highly variable. Carriage of viable mycoplasma by individual patients may last up to 3 months. As a result of this extended carriage and the relatively low rate of contagion, the period of spread in households may also last for months.

Pediatricians should regard *M. pneumoniae* as the most prominent single cause of pneumonia and of prolonged episodes of tracheobronchitis in schoolchildren and adolescents. This is particularly true in otherwise well children who do not have underlying chronic disorders. The infection is rarely severe enough to require hospitalization. However, children with sickle cell disease and other conditions may have severe and life-threatening pneumonias in which no other causative agents may be identified.

Mycoplasmal infection differs clinically from "typical" pneumococcal pneumonia in having a gradual onset with fever, sore throat, and cough as major complaints. Physical findings of pulmonary infection, rales, and rhonchi may be more severe than would be expected from the general examination. Radiological findings are generally those of bronchopneumonia involving the lower lobes unilaterally or bilaterally. Hospitalization generally is not required. Children with *M. pneumoniae* infection also may be seen initially with localized tracheobronchitis and with cough and rhonchi in the absence of pulmonary infiltrates.

Complications of *M. pneumoniae* infection (Table 21-5) have been reported with some frequency, although it is often difficult to obtain conclusive evidence linking the two events etiologically. Stevens-Johnson syndrome (erythema multiforme bullosa) is the most frequently observed complication and is firmly linked to *M. pneumoniae*. Neurological syndromes such as meningoencephalitis, transverse myelitis, and Guillain-Barré syndrome have been temporally

Table 21-5. Clinical manifestations of infection with *Mycoplasma pneumoniae*

Respiratory tract	Other
Coryza	Erythema multiforme, other
Pharyngitis	rashes
Tracheobronchitis	Meningoencephalitis,
Bullous myringitis	cerebellar ataxia
Pneumonia	Guillain-Barré syndrome
Pleural effusion	Myocarditis, pericarditis
	Autoimmune hemolytic
	anemia, thrombocytopenia
	Migratory polyarthritis,
	hepatitis

associated with clinically diagnosed atypical pneumonia. Seeking conclusive evidence of infection, particularly attempting to isolate *M. pneumoniae*, is indicated in the presence of potential neurological involvement.

Diagnostic tests for *M. pneumoniae* infection include tests for cold agglutinins, for complement-fixing antibody, and for isolation of the organism. Cold agglutinins develop early in the course of infection and are present at a titer of $\geq 1:64$ in approximately 50% of infected children. However, similar titers may be found during infection with respiratory viruses, particularly if cold agglutinins are sought using less specific bedside methods. Complement-fixing antibody may also lack specificity since cross-reactive antigens are found in other microorganisms. For clinical purposes, a fourfold or greater increase in complement-fixing antibody titer between acute and convalescent serum specimens provides reasonable evidence of infection. Such findings may be useful in guiding treatment of family and community contacts during the course of an outbreak.

M. pneumoniae is not part of the normal respiratory flora. To provide definitive diagnosis of respiratory infection with this agent, culture of pharyngeal swabs for mycoplasma may be done. Specific antisera are used for identification of compatible organisms grown in culture. Seeking such diagnostic support should be considered in unusually severe cases and particularly in those suspected of having neurological complications.

Erythromycin is effective in shortening the symptomatic course and promoting radiological resolution of mycoplasmal pneumonia. The oral dose is 50 mg/kg/day divided every 6 hours. Therapy should be given for 7 days. Clinically significant relapses are unusual, even though the organism may not be eradicated by this course of therapy.

In addition to causing a major portion of primary atypical pneumonia, *M. pneumoniae* can also give rise to inapparent infection, mild upper respiratory tract infection, bronchitis, bronchiolitis, bronchopneumonia, and myringitis bullosa. The incidence of *M. pneumoniae* infection in the children in any given locality may fluctuate widely over a period of years. For example, during 1957 to 1959 in Washington, D.C., *M. pneumoniae* was associated with 10% of all pediatric lower respiratory tract illnesses studied at the Children's Hospital, whereas 3 years later only 1% of these conditions were associated with *M. pneumoniae* (Chanock et al., 1963). *M. pneumoniae* plays a major role in respiratory tract disease of school-age children and young adults. Chanock (1965) reported serological evidence of *M. pneumoniae* infection in 55% of 530 marine recruits with pneumonia and in 28% of 141 recruits with febrile upper respiratory tract infections. Evans and Brobst (1961) found similar evidence of *M. pneumoniae* infection in 25% of 91 university students hospitalized for pneumonia. Although in most persons with cold agglutinin–positive pneumonia serological evidence of *M. pneumoniae* infection can be obtained, the converse is not true; for example, a sizable proportion of patients with *M. pneumoniae* pneumonia fail to develop cold agglutinins. Thus Chanock observed that among 239 marines with *M. pneumoniae* pneumonia, cold agglutinins formed in only 46% during convalescence.

Inflammation of the tympanic membrane was observed by Mufson et al. (1961) in four of 50 cases in a military outbreak of *M. pneumoniae* pneumonia. Myringitis with bullae and hemorrhage was observed in nine of 27 volunteers infected experimentally with *M. pneumoniae*. However, *M. pneumoniae* has not been identified as a cause of myringitis or middle ear disease in naturally infected children. *M. pneumoniae* is not known to invade beyond the lining mucosal cells of the respiratory tract, but disease may also be apparent at distant sites. The many clinical manifestations associated with infection are collected in Table 21-5.

Miscellaneous agents

Various mycotic infections, including *aspergillosis, candidiasis, coccidioidomycosis,* and *histoplasmosis,* are relatively common in certain parts of the world and may be manifested by an influenza-like illness or by atypical pneumonia. *Pneumocystis carinii* may cause an invasive pneumonia with bilateral alveolar disease. *P. carinii* pneumonia is extremely prevalent among patients with immunosuppressive conditions, including HIV infection (Chapters 1 and 11). The acquired forms of *toxoplasmosis,* caused by the protozoan parasite *Toxoplasma gondii,* include a syndrome characterized by fever, maculopapular rash, and pneumonia (Chapter 31). These infections have been noted more frequently as opportunistic respiratory pathogens among immunosuppressed hosts. Atypical pneumonia may accompany Q fever caused by *C. burnetii* (Chapter 30).

Many other organisms play an etiological role in respiratory tract infection; many of them are listed in Table 21-6. In immunocompromised patients or in normal hosts exposed to special geographical or ecological settings, fungi must be considered in the differential diagnosis. They include *Blastomyces, Cryptococcus, Histoplasma, Mucor, Coccidioides, Candida,* and *Aspergillus.* Other bacteria such as *Yersinia pestis* and *Francisella tularensis* may cause plague and tularemia, respectively, in patients who have been exposed to infected animal hosts *(F. tularensis)* or fleas from infected animals *(Y. pestis)* while camping or hunting. In recent years the gram-negative rods and Enterobacteriaceae have assumed an increasingly important role in pneumonias of children with immune suppression caused by underlying disease or therapeutic protocols and in patients on broad-spectrum antibiotics for other reasons. Aspiration pneumonias may have a predominance of mixed anaerobic bacteria. Infections with *Mycobacterium tuberculosis* are discussed in Chapter 32. More exotic causes must always be considered in the compromised host. Parasites, including *Ascaris, Pneumocystis, Toxoplasma,* and *Strongyloides,* have all been reported to cause pneumonias in such patients. Stagno et al. (1981) called attention to the role in pneumonia of infancy of a group of pathogens less often considered. They were cytomegalovirus, *Chlamydia, Pneumocystis,* and *U. urealyticum.*

CLINICAL SYNDROMES

This section describes the clinical signs and symptoms and treatment of acute respiratory tract infections. For clarity, these illnesses have been grouped into nine clinical syndromes and are listed together with their various causative agents in Table 21-6. This arbitrary division, made largely on anatomical grounds, is often inexact; for example, "pure" bronchiolitis without some extension of the process into the peribronchial tissues is probably a rare event. Nevertheless, the clinical picture of bronchiolitis is so distinct from that of pneumonia that it warrants separate discussion.

From a practical point of view, the question of whether or not to treat a patient with antimicrobial agents confronts every physician responsible for the care of persons with respiratory tract infections. The use of antimicrobial agents for viral infections is worthless and may be harmful because the sensitive bacteria will be eliminated, thereby promoting the growth of resistant organisms that may become the secondary bacterial invaders. On the other hand, the same antibiotics may be lifesaving when administered to a patient with severe bacterial pneumonia. The difficulties in making a precise etiological diagnosis have been discussed previously.

Common cold; coldlike illness; upper respiratory tract infection

These illnesses are grouped together under the same syndrome because their clinical manifestations overlap widely, and it would be difficult and serve little purpose to make a clinical distinction between them. Moreover the causes, albeit multiple, are mostly viral.

Clinical manifestations. The common cold is characterized by varying degrees of nasal congestion and discharge, conjunctivitis, sore throat, cough, and redness of the pharynx and tonsils without exudate. The incubation period is short; the average length is approximately 2 days, with a range of 1 to 6 days. The first symptom in some persons is a scratchy feeling or soreness of the throat. In others the cold starts with a nasal discharge that is typically thin, clear, and profuse; it may be mucoid or serous. Concomitantly, there is a feeling of fullness in the nasopharynx. Swelling of the nasal mucosa soon blocks one or both nostrils. Sneezing attacks are frequent. The eyes water. Some patients have a nonproductive cough. Headache or an uncomfortable feeling of fullness in the head is common. There may be slight fever, but the temperature rarely exceeds 38.3° C (101° F). Chilly sensations, malaise, and muscular aches are not uncommon at the beginning, but they are seldom prominent, nor do they persist in uncomplicated colds.

Examination shows variably inflamed and swollen nasal and pharyngeal mucous membranes. The nasal passages may be occluded. The senses of smell and hearing may be impaired. Enlarged nodules of lymphoid tissue may be seen on the posterior pharyngeal wall. The nasal discharge often becomes mucopurulent in 2 or 3 days, and at this time a postnasal drip may be evident. The cervical lymph nodes may be slightly enlarged or tender. Some persons are likely to develop cold sores caused by herpes simplex virus. Uncomplicated colds seldom last more than a week.

The cause of the vast majority of colds and coldlike illnesses is viral. Over 150 different viruses have been implicated, including rhinoviruses (100 or more types), coronaviruses, RSV, parainfluenza viruses, adenoviruses, and Coxsackie viruses A and B. In infants under 6 months of age group A streptococcus may cause febrile nasopharyngitis, and pertussis in the catarrhal stage may act like an upper respiratory tract infection.

Complications. The common cold may be complicated by an extension of the viral infection or by bacterial infections that include otitis media, sinusitis, tonsillitis, cervical adenitis, laryngitis, bronchitis, bronchiolitis, and pneumonia. Infants and children are particularly likely to develop otitis media; therefore the eardrums should be examined for this complication. Secondary infections may be caused by any pathogenic bacteria in the upper respiratory passages. Appropriate antimicrobial therapy has reduced the seriousness of these complications.

Diagnosis. The typical clinical pattern makes the diagnosis easy in most cases. Rhinitis, coryza, sneezing, scratchiness of the throat, and cough, all in the absence of pronounced constitutional symptoms, point to the common cold. There is no practical laboratory test by which the diagnosis can be confirmed. Similar clinical pictures may be presented by various other conditions. Allergic rhinitis may be clinically indis-

viruses is quite limited. As is true in adults with acute sinusitis, anaerobic bacteria are rarely present in the sinus aspirates. The organisms listed above have also been found in children with chronic sinusitis, although anaerobes may also be involved in some chronic cases. Nasopharyngeal and throat cultures are of little use in planning treatment since pathogens present in these locations frequently differ from those found in the sinus cavity. Thus the microbiology of acute sinusitis closely resembles that of acute otitis media. Treatment, as for ear infections, should be aimed at the major pathogens and their known patterns of drug resistance. Performing sinus aspiration rarely is needed for planning antimicrobial therapy for children with acute sinusitis; however, needle aspiration or endoscopic procedures may be essential in some children with chronic infection or with underlying disorders of host defenses.

Acute tonsillopharyngitis with exudate or membrane

Acute tonsillopharyngitis with exudate or membrane is characterized by fever, sore throat, tonsillar and pharyngeal reddening and edema, and the presence of an exudate or membrane. A varying degree of cervical lymph node enlargement may be present. A frequent cause is group A streptococcus (Chapter 28). A less common but very important cause is *C. diphtheriae* (Chapter 4). Membranous tonsillitis is also a frequent manifestation of infectious mononucleosis (p. 90) and is often seen in military recruits, infants, and children up to age 3 years with adenovirus infection. Antimicrobial therapy (discussed in detail on p. 484) is indicated for patients with exudative pharyngitis caused by group A hemolytic streptococcus.

Current experience indicates that a 10-day course of penicillin (or erythromycin or, possibly, an oral cephalosporin for patients who are allergic to penicillin) is most effective for routine use.

If the diphtheria bacillus is suspected or is proved the responsible agent, therapy with diphtheria antitoxin in addition to penicillin or erythromycin (p. 52) should be instituted. Antibiotics are of no value in the treatment of infectious mononucleosis or adenovirus infection.

Acute tonsillopharyngitis with vesicles or ulcers

Acute tonsillopharyngitis with vesicles or ulcers is characterized by fever, sore throat, and vesicles or shallow white ulcers 2 to 4 mm in diameter on the anterior fauces, palate, and buccal mucous membrane. It most commonly is caused by a virus, either herpes simplex virus or group A Coxsackie virus. A primary infection with herpes simplex virus is usually characterized by stomatitis and gingivitis rather than tonsillopharyngitis (Chapter 10). Gingivitis is not associated with herpangina, which is caused by group A Coxsackie virus. This syndrome is discussed in detail in Chapter 5. Antimicrobial agents are of no value in the treatment of these infections.

Infectious croup

Inflammatory obstruction of the airway produces the characteristic clinical picture in all forms of infectious croup. The severity and extent of the infectious process determine the sites of obstruction in the laryngotracheobronchial tree.

Mild laryngitis is characterized by hoarseness and a barking or croupy cough, which is likely to be worse at night. Low-grade fever, loss of appetite, and malaise may be the only constitutional signs. Difficulty in breathing is slight or absent; the condition responds promptly to appropriate treatment and subsides in a few days.

Acute laryngitis (croup). A more severe type of laryngitis begins in the same fashion as mild laryngitis but progresses rapidly to the stage of obstruction. The site of obstruction is usually the subglottic area. Hoarseness is more marked, and breathing becomes rapid and labored, with inspiratory stridor and inspiratory retraction of the suprasternal notch, the supraclavicular spaces, the substernal region, and even the intercostal spaces. The child grows restless, often in spite of high humidity and oxygen levels. For a few moments he may scramble about the crib desperately seeking relief and then lie still briefly, only to be roused again by air hunger. The cycle is repeated until the patient becomes exhausted. Cyanosis is sometimes evident in the nail beds and lips. If the obstruction is unrelieved, the patient's color becomes ashen gray, and he sinks into a relaxed, shocklike state as death approaches.

In patients whose infection is limited to the laryngeal area, auscultation of the chest reveals little beyond inspiratory stridor and generally diminished aeration. The pharynx is inflamed, and laryngoscopic examination shows little supraglottic involvement except in *H. influenzae* epiglottitis (discussed later). The main site of obstruction lies below the vocal cords where the soft subglottic tissues bulge to meet in the midline (Fig. 21-4). The mucosa appears deep red and velvety. A gummy mucopurulent exudate or dry yellow crusts add to the obstruction of the airway.

Acute laryngotracheitis and laryngotracheobronchitis (croup). In a patient with severe acute laryngitis the infection may descend rapidly to the trachea and sometimes the bronchi; this increases the patient's struggle for air, his prostration, and his fever. In laryngotracheobronchitis an expiratory wheeze and various types of bronchitic rales are heard on auscultation of the chest. Aeration of the lungs may be good at one moment and impaired the next. Finding localized areas of suppressed to absent breath sounds, bronchial breathing, and dullness to percussion indicates atelectasis resulting from the complete plugging of a bronchus with thick, tenacious exudate. If a main bronchus becomes plugged, air hunger, cyanosis, and restlessness are increased. The heart and mediastinum may be shifted to the affected side. In the presence of obstructive emphysema caused by partial blocking of a bronchus, the heart and mediastinum may be displaced to the opposite side. These various signs and the alarming dyspnea usually disappear after aspiration of the plugged bronchus.

The progression of symptoms and signs of acute laryngotracheitis has been described by Forbes (1961) as developing in the following four stages:

Stage 1
    Fever
    Hoarseness of voice
    Croupy cough
    Inspiratory stridor when distributed

Stage 2
    Continous respiratory stridor
    Lower-rib retraction
    Retraction of soft tissue of the neck
    Activation of accessory muscles of respiration
    Labored respiration

Stage 3
    Signs of anoxia and carbon dioxide retention
    Restlessness
    Anxiety
    Pallor
    Sweating
    Rapid respiration

Stage 4
    Intermittent cyanosis
    Permanent cyanosis
    Cessation of breathing

In patients with mild disease and those whose airway has been improved by treatment, croup rarely progresses beyond stage 1.

Acute epiglottitis. Acute epiglottitis is bacterial in etiology and nearly always is caused by *H. influenzae* type b. The site of the obstruction is supraglottic, in contrast with acute viral laryngotracheitis in which the obstruction is subglottic (Chapter 8).

Diagnosis. The typical picture of severe epiglottitis or croup is not soon forgotten. Croup begins as an ordinary upper respiratory tract infection. The child then acquires a hoarse voice and a barking cough. This is followed by dyspnea, inspiratory stridor, and retraction of the soft spaces of the thoracic cage. If obstruction is not relieved, the patient shows increasing restlessness, cyanosis, progressive air hunger, and prostration, ending in death.

First and foremost, it is important to identify *H. influenzae* epiglottitis because it is a medical emergency that requires immediate therapy. It is also important to consider the possibility of diphtheritic laryngitis, especially in unimmunized persons. This diagnosis is suggested by the presence of a faucial membrane and evidence of subglottic obstruction. However, even in the absence of a membrane in the pharynx, progression of inspiratory stridor over a 1- to 2-day period in a toxic patient may indicate the presence of diphtheritic laryngitis without evidence of pharyngeal involvement. The diagnosis may be confirmed by culture of the throat and tracheal aspirates.

Differential diagnosis

Spasmodic croup. Spasmodic croup may simulate infectious croup in many respects. It has been distinguished from infectious croup by (1) the absence or mildness of signs of inflammation,

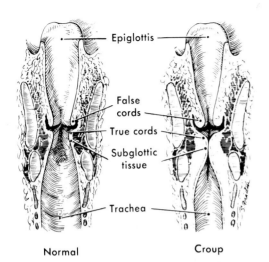

Epiglottis

False cords

True cords

Subglottic tissue

Trachea

Normal

Croup

Fig. 21-4. Schematic diagram of larynx and trachea in viral croup as compared with normal appearance.

(2) the typical remissions during the daytime, and (3) the history of previous attacks lasting for 2 or 3 days followed by uneventful recovery. Cramblett (1960) described a child with three typical attacks of acute spasmodic croup at 4, 11, and 29 months of age. Each attack was associated with an infection from a virus—parainfluenza virus type 2 in the first attack, influenza type A virus in the second, and ECHO virus type 11 in the third.

Foreign bodies. An awareness of the capacity of foreign bodies to reproduce the obstructive phenomena is essential. If there is a history of sudden onset of choking, paroxysmal coughing, and absence of signs of infection, fluoroscopic and roentgenographic examinations and endoscopy should clarify the diagnosis.

Retropharyngeal abscess. Retropharyngeal abscess may be mistaken for infectious croup. It occurs in infants and children and is marked by drooling, noisy and difficult mouth breathing, dysphagia, retraction of the head, and enlargement of the cervical lymph nodes. The diagnosis is established by a lateral roentgenogram of the neck and by finger palpation of a fluctuant mass on the posterior pharyngeal wall. Prompt institution of antibiotic therapy and controlled surgical drainage are the cornerstones of treatment.

Angioneurotic edema. Angioneurotic edema, seldom encountered in infants or young children, is characterized by supraglottic swelling in response to a specific food or some other allergen. The diagnosis is confirmed by finding pale red, rounded masses on either side of the superior isthmus of the larynx on direct laryn-

goscopic examination. Urticaria is an external sign pointing to the likely diagnosis. The rapid response to epinephrine is a good therapeutic test.

Complications. In the course of laryngotracheobronchitis the formation of exudate in the tracheobronchial tree contributes to the development of potentially life-threatening complications. Two factors are believed to promote this condition: (1) breathing air that is not saturated with moisture and (2) temporary alterations of function of the mucus-secreting glands of the respiratory tract. In any event, crusting of the exudate may lead to further obstruction of the airway and collapse of a segment of the lung. The cough reflex usually is diminished in these patients. Cyanosis develops or increases. Signs of consolidation may be mistaken for pneumonia.

Mediastinal emphysema and pneumothorax are common complications. Extraalveolar thoracic air may be produced through (1) the intrinsic route, in which minute perivascular ruptures occur in the alveoli, leading to pulmonary interstitial emphysema, mediastinal emphysema, pneumothorax, pneumoperitoneum, and subcutaneous emphysema, and (2) the extrinsic route, in which air enters the superior mediastinum behind the pretracheal fascia as a result of tracheostomy. From the superior mediastinum, air can penetrate adjacent areas. Both of these mechanisms may operate to produce mediastinal emphysema and pneumothorax. Tracheostomy is not the only factor nor even necessarily the most important factor since instances of extraalveolar thoracic air have been observed before or in the absence of tracheostomy.

The presence of pneumothorax may be suspected in a patient with absence of breath sounds and a hyperresonant percussion note on one side of the thorax and displacement of the heart and mediastinum to the opposite side. Roentgenographic examination shows the extent of the pneumothorax and is usually the means of detecting mediastinal emphysema. Subcutaneous emphysema produces a distinctive crackling or crepitus on palpation.

Interstitial bronchopneumonia probably is present in every case of severe croup because the disease process extends to the terminal bronchioles, peribronchial tissues, and alveoli. It is often impossible even by roentgenographic examination to distinguish between patchy areas of atelectasis and interstitial pneumonia. The combination of infection and atelectasis, if persistent, is conducive to bronchiectasis, which may be seen as an end result. Travis et al. (1977) have pointed out the occurrence of pulmonary edema in several patients with laryngotracheitis and epiglottitis.

Prognosis. The prognosis of patients with infectious croup is related to the character and extent of infection and to the amount of obstruction. As the disease progresses downward from simple laryngitis to laryngotracheobronchitis, the mortality rate has been reported to increase (Rabe, 1948). Only one death occurred among 262 patients with viral croup who did not have a tracheostomy. Of 35 patients with fatal cases, six had severe obstruction caused by crusted exudate in the trachea and bronchi (see Chapter 8).

Treatment. The keynote of treatment is to maintain the airway and to combat infection. The patient must be placed promptly in an atmosphere with a high humidity level. In the home this sometimes can be achieved by turning on the hot water taps in a closed bathroom. In the hospital the patient should be placed in a room or tent in which the air is supersaturated with moisture, preferably by means of a mechanical humidifier with 30% to 40% oxygen. The temperature should be 21.1° to 23.9° C (70° to 75° F). Higher temperatures, as generated in steam tents, are oppressive and not necessary. Cool mist may relieve stridor by decreasing local inflammation and edema. Alternatively, mist may also act centrally by altering central nervous system regulation of respiration.

The patient should have plenty to drink. If fluids cannot be given by mouth, they must be administered parenterally. Rest is of paramount importance. The patient should be spared all needless medical examinations, details of nursing care, and especially, a succession of diagnostic or therapeutic venipunctures, taking of blood for blood counts, taking of nose and throat cultures, and other tests. Every effort should be made not to disturb a sleeping child. Pulse oximetry offers a noninvasive method of continuously monitoring blood oxygen saturations. Expectorants have been tried and found wanting. Opiates and atropine are contraindicated.

In many cases, especially those in which infection is limited to the upper respiratory tract, a period of breathing supersaturated air, combined with rest, will be followed by no increase in the obstructive symptoms. Hoarseness, dyspnea, and inspiratory retraction or pulling are still present but are no worse. The child is not restless and sleeps from time to time. The color is good, with no cyanosis. Little by little the signs and symptoms disappear, and in a few days the patient progresses to complete recovery. Severe cases with a similar onset are likely not to pursue such a favorable course. The obstructive phenomena are aggravated until it is obvious that the child will suffocate unless an airway is established.

Indications for tracheostomy or intubation. The decision to perform a tracheostomy or intubation for a patient with croup and when to do it call for clinical judgment. If this procedure is indicated, it is best done before the patient becomes exhausted and before it must be done as an emergency, or last-ditch, procedure. If despite high humidity and oxygen levels, the patient shows increasing duskiness, dyspnea, inspiratory retraction, diminished air entry, and especially restlessness, increasing obstruction to the airway is present and is a clear indication for tracheostomy or intubation. Blood gas studies may show a falling partial pressure of oxygen (PO_2) with a normal partial pressure of carbon dioxide (PCO_2). The establishment of an airway is usually followed by immediate and dramatic relief, and the child falls asleep as the tube is being installed.

The teamwork of pediatrician, bronchoscopist, respiratory therapist, and nurse is vitally important for the proper care of the patient. The bronchoscopist should see the patient, if possible, when he is admitted to the hospital, even though there may be no indication for an artificial airway at the moment. Someone with experience should be in attendance at all times. Special nursing care is essential because the tube may become plugged at any time. Frequent aspiration of tracheobronchial secretions is usually necessary. A bronchoscopist should be quickly available to deal with sticky exudates or crusts that cannot be aspirated by a catheter and that give rise to obstruction and pulmonary collapse.

Specific chemotherapy. Since most cases of infectious croup are viral in origin, the indications for administering antimicrobial agents are specific only in patients with *H. influenzae* and *C. diphtheriae* infections.

Corticosteroid therapy. The advocates of corticosteroid therapy postulate that its anti-inflammatory effect will reduce edema and improve the airway. The opponents of this therapy point to the equivocal clinical trials and the extensive studies on laboratory animals supported by clinical experience indicating that cortisone enhances susceptibility to infection. Although there is no evidence of harmful effects after the use of these drugs for a period limited to 2 or 3 days, the value of corticosteroids in the treatment of croup remains controversial (Eden et al., 1967; Cherry, 1979; Leipzig et al., 1979). In the absence of a large randomized clinical trial, a meta-analysis of 10 previously published reports on the use of steroids supports their use in the treatment of children hospitalized with croup (Kairys et al., 1989). An increased proportion of the steroid-treated children had clinical improvement 12 and 24 hours after initiation of therapy. A reduced incidence of endotracheal intubation was also noted among steroid-treated children. A prudent approach would be to limit the use of steroids in croup to those children who both are hospitalized and have severe disease.

Other therapy. Nebulized racemic epinephrine has been helpful in the experience of some clinicians (Taussig et al., 1977; Westley et al., 1978). Treatments given at 2- to 4-hour intervals may produce acute beneficial results, but patients must continue under close observation because there may be a "rebound phenomenon," with relapse within several hours of the initial improvement. The dose is 0.5 ml of 2.25% racemic epinephrine in 2.5 ml of normal saline solution dispensed as a nebulized treatment. There is no added benefit to the use of an intermittent positive pressure breathing (IPPB) apparatus.

Acute bronchiolitis

Bronchiolitis usually begins as an ordinary upper respiratory tract infection with nasal discharge, cough, slight fever, fretfulness, and loss of appetite. In a day or so the infant gets rapidly worse and presents an alarming picture of rapid labored breathing, with retraction of the intercostal spaces, use of accessory respiratory muscles, cyanosis, and prostration. Increasing obstruction leads to progressive hypoxemia, which if unrelieved, may be followed by exhaustion and death. Respirations are rapid, shallow, difficult, and often wheezy, with a rate of 60 to 80 or more per minute. Inspiratory retraction is seen in the suprasternal notch and the intercostal and subcostal spaces. The cough is frequent, distressing, and often paroxysmal. Cyanosis appears or is intensified during coughing or crying and probably is continuous if the obstruction is severe. The patient is prostrate and takes little interest in his surroundings.

Physical findings, often changeable, are those of overinflated lungs; that is, the percussion note is hyperresonant, the diaphragm is depressed, and expiration is prolonged. Early, the breath sounds are diminished, and often no rales are heard. Later, fine, dry, or sibilant rales are audible. Fluoroscopic or roentgenographic examination of the chest shows the lung fields are abnormally transparent, with increased bronchovascular markings. The diaphragm is depressed, and the intercostal spaces are widened. Atelectatic areas are usually small and difficult to recognize in the roentgenogram. Occasionally, one or more segments are collapsed. Arterial blood gas determinations can be very helpful in assessing the patient's respiratory exchange, the need for further support, and the response to treatment. The anticipated findings are an initial hypoxemia, which may be followed by respiratory acidosis and hypercapnia as deterioration occurs.

The nonbacterial cause of bronchiolitis, long

suspected on clinical grounds, became more clearly defined as a result of the studies of Parrott et al. (1962). RSV is the most important single agent causing bronchiolitis, followed by parainfluenza virus types 3 and 1, adenoviruses, rhinoviruses, and influenza virus. Measles virus occasionally may cause bronchiolitis. In school-age children similar illnesses, wheezing-associated respiratory infections, are more often caused by *Mycoplasma pneumoniae* (Henderson et al., 1979b). RSV bronchiolitis and bronchopneumonia may be found as nosocomial infections among infants and children in nurseries and pediatric wards and may occur also among daycare center residents (Wenzel et al., 1977).

With the advent of specific antiviral therapy for lower respiratory infection secondary to RSV, timely determination of a causative agent is crucial. The agent responsible for an episode of bronchiolitis frequently can be determined by virus isolation or vital antigen detection. Virus isolation takes several days. Detection of viral antigen can be accomplished in several hours and thereby offers a means by which a rapid viral diagnosis can be ascertained. Techniques widely used for the detection of RSV antigen in respiratory epithelial cells include the indirect immunofluorescent method and the enzyme-linked immunosorbent assay. Immunofluorescence can also be applied for the detection of other viral antigens.

The treatment of acute bronchiolitis should aim at (1) relieving bronchiolar obstruction, (2) correcting hypoxemia and acidosis, (3) controlling potential cardiac complications, (4) providing supportive measures, and (5) combating any secondary bacterial infection.

The patient should breathe air well saturated with water vapor and high in oxygen content. The high humidity level is designed to render the exudates less sticky. Oxygen tends to dry bronchial secretions and therefore must be used only in conjunction with water vapor. Sometimes epinephrine (0.1 ml of 1:1000 solution given subcutaneously) or aminophylline seems to relieve bronchiolar spasm temporarily. Some groups have reported short-term improvement after the administration of racemic epinephrine by IPPB apparatus. Cardiovascular support and drugs may be required in the presence of manifestations of developing heart failure such as enlargement of the liver, gallop rhythm, change in quality of heart sounds, tachycardia, and pulmonary edema. If the patient has very severe bronchiolitis that progresses in spite of these measures, it may be necessary to provide assisted ventilation and all the support available in an intensive care unit.

Because of the viral cause of bronchiolitis, antimicrobial therapy is of no benefit. The routine prophylactic or therapeutic use of antimicrobial agents is contraindicated.

Ribavirin, a synthetic nucleoside with antiviral properties, has beneficial effects when administered by aerosol to infants with RSV bronchiolitis and pneumonia (Hall et al., 1983). Ribavirin should be considered for use in selected groups of infants hospitalized with lower respiratory tract disease caused by RSV. Infants with cardiopulmonary diseases, immunodeficiency diseases, or prematurity or severely ill infants should be considered candidates for ribavirin therapy.

Pneumonia

The term *pneumonia* is used to describe a variety of reactions of the lung to various infectious and noninfectious agents. This discussion is limited to infectious pneumonia, bacterial and nonbacterial, that affects chiefly infants and children. The clinical manifestations vary greatly, depending on the causative agent, the age of the patient, systemic reaction to the infection, the presence of any underlying compromise of host defense, and the degree of bronchial and bronchiolar obstruction.

Bacterial pneumonia. Most children with bacterial pneumonia are treated and recover without use of diagnostic procedures that would differentiate viral from bacterial pneumonia and document the specific bacterial cause. Nevertheless, viral pneumonia occurs far more frequently than bacterial pneumonia. Among bacterial causes, the pneumococcus and mycoplasma remain the most frequent agents of pneumonia. *H. influenzae* type b, *Str. pyogenes* (group A), and *S. aureus* are also important causes of pneumonia in otherwise normal children. Staphylococcal pneumonia may present as a nosocomial problem, particularly in neonates, or as a complication of other respiratory infections such as influenza.

The lack of availability of sputum or other materials for culture from the lower respiratory tract makes the causative diagnosis of bacterial pneumonia very difficult to establish with certainty in infants and young children. In most patients the diagnosis is based on clinical assessment and judgment. Occasionally, however, the following findings may be helpful: positive blood culture, empyema fluid available for sampling, positive bacterial antigen assay (latex agglutination test), or characteristic chest film such as pneumatoceles in patients with staphylococcal pneumonia. Leukocytosis with shift to the left, toxicity, grunting respirations, or splinting caused by pleural irritation may be clues to a bacterial cause. More invasive diagnostic procedures may be required in children who fail to respond to appropriate therapy and in those who are immunocompromised. These procedures include bronchoscopy with the flexible fiberoptic bronchoscope, bronchoalveolar lavage, lung aspiration, and open lung biopsy.

Pneumococcal pneumonia. The onset of pneumococcal pneumonia is typically sudden in a child who has been well or who has had an upper respiratory tract infection. In infants vomiting or a convulsion may be the first manifestation. An older child may complain of a headache, abdominal pain, or chest pain. Examination reveals a temperature of 38.9° to 40° C (102° to 104° F), rapid pulse, rapid shallow respirations, hot dry skin, and little else. In infants the possibility of central nervous system involvement must be considered, even in the absence of obvious neurological or meningeal signs. This also should be considered in those infants with high fever, convulsions, restlessness, stupor, stiff neck, bulging anterior fontanelle, or Brudzinski's sign; examination of the CSF often is required to differentiate meningismus from meningitis. The course of pneumococcal pneumonia in a 9-year-old child is shown in Fig. 21-5.

By about the second day of illness, cough, expiratory grunt, dilation of the nostrils, suppression of breath sounds, and inconstant rales over the involved portion of the lungs point

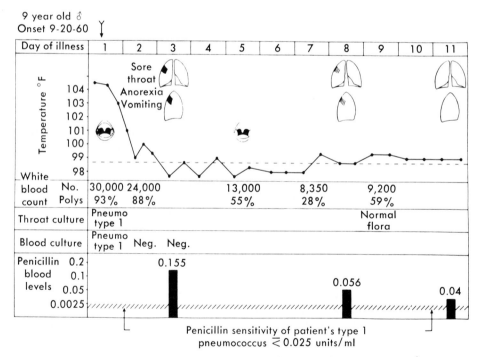

Fig. 21-5. Treatment of type 1 pneumococcal tonsillitis and pneumonia with a single injection of a penicillin preparation containing 600,000 units of aqueous procaine penicillin and 600,000 units of benzathine penicillin G. Note the dramatic subsidence of fever, the clearing of the exudative tonsillitis and pulmonary consolidation, and the rapid elimination of the type 1 pneumococci from the throat and blood. The penicillin blood level at 11 days (0.04 unit per milliliter) still exceeded the sensitivity of the patient's type 1 pneumococcus (<0.025 unit of penicillin per milliliter). (From Krugman S: Pediatr Clin North Am 1961; 8:1199.)

to the true nature of the disease. A pleural friction rub may be heard. Later, dullness and bronchial breathing indicate the area of consolidation, which may be confirmed by roentgenography. Resolution begins approximately 24 hours after appropriate antimicrobial treatment is started. Complications such as empyema, pericarditis, meningitis, arthritis, and peritonitis are seldom seen today. Otitis media is common but should be easily controlled. The causative diagnosis may be confirmed by culturing pneumococci from sputum, blood, or empyema fluid (Table 21-7). Antigen detection in pleural fluids has been positive for pneumococcal antigens, even when blood cultures have been negative (Siegel et al., 1978).

In evaluating children with pneumococcal pneumonia, it is important to remember that as many as 25% may have a predisposing underlying condition (Burman et al., 1985). These conditions include sickle cell disease, HIV infection, splenectomy, congenital heart disease, leukemia, immunoglobulin deficiency, asthma, galactosemia, and other metabolic disorders, especially in those children with hepatic damage. The peak incidence of pneumococcal disease is in the first 2 years of life, so some of these disorders may not yet have been detected.

Treatment. Pneumococcal pneumonia usually can be treated adequately by any one of a variety of antimicrobial agents, including penicillin, ampicillin, chloramphenicol, erythromycin, and the sulfonamides. Penicillin is the preferred drug (see Appendix A). The response to therapy usually is observed within 1 to 2 days. The treatment should be continued for at least 5 days or more if the clinical findings warrant it. Only one drug is necessary. Resistance in pneumococci and therapeutic considerations for patients infected with resistant organisms have been described previously.

Atypical pneumonia. The clinical manifestations of nonbacterial pneumonia (atypical pneumonia or viral pneumonia) are diverse. The onset is usually gradual but may be sudden. Systemic signs, especially fever, may be striking or inconspicuous. A mild respiratory tract illness usually precedes the more acute episode. Cough, fever, chilliness, headache, malaise, anorexia, listlessness, and irritability are common manifestations. Anorexia may be prominent. Cough appears early, is often severe and relentless, and interferes with sleep. Sputum, if obtainable, is mucoid or mucopurulent and may be blood streaked. Physical signs are variable; the child appears listless but only mildly or moderately ill. The temperature may be normal or elevated; respirations are usually normal. Chest findings are minimal, often limited to medium sticky rales and slight impairment of percussion note and breath sounds. The pneumonia frequently is discovered only on roentgenographic examination. The latter reveals a picture that also is not distinctive and varies from enlarged hilar shadows to patchy consolidation. Shifting areas of consolidation may be seen. The clinical course is irregular but usually benign, with complete recovery normally occurring in 1 to 3

Table 21-7. Some characteristics of pleural effusions

	Transudate	*Exudate*
Appearance	Light straw-colored serum ultrafiltrate	Cloudy, opaque, cellular
Specific gravity	<1.016	>1.016
pH	≥7.3	<7.2 (6-7)
Red blood cells	Up to 5,000	>100,000 (malignancy)
White blood cells	<1,000	>1,000 (usually >10,000)
Protein concentrate	<3 g	>3 g (>0.5 serum level)
Glucose	70-95 mg	<60 mg
Lactic dehydrogenase	<200	>300
Gram stain	Negative	Positive
Culture	Negative	Positive
Antigen detection	Negative	Positive
Cytology	Negative	Especially with malignancy

weeks. Laboratory findings include a normal or slightly increased WBC count. Standard bacteriological cultures are noncontributory.

Immunocompromised patients may develop pneumonias from unusual causes such as *Pneumocystis*, cytomegalovirus (Chapter 3), toxoplasmosis (Chapter 31), or tuberculosis (Chapter 32). Fungal pneumonias may also be associated with impaired host defenses or with exposure in endemic geographical areas. Blastomycosis has been reported in the valleys of the St. Lawrence, Ohio, and Mississippi rivers and in the southeastern United States. Histoplasmosis is endemic in certain parts of the United States, particularly the Ohio River valley. Coccidioidomycosis is endemic in the southwestern United States and in Argentina.

The wide spectrum of agents that may cause pneumonia in immunocompromised patients presents a serious diagnostic challenge. This diagnostic problem is of growing concern given the increasing incidence of the acquired immunodeficiency syndrome among children. Viral (cytomegalovirus, herpes simplex, parainfluenza), protozoal *(Pneumocystis)*, fungal *(Candida, Aspergillus, Cryptococcus*, Zygomycetes), and unusual bacterial (*Nocardia*, gram-negative bacilli, *Staphylococcus*) agents may be the causative culprits. Every case must be considered on its own individual features, but a precise diagnosis of pneumonia is often essential to successful intervention. Therefore performing invasive techniques, ranging from fiberoptic bronchoscopy to open lung biopsy, may be necessary if antigen detection and cultures of blood, sputum, or other sources are not helpful. Empiric therapy with amphotericin B, acyclovir, trimethoprim-sulfamethoxazole, and/or other drugs may be initiated on the basis of clinical clues before test results are received.

Treatment. Most atypical pneumonias are viral in origin and are not influenced by antimicrobial therapy. Some atypical pneumonias are caused by fastidious bacteria, including *Chlamydia* and *Mycoplasma*. Patients with pneumonia caused by *C. trachomatis* or *C. psittaci* should receive erythromycin or tetracycline. Erythromycin is recommended for *M. pneumoniae* pneumonia.

General therapeutic measures include bed rest and maintenance of fluid intake. Oxygen is indicated for patients who are cyanotic and dyspneic, and a moist atmosphere is helpful for those with obstructive bronchitis or bronchiolitis. Because of the lack of correlation between the results of upper respiratory tract cultures and the infecting flora of the lower respiratory tract, the etiology of pneumonia and other lower respiratory infections of infancy and childhood is often uncertain. The severity of illness, especially in infants, is often masked and the clinician is pressed to intervene with less than satisfying documentation of cause. For this reason antibiotics are often prescribed with a half-hearted zeal, "in case there is secondary bacterial invasion" superimposed on a likely viral infection.

The small infant has a number of liabilities that predispose him to respiratory failure with an infection that in an older child might be relatively benign (Pagtakhan and Chernick, 1982). These liabilities include the following: obligatory nasal breathing, immature musculature of the chest wall, tiny diameters and collapsibility of airways, limited collateral ventilatory pathways, increased tendency for parenchymal collapse, fragility of metabolic and energy balances, and easy fatigability.

The survival of infants with bronchopulmonary dysplasia has augmented the population of infants for whom a "minor respiratory infection" may become life threatening and who may require a temporary period of mechanical ventilatory support. Similarly at high risk are infants with congenital heart disease (MacDonald et al., 1982) and with severe asthma.

Unusual pneumonias such as those of fungal or protozoal origin require the use of drugs with special problems of toxicity. Amphotericin B, which is effective for many of the fungi, should be used only with careful attention to its potential for nephrotoxicity, febrile reactions, anemia, hypokalemia, cardiac arrhythmias, and other adverse effects. Newer agents such as fluconazole may be less toxic but do not yet have clearly defined indications in the initial treatment of most severe fungal infections. *P. carinii* pneumonia generally responds well to treatment with trimethoprim-sulfamethoxazole, although patients who do not respond well or who are sensitive to this combination may require therapy with pentamidine isothionate. Patients with

HIV infection have higher rates of adverse reactions to therapy with either trimethoprim-sulfamethoxazole or pentamadine isothionate.

Influenza-like illness

The syndrome termed *influenza-like illness* is characterized by sudden onset, chills or chilliness, fever, headache, marked prostration, muscular pains in the back and extremities, respiratory symptoms, and lack of any clear-cut abnormal physical findings outside the upper respiratory tract.

This syndrome may be caused by several viruses in addition to the influenza viruses A and B: parainfluenza virus types 1, 2, and 3; adenoviruses; Coxsackie viruses group A and group B; and lymphocytic choriomeningitis virus.

The incubation period is short, usually 24 to 72 hours. The onset of illness is sudden, with chills or feelings of chilliness, fever, headache, aches and pains in the back and legs, malaise, anorexia, and prostration. Nausea and vomiting may occur. Pain or a burning sensation in the eyes may be present. Constitutional symptoms are more prominent, as a rule, than are respiratory symptoms. There is commonly a hacking cough accompanied by substernal soreness, which suggests tracheobronchitis. Dryness or scratchiness of the throat may occur together with hoarseness. Rhinitis, sneezing, and nasal discharge usually appear later.

The physical findings are characteristically scanty and ill defined. In those patients who have fever, the temperature may go as high as 39.4° to 40° C (103° to 104° F). The temperature more likely will be higher in children than in adults. The pulse rate is usually in proportion to the degree of fever. The face may appear flushed, and the conjunctivae may be injected. The throat may look normal, or it may be reddened and show glistening hypertrophied lymphoid nodules on the posterior pharyngeal wall. The lungs are usually clear. Signs of consolidation are not present in uncomplicated influenza-like illness.

The clinical laboratory findings are usually normal. The WBC count occasionally shows moderate leukopenia. The sedimentation rate is increased. Blood cultures are sterile. Results of roentgenographic examination of the chest are usually normal.

Like most other viral diseases, influenza-like illness is a self-limited infection. The course of the disease is usually one of rapid and progressive improvement. After severe infections, some patients tend to show persistent prostration and sweating, and they are easily tired for several days after the temperature comes down to normal. Prompt and complete recovery is the rule in ordinary epidemics, and complications rarely are seen outside a pandemic. When complications do occur, they most frequently arise in the respiratory tract, manifesting as either otitis media or pneumonia. The pneumonia may be either viral or due to secondary bacterial superinfection. Other complications of influenza include myositis, myocarditis, Reye syndrome, and Guillain-Barré syndrome.

Amantadine is an oral antiviral drug that inhibits the uncoating of influenza A virus. The clinical usefulness of amantadine is limited to influenza type A and does not extend to treatment of illness caused by influenza type B. When administered early in the course of influenza type A disease, amantadine shortens the illness and alleviates symptoms in patients; however, there is no evidence to suggest that therapy with amantadine is effective in preventing complications of influenza type A infection. Treatment with amantadine should be considered for patients with severe disease or for those with an underlying condition that puts them at high risk of having a severe or complicated course. The dose of amantadine for children 9 years or younger or for children who weigh less than 45 kg is 4 to 8 mg/kg/day given orally in one or two doses (not to exceed 150 to 200 mg/day). For older children and for children who weigh more than 45 kg, it is 200 mg/day in two divided doses. Treatment should be started as soon as possible after the onset of symptoms and should be continued for 2 to 7 days, depending on the clinical response.

Otherwise, treatment of influenza-like illness is largely symptomatic. Bed rest is recommended. Complications rarely are encountered and are best dealt with as they arise. The routine prophylactic use of antibacterial agents is discouraged. Antipyretics are usually effective in alleviating symptoms. Salicylates should be avoided because of the increased risk of Reye syndrome in children with influenza. Fluids

4. Household members (including children) of high-risk persons.

VACCINATION OF OTHER GROUPS
General population

Physicians should administer influenza vaccine to any person who wishes to reduce the chance of acquiring influenza infection. Persons who provide essential community services and students or other persons in institutional settings (e.g., schools and colleges) may be considered for vaccination to minimize the disruption of routine activities during outbreaks.

Pregnant women

Influenza-associated excess mortality among pregnant women has not been documented except in the pandemics of 1918-1919 and 1957-1958. However, pregnant women who have other medical conditions that increase their risks for complications from influenza should be vaccinated, as the vaccine is considered safe for pregnant women. Administering the vaccine after the first trimester is a reasonable precaution to minimize any concern over the theoretical risk of teratogenicity. However, it is undesirable to delay vaccination of pregnant women who have high-risk conditions and who will still be in the first trimester of pregnancy when the influenza season begins.

Persons infected with HIV

Little information exists regarding the frequency and severity of influenza illness among human immunodeficiency virus (HIV)-infected persons, but recent reports suggest that symptoms may be prolonged and the risk of complications increased for HIV-infected persons. Because influenza may result in serious illness and complications, vaccination is a prudent precaution and will result in protective antibody levels in many recipients. However, the antibody response to vaccine may be low in persons with advanced HIV-related illnesses; a booster dose of vaccine has not improved the immune response for these individuals.

Foreign travelers

Increasingly, the elderly and persons with high-risk medical conditions are embarking on international travel. The risk of exposure to influenza during foreign travel varies, depending on season and destination. In the tropics, influenza can occur throughout the year; in the southern hemisphere, the season of greatest activity is April-September. Because of the short incubation period for influenza, exposure to the virus during travel can result in clinical illness that also begins while traveling, an inconvenience or potential danger, especially for persons at increased risk for complications. Persons preparing to travel to the tropics at any time of year or to the southern hemi-sphere during April-September should review their influenza vaccination histories. If they were not vaccinated the previous fall/winter, they should consider influenza vaccination before travel. Persons among the high-risk categories should be especially encouraged to receive the most currently available vaccine. High-risk persons given the previous season's vaccine before travel should be revaccinated in the fall/winter with current vaccine.

PERSONS WHO SHOULD NOT BE VACCINATED

Inactivated influenza vaccine should not be given to persons known to have anaphylactic hypersensitivity to eggs (see Side Effects and Adverse Reactions).

Persons with acute febrile illnesses usually should not be vaccinated until their symptoms have abated.

SIDE EFFECTS AND ADVERSE REACTIONS

Because influenza vaccine contains only noninfectious viruses, it cannot cause influenza. Respiratory disease after vaccination represents coincidental illness unrelated to influenza vaccination. The most frequent side effect of vaccination is soreness at the vaccination site that lasts for up to 2 days; this is reported for fewer than one-third of vaccinees. In addition, two types of systemic reactions have occurred:

1. Fever, malaise, myalgia, and other systemic symptoms occur infrequently and most often affect persons who have had no exposure to the influenza virus antigens in the vaccine (e.g., young children). These reactions begin 6-12 hours after vaccination and can persist for 1 or 2 days.

2. Immediate—presumably allergic-reactions (such as hives, angioedema, allergic asthma, or systemic anaphylaxis) occur rarely after influenza vaccination. These reactions probably result from hypersensitivity to some vaccine component—most likely residual egg protein. Although current influenza vaccines contain only a small quantity of egg protein, this protein presumably induces immediate hypersensitivity reactions among persons with severe egg allergy. Persons who have developed hives, have had swelling of the lips or tongue, or experienced acute respiratory distress or collapse after eating eggs should not be given the influenza vaccine. Persons with documented immunoglobulin E (IgE)-mediated hypersensitivity to eggs—including those who have had occupational asthma or other allergic responses from exposure to egg protein—may also be at increased risk for reactions from influenza vaccine. The protocol for influenza vaccination developed by Murphy and Strunk may be considered for patients who have

egg allergies and medical conditions that place them at increased risk for influenza infection or its complications.

Unlike the 1976 swine influenza vaccine, subsequent vaccines prepared from other virus strains have not been clearly associated with an increased frequency of Guillain-Barré syndrome. Although influenza vaccination can inhibit the clearance of warfarin and theophylline, studies have failed to show any adverse clinical effects attributable to these drugs among patients receiving influenza vaccine.

SIMULTANEOUS ADMINISTRATION OF OTHER VACCINES, INCLUDING CHILDHOOD VACCINES

The target groups for influenza and pneumococcal vaccination overlap considerably. Both vaccines can be given at the same time at different sites without increasing side effects. However, influenza vaccine must be given each year; with few exceptions, pneumococcal vaccine should be given only once.

Children at high risk for influenza-related complications may receive influenza vaccine at the same time as measles-mumps-rubella, *Haemophilus* b, pneumococcal, and oral polio vaccines. Vaccines should be given at different sites. Influenza vaccine should not be given within 3 days of vaccination with pertussis vaccine.

TIMING OF INFLUENZA VACCINATION ACTIVITIES

Beginning each September, when vaccine for the upcoming influenza season becomes available, high-risk persons who are hospitalized or who are seen by health-care providers for routine care should be offered influenza vaccine. Except in years of pandemic influenza (e.g., 1957 and 1968), high levels of influenza activity rarely occur in the contiguous 48 states before December. Therefore, November is the optimal time for organized vaccination campaigns for high-risk persons. In facilities such as nursing homes, it is particularly important to avoid administering vaccine too far in advance of the influenza season because antibody levels begin declining within a few months. Vaccination programs may be undertaken as soon as current vaccine is available if regional influenza activity is expected to begin earlier than December.

Children <9 years of age who have not previously been vaccinated should receive two doses of vaccine at least a month apart to maximize the chance of a satisfactory antibody response to all three vaccine antigens. The second dose should be given before December, if possible. Vaccine should be offered to both children and adults up to and even after influenza

virus activity is documented in a community, as late as April in some years.

STRATEGIES FOR IMPLEMENTING INFLUENZA VACCINE RECOMMENDATIONS

Despite the recognition that optimum medical care for both adults and children includes regular review of vaccination records and administration of vaccines as appropriate, <30% of persons among high-risk groups receive influenza vaccine each year. More effective strategies are needed for delivering vaccine to high-risk persons, their health-care providers, and their household contacts.

In general, successful vaccination programs have combined education for health-care workers, publicity and education targeted toward potential recipients, a plan for identifying (usually by medical-record review) persons at high-risk, and efforts to remove administrative and financial barriers that prevent persons from receiving the vaccine.

Persons for whom influenza vaccine is recommended can be identified and vaccinated in the settings described below.

Outpatient clinics and physicians' offices

Staff in physicians' offices, clinics, health-maintenance organizations, and employee health clinics should be instructed to identify and label the medical records of patients who should receive vaccine. Vaccine should be offered during visits beginning in September and throughout the influenza season. Offer of vaccine and its receipt or refusal should be documented in the medical record. Patients among high-risk groups who do not have regularly scheduled visits during the fall should be reminded by mail or telephone of the need for vaccine. If possible, arrangements should be made to provide vaccine with minimal waiting time and at the lowest possible cost.

Facilities providing episodic or acute care (e.g., emergency rooms, walk-in clinics)

Health-care providers in these settings should be familiar with influenza vaccine recommendations and should offer vaccine to persons among high-risk groups or should provide written information on why, where, and how to obtain the vaccine. Written information should be available in language(s) appropriate for the population served by the facility.

Nursing homes and other residential long-term–care facilities

Vaccination should be routinely provided to all residents of chronic-care facilities with the concurrence of attending physicians rather than by obtaining individual vaccination orders for each patient. Consent for vaccination should be obtained from the resident or a family member at the time of admission to the facility, and all residents should be vaccinated at one time immediately preceding the influenza season. Residents admitted during the winter months after completion of the vaccination program should be vaccinated when they are admitted.

Acute-care hospitals

All persons ≥65 years of age and younger persons (including children) with high-risk conditions who are hospitalized from September through March should be offered and strongly encouraged to receive influenza vaccine before they are discharged. Household members and others with whom they will contact should receive written information about why and where to obtain influenza vaccine.

Outpatient facilities providing continuing care to high-risk patients (e.g., hemodialysis centers, hospital specialty-care clinics, outpatient rehabilitation programs)

All patients should be offered vaccine in one period shortly before the beginning of the influenza season. Patients admitted to such programs during the winter months after the earlier vaccination program has been conducted should be vaccinated at the time of admission. Household members should receive written information regarding the need for vaccination and the places to obtain influenza vaccine.

Visiting nurses and others providing home care to high-risk persons

Nursing-care plans should identify high-risk patients, and vaccine should be provided in the home if necessary. Care givers and others in the household (including children) should be referred for vaccination.

Facilities providing services to persons ≥65 years of age (e.g., retirement communities, recreation centers)

All unvaccinated residents/attendees should be offered vaccine on site at one time period before the influenza season; alternatively, education/publicity programs should emphasize the need for influenza vaccine and should provide specific information on how, where, and when to obtain it.

Clinics and others providing health care for travelers

Indications for influenza vaccination should be reviewed before travel and vaccine offered if appropriate (see Foreign Travelers).

Health-care workers

Administrators of all health-care facilities should arrange for influenza vaccine to be offered to all personnel before the influenza season. Personnel should be provided with appropriate educational materials and strongly encouraged to receive vaccine, with particular emphasis on vaccination of persons who care for high-risk persons (e.g., staff of intensive-care units, including newborn intensive-care units; staff of medical/surgical units; and employees of nursing homes and chronic-care facilities). Using a mobile cart to take vaccine to hospital wards or other work sites and making vaccine available during night and weekend work shifts may enhance compliance, as may a follow-up campaign if an outbreak occurs in the community.

PNEUMOCOCCAL POLYSACCHARIDE VACCINE

The current pneumococcal vaccine (Pneumovax® 23, Merck Sharp & Dohme, and Pnu-Imune® 23, Lederle Laboratories) is composed of purified capsular polysaccharide antigens of 23 types of *S. pneumoniae* (Danish types 1, 2, 3, 4, 5, 6B, 7F, 8, 9N, 9V, 10A, 11A, 12F, 14, 15B, 17F, 18C, 19F, 19A, 20, 22F, 23F, 33F). It was licensed in the United States in 1983, replacing a 14-valent vaccine licensed in 1977. Each vaccine dose (0.5 ml) contains 25 μg of each polysaccharide antigen. The 23 capsular types in the vaccine cause 88% of the bacteremic pneumococcal disease in the United States. In addition, studies of the human antibody response indicate that cross-reactivity occurs for several types (e.g., 6A and 6B) that cause an additional 8% of bacteremic disease.

Most healthy adults, including the elderly, show a twofold or greater rise in type-specific antibody, as measured by radioimmunoassay, within 2–3 weeks of vaccination. Similar antibody responses have been reported in patients with alcoholic cirrhosis and diabetes mellitus requiring insulin. In immunocompromised patients, the response to vaccination may be less. In children <2 years old, antibody response to most capsular types is generally poor. In addition, response to some important pediatric pneumococcal types (e.g., 6A and 14) is decreased in children <5 years old.

Following vaccination of healthy adults with polyvalent pneumococcal vaccine, antibody levels for most pneumococcal vaccine types remain elevated at least 5 years; in some persons, they fall to prevaccination levels within 10 years. A more rapid decline in antibody levels may occur in children. In children who have undergone splenectomy following trauma and in those with sickle cell disease, antibody titers for some types can fall to prevaccination levels 3–5 years after vaccination. Similar rates of decline can occur in children with nephrotic syndrome.

Patients with AIDS have been shown to have an impaired antibody response to pneumococcal vaccine. However, asymptomatic HIV-infected men or those with persistent generalized lymphadenopathy respond to the 23-valent pneumococcal vaccine.

VACCINE EFFICACY

In the 1970s, pneumococcal vaccine was shown to reduce significantly the occurrence of pneumonia in young, healthy populations in South Africa and Papua New Guinea, where incidence of pneumonia is high. It was also demonstrated to protect against systemic pneumococcal infection in hyposplenic patients in the United States. Since then, studies have attempted to assess vaccine efficacy in other U.S. populations (CDC, unpublished data) (Table 21-9). A prospective, ongoing case-control study in Connecticut has shown an overall protective efficacy of 61% against pneumococcal bacteremia caused by vaccine and vaccine-related serotypes. The protective efficacy was 60% for patients with alcoholism or chronic pulmonary, cardiac, or renal disease and 64% for patients ≥55 years old without other high-risk chronic conditions. In another multicenter case-control study, vaccine efficacy in immunocompetent persons ≥55 years old was 70%.

A smaller case-control study of veterans failed to show efficacy in preventing pneumococcal bacteremia, but determination of the vaccination status was judged to be inadequate and the selection of controls was considered to be potentially biased.

Studies based on CDC's pneumococcal surveillance system suggest an efficacy of 60%–64% for vaccine-type strains in patients with bacteremic disease. For all persons ≥65 years of age (including persons with chronic heart disease, pulmonary disease, or diabetes mellitus), vaccine efficacy was 44%-61% (CDC, unpublished data). In addition, estimates of vaccine efficacy for serologically related types were 29%–66%. Limited data suggest that clinical efficacy may decline ≥6 years after vaccination (CDC, unpublished data).

A randomized, double-blind, placebo-controlled trial among high-risk veterans showed no vaccine efficacy against pneumococcal pneumonia or bronchitis; however, case definitions used were judged to have uncertain specificity. In addition, this study had only a 6% ability to detect a vaccine efficacy of 65% of pneumococcal bacteremia. In contrast, a French clinical trial found pneumococcal vaccine to be 77% effective in reducing the incidence of pneumonia in nursing home residents.

Despite conflicting findings, the data continue to

Table 21-9. Clinical effectiveness of pneumococcal vaccination in U.S. populations

Location	Method	No. persons	Type infection	Vaccine efficacy (%)	95% C.I.
Connecticut	Case-control*	543 cases 543 controls	VT,† VT-related	61	42, 73
Philadelphia	Case-control*	122 cases 244 controls	All serotypes	70	37, 86
Denver	Case-control*	89 cases 89 controls	All serotypes	−21	−221, 55
CDC-1	Epidemiologic*	249 vaccinated 1638 unvaccinated	VT	64	47, 76
CDC-2	Epidemiologic*	240 vaccinated 1527 unvaccinated	VT	60	45, 70
VA cooperative study	Randomized controlled trial‡	1145 vaccinated 1150 controls	All serotypes VT	−34§ −19§	−119, 18§ −164, 47§
Connecticut	Prospective surveillance case-control	1054 cases 1054 controls	All serotypes VT	56	42, 67

*Only patients with isolates from normally sterile body sites were included.
†Vaccine-type pneumococcal infection.
‡Pneumococcal pneumonia and bronchitis were diagnosed primarily by culture of respiratory secretions.
§Values calculated from the published data.

support the use of the pneumococcal vaccine for certain well-defined groups at risk.

RECOMMENDATIONS FOR VACCINE USE
Adults

1. Immunocompetent adults who are at increased risk of pneumococcal disease or its complications because of chronic illnesses (e.g., cardiovascular disease, pulmonary disease, diabetes mellitus, alcoholism, cirrhosis, or cerebrospinal fluid leaks) or who are ≥65 years old.
2. Immunocompromised adults at increased risk of pneumococcal disease or its complications (e.g., persons with splenic dysfunction or anatomic asplenia, Hodgkin's disease, lymphoma, multiple myeloma, chronic renal failure, nephrotic syndrome, or conditions such as organ transplantation associated with immunosuppression).
3. Adults with asymptomatic or symptomatic HIV infection.

Children

1. Children ≥2 years old with chronic illnesses specifically associated with increased risk of pneumococcal disease or its complications (e.g., anatomic or functional asplenia [including sickle cell disease], nephrotic syndrome, cerebrospinal fluid leaks, and conditions associated with immunosuppression).
2. Children ≥2 years old with asymptomatic or symptomatic HIV infection.
3. The currently available 23-valent vaccine is **not** indicated for patients having only recurrent upper respiratory tract disease, including otitis media and sinusitis.

Special groups

Persons living in special environments or social settings with an identified increased risk of pneumococcal disease or its complications (e.g., certain Native American populations).

ADVERSE REACTIONS

Approximately 50% of persons given pneumococcal vaccine develop mild side effects, such as erythema and pain at the injection site. Fever, myalgia, and severe local reactions have been reported in <1% of those vaccinated. Severe systemic reactions, such as anaphylaxis, rarely have been reported.

PRECAUTIONS

The safety of pneumococcal vaccine for pregnant women has not been evaluated. Ideally, women at high risk of pneumococcal disease should be vaccinated before pregnancy.

TIMING OF VACCINATION

When elective splenectomy is being considered, pneumococcal vaccine should be given at least 2 weeks before the operation, if possible. Similarly, for planning cancer chemotherapy or immunosuppressive therapy, as in patients who undergo organ transplantation, the interval between vaccination and initiation of chemotherapy or immunosuppression should also be at least 2 weeks.

REVACCINATION

In one study, local reactions after revaccination in adults were more severe than after initial vaccination when the interval between vaccinations was 13 months (Table 21-10). Reports of revaccination after longer intervals in children and adults, including a large group of elderly persons revaccinated at least 4 years after primary vaccination, suggest a similar incidence of such reactions after primary vaccination and revaccination (unpublished data).

Without more information, persons who received the 14-valent pneumococcal vaccine should not be routinely revaccinated with the 23-valent vaccine, as increased coverage is modest and duration of protection is not well defined. However, revaccination with the 23-valent vaccine should be strongly considered for persons who received the 14-valent vaccine if they are at highest risk of fatal pneumococcal infection (e.g., asplenic patients). Revaccination should also be considered for adults at highest risk who received the 23-valent vaccine ≥6 years before and for those shown to have rapid decline in pneumococcal antibody levels (e.g., patients with nephrotic syndrome, renal failure, or transplant recipients). Revaccination after 3–5 years should be considered for children with nephrotic syndrome, asplenia, or sickle cell anemia who would be ≤10 years old at revaccination.

STRATEGIES FOR VACCINE DELIVERY

Recommendations for pneumococcal vaccination have been made by the ACIP, the American Academy of Pediatrics, the American College of Physicians, and the American Academy of Family Physicians. Recent analysis indicates that pneumococcal vaccination of elderly persons is cost-effective. The vaccine is targeted for approximately 27 million persons aged ≥65 years and 21 million persons aged <65 years with high-risk conditions. Despite Medicare reimbursement for costs of the vaccine and its administration, which began in 1981, annual use of pneumococcal vaccine has not increased above levels observed in earlier years. In 1985, <10% of the 48 million persons

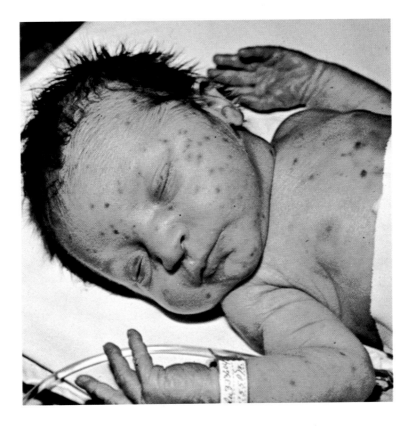

Plate 5
A 3-day-old infant with generalized macular lesions characteristic of neonatal purpura resulting from congenital rubella. His jaundice is caused by rubella hepatitis. (Courtesy Dr. Kenneth Schiffer, Albert Einstein College of Medicine, New York, NY; from Cooper LZ et al.: Am J Dis Child 1965;110:416.)

Table 21-10. Reactions to revaccination with pneumococcal vaccine

| Study | Vaccinees | | | Revaccination period | Reactions |
	Condition	Age	No.		
Borgono, et al. 1978	Normal	Adults	7	13 mos	Increase in local reactions
Carlson, et al. 1979	Normal	21-62 yrs	23	12-18 mos	Increase in local reactions
Rigau-Perez, et al. 1983	Sickle cell disease	≥3 yrs	28	28-35 mos	No increase in reactions compared with primary vaccination
Lawrence, et al. 1983	Normal	2-5 yrs	52	35 mos (mean)	Increase in local reactions
Mufson, et al. 1984	Normal	23-40 yrs	12	24-48 mos	No increase in reactions compared with primary vaccination
Weintrub, et al. 1984	Sickle cell disease	10-27 yrs	17	8-9 yrs	No "serious" local reactions
Kaplan, et al. 1986	Sickle cell disease	4-23 yrs	86	37-53 mos	Four "severe" reactions*

*Severe reaction was defined as presence of local pain, redness, swelling, and axillary temperature >100 F (37.8 C); two patients aged 21 and 23 years had temperatures of 102 F (38.9 C).

considered to be at increased risk of serious pneumococcal infection were estimated to have ever received pneumococcal vaccine.

Opportunities to vaccinate high-risk persons are missed both at time of hospital discharge and during visits to clinicians' offices. Two thirds or more of patients with serious pneumococcal disease had been hospitalized at least once within 5 years before their pneumococcal illness, yet few had received pneumococcal vaccine. More effective programs for vaccine delivery are needed, including offering pneumococcal vaccine in hospitals (at the time of discharge), clinicians' offices, nursing homes, and other chronic-care facilities. Many patients who receive pneumococcal vaccine should also be immunized with influenza vaccine, which can be given simultaneously at a different site. In contrast to pneumococcal vaccine, influenza vaccine is given annually.

VACCINE DEVELOPMENT

A more immunogenic pneumococcal vaccine preparation is needed, particularly for children <2 years old. The development of a protein-polysaccharide conjugate vaccine for selected capsular types holds promise.

REFERENCES

Adair JC, Ring WH. Management of epiglottitis in children. Anesth Analg 1975;54:622.

Adams JM, Imagawa DT, Zide K. Epidemic bronchiolitis and pneumonitis related to respiratory syncytial virus. JAMA 1961;176:1037.

Almeida JD, Tyrrell DAJ. The morphology of three previously uncharacterized human respiratory viruses that grow in organ culture. J Gen Virol 1967;1:175.

Amman AJ, et al. Polyvalent pneumococcal-polysaccharide immunization of patients with sickle-cell anemia and patients with splenectomy. N Engl J Med 1977;297:897.

Anas N, Boettrich C, Hall CB, et al. The association of apnea and respiratory syncytial virus infection. J Pediatr 1982;101:65.

Anderson KC, Maurer MJ, Dajani AS. Pneumococci relatively resistant to penicillin: a prevalence survey in children. J Pediatr 1980;97:939.

Anderson LJ, et al. Antigenic characterization of respiratory syncytial virus strains with monoclonal antibodies. J Infect Dis 1985;151:626-633.

Anderson LJ, et al. Multicenter study of strains of respiratory syncytial virus. J Infect Dis 1991;163:687-692.

Andiman WA, McCarthy P, Markowitz RL, et al. Clinical, virologic, and serologic evidence of Epstein-Barr virus infection in association with childhood pneumonia. J Pediatr 1981;99:880.

Andrewes CH. The taxonomic position of common cold viruses and some others. Yale J Biol Med 1961-1962;34:200.

Andrewes CH, Bang FB, Chanock, RM, Zhdanov VM. Para-influenza virus 1, 2, 3: suggested names for recently isolated myxoviruses. Virology 1959;8:129.

Arth C, Von Schmidt BV, Grossman M, Schachter J. Chlamydial pneumonitis. J Pediatr 1978;93:447.

Austrian R. Pneumococcal infection and pneumococcal vaccine N Engl J Med 1977;297:938.

Austrian R, et al. Prevention of pneumococcal pneumonia by vaccination. Trans Assoc Am Phys 1976;89:184.

Beale J, McLeod DL., Stackiw W, Roads AJ. Isolation of cytopathic agents from respiratory tract in acute laryngotracheobronchitis. Br Med J 1958;1:302.

Beare AS, Craig JW. Virulence for man of a human influenza A virus antigenically similar to "classical" swine viruses. Lancet 1960;2:4.

Beaty HN, et al. Legionnaires' disease in Vermont, May to October 1977. JAMA 1978;240:127.

Beem M, et al. Association of the chimpanzee coryza agent with acute respiratory disease in children. N Engl J Med 1960;263:523.

Beem MP, Saxon EM. Respiratory tract colonization and a distinctive pneumonia syndrome in infants infected with Chlamydia trachomatis. N Engl J Med 1977;296:306.

Benfield GFA. Recent trends in empyema thoracis. Br J Dis Chest 1981;75:358.

Beschamps GJ, Lynn HB, Wenzl JE. Empyema in children: review of Mayo Clinic experience. Mayo Clin Proc 1970;45:43.

Bloom HH, Forsyth BR, Johnson KM, Chanock RM. Relationship of rhinovirus infection to mild upper respiratory disease. I. Results of a survey in young adults and children. JAMA 1963;186:38.

Bloom HH, Johnson KM, Jacobsen R, Chanock RM: Recovery of parainfluenza viruses from adults with upper respiratory illnesses. Am J Hyg 1961;74:50.

Bock BV, et al. Legionnaires' disease in renal-transplant recipients. Lancet 1978;1:410.

Bradburne AS, Tyrrell DA. Coronaviruses of man. In Melnick JL, ed. Progress in medical virology, vol. 12. New York: S Karger, 1970.

Brandt CD, et al. Infections in 18,000 infants and children in controlled study of respiratory tract disease. I. Adenovirus pathogenicity in relation to serologic type and illness syndromes. Am J Epidemiol 1969;90:484.

Bryson YJ. The use of amantadine in children for prophylaxis and treatment of influenza A infections. Pediatr Infect Dis 1982;1:44-46.

Burman, LA, Norrby R, Trollfors B. Invasive pneumococcal infections; incidence, predisposing factors, and prognosis. Rev Infect Dis 1985;7:133.

Burrows B, Knudson RG, Lebowitz MD. The relationship of childhood respiratory illness to adult obstructive airway disease. Am Rev Respir Dis 1977;115:751.

Carson JL, Collier AM, Clyde WA Jr. Ciliary membrane alterations occurring in experimental *Mycoplasma pneumoniae* infection. Science 1979;206:349.

Carson JL, Collier AM, Hu SS. Acquired ciliary defects in nasal epithelium of children with acute viral upper respiratory infections. N Engl J Med 1985;312:463.

Cates KL, et al. A penicillin-resistant pneumococcus. J Pediatr 1978;93:624.

Cattaneo SM, Kolman JW. Surgical therapy of empyema in children. Arch Surg 1973;106:564.

Centers for Disease Control. Multiple-antibiotic resistance of pneumococci- South Africa. MMWR 1977;26:285.

Chandler FW, Hicklin MD, Blackmon JA. Demonstration of the agent of Legionnaires' disease in tissue. N Engl J Med 1977;297:1218.

Chanock RM. Mycoplasma infections of man. N Engl J Med 1965;273:1199.

Chanock RM, Bell JA, Parrott RH. Natural history of parainfluenza infection. In Pollard M ed. Perspectives in virology, vol 2. Minneapolis: Burgess Publishing Co. 1961, p 126.

Chanock RM, Finberg L. Recovery from infants with respiratory illness of a virus related to chimpanzee coryza agent (CCA). II. Epidemiologic aspects of infection in infants and young children. Am J Hyg 1957;66:291.

Chanock RM, Hayflick L, Barile MD. Growth on artificial medium of an agent associated with atypical pneumonia and its identification as a PPLO. Proc Natl Acad Sci USA 1962;48:41.

Chanock RM, et al. Respiratory syncytial virus. I. Virus recovery and other observations during 1960 outbreak of bronchiolitis, pneumonia, and minor respiratory diseases in children. JAMA 1961;176:647.

Chanock RM, et al. Biology and ecology of two major lower respiratory tract pathogens—RS virus and Eaton PPLO. In Pollard M (ed). Perspectives in virology, vol 3. New York: Harper & Row, 1963, p 257.

Chanock RM, et al. Possible role of immunologic factors in pathogenesis of RS virus lower respiratory tract disease. In Pollard M (ed). Perspectives in virology, vol 4. New York: Academic Press, 1969, pp 125-139.

Chanock RM, et al. Influence of immunological factors in respiratory syncytial virus disease. Arch Environ Health 1970;21:347.

Chany C, et al. Severe and fatal pneumonia in infants and young children associated with adenovirus. Am J Hyg 1958;67:3967.

Chaudhary S, Bilisnky SA, Hennessy JL, et al. Penicillin V and rifampin for the treatment of group A streptococcal pharyngitis. J Pediatr 1985;106:481.

Cherry JD. The treatment of croup: continued controversy due to failure of recognition of historic, ecologic, etiologic and clinical perspectives. J Pediatr 1979;94:352.

Committee on Infectious Diseases. Report, ed 22. Elk Grove Village, IL: American Academy of Pediatrics, 1991.

Cowan MH, et al. Pneumococcal polysaccharide immunization in infants and children. Pediatrics 1978;62:721.

Cradock-Watson JE, McQuillin J, Gardner PS. Rapid diagnosis of respiratory syncytial virus infection in children by the immunofluorescent technique. J Clin Pathol 1971;24:347.

Cramblett HG. Croup—present day concept. Pediatrics 1960;25:1071.

Dees SC, Asthma. In Kendig E (ed). Disorders of the respiratory tract in children. Philadelphia: WB Saunders, 1977, p 820.

Denny FW, Clyde WA. Acute lower respiratory tract infections in nonhospitalized children. J Pediatr 1986;108:635-646.

Denny FW, Clyde WA Jr, Glezon WP. *Mycoplasma pneumoniae* disease: clinical spectrum pathophysiology, epidemiology, and control. J Infect Dis 1971;123:74.

Dolin R, et al. A controlled trial of amantadine and rimantadine in the prophylaxis of influenza A infection. N Engl J Med 1982;307:580-583.

Eaton MD, Meiklejohn G, van Herrick WJ. Studies on etiology of primary atypical pneumonia: filtrable agent transmissible to cotton rats, hamsters, and chick embryos. J Exp Med 1944;79:649.

Eden AN, Kaufman A, Yu R. Corticosteroids and croup: controlled double blind study. JAMA 1967;200:133.

Edwards KM, Thompson J, Paolini BS, Wright PF. Adenovirus infections in young children. Pediatrics 1985; 76:420-424.

Eliasson R, Mossberg B, Camner R, Afzelius BA. The immotile cilia syndrome. N Engl J Med 1977;297:1.

Escobar JA, et al. Etiology of respiratory tract infections in children in Cali, Colombia. Pediatrics 1976;57:123.

Evans AS, Brobst M. Bronchiolitis, pneumonitis, and pneumonia in University of Wisconsin students. N Engl J Med 1961;265:401.

Faden HS. Treatment of *Haemophilus influenza* type b epiglottitis. Pediatrics 1979;63:402.

Fernald GW, Collier AM, Clyde WA Jr. Respiratory infections due to *Mycoplasma pneumoniae* in infants and children. Pediatrics 1975;55:327.

Finland M. Pneumonia and pneumococcal infections, with special reference to pneumococcal pneumonia. Am Rev Respir Dis 1979;120:481.

Fogel JM, Berg IJ, Gerber MA, Sherter CB. Racemic epinephrine in the treatment of croup: nebulization alone versus nebulization with intermittent positive pressure breathing. J Pediatr 1982;101:1028-1031.

Forbes JA. Croup and its management. Br Med J 1961; 1389.

Forfar JO. Demography, vital statistics, and the pattern of disease in childhood. In Forfar JO, Arneil GC eds. Textbook of paediatrics, London: Churchill Livingstone, 1984, pp. 9-16.

Fox JP, Cooney, MK, Hall CE. The Seattle virus watch. V. Epidemiologic observations of rhinovirus infections in families with young children. Am J Epidemiol 1975; 101:122.

Fox JP, et al. The virus watch program: a continuing surveillance of viral infections in metropolitan New York families. VI. Observations of adenovirus infections: virus excretion patterns, antibody response, efficiency of surveillance, patterns of infection and relation to illness. Am J Epidemiol 1969;89:25.

Francis T Jr. Factors conditioning resistance to epidemic influenza. Harvey Lect 1942;37:39.

Fraser DW, et al. Legionnaires' disease. Description of an epidemic of pneumonia. N Engl J Med 1977;296:1150.

Freij BJ, Kusmiesz H, Nelson JD et al. Parapneumonic effusions and empyema in hospitalized children: a retrospective review of 227 cases. Pediatr Infect Dis 1984;3:578.

Friis B, Andersen P, Brenoe E, et al. Antibiotic treatment of pneumonia and bronchiolitis: a perspective randomized study. Arch Dis Child 1984;59:1038.

Frommell G, Bruhn FW, Schwartzman JD. Isolation of Chlamydia trachomatis from infant lung tissue. N Engl J Med 1977;296:1150.

Gardner PS. How etiologic, pathologic and clinical diagnoses can be made in a correlated fashion. Pediatr Res 1977;11:254.

Gardner PS, McQuillin J, Court SDM. Speculation on pathogenesis in death from respiratory syncytial virus infection. Br Med J 1970;1:327.

Gardner PS, et al. Death associated with respiratory tract infections in children. Br Med J 1967;4:316.

Gaston MH, Verter JI, Woods G, et al and the Prophylactic Penicillin Study Group. Prophylaxis with oral penicillin in children with sickle cell anemia: a randomized trial. N Engl J Med 1986;314:1593-1599.

Ginsberg CM, Howard JB, Nelson JD. Report of 65 cases of *Hemophilus influenzae* b pneumonia. Pediatrics 1979;64:283.

Glezen WP. Pathogenesis of bronchiolitis-epidemiologic considerations. Pediatr Res 1977;11:234.

Glezen WP, Denny FW. Epidemiology of acute lower respiratory disease in children. N Engl J Med 1973;228:498.

Glezen WP, Frank AL, Taber LH, Kasel JA. Parainfluenza virus type 3: seasonality and risk of infection and reinfection in young children. J Infect Dis 1984;150:851-857.

Glezen WP, Paredes A, Allison JE, et al. Risk of respiratory syncytial virus infection for infants from low-income families in relationship to age, sex, ethnic group, and maternal antibody level. J Pediatr 1981;98:708.

Glezen WP, Taber LH, Frank AL, Kasel JA. Risk of primary infection and reinfection with respiratory syncytial virus. Am J Dis Child 1986;140:543-546.

Glezen WP, Wilfert CM. Your role in the war against flu. Contemp Pediatr 1988;86-98.

Glezen WP, et al. Epidemiologic patterns of acute lower respiratory disease in children in a pediatric group practice. J Pediatr 1971;78:397.

Glicklich M, Cohen RD, Jona JZ. Steroids and bag and mask ventilation in the treatment of acute epiglottitis. J Pediatr Surg 1979;14:247.

Goldman AS, Schochet SS Jr, Howell JT: The discovery of defects in respiratory cilia in the immotile cilia syndrome. J Pediatr 1980;96:244.

Graham NM et al. Adverse effects of aspirin, acetaminophen, and ibuprofen on immune function, viral shedding, and clinical status in rhinovirus-infected volunteers. J Infect Dis 1990;162:1277-1282.

Graman PS, Hall CB. Nosocomial viral respiratory infections. Sem Resp Infect 1989;4:253-260.

Gray BM, Converse GM III, Dillon HC Jr. Serotypes of Streptococcus pneumoniae causing disease. J Infect Dis 1980;140:979.

Groothuis JR, Gutierrez KM, Lauer BA. Respiratory syncytial virus infection in children with bronchopulmonary dysplasia. Pediatrics 1988;82:199-203.

Hall CB, Douglas RG. Modes of transmission of respiratory syncytial virus. J Pediatr 1981;99:100-103.

Hall CB, Hall WJ, Gala CL, et al. Long term prospective study in children after respiratory syncytial virus infection. J Pediatr 1984;105:358.

rotavirus in respiratory secretions of children with pneumonia. J Pediatr 1983;103:583.

Sanyal SK, Mariencheck WC, Hughes WT, et al: Course of pulmonary dysfunction in children surviving *Pneumocystis carinii* pneumonitis: a prospective study. Am Rev Respir Dis 1981;124:161.

Schachter J. Chlamydial infections. N Engl J Med 1978;298:428, 490, 540.

Schachter J, Sugg N, Sung M. Psittacosis—the reservoir persists. J Infect Dis 1978; 137:44.

Schachter J, et al. Pneumonitis following inclusion blennorrhea. J Pediatr 1975;87:779.

Schachter J, et al. Prospective study of chlamydial infections in neonates. Lancet 1979;2:377.

Schaefer C, Harrison R, Boyce WT, et al. Illnesses in infants born to women with *Chlamydia trachomatis* infection. Am J Dis Child 1985;139:127.

Shands KN, Ho JL, Meyer RD, et al. Potable water as a source of Legionnaires' disease. JAMA 1985;253:1412.

Shapiro ED, Berg AT, Austrian R, et al. The protective efficacy of polyvalent pneumococcal polysaccharide vaccine. N Engl J Med 1991;325:1453-1460.

Shope RE. The influenza of swine and man. Harvey Lect 1935-1936;31:183.

Siegel JD, Gartner JC, Michaels RH. Pneumococcal empyema in childhood. Am J Dis Child 1978;132:1094.

Siegel ST, Wolff LJ, Baehner RL, et al. Treatment of *Pneumocystis carinii* pneumonitis. Am J Dis Child 1984; 138:1051.

Skolnik NS. Treatment of croup: a critical review. Am J Dis Child 1989;143:1045-1049.

Smit P, et al. Protective efficacy of pneumococcal polysaccharide vaccines. JAMA 1977;238:2613.

Smith CB, Purcell RH, Bellanti JA, Chanock RM. Protective effect of antibody to parainfluenza type 1 virus. N Engl J Med 1966;275:1145.

Smith W, Andrewes CH, Laidlaw PO. A virus obtained from influenza patients. Lancet 1933;2:66.

Stagno S, Brasfield DM, Brown MB, et al. Infant pneumonitis associated with cytomegalovirus, chlamydia, *Pneumocystis*, and *Ureaplasma*: a prospective study. Pediatrics 1981;68:322.

Stagno S, Pifer LL, Hughes WT, et al. *Pneumocystis carinii* pneumonitis in young immunocompetent infants. Pediatrics 1980;66:56-62.

Steen-Johnsen J, Orstavik I, Attramadal A. Severe illnesses due to adenovirus type 7 in children. Acta Paediatri Scand 1969;58:157.

Steigman AJ, Lipton MM, Brapennicke H. Acute lymphonodular pharyngitis: a newly described condition due to coxsackie A virus. Am J Dis Child 1962;102:713.

Stiles QR, Lindesmith GG, Tucker BL, et al. Pleural empyema in children. Ann Thorac Surg 1970;10:37.

Stuart-Harris C. Swine influenza virus in man. Lancet 1976;2:31.

Sturm R, Staneck JL, Myers JP, et al. Pediatric Legionnaires' disease diagnosis by direct immunofluorescent staining of sputum. Pediatrics 1981;68:539.

Sussman SJ, Magoffin RL, Lennette EH, Schieble J. Cold agglutinins, Eaton agent, and respiratory infections of children. Pediatrics 1966;38:571.

Taussig LM, Castro O, Beaudry PH, et al. Treatment of laryngotracheobronchitis (croup): use of intermittent positive-pressure breathing and racemic epinephrine. Am J Dis Child 1975;129:790-793.

Taussig LM, et al. Treatment of laryngotracheobronchitis (croup). Am J Dis Child 1977;238:2613.

Taylor-Robinson D, Tyrrell DA. Serotypes of viruses (rhinoviruses) isolated from common colds. Lancet 1962; 1:452.

Terranova W, Cohen MI, Fraser DW. 1974 outbreak of Legionnaires' disease diagnosed in 1977, clinical and epidemiological features. Lancet 1978;2:122.

Travis KW, Todrez ID, Shannon DC. Pulmonary edema associated with croup and epiglottitis. Pediatrics 1977; 59:695.

Turner JAP, Corkey CWB, Lee JYC, et al. Clinical expressions of immotile cilia syndrome. Pediatrics 1981;67:805.

Turner RB, Hayden FG, Hendley JO. Counterimmunoelectrophoresis of urine for diagnosis of bacterial pneumonia in pediatric outpatients. Pediatrics 1983;71:780.

Unger A, Tapia L, Mimnich LL, et al. Atypical neonatal respiratory syncytial virus infection. J Pediatr 1982; 100:762.

Valenti WM, Clarke TA, Hall CB, et al. Concurrent outbreaks of rhinovirus and respiratory syncytial virus in an intensive care nursery: epidemiology and associated risk factors. J Pediatr 1982;100:722.

Van der Veen J, Oei KG, Abarbanal MFW. Patterns of infections with adenovirus types 4, 7, and 21 in military recruits during a 9-year survey. J Hyg (Camb) 1969; 67:255-268.

Wald ER, Milmoe GJ, Bowen A, et al. Acute maxillary sinusitis in children. N Engl J Med 1981;304, 749-754.

Wang EL, Prober CG, Manson B, et al. Association of respiratory viral infections with pulmonary deterioration in patients with cystic fibrosis. N Engl J Med 1984;311:1653.

Weber ML, et al. Acute epiglottitis in children—treatment with nasotracheal intubation. Pediatrics 1976;57:152.

Welliver RC. Detection, pathogenesis, and therapy of respiratory syncytial virus infections. Clin Micro Rev 1988;1:27-39.

Welliver RC, Kaul A, Ogra PL. Cell-mediated immune response to respiratory syncytial virus infection: relationship to the development of reactive airway disease. J Pediatr 1979;94:370.

Welliver RC, Sun M, Rinaldo D, Ogra PL. Predictive value of respiratory syncytial virus specific IgE responses for recurrent wheezing following bronchiolitis. J Pediatr 1986;109:776-780.

Welliver R, Wong DT, Choi TS, Ogra PL. Natural history of parainfluenza virus infection in childhood. J Pediatr 1982;101:180-187.

Welliver RC, et al. Role of parainfluenza virus specific IgE in pathogenesis of croup and wheezing subsequent to infection. J Pediatr 1982;101:889-896.

Wenzel RP, et al. Hospital-acquired viral respiratory illness on a pediatric ward. Pediatrics 1977;60:367.

Westley CR, Cotton EK, Brooks JG. Nebulized racemic epinephrine by IPPB for the treatment of croup. Am J Dis Child 1978;132:484.

Winterbauer RH, Dreis DF. Thoracic empyema: handling a dangerous infection wisely. J Respir Dis 1983;116.

Wolfe WG, Spock A, Bradford WD. Pleural fluid in infants and children. Am Rev Respir Dis 1968;98:1027.

Yunis EJ, et al. Adenovirus and ileocecal intussusception. Lab Invest 1975;33:347.

Zollar LM, Krause HE, Mufson MA. Microbiologic studies on young infants and lower respiratory tract disease. Am J Dis Child 1973;126:56.

Zuravleff JJ, Yu VC, Shonnard JW, et al. Diagnosis of legionnaires' disease. JAMA 1983;250:1981.

22

ROSEOLA INFANTUM (EXANTHEM SUBITUM)

Roseola infantum is a common benign infectious disease of infancy characterized by 3 to 5 days of high fever associated with a paucity of physical findings. The temperature falls to normal by crisis and may be accompanied by a morbilliform rash. Virological and immunological findings of the past several years have clarified the etiology of this clinical syndrome, thereby permitting more precise definitions so that it can be separated from the many febrile rash illnesses caused by other agents such as the enteroviruses and adenoviruses. Zahorsky (1910) is credited with an initial description of the clinical illness.

ETIOLOGY

For more than 75 years roseola infantum was considered a viral infection, but its cause remained obscure. The successful human transmission of the infection was reported by Kempe et al. in 1950 and by Hellström and Vahlquist in 1951. The viral cause of roseola infantum was established by Yamanishi et al. (1988) who demonstrated human herpes virus type 6 (HHV-6) in the blood of infants with the clinical syndrome. This newer member of the herpes family had been first reported in peripheral blood mononuclear cells of patients with lymphoreticular disorders (Salahuddin et al., 1986). Originally labeled *human B lymphotropic virus (HBLV)*, it was renamed once it was verified as a herpes virus with tropism for T lymphocytes. HHV-6 is a typical herpesvirus with an icosahedral capsid of 162 capsomers, a virion diameter of 145 to 200 nm, and a large double-stranded DNA genome of approximately 170 kilobases. There is little immunological cross-reactivity with the other human herpesviruses (herpes simplex types 1 and 2, cytomegalovirus, varicella-zoster virus, and Epstein-Barr virus). The availability of serological markers enhanced further investigations that have clarified the following features of HHV-6 infection.

1. Nearly all newborns have transplacentally acquired specific IgG antibodies to HHV-6, which are catabolized rapidly in the first months of life.
2. After the loss of passively acquired maternal antibody, there is rapid acquisition of active immunity, with 90% of children seropositive by age 2 years and nearly 100% by 3 years of age (Brown et al., 1988; Yoshikawa et al., 1989).
3. Primary infection may be occult or an undifferentiated febrile illness or, in less than one third of the children, the full picture of exanthem subitum (Asano et al., 1989b; Asano et al., 1991; Suga et al., 1989; Yoshiyama et al., 1990).
4. Primary infection results initially in the appearance of specific IgM antibody, followed soon by an IgG response that persists as IgM wanes.

Less certain are the details about probable viral persistence in peripheral blood mononuclear cells, latency, reactivation, and the role of HHV-6 in the pathogenesis of other disorders (Carrigan et al., 1991; Linde et al., 1988; Okuno et al., 1990).

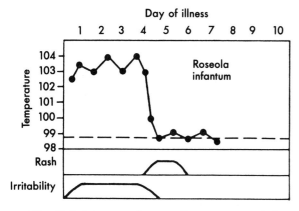

Fig. 22-1. Schematic diagram illustrating typical clinical course of roseola infantum. Between the third and fourth days the temperature drops to normal, and a maculopapular eruption may appear.

CLINICAL MANIFESTATIONS
Incubation period

The incubation period is difficult to determine because the contact is rarely known. The experimental disease produced by intravenous injection of serum had an incubation period of 9 days. In the epidemics reported by Cushing (1927) and by Barenberg and Greenspan (1939), this period appeared to range between 10 and 15 days.

Course

The typical course of roseola infantum is illustrated in Fig. 22-1. The temperature rises abruptly to approximately 40° to 40.6° C (104° to 105° F). The infant may be anorexic and irritable and usually shows no evidence of coryza, conjunctivitis, or cough. The fever persists for approximately 3 to 5 days and then falls by crisis coincidental with the appearance of the rash. Most infants with this disease do not appear as acutely ill as their temperature chart seems to suggest. Occasionally, they may be listless and irritable during periods of hyperpyrexia. It is not uncommon for a febrile convulsion to accompany the disease.

Fever

The characteristic temperature curve is illustrated in Fig. 22-1. The fever is typically high and continuous, persisting for 3 or 4 days. Administration of antipyretics causes a temporary drop that is followed by a rapid rise to the same high levels as before. In some patients the temperature is of the intermittent type, being normal or slightly elevated in the morning and very high in the evening. On either the third or the fourth day it drops precipitously back to normal levels. In rare instances the fever may persist for more than 5 days, but the diagnosis under these circumstances may be questionable. Also, occasionally the temperature may fall by rapid lysis rather than by crisis. Hall et al. (1991) in studies at the University of Rochester, New York found that 12% of emergency room visits for acute febrile illness in children less than 3 years of age were caused by HHV-6 infections.

Rash

As indicated in Fig. 22-1, the appearance of the rash often coincides with the subsidence of the fever on the third or fourth day. Occasionally, it may not be apparent until after 1 day of normal temperature, or it may emerge before the fever has subsided. The lesions are discrete, rose-pink macules or maculopapules, 2 to 3 mm in diameter, that fade on pressure, rarely coalesce, and are similar in appearance to those of rubella. The rash characteristically appears on the trunk first and then spreads to the neck, upper extremities, face, and lower extremities. Occasionally, the rash may be limited to the trunk. The duration of the eruption is usually 1 to 2 days; occasionally, it may be evanescent, disappearing in a matter of hours. There is usually no evidence of pigmentation or desquamation.

Other clinical features

The most significant clinical manifestation of roseola infantum is the striking contrast between the infant's general appearance and the febrile course. In spite of a persistently elevated temperature, the patient may be alert and playful and may not look acutely ill. The physical findings are rather nonspecific. The pharynx is usually mildly inflamed. The tonsils, if present, are usually reddened and occasionally are covered with a follicular exudate. Mild catarrhal otitis media may be present. Lymphadenopathy, particularly of the occipital, cervical, and postauricular groups, is a common finding. All these manifestations are caused by the primary infection and not by secondary bacterial invaders.

DIAGNOSIS

A diagnosis of roseola infantum is made chiefly on the basis of clinical manifestations. Specific serological and virological tests for confirmation of the diagnosis of the acute illness are not readily available (Ueda et al., 1989). The white blood cell count is usually low, but as a rule leukopenia does not develop until the third day of illness. Indeed, during the first 2 days there may be leukocytosis with an increase in polymorphonuclear leukocytes. As leukopenia develops, the percentage of lymphocytes and monocytes increases. The development of a rash and leukopenia in an infant who has been febrile for the previous 3 or 4 days should strongly suggest roseola infantum as the most probable diagnosis.

DIFFERENTIAL DIAGNOSIS

Differential diagnosis is discussed in Chapter 36.

COMPLICATIONS

The most common complication of roseola infantum seen in hospital practice is convulsive seizures. Most infants, however, are treated at home. Consequently, a more accurate estimate of the incidence of this complication can be obtained from surveys in general practice rather than in hospital practice. In general, the incidence would probably parallel that of febrile convulsions. Spinal taps have been performed on many patients, with completely normal results.

Encephalitis and other complications of the central nervous system have been reported, but their confirmation is lacking in the era of specific serological or virological tests.

PROGNOSIS

The prognosis is uniformly excellent even for those cases complicated by seizures. The period of high, unresponsive fever may be a harrowing experience for both the parents and the physician. With subsidence of the fever and appearance of the rash, however, the diagnosis becomes obvious, and a complete recovery ensues for the infant.

IMMUNITY

One attack probably confers permanent immunity. The rarity of the disease in infants less than 6 months of age attests to the demonstration that nearly all adults are immune (Brown et al., 1988; Linde et al., 1988) and that transplacental HHV-6–specific IgG antibodies are efficacious in preventing infection. The detection of HHV-6 antibody using the indirect immunofluorescence method is evidence of past infection (Ueda et al., 1989).

EPIDEMIOLOGICAL FACTORS

The age incidence of patients with roseola infantum is very striking. The vast majority of cases, more than 95%, occur in infants 6 months to 3 years of age. The disease has occasionally been described in older children and in adults. Both sexes are equally susceptible.

The disease occurs the year round, with a concentration of cases in the spring and autumn months.

Roseola infantum is the most common exanthem seen in infants under 2 years of age. An estimated 30% of all children develop the apparent disease. In the majority of infants HHV-6 occurs as either an inapparent infection or a febrile illness without rash.

Roseola infantum does not seem to have the contagious characteristics of measles, rubella, or chickenpox. It is rare for children to acquire the overt disease from a sibling, even when they are less than 3 years of age. Epidemics in foundling homes have been reported, but they are exceptional. For many years patients with illnesses diagnosed as roseola infantum have been routinely admitted to the authors' general infants' ward without any clinical evidence of spread. However, some of the unexplained febrile episodes associated with hospitalization of infants may represent unsuspected nosocomial spread of HHV-6. Virus has been detected in saliva, which may provide a possible mode of transmission.

TREATMENT

There is no specific treatment for patients with roseola infantum. Acetaminophen may be given for its antipyretic effect. Elixir of phenobarbital may be given to infants with a history of convulsive seizures during either the current or previous illnesses.

Antimicrobial agents do not alter the course of the infection. Since the diagnosis is established only after the patient has recovered, the physician may have a dilemma. Should he treat or not treat with antimicrobial agents? Treatment justifiably may be withheld if an infant (1) appears well and shows no abnormal physical findings despite continued hyperpyrexia and (2) has a normal or low white blood cell count. On the other hand, treatment might be indicated if high fever is accompanied by one or more of the following manifestations: (1) inflammatory exudate on the tonsils and pharynx, (2) catarrhal otitis media, and (3) leukocytosis.

The management of an infant whose disease is ushered in by high fever and convulsions should be the same as that for any initial febrile convulsion.

REFERENCES

Asano Y, Yoshikawa T, Suga S, et al. Viremia and neutralizing antibody response in infants with exanthem subitum. J Pediatr 1989a;114:535-539

Asano Y, Suga S, Yoshikawa T, et al. Human herpesvirus type 6 infection (exanthem subitum) without fever. J Pediatr 1989b;115:264-265.

Asano Y, Nakashima T, Yoshikawa T, et al. Severity of human herpesvirus-6 viremia and clinical findings in infants with exanthem subitum. J Pediatr 1991;118:891-895.

Barenberg LH, Greenspan L. Exanthem subitum (roseola infantum). Am J Dis Child 1939;58:983.

Berenberg W, Wright S, Janeway CA: Roseola infantum (exanthem subitum). N Engl J Med 1949;241:253.

Brown NA, Sumaya CV, Liu CR, et al: Fall in human herpesvirus 6 seropositivity with age. Lancet 1988;2:396.

Carrigan DR, Drobyski WR, Russler SK, et al. Interstitial pneumonitis associated with human herpesvirus-6 infection after marrow transplantation. Lancet 1991;338:147-149.

Clemens HH. Exanthem subitum (roseola infantum): report of 80 cases. J Pediatr 1945;26:66.

Cushing HB. An epidemic of roseola infantum. Can Med Assoc J 1927;17:905.

Fox JD, Briggs M, Ward PA, et al. Human herpesvirus 6 in salivary glands. Lancet 1990;336:590-593.

Hall CB, Pruksananonda P, Insel RA, et al. Human herpes virus 6 (HHV-6) infection in children. Pediatr Res 1991;29:173A.

Hellström B, Vahlquist B. Experimental inoculation of roseola infantum. Acta Paediatr 1951;40:189.

Irving WL, Cunningham AL. Serological diagnosis of infection with human herpesvirus type 6. Br Med J 1990;300:156-159.

Juretić M. Exanthem subitum: a review of 243 cases. Helv Paediatr Acta 1963;18:80.

Kempe CH, Shaw EB, Jackson JR, Silver HK. Studies on the etiology of exanthem subitum (roseola infantum). J Pediatr 1950;37:561.

Knowles WA, Gardner SD. High prevalence of antibody to human herpesvirus-6 and seroconversion associated with rash in two infants, Lancet 1988;2:912-913.

Levy JA, Ferro F, Greenspan D, et al. Frequent isolation of HHV-6 from saliva and high seroprevalence of the virus in the population. Lancet 1990;335:1047-1050.

Linde A, Dahl H, Wahren B, et al. IgG antibodies to human herpesvirus-6 in children and adults both in primary Epstein-Barr virus and cytomegalovirus infections. J Virol Methods 1988;21:117-123.

Okuno T, Takahashi K, Balachandra K, et al. Seroepidemiology of human herpesvirus 6 infection in normal children and adults. J Clin Microbiol 1989;27:651-653.

Okuno T, Higashi K, Shiraki K, et al. Human herpesvirus 6 infection in renal transplantation. Transplantation 1990;49:519-522.

Salahuddin SZ, Ablashi DV, Markham PD, et al. Isolation of a new virus, HBLV, in patients with lymphoproliferative disorders. Science 1986;234:596-601.

Suga S, Yoshikawa T, Asano Y, et al: Human herpesvirus-6 infection (exanthem subitum) without rash. Pediatrics 1989;83:1003-1006.

Ueda K, Kusuhara K, Hirose M, et al: Exanthem subitum and antibody to human herpesvirus-6. J Infect Dis 1989;159:750-752.

Yamanishi K, Okuno T, Shiraki K, et al. Identification of human herpesvirus-6 as a causal agent for exanthem subitum. Lancet 1988;1:1065-1067.

Yoshikawa T, Suga S, Asano Y, et al. Distribution of antibodies to a causative agent of exanthem subitum (human herpervirus-6) in healthy individuals, Pediatrics 1989; 84:675-677.

Yoshiyama H, Suzuki E, Yoshida T, et al. Role of human herpesvirus 6 infection in infants with exanthema subitum, Pediatr Infect Dis J 1990;9:71-74.

Zahorsky JG. Roseola infantilis. Pediatrics 1910;22:60-64.

23

RUBELLA (GERMAN MEASLES)

Rubella is an acute infectious disease characterized by minimal or absent prodromal symptoms, a 3-day rash, and generalized lymph node enlargement, particularly of the postauricular, suboccipital, and cervical lymph nodes. Before 1941 rubella was important chiefly because it was responsible for epidemics in schools and military installations and because it was frequently confused with measles and scarlet fever. Since 1941 a great deal of interest has been focused on this disease because of the association of rubella during pregnancy with an increased incidence of congenital malformations.

ETIOLOGY

Rubella is caused by a specific virus that is present in the blood and nasopharyngeal secretions of patients with the disease. In 1914 Hess postulated, because of his transmission studies with rhesus monkeys, that rubella was caused by a virus. This observation was not confirmed until 1938 when Hiro and Tasaka produced the disease in children by inoculating them with filtered nasal washings obtained from patients during the acute phase of rubella. Habel et al., in 1942, also successfully transmitted rubella to the rhesus monkey, using nasal washings and blood. Reports by Anderson in 1949 and by Krugman et al. in 1953 confirmed Hiro and Tasaka's findings. Krugman et al. (1953) and Krugman and Ward (1954) also demonstrated that virus was present in the blood 2 days before and on the first day of rash and proved conclusively that rubella can occur without a

rash. The cultivation of rubella virus in tissue culture was reported independently and simultaneously by two groups. Weller and Neva in 1962 observed a cytopathic effect in human amnion cells. At the same time, Parkman et al. (1962) isolated the virus in cultures of African green monkey kidney tissue. Cells infected with rubella virus remained normal in appearance in spite of challenge with ECHO virus type 11, which characteristically causes a cytopathic effect.

Rubella virus is a moderately large virus. Its genome consists of single-stranded RNA. Its nucleocapsid is 30 nm in diameter, and it is surrounded by a lipid envelope, 60 to 70 nm in diameter, containing glycoproteins. The nucleocapsid protein consists of four polypeptides. The envelope glycoprotein consists of E1 and E2 glycopeptides. Hemagglutination inhibition and neutralizing antibodies react with the E1 peptides (Dorsett et al., 1985).

Rubella virus is highly sensitive to heat, to extremes of pH, and to a variety of chemical agents. It is rapidly inactivated at 56° C and at 37° C. However, at 4° C the virus titer is relatively stable for 24 hours. For long-term preservation of the virus, a temperature of $-60°$ C is much better than the usual deep-freeze temperature of $-20°$ C. It is inactivated by a pH below 6.8 or above 8.1, ultraviolet irradiation, ether, chloroform, formalin, β-propiolactone, and other chemicals. It is resistant to thimerosal (Merthiolate) (1:10,000 solution) and antibiotics. Viral replication is not inhibited by 5-iodo-2′-

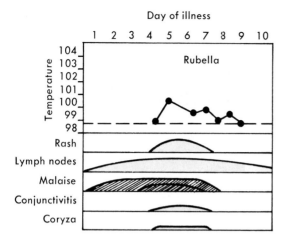

Fig. 23-1. Schematic diagram illustrating typical course of rubella in children and adults. Lymph nodes begin to enlarge 3 to 4 days before rash. Prodromal symptoms (malaise) are minimal in children *(shaded area)*. In adults there may be a 3- to 4-day prodrome *(hatched area)*. Conjunctivitis and coryza, if present, are usually minimal and accompany the rash.

deoxyuridine (IDU) but is inhibited by amantadine. On the basis of its biochemical, biophysical, and ultrastructural properties, rubella virus is classified in the togavirus group, which includes most of the arboviruses. Its clinical and laboratory behavior, however, is more like that of the paramyxoviruses.

Rubella virus has been cultivated in a variety of tissue cultures. In general, the virus produces interference without a cytopathic effect in the following primary tissue culture cells: African green monkey kidney, bovine embryo kidney, guinea pig kidney, rabbit kidney, human amnion, and human embryonic kidney. Interference without a cytopathic effect has also been observed in rhesus monkey and human diploid cell lines. Cytopathic effect has been observed in a variety of continuous cell lines, including rabbit kidney (RK_{13}), rabbit cornea, and hamster (BHK-21). Rubella virus strains belong to one serological type. Hemagglutination and complement-fixing antigens have been prepared in several tissue culture systems. The inhibition of these antigens by specific rubella antisera has formed the basis for practical serological tests.

POSTNATALLY ACQUIRED RUBELLA
Clinical manifestations

The first symptoms of rubella occur after an incubation period of approximately 16 to 18 days, with a range of 14 to 21 days. The typical clinical course is illustrated in Fig. 23-1. In the child the first apparent sign of illness is the appearance of the rash. In adolescents and adults, however, the eruption is preceded by a 1- to 5-

day prodromal period characterized by low-grade fever, headache, malaise, anorexia, mild conjunctivitis, coryza, sore throat, cough, and lymphadenopathy. These symptoms rapidly subside after the first day of rash. The enanthem of rubella, described by Forchheimer in 1898, may be observed in many patients during the prodromal period or on the first day of rash. It consists of reddish spots, pinpoint or larger in size, located on the soft palate. In patients with scarlet fever the soft palate may be covered with punctate lesions, and in patients with measles it may have a red, blotchy appearance; these lesions are indistinguishable from the enanthem of rubella. Obviously, the so-called Forchheimer spots are not pathognomonic for rubella and do not have the same diagnostic significance as Koplik's spots in measles.

Lymph node involvement. Observations made of patients with experimentally induced rubella or during epidemics indicate that lymph node enlargement may begin as early as 7 days before onset of rash (Fig. 23-2). There is generalized lymphadenopathy, but the suboccipital, postauricular, and cervical nodes are most commonly involved. The swelling and tenderness are most apparent and severe on the first day of rash. Subsequently, the tenderness subsides within 1 or 2 days, but the palpable enlargement of the nodes may persist for several weeks or more. As indicated in Table 23-1, the extent of the lymphadenopathy may be extremely variable; occasionally, it may even be absent. At times, splenomegaly also may be noted during the acute stage of the disease.

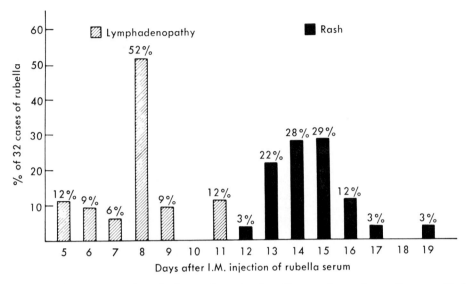

Fig. 23-2. Time of onset of lymphadenopathy and rash in 32 cases of experimentally transmitted rubella. Note appearance of lymphadenopathy 5 to 7 days before onset of rash. (From Green RH, et al.: Am J Dis Child 1965;110:348.)

Table 23-1. Clinical aspects of experimental rubella in children

Patient	Maximum temperature (F°)	Rash	Lymph node enlargement	Leukopenia
C.R.	100.4	+	+ +	0
J.G.	101.6	0	+	0
P.K.	100.8	0	+ +	+ +
N.K.	99.6	+ +	+	+ +
E.T.	101.6	+ + +	+ + +	0
K.L.	100.4	+ +	+	+
J.S.	99.0	+ +	+	0
S.E.	99.4	+ +	0	0
G.O.	99.8	+ +	+ +	0
C.N.	99.4	+ + +	+ + +	—
P.A.	99.6	+ + +	+ +	—
T.B.	99.2	+	+	—
M.I.	99.4	+ +	+ + +	—

From Krugman S, Ward R: J Pediatr 1954;44:489.
Key: +, mild; + +, moderate; + + +, marked; 0, none; —, not done.

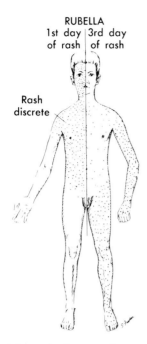

RUBELLA
1st day | 3rd day
of rash | of rash

Rash
discrete

Fig. 23-3. Schematic drawing illustrating development and distribution of rubella rash.

Nevertheless, involvement of the suboccipital, postauricular, and cervical lymph nodes is not pathognomonic for rubella. Lymphadenopathy is associated with diseases such as measles, chickenpox, adenovirus infections, infectious mononucleosis, and many others.

Exanthem. The rash, particularly in children, may be the first obvious indication of illness. It appears first on the face and then spreads downward rapidly to the neck, arms, trunk, and extremities. The eruption appears, spreads, and disappears more quickly than does the rash of measles (Fig. 23-3). By the end of the first day, the entire body may be covered with the discrete pink-red maculopapules. On the second day, the rash begins to disappear from the face, and the lesions on the trunk may coalesce to form a uniform red blush that may resemble the rash of mild scarlet fever. The lesions on the extremities, however, remain discrete and generally do not coalesce. By the end of the third day in the typical case, the rash has disappeared. If the eruption has been intensive, there may be some fine, branny desquamation; usually there is none.

The characteristic pink-red lesions of rubella differ from the purple-red lesions of measles and the yellow-red lesions of scarlet fever. In rubella the lesions are generally discrete and may or may not coalesce; if they do, a diffuse erythematous blush results. In contrast, the lesions of measles, particularly around the head and neck, tend to coalesce and form irregular blotches with crescentic margins. The similarities and differences between the eruptions of rubella and those of scarlet fever have been referred to previously. The circumoral area also differs in these two diseases; in rubella the rash involves this area, and in scarlet fever there is circumoral pallor.

The duration and extent of the rash may be variable. The eruption, which as a rule lasts for 3 days, may persist for 5 days or may be so evanescent that it disappears in less than a day. In an unknown number of instances rubella may even occur without a rash. The existence of rubella without rash has been established. In 13 cases of experimentally induced rubella that the authors studied in 1954 (Table 23-1), the rash was extensive in three, moderate in six, mild in two, and absent in two. In 1965 Green et al. studied 24 children who were intimately exposed to rubella. A rise in rubella virus–neutralizing antibody titer was observed in 22 of the children. Rubella without rash occurred in eight of the 22 infected children. These two studies suggest that the incidence of subclinical rubella infections is approximately 25%.

Fever. In children the temperature may be either normal or slightly elevated. Fever, if present, rarely persists beyond the first day of rash and is usually low grade. A typical temperature course is illustrated in Fig. 23-1. During epidemics, patients with rubella occasionally have temperatures as high as 40° C (104° F). In adolescents and adults there may be low-grade fever during both the prodromal period and the first day of rash. The maximal temperature in a group of 13 children with experimentally induced rubella is listed in Table 23-1; in eight it was normal, and in five it ranged between 38° and 38.7° C (100.4° and 101.6° F).

Blood picture. Generally, the white blood cell count is low. As indicated in Table 23-1, however, the white blood cell count may be normal. An increased number of plasma cells and Türk cells also have been described in rubella. Oc-

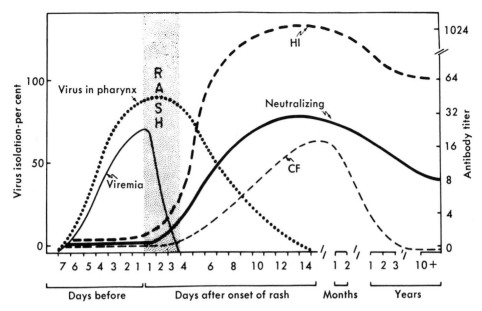

Fig. 23-4. Natural history of postnatal rubella. Pattern of virus excretion and antibody response. (Modified from Cooper LZ, Krugman S: Arch Ophthalmol 1967;77:434.)

casionally, there may be an increased percentage of abnormal lymphocytes or a decrease in platelets.

Diagnosis

Confirmatory clinical factors. A diagnosis of rubella is suggested by the appearance of a maculopapular eruption beginning on the face, progressing rapidly downward to the trunk and extremities, and subsiding within 3 days. Prodromal symptoms are minimal or absent, fever is low grade or absent, and lymphadenopathy precedes the appearance of the rash. A history of exposure, if available, is helpful.

Detection of causative agent. As indicated in Fig. 23-4, rubella virus may be recovered from the pharynx as early as 7 days before the onset of rash and as late as 14 days after onset of rash. The availability of virus isolation procedures has provided an important laboratory tool for the precise diagnosis of rubella. As indicated in Fig. 23-4, virus may be recovered from the pharynx with regularity within 5 days after the onset of rash; in contrast, viremia that is present before the onset of rash is rarely observed after the onset of rash.

Serological tests. The pattern of appearance and persistence of rubella virus–neutralizing,

complement-fixing (CF), and hemagglutination-inhibition (HI) antibody is shown in Fig. 23-4. Antibody is usually detectable by the third day of rash, and peak levels are reached approximately 1 month later. CF antibody may be short lived, declining to nondetectable levels within a year or more after infection. Neutralizing and HI antibodies usually persist for life. The HI antibody test has the advantages of high sensitivity and speed with which results are obtained. A serological diagnosis is possible if acute- and convalescent-phase serum specimens are obtained. The acute-phase serum should be obtained as early as possible after onset of rash; convalescent-phase serum should be collected 2 to 4 weeks later. Evidence of a fourfold or greater rise in rubella antibody titer is indicative of a recent infection.

Differential diagnosis is discussed in Chapter 36.

Complications

Rubella in childhood is rarely followed by complications. Secondary bacterial infections, which are so common in measles, are not encountered in rubella. The following complications have been observed, especially during epidemics.

Arthritis. Joint involvement in adolescents and adults with rubella is much more common than is generally appreciated. It usually develops just as the rash is fading on the second to third day of illness. Either one or more of the larger and smaller joints may be involved. The arthritis may be manifested by a return of fever and either transient joint pain without swelling or massive effusion into one or more joint spaces. These manifestations usually clear spontaneously within 5 to 10 days. Rubella arthritis, with involvement of the knees, ankles, or elbows, may simulate the polyarthritis of rheumatic fever. When there is fusiform swelling of the fingers, it may resemble rheumatoid arthritis. In 1958 Johnson and Hall studied 10 female patients with rubella arthritis of the small- and medium-sized joints that lasted 1 week. Positive latex fixation tests for rheumatoid factor were demonstrated in 9 of the 10 patients with arthritis as compared with only 2 of 7 patients who had rubella without arthritis. On the other hand, the euglobulin-sensitized sheep cell agglutination test was negative in 14 women with rubella arthritis observed by Kantor and Tanner (1962). None showed any clinical manifestations suggesting rheumatoid disease over a 2- to 5-year follow-up period. During an epidemic of rubella in a London suburb, Fry et al. (1962) observed arthritis in 15% of 74 adults who acquired the disease; they detected arthritis in 33% of 40 females and in 6% of 34 males. During an epidemic of rubella in Bermuda in 1971, joint manifestations were observed in 25% of children under the age of 11 years and in 52% of patients 11 years of age or older (Judelsohn and Wyll, 1973).

Encephalitis. Complications of rubella in the central nervous system (CNS) are extremely rare. Encephalitis is less commonly encountered after this disease than after measles or varicella. The incidence usually cited is 1 in 6000 cases of rubella. The clinical manifestations are similar to those observed in other types of postinfectious encephalitis. Complete recovery is generally the rule, but fatalities have been reported. Observations by Kenny et al. in 1965 indicated that demyelinization apparently is not a feature of rubella encephalopathy. Neurological abnormalities are minor and occur infrequently, and intellectual function is generally unaffected if the patient survives. Electroencephalographic abnormalities, however, are relatively common and persistent.

Purpura. Thrombocytopenic and nonthrombocytopenic purpura may, in rare instances, complicate rubella. In addition to a reduction in platelet count, when present, there is usually prolonged bleeding time and increased capillary fragility. In some reported cases the clinical manifestations have included one or more of the following disorders: cutaneous hemorrhages, epistaxis, bleeding gums, hematuria, bleeding from the intestinal tract, and, rarely, cerebral hemorrhage. Most patients become symptom free within 2 weeks, and the platelet count returns to normal values.

Prognosis

The prognosis is almost uniformly excellent. Rubella is one of the most benign of all infectious diseases in children. The extremely rare complications of encephalitis and thrombocytopenic purpura may alter the prognosis. Many reported deaths attributed to rubella infection reflect errors in diagnosis.

Immunity

Active immunity. One attack of rubella is generally followed by permanent immunity. Many of the so-called second attacks represent errors in diagnosis. Active immunity is induced by infection after natural or artificial exposure. As indicated in Fig. 23-4, rubella-neutralizing antibody may persist for many years after infection.

Passive immunity. Neutralizing antibodies for rubella are present in gamma globulin and in convalescent-phase serum. Rubella, like measles and mumps, is rarely observed in the early months of life because of transplacentally acquired immunity.

Epidemiological factors

Rubella is worldwide in distribution. It is endemic in most large cities. Localized epidemics occur at irregular intervals in contrast to the fairly consistent periodicity of measles. During the prevaccine era, major epidemics occurred at 6- to 9-year intervals. Rubella outbreaks usually occur during the spring months in the temperate zones.

The extensive and routine use of live attenuated rubella vaccine since licensure in 1969 has had a major impact on the epidemiology of the disease. The last epidemic occurred in 1964. During the subsequent 28 years there was a progressive decrease in the number of reported cases of rubella. Major epidemics of the disease have been eliminated in the United States.

The age distribution of rubella during the prevaccine era was striking. It was rare in infancy and uncommon in preschool-age children. There was an unusually high incidence of the disease in older children, adolescents, and young adults. Rubella was a constant problem in boarding schools, colleges, and military installations. A significant number of man-days were lost as a result of outbreaks among military personnel.

Rubella is probably spread via the respiratory route. Studies of human volunteers have confirmed this impression. The disease has been transmitted with nasopharyngeal secretions obtained from patients with rubella on the first day of the rash. The period of infectivity probably extends from the latter part of the incubation period to the end of the third day of the rash.

Isolation and quarantine

Isolation and quarantine precautions generally are not warranted. However, outbreaks of rubella have been a problem in hospital and medical personnel in several states, including New York (McLaughlin and Gold, 1979), California, and Colorado (Edell et al., 1979). During the New York experience a male physician with rubella exposed 170 persons, including susceptible pregnant patients. These episodes create a difficult problem for institutions and staff—a problem that can be prevented by routine screening of both male and female medical personnel caring for patients who may be pregnant and by immunization of those with no detectable rubella antibody.

Treatment

Symptomatic treatment. Rubella in many instances is asymptomatic, and no treatment at all is required. Even if the child has a low-grade fever, bed rest may be unnecessary. Headache, malaise, and pain in the lymph nodes can be easily controlled with acetaminophen.

Treatment of complications. Arthritis is usually well controlled by aspirin. Bed rest is advised if there is fever or involvement of the weight-bearing joints. A patient with encephalitis should be treated in the same way as a patient with measles encephalitis (p. 235). Corticosteroid therapy and platelet transfusions may be indicated in severe cases of thrombocytopenic purpura.

CONGENITAL RUBELLA

Congenital rubella was identified as a clinical entity more than a century after the disease was first recognized. In 1941 Gregg reported the occurrence of congenital cataracts among 78 infants born after maternal rubella infection acquired during the 1940 epidemic in Australia. More than half of these infants had congenital heart disease. Since 1941, Gregg's report of the rubella syndrome has been amply confirmed. The occurrence of rubella during the first trimester of pregnancy has been associated with a significantly increased incidence of congenital malformations, stillbirths, and abortions. The epidemic of rubella in the United States in 1964 was followed by the birth of many thousands of infants with the congenital rubella syndrome.

Pathogenesis

Studies by many investigators have provided evidence to support the following concept of the natural history of congenital rubella. As indicated in Fig. 23-4, viremia is present for several days before onset of rash. Maternal viremia may be followed by a placental infection and subsequent fetal viremia leading to a disseminated infection involving many fetal organs. Timing is the crucial element in the pathogenesis of congenital rubella. A fetal infection probably will be chronic and persistent if it is acquired during the early weeks and months of pregnancy. However, after the fourth month of gestation, the fetus apparently is no longer susceptible to the chronic infection that is characteristic of intrauterine rubella during the first 8 to 12 weeks.

The pathogenesis of rubella embryopathy is not entirely clear. Studies in human embryonic tissue culture cells have indicated that rubella infection was associated with inhibition of mitosis and an increased number of chromosomal breaks (Plotkin et al., 1965). Autopsies of infants with congenital rubella revealed hypoplastic organs with a subnormal number of cells (Naeye and Blanc, 1965). Consequently, it is likely that rubella embryopathy may be caused by (1) inhibition of cellular multiplication; (2) chronic, persistent infection during the crucial period of organogenesis; or (3) a combination of both factors.

Clinical manifestations

The classic rubella syndrome described by Gregg and others in the 1940s was characterized by intrauterine growth retardation, cataracts, microcephaly, deafness, congenital heart disease, and mental retardation. Extensive studies of this syndrome during the 1964 rubella epidemic in the United States shed new light on this problem. The availability of specific virus isolation and serological techniques provided information that revealed a broader spectrum of this disease. Intrauterine rubella infection may be followed by spontaneous abortion of the infected fetus, a stillbirth, live birth of an infant with single or multiple malformations, or birth of a normal infant. The various manifestations of congenital rubella are listed in the box. It is clear that the consequences of rubella infection during pregnancy are varied and unpredictable. Virtually every organ may be involved—singly, multiply, transiently, or progressively and permanently.

Neonatal manifestations. A variety of clinical manifestations may be present during the first weeks of life. Low birth weight in relation to period of gestation is common. Thrombocytopenic purpura characterized by a petechial and purpuric eruption may occur in association with other transient conditions such as hepatosplenomegaly, hepatitis, hemolytic anemia, bone lesions (metaphyseal rarefaction), and bulging anterior fontanelle with or without pleocytosis in the cerebrospinal fluid (CSF). These transient manifestations may occur in association with the classic cardiac, eye, hearing, and CNS defects. An infant with neonatal thrombocytopenic purpura characterized by the typical "blueberry muffin" skin lesions is shown in Plate 5.

Cardiac defects. Patent ductus arteriosus, with or without pulmonary artery stenosis, and atrial and ventricular septal defects are the most common cardiac lesions. Clinical evidence of congenital heart disease may be present at birth or delayed for several days. Other cardiac manifestations include myocardial involvement as indicated by electrocardiographic findings and necropsy evidence of extensive necrosis of the myocardium. Many infants have tolerated the

---

MANIFESTATIONS OF CONGENITAL RUBELLA

Growth retardation (low birth weight)
Eye defects
  Cataracts
  Glaucoma
  Retinopathy
  Microphthalmia
Deafness
Cardiac defects
  Patent ductus arteriosus
  Ventricular septal defect
  Pulmonary stenosis
  Myocardial necrosis
Central nervous system defects
  Psychomotor retardation
  Microcephaly
  Encephalitis
  Spastic quadriparesis
  Cerebrospinal fluid pleocytosis
  Mental retardation
  Progressive panencephalitis
Hepatomegaly
Hepatitis
Thrombocytopenic purpura
Splenomegaly
Bone lesions
Interstitial pneumonitis
Diabetes mellitus
Psychiatric disorders
Thyroid disorders
Precocious puberty

---

cardiac lesions with little difficulty; others have developed congestive heart failure in the first months of life.

Eye defects. Cataracts, unilateral or bilateral, are common consequences of congenital rubella. They appear as pearly white nuclear lesions, frequently associated with microphthalmia. The cataracts may be too small at birth to be visible on casual examination. A careful ophthalmoscopic examination with a $+8$ lens held 15 to 20 cm from the eye may reveal an early cataract.

Rubella glaucoma is a less common eye lesion, and it may be clinically indistinguishable from hereditary infantile glaucoma. It may be present at birth, or it may appear after the neonatal period. The cornea is enlarged and hazy, the anterior chamber is deep, and ocular tension is increased. Glaucoma that requires prompt surgical therapy must be differentiated from transient corneal clouding.

Retinopathy is the most common eye manifestation of congenital rubella. It is characterized by discrete, patchy, black pigmentation that is variable in size and location. Retinopathy does not affect visual acuity if the lesions do not involve the macular area. The presence of this lesion is a valuable aid in the clinical diagnosis of congenital rubella.

Hearing loss. Deafness may be the only manifestation of congenital rubella. It may be unilateral but is usually bilateral. It is probably caused by maldevelopment and possibly by degenerative changes in the cochlea and organ of Corti. Hearing loss may be severe or so mild that it is overlooked unless detected by an audiometric examination. Severe bilateral hearing loss is responsible for speech defects.

Central nervous system involvement. Psychomotor retardation is a common manifestation of congenital rubella. In severe cases the brain is the site of a chronic, persistent infection, as indicated by the presence of pleocytosis, increased concentration of protein, and rubella virus in the CSF for as long as 1 year after birth. Microcephaly is a well-known manifestation (Desmond et al., 1967). The most common consequence of CNS involvement is mental retardation (mild or profound). Behavioral disturbances and manifestations of minimal cerebral dysfunction also are common. Less common are severe spastic diplegia and autism.

Progressive rubella panencephalitis has been described in four patients with congenital rubella (Townsend et al., 1975; Weil et al., 1975). Severe, progressive neurological deterioration was noted during the second decade of life. In two patients there was progression of spasticity, ataxia, intellectual deterioration, seizures, and subsequent fatality. Other findings included high levels of rubella antibody in serum and CSF, increased CSF protein and gamma globulin levels, histopathological changes in the brain, and isolation of rubella virus from a brain biopsy of one of the patients. This syndrome in some ways resembled subacute sclerosing panencephalitis, a rare complication of measles.

Diagnosis

The presence of congenital rubella should be suspected under the following circumstances: (1) a history of possible rubella or exposure to rubella during the first trimester of pregnancy and (2) the presence of one or more of the various manifestations of congenital rubella listed in the box on p. 388. However, final confirmation of the diagnosis is dependent on virus isolation and/or immunological procedures.

Virus isolation. Rubella virus has been cultured from pharyngeal secretions, urine, CSF, and virtually every tissue and organ in the body. Infants with congenital rubella may remain chronically infected for many weeks or months. As indicated in Fig. 23-5, the incidence of virus shedding decreases with advancing age. Most infants with congenital rubella are no longer shedding virus and have a normal pattern of serum immunoglobulins by 1 year of age. However, infants with severe dysgammaglobulinemia may shed virus for a more prolonged period. Isolation of virus from the blood is very rare. Viremia has been observed chiefly in infants with immunological disorders.

Immunological response. The response to an intrauterine infection is shown in Fig. 23-6. It differs significantly from the response to rubella acquired postnatally. The chief difference lies in the pattern of virus excretion and antibody response. In rubella acquired after birth, virus excretion is transient, rarely persisting for more than 2 or 3 weeks (Fig. 23-4); in contrast, virus shedding may persist for many months after birth in congenital rubella.

As indicated in Fig. 23-6, the serum of an infant with congenital rubella contains actively acquired IgM-specific antibody and passively acquired maternal IgG antibody. Several months later, transplacentally acquired IgG is no longer detectable, and high levels of IgM may be present. By the end of 1 year, actively acquired IgG apparently is the dominant rubella antibody. Consequently, the presence and persistence of rubella antibody in the serum of an infant 5 to 6 months of age or older and the identification of the antibody in early infancy as IgM are indicative of congenital rubella infection.

The pattern of persistence of HI antibody following congenital rubella is different from that following naturally acquired infection. Detectable levels of antibody persist for many years in most children after a natural rubella infection. However, approximately 20% of children with

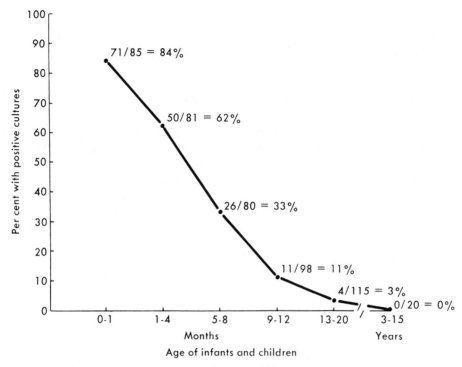

Fig. 23-5. Incidence of rubella virus excretion by age in infants with congenital rubella. (From Cooper LZ, Krugman S: Arch Ophthalmol 1967;77:434.)

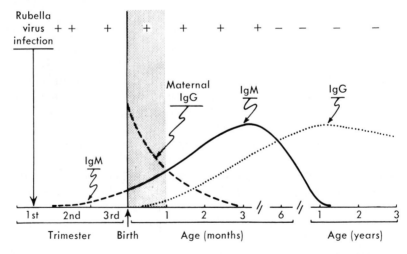

Fig. 23-6. Natural history of congenital rubella. Pattern of virus excretion and antibody response.

congenital rubella by age 5 years may no longer have detectable rubella HI antibody (Cooper et al., 1971).

Differential diagnosis

Cytomegalovirus infection, congenital toxoplasmosis, and congenital syphilis also may be characterized by the following manifestations of congenital rubella: thrombocytopenic purpura, jaundice, hepatosplenomegaly, and bone lesions. Herpes simplex virus infection shows the same manifestations with the exception of bone lesions and a vesicular skin rash. The diagnosis may be clarified by the presence of other findings more compatible with congenital rubella such as congenital cataract, glaucoma, patent ductus arteriosus, or maternal history of rubella. The precise diagnosis should be confirmed by specific laboratory tests.

Prognosis

Neonatal thrombocytopenic purpura carries a bad prognosis. The mortality rate exceeded 35% after the first-year follow-up of a large group of infants (Cooper and Krugman, 1967). The usual causes of death were sepsis, congestive heart failure, and general debility. In the absence of purpura, the mortality rate was approximately 10%. Deaths usually occurred during the first 6 months of life. The prognosis is excellent for children with minor defects.

There has been a long-term follow-up of approximately 500 children born with the congenital rubella syndrome in New York City during the epidemic of 1964 to 1965. These patients, now in their twenties, can be divided into three groups: approximately one third that is relatively normal; one third that is mildly to moderately incapacitated; and the remainder that is profoundly handicapped and requires institutional care. Patients with congenital rubella syndrome have had difficulty in developing social skills, especially after leaving special educational units as young adults. Suicide attempts have not been uncommon. Approximately 15% of patients with congenital rubella syndrome have developed insulin-dependent diabetes.

Epidemiological factors

The incidence of congenital rubella is dependent on the immune status of women of childbearing age and the occurrence of significant epidemics. In the United States approximately 15% of young women have no detectable rubella antibody. During the 1964 epidemic, 3.6% of pregnant women had rubella; in contrast, the infection rate was 0.1% to 0.2% during interepidemic years (Sever, 1967).

Congenital rubella is a contagious disease. The infected newborn infant may disseminate the virus to close contacts for many months. This reservoir may provide a source for maintaining the virus in nature from year to year.

The risk associated with maternal rubella infection has been variously estimated. An evaluation of several prospective studies indicates that the risk of congenital malformations after maternal rubella is as follows: (1) 30% to 50% during the first 4 weeks of gestation, (2) 25% during the fifth to eighth weeks of gestation, and (3) 8% during the ninth to twelfth weeks of gestation. The overall risk of malformations from rubella during the first trimester is approximately 20%. There is a slight risk of deafness when rubella occurs during the thirteenth to sixteenth weeks.

Isolation and quarantine

Isolation of infants with congenital rubella. The primary aim of isolation procedures is to prevent rubella infection in susceptible pregnant women. Infants with congenital rubella may shed virus for many weeks or months after birth. Intimate contact is generally required for the transmission of rubella. The risk of infection by the airborne route is probably inconsequential. Accordingly, potentially susceptible pregnant women should avoid close exposure to these infants.

Isolation in the hospital. Infants suspected of having congenital rubella should be admitted to a separate room designated as the isolation unit. Personnel assigned to this area should be selected on the basis of their childbearing potential and immune status. If appropriate laboratory facilities are available, it would be wise to screen all staff members for presence of rubella antibody. Isolation should be continued until the infant is ready to go home.

Isolation in the home. No special precautions are necessary for the parents and young sibling contacts. Potentially susceptible female visitors to the home should avoid physical contact with the infant during the contagious period. If laboratory facilities are available for identification of rubella virus, infants should be considered contagious until negative cultures have been obtained. As indicated in Fig. 23-5, evidence of virus shedding may disappear by 1 month of age in some infants; on the other hand, it may persist for a year or more in a small number of infants. If laboratory facilities are not available, the data shown in Fig. 23-5 may be used as a guide for the estimation of period of contagion. In general, there is some correlation between the severity of the infection and the duration of virus shedding. Infants with severe involvement usually will shed virus much longer than infants with minimal involvement.

PREVENTIVE MEASURES

The following guidelines for the use of the currently licensed rubella vaccine are extracted from the recommendations of the Immunization Practices Advisory Committee (ACIP) (MMWR 1990;39:3-18).

LIVE RUBELLA VIRUS VACCINE

The live rubella virus vaccine* currently distributed in the United States is prepared in human diploid cell culture. In January 1979, this vaccine (RA 27/3) replaced the HPV-77:DE-5 vaccine grown in duck embryo cell culture becaue it induced higher seroresponse, greater resistance to reinfection, and lower reaction rate. Although both subcutaneous and intranasal administration of the vaccine have been studied, the vaccine is licensed only for subcutaneous administration. The vaccine is produced in monovalent form (rubella only) and in combinations: measles-rubella (MR), rubella-mumps, and measles-mumps-rubella (MMR) vaccines.

In clinical trials, ≥95% of susceptible persons who received a single dose of rubella vaccine when they were ≥12 months of age developed antibody. Clinical efficacy and challenge studies have shown that >90% of vaccinees have protection against both clinical rubella and viremia for at least 15 years. Available follow-up studies indicate that vaccine-induced protection is long-term, probably lifelong; therefore, a history of vaccination can be considered presumptive evidence of immunity.

Although vaccine-induced titers are generally lower than those stimulated by rubella infection, vaccine-induced immunity usually protects against both

clinical illness and viremia after natural exposure. In studies that have attempted to reinfect persons artificially who received RA 27/3 vaccine, vaccinees demonstrated a resistance to reinfection similar to the resistance that follows natural infection. A small number of reports have indicated that viremic reinfection following exposure may occur in vaccinated individuals with low levels of detectable antibody. The frequency and consequences of this phenomenon are currently unknown but believed to be rare. These reports are to be expected, because there are also rare reports of clinical reinfection and fetal infection following disease-induced immunity.

Some vaccinees intermittently shed small amounts of virus from the pharynx 7-28 days after vaccination. However, studies of >1,200 susceptible household contacts and experience gained over 20 years of vaccine use failed to identify transmission of vaccine virus. These findings indicate that vaccinating susceptible children whose mothers or other household contacts are pregnant does not present a risk. Rather, vaccination of such children provides protection for these pregnant women.

VACCINE USE
Rubella immunity

Persons can be considered immune to rubella only if they have documentation of (a) laboratory evidence of rubella immunity or (b) adequate immunization with at least one dose of rubella vaccine on or after the first birthday. Many persons will receive two doses of rubella vaccine as a result of the new two-dose schedule for MMR vaccination, which is recommended to improve control of measles. Clinical diagnosis of rubella is unreliable and should not be considered in assessing immune status.

General recommendations

Persons ≥12 months of age should be vaccinated, unless they are immune. All children, adolescents, and adults—particularly females—are considered susceptible and should be vaccinated if there are no contraindications (see section on PRECAUTIONS AND CONTRAINDICATIONS). Those who should be vaccinated include persons who may be immune to rubella but who lack adequate documentation of immunity. All vaccinations should be documented in the patient's permanent medical record.

Vaccinating susceptible individuals both protects them against rubella and prevents their spreading the virus. Vaccinating susceptible postpubertal females confers individual protection against rubella-induced fetal injury. Vaccinating adolescents or adults in high-risk population groups, such as those in colleges, places of employment, or military bases, protects them against rubella and reduces the chance of epidemics.

---

*Official name: rubella virus vaccine, live.

Dosage

The dose of 0.5 ml of reconstituted vaccine (whether as a monovalent product or, preferably, in combination with measles and mumps antigens) should be administered subcutaneously.

Age at vaccination

Live rubella virus vaccine is recommended for all children ≥12 months of age. It should not usually be given to younger infants, because persisting maternal antibodies may interfere with seroconversion. When the rubella vaccine is part of a combination that includes the measles antigen, the combination vaccine should generally be given to children at ≥15 months of age to maximize measles seroconversion. A second dose of MMR is recommended at school entry, although in some localities the decision may be made to administer the second dose at older ages (e.g., entry to middle or junior high school). Initial vaccination with MMR may be given at 12 months of age to children living in areas at high risk for measles transmission among preschool-age children (i.e., a county with >5 cases among preschool-age children during each of the last 5 years, a county with a recent outbreak among unvaccinated preschool-age children, or a county with a large inner-city, urban population). These recommendations may be implemented for an entire county or in smaller, defined, high-risk areas. MMR may be administered to children before their first birthday if monovalent measles vaccine is not readily available. Infants vaccinated with MMR before the first birthday should be considered unvaccinated for purposes of determining the need for further vaccination. They should be revaccinated with rubella, measles, and mumps vaccines, preferably by starting the two-dose schedule of MMR with a first dose given generally at 15 months of age.

Older children who have not received rubella vaccine should be vaccinated promptly. Because a history of rubella illness is not a reliable indicator of immunity, all children should be vaccinated unless there are contraindications (see section on PRECAUTIONS AND CONTRAINDICATIONS).

Vaccination of women of childbearing age

The Immunization Practices Advisory Committee (ACIP) has weighed several factors in developing recommendations for vaccinating women of childbearing age against rubella. Although there may be concern about giving rubella vaccine during pregnancy, available data on previously and currently available rubella vaccines indicate that the risk of teratogenicity from live rubella vaccines is small. From January 1971 to April 1989, CDC followed to term 321 known rubella-susceptible pregnant women who had been vaccinated with live rubella vaccine within 3 months before or 3 months after conception. Ninety-four women received HPV-77 or Cendehill vaccines, one received vaccine of unknown strain, and 226 received RA 27/3 vaccine. None of the 324 infants (three of the mothers receiving RA 27/3 vaccine delivered twins) had malformations compatible with congenital rubella infection. This total included the five infants who were born to these susceptible women and who had serologic evidence of subclinical infection. (Three of the infants were exposed to HPV-77 or Cendehill vaccine; two were exposed to RA 27/3 vaccine.)

On the basis of the experience to date, the estimated risk of serious malformations attributable to RA 27/3 rubella vaccine, derived from the binomial distribution with 95% confidence limits, is from 0% to 1.6%. (If the susceptible infants exposed to other rubella vaccines are included, the risk is from 0% to 1.2%.) This risk is substantially less than the ≥20% risk of CRS associated with maternal infection during the first trimester of pregnancy. Moreover, the observed risk with both the HPV-77 or Cendehill and RA 27/3 strains of vaccine is zero.

Rubella vaccine virus has been isolated from aborted tissue from one (3%) of 35 susceptible women who had been given RA 27/3 vaccine while pregnant, whereas virus was isolated from aborted tissue from 17 (20%) of 85 susceptible women who had been given HPV-77 or Cendehill vaccines while pregnant. This finding provides additional evidence that the RA 27/3 vaccine poses no greater risk of teratogenicity than did the HPV-77 or Cendehill vaccines.

The risk of vaccine-associated defects is negligible and should not ordinarily be a reason to consider interruption of pregnancy. Because birth defects, one-third of which are serious, are noted in 3% of all births, confusion about the etiology of birth defects may result if vaccine is administered during pregnancy.

As of April 30, 1989, CDC discontinued accepting new enrollees into its registry of women vaccinated with rubella vaccine during pregnancy. However, all suspected cases of CRS, whether presumed to be due to wild-virus or vaccine-virus infection, should continue to be reported through state and local health departments.

The continuing occurrence of rubella among women of childbearing age and the lack of evidence for teratogenicity from the vaccine strongly indicate the need to continue vaccination of susceptible adolescent and adult females of childbearing age. However, because of concern about risk for the fetus, women of childbearing age should receive vaccine only if they state that they are not pregnant and are counseled not to become pregnant for 3 months after vaccination. In view of the importance of protecting this age group against rubella, reasonable practices in a rubella immunization program include (a) asking women if they are pregnant, (b) excluding those who state that they are, (c) explaining the concern about risk for the fetus to the others, and (d) explaining the importance of not becoming pregnant during the 3 months following vaccination.

Use of vaccine following exposure to rubella

There is no conclusive evidence that giving live rubella virus vaccine following exposure will prevent illness. However, a single exposure may not cause infection. Because postexposure vaccination will protect an individual exposed in the future, and because there is no evidence that vaccinating an individual who is incubating rubella is harmful, vaccination is still recommended, unless otherwise contraindicated.

Use of human immune globulin following exposure to rubella

Immune globulin (IG) given after exposure to rubella will not prevent infection or viremia, but it may modify or suppress symptoms and create an unwarranted sense of security. The routine use of IG for postexposure prophylaxis of rubella in early pregnancy is not recommended. Infants with congenital rubella have been born to women who were given IG shortly after exposure. The only instance in which IG might be useful would be when a pregnant woman who has been exposed to rubella would not consider termination of pregnancy under any circumstances.

Recent administration of IG

Vaccine should be administered approximately 2 weeks before or deferred for approximately 3 months after receipt of IG, because passively acquired antibodies might interfere with the response to the vaccine. However, previous administration of anti-Rho (D) IG (human) or blood products does not generally interfere with an immune response and is not a contraindication to postpartum vaccination. In this situation, persons who have received the globulin or blood products should be serologically tested 6-8 weeks after vaccination to assure that seroconversion has occurred. Obtaining laboratory evidence of seroconversion in other vaccinees is not necessary.

Vaccine shipment and storage

During storage, before reconstitution, rubella vaccine must be kept at a temperature of 2 C-8 C (35.6 F-46.4 F) or colder. It must also be protected from light, which may inactivate the virus. Reconstituted vaccine should be discarded if not used within 8 hours. Vaccine must be shipped at 10 C (50 F) or colder and may be shipped on dry ice.

ADVERSE EVENTS

Vaccinees can develop low-grade fever, rash, and lymphadenopathy after vaccination. Arthralgia and transient arthritis occur more frequently in suscep-

tible adults than in children, and more frequently in susceptible postpubertal females than in susceptible men. Arthralgia or arthritis are rare following vaccination of children with RA 27/3 vaccine. By contrast, approximately 25% of susceptible postpubertal females develop arthralgia following RA 27/3 vaccination, and approximately 10% have been reported to have arthritis-like signs and symptoms. Rarely, transient peripheral neuritic complaints, such as paresthesias and pain in the arms and legs, have occurred.

When joint symptoms occur, or when pain and/or paresthesias not associated with joints occur, they generally begin 1-3 weeks after vaccination, persist for 1 day-3 weeks, and rarely recur. Adults with joint symptoms following rubella vaccination usually have not had to disrupt work activities. Infrequently, susceptible vaccinees, primarily adult females, reportedly have developed chronic or recurrent arthralgias, sometimes with arthritis or neurologic symptoms including paresthesias, carpal tunnel syndrome, and blurred vision. Onset of these symptoms occurred within 1 month of initial vaccination. One group of investigators has reported the frequency of chronic joint symptoms and signs in adult females to be as high as 5%-11%; however, other data from the United States and experience from other countries that use the RA 27/3 strain suggest that such occurrences are rare. In comparative studies, the frequency of chronic joint complaints is substantially higher following natural infection than following vaccination.

The mechanism for joint abnormalities after vaccination is unclear. Joint destruction rarely has been reported. One group of investigators has reported that viral persistence in peripheral blood lymphocytes has occurred among a substantial number of these patients. This same group has postulated that defective immunity, in the form of partial antibody, detected by an enzyme immunoassay (EIA) kit but not by hemagglutination-inhibition (HI) assay, may facilitate viral persistence. No conclusive evidence has shown that immune complexes play a role in disease pathogenesis. Rubella virus has been isolated from both peripheral blood lymphocytes and synovial cells from children with chronic arthritis, primarily juvenile rheumatoid arthritis; however, a causal relationship has not been proven.

Available published data indicate that only susceptible vaccinees have side effects of vaccination. There is no conclusive evidence of an increased risk of these reactions for persons who are already immune when vaccinated.

PRECAUTIONS AND CONTRAINDICATIONS
Pregnancy

Pregnant women should not be vaccinated with rubella vaccine. If a pregnant woman is vaccinated or if she becomes pregnant within 3 months after vaccination, she should be counseled about the concern for the fetus, but rubella vaccination during pregnancy should not ordinarily be a reason to consider interruption of pregnancy.

Febrile illness

Vaccination of persons with severe febrile illness should be postponed until recovery. However, susceptible children with mild illnesses, such as upper respiratory infection, should be vaccinated. Considering the importance of protecting against rubella, medical personnel should use every opportunity to vaccinate susceptible individuals.

Allergies

Hypersensitivity reactions rarely follow the administration of live rubella vaccine. Most of these reactions are considered minor and consist of wheal and flare or urticaria at the injection site.

Live rubella vaccine is produced in human diploid cell culture. Consequently, a history of anaphylactic reactions to egg ingestion needs to be taken into consideration only if measles or mumps antigens are to be included with rubella vaccine.

Since rubella vaccine contains trace amounts of neomycin (25 μg), persons who have experienced anaphylactic reactions to topically or systemically administered neomycin should not receive rubella vaccine. Most often, neomycin allergy is manifested as a contact dermatitis, which is a delayed-type (cell-mediated) immune response, rather than anaphylaxis. In such individuals, the adverse reaction, if any, to neomycin in the vaccine would be an erythematous, pruritic nodule or papule at 48-96 hours. A history of contact dermatitis to neomycin is not a contraindication to receiving rubella vaccine. No preparations of live rubella vaccine contain penicillin.

Altered immunocompetence

Replication of vaccine viruses can be enhanced in persons with immune deficiency diseases and in persons with immunosuppression, as occurs with leukemia, lymphoma, generalized malignancy, or resulting from therapy with alkylating agents, antimetabolites, radiation, or large doses of corticosteroids. Although there is no evidence that wild rubella or rubella vaccine virus causes serious illness in immunocompromised persons, concern exists about the risk of any live virus vaccine, including rubella vaccine, for such persons. Therefore, such patients should not be given live rubella virus vaccine—except persons with symptomatic infection with human immunodeficiency virus (HIV), who can receive MMR (see below).

Patients with leukemia in remission who have not received chemotherapy for at least 3 months may be vaccinated with live virus vaccines. Short-term (<2

weeks), low- to moderate-dose systemic corticosteroid therapy, topical steroid therapy (e.g., nasal, skin), long-term alternate-day treatment with low to moderate doses of short-acting systemic steroids, and intraarticular, bursal, or tendon injection of corticosteroids are not immunosuppressive in their usual doses and do not contraindicate rubella vaccine administration.

The growing number of infants and preschoolers with HIV infection has directed special attention to the appropriate immunization of such children. Asymptomatic children do not need to be evaluated and tested for HIV infection before decisions concerning vaccination are made. Asymptomatic HIV-infected persons in need of MMR should receive it. MMR should be considered for all symptomatic HIV-infected children, including children diagnosed as having acquired immunodeficiency syndrome (AIDS), because measles disease in these children can be severe. Limited data on MMR vaccination among asymptomatic and symptomatic HIV-infected children indicate that MMR has not been associated with serious or unusual adverse events, although antibody responses have been variable.

The administration of high-dose intravenous immune globulin (IVIG) to HIV-infected children at regular intervals is being studied to determine whether it will prevent a variety of infections. For those children who have received IVIG within the 3 months preceding vaccination, MMR vaccine may be ineffective.

SIMULTANEOUS ADMINISTRATION OF CERTAIN LIVE VIRUS VACCINES

In general, the simultaneous administration of the most widely used live and inactivated vaccines does not impair antibody responses or increase rates of adverse reactions. The administration of MMR vaccine yields results similar to that of individual measles, mumps, and rubella vaccines at different sites or at different times.

Equivalent antibody responses and no clinically important increases in the frequency of adverse events occur when diphtheria-tetanus-pertussis vaccine (DTP), *Haemophilus influenzae* b conjugate vaccine (HbCV), oral polio vaccine (OPV), or inactivated polio vaccine (IPV) are administered with MMR either simultaneously at different sites or at separate times. Routine simultaneous administration of MMR, DTP, HbCV, and OPV (or IPV) to all children ≥15 months who are eligible to receive these vaccines is recommended. Vaccination with MMR and HbCV at 15 months, followed by DTP and OPV (or IPV) at 18 months remains an acceptable alternative for children whose parents/caregivers are known generally to follow health-care recommendations. If the child might not be brought back for future immunizations, simultaneous administration of all vaccines (including

DTP, OPV, MMR, and HbCV) appropriate to the age and previous vaccination status of the recipient is recommended.

REPORTING OF ADVERSE EVENTS

The National Childhood Vaccine Injury Act of 1986 requires physicians and other health-care providers who administer vaccines to maintain permanent immunization records and to report occurrences of adverse events specified in the Act. These adverse events, as well as other adverse events that require medical attention, must be reported to the U.S. Department of Health and Human Services. Until November 1, 1990, separate systems for reporting adverse events existed for vaccines purchased with public funding and for vaccines purchased in the private sector. After November 1, 1990, all reportable events should be reported to the Vaccine Adverse Events Reporting System (VAERS). Adverse events other than those specified in the Act, especially events that are serious or unusual, should also be reported to VAERS. VAERS forms and instructions are available in the Food and Drug Administration's *FDA Drug Bulletin* and the *Physicians' Desk Reference,* or they may be obtained by calling VAERS at 1-800-822-7967.

STRATEGIES FOR ELIMINATING CRS

The widespread vaccination of school-age children since 1969 has effectively prevented major epidemics of rubella and congenital rubella in the United States. With continued vaccination of children at levels approaching 100%, an immune birth cohort will eventually replace the 6%-25% of persons of childbearing age currently susceptible to rubella, and rubella can be expected to disappear. Recent data suggest that the rates of rubella susceptibility among postpubertal females and in reported cases of rubella continue to decline. Because the process of replacing the adult cohort with immune persons will take years, cases of CRS can still be expected to occur.

Elimination of CRS can be hastened by expanding existing efforts to vaccinate susceptible adolescents and young adults, particularly females of childbearing age, along with continuing routine vaccination of children. In 1985-1988, 40%-60% of the rubella cases occurred in older, postadolescent populations, clearly indicating that rubella in postpubertal populations still occurs. Effective vaccination of all susceptible children in junior and senior high schools can be expected to contribute greatly to the elimination of CRS. Such efforts have resulted in decreases in the reported incidence of rubella in all persons and in the incidence of reported CRS.

The major components of a strategy to eliminate CRS are achieving and maintaining high immunization levels, accurate surveillance of rubella and CRS, and prompt outbreak-control measures. The following recommendations are presented to help preserve the level of rubella and CRS control already achieved and to bring about the further reduction in susceptibility that will be required to eliminate CRS.

Ongoing programs

The primary strategy for eliminating CRS in the United States is to interrupt rubella transmission by achieving and maintaining high immunization levels among all children. Official health agencies should take steps, including developing and enforcing immunization requirements, to ensure that all students in grades kindergarten through 12 are protected against rubella, unless vaccination is contraindicated. School-entry laws should be vigorously enforced. States that do not require proof of immunity of students at all grade levels should consider expanding existing laws or regulations to include the age groups not yet protected.

Recent age-specific data indicate that preschool-age children account for an important proportion of reported rubella cases. Proof of rubella immunity for attendance at day-care centers should be required and enforced. Licensure should depend on such requirements.

To hasten the elimination of CRS, continued effort should be directed toward vaccinating susceptible women of childbearing age. A multifaceted approach is necessary.

General principles

- Voluntary vaccination programs have been less successful than mandatory programs. The military services require rubella immunity of recruits and have essentially eliminated rubella from military bases. In all settings where young adults congregate, men and women should be included in vaccination programs, because men may transmit disease to susceptible women.
- If it is practical and if reliable laboratory services are available, women of childbearing age who are potential candidates for vaccination can have serologic tests to determine susceptibility to rubella. However, with the exception of premarital and prenatal screening, routinely performing serologic tests for all women of childbearing age to determine susceptibility (so that vaccine is given only to proven susceptible women) can be effective but is expensive. Also, two visits to the health-care provider would be necessary—one for screening and one for vaccination. Accordingly, rubella vaccination of a woman who is not known to be pregnant and has no history of vaccination is justifiable without serologic testing—and may be preferable, particularly when costs of serology are high and follow-up of identified susceptible women for vaccination is not assured.

Vaccinated women should be counseled to avoid becoming pregnant for a 3-month period following vaccination. Routine serologic screening of men is not recommended.

- Vaccine should be administered only if there is no contraindication to vaccination.
- Health-care providers are encouraged to use MMR in routine childhood-vaccination programs and whenever rubella vaccine is to be given to persons also likely to be susceptible to measles and/or mumps.

Premarital screening and vaccination

Routine premarital testing for rubella antibody identifies many susceptible women before pregnancy. Documented histories of rubella vaccination or serologic evidence of immunity should be considered acceptable proof of immunity. To ensure a significant reduction in susceptibility through premarital screening, more aggressive follow-up of women found to be susceptible is required.

Postpartum vaccination

Prenatal screening should be carried out on all pregnant women not known to be immune. Women who have just delivered babies should be vaccinated before discharge from the hospital, unless they are known to be immune. Although such women are unlikely to become pregnant, counseling to avoid conception for 3 months following vaccination is still necessary. It is estimated that postpartum vaccination of all women not known to be immune could have prevented approximately 40% of recent CRS cases. Breast-feeding is not a contraindication to vaccination, even though virus may be excreted in breast milk, and infants may be infected. Women attending abortion clinics should be vaccinated after termination of pregnancy.

Routine vaccination in any medical setting

Vaccination of susceptible women of childbearing age should be part of routine general medical and gynecologic outpatient care, should take place in all family-planning settings, and should become routine before discharge from a hospital for any reason, if there are no contraindications (see section on PRECAUTIONS AND CONTRAINDICATIONS). Vaccination should be offered to adults, especially women of childbearing age, any time that contact is made with the health-care system, including when children are undergoing routine examinations or immunizations.

Vaccination of medical personnel

Medical personnel, both male and female (e.g., volunteers, trainees, nurses, physicians), who might transmit rubella to pregnant patients or other personnel, should be immune to rubella. Consideration should be given to making rubella immunity a condition for employment. All medical personnel who have patient contact and who are beginning employment should have proof of rubella immunity or prior vaccination.

Vaccination of workers

Ascertainment of rubella-immune status and availability of rubella immunization should be components of the health-care program in places employing women of childbearing age (e.g., day-care centers, schools, colleges, prisons, companies, government offices, and industrial sites).

Vaccination for college entry

Colleges are high-risk areas for rubella transmission because of large concentrations of susceptible persons. Proof of rubella as well as measles immunity should be required for attendance for both male and female students. All students born in or after 1957 who enter institutions of post-high-school education should have documentation of receipt of two doses of measles vaccine (preferably given as MMR) and at least one dose of rubella vaccine or other evidence of measles and rubella immunity.

Outbreak control

Outbreak control will continue to play an important role in eliminating CRS. Aggressive responses to outbreaks may interrupt chains of transmission and will increase vaccination coverage among persons who might otherwise not be protected. Although methods for controlling rubella outbreaks are evolving, the main strategy should be to define target populations, ensure that susceptible persons are vaccinated rapidly (or excluded from exposure if a contraindication exists), and maintain active surveillance to permit modification of control measures if the situation changes.

Laboratory confirmation of rubella cases is important; however, control measures should be implemented **before** serologic confirmation. This approach is especially important in any outbreak setting involving pregnant women (e.g., obstetric-gynecologic and prenatal clinics). All persons at risk who cannot readily provide laboratory evidence of immunity or a documented history of vaccination on or after their first birthday should be considered susceptible and should be vaccinated if there are no contraindications.

An effective means of terminating outbreaks and increasing rates of immunization quickly is to exclude from possible contact individuals who cannot provide valid evidence of immunity. Experience with measles-outbreak control indicates that almost all students who are excluded from school because they lack evidence of measles immunity quickly comply with requirements and are promptly readmitted to school.

All persons who have been exempted from rubella vaccination because of medical, religious, or other reasons should also be excluded from attendance. Exclusion should continue until 3 weeks after the onset of rash of the last reported case in the outbreak setting. Less rigorous approaches, such as voluntary appeals for vaccination, have not been effective in terminating outbreaks.

Mandatory exclusion and vaccination of adults should be practiced in rubella outbreaks in medical settings because pregnant women may be exposed. This approach may be successful in terminating, or at least limiting, outbreaks. Vaccination during an outbreak has not been associated with substantial personnel absenteeism. Vaccination of susceptible persons before an outbreak occurs is preferable, because vaccination causes far less absenteeism and disruption of routine work activities than does rubella infection.

SURVEILLANCE

Surveillance of rubella and CRS has three purposes: (a) to provide important data on program progress and long-term trends, (b) to help define groups in greatest need of vaccination and in turn provide information for formulation of new strategies, and (c) to evaluate vaccine efficacy, duration of vaccine-induced immunity, and other issues related to vaccine safety and efficacy.

As the rates of rubella and CRS decline in the United States, effective surveillance becomes increasingly important. Known or suspected rubella cases should be reported immediately to local health departments. Because an accurate assessment of CRS elimination can be made only through aggressive case finding, surveillance of CRS will have to be intensified.

Surveillance of rubella is complicated by the fact that the symptoms of the clinical disease are not distinctive and can be confused with a number of other illnesses. Thus, cases should be laboratory confirmed, particularly outside of the outbreak setting. Similarly, laboratory confirmation of suspected cases of CRS is also necessary, because the constellation of findings of CRS may not be specific.

Laboratory diagnosis

Rubella serologic testing for evidence ot immunity. Until recently, HI antibody testing was the most frequently used method of screening for the presence of rubella antibodies. However, the HI test has been supplanted in many settings by a number of equally or more sensitive commercial assays to determine rubella immunity. EIAs are the most commonly used of these newer commercial assays, but latex agglutination, immunofluorescence assay (IFA), passive hemagglutination, hemolysis-in-gel, and virus neutralization tests are also available.

When adults who have not produced detectable HI antibodies following vaccination have been examined more closely, almost all have had detectable antibody by a specific but more sensitive test. Similarly, a small number of children who initially seroconverted have subsequently lost detectable HI antibody during up to 16 years of follow-up. However, almost all had detectable antibody by more sensitive tests. Immunity in a number of these children was confirmed by documenting a booster response (i.e., absence of immunoglobulin M [IgM] antibody and a rapid rise in immunoglobulin G [IgG] antibody) following revaccination.

Although some individuals have antibody levels following previous vaccination or infection that are below levels detectable by HI antibody testing, the clinical significance of such low-level antibody has not been as well documented as that of higher levels of antibody. Limited data suggest that, on rare occasions, infection with viremia can occur in persons with low antibody levels. CRS following reinfection has been documented, although such instances have been rare. Further study is warranted to assess the appropriate interpretation of antibodies detectable only by these more sensitive tests. Nevertheless, available data continue to support the presumption that any antibody level that is measured by a licensed assay and is above the standard positive cutoff value for that assay can be considered evidence of immunity.

Rubella. The diagnosis of acute rubella should be confirmed serologically. The presence of IgM antibody or a significant rise in IgG or total antibody levels is evidence of acute rubella infection. For HI assays, a fourfold rise in the titer of antibody indicates recent infection; for other types of assays, the criteria for a significant rise in antibody level vary by type of assay and by laboratory. The acute-phase serum specimen should be drawn as soon after rash onset as possible, preferably within the first 7 days. The convalescent-phase serum specimen should be drawn 10 or more days after the acute-phase serum specimen. If the acute-phase serum specimen is drawn more than 7 days after rash onset, a significant rise in antibody titer may not be detected by most commonly used tests. In this case, complement fixation (CF) testing may be especially useful, because CF antibodies appear in serum later than HI, EIA, or IFA antibodies. The acute- and convalescent-phase serum specimens should be tested simultaneously in the same laboratory.

Occasionally, significant rises may not be detected, even if the first specimen is drawn within the first 7 days after rash onset. Rubella infection may also be serologically confirmed by demonstrating rubella-specific IgM antibody. If IgM is to be determined, one serum specimen should be drawn between 1 week and 2 weeks after rash onset. Although rubella-specific IgM antibody may be detected shortly after rash onset, IgM antibody is less likely to be detected if the specimen is drawn earlier than 1 week or later than 4-5 weeks following rash onset. False-negative IgM antibody test results may sometimes occur even when the specimen is appropriately drawn. False-positive IgM test results may also occur.

In the absence of rash illness, the diagnosis of subclinical cases of rubella can be facilitated by obtaining the acute-phase serum specimen as soon as possible after **exposure.** The convalescent-phase specimen should then be drawn 28 or more days after exposure. If acute- and convalescent-phase paired sera provide inconclusive results, rubella-specific IgM antibody testing can be performed, but results should be interpreted cautiously. Expert consultation may be necessary to interpret the data.

Confirmation of rubella infection in pregnant women of unknown immune status following rash illness or exposure may be difficult. A serum specimen should be obtained as soon as possible. Unfortunately, serologic results are often nonconfirmatory. Such situations can be minimized by performing prenatal serologies routinely. In addition, health providers should request that laboratories performing prenatal screening retain such specimens until delivery so that retesting, if necessary, can be done.

Congenital rubella. Suspected cases of CRS should be managed with contact isolation (see CDC "Guidelines for Isolation Precautions in Hospitals"). While diagnostic confirmation is pending, children with suspected CRS should be cared for only by personnel known to be immune. Confirmation by attempting virus isolation can be done by using nasopharyngeal and urine specimens. Serologic confirmation can be cbtained by testing cord blood for the presence of rubella-specific IgM antibodies. An alternative but less rapid serologic method is to document persistence of rubella-specific antibody in an infant with suspected CRS, age 3 months or older, at a level beyond that expected from passive transfer of maternal antibody, i.e., a rubella antibody level in the infant that does not decline at the expected rate (the equivalent of one twofold dilution in HI titer per month). However, some infected infants may lose antibody because of agammaglobulinemia or dysgammaglobulinemia.

In some infants with CRS, virus can persist and be isolated for the first year of life. CRS precautions need to be exercised through the first year of life, unless nasopharyngeal and urine cultures are negative for rubella virus.

INTERNATIONAL TRAVEL

Persons without evidence of rubella immunity who travel abroad should be vaccinated against rubella because rubella is endemic and even epidemic in many countries throughout the world. No immunization or record of immunization is required for entry into the United States. However, international travelers should have immunity to rubella (i.e., laboratory evidence of rubella antibodies or verified rubella vaccination on or after the first birthday). Protection is especially important for susceptible women of childbearing age, particularly those planning to remain out of the country for a prolonged period.

ACIP recommendations for use of measles-mumps-rubella vaccine (MMR) can be found on p. 235.

REFERENCES

Anderson SG. Experimental rubella in human volunteers. J Immunol 1949;62:29.

Best JM, Banatvala JE, Bowen JM. New Japanese rubella vaccine: comparative trials. Br Med J 1974;3:221.

Boué A, Nicolas A, Montagnon B. Reinfection with rubella in pregnant women. Lancet 1971;1:1251.

Brody JA, et al. Rubella epidemic on St. Paul Island in the Pribilofs, 1963. JAMA 1965;191:619.

Burke JP, Hinman AR, Krugman S (eds). International symposium on prevention of congenital rubella infection. Rev Infect Dis 1985;7(Suppl 1):1.

Buser F, Nocolas A. Vaccination with RA 27/3 rubella vaccine. Am J Dis Child 1971;122:53.

Cooper LZ, Florman AL, Ziring PR, Krugman S. Loss of rubella hemagglutination inhibition antibody in congenital rubella. Am J Dis Child 1971;122:397.

Cooper LZ, Krugman S. Clinical manifestations of postnatal and congenital rubella. Arch Ophthalmol 1967;77:434.

Cooper LZ, et al. Neonatal thrombocytopenic purpura and other manifestations of rubella contracted in utero. Am J Dis Child 1965;110:416.

Cooper LZ, et al. Transient arthritis after rubella vaccination. Am J Dis Child 1969;118:218.

Davis WJ, et al. A study of rubella immunity and resistance to reinfection. JAMA 1971;215:600.

Desmond MM, et al. Congenital rubella encephalitis. J Pediatr 1967;71:311.

Dorsett PH, Miller DC, Green KY, et al. Structure and function of rubella virus proteins. Rev Infect Dis 1985;7:S150.

Edell TA, et al. Rubella in hospital personnel and patients, Colorado. MMWR 1979;28:325.

Enders JF. Rubella vaccination. N Engl J Med 1970;283:161.

Fleet WF Jr, et al. Exposure of susceptible teachers to rubella vaccines. Am J Dis Child 1972;123:28.

Fleet WF Jr, et al. Fetal consequences of maternal rubella immunization. JAMA 1974;227:621.

Forchheimer F. Enanthem of German measles. Philadelphia Med 1898;2:15.

Fry J, Dillane JB, Fry L. Rubella, 1962. Br Med J 1962;2:833.

Grayston JT, Watten RH. Epidemic rubella in Taiwan, 1957-1958. III. Gamma globulin in the prevention of rubella. N Engl J Med 1959;261:1145.

Green RH, et al. Studies on the natural history and prevention of rubella. Am J Dis Child 1965;110:348.

Gregg NM. Congenital cataract following German measles in the mother. Trans Ophthalmol Soc Aust 1941;3:35.

Gregg NM, et al. Occurrence of congenital defects in children following maternal rubella during pregnancy. Med J Aust 1945;2:122.

Guyer B, et al. The Memphis State University rubella outbreak. JAMA 1974;227:1298.

Habel K, et al. Transmission of rubella to *Macacus mulatta* monkeys. Public Health Rep 1942;57:1126.

Halstead S, Diwan AR. Failure to transmit rubella virus vaccine—a close contact study in adults. JAMA 1971;215:634.

Hermann KL, et al. Rubella immunization: persistence of antibody four years after a large-scale field trial. JAMA 1976;235:2201.

Hess AF. German measles (rubella): an experimental study. Arch Intern Med 1914;13:913.

Hill AB, Doll R, Galloway T McL, Hughes JPW. Virus diseases in pregnancy and congenital defects. Br J Prev Soc Med 1958;12:1.

Hiro Y, Tasaka S. Die Röteln sind eine Virus-krankheit. Monatsschr Kinderheilkd 1938;76:328.

Horstmann DM, et al. Rubella: reinfection of vaccinated and naturally immune persons exposed in an epidemic. N Engl J Med 1970;283:771.

Houser HG, Schalet N. Prevention of rubella with gamma globulin. Clin Res 1958;6:281.

Ingalls TH. Progress in pediatrics: German measles and German measles in pregnancy. Am J Dis Child 1957;93:555.

Jackson ADM, Fisch L. Deafness following maternal rubella, results of a prospective investigation. Lancet 1958;2:1241.

Johnson RE, Hall AP. Rubella arthritis; report of cases studied by latex tests. N Engl J Med 1958;258:743.

Judelsohn RG, Wyll SA. Rubella in Bermuda: termination of an epidemic by mass vaccination. JAMA 1973;223:401.

Kantor TG, Tanner M. Rubella arthritis and rheumatoid arthritis. Arthritis Rheum 1962;5:378.

Kenny FM, Michaels RH, Davis KS. Rubella encephalopathy: later psychometric, neurologic and encephalographic evaluation of seven survivors. Am J Dis Child 1965;110:374.

Kilroy AW, et al. Two syndromes following rubella immunization: clinical observations and epidemiological studies. JAMA 1970;214:2287.

Klock LE, et al. A clinical and serological study of women exposed to rubella vaccinees. Am J Dis Child 1972;123:465.

Korns RF. Prophylaxis of German measles with human serum globulin. J Infect Dis 1952;90:183.

Korones SB, et al. Congenital rubella syndrome: study of 22 infants. Am J Dis Child 1965;110:434.

Krugman S. (ed). Proceedings of the International Conference on Rubella Immunization. Am J Dis Child 1969;118:1.

Krugman S. Present status of measles and rubella immunization in the United States: a medical progress report. J Pediatr 1971;78:1; J Pediatr 1977;90:1.

Krugman S, Ward R. The rubella problem. J Pediatr 1954;44:489.

Krugman S, Ward R, Jacobs KG, Lazar M. Studies on rubella immunization. I. Demonstration of rubella without rash. JAMA 1953;151:285.

Landrigan PJ, Stoffels MA, Anderson E, Witte JJ. Epidemic rubella in adolescent boys. JAMA 1974;227:1283.

Levin MJ, et al. Diagnosis of congenital rubella in utero. N Engl J Med 1974;290:1187.

Lock FR, Gatling HB, Mauzy CH, Wells HB. Incidence of anomalous development following maternal rubella. Am J Obstet Gynecol 1961;81:451.

Lündström R. Rubella during pregnancy. A follow-up study of children born after an epidemic of rubella in Sweden, 1951, with additional investigations on prophylaxis and treatment of maternal rubella. Acta Paediatr 1962;51 (Suppl 133):1-110.

MacFarlane DW, Boyd RD, Dodrill CB, Tufts E. Intrauterine rubella, head size, and intellect. Pediatrics 1975;55:797.

McLaughlin MD, Gold LH. The New York rubella incident: a case for changing hospital policy regarding rubella testing and immunization. Am J Public Health 1979;69:287.

Menser MA, Forrest JM, Bransby RD. Rubella infection and diabetes. Lancet 1978;1:57.

Meyer HM, Parkman PD. Rubella vaccination—a review of practical experience. JAMA 1971;215:613.

Meyer HM Jr, Parkman PD, Panos TC. Attenuated rubella virus. II. Production of an experimental live-virus vaccine and clinical trial. N Engl J Med 1966;275:575.

Michaels RH, Mellin GW. Prospective experience with maternal rubella and the associated congenital malformations. Pediatrics 1960;26:200.

Modlin JF. Surveillance of the congenital rubella syndrome, 1969-73. J Infect Dis 1974;130:316.

Modlin JF, et al. A review of five years experience with rubella vaccine in the United States. Pediatrics 1975; 55:20.

Naeye RL, Blanc W. Pathogenesis of congenital rubella. JAMA 1965;194:1277.

Neff JM, Carver DH. Rubella immunization: reconsideration of our present policy. Am J Epidemiol 1970;92:162.

Parkman PD, Buescher EL. Artenstein MS. Recovery of rubella virus from army recruits. Proc Soc Exp Biol Med 1962;111:225.

Parkman PD, Meyer HM Jr, Kirschstein RL, Hopps HE. Attenuated rubella virus. I. Development and laboratory characterization. N Engl J Med 1966;275:569.

Pitt DB. Congenital malformations and maternal rubella. Med J Aust 1957;1:233.

Plotkin SA, Boué A, Boué JG. The in vitro growth of rubella virus in human embryonic cells. Am J Epidemiol 1965;81:71.

Schiff GM, Donath R, Rotte T. Experimental rubella studies. I. Clinical and laboratory features of infection caused by the Brown strain rubella virus. II. Artificial challenge studies of adult rubella vaccinees. Am J Dis Child 1969;118:269.

Schiff GM, et al. Rubella vaccines in a public school system. Am J Dis Child 1974;128:180.

Shaffner W, et al. Polyneuropathy following rubella immunization. Am J Dis Child 1974;127:684.

Scott HD, Byrne EB. Exposure of susceptible pregnant women to rubella vaccinees; serologic findings during the

Rhode Island immunization campaign. JAMA 1971; 215:609.

Sennett RA, Copeman WSC. Notes on rubella, with special reference to certain rheumatic sequelae. Br Med J 1940;1:924.

Seppala M, Vaheri A. Natural rubella infection of the female genital tract. Lancet 1974;1:46.

Siegel M. Unresolved issues in the first five years of the rubella immunization program. Am J Obstet Gynecol 1976;124:327.

Sever JL. Epidemiology of rubella. Washington DC: Pan American Health Organization, World Health Organization, May 1967, Scientific Publication No 147, p 366.

Stewart GL, et al. Rubella virus hemagglutination-inhibition test. N Engl J Med 1967;276:554.

Tingle AJ, Allen M, Petty RE. Rubella-associated arthritis. I. Comparative study of joint manifestations associated with natural rubella and RA 27/3 rubella immunization. Ann Rheum Dis 1986;45:110-114.

Townsend JJ, et al. Progressive rubella panencephalitis: late onset after congenital rubella. N Engl J Med 1975; 292:990.

Vesikari T, Buimovici-Klein E. Lymphocyte responses to rubella antigen and phytohemagglutinin after administration of the RA 27/3 strain of live attenuated rubella vaccine. Infect Immunol 1975;11:748.

Warkany J, Kalter H. Congenital malformations. N Engl J Med 1961;265:1046.

Weil ML, et al. Chronic progressive panencephalitis due to rubella virus stimulating SSPE. N Engl J Med 1975;292:994.

Weller TH, Neva FA. Propagation in tissue culture of cytopathic agents from patients with rubella-like illness. Proc Soc Exp Biol Med 1962;111:215.

Wesselhoeft C. Rubella (German measles). N Engl J Med 1947;236:943, 978.

Wilkins J, Leedon JM, Portnoy B, Salvatore MA. Reinfection with rubella virus despite live vaccine-induced immunity. Am J Dis Child 1969;118:275.

Ziring PR, Florman AF, Cooper LZ. The diagnosis of rubella. Pediatr Clin North Am 1971;18:87.

24

SEPSIS IN THE NEWBORN

SAMUEL P. GOTOFF

The incidence of sepsis in the neonate is greater than at any other period of life and varies from hospital to hospital, depending on rates of prematurity, prenatal care, conduct of labor, and environmental conditions in nurseries. Attack rates of neonatal sepsis increase significantly in low-birth-weight infants and in the presence of obstetrical risk factors such as prolonged rupture of membranes, maternal intrapartum fever, and chorioamnionitis. Reliable statistics are not available because sepsis of the newborn is poorly defined and is not a reportable disease. Estimates of incidence range from one to four per 1,000 live births.

The terms *sepsis* and *septicemia* are synonymous and are not used consistently in the literature. In older children and adults sepsis is a syndrome, a constellation of signs and symptoms, caused by microorganisms or their toxic products in the circulation. The causative agents are usually bacteria, and bacteremia (bacteria in the blood) is usually demonstrated; but other microorganisms can produce the syndrome, and bacterial infection can be present without a positive blood culture. Bacterial products from gram-negative organisms (endotoxin), gram-positive cocci (teichoic acids), and staphylococci (toxic shock syndrome toxin) can produce septic shock. The inciting bacterial infection may be localized (e.g., pneumonia, peritonitis, pyelonephritis) or without a focus. Some authors use *sepsis* in the newborn to describe any symptomatic infant with bacteremia.

Bone et al. (1989) have described the septic syndrome in adults, and these criteria have been used to study septic shock in infants and children (Jacobs et al., 1990). The criteria for septic syndrome include the presence of infection, with fever or hypothermia, tachycardia, tachypnea, and evidence of impaired organ system perfusion manifested by hypoxemia, acidosis, oliguria, or altered mental status. It may be necessary to modify these criteria for the newborn, but the differentiation of sepsis and infection may become important because new modalities of therapy directed at the mediators of sepsis in addition to the microorganisms are already in clinical trials (Ziegler et al., 1991).

The Centers for Disease Control (CDC) has published criteria for primary bloodstream nosocomial infection in neonates (Garner et al., 1988). Primary bloodstream infection includes laboratory-confirmed bloodstream infection and clinical sepsis. *Laboratory-confirmed bloodstream infection* must meet one of the criteria in the box, "Laboratory-Confirmed Bloodstream Infection" (p. 404). *Clinical sepsis* must meet either of the criteria in the box on p. 404. These criteria have been used by hospitals participating in the CDC National Nosocomial Infections Surveillance System since January 1988. The problem with these criteria is that fever may not be caused by infection or may be caused by infection without sepsis, and there are other explanations of these signs. These criteria should be considered in the context of each individual patient.

Table 24-1. Patterns of neonatal sepsis

Characteristics	Early onset	Late onset — Community	Late onset — Nosocomial
Onset	Birth to 1 week (usually 72 hr)	1 wk to 1 mo	1 wk to discharge
Gestation	50% premature	Usually full-term	Usually premature
Risk factors	Amnionitis, premature rupture of membranes	None	Endotracheal tube, vascular catheter, surgery
Transmission	Vertical	Horizontal, vertical	Horizontal
Common pathogens	Group B streptococci (all), *Escherichia coli*, *Klebsiella*, *Listeria monocytogenes*, enterococci, *Streptococcus pneumoniae*, nontypeable *Haemophilus influenzae*	Group B streptococcus type III, *E. coli* K1, *L. monocytogenes*, herpes simplex virus (HSV), enterovirus	Coagulase-negative staphylococci, *Staphylococcus aureus*, *Candida albicans*, *Pseudomonas aeruginosa*, *Klebsiella*, *Serratia*, *E. coli*
Clinical clues	Rash (*Listeria*)	Vesicular rash (HSV), bacterial meningitis	Thrush, candida dermatitis, ecthyma gangrenosum, pustules, abscesses

ETIOLOGY

The syndrome of neonatal sepsis is caused by bacteria, viruses, fungi, or protozoa.

Bacteria

The predominant bacterial causes of sepsis have changed over time (Gladstone et al., 1990) and may vary from hospital to hospital. Less mature infants are susceptible to systemic infection with less virulent organisms. The most common organisms associated with neonatal infections are shown in Table 24-1, according to the timing of infection and geographical location. The causative agents of early-onset infections are found in the maternal genital and gastrointestinal tracts. Late-onset infections in the nursery are nosocomial: acquired from other infants, personnel, or fomites and contaminated equipment. Late-onset infections occurring after hospital discharge may be acquired from the mother or other members of the household and from nosocomial sources.

All serotypes of group B streptococci (GBS) and *Escherichia coli* K1 account for approximately 75% of early-onset sepsis. The less vir-

ulent organisms such as coagulase-negative staphylococci, α-hemolytic streptococci, and *Haemophilus* species (not type b) have been repeatedly incriminated as neonatal pathogens and may produce sepsis. Gram-negative enteric organisms such as *Klebsiella* and *Enterobacter*, *Pseudomonas* species, *Serratia*, and *Staphylococcus aureus* can also produce sepsis. The widespread use of antibiotics in the neonatal intensive care unit (NICU) has led to the selection of resistant organisms such as aminoglycoside-resistant gram-negative enteric bacilli and methicillin-resistant staphylococci. Coagulase-negative staphylococci are the major cause of nosocomial infections in children and account for 31% of all nosocomial infections in NICU patients (Jarvis et al., 1985). Although coagulase-negative staphylococci are common skin organisms and contamination of blood cultures can result during venipuncture if aseptic technique is not followed, organ system infections caused by commensal species are well documented. Endocarditis (Noel et al., 1988), meningitis (Gruskay et al., 1989), pneumonia (Hall et al., 1987), enterocolitis (Gruskay et al., 1986), and cathe-

LABORATORY-CONFIRMED BLOODSTREAM INFECTION

- Recognized pathogen isolated from blood culture AND pathogen is not related to infection at another site (e.g., pneumonia)
- One of the following: fever (>38° C [100.4° F]), chills, or hypotension AND any of the following:

  Common skin contaminant isolated from two blood cultures drawn on separate occasions AND organism is not related to infection at another site

  Common skin contaminant isolated from blood culture from patient with intravascular access device AND physician institutes appropriate antimicrobial therapy

  Positive antigen test on blood AND organism is not related to infection at another site
- Patient ≤12 months of age has one of the following: fever (>38° C), hypothermia (<37° C [98.6° F]), apnea, or bradycardia AND any of the following:

  Common skin contaminant isolated from two blood cultures drawn on separate occasions AND organism is not related to infection at another site

  Common skin contaminant isolated from blood culture from patient with intravascular access device AND physician institutes appropriate antimicrobial therapy

  Positive antigen test on blood AND pathogen is not related to infection at another site

CLINICAL SEPSIS

- One of the following clinical signs or symptoms with no other recognized cause: fever (>38° C), hypotension, or oliguria (<20 ml/hr) AND all of the following:

  Blood culture not done or no organism or antigen detected in blood

  No apparent infection at another site

  Institution of appropriate antimicrobial therapy for sepsis by physician
- Patient ≤12 months of age with one of the following clinical signs or symptoms and no other recognized cause: fever, hypothermia, apnea, or bradycardia AND all of the following:

  Blood culture not done or no organism or antigen detected in blood

  No apparent infection at another site

  Institution of appropriate antimicrobial therapy for sepsis by physician

ter-associated bacteremia (Valvano et al., 1988) may lead to the sepsis syndrome.

Less commonly, coagulase-negative staphylococci cause early-onset sepsis. Vaginal colonization with coagulase-negative staphylococci was reported in approximately 50% of 465 women cultured (Hall et al., 1990). Vertical transmission of coagulase-negative staphylococci to newborn infants occurred in 29%. In autopsies of premature fetuses from mothers with chorioamnionitis, coagulase-negative staphylococci were recovered from placenta, lung, and liver in 18%, suggesting that coagulase-negative staphylococci may cause early-onset disease (Madan et al., 1988). Further discussion of staphylococcal infections can be found in Chapter 27.

Fungi

Candida species, particularly *C. albicans*, are important causes of late-onset sepsis in the NICU. Broad-spectrum antibiotics, indwelling vascular catheters, very-low-birth-weight (<1500 g), and parenteral nutrition are the principal predisposing risk factors. The incidence is 2% to 5% in very-low-birth-weight infants. The presence of mucous membrane (thrush) or cutaneous manifestations, present in 50% of cases, suggests a related systemic infection. Otherwise, the clinical signs are similar to those of bacterial sepsis. Clinical signs of meningeal involvement are less common than cerebrospinal fluid abnormalities. CSF cultures are positive in approximately one third of infants with systemic disease. Urine cultures are often positive; and urinary tract infection may lead to renal insufficiency or filling defects apparent on ultrasonography. Endocarditis may result from an indwelling intracardiac catheter. Echocardiography may demonstrate valvular lesions, thrombosis, or intracardiac fungal mass. Endophthalmitis, hepatic or splenic abscesses, arthritis, and osteomyelitis have been associated with *Candida* sepsis.

It is important to distinguish between catheter-associated transient candidemia and disseminated candidiasis. The former is characterized by positive blood cultures, resulting from contamination of in situ intravascular catheters, but there is no evidence of focal or disseminated disease, and it is treated by removing the catheter. Disseminated candidiasis is characterized by involvement of one or more organ systems, positive cultures of *Candida* from a normally sterile fluid or tissue, or a positive blood culture in the absence of an intravascular catheter. Candidal sepsis is frequently indolent. Untreated patients may be fungemic for 2 to 3 days; occasionally, they appear to improve spontaneously only subsequently to develop shock, meningitis, and osteoarticular infection, leading to death. Blood cultures positive for *Candida* should be repeated and should be considered representative of infection rather than of a contaminant.

Other organisms that may be responsible for neonatal infections, in some cases causing an illness resembling acute bacterial sepsis, are discussed in sections of Chapter 3 (cytomegalovirus), 5 (enteroviruses), 10 (herpes simplex virus), 25 *(Treponema pallidum)*, 28 (streptococci), 30 *(Borrelia burgdorferi)*, and 31 *(Toxoplasma)*.

PATHOLOGY

In most cases and with large numbers of microorganisms in the bloodstream, the infection becomes generalized rapidly, often leaving little evidence of an initial focus. Inflammatory processes can develop in any organ or part of the body, resulting in meningitis, pneumonia, empyema, pericarditis, myocarditis, endocarditis, peritonitis, hepatitis, pyelonephritis, otitis media, osteomyelitis, pyarthrosis, and miliary abscesses in the soft tissues.

Group B streptococcal early-onset disease readily demonstrates the characteristic features of such overwhelming bacterial infection. Large numbers of organisms can be found in virtually every tissue from the central nervous system (CNS) to the lungs, liver, and spleen. The inflammatory response is often minimal, even at the time of death, which frequently occurs in 2 to 3 days. In this specific setting the pathological features tend to substantiate the in vitro observation of decreased chemotaxis of polymorphonuclear (PMN) leukocytes and the clinical finding of neutrophil storage pool depletion.

Meningitis is the most important complication of sepsis in the newborn infant. Infants with early-onset sepsis and meningitis may have a minimal inflammatory response in the CSF and meninges at autopsy. Late-onset meningitis is more often accompanied by a significant inflammatory response. In addition to the inflammatory reaction in the meninges, widespread, devastating infectious vasculitis, sometimes hemorrhagic, results in severe cerebral cortical changes in many cases.

PATHOGENESIS
Local factors

Infection in the first week of life (usually in the first 72 hours) is referred to as *early-onset disease*. Neonatal sepsis may have its onset in utero, secondary to maternal hematogenous infection or, more often, chorioamnionitis. Inhalation of infected amniotic fluid can produce pneumonia and sepsis in utero, manifested by fetal distress or neonatal asphyxia; in addition, aspiration of infected amniotic fluid or secretions in the birth canal can produce pneumonia and sepsis. Other portals of entry include the skin, umbilical cord, nasopharynx, gastrointestinal tract, and urinary tract. Based on studies of group B streptococcal infections, two thirds of early-onset infections are associated with maternal risk factors, infection, or premature delivery (Boyer et al., 1983). Early-onset disease is transmitted vertically. Approximately 50% of infants whose mothers are colonized with group B streptococci will become colonized; however, only one in 50 to 75 colonized infants will develop invasive disease. The risk of colonization and disease in the infant is related to the size of the inoculum (Dillon et al., 1987). However, women who are not heavily colonized (i.e., require special broth media to detect bacteria) may have infants who have early-onset group B streptococcal disease (Morales and Lim, 1987).

Late-onset infections occur in premature or sick infants in the NICU or in the healthy, full-term infant after discharge from the nursery. In the former setting the risk of infection and sepsis is affected by the degree of prematurity, coexisting disease, and use of antibiotics and invasive life-supportive measures such as endotracheal tubes and indwelling vascular catheters. In healthy newborn infants the virulence of the microorganism becomes more important. Encapsulated bacteria with unique antigenic specificity such as *E. coli* K1, type III group B streptococci, pneumococci, and *Haemophilus influenzae* are usually implicated. The capsule enables these strains to inhibit alternative complement pathway activation and resist phagocytosis in the absence of specific antibody.

Host factors

Immunoglobulins. The impaired humoral defenses of the newborn play a significant role in the pathogenesis of neonatal sepsis. Transplacental transmission of IgG antibodies confers a spectrum of passively acquired antibody dependent on the distribution of maternal IgG antibodies. The neonate receives no immunoglobulins of the IgA or IgM classes. Because the normal newborn has not been challenged with antigens in utero, these antibodies are not yet synthesized, although the fetus is capable of synthesizing IgM and IgA early in intrauterine life. Thus the presence of IgM and IgA antibodies in cord blood may be diagnostic of a number of intrauterine infections (e.g., syphilis, toxoplasmosis, rubella). Specific bactericidal and opsonic antibodies against gram-negative bacteria are predominantly in the IgM class; thus the newborn infant lacks optimal humoral protection from infection with enteric organisms.

Most adult women have low or undetectable levels of IgG antibodies to the type-specific capsular polysaccharide of group B streptococci. These antibodies are protective in experimental models of infection, promote opsonophagocytosis in vitro, and are uniformly lacking in the sera of infected newborn infants. Thus type-specific antibody deficiency contributes to the susceptibility to group B streptococcal infection.

Cord-serum IgG levels in full-term infants are comparable to or slightly greater than maternal levels. In premature infants cord IgG levels are directly proportional to gestational age. One group of infants between 25 and 28 weeks' gestation had a mean plasma IgG concentration of 251 mg/dl in the first week of life (Ballow et al., 1986). Infants with birth weights below 1500 g become profoundly hypogammaglobulinemic during the first few months of life. Studies of type-specific IgG antibodies to group B streptococci have shown that the ratio of cord to maternal serum concentrations is 1.0, 0.5, and 0.3 at term, 32 weeks, and 28 weeks gestation, respectively (Gotoff et al., 1986). Thus those women with sufficiently high levels of IgG antibody (e.g., as a result of immunization) could provide transplacental immunity to a premature infant.

The IgG and IgM antibody response to infectious agents is variable in the newborn and is generally diminished in comparison with the adult. This relative deficiency may affect recovery and protection from subsequent infection.

Complement. The complement system plays an integral role in host defense against infection. Complement's protective functions are particularly directed against extracellular pathogens, including gram-positive pyogenic bacteria and gram-negative enteric organisms. The organisms that can resist phagocytosis in the absence of antibody tend to be capable of acting as invasive pathogens. GBS and *E. coli* K1, significant pathogens in this age group, contain sialic acid in their capsules, which inhibits the binding of the complement fragment C3b by the alternative pathway. Antibody is required for effective opsonization. Complement and/or antibody opsonizes bacteria, which allows phagocytosis to occur.

Complement activation is classically initiated by antigen-antibody interactions. The components "fix" or join the cascade in the sequence 1, 4, 2, 3, 5, 6, 7, 8, 9. The second, or alternative, pathway apparently is triggered by formation of C3b, the major fragment of C3. Generation of C3b continuously occurs at a low level unless a microorganism or other target particle enters the picture and fixes C3b. Then amplification of fixation occurs with C3b plus B (Bb) acting as an enzyme. Activation of either the classic pathway or the alternative pathway fixes C3b to the bacterium and results in its opsonization. Activation of the complement cascade by either pathway also promotes vasodilation by release of C3a and C5a, releases the major chemotactic factor, which is a split product of C5, and fixes late-acting components to the organism, which then induces lysis.

There is essentially no transfer of complement from the maternal circulation. The fetus synthesizes complement components as early as the first trimester. Full-term newborn infants have slightly diminished classic pathway complement activity and moderately diminished alternative pathway activity. There is considerable variability in both concentration of complement components and activity. The alternative pathway components (B and P) are usually 35% to 60% of normal. Premature infants have lower levels of complement components and less activity than full-term newborns. These deficiencies contribute to diminished complement-derived chemotactic activity and to diminished ability to opsonize certain organisms in the absence of antibody. Many studies have been performed with different strains of microorganisms and different conditions, examining both classic and alternative pathways. In general, opsonization of S. aureus is normal in neonatal sera, but varying degrees of impairment have been noted with group B streptococci and E. coli.

Fibronectin. Fibronectin is a glycoprotein found in plasma and tissues that contributes to adhesion of neutrophils and monocytes and binds to certain bacteria such as group B streptococci with or without antibody and complement. Plasma fibronectin levels are decreased in neonates and further diminished in premature newborns and newborns with sepsis, birth asphyxia, and respiratory distress syndrome.

Monocyte-macrophage system. The monocyte-macrophage system consists of circulating monocytes and tissue macrophages of the reticuloendothelial system (RES). The number of circulating monocytes in neonatal blood is normal, but the mass or function of the macrophages in the RES apparently is diminished in the newborn and particularly in the premature infant as estimated by the relative increase in the number of damaged erythrocytes (pocked cells) in the circulation. In both term and premature infants chemotaxis of monocytes is impaired, affecting the inflammatory response in tissues and delayed hypersensitivity skin tests. Monocytes from neonates ingest and kill microorganisms as well as monocytes from adults. Comparable amounts of interferon and tumor necrosis factor (TNF) are synthesized by neonatal and adult monocytes.

Neutrophils. The number of circulating neutrophils is elevated in the premature and term infant after birth, with a peak at 12 hours returning to adult levels by 72 hours. Band neutrophils are below 15% in the normal newborn. Increased numbers of immature neutrophils may be seen in newborns with sepsis, as may asphyxia and other stress responses. Neutropenia occurs in some patients with sepsis. It may

reflect increased margination of circulating cells or depletion of the neutrophil storage pool. A bone marrow examination that reveals neutrophil storage pool depletion is often associated with a fatal outcome (Christensen et al., 1982).

Chemotaxis. In most studies chemotaxis of neonatal neutrophils is significantly less than in adults. In contrast, phagocytosis and killing by PMN leukocytes from healthy newborn infants have usually been comparable to those from adults. However, microbicidal activity is impaired in sick infants with sepsis, respiratory distress, hyperbilirubinemia, and hypoglycemia (Shigeoka et al., 1979). In experiments using high ratios of bacteria to PMN leukocytes (Mills et al., 1979) or a limited source of opsonins (Marodi et al., 1985), phagocytosis and killing may be impaired.

CLINICAL MANIFESTATIONS

The clinical signs of infection in the newborn infant vary from mild to severe. Signs suggestive of sepsis are listed in the box on p. 408. Variables include the duration of infection, virulence of the causative agent, and degree of maturity of host defense mechanisms. Asymptomatic bacteremia has been demonstrated in infants born to women with risk factors (Roberts, 1976; Ramsey and Zwerdling, 1977). Overwhelming infection may be apparent at birth as a result of an intrauterine infection. In some cases there are localized findings such as pneumonia, meningitis, or cutaneous involvement. In other infants the initial presentation may be apnea, bradycardia, hypotension, or hypothermia. In infants whose signs of infection develop after birth, the earliest manifestations of infection are often subtle and nonspecific. Inability to tolerate feedings, irritability, or lethargy may be the initial sign of infection. Signs consistent with infection may also be explained by noninfectious diseases of other organs. Interpretation of abnormal signs is frequently difficult because of coexisting noninfectious disease in the infant such as hyaline membrane disease.

Thermal instability

Fever in newborn infants does not always signify infection but may be due to elevated environmental temperature, dehydration, or hematoma. In contrast to older children and adults, about half of infected new-born infants

MANIFESTATIONS OF NEONATAL SEPSIS

General

Fever or hypothermia (>38° C [100.4° F]), <37° C [98.6° F])

Bleeding from disseminated intravascular coagulation

Oliguria

Respiratory

Apnea

Tachypnea with retractions

Flaring, grunting

Cyanosis

Circulatory

Bradycardia

Tachycardia

Pallor, mottling; cold, clammy skin

Hypotension

Poor capillary filling

Central nervous system

Irritability, lethargy, coma

Irregular respirations

Hypotonia, hyporeflexia

Laboratory

Neutrophil storage pool depletion

Thrombocytopenia

Metabolic acidosis

Hypoxia

Elevated blood urea nitrogen (BUN) and creatinine levels

Prolonged prothrombin time (PT) and partial thromboplastin time (PTT)

Hypofibrinogenemia, hypoalbuminemia

Hyperbilirubinemia

Elevated liver enzymes

---

will have elevated temperatures (>100° F, axillary). A single temperature elevation is rarely associated with infection, but a sustained elevation (i.e., more than 1 hour) is highly predictive. Infected febrile infants will usually have other signs of infection.

A study of full-term infants in Cook County, Illinois, Children's Hospital showed that 100 babies, or 1% of all babies born during an 18-month period, had a temperature of 37° to 38° C (98.6° to 100.4° F) during the first 4 days of life (Voora et al., 1982). Forty-eight of these babies had other symptoms compatible with sep-

sis. Ten percent had culture-proved bacterial disease. Eight of the 10 had other signs, and two had no other signs. Only one infant of 9,900 afebrile term infants had culture-proved bacterial disease. Thus an elevated temperature probably is a manifestation of infection in term infants, and sepsis is increasingly probable if other signs or symptoms are also present. This study excluded preterm infants and term infants requiring immediate intensive care for reasons other than fever. The former group of infants may exhibit fever, temperature instability, or subnormal temperature in response to infection. In premature infants with sepsis, subnormal temperatures and irregular fluctuations are observed as often as fever.

Gastrointestinal signs

Lack of interest in feeding, poor sucking, and failure to tolerate feedings by gastrointestinal intubation are common early signs that may be due to infection. Vomiting and diarrhea may be observed. Abdominal distention, also a frequent finding, is probably secondary to paralytic ileus related to generalized infection. Jaundice is common in sepsis of the newborn infant and may be the initial sign in some patients. Usually, hyperbilirubinemia is indirect; and in the first few days of life it may be difficult to distinguish from "physiological" jaundice or hemolytic disease. Stage III necrotizing enterocolitis includes peritonitis, usually resulting in sepsis.

Respiratory signs

Cyanosis, irregular breathing, tachypnea, retractions, and apnea occur frequently in premature infants and infants born after difficult delivery but may be signs of sepsis. It is frequently impossible to distinguish respiratory distress syndrome from pneumonia, especially from that caused that group B streptococci in premature infants. Increased respiratory effort may reflect the response to metabolic acidosis, congestive heart failure, or shock.

Cardiovascular signs

Cardiac manifestations may be due to myocarditis, endocarditis, pericarditis, or sepsis. Tachycardia, bradycardia, arrhythmias, hypotension, and poor peripheral perfusion are among the more common signs of sepsis. Congenital heart disease, particularly hypoplastic left-heart syndrome, and acquired isolated heart disease (e.g., myocarditis) should be considered in the differential diagnosis.

Central nervous system signs

Meningitis and cerebral vasculitis often result from high-level bacteremia and are found in approximately a third of newborn infants with sepsis (Nyhan and Fousek, 1958). In one study of *E. coli* bacteremia, meningitis occurred only in infants with colony counts greater than 1,000/ml of blood (Dietzman et al., 1974).

The conventional signs of meningitis seen in older children such as stiff neck, hyperactive reflexes, and Brudzinski's sign are infrequent in the newborn. Newborn infants will demonstrate lethargy and/or irritability. Some will have a full fontanelle, seizures, or focal neurological findings. Some of these signs may be associated with hypoxia, intracranial hemorrhage, hypoglycemia, hypocalcemia, intrauterine exposure to cocaine or related drugs, and other CNS disorders.

Because of the nonspecific character of the initial features of both meningitis and sepsis of the newborn infant, examination of the CSF is crucial in establishing the diagnosis.

Complications and sequelae of neonatal meningitis include subdural effusion, brain abscess, hydrocephalus, encephalopathy, and cerebral infarcts. Poor outcome is directly correlated with the presence of ventriculitis, persistence of positive CSF cultures, a CSF cell count greater than 10,000/ml, and a CSF protein count greater than 500 mg/dl.

Cutaneous and mucous membrane signs

Skin or mucous membrane manifestations associated with sepsis are present in a minority of patients but provide visible evidence of infection. A recognizable focus of infection may be impetigo, cellulitis or a subcutaneous abscess, mastitis, omphalitis, or conjunctivitis. The presence of small salmon-pink papules may suggest *Listeria monocytogenes* sepsis. A vesicular rash may be a sign of herpes simplex virus infection. There are multiple mucocutaneous lesions of *Candida albicans* that may represent local disease or a component of systemic infection. Thrush is characterized by white curdlike plaques on an erythematous base located on the tongue, gums, or buccal mucosa. The rash may be seen initially as erythematous maculopapular or vesicular scaling lesions that frequently coalesce and often form satellite lesions. Intertriginous areas are usually involved. Occasionally, evidence of embolic bacterial disease may be present. The skin lesion, ecthyma gangrenosum, is indicative of *Pseudomonas* sepsis. Nonspecific cutaneous pathology suggestive of infection includes petechiae and purpura. Bleeding from disseminated intravascular coagulation (DIC) is highly indicative of sepsis.

Miscellaneous manifestations

The bacteremic infant should be investigated for possible localized infection. Group B streptococci commonly cause pneumonia and meningitis and also may produce otitis media or disseminate to skin, bones, joints, or the urinary tract. These organisms less often cause infections in other tissues. *E. coli* and other gram-negative organisms gain access to the blood from the gastrointestinal tract and may disseminate to any of multiple locations, including the CNS, urinary tract, bones and joints, liver, and peritoneal cavity.

DIAGNOSIS

The newborn infant responds similarly to a variety of stresses, regardless of their nature or location. Therefore the possibility of infection or sepsis in the newborn infant must be considered with any clinical deterioration unless the setback is readily explained otherwise and corrected promptly.

The early recognition of infection in the newborn infant hinges on suspecting it in the presence of a variety of subtle or seemingly unlikely nonspecific signs and symptoms. Rapid identification of the septic infant is important for effective therapy. Recognition of a potentially infected mother before delivery of her infant should alert the obstetrician and pediatrician to the possible danger to the infant.

Ideally, the mother should be evaluated and appropriate specimens obtained if she is suspected of having an infection. This should include Gram stain and bacterial cultures of materials such as blood, amniotic fluid, and urine. The presence of prolonged rupture of membranes or malodorous amniotic fluid indicates the infant should be evaluated thoroughly and appropriate cultures obtained. PMN leukocytes and bacteria in a stained smear of gastric aspirate or from the external ear canal may reflect infection of amniotic fluid swallowed before delivery

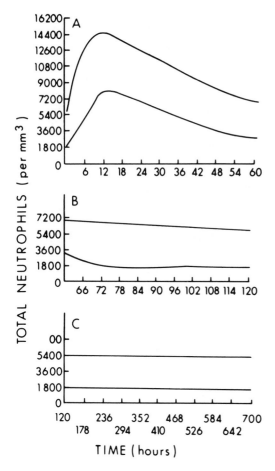

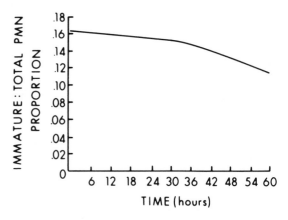

Fig. 24-2. Reference range for the proportion of immature to total neutrophils in the first 60 hours of life. (Modified from Manroe et al. J Pediatr 1978;95:89.)

Fig. 24-1. Total neutrophil count reference range. **A,** First 60 hours of life; **B,** 60 to 120 hours of life; **C,** 120 hours to 28 days. (Modified from Manroe BL et al. J Pediatr 1978;95:89.)

or of contents of the birth canal. This information may be helpful since amnionitis is a risk factor for neonatal infection.

The most reliable indirect indicator of bacterial infection is the peripheral white blood cell (WBC) count. An absolute neutrophil count outside the normal range (Fig. 24-1) with a ratio of immature to total neutrophils higher than the established norm for age (Fig. 24-2) is suggestive of bacterial infection. This test is somewhat insensitive and may be abnormal in noninfectious conditions. Preterm infants are more likely to have neutropenia (<1,500 cells/ml) than term infants. Neutropenia may be transient or reflect neutrophil storage pool depletion (<7% of nucleated bone marrow cells composed of PMN leukocytes plus band forms plus metamyelocytes).

Thrombocytopenia from bone marrow suppression or DIC may be present. Other indirect measurements, including C-reactive protein, erythrocyte sedimentation rate (ESR), haptoglobin, IgM, leukocyte alkaline phosphatase, buffy coat smear, nitroblue tetrazolium dye reduction test, and endotoxin detection by limulus lysate test, are unreliable individual tests. Cytokines such as interleukin-1 (IL-1), IL-6, TNF, and platelet activating factor (PAF) may be elevated in plasma and in CSF of older children and adults with sepsis. Studies of these mediators of inflammation in newborn infants are in progress.

Identification of infecting bacteria or other organisms by Gram stain and culture of normally sterile body fluids is essential. Blood cultures from the infant should be obtained from a peripheral vein after skin cleansing with iodine and alcohol. Infant blood cultures from peripheral veins have a lower incidence of contamination than do cord blood cultures. Quantitative cultures performed on babies with *E. coli* bacteremia have demonstrated that one half of the infants had colony counts of less than 50 organisms/ml. When colony counts were in excess of 1,000/ml, the incidence of associated meningitis increased, and the mortality rate was high (Dietzman, Fischer, and Schoenknecht, 1974). These quantitative studies prompted additional work to define the quantity of blood necessary to detect bacteremia in infants. Using a rabbit model with *E. coli* and simulating the colony counts defined in infants, 2 ml of blood placed in a commercial 50-ml bottle of trypticase soy broth allowed detection of all bacteremias (Fischer et al., 1974). If the colony count exceeded 5 organisms/ml of blood, the bacteremias would be detected in 0.2 ml of blood when cultured in broth bottles. No quantity of blood from an infant is too small to culture for suspected bacteremia. If possible, a second blood culture from another site should be obtained to increase the yield and to provide confirmation if a commensal skin organism is isolated.

Diagnostic evaluations may be indicated for asymptomatic infants because of maternal risk factors. The probability of neonatal infection and subsequent neonatal sepsis correlates with the degree of prematurity and bacterial contamination of amniotic fluid. In an asymptomatic term infant whose mother has chorioamnionitis, two blood cultures and a gastric aspirate should be examined to confirm the maternal diagnosis and identify presumptively the organisms by Gram stain. If the blood culture is positive or if the infant becomes symptomatic, lumbar puncture should be performed. Prolonged rupture of membranes for longer than 18 hours suggests the need for blood cultures in premature infants but not necessarily in asymptomatic term infants without signs of fetal distress.

Antigen detection by methods such as countercurrent immunoelectrophoresis (CIE), latex agglutination, or coagglutination with *Staphylococcus* protein A can provide specific diagnoses of group B streptococci, *H. influenzae* type b, many *Streptococcus pneumoniae* strains, *Neisseria meningitidis* (A, B, C, X, Y, Z), and *E. coli* K1 (cross-reaction with group B *N. meningitidis*) within minutes to an hour of performing the test, depending on the method chosen. The use of antigen-detection tests is indicated if the mother or infant has received antibiotics or if blood culture–negative sepsis is suspected for other reasons. Testing serum, CSF, and concentrated urine can detect the antigens of group B streptococci in the vast majority of newborn patients infected with this organism. Misleading positive test results for group B streptococcal antigen are not infrequent. In particular, urine samples collected in bags may be contaminated by organisms from the skin (Sanchez et al., 1990). Thus a positive antigen test result is not reliable for making the diagnosis without consistent clinical findings. Antigen detection is useful in certain circumstances mentioned above but should not take the place of culture. Negative antigen determinations do not rule out bacterial infection.

Pneumonia has been demonstrated at autopsy in infants who had negative blood cultures (Squire et al., 1979). Sepsis associated with necrotizing enterocolitis, peritonitis, and meningitis can occur with negative blood cultures. Thus blood culture–negative sepsis must be considered when clinical criteria are present, although uncertainty may exist. At times, the clinical course will resolve the issue.

The diagnosis of mucocutaneous infection is confirmed by scraping the membrane or skin lesion and demonstrating hyphae, pseudohyphae, or yeast forms. Diagnosis of invasive disease is made by culturing *Candida* from normally sterile body fluids. Blood cultures should be labeled to notify the laboratory that fungemia is expected so special media can be used and incubation prolonged. Methylene blue or Gram stain of exudates or buffy coat may provide presumptive evidence of disease. Demonstration of a fungal antigen may be useful in the future, but this technique requires further study. Serological methods are not helpful. The WBC counts are variable; marked leukocytosis may be noted. Thrombocytopenia is a common early finding. Elevation of blood urea nitrogen (BUN), creatinine, bilirubin, and liver enzymes may occur in the course of systemic candidiasis. Ultrasound of catheter-tip sites (to rule out infected thrombi), kidney, heart, and the CNS should be performed. Formal ophthalmological consultation for indirect funduscopic examination is necessary to rule out chorioretinitis or endophthalmitis, which may threaten vision.

PROGNOSIS

Despite advances in antimicrobial therapy, the outlook for infants with neonatal septicemia remains poor. Furthermore, it is unlikely that newer antibiotics will reduce further the mortality or morbidity of established infection. Drugs to which organisms are sensitive and reach all tissues, including the CNS, are available. All too often the immature immune function of the neonate is unable effectively to eradicate the infection, and irreversible damage is sustained. Collected experiences over the past four decades show an overall decline in case fatality rates from approximately 90% to 26%, which probably is due to improved supportive measures and optimal antimicrobial therapy.

Important factors influencing the outcome of sepsis in the newborn infant are the causative agent, the prompt recognition and initiation of optimal therapy, complications of sepsis, gestational age, and the severity of coexistive disease. Early diagnosis and the initiation of specific antimicrobial therapy are helpful in improving the prognosis. Unfortunately, even prompt, early therapy has not been able to prevent the mortality or eliminate morbidity.

Meningitis is the most serious infection in respect to both mortality and sequelae. Meningitis caused by gram-negative organisms still carries a mortality rate of approximately 30%, and one third of the survivors have sequelae. Mortality is greater for preterm infants than for full-term infants. Gram-positive organisms causing meningitis are primarily group B streptococci, and the mortality rate varies from 25% with early-onset disease to 20% with late-onset disease. Long-range sequelae are present in an estimated 30% of the survivors.

EPIDEMIOLOGICAL FACTORS

Clusters and outbreaks of neonatal infection have been recorded within the nursery setting. Antibiotics are an essential part of the supportive therapy in the nursery, but their use selects for survival of resistant organisms. Outbreaks of infection with gram-negative organisms, including *Klebsiella* species, *Pseudomonas* species, *Serratia marcescens*, and *Citrobacter diversus*, have occurred in intensive care nurseries. Many of the supportive measures are of necessity invasive to the newborn and may carry a previously unrecognized risk of infection.

TREATMENT

If neonatal infection is suspected, treatment should be initiated as rapidly as possible after specimens for diagnostic studies have been obtained. Initial treatment depends on clinical findings and epidemiological and microbiological considerations (see Table 24-1). There may be clinical signs suggesting a specific cause (see "Cutaneous and mucous membrane signs," p. 409). Epidemiological considerations include age at onset, maternal colonization, obstetrical risk factors, neonatal interventions, and probable source (cutaneous, respiratory, or gastrointestinal). In the absence of clinical signs or rapid diagnostic information (Gram stain, Tzanck preparation for herpesviruses, antigen detection), the selection of antimicrobial agents is empiric. The choice is based on the most likely pathogens and their antibiotic sensitivity patterns. With the heavy use of antibiotics in special care nurseries, antibiotic resistance to synthetic penicillins and aminoglycosides is common, and physicians should be aware of the sensitivity patterns of the organisms colonizing the infants in their nurseries.

It is important to remember that nonbacterial infectious agents can produce the syndrome of neonatal sepsis. Herpes simplex virus infection requires specific treatment with acyclovir and *Candida* infection with amphotericin and possibly flucytosine.

Table 24-2. Antimicrobial therapy of newborn sepsis

Organism	Antibiotics
Group B streptococci	Penicillin
Group D streptococci (enterococci)	Ampicillin plus aminoglycoside
Listeria monocytogenes	Ampicillin
Staphylococci, coagulase positive	Nafcillin oxacillin
Staphylococcus epidermidis	Vancomycin
Enterobacteriaceae (*Escherichia coli, Klebsiella, Enterobacter, Serratia*)	Ampicillin plus aminoglycoside or cefotaxime
Anaerobic enteric organisms	Clindamycin or metronidazole
Pseudomonas species	Ceftazidime or gentamicin plus ticarcillin
Unknown bacteria	Ampicillin plus gentamicin or cefotaxime
Herpes simplex virus	Acyclovir
Candida species	Amphotericin with or without flucytosine

The initial empiric treatment of early-onset infections (group B streptococci, *E. coli, Listeria*) should consist of ampicillin and an aminoglycoside (usually gentamicin) by the intravenous or intramuscular route. Cefotaxime may be substituted for the aminoglycoside. Late-onset infections acquired in the NICU are more likely to occur with staphylococci, a variety of Enterobacteriaceae, *Pseudomonas*, or *Candida*. Thus an antistaphylococcal drug, nafcillin for *S. aureus* or vancomycin for coagulase-negative staphylococci, should be substituted for ampicillin. A history of recent antimicrobial therapy or antibiotic-resistant infections in the NICU should lead to the consideration of a different aminoglycoside agent and vancomycin for methicillin-resistant staphylococcal infection. The commonly used antibiotics are shown in Table 24-2. Dosages are listed in Appendix A. When the history or the presence of necrotic skin lesions suggests the possibility of *Pseudomonas* infection, initial therapy should be ticarcillin and gentamicin or ceftazidime. If sepsis is secondary to necrotizing enterocolitis, an agent effective against anaerobic organisms, clindamycin or metronidazole, should be added.

Once the pathogen has been identified and the antibiotic sensitivities determined, the most appropriate drug(s) should be selected. The morbidity and mortality of gram-negative sepsis and meningitis remain a significant problem. It takes longer to sterilize CSF, and studies of intrathecal and intraventricular gentamicin have not demonstrated any improvement in clinical or bacteriological outcome (McCracken and Mize, 1976; McCracken et al., 1980). For most of the gram-negative enteric bacteria, a third-generation cephalosporin (cefotaxime or ceftazidime) should be used. Enterococcus should be treated with both a penicillin (ampicillin) and an aminoglycoside since synergism has been demonstrated with this combination of antibiotics in a substantial proportion of the strains. Ampicillin alone is adequate for treating *Listeria*, whereas penicillin will suffice for group B streptococcus. Clindamycin or metronidazole is appropriate for anaerobic infections.

Third-generation cephalosporins such as cefotaxime are valuable additions for treating documented neonatal sepsis and meningitis because (1) the minimal inhibitory combinations for gram-negative enteric bacilli are much lower than for the aminoglycosides; (2) there is excellent penetration into CSF in the presence of inflamed meninges; and (3) much higher doses than those of the aminoglycosides can be given since toxicity is quite limited. The end result is much higher bactericidal titers in serum and CSF than are achievable with ampicillin/aminoglycoside combinations. However, these cephalosporins should not be used indiscriminately since they have only modest activity against *S. aureus* and *Listeria* and enterococci are resistant to both drugs. Since emergence of resistant organisms has been reported, these agents should probably not be used alone for treatment of serious infections (Heusser et al., 1990). Because ceftriaxone may contribute to hyperbilirubinemia, its use should be avoided in the neonatal period.

Therapy should be continued for a total of 10 to 14 days or for at least 5 to 7 days after clinical response when there is no evidence of deep-tissue involvement or abscess formation. Blood culture 24 to 48 hours after initiation of therapy should be negative. If the culture is positive, change in therapy may be indicated, and the possibility of an infected indwelling catheter, endocarditis, or an occult abscess should be considered.

Aminoglycosides and vancomycin are potentially nephrotoxic and ototoxic. Infants receiving these drugs for longer than 72 hours should have peak and trough levels determined. Desirable peaks for gentamicin and tobramycin are 6 to 10 mg/L; for amikacin, 15 to 25 mg/L; and for vancomycin, 25 to 40 mg/L. Trough levels should be less than 2 mg/L for gentamicin and tobramycin and less than 10 mg/L for amikacin and vancomycin. Serum BUN and creatinine levels should also be monitored.

Herpes simplex virus. Early antiviral therapy for herpes simplex virus infection appears to improve morbidity and mortality. Acyclovir in an intravenous dose of 30 mg/kg/day in three divided doses for 3 weeks is currently recommended (see Chapter 10).

Candidiasis. The choice of treatment of neonates with systemic candidiasis is controversial. Most authorities use amphotericin B alone, whereas others combine intravenous amphotericin with oral flucytosine. Despite frequent resistance to flucytosine, its combination with amphotericin is synergistic against *Candida*. Amphotericin B is usually given in an initial dose of 0.25 mg/kg, with increments every 24 to 48 hours up to a maximum of 1 mg/kg/24 hours. Amphotericin is administered in a 5% to 10% dextrose concentration in water infusion, without electrolytes, over 4 to 6 hours. Catheter-associated candidemia has been treated with a total dose of 10 to 15 mg/kg. Removal of the catheter is recommended, if possible, because *Candida* is difficult to eradicate from colonized central lines; the total dose of amphotericin B may be reduced to 5 to 10 mg/kg if the catheter is removed, the fungemia is rapidly cleared, and there is no evidence of metastatic infection. Disseminated candidiasis requires a total amphotericin dose of as much as 25 to 35 mg/kg. Toxicity from amphotericin occurs in approximately half of treated infants, with elevations of BUN and creatinine, oliguric renal failure, and hypokalemia. Potassium supplementation and adjustment in daily dosage or alternate-day antifungal therapy may be necessary. Bone marrow suppression and hepatotoxicity are less common. Toxicity is diminished in patients treated with 0.5 mg/kg/24 hours of amphotericin and 100 mg/kg/24 hours of flucytosine. Toxic effects of flucytosine include gastrointestinal dysfunction, hepatotoxicity, and bone marrow suppression.

Supportive therapy. Supportive therapy is important in the management of neonatal sepsis. Fluids and electrolytes should be carefully monitored, with correction of hypovolemia, hyponatremia, hypocalcemia, and limitation of fluids if there is inappropriate antidiuretic hormone secretion. Shock, hypoxia, and metabolic acidosis should be identified and managed accordingly. Adequate oxygenation of tissues should be maintained; ventilatory support is frequently necessary. Hypoglycemia should be treated promptly. Hyperbilirubinemia should be monitored and treated with exchange transfusion since the risk of kernicterus increases in the presence of sepsis. Parenteral nutrition should be considered for infants who cannot sustain enteral feedings.

DIC may complicate neonatal septicemia. Platelet counts, hemoglobin, prothrombin and partial thromboplastin times, and fibrin-split products should be monitored. DIC may be treated with fresh frozen plasma, platelet transfusions, or whole blood.

Adjunctive therapy. Neutropenia caused by neutrophil storage pool depletion has been associated with a poor prognosis (Christensen et al., 1982). A number of clinical trials of PMN leukocyte replacement therapy have been carried out with variable results (Baley, 1988; Cairo, 1989b). The logistics of obtaining PMN suspensions are difficult, and screening donors for viral infection (human immunodeficiency virus, hepatitis B virus, and cytomegalovirus) is imperative. Thus few centers use this form of adjunctive therapy. The use of granulocyte and granulocyte-monocyte stimulating factors (G-CSF and GM-CSF) is under study at this time. This treatment has been successful in other neutropenic conditions (Cairo, 1989a). Furthermore, as discussed earlier ("Host Factors"), phagocytosis is very inefficient in the absence of opsonins.

Treatment of neonatal sepsis with intravenous immunoglobulins (IVIGs) containing specific antibodies is currently under investigation. Although PMNs, antibody, and complement are present in whole blood, the limitations of volume appear to limit the amounts of each component, which is why component therapy is under study.

Therapeutic dilemmas. There are two situations in which the clinical status may be uncertain, cultures of the infant are negative, and the physician must decide how long to continue antimicrobial therapy. The first concerns the infant whose mother was treated with antibiotics for proven or suspected infection or for risk factors (see "Prevention"). The second concerns the infant who was treated for presumptive infection or sepsis and whose cultures are negative. Since bacterial infection may be present without documented bacteremia, a negative culture does not exclude the possibility of bacterial infection. Squire et al. (1979) reported negative blood cultures in 18% (seven of 39 newborn infants) who had proven infection at autopsy. Tests for antigenuria or antigenemia may be helpful in these situations. After waiting 3 days for culture results, the decision to continue treatment should depend on the clinical course. If another explanation for clinical signs is established or if the infant is well, antibiotics can be discontinued. If the clinical condition is consistent with infection, therapy should be continued.

PREVENTION

Aggressive obstetrical management of suspected maternal chorioamnionitis with antibiotics and rapid delivery of the newborn infant appears to have decreased the morbidity and mortality of early-onset neonatal sepsis (Gibbs et al., 1988).

A number of approaches have been tried to prevent group B streptococcal early-onset infections. With a colonization rate as high as 30% among pregnant women, eradication of group B streptococci poses a formidable task and a significant risk of penicillin reactions. Treatment of colonized pregnant women was apparently successful in preventing colonization of the newborn if treatment was continued until the time of delivery (Merenstein et al., 1980). Recolonization rates as high as 65% have been observed between the time of cessation of treatment and the time of delivery. Nevertheless, treatment of certain colonized women such as those with a previously infected premature infant may be appropriate.

Controlled trials of penicillin administered in the first hour of life have been carried out in Dallas and Chicago. The Dallas study showed a significantly lower rate of group B streptococcal infection (0.6 of 1,000) compared to controls (1.7 of 1,000) in 18,738 newborn infants (Siegel et al., 1980). At Chicago's Cook County Hospital, infants under 2,000 g were enrolled in a controlled study of penicillin prophylaxis after blood cultures were obtained (Pyati et al., 1983). The number of infants in the early treatment group who had disease (10 of 589) was similar to that in the control group (14 of 598). Fatality rates were the same in both groups.

Infants with positive blood cultures at birth have intrauterine infections that obviously are not prevented by postnatal administration of penicillin. Excluding these infants, selective intrapartum chemoprophylaxis may effectively prevent group B streptococcal infections that are acquired during birth.

Since the majority of infants with early-onset group B streptococcal infections are symptomatic during the first 24 hours of life Boyer and Gotoff (1986, 1988) investigated the use of intrapartum ampicillin to prevent early-onset disease. To limit the number of allergic reactions and the cost of treatment, the selection of women for ampicillin chemoprophylaxis was based on a positive prenatal culture and the presence of a risk factor—either premature labor (<37 weeks) or prolonged ruptured membranes (>18 hours). Women with chorioamnionitis were treated with ampicillin and were excluded from the study. Twenty of the 1,825 infants born to prenatally colonized women developed group B streptococcal early-onset disease. None of the 320 infants born to ampicillin-treated mothers developed early-onset infection. Attack rates of bacteremic group B streptococcal obstetrical infection were also reduced significantly by intrapartum chemoprophylaxis. Tupperainen and Hallman (1989) selected patients with heavy vaginal colonization detected by a rapid latex agglutination test during labor. Of 94 randomized parturient women, 36 received intrapartum penicillin, and 58 did not. Seven of the 58 babies whose mothers were untreated developed early-onset group B streptococcal disease. In a similar study with a rapid coagglutination test for antigen on a vaginal swab obtained at the time of hospital admission, Morales and Lim (1987) prevented chorioamnionitis and neonatal sepsis in the ampicillin-treated patients. In the control group there were 11 cases of chorioamnionitis (23%) and 13 cases of neonatal sepsis (27%) caused by group B streptococci. Although the risk of infection was higher in women with heavy colonization, light colonization resulted in a 14% rate of maternal infection and a 16% rate of neonatal infection. Light colonization was not detected by the rapid test for antigen. The limited sensitivity and logistical problems of screening for colonization with antigen-detection tests at the onset of labor must be weighed against the drawbacks of using prenatal cultures, which include late acquisition of group B streptococci in 7% of women.

In summary, the decision to use preventive measures depends on the incidence of group B streptococcal early-onset disease in the community. Attack rates above one per 1,000 may be an appropriate indication. Limiting prophylaxis to premature infants could miss approximately half of the infants with group B streptococcal early-onset disease. The addition of infants whose mothers have chorioamnionitis or prolonged membrane rupture will identify about 70% of those infants who could be expected to develop early onset GBS disease. The remaining

30%, full-term infants without risk factors who develop early-onset group B streptococcal infections, have a better outcome. Disease may be prevented in these infants by penicillin administration in the delivery room (Siegel et al., 1980). When a group B streptococcal vaccine becomes licensed (Baker et al., 1988), clinical trials will determine whether early-onset and late-onset infections are preventable.

Prevention of nosocomial infections is based on appropriate design of nurseries and following the policies of neonatal care published by the American Academy of Pediatrics. Careful hand-washing technique is most important. Gloves should be worn when handling infants with congenital syphilis, necrotizing enterocolitis, and staphylococcal infections. Bathing of infants with hexachlorophene-containing soap decreases skin colonization with staphylococci but may not control epidemics. Nasal antibiotics have also been used to reduce colonization. Control of epidemics in NICUs usually requires cohorting of infected and colonized infants.

REFERENCES

Baker C, Edwards MS. Group B streptococcal infections. In Remington JS, Klein JO (eds). Infectious disease of the fetus and newborn infant. Philadelphia: WB Saunders, 1990, p 742.

Baker C, Rench MA, Edwards MS, et al. Immunization of pregnant women with a polysaccharide vaccine of group B streptococcus. N Engl J Med 1988;319:1180.

Baley JE. Neonatal sepsis: The potential for immunotherapy. Clin Perinatol 1988;15:755.

Baley JE, Kliegman RM, Fanaroff AA. Disseminated fungal infections in very low birth weight infants: clinical manifestations and epidemiology. Pediatrics 1984;73:144.

Ballow M, Cates LK, Rowe JC, et al. Development of the immune system in very low birth weight (less than 1500 g) premature infants: concentrations of plasma immunoglobulins and patterns of infections. Pediatr Res 1986;20:899.

Bell WE, McGuinness GA. Suppurative central nervous system infections in the neonate. Semin Perinatol 1982;6:1.

Berman PH, Banker BQ. Neonatal meningitis: a clinical and pathological study of twenty-nine cases. Pediatrics 1966;38:6.

Bone RC, Fisher CJ, Clemmer TP, et al. Sepsis syndrome: A valid clinical entity. Crit Care Med 1989;17:389.

Bortolussi R, Fischer GW. Opsonic and protective activity of immunoglobulin, modified immunoglobulin and serum against neonatal Escherichia coli K1 infection. Pediatr Res 1986;20:175.

Boyer KM, Gadzala CA, Burd LI, et al. Selective intrapartum chemoprophylaxis of neonatal group B streptococcal early-onset disease: I. Epidemiologic rationale. J Infect Dis 1983;148:795.

Boyer KM, Gotoff SP. Antimicrobial prophylaxis of neonatal group B streptococcal sepsis. Clin Perinatol 1988;15:831.

Boyer KM, Gotoff SP. Prevention of early-onset neonatal group B streptococcal disease with selective intrapartum chemoprophylaxis. N Engl J Med 1986;314:1665.

Butler KM, Baker CJ. Candida: an increasingly important pathogen in the nursery. Pediatr Clin North Am 1988;35:543.

Cairo MS. Review of G-CSF and GM-CSF effects on neonatal neutrophil kinetics. Am J Pediatr Hematol Oncol 1989a;11(2):2983.

Cairo MS. Review of G-CSF and GM-CSF effects on neonatal neutrophil kinetics. Am J Pediatr Hematol Oncol 1989a;11(2):2983.

Cairo MS. Neutrophil transfusions in the treatment of neonatal sepsis. Am J Pediatr Hematol Oncol 1989b; 11(2):227.

Cates KL, Goetz C, Rosenberg N, et al. Longitudinal development of specific and functional antibody in very low birth weight premature infants. Pediatr Res 1988;23:14.

Christensen RD, Rothstein G, Anstall HB, Bybee B. Granulocyte transfusions in neonates with bacterial infection, neutropenia, and depletion of mature marrow neutrophils. Pediatrics 1982;70:1.

Cross AS, Gemski P, Sadoff JC, et al. The importance of the K1 capsule in invasive infections caused by E. coli. J Infect Dis 1984;149:184.

deLouvois J, Harvey D. Antibiotic therapy of the newborn. Clin Perinatol 1988;18:175.

Dietzman DE, Fischer GW, Schoenknecht FD. Neonatal E. coli septicemia—bacterial counts in blood. J Pediatr 1974;85:128.

Dillon HC, Khare S, Gray BM. Group B streptococcal carriage and disease: a six-year prospective study. J Pediatr 1987;110:31.

Dobson SRM, Baker CJ. Enterococcal sepsis in neonates: features by age at onset and occurrence of focal infection. Pediatrics 1990;85:165.

Eisenfeld L, Ermocilla R, Wirtschafter D, Cassady G. Systemic bacterial infections in neonatal deaths. Am J Dis Child 1983;137:645.

Fischer GW, Crumrine MH, Jennings PB. Experimental E. coli sepsis in rabbits. J Pediatr 1974;85:117.

Friesen CA, Cho CT. Characteristic features of neonatal sepsis due to Haemophilus influenzae. Rev Infect Dis 1986;8:777.

Garner JS, Jarvis WR, Emori TG. CDC definitions for nosocomial infections, 1988. Am J Infect Control 1988;16:128.

Gibbs RS, Dinsmoor MJ, Newton ER, Ramamurthy RS. A randomized trial of intrapartum versus immediate postpartum treatment of women with intra-amniotic infection. Obstet Gynecol 1988;72:823.

Girardin E, Gran GE, Dayer J-M, et al. Tumor necrosis factor and interleukin-1 in the serum of children with severe infections purpura. N Engl J Med 1988;319:397.

Gladstone IM, Ehrenkranz RA, Edberg SC, Baltimore RS. A ten-year review of neonatal sepsis and comparison with the previous fifty-year experience. Pediatr Infect Dis J 1990;9:819.

Gotoff SP, Boyer KM. Prevention of group B streptococcal early onset sepsis: 1989. Pediatr Infect Dis J 1989;8:268.

Gotoff SP, Odell C, Papierniak CK, et al. Human IgG antibody to group B streptococcus type III: comparison of protective levels in a murine model with levels in infected human neonates. J Infect Dis 1986;153:511.

Gruskay J, Harris MC, Costarino AT, et al. Neonatal *Staphylococcus epidermidis* meningitis with unremarkable CSF examination results. Am J Dis Child 1989;143:580.

Gruskay J, Abbasi S, Anday E, et al. *Staphylococcus epidermidis*-associated enterocolitis. J Pediatr 1986;109:520.

Hall RT, Kurth CG, Hall SL. Ten-year survey of positive blood cultures among admissions to a neonatal intensive care unit. J Perinatol 1987;7:122.

Hall RT, Hall SL, Barnes WG, et al. Characteristics of coagulase-negative staphylococci from infants with bacteremia. Pediatr Infect Dis J 1987;6:377.

Hall SL, Hall RT, Barnes WG, et al. Relationship of neonatal to maternal vaginal colonization with coagulase-negative staphylococci. Am J Perinatol 1990;7:384.

Heusser MF, Patterson JE, Kuritza AP, et al. Emergence of resistance to multiple beta-lactams in *Enterobacter cloacae* during treatment for neonatal meningitis with cefotaxime (CFX). Pediatr Infect Dis J 1990;9:509.

Hill HR. Host defenses in the neonate: prospects for enhancement. Semin Perinatol 1985;9:2.

Jacobs RF, Sowell MK, Moss MM, Fiser DH. Septic shock in children: bacterial etiologies and temporal relationships. Pediatr Infect Dis J 1990;9:196.

Jarvis WR, Thornsberry C, Boyce J, et al. Methicillin-resistant *staphylococcus aureus* at children's hospital in the United States, Pediatr Infect Dis J 1985;4:651.

Jason JM. Infectious disease-related deaths of low birth weight infants, United States, 1968 to 1982. Pediatrics 1989;84:296.

Klein JO, Feigin RD, McCracken GH. Report of the task force on diagnosis and management of meningitis. Pediatrics 1986;78:958.

Kovatch AL, Wald ER. Evaluation of the febrile neonate. Semin Perinatol 1985;9:12.

Madan E, Meyer MP, Amortequi A. Chorioamnionitis: a study of organisms isolated in perinatal autopsies. Ann Clin Lab Sci 1988;18:39.

Manroe BL, Weinberg AG, Rosenfeld CR, Browne R. The neonatal blood count in health and disease. I. Reference values for neutrophilic cells. J Pediatr 1978;95:89.

Markowitz LE, Steere AC, Benach JL, et al. Lyme disease during pregnancy. JAMA 1986;255:3394.

Marodi L, Leijh PCJ, Braat A, et al. Opsonic activity of cord blood sera against various species of microorganism. Pediatr Res 1985;19:433.

McCracken GH Jr, Mize SG, Threlkeld N. Intravesicular gentamicin therapy in gram-negative bacillary meningitis in infancy. Lancet 1980;1:787.

McCracken GH Jr, Mize SG. A controlled study of intrathecal antibiotic therapy in gram-negative enteric meningitis in infancy. Report of the neonatal meningitis cooperative study group. J Pediatr 1976;89:66.

Merenstein GB, Todd WA, Brown G, et al. Group B β-hemolytic streptococcus: randomized controlled treatment study at term. Obstet Gynecol 1980;55:315.

Mills EL, Thompson T, Bjorksten B, et al. The chemiluminescence response and bactericidal activity of polymorphonuclear neutrophils from newborns and their mothers. Pediatrics 1979;63:429.

Morales WJ, Lim DV. Reduction of group B streptococcal maternal and neonatal infections in preterm pregnancies

with premature rupture of membranes through a rapid identification test. Am J Obstet Gynecol 1987;157:13.

Morales WJ, Lim DV, Walsh AF. Prevention of neonatal group B streptococcal sepsis by the use of a rapid screening test and selective intrapartum chemoprophylaxis. Am J Obstet Gynecol 1986;155:979.

Noel GJ, Laufer DA, Edelson PJ. Anaerobic bacteremia in a neonatal intensive care unit: an eighteen-year experience, Pediatr Infect Dis J 1988;7:858.

Noel GJ, O'Loughlin JE, Edelson PJ. Neonatal *Staphylococcus epidermidis* right-sided endocarditis: description of five catheterized infants. Pediatrics 1988;82:234.

Nora FJ, Baker CJ. Intravenously administered immune globulin for premature infants: a time to wait. J Pediatr 1989;115:970.

Nyhan WL, Fousek MD. Septicemia of the newborn. Pediatrics 1958;22:268.

Patrick CC. Coagulase-negative staphylococci: pathogens with increasing clinical significance. J Pediatr 1990; 116:497.

Peter G, Cashore WJ. Infection acquired in the nursery: epidemiology and control. In Remington JS, Klein JO: Infectious diseases of the fetus and newborn infant. Philadelphia: WB Saunders, 1990.

Pierce JR, Merenstein GB, Stocker JT. Immediate postmortem cultures in an intensive care nursery. Pediatr Infect Dis 1984;3:510.

Pyati SP, Pildes RS, Jacobs NW, et al. Penicillin in infants weighing two kilograms or less with early-onset group B streptococcal disease. N Engl J Med 1983;308:1383.

Ramsey PG, Zwerdling R. Asymptomatic neonatal bacteremia. N Engl J Med 1977;295:225.

Roberts KB. Persistent group B streptococcus bacteremia without clinical "sepsis" in infants. J Pediatr 1976;88:1059.

Sanchez PJ, Siegel JD, Cushion NB, Threlkeld N. Significance of a positive urine group B streptococcal latex agglutination test in neonates. J Pediatr 1990;116:601.

Schuchat A, Oxtoby M, Cochi S, et al. Population-based risk factors for neonatal group B streptococcal disease: results of a cohort study in metropolitan Atlanta. J Infect Dis 1990;162:672.

Shigeoka AO, Santos JI, Hill HR. Functional analysis of neutrophil granulocytes from healthy, infected and stressed neonates. J Pediatr 1979;95:454.

Siegel JD, McCracken GH, Threlkeld N, et al. Single-dose penicillin prophylaxis against neonatal group B streptococcal infection. N Engl J Med 1980;303:769.

Silver RP, Aaronson W, Vaun WF. The K1 capsular polysaccharide of *Escherichia coli*. Rev Infect Dis 1988; 10:5282.

Squire E, Favara B, Todd J. Diagnosis of neonatal bacterial infection: hematologic and pathologic findings in fatal and nonfatal cases. Pediatrics 1979;64:60.

Teberg AJ, Yonekura ML, Salminen C, et al. Clinical manifestations of epidemic neonatal listeriosis. Pediatr Infect Dis 1987;6:817.

Tuppurainen N, Hallman M. Prevention of neonatal group B streptococcal disease: intrapartum detection and chemoprophylaxis of heavily colonized parturients. Obstet Gynecol 1989;73:583.

Valvano MA, Hartstein AI, Morthland VH, et al. Plasmid DNA analysis of *Staphylococcus epidermidis* isolated from blood and colonizing cultures in very low birth weight neonates. Pediatr Infect Dis 1988;7:116.

Voora S, Srinivasan G, Lilien LD, et al. Fever in full term newborns in the first four days of life. Pediatrics 1982;69:40.

Weese-Mayer DE, Fondriest DW, Brouillette RT, Shulman ST. Risk factors associated with candidemia in the neonatal intensive care unit: a case-control study. Pediatr Infect Dis 1987;6:190.

Wilson CB. Developmental immunology and role of host defenses in neonatal susceptibility. In Remington JS, Klein JO (eds): Infectious disease of the fetus and newborn infant. Philadelphia: WB Saunders, 1990, p 17.

Wood BM, Klein JO. Therapy of bacterial sepsis and meningitis in infants and children. Pediatr Infect Dis 1989;8:635.

Ziegler E, Fisher C, Sprung C, et al. Treatment of gram-negative bacteremia and septic shock with HA-IA human monoclonal antibody against endotoxin. N Engl J Med 1991;324:429.

25

SEXUALLY TRANSMITTED DISEASES

MARGARET R. HAMMERSCHLAG
SARAH A. RAWSTRON

Sexually transmitted diseases (STDs) comprise a wide range of infections and conditions that are transmitted mainly by sexual activity. The "classic" STDs, gonorrhea and syphilis, currently are being overshadowed by a new set of STDs that are not only more common, but more difficult to diagnose and treat. These "new" STDs include infections caused by *Chlamydia trachomatis*, human papilloma virus, and human immunodeficiency virus (HIV). Physicians are confronted by particularly complex social and clinical problems caused by STDs in neonates and infants, in abused older children, and in adolescents. Rapid application of new technology to the diagnosis of STDs has led to a growing array of diagnostic laboratory tests that require critical evaluation by clinicians.

This chapter presents a comprehensive overview of STDs in neonates, infants, older children, and adolescents.

GONORRHEA

Gonorrhea is the most frequently reported infectious disease in the United States. The World Health Organization estimates that there are approximately 100 million gonorrheal infections each year throughout the world. The reported number of cases of gonorrhea in the United States exceeds 1 million annually, and it is estimated that more than 2½ million cases occur. Many cases escape detection and contribute to the silent reservoir of infection in males and females. The reported age-specific rate for gonococcal disease in children up to 14 years was 10.6 per 100,000 for males and 30.6 per 100,000 for females in 1982 (Centers for Disease Control, 1989).

Gonorrhea is an inflammatory disease of the mucous membranes of the genitourinary tract that occurs only in humans. It is caused by *N. gonorrhoeae*, which first was described by Neisser in 1879. The most common portal of entry is the genitourinary tract, and the organism may then cause various inflammatory diseases of adjacent tissues such as cervicitis, salpingitis, and vulvovaginitis in children. The newborn may acquire the organism during delivery when direct contact with contaminated vaginal secretions leads to conjunctivitis. Bacteremia may occur and most often causes cutaneous lesions and arthritis, rarely endocarditis and meningitis. Children may present with gonococcal proctitis and pharyngitis and asymptomatic presence of gonococci in the rectum, pharynx, and genitourinary tract.

Bacteriology

N. gonorrhoeae is a nonmotile non–spore-forming, gram-negative coccus that characteristically grows in pairs, with flattened adjacent sides in the configuration of "coffee beans." All *Neisseria* species, including *N. meningitidis*, rapidly oxidize dimethyl- or tetramethyl-para-phenyline diamine, the basis of the diagnostic oxidase test.

The cell envelope of *N. gonorrhoeae* is similar to that of other gram-negative bacteria. Specific surface components of the envelope have been related to adherence, tissue and cellular penetration, cytoxicity, and evasion of host defenses, both systemically and at the mucosal level.

Pili. Pili are filamentous projections that traverse the outer membrane of the organism and are composed of repeating protein subunits. When *N. gonorrhoeae* is grown on translucent agar, various morphology of the colony can be seen. Fresh clinical isolates initially form colony types P+ and P++ (formerly called *T1* and *T2*). The organisms have numerous pili extending from the cell surface. After 20 to 24 hours, P− (formerly T3 and T4) colonies, in which the cells are nonpiliated, predominate. These nonpiliated organisms are not virulent. The shift between P+ or P++ and P− colony types is termed *phase variation* and is mediated by chromosomal rearrangement. The protein that constitutes pili (pilin) has regions of considerable antigenic variability between strains of *N. gonorrhoeae*. Single strains of *N. gonorrhoeae* also can produce pili of different antigenic composition. It was originally thought that a pilus-based vaccine against *N. gonorrhoeae* would be feasible, but recognition of these antigenic variations has made this possibility unlikely. Piliated gonococci are better able to attach to human mucosal surfaces than nonpiliated organisms. Pili also contribute to killing by neutrophils (Britigan et al., 1985).

Outer membrane. The gonococcus has a cell envelope like other gram-negative bacteria. The envelope consists of three layers: an inner cytoplasmic membrane, a middle peptidoglycan cell wall, and an outer membrane. The outer membrane contains lipooligosaccharide (LOS), phospholipid, and a variety of proteins. One of them is protein I, which functions as a porin and is believed to play an important role in pathogenesis. Preliminary data suggest it may facilitate endocytosis of the organism or otherwise trigger invasion. Protein I is also the basis of the most commonly used gonococcal serotyping system because there is consistent antigenic variation between different strains. Certain *N. gonorrhoeae* protein I serovars are associated with resistance of the organism to the bactericidal effect of normal nonimmune serum and an increased propensity to cause bacteremia. Gonococcal LOS is an endotoxin that differs from the polysaccharide of most gram-negative bacteria. Some components of LOS are also related to resistance of *N. gonorrhoeae* to serum bactericidal activity. LOS also demonstrates interstrain antigenic variations, which are the basis of another serotyping system (Apicella, 1976).

Strain typing. Characterization of gonococcal strains recently has been based on two primary methods, auxotyping and serology. Auxotyping is based on the differing requirements for specific nutrient or cofactors. It is done by examining the ability of strains of the organism to grow on chemically defined media that lack these factors (Catlin, 1973). More than 30 auxotypes have been identified. Common types include prototrophic (Proto) strain, also known as *zero* or *wild type* strain; proline-requirement (Pro-)strain; and strains that require arginine, hypoxanthine, and uracil.

The most widely based serotyping system is based on protein I as described previously. There are two major subgroups, IA and IB, which can be classified further into serovars based on coagglutination with a panel of monoclonal antibodies. Combining typing strains with auxotyping and serology has been helpful in studying the epidemiology of gonococcal infection both geographically and temporally. It has been especially helpful in analyzing patterns of antibiotic resistance (Hook et al., 1987).

Genetics. Many strains of *N. gonorrhoeae* possess a 24.5 MD conjugative plasmid. Many strains now carry a plasmid that specifies production of a TEM-1 type β-lactamase. This plasmid is similar to those found in *Haemophilus* species, including *H. ducreyi*. In fact, *N. gonorrhoeae* may have acquired the plasmid from *H. ducreyi*. The plasmid may also code for high-level resistance to tetracycline, minimum inhibitory concentration (MIC) greater than 16 mg/L, which can be readily transferred to other gonococci. This resistance factor, called the *tctM determinant*, functions by encoding for a protein that protects ribosomes from the effect of tetracycline.

Antibiotic resistance in *N. gonorrhoeae* also may be mediated by chromosomal mutations. Chromosomal resistance to β-lactam antibiotics and the tetracyclines appears to result from a series of minor mutations that reduce the permeability of the outer membrane or alter penicillin-binding protein-2, reducing its affinity for penicillin.

Diagnosis. Gram stain of synovial fluid, urethral discharge, or urinary sediment in the male may reveal the characteristic gram-negative diplococci. The female adult cervix and the vagina of prepubertal children may be colonized with other *Neisseria* species, rendering the Gram stain less reliable.

In younger children, because of medical-legal implications, the importance of an accurate microbiological diagnosis cannot be overemphasized. Gram stain of the vaginal discharge in a child with suspected gonorrhea is not accurate and has a poor predictive value for the diagnosis of gonorrhea. Diagnostic specimens of the pharynx, rectum, and vagina/urethra should be taken and immediately plated onto selective media appropriate for isolation of *N. gonorrhoeae* (e.g., chocolate blood agar and Thayer-Martin agar). The plates should then be placed in an atmosphere enriched with carbon dioxide, which is done most easily by using an extinction candle jar. *N. gonorrhoeae* are gram-negative, oxidase-positive diplococci, and their presence should be confirmed with additional tests, including rapid carbohydrate tests, enzyme-substrate tests, and rapid serological tests. Failure to perform appropriate confirmatory tests may lead to misidentification of other organisms as *N. gonorrhoeae*. Whittington et al. (1988) found that 14 of 40 presumptive gonococcal isolates sent to the Centers for Disease Control (CDC) for confirmation had been misidentified as *N. gonorrhoeae*. They included other *Neisseria* species, *Moraxella catarrhalis*, and *Kingella denitrificans*. The CDC recommends that confirmation of an organism as *N. gonorrhoeae* should include at least two procedures that use different principles (e.g., biochemical and enzyme-substrate or serological).

Pathology and pathogenesis

Stratified squamous epithelium can resist invasion by the gonococcus, whereas columnar epithelium is susceptible to it. This difference accounts for the absence of lesions in the adult vagina and on the external genitalia of both sexes. The susceptibility of columnar epithelium leads to infection of the urethra, prostate gland, seminal vesicles, and epididymis in males. In females infection occurs primarily in the urethra, Skene's and Bartholin's glands, cervix, and fallopian tubes. Gonorrhea can occur in males or females without signs or symptoms (Amstey and Steadman, 1976). The primary infection can occur in the rectal or pharyngeal mucosa of either sex. The alkaline pH of secreted mucus and the lack of estrogen permit vaginal infections with overt vulvovaginitis to occur in the prepubertal girl (Hook and Holmes, 1985).

Gonococci penetrate the surface cell layers through the intracellular spaces and reach the subepithelial connective tissue by the third or fourth day of infection. An inflammatory exudate quickly forms beneath the epithelium. In the acute phase of infection numerous leukocytes, many with phagocytosed gonococci, are present in the lumen of the urethra, causing a characteristic profuse yellow-white discharge in males. In the absence of specific treatment, the inflammatory exudate in the subepithelial connective tissue is replaced by fibroblasts and eventually by fibrous tissue around the urethra, with ensuing stricture of the urethra.

Direct extension occurs through the lymphatic vessels and less often through the blood vessels. Infection spreads to the posterior urethra, Cowper's glands, seminal vesicles, prostate, and epididymis, which leads to perineal, perianal, ischiorectal, or periprostatic abscesses. In teenage and adult males acute prostatitis can result in prostatic abscess or chronic prostatitis, and epididymitis is the most frequent complication. After healing has taken place, scar formation may destroy the lumen of the epididymis, and azospermia may result from bilateral involvement. Antimicrobial treatment usually prevents these complications. As many as 50% of untreated teenage and adult males become asymptomatic but remain infectious for periods up to 6 months.

In females primary infection most frequently affects the columnar epithelium of the postpubertal cervix, and the histopathological appearance resembles that of the male urethra. Spread of infection to the fallopian tubes may be acute or subacute, without signs and symptoms, and sometimes it is extremely difficult to diagnose. Acute stages can result in peritonitis. As a rule, the infection is confined to the pelvis. The end result of untreated or inadequately treated salpingitis is complete or partial obstruction of the tubes, which often leads to tubal pregnancy or sterility. Pelvic inflammatory disease (PID) is an especially common complication of gonorrhea in female adolescents, and when it occurs in this age range, it is especially likely to result in infertility (see "Pelvic Inflammatory Disease and Salpingitis," p. 426) (Hook and Holmes, 1985).

Clinical manifestations

In pregnancy. The effects of gonococcal disease on the infant may begin before delivery since there is evidence that gonococcal disease in pregnant women may have an adverse effect on both the mother and the infant. Edwards et al. (1978) observed 19 women with intrapartum gonorrhea. They had a significantly greater occurrence of premature rupture of membranes, prolonged rupture of membranes, chorioamnionitis, and premature delivery. Other studies have shown an alarming incidence of perinatal deaths and abortions. In addition to the effect on the fetus, postpartum complications in the mother are common. Therefore the diagnosis of gonococcal disease should be sought and controlled during pregnancy. To obtain control, the following issues should be considered:

1. Recurrent infection after an initial episode during pregnancy is very common. Therefore specimens for culture should be obtained in later pregnancy from the woman who is infected in early pregnancy.
2. Many mothers conceive their first child while they are teenagers, an age range in which gonococcal disease has a particularly high prevalence and in which the young women may look to their pediatrician for medical care.
3. Gonococcal disease is especially dangerous to women because PID is a relatively frequent complication (see "Pelvic Inflammatory Disease and Salpingitis," p. 425).

In infancy

Ophthalmia neonatorum. Gonococcal ophthalmia is the most common form of gonorrhea in infants and results from perinatal contamination of infants by their infected mothers during parturition. An initially nonspecific conjunctivitis with serosanguinous discharge is rapidly replaced by a thick, purulent exudate. Corneal ulceration and iridocyclitis appear unilaterally or bilaterally. Unless therapy is initiated promptly, perforation of the cornea may occur, leading to blindness.

Ophthalmia neonatorum, formerly a leading cause of blindness, has been controlled by prophylaxis with silver nitrate or with antimicrobial agents such as erythromycin and tetracycline. Crede's original study in 1888 reported that use of 2% silver nitrate prophylaxis reduced the incidence of gonococcal ophthalmia from 10% to 0.3%.

Neonatal ocular prophylaxis is not 100% effective; failures do occur (Rothenberg, 1979; Bernstein et al., 1983). The infant possibly is more likely to acquire the infection despite prophylaxis if there has been premature rupture of membranes (Handsfield et al., 1973). A recent study of neonatal ocular prophylaxis in the United States suggests that prenatal screening and treatment of pregnant women has had a significant impact on the prevention of gonococcal ophthalmia (Hammerschlag et al., 1989). Bacitracin and sulfonamides are known as ineffective prophylactics (Rothenberg, 1979).

In young children. Gonococcal vulvovaginitis is the most common gonococcal disease in children. It must be distinguished bacteriologically from vulvovaginitis caused by other agents by isolating *N. gonorrhoeae* from a vaginal swab; an endocervical culture is not necessary. In preadolescent females the vaginal exudate may be minimal and may be confused with a benign discharge. Symptoms referable to the urinary tract may predominate.

N. gonorrhoeae is the most common sexually transmitted disease found in sexually abused children (Schwarz and Whittington, 1990); a positive culture for *N. gonorrhoeae* from any site in a child without prior peer sexual activity is strongly suggestive of sexual abuse. *N. gonorrhoeae* rarely may be spread by sexual play among children, but the index case has usually been a victim of abuse (Potterat et al., 1986). *N. gonorrhoeae* has been found in approximately 5% of children suspected of having been sexually abused (Table 25-1). It may cause purulent vulvovaginitis in girls or urethritis in boys. Gonococcal ophthalmia may also occur as a result of autoinoculation from a genital site. However, as many as 20% to 25% of children with genital cultures containing *N. gonorrhoeae* may be asymptomatic, and an even higher number of rectal and pharyngeal infections are asymptomatic (Groothius et al., 1983; De Jong, 1986; McClure et al., 1986).

Ascending pelvic infection may occur in prepubertal females, and it may occur in the absence of significant vaginal discharge. The main signs of early disease are dysuria and vaginal discharge. When gonococcal infection spreads from the cervix into the fallopian tubes, it is characterized by lower abdominal pain. The onset of acute salpingitis, or PID, may be abrupt

Table 25-1. Prevalence of syphilitic, gonorrheal, and chlamydial infections in sexually abused children

Study (year)	Number tested	Number (%) positive		
		Syphilis	Gonorrhea	Chlamydia
Tilelli, et al. (1980)	103	NS*	3 (3)	NS
Rimsza and Niggerman (1982)	285	0	21 (7)	NS
White et al. (1983)	409	6 (1)	46 (11)	NS
De Jong (1986)	532	1 (0.2)	25 (5)	NS
Hammerschlag et al. (1984)	51	0	5 (10)	2 (4)
Ingram et al. (1984)	50	NS	10 (20)	3 (6)

*NS, Not studied.

and must be distinguished from acute appendicitis, cystitis, pyelonephritis, cholecystitis, and ectopic pregnancy (see "Pelvic Inflammatory Disease and Salpingitis").

In teenage males the onset of gonococcal urethritis is marked by sudden burning on urination occurring 2 days to 2 weeks after sexual exposure, similar to the presentation in adult males. This is followed by a mucopurulent discharge from the urethra. Involvement of the prostate gland is manifested by retention of urine, pain, and fever. Epididymitis is characterized by severe pain, tenderness, and swelling. Asymptomatic infection also occurs in approximately 50% of teenage and adult females (Hein et al., 1977).

Extragenital manifestations

Disseminated gonococcal infection. Disseminated gonococcal infection (DGI) results from gonococcal bacteremia and occurs in 0.5% to 3% of patients with gonorrhea (Holmes et al., 1971). The strains of *N. gonorrhoeae* associated with DGI are very susceptible to penicillin, are resistant to the bactericidal action of nonimmune serum, have the AHU-auxotype, and belong to several specific protein 1A serovars (Knapp and Holmes, 1975). Individuals with deficient terminal components of complement (C5, C6, C7, or C8) are more susceptible to disseminated gonococcal infection and meninogoccal bacteremia (Petersen et al., 1979). Approximately 5% of patients with disseminated gonococcal infection

have this deficiency. Other host risk factors apparently associated with an increased risk of dissemination include female sex, menstruation, pharyngeal gonorrhea, and pregnancy (Holmes et al., 1971).

The most common clinical manifestation of disseminated gonococcal infection is the arthritis-dermatitis syndrome. The patients first complain of arthralgias that may be migratory. The knees, elbows, and more distal joints usually are involved. Physical examination will demonstrate arthritis or periarticular inflammation (e.g., tenosynovitis) in two or more joints. A characteristic rash consisting of discrete papules and pustules, often with a hemorrhagic or necrotic component, will also be present in 75% of patients. Usually five to 40 lesions are present, occurring primarily on the extremities. The polyarthropathy and dermatitis frequently resolve spontaneously if not treated. However, arthritis may persist and progress, usually in one or two joints, most commonly the knee, ankle, elbow, or wrist. At this stage the clinical picture is that of septic arthritis. Disseminated gonococcal infection is the leading cause of infective arthritis in young adults.

Studies of septic arthritis in children have found *N. gonorrhoeae* is the third most frequent organism in children over 3 years of age and the most frequent in children over 11 years of age (Nelson, 1972). Some patients can develop gonococcal septic arthritis without prior polyarthritis or dermatitis.

Most clinical manifestations of disseminated gonococcal infection are secondary to the bacteremia, although immune complexes and other immunological mechanisms may be contributory to some cases. Patients usually will have fever and some systemic toxicity, which is frequently mild and often absent. Gonococci frequently can be recovered from blood cultures during the polyarthritis-dermatitis stage. The organism may also be detected by immunochemical methods in biopsy specimens from the skin lesions, but cultures are usually negative. Gram-stained smears and cultures of pustular skin lesions are also usually negative. Overall, approximately 50% of patients with disseminated gonococcal infection will have positive cultures of the blood or synovial fluid, but N. gonorrhoeae can be recovered from a mucosal site (e.g., pharynx, rectum) in at least 80% of patients—an important consideration when evaluating a child with suspected septic arthritis.

The differential diagnosis of disseminated gonococcal infection includes meningococcemia, other infectious arthritis, and an entire range of inflammatory arthritides, including Reiter's syndrome. Infrequent but serious complications of disseminated gonococcal infection include infective endocarditis, meningitis, osteomyelitis, and pneumonia.

Perihepatitis. Gonococcal perihepatitis (Fitz-Hugh-Curtis syndrome) results from extension of infection from salpingitis to the capsule and outer surface of the liver. It should be considered in females with right upper quadrant pain, palpable liver, abnormal liver function tests, and adnexal and uterine cervical tenderness. A positive endocervical culture for N. gonorrhoeae supports the diagnosis.

Conjunctivitis. Conjunctivitis beyond the newborn period follows direct spread of the gonococcus, usually via fingers contaminated with gential secretions. It rarely results from gonococcemia.

Oropharyngitis. Gonococcal oropharyngitis is common among homosexuals and among children who are victims of sexual abuse. Infection follows orogenital contact and may simulate streptococcal pharyngitis, with swollen tonsils, exudate, and enlarged cervical lymph nodes, or it may be asymptomatic. Temporomandibular arthritis has been reported as a complication of gonococcal pharyngitis (Weisner et al., 1973).

Treatment

During the 20 years before 1976, all N. gonorrhoeae were sensitive to penicillin, but a gradual increase had been noted in the mean MIC. In March 1976 reports appeared of the first clinical isolations of penicillinase-producing N. gonorrhoeae (PPNG) arising in the Far East. PPNG currently may account for more than 30% of isolates of N. gonorrhoeae in the United States (Schwarcz et al., 1990). There has also been a similar increase in tetracycline-resistant N. gonorrhoeae (TRNG). Recent studies have demonstrated a parallel increase of infections caused by PPNG among children with gonorrhea, which should not be surprising since these infections are acquired from adults (Rawstron et al., 1989). The CDC (1989) defines any area that has a rate of PPNG higher than 3% over a 3-month period as a hyperendemic area for PPNG and recommends that all infections be treated with penicillinase-resistant antibiotics. These resistant strains cause the same disease spectrum as penicillin-sensitive organisms. In 1983 an outbreak of chromosomally mediated penicillin-resistant gonococci was reported from North Carolina; subsequently, it has occurred in other areas of the country (Hook et al., 1987). These organisms, which do not produce penicillinase, are rare in children.

Prevention of neonatal infection. Endocervical cultures for gonococci should be obtained from all pregnant women as an integral part of prenatal care at the first prenatal visit. A second culture late in pregnancy should be obtained from women who are at high risk of gonococcal infection.

Prevention of gonococcal ophthalmia. Routine preventive prophylaxis of gonococcal ophthalmia includes (1) 1% silver nitrate (with no irrigation with saline solution, which might reduce efficacy) or (2) ophthalmic ointments containing tetracycline or erythromycin. Use of bacitracin ointment (not effective) and penicillin drops (sensitizing) is not recommended.

Management of infants born to mothers with untreated gonococcal infection. The infant born to a mother with untreated gonorrhea should have orogastric and rectal cultures taken routinely and blood cultures taken if the infant is symptomatic. A term infant should receive a single injection of ceftriaxone (50 mg/kg intravenously [IV] or intramuscularly [IM], not to exceed 125 mg). Although ceftriaxone is not usually given to newborn infants, it is indicated in this specific setting.

Neonatal disease

Gonococcal ophthalmia. Infants with gonococcal ophthalmia should be hospitalized. They should receive ceftriaxone (25 to 50 mg/kg/day IV or IM in a single dose) or cefotaxime (25 mg/kg IV or IM every 12 hours for 7 days). However, some data suggest that uncomplicated gonococcal ophthalmia can be cured with a *single* injection of ceftriaxone (50 mg/kg, up to 125 mg) (Laga et al., 1986). Infants with gonococcal ophthalmia should receive eye irrigations with buffered saline solution until the discharge is cleared. Additional topical therapy is not indicated. Simultaneous infection with *C. trachomatis* has been reported and should be considered in infants who do not respond satisfactorily. Both mother and infant should be tested for chlamydial infection.

Complicated infection. Infants with arthritis, abscess, and septicemia should be treated by hospitalization and administration of ceftriaxone for 7 days. Meningitis should be treated with ceftriaxone for 10 to 14 days.

Childhood disease beyond infancy. Children with gonorrhea should be hospitalized and treated with ceftriaxone (125 mg IM once if <45 kg and 250 mg if >45 kg). Children who cannot tolerate ceftriaxone may be treated with spectinomycin (40 mg/kg IM once) (Nelson et al., 1976). Spectinomycin is not as effective in treating rectal or pharyngeal gonorrhea. The source of the infection must be identified.

Children with disseminated gonococcal infection (bacteremia or arthritis) should be treated with ceftriaxone (50 mg/kg, maximum 1 g, once daily for 7 days). All children with rectogenital gonorrhea should also be evaluated for coinfection with chlamydia. If the infection has not been confirmed as PPNG, amoxicillin (50 mg/kg orally) as a single dose plus probenecid (25 mg/kg) may be administered (Nelson et al., 1976). The newer expanded-spectrum oral cephalosporins such as cefixime are effective as a single dose (oral) in adults but have not yet been evaluated in children.

Gonococcal infections in adolescents. Single-dose efficacy is a major consideration in treatment of gonococcal infections, especially in adolescents. Another important factor is coinfection with *C. trachomatis*, which can be documented in up to 45% of adolescents with gonorrhea in some populations. For teenagers more than 12 years of age, treatment should follow the recommended regimens for adults with one exception: quinolones are not approved for use in children up to 18 years of age.

The first-line regimen recommended by the CDC is single-dose ceftriaxone (250 mg IM) *plus* doxycycline (100 mg orally two times a day for 7 days) (Judson, Ehret, and Handsfield, 1985). The latter is necessary to treat possible coinfection with *C. trachomatis* (Stamm et al., 1984).

Alternative regimens for individuals who cannot tolerate ceftriaxone are spectinomycin (2 g IM in a single dose) plus doxcycline; cefotaxime (1 g IM once); cefuroxime axetil (1 g orally) plus probenecid (1 g); and ceftizoxime (500 mg IM once). Experience is less extensive with these regimens. If the adolescent is more than 16 years old, ciprofloxacin (500 mg orally once) or norfloxacin (800 mg orally once) can be used. All these regimens should be followed by a 7-day course of doxycycline. Tetracyclines cannot be used as a single drug for gonorrhea and chlamydia because of the increasing prevalence of TRNG strains.

PELVIC INFLAMMATORY DISEASE AND SALPINGITIS

Vaginal infection of females who are adolescent or younger may progress to involve the fallopian tubes or may disseminate to the pelvis. Pelvic inflammatory disease (PID) comprises a spectrum of inflammatory disorders of the upper genital tract in women and may include endometritis, salpingitis, tuboovarian abscess, and pelvic peritonitis. *N. gonorrhoeae* and *C. trachomatis* are implicated in most cases; however, endogenous organisms such as anaerobes, gram-negative rods, streptococci, and mycoplasmas may also be causative agents of disease (Eschenbach et al., 1975; Mardh, 1980). PID in adolescents is particularly likely to result in infertility and is the single most common cause of infertility in young women (Shafer et al., 1982; Westrom, 1980; Gates, 1984).

A confirmed diagnosis of salpingitis and a more accurate bacteriological diagnosis are made by laparoscopy. Since laparoscopy is not always available, the diagnosis of PID is often based on imprecise clinical findings and culture of specimens from the lower genital tract. Cultures of women with acute PID have recovered

N. gonorrhoeae from the endocervix from approximately 35% to 80% of cases and from a smaller proportion of samples of fallopian tube aspirates (Eschenbach et al., 1975).

Risk factors for PID and acute salpingitis include young age at acquisition of gonococcal disease, a history of previous PID, multiple sexual partners, and use of an intrauterine device (IUD) for contraception. Approximately 15% of teenagers who develop gonorrhea will progress to PID (Westrom, 1980).

Diagnosing PID may be difficult, and the differential diagnosis includes numerous other conditions of the lower abdomen, including appendicitis, ectopic pregnancy, cholecysitis, mesenteric adenitis, pyelonephritis, and septic abortion. Misdiagnosis of PID is common, and it is one of the more common causes of medically nonindicated laparotomy. As mentioned previously, laparoscopy assists in establishing a diagnosis. Recommendations by Shafer et al. (1982) suggest that a clinical diagnosis of PID be supported by presence of lower abdominal pain and tenderness, cervical motion tenderness, and adnexal tenderness. Fever, leukocytosis, elevated sedimentation rate, and adnexal mass observed through abdominal ultrasound support the diagnosis. Culdocentesis, if performed, may reveal evidence of purulent reaction in the peritoneal cavity. The outcome for fertility probably is improved with prompt and vigorous therapy. Indications for hospitalization for therapy of PID include the following:

1. All adolescents
2. Diagnostic uncertainty
3. Failure to respond to prior regimen
4. Pregnancy
5. Fever and peritoneal signs
6. Adnexal mass
7. IUD use
8. Noncompliance

Other complications such as meningitis, endocarditis, pericarditis, and, in adults, uveitis and liver abscesses are rare.

Treatment and prevention of salpingitis and pelvic inflammatory disease

Coinfection with both chlamydiae and gonococci is common in both children and adults. In female adolescents treatment of gonorrhea with drug regimens that are effective against gonococci but not chlamydiae has led to a high incidence of residual salpingitis and in males of urethritis, both associated with continued disease caused by chlamydia (Stamm et al., 1984). The detailed recommendations are contained in the "Sexually Transmitted Diseases Treatment Guidelines," published by the CDC as a supplement to the *Morbidity and Mortality Weekly Report*. The last edition was published in 1989, and the following recommendations are based on this edition. The preferred regimens for treatment of PID should include a drug effective against gonorrhea and against endogenous bacteria, including anaerobes, and a course of therapy for chlamydia. Regimens include cefoxitin or clindamycin and gentamicin plus a course of doxycycline. For children less than 8 years of age, erythromycin is substituted for the doxycycline. These regimens are effective in adolescent and adult women (Wasserheit et al., 1986; Wolner-Hanssen et al., 1986; Walters and Gibbs, 1990).

Follow-up. Follow-up urethral specimens should be obtained from males 7 days after treatment is completed, and cervical and rectal specimens should be obtained from females 7 to 14 days after treatment is completed.

SYPHILIS

Primary syphilis and secondary syphilis have again reached epidemic proportions in the United States. The incidence of 20 cases per 100,000 persons in 1990 was a 75% increase from 1985, the highest incidence since 1949. The number of babies with congenital syphilis is known to parallel closely the rates of primary and secondary syphilis among women of childbearing age. Indeed, the number of babies with congenital syphilis reported to the CDC has risen steadily from a low of 115 in 1978 to 2,889 in 1990 (CDC, 1990). In the past the number of reported cases of congenital syphilis was considered an underestimate of true disease (Rathbun, 1983). However, in 1988 the reporting definitions for congenital syphilis recommended by the CDC were changed (see definition in the box on p. 437). Therefore numbers of babies with congenital syphilis increased after 1988, partly because of the change in definition (Cohen et al., 1990) and partly from a true increase in numbers. Statistics after 1988, using the new definition, have continued to rise for the number of babies with congenital syphilis.

The epidemiology of syphilis has also changed recently. The rates of early syphilis have increased most for heterosexual minorities, predominantly blacks. One reason for this increase of syphilis has been the increases of crack/cocaine use among the urban poor, with an associated exchange of sex for drugs (CDC, 1988b). Unfortunately, because much of this sexual activity is anonymous, contact tracing and treatment of sexual partners, the usual methods of containing syphilis, have become increasingly difficult, undoubtedly impeding control of this disease.

Children of any age can have syphilis, which may be congenital or acquired. Physicians taking care of children should be aware of the signs and symptoms of acquired and congenital syphilis.

Bacteriology

Treponema pallidum is the causative agent of syphilis. It is a thin, delicate organism, varying in length from 5 to 15 μm, with a width of 0.15 μm, which means it is not visible by light microscopy. *T. pallidum* has tight spirals every 1.1 μm along its length, appearing like a helical coil (Hovind-Hougen, 1983). When seen through dark-field microscopy, it exhibits a spiral movement, with flexion around its midportion. The organism divides slowly, only every 30 hours, and cannot be cultured on artificial media. Tissue culture does not sustain the growth of *T. pallidum* for long periods (Jenkin and Sander, 1983), and inoculation into rabbits is the only reliable means for cultivating this organism. Humans are the only natural host, although several mammals (including rabbits and monkeys) can be infected.

Pathogenesis

The central problem in understanding the pathogenesis of syphilis is that, although there is a vigorous host response to infection, treated disease has a minimal effect on resistance to reinfection, and the infection may persist for life. The treponemes initially invade the body through microscopic abrasions produced by sexual intercourse. Approximately one third of people having sex with infected partners will become infected. The treponemes attach to the cells by one end, although no specialized receptor site has been seen on electron microscopy (Hovind-Hougen, 1983). Once inside the epi-

thelial layer, the organisms replicate locally. The host responds first with an influx of polymorphonuclear neutrophil leukocytes (PMNs). The *T. pallidum* undergoes rapid phagocytosis (Musher et al., 1983), probably because host IgG is present on the surface of the organism (Alderete and Baseman, 1979). Lymphocytes soon replace the PMNs (Baker-Zander and Sell, 1980).

By the time the patient comes to clinical attention, a variety of antibodies usually are detected. However, the occurrence of secondary syphilis at the same time that the antibody titers are their highest indicates that the host response to infection is not effective since the localized disease comes under control at the same time that the manifestations of generalized infection appear. However, at this time the host is immune to intradermal challenge with *T. pallidum* (Musher, 1984). The host eventually suppresses the infection, and there are no clinically apparent lesions, although the organism is not necessarily eradicated from the body since *T. pallidum* can be isolated from patients years after infection.

Acquired syphilis

Acquired syphilis in childhood appears to follow a course similar to that in adults. Although most recognized syphilitic disease of children is congenital, syphilis can be acquired at any age. Acquired syphilis in preadolescent children almost always represents the result of sexual abuse or assault, although sexually active adolescents may acquire the disease through consenting sexual activity.

Primary syphilis. Primary syphilis is characterized by a painless chancre that appears at the site of contact 10 to 90 days after exposure (average, 21 days). A chancre looks like a rounded, firm ulcer with a rubbery base and well-defined margins. The lesion is usually single and most commonly is found on the glans penis of the male and on the cervix or external genitalia of the female. It can also be found on the scrotum, anus, rectum, lips, tongue, tonsil, nipple, and fingers. Primary lesions in women often go unnoticed since they may not be visible. Chancres persist for 3 to 6 weeks, then heal spontaneously. They usually are accompanied by regional lymphadenopathy. The lymph nodes are painless, not fluctuant, not tender, rubbery in consistency, and often bilaterally enlarged with genital lesions.

The diagnosis of primary syphilis can be made definitively by a positive dark-field examination or a positive direct fluorescent antibody test for *T. pallidum* (DFA-TP). In addition, serological tests for syphilis should be performed. However, nontreponemal serological tests are positive in only approximately 80% of patients presenting with primary syphilis. The treponemal tests (eg., FTA-ABS) become positive earlier, with approximately 90% of patients initially seen with primary syphilis having positive tests (Duncan et al., 1974). Therefore, if primary syphilis is suspected, the laboratory should be instructed to perform the treponemal test even if the nontreponemal or reagin test, usually the VDRL, is nonreactive.

Secondary syphilis. The secondary manifestations usually appear 3 to 6 weeks after the appearance of the chancre and 6 weeks to several months after the initial contact. The primary lesion may still be evident or may have healed when the secondary lesions appear. Signs and symptoms commonly include local or generalized rash, generalized adenopathy, malaise, fever, headache, and pharyngitis. Less common manifestations are condylomata lata, mucous patches of the mouth, and alopecia. This is a systemic infection, and it is not unusual to find pleocytosis or increased protein in the cerebrospinal fluid (CSF) of patients with secondary syphilis. Lukehart et al. (1988) isolated *T. pallidum* from 10 (30%) of 33 patients with secondary syphilis, with four of these patients having normal CSF values. Therefore patients with central nervous system (CNS) involvement with *T. pallidum* can have normal CSF values. Nevertheless, it is neither routine nor recommended to perform lumbar punctures on patients with secondary syphilis since CNS involvement is so common it is considered a part of the disease.

The skin rash is usually macular or maculopapular and rarely pustular. The rose-pink rash spreads to involve the whole body, including palms and soles, and darkens to a dull red color; it is usually not pruritic. *T. pallidum* can be demonstrated in any mucous or cutaneous lesion but is found most easily in moist lesions. The diagnosis is usually made by serology during this stage, and serological tests are virtually always positive with high titers (>1:16). Secondary syphilitic manifestations usually resolve in 3 to 12 weeks.

Other conditions that may resemble primary and secondary syphilis include carcinoma, scabies, lichen planus, psoriasis, drug reactions, Behcet's syndrome, Reiter's syndrome, pityriasis rosea, and tinea versicolor.

Latent syphilis. After the secondary lesions resolve, the stage of latent syphilis begins. The latent stage is arbitrarily divided into early latency (syphilis of less than 1 year's duration), and late latency (syphilis of more than 1 year's duration). During early latency approximately 25% of patients with untreated syphilis will have relapses of secondary syphilis. Late latency is the stage during which tertiary manifestations can occur. By definition, latent syphilis is clinically inapparent, and the diagnosis is usually made by finding a positive serology in the absence of any primary or secondary symptoms. All untreated cases of syphilis are latent at some time during the course of the disease; indeed, the disease may be latent for the duration of the infection or the life of the patient. Approximately one third of infected untreated individuals will develop late syphilitic manifestations, with characteristic CNS, cardiovascular, or gummatous lesions. Approximately two thirds of untreated, infected individuals will not have any problems later, although more than half will remain serologically positive. However, these patients do have a shorter-than-normal life expectancy. Patients who have latent syphilis for more than 4 years are rarely contagious to their sexual partners, but pregnant women can transmit the disease to the fetus even after having latent syphilis for many years.

Late syphilis. Late syphilis is an uncommon entity in the postantibiotic era among adults and is extremely uncommon in children. Late syphilis is asymptomatic in the majority of people but may present as neurosyphilis, cardiovascular syphilis, or gummas. Gummas probably represent a hypersensitivity phenomenon. The other lesions of late syphilis are those of a vascular disease, with obliterative endarteritis of terminal arterioles and small arteries, which results in inflammatory and necrotic changes. Patients can have more than one late manifestation of syphilis.

Neurosyphilis. The essential pathological process of all types of neurosyphilis is obliterative endarteritis, usually of terminal vessels, with associated parenchymatous degeneration. Neurosyphilis may be divided into the following groups, depending on the type and degree of CNS pathological condition: asymptomatic; meningeal; meningovascular; and parenchymatous, consisting of paresis or tabes dorsalis.

Optic atrophy is a serious complication of neurosyphilis and is detected by examination of the peripheral visual fields. Pupillary changes may be seen in late neurosyphilis; the classic change is the Argyll Robertson pupil, which is small and irregular, fails to react to light, but responds normally to accommodation effort.

Asymptomatic neurosyphilis. The patient with asymptomatic neurosyphilis is usually seen because of a positive serology without signs or symptoms of CNS involvement. However, the CSF shows an increase in number of cells and total amount of protein and a reactive CSF VDRL for syphilis.

Meningeal neurosyphilis. Acute syphilitic meningitis usually appears within a year of infection as acute hydrocephalus, cranial nerve palsies, or focal cerebral involvement. The CSF shows pleocytosis, increased protein, and a positive CSF VDRL.

Meningovascular neurosyphilis. In patients with meningovascular neurosyphilis definite signs and symptoms of CNS damage are present, indicating cerebrovascular occlusion, infarction, and encephalomalacia with focal neurological signs, depending on the size and location of the lesion. The CSF is always abnormal, with pleocytosis, increase in amount of protein, and a reactive CSF VDRL.

Parenchymatous neurosyphilis. This form of neurosyphilis appears as paresis or tabes dorsalis. The manifestations of paresis can be myriad and are always indicative of widespread damage to the parenchyma. Personality changes range from minor ones to obvious psychosis. Focal neurological signs are uncommon. Results of the CSF studies are invariably abnormal; the number of cells and the concentration of protein are increased; and the CSF VDRL is positive.

Cardiovascular syphilis. The damage in patients with cardiovascular syphilis is caused by medial necrosis of the aorta, with aortic dilation often extending into the valve commissures. The essential signs are those of aortic insufficiency or saccular aneurysm of the thoracic aorta.

Syphilitic gummas. Gummas are nonspecific granulomatous-like lesions. They most commonly are found in skin or bone and less commonly in mucosae, viscera, and muscle. They are usually benign, although they may cause serious problems if located in vital areas.

Congenital syphilis

Congenital syphilis results from transplacental infection of the developing fetus from a mother with spirochetemia. An untreated syphilitic pregnant woman can transmit infection to the fetus at any clinical stage of her disease, although transmission is more likely with early infection. Fiumara et al. (1952) found that 50% of mothers with untreated primary or secondary syphilis had babies with congenital syphilis. The transmission to the fetus declined to 40% in early latent syphilis and 10% in late latent syphilis. Stillbirth is a frequent outcome of untreated syphilitic pregnancies. Wendel (1988) found that one half of babies with congenital syphilis were stillborn. However, evidence of fetal damage such as abortion is rare before the eighteenth week of gestation. Pathological examination of tissues obtained from therapeutic abortions before 12 weeks of gestation have shown that treponemal organisms were present in fetuses from mothers who had untreated syphilis (Harter and Benirschke, 1976). No inflammatory response has been seen unless gestation was 15 weeks or more in duration. Fetal immunoimmaturity and the inability to recognize *T. pallidum* antigens are probably responsible for the lack of damage caused by syphilis in fetuses less than 18 weeks' gestation.

Babies have congenital syphilis usually because of lack of prenatal care in the mother (Mascola et al., 1984). This is a preventable disease if the mother receives appropriate therapy early in pregnancy. However, treatment does not guarantee that the baby will not be infected, particularly if therapy is given late in pregnancy (Mascola et al., 1984). A woman who has been adequately treated with penicillin and followed with quantitative serology and has no evidence of reinfection does not need retreatment with each subsequent pregnancy. However, if any doubt exists about the adequacy of previous treatment or the presence of active infection, a course of treatment should be given to prevent congenital syphilis. Women who have been treated for syphilis in the past may become reinfected, and their babies can develop congenital syphilis.

The signs and symptoms of congenital syphilis are divided arbitrarily into early manifestations, which appear in the first 2 years of life, and late manifestations, which emerge anytime thereafter. The outcome of untreated fetal infection is variable. Intrauterine death (stillbirth) occurs in an estimated 25% to 50% of infections. Historically, perinatal death may occur in another 25% to 30% of untreated infected babies, although perinatal death is less common now since many deaths in the past were due to prematurity (Wendel, 1988). Those infants who survive have a broad spectrum of manifestations.

Early congenital syphilis. The abnormal physical and laboratory findings in patients with early congenital syphilis are varied. The onset may be before birth to approximately 3 months of age, with most cases occurring within the first 5 weeks of age. Some babies are so severely infected that they are stillborn, and some die in the early neonatal period despite the use of antibiotics. However, not all babies become symptomatic. A baby with congenital syphilis may appear normal at birth only to appear later with multi-organ system involvement (Taber and Huber, 1975). Some neonates have only hepatosplenomegaly, with or without jaundice, and some are totally asymptomatic but have evidence of bone involvement on roentgenograms or abnormal lumbar puncture results. Since most congenital syphilis is now discovered during the newborn hospital stay because of suspicion raised by positive serology in the mother or baby, the current presentation of congenital syphilis is a little different than that described formerly in the literature (Fiumara, 1975). More babies who are asymptomatic but have abnormal tests indicative of infection are found. In the past these infants probably would have presented later with symptoms.

Skeletal system. The roentgenographic changes in the bones are of diagnostic value because of their frequency and early appearance. They are present in approximately 50% to 95% of babies with congenital syphilis (Hira et al., 1985). The changes often are present at birth but may not appear until the first few weeks of life. The bony changes include osteochondritis and periostitis; metaphyseal changes are most common. The findings are symmetrical and self-limited and heal in approximately 6 months, with or without therapy. The skeletal lesions are usually asymptomatic but are occasionally painful, so much so that the child will refuse to move the affected limb (pseudoparalysis of Parrot).

The femur and tibia are most often involved, and an x-ray study of the knee is recommended when screening for syphilis. On x-ray films the earliest changes are revealed in the metaphysis and are seen as transverse, saw-tooth, radiodense bands of provisional calcification, with an underlying zone of osteoporosis, which is seen as radiolucent bands. Irregular areas of increased density and rarefaction produce the moth-eaten appearance of the x-ray film. The classic Wimberger's sign consists of a focal defect in the medial proximal tibial epiphysis and is caused by destructive osteitis. Periostitis appears later than osteochondritis and is seen on x-ray films as multiple layers of periosteal new bone formation. X-ray findings in patients with congenital syphilis are shown in Figs. 25-1, 25-2, and 25-3.

Rhinitis. Rhinitis was a common manifestation historically but is uncommon now. It is not usually present at birth but appears after the first week of life. It initially is seen as severe and intractable rhinorrhea, which is often bloody and may be associated with a hoarse cry caused by laryngitis.

Rash. Historically, the syphilitic rash typically appeared 1 or 2 weeks after the rhinitis, but it is more common now to see the rash without preceding rhinitis. The typical eruption is maculopapular and consists of small, dark-red spots, but bullous eruptions can also occur. The rash commonly is present on the back, perineum, extremities, palms, and soles. The rash lasts 1 to 3 months without treatment, and the lesions may be covered by a fine, silvery scale and be followed by desquamation. The rash usually fades to leave coppery residual pigmentation.

Constitutional symptoms. The most common finding with early congenital syphilis is hepatosplenomegaly. Jaundice may be associated with it because of hepatic dysfunction, which is manifest by an increase in conjugated bilirubin (Srinivasan et al., 1983). Generalized lymphadenopathy may occur, although it is more com-

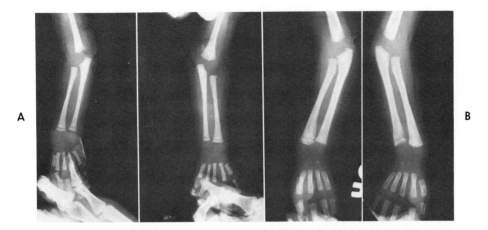

Fig. 25-1. Congenital syphilis. **A,** Typical wide horizontal metaphyseal radiolucent bands. **B,** Destructive syphilitic metaphysitis of the radius and ulna in a 6-week-old infant. Note subperiosteal reaction.

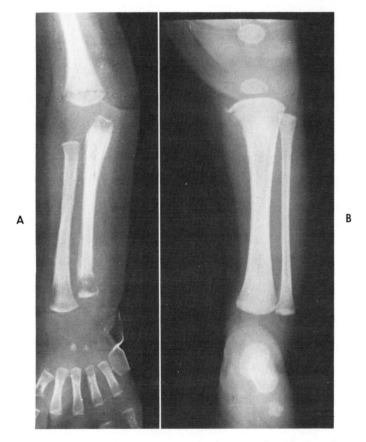

Fig. 25-2. Congenital syphilis. **A,** Panosteitis in an infant 9 weeks old. Metaphysitis is present and subperiosteal bone is appearing. **B,** Radiolucent area of the medial aspect of the proximal tibial metaphyses. This is called *Wimberger's sign*.

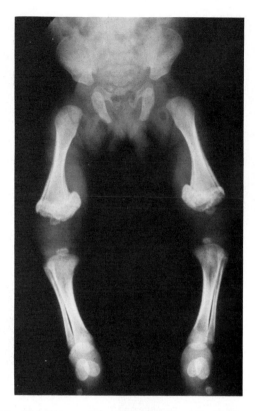

Fig. 25-3. Congenital syphilis. Diaphysitis with abundant callus formation secondary to pathological fractures through the metaphyseal lesions. The lesions healed, and there were no sequelae.

mon in historical cases. Infants may have fevers and occasionally nephrosis or nephritis. Choroiditis and iritis are uncommon.

The laboratory findings include a Coombs-negative hemolytic anemia with leukopenia or leukocytosis and thrombocytopenia. Congenital syphilis is one of the causes of a leukemoid reaction. Lumbar puncture may reveal a positive CSF VDRL, with increased protein and pleocytosis, although most babies clinically have no findings of CNS involvement. Sanchez et al., (1991) recently described five infants with congenital syphilis, four of whom had *T. pallidum* recovered from the CSF by rabbit infectivity tests. Three of the babies had a positive CSF VDRL, but one asymptomatic baby had normal CSF findings, although *T. pallidum* had been recovered from the CSF.

The congenital syphilis of neonates and infants may resemble other intrauterine infections, including toxoplasmosis, rubella, cytomegalovirus, and herpes simplex virus. Other conditions

that may resemble congenital syphilis in newborns include bacterial sepsis, blood group incompatibility, battered child syndrome, "periostitis" of prematurity, neonatal hepatitis, and osteomyelitis.

The placenta is a useful organ to examine when looking for congenital syphilis. The presence of necrotizing funisitis suggests congenital syphilis (Fojaco et al., 1989). The placenta may also be large and bulky and have the characteristic findings of focal villitis, endovascular and perivascular proliferation of vessels, and relative immaturity of villi (Russell and Altshuler, 1974). *T. pallidum* seen in tissue specimens confirms the diagnosis of congenital syphilis.

Late congenital syphilis. Late manifestations of congenital syphilis are the result of scarring from the early systemic disease and include involvement of the teeth, bones, eyes, and eighth nerve (Fiumara and Lessell, 1983); gummas in the viscera, skin, or mucous membranes; and neurosyphilis. Late syphilis is very rare nowadays.

Teeth. Characteristic changes are found in the permanent upper-central incisors, which present a notched appearance of the biting edges; these are called *Hutchinson's teeth*. First molars with maldevelopment of the cusps are known as *mulberry* or *Moon's molars* (Figs. 25-4 and 25-5).

Interstitial keratitis. Interstitial keratitis is the most common late lesion. It may appear at any age between 4 and 30 years or later, but characteristically it appears when the patient is close to puberty. It first is seen as unilateral photophobia, pain, and blurred vision. A ground-glass appearance may develop in the cornea, accompanied by vascularization of the adjacent sclera. These changes become bilateral and lead to blindness. Penicillin treatment is ineffective, but steroid treatment can help prevent loss of vision.

Eighth nerve deafness. Hearing loss is usually sudden and appears around 8 to 10 years of age. Hutchinson's triad consists of interstitial keratitis accompanied by neural deafness and typical Hutchinson's teeth.

Neurosyphilis. The same manifestations of neurosyphilis seen in patients with acquired syphilis can occur in those with congenital syphilis, although symptomatic neurosyphilis is very rare. Paresis is seen more frequently and tabes

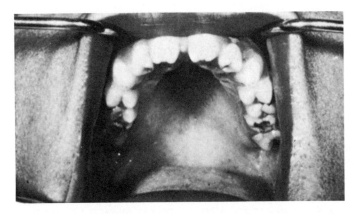

Fig. 25-4. Hutchinson's teeth. Note the notched edges and screwdriver shape of the central incisors.

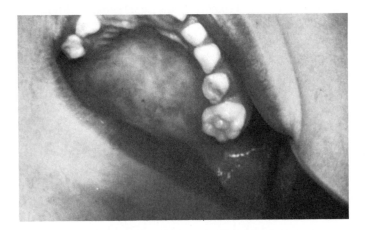

Fig. 25-5. Mulberry or Moon's molar.

dorsalis less frequently in the congenital form than in the acquired form of the disease.

Bone changes. Bone changes include sclerosing lesions, saber shins, frontal bossing, and the gummatous or destructive lesion of saddle nose. Perforation of the hard palate is almost pathognomonic of congenital syphilis.

Clutton's joint. Clutton's joint is painless arthritis of the knees and, rarely, other joints. It usually is first seen around puberty.

Cutaneous lesions. Rhagades represent scarring from persistent rhinitis during infancy and are rarely seen today.

Laboratory procedures in the diagnosis of syphilis

There are two main ways of diagnosing syphilis. The first is to detect treponemes, using dark-field or immunofluorescent methods. The second is to detect antibodies formed in response to a treponemal infection, using nontreponemal and treponemal antibody tests.

Detection of T. pallidum

Dark-field examination. The diagnosis of syphilis can be made by a positive dark-field examination of appropriate specimens. This test requires a compound microscope equipped with a dark-field condenser with which the specimen is illuminated by reflected light against a dark background. A positive diagnosis can be made by an experienced worker on the basis of characteristic morphological aspects and motility.

Dark-field examination is most productive during primary, secondary, and early congenital syphilis when lesions are present. Gloves should be worn when examining suspected syphilitic lesions and when performing dark-field examinations. Lesions should be cleaned thoroughly with physiological saline solution with no additives. The lesion should then be squeezed and scraped firmly to collect serum rather than blood. Aspirated material from involved regional lymph nodes also can be examined for *T. pallidum*. The specimen must be viewed within 5 to 10 minutes to detect motile treponemes. If the result of the initial dark-field examination is negative, it should be repeated on at least 2 successive days to confirm a negative result.

Immunofluorescent antigen detection. Alternative methods to detect *T. pallidum* in lesions are direct and indirect fluorescent antibody tests for *T. pallidum*. These tests use either monoclonal or polyclonal antibodies against *T. pallidum* that are directly fluorescein tagged or use a second fluorescein-tagged antibody to detect the antigen-antibody complex (Yobs et al., 1964). The advantage of this method is that slides are more permanent and can be mailed to reference laboratories for review by experts if the volume of patients seen is too small to warrant having a dark-field microscope.

Serological tests. The serological diagnosis of syphilis uses two general types of tests: reaginic and treponemal.

Reaginic tests. The reaginic tests use cardiolipin and lecithin as antigen. The antibody measured has been termed *reagin,* which has no relationship to the reaginic IgE in allergic patients. Antibody appears in the blood 1 to 3 weeks after the chancre appears or approximately 4 to 6 weeks after the infection.

The reaginic tests commonly used today are the VDRL test, rapid plasma reagin (RPR) test, and automated reagin (ART). The RPR test and ART use a modified VDRL antigen. These two tests are very useful when large numbers of sera are screened and speed is essential. The tests are inexpensive, can be well controlled, and are quantitated. The height of the titer tends to correlate with disease activity, rising with new infection and falling after treatment. A change of one doubling dilution is within laboratory error and therefore not significant. Changes of two dilutions (fourfold changes) are considered significant when assessing disease activity. However, these tests are not specific for syphilis and may also be reactive in patients with collagen-vascular disease, liver disease, and other conditions.

A positive serology will be found in approximately 80% of patients with primary syphilis, in 100% of patients with secondary syphilis, in 95% of those with early latent syphilis, but in only 70% of patients with late latent or late (tertiary) syphilis (Sparling, 1971). Thus false-negative serology using reaginic tests is a problem in very early and again in later stages of untreated syphilis.

With adequate treatment, the reaginic tests should become nonreactive 6 to 12 months after primary syphilis and 12 to 24 months after secondary syphilis (Fiumara, 1980). Patients with later stages of syphilis who are treated take longer for their titers to fall and may never revert to nonreactive on nontreponemal tests; thus they may remain with low titers for life or "serofast."

Treponemal tests. The fluorescent treponemal antibody absorption (FTA-ABS) test is an indirect antibody test that uses *T. pallidum* as the antigen. The FTA-ABS test is quite sensitive and specific (Deacon et al., 1966). It is technically more difficult than the nontreponemal tests and is used for confirmation of positive nontreponemal tests. The results of this test are reported as positive or negative, and they are not quantitated. The treponemal tests become reactive earlier in primary syphilis than do nontreponemal tests and once positive, normally remain so for life, even after appropriate therapy.

The microhemagglutination assay for antibodies to *T. pallidum* (MHA-TP) is a qualitative hemagglutination test that uses sheep erythrocytes as carriers for the *T. pallidum* antigen. False-positive tests are very uncommon with both FTA-ABS and MHA-TP. However, patients with lupus may have false-positive FTA-ABS, MHA-TP, and nontreponemal tests.

Another treponemal test, the *Treponema pallidum* immobilization (TPI) test, has been used in the past but is presently available for research purposes only. The test uses live *T. pallidum* and complement; when serum containing specific antibody is present, the *T. pallidum* is immobilized.

IgM tests. *T. pallidum* IgM tests are useful in diagnosing congenital syphilis since, unlike IgG, IgM does not cross the placenta. Therefore detection of specific IgM in a baby is a strong indication of infection. There are various kinds of *T. pallidum* IgM tests, but none is widely available. The original *T. pallidum* IgM test described by Scotti and Logan (1968) had too many false-positive (10%) and false-negative (up to 35%) results for widespread clinical use (Kaufman et al., 1974). A newer IgM-FTA test is performed by the CDC, although its usefulness has not been evaluated fully. Western blot tests have been used for research purposes and apparently are sensitive and specific for evaluating babies with congenital syphilis, although only small numbers of babies have been evaluated using this technique (Sanchez et al., 1989). None of these IgM tests will detect all babies with syphilis since some babies are so recently infected that they have no IgM present at delivery. Antigen detection tests may be more useful in identifying them.

Diagnosis of congenital syphilis

The diagnosis of congenital syphilis in the newborn period can be difficult. Both the nontreponemal and treponemal tests measure IgG antibody and therefore do not distinguish disease in the infant from maternally derived antibody. The minority of babies with congenital syphilis are symptomatic at birth. Although some infants will develop symptoms later if left untreated, some may never become symptomatic. Unfortunately, there is no "gold standard" test for congenital syphilis. A combination of physical findings, x-ray results, laboratory tests, and ancillary tests is used to screen for and diagnose congenital syphilis. In the past clinicians waited for the development of symptoms, but in present-day practice this is unwise because of the high probability of losing the patient to follow-up. In the diagnosis of congenital syphilis, therefore, it is best to err on the side of overdiagnosis and overtreatment (see the 1989 CDC guidelines for the diagnosis of congenital syphilis in the box on p. 437). The 1989 CDC guidelines recommend that infants should be evaluated for congenital syphilis if they are born to mothers with positive nontreponemal and treponemal tests and the mothers fit any of the following criteria:

1. Have untreated syphilis
2. Were treated for syphilis less than 1 month before delivery
3. Were treated for syphilis during pregnancy with a nonpenicillin regimen (e.g., erythromycin)
4. Did not have the expected decrease in nontreponemal titers after treatment of syphilis (fourfold decline by 3 months with primary or secondary syphilis or by 6 months in early latent syphilis)
5. Did not have a well-documented history of treatment for syphilis
6. Were treated but had insufficient serological follow-up during pregnancy to assess disease activity

It is also recommended that an infant not be released from the hospital until the serological status of its mother is known because one third of babies born to mothers with positive serology have nonreactive cord blood serology (Miller et al., 1960). Therefore maternal serology is preferred over cord blood serology in screening for congenital syphilis at delivery.

Infants whose mothers fit the criteria listed above should be evaluated with a physical examination, looking for evidence of congenital syphilis. They should have a nontreponemal antibody titer evaluation and a lumbar puncture, with analysis for CSF VDRL, cells, and protein. They should also have long-bone x-ray studies performed. Roentgenograms of the knee are preferred for screening. Treponemal IgM tests should be performed if available. Although not specifically recommended by the CDC, a complete blood count and a serum alanine aminotransferase (ALT) level to screen for hepatitis are useful when trying to determine if infection is present in an asymptomatic baby.

Treatment

T. pallidum is exquisitely sensitive to penicillin with an MIC of 0.005 to 0.01 µg/ml as defined by rabbit experimentation (Eagle et al., 1950). Effective therapy of syphilis has been aimed at maintaining an MIC of 0.03 units/ml (0.018 µg/ml) for 7 to 10 days (Idsoe et al., 1972) because of the slow dividing time of *T. pallidum* (every 30 hours). Thus therapy is designed to achieve and maintain several times the necessary inhibitory levels. Penicillin remains the drug of choice because there is no evidence of resistance of *T. pallidum* to penicillin, and it has minimal toxicity and established efficacy in treating syphilis.

Congenital syphilis

Who should be treated. The decision to treat rests on the results of the evaluation described previously. Infants diagnosed with either confirmed or presumptive congenital syphilis (see

SURVEILLANCE CASE DEFINITION FOR CONGENITAL SYPHILIS

For reporting purposes, congenital syphilis includes cases of congenitally acquired syphilis in infants and children, as well as syphilitic stillbirths.

A CONFIRMED CASE of congenital syphilis is an infant in whom *Treponema pallidum* is identified by darkfield microscopy, fluorescent antibody, or other specific stains in specimens from lesions, placenta, umbilical cord, or autopsy material.

A PRESUMPTIVE CASE of congenital syphilis is either of the following:

A. Any infant whose mother had untreated or inadequately treated* syphilis at delivery, regardless of findings in the infant;

OR

B. Any infant or child who has a reactive treponemal test for syphilis and any one of the following:

1. Any evidence of congenital syphilis on physical examination†; or
2. Any evidence of congenital syphilis on long-bone radiograph; or
3. Reactive cerebrospinal fluid (CSF) VDRL‡; or
4. Elevated CSF cell count or protein (without other cause)‡; or
5. Quantitative nontreponemal serologic titers which are fourfold higher than the mother's (both drawn at birth); or
6. Reactive test for FTA-ABS-19S-IgM antibody.‡

A SYPHILITIC STILLBIRTH is defined as a fetal death in which the mother had untreated or inadequately treated syphilis at delivery of a fetus after a 20-week gestation or of a fetus weighing >500 g.

From MMWR 1989;38:828.

*Inadequate treatment consists of any nonpenicillin therapy or penicillin given <30 days prior to delivery.

†Signs in an infant (<2 years of age) may include hepatosplenomegaly, characteristic skin rash, condyloma lata, snuffles, jaundice (syphilitic hepatitis), pseudoparalysis, or edema (nephrotic syndrome). Stigmata in an older child may include: interstitial keratitis, nerve deafness, anterior bowing of shins, frontal bossing, mulberry molars, Hutchinson's teeth, saddle nose, rhagades, or Clutton's joints.

‡It may be difficult to distinguish between congenital and acquired syphilis in a seropositive child after infancy. Signs may not be obvious and stigmata may not yet have developed. Abnormal values for CSF VDRL, cell count, and protein, as well as IgM antibodies, may be found in either congenital or acquired syphilis. Findings on long-bone radiographs may help, since these would indicate congenital syphilis. The decision may ultimately be based on maternal history and clinical judgment; the possibility of sexual abuse also needs to be considered.

---

definitions in box above should be treated. Even when the diagnosis is "normal," babies should be treated if their mothers had untreated syphilis at delivery or have evidence of relapse or reinfection after treatment, as shown by a rising nontreponemal titer or a titer that has not fallen within an appropriate time. If the infants do not undergo a full evaluation, it is recommended they be treated as if they had congenital syphilis.

How they should be treated. Treatment of congenital syphilis is the same regardless of whether there are CSF abnormalities or not since patients can have neurosyphilis and normal CSF values. Treatment should be with aqueous crystalline penicillin G (50,000 units/kg/dose) administered every 8 to 12 hours (100,000 to 150,000 units/kg/day). This dose is increased compared with previous recommendations. An alternative,

which perhaps is preferable because of its ease of administration, is procaine penicillin (50,000 units/kg/day), given as one intramuscular dose daily (McCracken and Kaplan, 1974). The length of therapy for both regimens is 10 to 14 days. If more than 1 day of therapy is missed, the entire therapy should be restarted.

There is a small group of infants who are at low risk of infection but who should receive therapy if their follow-up cannot be assured. Babies who fit the criteria for evaluation but do not fit the criteria for congenital syphilis should be treated if they cannot be followed. For these babies one dose of benzathine penicillin G (50,000 units/kg) is recommended by the CDC. Some experts, however, do not like to use benzathine penicillin G in babies with congenital syphilis since CSF levels are subtherapeutic (Speer et al., 1977) and treatment failures, although not common, have been documented (Beck-Sague and Alexander, 1987). If follow-up of these patients is a problem, they should be treated with procaine penicillin for 10 days.

Treatment beyond the newborn period. After the newborn period, all children with syphilis should have a lumbar puncture performed. Any child who is thought to have congenital syphilis or who has neurological involvement should be treated with aqueous crystalline penicillin G (50,000 units/kg/dose) every 4 to 6 hours for 10 to 14 days. Older children with acquired syphilis and normal neurological results may be treated with benzathine penicillin G (50,000 units/kg IM) up to the adult dose of 2.4 million units. If the child has latent syphilis of unknown duration, three doses of benzathine penicillin (50,000 units/kg/dose [maximum 2.4 million units per dose]) at weekly intervals should be given. Penicillin is the only recommended treatment for children with syphilis; therefore if there is a history of penicillin allergy, children should be skin tested and desensitized if necessary (Zenker and Rolfs, 1990).

Adolescents with syphilis. Adolescents with syphilis should be treated similarly to adults with the same stage of disease. Primary, secondary, and early latent syphilis of less than 1 year's duration should be treated with benzathine penicillin G (50,000 units/kg), with a maximum of 2.4 million units IM in one dose. Alternative regimen for penicillin-allergic patients is doxycycline (100 mg orally twice a day for 2 weeks).

Adolescents with late latent syphilis of more than 1 year's duration should be treated with benzathine penicillin G (150,000 units/kg total, with a maximum of 7.2 million units total) administered as three doses of 50,000 units/kg IM (maximum of 2.4 million units) given 1 week apart for 3 consecutive weeks. Alternative therapy for penicillin-allergic patients is doxycycline in the same doses used for patients with early syphilis but given for 4 weeks instead of 2 weeks.

Neurosyphilis. Recommended treatment for neurosyphilis in adults is aqueous penicillin G, 2 to 4 million units every 4 hours intravenously (12 to 24 million units per day) for 10 to 14 days. Alternative therapy is procaine penicillin (2 to 4 million units IM daily) with probenicid (500 mg orally four times a day) for 10 to 14 days. Many experts also recommend benzathine pen-

icillin G (2.4 million units IM weekly for three doses) after finishing either of the above treatment regimens.

Jarisch-Herxheimer reaction

Jarisch-Herxheimer reaction is an acute febrile reaction that may occur after any therapy for syphilis. The reaction consists of a fever, which is usually accompanied by headache and myalgia, that commonly lasts less than 24 hours. Pregnant women may have associated contractions and should be warned about this possibility. There is no treatment recommended except for antipyretics if necessary.

Follow-up

Infants with congenital syphilis should be followed with serological tests at 3, 6, and 12 months of age. If the baby did not receive therapy, follow-up should also include serology at 1 and 2 months to assure that titers are falling. Nontreponemal titers usually disappear by 6 months of age in the absence of infection. If titers are stable or increasing, the child should be reevaluated and retreated. Treponemal titers are usually negative by 1 year of age in the absence of infection. If the treponemal titers are still positive at 12 months, this is strong evidence that the child was truly infected with syphilis. If the child received adequate therapy in the newborn period and the nontreponemal titer is nonreactive, the child does not need retreatment. Infants who were never treated for congenital syphilis should be evaluated, including performance of a lumbar puncture, and treated. Lumbar punctures should be repeated every 6 months for 3 years or until the CSF examination is normal in infants with a positive CSF VDRL in the newborn period.

Syphilis and HIV disease

There have been reports of adult patients with neurosyphilis and HIV disease and of one case of a patient with secondary syphilis who had a nonreactive VDRL test result on several occasions before the result became positive. Musher et al. (1990) found that HIV coinfection with syphilis has caused the following: failure to respond to treatment within the expected time; relapse after treatment; and the frequent appearance of early neurosyphilis, especially after conventional doses of benzathine penicillin.

There have been no documented treatment failures among either pregnant women who are HIV positive with syphilis or their offspring. At this time, the CDC recommends no change in therapy for patients with early syphilis in HIV-infected patients, although some experts have recommended CSF examination and treatment appropriate for neurosyphilis for all patients with HIV and syphilis (Musher, 1990). Recommended penicillin regimens do not always attain treponemicidal CSF levels (Dunlop et al., 1979; Frenz et al., 1984), although most patients do well with these regimens. These patients should be followed very closely for signs of treatment failure. Any patient with syphilis should have HIV testing because both of these diseases may be present in the same patient.

Syphilis and sexual abuse

Syphilis is not commonly found among sexually abused children (see Table 25-1). However, it has been reported in a few instances. White et al. (1983) detected six cases among 108 of 409 prepubertal children on whom serological tests were performed. Five children were asymptomatic and had additional sexually transmitted disease, and only one was symptomatic with chancres. De Jong (1986) found only one out of 532 abused children had a positive serological test for syphilis. Children are seen with the same signs and symptoms as adults with syphilis. Ginsberg (1983) described three patients with acquired syphilis, one of whom was initially seen with a primary chancre and two with rashes of secondary syphilis. Similar findings have been described by Ackerman et al. (1972), who observed three abused children first seen with rashes of condylomata lata of secondary syphilis. It is recommended that a serological test for syphilis be performed on every child suspected of being sexually abused and that the test also be repeated after 12 weeks.

CHLAMYDIA TRACHOMATIS

The genus *Chlamydia* comprises a group of obligate intracellular parasites with a unique developmental cycle with morphologically distinct infectious and reproductive forms. All members of the genus have a gram-negative envelope without peptidoglycan, share a genus-specific lipopolysaccharide antigen, and use host adenosine triphosphate (ATP) for the synthesis of chlamydial protein. The genus now contains three species, *Chlamydia trachomatis*, *C. psittaci*, and the recently described *C. pneumoniae* (TWAR strain). There are 15 known serotypes of *C. trachomatis* (Table 25-2).

The chlamydial developmental cycle involves an infectious, metabolically inactive extracellular form (elementary body [EB]) and a noninfectious, metabolically active intracellular form (reticulate body) (Fig. 25-6). EBs, 200 to 400 nm in diameter, attach to the host cell by a process of electrostatic binding and are taken into the cell by endocytosis that is not dependent on the

Table 25-2. Serovars of *Chlamydia trachomatis*

Serovar	Disease
A, B, Ba, C	Hyperendemic blinding trachoma
D, E, F, G, H, I, J, K	Neonatal inclusion conjunctivitis
	Infantile pneumonitis
	Nongonococcal urethritis
	Mucopurulent cervicitis and salpingitis
	Proctitis
	Epididymitis
L1, L2, L3	Lymphogranuloma venereum

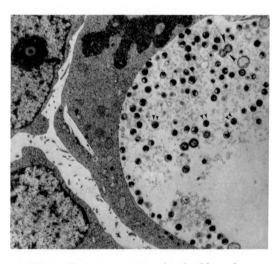

Fig. 25-6. Electron micrograph of *Chlamydia trachomatis* inclusions at 48 hours, demonstrating reticulate body undergoing binary fission (*arrows*) and elementary bodies (*double arrows*).

microtubule system. Within the host cell, the EB remains within a membrane-lined phagosome. Fusion of the phagosome with the host cell lysosome does not occur. The EBs then differentiate into reticulate bodies that undergo binary fission. After approximately 36 hours, the reticulate bodies differentiate into EBs. At approximately 48 hours, release may occur by cytoloysis or by a process of exocytosis or extrusion of the whole inclusion, leaving the host cell intact. Thus there is a biological basis for the prolonged subclinical infection, which is a hallmark of human chlamydial disease. Because the organisms are obligate intracellular parasites, they are actively infecting cells rather than simple colonizers, which have no interaction with the host cells.

C. trachomatis is probably the most prevalent sexually transmitted infection in the United States today. The CDC estimates that the number of new *C. trachomatis* infections exceeds 4 million annually. The prevalence of chlamydial infection is more weakly associated with socioeconomic status, urban or rural residence, and race or ethnicity than gonorrhea and syphilis. Prevalences of *C. trachomatis* infection are consistently greater than 5% among sexually active, adolescent, young adult women attending outpatient clinics, regardless of the region of the country, location of the clinic (urban or rural),

or the race or ethnicity of the population (Table 25-3). Prevalences commonly exceed 10%. Decreasing age at first intercourse and increasing age of marriage have contributed much to the higher prevalence of *C. trachomatis* infection. Infection with *C. trachomatis* is usually asymptomatic and of long duration. If a pregnant woman has active infection during delivery, the infant can acquire the infection and is at risk to develop either conjunctivitis or pneumonia (Alexander and Harrison, 1983). Rarely, children acquire chlamydial infection as a result of sexual abuse.

Infections in adolescents and adult males

C. trachomatis is the single most frequently identifiable cause of nongonococcal urethritis in men, accounting for 30% to 40% of all episodes, or 1.5 million episodes annually. The usual incubation period is 5 to 10 days. Nongonococcal urethritis generally causes less dysuria and less profuse, less purulent urethral exudate than gonorrhea. However, in the individual patient it may be difficult to differentiate between chlamydial and gonococcal infection (Chacko and Lovchik, 1984). Most men develop symptoms after *C. trachomatis* infection, but a large proportion may have prolonged, clinically inapparent infection. The presence of four or more PMNs per high-power field (hpf) on a Gram stain

Table 25-3. Studies on prevalence of STDs in adolescents

Study (date)	Location	Infection	Sex	Number infected (%)
Chacko and Lovchik (1984)	Baltimore	*C. trachomatis*	M	35
			F	23
Golden et al. (1984)	Brooklyn	*C. trachomatis*	F	10.2
		Gonorrhea	F	9.7
		Syphilis	F	3
Saltz et al. (1981)	Cincinnati	*C. trachomatis*	F	22
		Gonorrhea	F	3
Fraser et al. (1982)	Oklahoma City	*C. trachomatis*	F	8
		Gonorrhea	F	12
Fisher et al. (1987)	Suburban New York City	*C. trachomatis*	F	14.5
Chambers et al. (1987)	San Francisco	*C. trachomatis*	M	30
		Gonorrhea	M	4
Blythe et al. (1988)	Indianapolis	*C. trachomatis*	F	25
		Gonorrhea	F	5.5
Moscicki et al. (1990)	San Francisco	*C. trachomatis*	F	8
		HPV	F	18

of an intraurethral smear or more than 15 PMNs per hpf in the sediment of a first-voided urine specimen is evidence of urethritis even in the absence of frank discharge (Chambers et al., 1987).

C. trachomatis can also cause proctitis among homosexual men. If the infection is due to a lymphogranuloma venereum strain, the individual may develop proctocolitis that is difficult to differentiate from Crohn's disease both clinically and histopathologically.

C. trachomatis can also cause epididymitis in young men. It has been estimated that one diagnosed case of epididymitis caused by *C. trachomatis* occurs for every 18 diagnosed episodes of uncomplicated chlamydia-related urethritis in men aged 15 to 34 years. Overall, *C. trachomatis* causes 50% of epididymitis among men 15 to 34 years of age (Hammerschlag, 1989).

Infections in adolescent and adult females

Nonpregnant women. Most cervical infections with *C. trachomatis* in women are asymptomatic and of long duration (Eagar et al., 1985). Sexually active adolescent women have one of the highest reported rates of chlamydial infection, often exceeding 10% to 15%. Although *C. trachomatis* has been associated with mucopurulent cervicitis, the majority of women will have no specific physical clinical findings.

Among the many possible complications of chlamydial infection, the most important in female patients is acute salpingitis. Several studies and histopathological reports from Scandinavia indicate a very strong causal association between *C. trachomatis* and salpingitis (Mardh, 1980). Later clinical and animal studies from the United States, using aggressive culture methods, including cultures from the fallopian tubes, have confirmed the European experience (Patton, 1985; Bowie and Jones, 1981; Wasserheit et al., 1986). The organism is probably responsible for at least 20% of salpingitis cases in the United States. Studies from Sweden and the United States indicate that approximately one in four patients admitted to the hospital with acute salpingitis has upper genital tract infection with *C. trachomatis*, confirmed by isolation of the organism from the fallopian tubes. The presence of *C. trachomatis* in the cervix of a woman with PID does not necessarily imply that the organism will be present in the tubes, but it is very suggestive. Investigators from Sweden found that 19 of 53 women with salpingitis had cervical chlamydial infection and that of those who had cervical infection and laparoscopy, six of seven grew *C. trachomatis* from the fallopian tubes (Mardh, 1980). Why ascending infection develops in some women with cervical infection is not known. Salpingitis is 10 times more likely to occur in a sexually active 15-year-old girl than in a sexually active 25-year-old woman (Westrom, 1980).

In addition to being more prevalent than gonococcal infections, chlamydial salpingitis apparently has a more severe clinical outcome. Compared with patients with gonococcal salpingitis or non-chlamydial, nongonococcal salpingitis, patients with chlamydial salpingitis have a less acute presentation, are less often febrile, have a longer history of symptoms, have a higher erythrocyte sedimentation rate, and have more tubal inflammation (Cromer and Heald, 1987). In addition, chlamydial salpingitis is more likely to lead to infertility. Infertility rates of 13% after one episode of salpingitis, 36% after two episodes, and 75% after three or more episodes have been reported (Westrom, 1980). Case-control studies have documented a consistent association between high titers of antibody to *C. trachomatis* and tubal obstruction (Westrom, 1980; Brunham et al., 1986). Studies in animals have shown that *C. trachomatis* infects and subsequently destroys the tubal mucosa (Patton, 1985). A similar microscopic and pathological appearance of the tubes has been found in several patients from whom *C. trachomatis* was isolated. This pattern of repeated infections leading to fibrosis and eventual scarring is also seen in another human chlamydial infection, trachoma.

Another serious complication of chlamydial salpingitis is an increased risk of ectopic pregnancy, which is related directly to the oviduct damage. Many women who have had an ectopic pregnancy give no history of PID, but over 20% have histopathological and serological evidence of chlamydial infection (Brunham et al., 1986).

Pregnant women. In the United States the prevalence of *C. trachomatis* infection in pregnant women ranges from a low of 2% to more than 30%, depending on the population studied (Hammerschlag, 1989). Chlamydial infection during pregnancy has been inconstantly linked to prematurity. The overall relationship, when found, has been weak, and the mechanism is not understood (Harrison et al., 1983). Late (72 + hours) endometritis occurs consistently in 10% to 30% of women with chlamydial infections after induced abortion. *C. trachomatis* apparently is an important cause of postabortion complications.

Infections in infants

Pregnant women who have cervical infection with *C. trachomatis* can transmit the infection to their infants who may subsequently develop neonatal conjunctivitis and/or pneumonia. Epidemiological evidence strongly suggests that the infant acquires chlamydial infection from the mother during vaginal delivery (Alexander and Harrison, 1983). Infection after cesarean section is rare and usually occurs after early rupture of the amniotic membrane. No evidence supports the idea of postnatal acquisition from the mother or other family members. Approximately 50% to 75% of infants born to infected women will become infected at one or more anatomical sites, including the conjunctiva, nasopharynx, rectum, and vagina.

Conjunctivitis. Inclusion conjunctivitis, or inclusion blennorrhea, is probably the major clinical manifestation of perinatally acquired chlamydial infection. The risk of developing chlamydial conjunctivitis after vaginal delivery in an infant born to a mother with active cervical chlamydial infection ranges from 20% to 50% (Alexander and Harrison, 1983). *C. trachomatis* is also the most common identifiably infectious cause of neonatal conjunctivitis in the United States, accounting for 17% to more than 40% of cases.

The incubation period is usually 5 to 14 days but may be shorter if the membranes ruptured prematurely. The clinical presentation is variable, ranging from minimal conjunctival injection with scant mucopurulent discharge to a more severe presentation with chemosis, pseudomembrane formation, and marked palpebral swelling. The conjunctivae are frequently very friable and may bleed when stroked with a swab. Although conjunctivitis may initially be unilateral, it frequently becomes bilateral. If not treated, the infection may persist for weeks. Chlamydial conjunctivitis in infants is not a follicular conjunctivitis as seen in classic endemic trachoma. Approximately 50% of infants with chlamydial conjunctivitis will also be infected in the nasopharynx.

Pneumonia. The nasopharynx is the most frequent site of perinatally acquired chlamydial infection. Approximately 70% of infected infants have positive cultures at that site. Most of these nasopharyngeal infections are asymptomatic and may persist for 3 years or more.

Chlamydial pneumonia develops in approximately 30% of infants with nasopharyngeal infection. In those who develop pneumonia the presentation and clinical findings are very characteristic. The children usually are initially seen at 4 to 12 weeks of age. A few cases have been

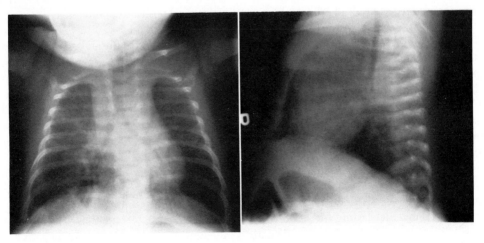

Fig. 25-7. Roentgenographic findings of a child with chlamydial pneumonia demonstrating hyperinflation and atelectasis.

seen initially as early as 2 weeks of age, but no infant cases have been seen beyond 4 months. The infants frequently have a history of cough and congestion, with an absence of fever. On physical examination the infant is tachypneic, and rales are heard on auscultation of the chest; wheezing is distinctly uncommon. There are no specific radiographic findings except hyperinflation (Fig. 25-7) (Beem and Saxon, 1977; Harrison et al., 1978). A review of chest films of 125 infants with chlamydial pneumonia found bilateral hyperinflation and diffuse infiltrates, with a variety of radiographic patterns, including interstitial, reticular, and nodular ones, atelectasis, and bronchopneumonia. Lobar consolidation and pleural effusions were not seen (Radkowski et al., 1981). Significant laboratory findings include peripheral eosinophilia (>300 cells/cm^3) and elevated serum immunoglobulin levels.

C. trachomatis is rarely isolated from the lungs of infants with chlamydia pneumonia, leading some to believe that an immune mechanism is involved in pathogenesis (Alexander and Harrison, 1983). Histopathological studies have not revealed any characteristic features. Biopsy material has shown pleural congestion and near-total alveolar and partial bronchiolar mononuclear consolidation with occasional eosinophils, granular pneumocytes, and focal aggregations of neutrophils. Marked necrotic changes are evident in the bronchioles. Follow-up studies have suggested that infantile chlamydial pneumonia may be associated with pulmonary function test abnormalities and respiratory symptoms 7 to 8 years after recovery from the acute illness (Weiss et al., 1986).

Infections in older children

C. trachomatis has not been associated with any specific clinical syndrome in older infants and children. It has been suggested that the isolation of C. trachomatis from a rectal or genital site in children without prior sexual activity may be a marker of sexual abuse. Although evidence for other modes of spread such as through fomites is lacking for this organism, perinatal maternal-infant transmission resulting in vaginal and/or rectal infection has been documented, with prolonged infection lasting for periods up to 2 years. Pharyngeal infection for up to 3 years has also been observed. Schachter et al. (1986a) have detected subclinical rectal and vaginal in-

fection in 14% of infants born to chlamydia-positive women; some infants were still culture positive at 18 months of age.

Reporting of vaginal infection with C. trachomatis in prepubertal children was uncommon before 1980. The possibility of sexual contact frequently was not discussed. In 1981 Rettig and Nelson reported concurrent or subsequent chlamydial infection in 9 of 33 (27%) prepubertal children with gonorrhea. This rate compares with those of 11% to 62%, depending on the study, of concurrent infection in men and women. C. trachomatis was not found in any of 31 children presenting with urethritis or vaginitis that was not gonococcal. No information was given about possible sexual activity.

Recent studies have identified rectogenital chlamydial infection in 4% to 13% of sexually abused children when the children were routinely cultured for the organism (see Table 25-1). Most of those with chlamydial infection were asymptomatic. In two studies that had control groups, similar percentages of control patients were infected (Hammerschlag et al., 1984; Ingram et al., 1984). The control group in one study comprised children who were referred also for evaluation of possible sexual abuse but were found to have no history of sexual contact and siblings of abused children. The mean age of this group was 4½ years as compared to 7½ years for the group with a history of sexual contact, thus suggesting a bias related to the inability to elicit a history of sexual contact from young children. In the second study the control group was selected from a well-child clinic. Three girls in this group had positive chlamydial cultures; two who had positive vaginal cultures were sisters who had been sexually abused 3 years previously and had not received interim treatment with antibiotics. The implication of this observation was that these children were infected for at least 3 years and were totally asymptomatic. The remaining control child had C. trachomatis isolated from her throat and rectum; no history of sexual contact could be elicited.

The possibility of prolonged vaginal or rectal carriage in the sexually abused group was minimized in the study of Hammerschlag et al. (1984) since the chlamydial cultures obtained at the initial examination were negative and the infection was detected only at follow-up examination 2 to 4 weeks later. However, the two abused girls who developed chlamydial infection were victims of a single assault by a stranger. In the setting of repeated abuse by a family member over long periods of time, development of infection would be difficult to demonstrate.

Lymphogranuloma venereum. Lymphogranuloma venereum (LGV) is a systemic, sexually transmitted disease caused by the LGV biovars of *C. trachomatis* (L1, L2, L3). Approximately 20 cases of LGV have been reported in children. Fewer than 1,000 cases are reported in adults in the United States each year. Unlike the trachoma biovar, LGV stains have a predilection for lymph node involvement. The clinical course of LGV can be divided into three stages: (1) the primary lesion, a painless papule on the genitals, which usually is very transient; (2) lymphadenitis or lymphadenopathy; and (3) the tertiary stage. Most patients present during the second stage with enlarging, painful buboes, usually in the groin. The nodes may break down and drain. Males are more likely to have this presentation. In females the lymphatic drainage of the vulva is to the retroperitoneal nodes. Fever, myalgia, and headache are also common. The tertiary stage includes the genitoanorectal syndrome, with rectovaginal fistulas, rectal strictures, and urethral destruction. Diagnosis can be made by culture of *C. trachomatis* from a bubo aspirate or serologically. Most patients with LGV will have complement fixation (CF) titers greater than 1:16. The recommended therapy is 2 to 3 weeks of either tetracycline or sulfisoxazole.

Diagnosis

The definitive diagnosis of genital chlamydial infection in adolescents and adults is isolation of the organism in tissue culture—from the urethra in men and the endocervix in women. Care should be taken to obtain *cells*, not discharge. The most commonly used tissue culture system is McCoy cells treated with cyclohex-imide. After a 48- to 72-hour incubation period, the cultures are confirmed by staining the inclusions, preferably with a fluorescein-conjugated monoclonal antibody, although iodine can also be used. Characteristic intracytoplasmic inclusions should be visible. Alternately, one of the recently developed nonculture antigen-detection methods can be used. The types currently available are a direct fluorescent antibody (DFA) test, in which chlamydial EBs are iden-

tified directly on a specimen smear stained with a conjugated anti-chlamydial monoclonal antibody, the enzyme immunoassay (EIA) test, and DNA probes. These types of test are best for screening in high-prevalence populations (prevalence of infection >7%) (Chernesky et al., 1986). There are very few reports on the performance of the DNA probe.

Serology is not helpful for the diagnosis of chlamydial infections in adults. Since most infections in adolescents and adults are asymptomatic, it would be difficult to demonstrate either seroconversion or rises in titers. Serosurveys of populations of sexually active adults have found prevalences of antichlamydial antibody in more than 20% of individuals. The most widely available serological test is the complement fixation (CF) test. This genus-specific test is most useful for the diagnosis of LGV. Unfortunately, it is not sensitive enough for use in oculogenital infections caused by the trachoma biovar in adults or children. The microimmunofluoresence (MIF) test is species specific and sensitive but is available only at a limited number of research laboratories.

Chlamydial conjunctivitis and pneumonia in infants. Culture of chlamydia from the conjunctivae or nasopharynx is diagnostic. The nasopharyngeal specimens can be obtained with a posterior swab or by aspirate. The use of dacron-tipped swabs with either wire or plastic shafts is preferred. The diagnosis of conjunctivitis can be made by examination of Giemsa-stained conjunctival scrapings, but this method has only had a 30% sensitivity compared to that of culture in several studies. The DFA and EIA tests can also be used for conjunctival and nasopharyngeal specimens. These tests apparently perform very well at these sites (Hammerschlag et al., 1987; Roblin et al., 1989). Diagnosis of chlamydial pneumonia also can be made serologically; an IgM titer greater than 1:32 with the MIF test is very suggestive (Harrison et al., 1978).

Chlamydial infections in older children. Because of the medical and legal implications, culture is the only approved method for the diagnosis of rectal and genital chlamydial infections in prepubertal children. Culture means isolation of the organism in tissue culture with confirmation by visual identification of the characteristic inclusions, preferably with fluorescent antibody (FA) staining. Non-culture methods cannot be used in this setting. Very little data are available about the use of these tests in rectal and genital specimens from prepubertal children, and what is available suggests that they are neither sensitive or specific (Hammerschlag et al., 1988; Hauger et al., 1988; Porder et al., 1989).

Treatment

Because of its long growth cycle, treatment of chlamydial infections requires multiple-dose regimens. None of the currently recommended single-dose regimens for gonorrhea are effective against *C. trachomatis*.

Uncomplicated genital infection in adolescent and adult males and nonpregnant women. The treatment of choice is doxycycline (100 mg orally, twice a day for 7 days). An alternative regimen for those who cannot tolerate doxycycline is erythromycin base (500 mg four times a day orally for 7 days).

As of this writing, an investigational drug, azithromycin, a long-acting azalide similar to macrolides, holds promise as a single-dose regimen for treating uncomplicated genital chlamydial infections. Azithromycin has a 30-hour half-life in serum. Preliminary studies suggest that 1 g of azithromycin given as a single oral dose, is equivalent to 7 days of doxycycline for the treatment of uncomplicated genital chlamydial infection in men and nonpregnant women.

C. trachomatis in pregnancy. The CDC currently recommends four different erythromycin regimens, none of which have been extensively evaluated, for treating *C. trachomatis* in pregnant women. Poor tolerance may reduce the compliance to 50% or less in some populations (Schachter, 1986b).

The primary regimen is erythromycin base, 500 mg four times a day orally for 7 days. If not tolerated, the dose can be reduced to 250 mg four times a day, orally, for 14 days. If erythromycin is not tolerated, limited data suggest amoxicillin (500 mg three times a day, orally, for 7 days) may be effective.

Chlamydial conjunctivitis and pneumonia in infants. Oral erythromycin suspension (ethylsuccinate or stearate); 50 mg/kg/day for 10 to 14 days) is the therapy of choice for chlamydial conjunctivitis and pneumonia in infants. It provides better and faster resolution of the conjunctivitis and treats any concurrent nasopha-

ryngeal infection, which will prevent the potential development of pneumonia. Additional topical therapy is not needed (Heggie et al., 1985). Erythromycin administered at the same dose for 2 to 3 weeks is the treatment of choice for pneumonia and results in clinical improvement and elimination of the organism from the respiratory tract.

Although an initial study suggested that neonatal ocular prophylaxis with erythromycin ointment would prevent the development of chlamydial ophthalmia, subsequent studies have not confirmed this (Bell et al., 1987; Hammerschlag et al., 1989). It appears that neither ocular prophylaxis with silver nitrate nor erythromycin and tetracycline ointments or drops are effective for the prevention of neonatal chlamydial conjunctivitis or pneumonia. The identification and treatment of pregnant women before delivery is the optimal method of prevention of chlamydial infection in infants.

Older children. Chlamydial infections in older children can be treated with oral erythromycin (50 mg/kg/day, four times a day, orally, to a maximum of 2 g/day for 7 to 14 days). Children older than 8 years of age may be treated with doxycycline (2 to 4 mg/kg/day divided into two doses, orally, for 7 days).

BACTERIAL VAGINOSIS

Bacterial vaginosis (nonspecific vaginitis) is a polymicrobial infection apparently caused by the interaction of *Gardnerella vaginalis* and several anaerobic bacteria. The diagnosis of bacterial vaginosis is made by examination of the vaginal secretions for clue cells (vaginal epithelial cells heavily covered with bacteria) (Fig. 25-8, *A* and *B*), the development of a fishy odor after the addition of 10% potassium hydroxide to vaginal secretions ("whiff test"), and a vaginal pH greater than 4.5 (Amsel et al., 1983; Thomason et al., 1990).

Although bacterial vaginosis is very common in adult women, it has been diagnosed infrequently in children (Table 25-4). One possible reason is that prior studies of pediatric populations have concentrated on the isolation of *G. vaginalis* and have not routinely examined vaginal secretions for clue cells or odor. The CDC has stated that cultures for *G. vaginalis* are not useful and are not recommended for the diagnosis of this syndrome. Studies in children have suggested that *G. vaginalis* may be part of the

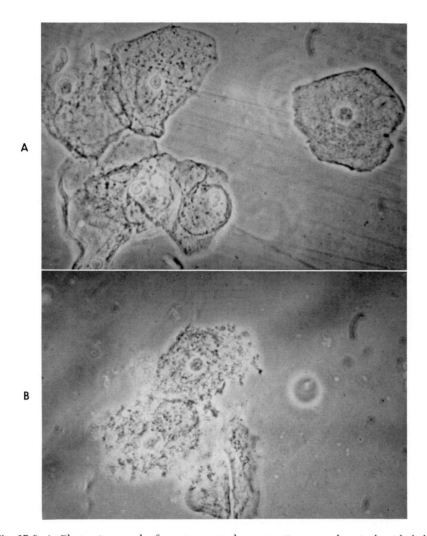

Fig. 25-8. A, Photomicrograph of a wet mount, demonstrating normal vaginal epithelial cells. **B,** Photomicrograph of wet mount containing clue cells, which are epithelial cells studded with bacteria.

Table 25-4. Prevalence of trichomoniasis and bacterial vaginosis in sexually abused children

Study (year)	Number tested	Cause	Number (%) positive
White et al. (1983)	409	Trichomoniasis	4 (1)
De Jong (1983)	25*	Trichomoniasis	0
		Bacterial vaginosis	3 (12)
Hammerschlag et al. (1985)	31	Trichomoniasis	2 (6)
		Bacterial vaginosis	6 (19)

*Only patients with signs suggestive of vaginitis were evaluated.

normal vaginal flora (Hammerschlag et al., 1985).

Bartley et al. (1987) examined a group of sexually abused children and a group of control children. Although *G. vaginalis* was isolated from the vaginal cultures of 14.6% of the abused girls, it was also found in 4.2% of the controls. Presence of *G. vaginalis* was not associated with vaginal discharge in these children. Another study reported finding *G. vaginalis* in vaginal specimens from 37% of non-sexually active postmenarcheal girls (median age, 15.9 years; range, 13 to 21 years) (Shafer et al., 1985). Although some practitioners have suggested that the presence of *G. vaginalis* is an indicator of sexual abuse, the preceding data suggest otherwise.

Data from adults suggest that acquisition of bacterial vaginosis is related to sexual activity. In a major study Amsel et al. (1983) diagnosed bacterial vaginitis in 69 of 397 females consecutively coming to a student health center gynecology clinic. They failed to demonstrate the disease among 18 patients who had no history of previous sexual intercourse. Four of these sexually inexperienced patients had positive vaginal cultures for *G. vaginalis*, which suggests that other organisms or factors are involved in the sexual transmission of bacterial vaginitis. Other investigators have found that male partners of women with bacterial vaginosis have a high prevalence of urethral colonization with *G. vaginalis*.

Minimal data exist on the prevalence of bacterial vaginosis in sexually abused female children. Hammerschlag et al. (1985) obtained paired vaginal wash specimens from 31 girls within 1 week and 2 or more weeks after sexual assault. None had bacterial vaginosis as defined by the presence of both clue cells and a positive whiff test at the initial examination. Vaginal pH was not used as a diagnostic criterion because the normal pH range in prepubertal girls is not well defined. At follow-up examination, four (13%) of the 31 girls had bacterial vaginosis. Two girls were asymptomatic. Treatment with metronidazole was followed by clinical improvement. None of the 23 controls (nonabused children) had bacterial vaginosis.

Bacterial vaginosis apparently is also a common cause of vaginal discharge in children without sexual contact. Samuels et al. (1985) examined vaginal washes from 29 girls, 3 months to 1 year of age, with symptomatic vulvovaginitis. Bacterial vaginosis was diagnosed in nine (31%) of these children. All had a discharge, which was uniformly thin and ranged from grey-white to yellow in color, and only three (33%) of these girls had a history of sexual abuse; *N. gonorrhoeae* also was isolated from a pharyngeal culture from one child. Treatment with metronidazole resulted in reversion of the vaginal secretions to normal on follow-up examination. The relatively common occurrence of bacterial vaginosis in children may be due, in part, to the frequent colonization of the prepubertal vagina with anaerobes, especially *Bacteroides* species.

Treatment

Oral metronidazole (15 mg/kg/day, three times a day for 7 days) apparently is effective for the treatment of bacterial vaginosis in children. Ampicillin or amoxicillin have been recom-

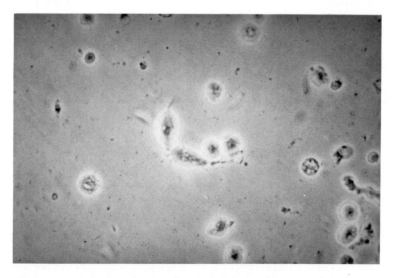

Fig. 25-9. Photomicrograph of wet mount, demonstrating *Trichomonas vaginalis* trophozoites.

mended as alternative regimens when the use of metronidazole is contraindicated, but they are less effective. The combination of amoxicillin and clavulanate (Augmentin) may be effective since it offers better coverage for anaerobic bacteria, especially *Bacteroides* species.

TRICHOMONIASIS

Trichomonas vaginalis is a flagellated protozoan that inhabits the urogenital systems of both males and females and is considered a pathogen (Fig. 25-9). The trophozoites (the only stage) are found in the urine of both sexes, in vaginal secretions, and in prostatic secretions. Approximately 5 million women in the United States have trichomoniasis, and roughly 1 million men may harbor the parasite. The infection in males is generally asymptomatic, but 25% to 50% of infected women exhibit symptoms, which include dysuria, vaginal itching and burning, and in severe infections, a foamy, yellowish-green discharge with a foul odor.

Although nonsexual transmission of *T. vaginalis* has been reported between infected mothers and their infants at delivery, the exact risk of the infant's acquiring the infection is unknown (Al-Salihi et al., 1974). The presence of this organism in vaginal specimens from prepubertal girls strongly suggests sexual abuse; but as with other sexually transmitted diseases, perinatally acquired infection can be an important confounding variable. The duration of perinatally acquired trichomoniasis has been assumed to be very short—2 to 3 months after birth. Recently, the authors saw two female infants with well-documented neonatal trichomonal infection that persisted for 6 and 9 months before the infants were finally treated. In most reports of infection with *T. vaginalis* in prepubertal children published before 1978, the possibility of sexual activity or abuse is not discussed (Neinstein et al., 1984). In one study of unselected girls who went to a well-child clinic, *T. vaginalis* was identified in two girls; both were postmenarcheal, and one was sexually active. They both were symptomatic (Hammerschlag et al., 1978).

In most reported studies wet mount examinations have been performed infrequently in asymptomatic sexually abused children and often are not performed in abused girls who have not had a vaginal discharge. Patients with trichomoniasis may be asymptomatic and have negative results from wet mount preparations (Wolner-Hanssen et al., 1989). In one study in which both wet mount examinations and cultures were used, trichomoniasis was found in two of 31 abused children at follow-up, but not at an initial examination (see Table 25-4). *T. vaginalis* was not identified in the children who served as controls. Trichomonads are not infrequently seen in urine collected for other purposes. If the specimen was obtained with a urinary collection bag, as is done frequently in young children, especially girls, the trichomads may have originated in the vagina or may represent fecal contamination.

T. hominis, a commensal species that can inhabit the colon, is considered nonpathogenic. The only way the two species can be differentiated is by the presence of an undulating membrane that extends most of the length of the organism in *T. hominis* but only half the length of the organism in *T. vaginalis*. Old urine specimens may also be contaminated with *Bodo* species or other free-living flagellates, especially if the urinary collection vessel is open to the air and is not sterile. The presence of a trichomonad in a vaginal specimen has greater significance.

Diagnosis

Although some workers believe wet mount examinations are as efficient as culture for the diagnosis of *T. vaginalis* infection, current evidence suggests that cultivation methods are superior (Fouts and Kraus, 1980). Several culture media are available commercially. A conjugated monoclonal antibody stain has been developed that apparently is both sensitive and specific, but available clinical data are limited. It has not been evaluated as yet as an assay for the diagnosis of trichomoniasis in children (Kruger et al., 1988).

Treatment

Trichomoniasis in adult women can be successfully treated with a single oral dose (2 g) of metronidazole or with 250 mg by mouth given three times daily for 7 days, but there are no published studies of its use in children. The few cases of trichomoniasis in prepubertal girls reported in the literature were treated with 7-day courses of oral metronidazole (15 to 35 mg/kg/day) (Jones et al., 1985).

HUMAN PAPILLOMA VIRUS INFECTION

Human papilloma virus (HPV), a double-stranded DNA virus, is the organism responsible for common warts and venereal warts, or condylomata acuminata. Genital papillomas in adults are transmitted by sexual intercourse. The majority is caused by human papilloma virus type 6 (HPV-6) or type 11 (HPV-11); and smaller numbers are caused by types 16 (HPV-16) and 18 (HPV-18). Common skin warts and genital warts do not share HPV types.

HPV is becoming recognized as one of the most frequently occurring STDs. In the San Francisco Bay area Moscicki et al. (1990) reported that 18% of sexually active females tested positive for HPV DNA. HPV represented the most common STD in that age group, followed by *C. trachomatis*, with a prevalence rate of 8%. A similar study of adolescents in New York City reported an HPV prevalence rate of 33%. More than 80% of male partners of females with HPV are infected with HPV; most of these infections are subclinical. The cause of genital papillomas in children is less well studied, but sexual abuse by an infected adult or, less likely, contact with warts at other body sites has been suggested. Human papilloma viruses can also be transmitted to infants at birth, causing laryngeal papilloma (Boyd, 1990). The condylomata may affect the vulva, perineum, vaginal introitus, and periurethral areas. Girls apparently are affected twice as frequently as boys, although this may reflect a difference in patterns of reporting rather than a true epidemiological observation (Davis and Emans, 1989; Boyd, 1990).

Clinical manifestations

The lesions of condylomata acuminata are usually flesh-colored to purple papillomatous growths. These warts are often multiple and commonly coalesce into larger masses. In females condylomata acuminata lesions usually occur at the posterior part of the introitus, the adjacent labia minora, and the rest of the vestibule. Less commonly, they can be found on the clitoris, perineum, vagina, cervix, anus, and rectum.

In males venereal warts are usually localized to the penis, including the shaft, prepuce, frenulum, corona, and glans. The meatus, anus, and scrotum may also be involved. Anal warts are seen most commonly in patients who have engaged in anal intercourse. In contrast, many females with anal warts report no history of anal sex, suggesting autoinoculation as a mode of transmission. The anatomical distribution may be different in prepubertal children, especially males. Male children are less likely to have involvement of the penile shaft, prepuce, or glans—3% vs. 18% to 52%—and are more likely to have perianal disease—77% vs. 8% (Boyd, 1990). Female disease patterns show fewer age-related differences.

Recently, a new clinical and histological type of HPV infection has been described as subclinical HPV infection. The lesions with this type cannot be seen with the naked eye and require colposcopy, aceto-whitening, or cytological studies for diagnosis. They can occur anywhere in the anogenital tract. In women they occur predominantly on the cervix; in males they can occur anywhere on the penis and on the perianal area, scrotum, and urethra. Recently, increasing attention has been focused on the association between HPV infection and the various genital carcinomas, particularly cervical carcinoma in women. HPV structural antigens and DNA have been found in the lesions of cervical intraepithelial neoplasia, which precedes the development of frank cervical carcinoma. HPV antigens and DNA have also been found in invasive carcinoma specimens and in specimens of anal, vulvar, vaginal, and penile carcinomas. Studies of adolescents in San Francisco have found infection with oncogenic-related HPV types is very common (Moscicki et al., 1990).

The risk of developing genital warts in sexually abused children has not been adequately assessed because no studies have included data on long-term follow-up. However, one half of the cases of genital warts in children reported since 1976 was related to sexual abuse (Seidel et al., 1979; De Jong et al., 1982; Neinstein et al., 1984). Rock et al. (1986) examined by molecular hybridization the genital tract papillomas in five children for the presence of HPV DNA. Papilloma virus DNA was detected in each sample and contained either HPV-6, HPV-11, or HPV-16. These types are the same as those responsible for genital warts in adults. Sexual abuse was thought likely to have occurred in three of these children. Although there was no history of maternal condylomata at the time of birth in the remaining two children, many congenital infections in women are subclinical, and flat warts of the vulva and vagina may go unnoticed by the affected individual and the physician (Bender, 1986).

It is very unlikely that hand or common warts are transmitted from caretakers to children to cause genital warts. Modern HPV typing has not revealed HPV types 1 and 2, which are the types associated with common warts in the anogenital area. Studies have found no correlation between the frequency of hand warts and that of genital warts.

The major confounding variable in linking the presence of genital warts with sexual abuse is ruling out perinatal acquisition. Maternal HPV infection may be more common than previously thought. One study found evidence of HPV, as defined by DNA probes, in 4% of male infants undergoing routine circumcision. The prolonged incubation period, or period of latency, before clinical condylomata are evident further complicates this issue. It is impossible to define the longest latency period between viral infection at delivery and the presence of clinical disease. The average latency period apparently is approximately 3 months, but it may range up to 2 years. A child who is first found to have perianal condylomata at 20 months of age may have had visible disease that could have been detected on close inspection (with colposcopy) 6 months earlier. Most cases of childhood condylomata occurring beyond the plausible incubation period (2 years) after acquisition at delivery probably are due to child abuse. Other means of transmission are unlikely. It is theoretically possible to transfer anogenital condylomata inadvertently from caretakers during activities such as shared bathing, but this has never been proven conclusively. The prolonged incubation period would also make it difficult to determine when abuse occurred.

Diagnosis

Until the recent recognition that HPV infection can be inapparent, the diagnosis of condylomata acuminata was usually based on the history and appearance of the lesions. Anogenital warts must be differentiated from other papillomatous lesions, including benign and malignant neoplasms, anatomical variants, and other infectious conditions. Of the latter, the most important lesions to differentiate are condylomata

lata of secondary syphilis. Because both may coexist, obtaining serological tests for syphilis and dark-field microscopy of suspicious or ulcerating lesions is strongly recommended. Genital lesions of molluscum contagiosum also can be confused with genital warts.

In adolescents and women the Papanicolaou (Pap) test commonly is used to diagnose HPV infection. The koilocyte ("balloon cell") can be seen on a Pap smear and is pathognomic for HPV. However, there is a subjective component to reading smears, and the sampling error presents a problem. A negative Pap smear result does not rule out HPV infection. Performing a biopsy should be considered for any puzzling lesion.

Electron microscopy can be used to identify HPV particles in biopsy specimens and may be especially useful in identifying lesions from children. More recently, antigen detection and molecular hybridization techniques have shown promise in detecting HPV in scrapings and biopsies of lesions (Bauer et al., 1991). However, the same problems encountered with Pap smears occur with these newer methods. Their diag-

---

LABORATORY STUDIES INDICATED AS PART OF EVALUATION OF SEXUALLY ASSAULTED CHILDREN AT INITIAL AND FOLLOW-UP EXAMINATIONS*

Gram stain of any genital or anal discharge
Cultures for *N. gonorrhoeae* and *C. trachomatis*, if available*
Serological tests for syphilis
Wet mount preparation for trichomonads and clue cells (girls)
Whiff test (girls)
Vaginal culture for *T. vaginalis*, if available (girls)
Serum sample (save frozen)
Cultures of lesions for herpes simplex virus
Hepatitis B surface antigen†
Human immunodeficiency virus antibody†
All studies should be repeated seven days later, except for syphilis and hepatitis B serologies which should be obtained 12 weeks later.

---

*Systematic genital and extragenital cultures should be obtained from all children.

†Obtain if there is supportive epidemiological evidence.

nostic use may be compromised because of sampling error, insufficient material, or interference by large numbers of red or white blood cells that obscure visualization of the cervical epithelial cells. None of these methods have been evaluated in prepubertal children.

Treatment

None of the currently available therapies is completely satisfactory for the treatment of genital warts in adults, and less information is available about treatment for children. Children have been treated with local application of podophyllin, cryosurgery, electrosurgery, ablation with carbon dioxide laser, and 75% trichloroacetic acid. Treatment of genital warts in children can be complicated and should be carried out in consultation with an expert.

SEXUALLY TRANSMITTED DISEASES AND SEXUAL ABUSE OF CHILDREN

Sexual assault is a violent crime that affects men, women, and children of all ages. STDs can be transmitted during sexual assault. In children the isolation of a sexually transmitted organism may be the first indication that abuse has occurred. However, most sexually abused children are not initially seen with genital complaints. Unfortunately, the presence of an STD is frequently viewed as a shortcut to prove abuse. Although the presence of a sexually transmissible agent in a child beyond the neonatal period is suggestive of sexual abuse, exceptions do occur. For example, rectal and genital infection with *C. trachomatis* in young children may be due to persistent perinatally acquired infection, which may persist for up to 3 years. The use of STDs as indicators of sexual abuse is further complicated by inappropriate use of certain diagnostic tests such as tests for *C. trachomatis* antigen or misidentification of other bacteria as *Neisseria gonorrhoeae*. A much higher standard of accuracy must be used for children than for adults since identification of an STD in a child will have legal and social as well as medical implications.

Epidemiology of sexual abuse in children

The incidence and prevalence of sexual abuse of children are difficult to estimate, in major part because much sexual abuse in childhood escapes detection. Several relatively extensive studies of sexual abuse of children in the United States have examined sex, race, and age-dependent variables. Patterns of childhood sexual abuse appear to depend on the sex and age of the victim (Glaser et al., 1989). Approximately 80% to 90% of abused children are female, with mean ages of 7 to 8 years. Most, 75% to 85%, were abused by a male assailant, adult or minor, known to the child. This individual is most likely a family member, especially the father or father substitute (stepfather, mother's boyfriend), uncles, and other male relatives (Rimsza and Niggemann, 1982). Victims of unknown assailants usually are older than the children abused by a known person, and the abuse usually involves only a single episode. In contrast, abuse by family members or acquaintances usually involves multiple episodes over periods of time ranging from 1 week to years.

Most victims describe a single type of sexual activity, but more than 20% have experienced multiple types of forced sexual acts. Vaginal penetration occurs in approximately 50% and anal penetration in one third of female victims. More than 50% of male victims have experienced anal penetration. Other types of sexual activity include orogenital contact in 20% to 50% of victims and fondling. Children who are abused by a known assailant usually experience less trauma than victims of assault by a stranger.

Risk of infection

An accurate determination of the risk of sexually transmitted conditions in victims of sexual abuse has been hindered by a variety of factors. First, the prevalence of sexually transmitted infections may vary regionally and among different populations within the same region. Second, few studies have attempted to differentiate between infections existing before the abuse. The presence of preexisting infection in adults is usually related to prior sexual activity (Jenny et al., 1990). In children preexisting infection may be related to prolonged colonization after perinatal acquisition, inadvertant nonsexual spread, prior peer sexual activity, or prior sexual abuse (Glaser et al., 1989). Finally, incubation periods for STDs range from a few days for *N. gonorrhoeae* to several months for human papilloma virus. The incubation periods and timing of an examination after an episode of abuse are critically important in detecting infections. Multiple episodes of abuse increase the risk of infection, probably by increasing the number of contacts with an infected individual. In most cases the site of infection is consistent with the child's history of assault (Rimsza and Niggemann, 1982). Rates of infection also vary with the type of assault initially described. Vaginal or rectal penetration is more likely to lead to detectable infection than fondling (Tilelli et al., 1980; White et al., 1983). However, the majority of children who are abused will have no physical complaints related to either trauma or infection.

OTHER INFECTIONS

Several other STDs deserve mention. Chancroid is caused by *H. ducreyi*, a small, nonmotile, gram-negative, non–spore-forming rod. Clinically, chancroid usually is seen initially as a small, inflammatory papule on the preputial orifice or frenulum in men and on the labia, fourchette, or perianal region in women. The lesion becomes pustular and ulcerative within 2 to 3 days. An associated painful, tender inguinal adenopathy occurs in over 50% of cases. Unlike that of lymphogranuloma venereum, the characteristic ulcer of chancroid is concurrent with lymphadenopathy. Recently, reported cases of chancroid have increased dramatically in the United States, especially in urban areas such as Los Angeles, New York, and Miami (Schmid, 1990). Although no reports of chancroid in children have been found in the literature, chancroid may appear with the increasing incidence in reports about the adult population.

Infection with hepatitis B virus (HBV) is also a sexually transmitted disease and may be a complication of sexual abuse (Szmuness et al., 1975) (Chapter 9). It has been recommended that male victims of homosexual rape be screened for HBV infection. Although homosexual behavior is a well-recognized risk factor for acquiring HBV infection, a similar increased risk exists among heterosexuals with multiple sex partners. Screening for HBV probably should also be included in the medical evaluation of the child victim of sexual assault.

Consideration should also be given to screening for HIV infection in victims of sexual assault, including children (Gellert et al., 1990). Although no available studies document the risks of transmission in this situation, individual reports have noted acquisition of HIV infection through sexual assault (Leiderman and Grimm, 1986; Gutman et al., 1991). Since HIV, like HBV, can be transmitted through homosexual or heterosexual activity, screening for infection may be indicated in both instances.

Investigators in Newark, New Jersey, have reported some children with probable perinatally acquired HIV first seen with the infection at 8 to 9 years of age. Although the apparent usual incubation period is 18 months, it is possible that it may extend for years in some individuals. The group in Newark now screens all sexually abused children for HIV—not for forensic purposes, but because they believe that sexual abuse is an epidemiological risk factor for HIV infection in their population.

Laboratory studies that are indicated as part of the evaluation of sexually assaulted children at initial and follow-up examinations are presented in the box on p. 449.

REFERENCES

Sexually transmitted diseases and sexual abuse (general)

Centers for Disease Control: 1989 sexually transmitted diseases treatment guidelines. MMWR 1989;38:No. S-8.

DeJong AR. Sexually transmitted diseases in sexually abused children. Sex Transm Dis 1986;13:123-126.

Glaser JB, Hammerschlag MR, McCormack WM. Epidemiology of sexually transmitted diseases in rape victims. Rev Infect Dis 1989;11:246-254.

Hammerschlag MR. Sexually transmitted diseases in sexually abused children. Adv Pediatr Infect Dis 1988; 3:1-18.

Hammerschlag MR, Alpert S, Rosner I et al. Microbiology of the vagina in children: normal and potentially pathogenic organisms. Pediatrics 1978;62:57-62.

Jenny C, Hooton TM, Bowers A, et al. Sexually transmitted diseases in victims of rape. N Engl J Med 1990;322:713-716.

Neinstein LS, Goldenring J, Carpenter S. Non-sexual transmission of sexually transmitted diseases: an infrequent occurrence. Pediatrics 1984;74:67-75.

Rimsza ME, Niggemann EH. Medical evaluation of sexually abused children: a review of 311 cases. Pediatrics 1982;69:8-14.

Schwarcz SK, Whittington WL. Sexual assault and sexually transmitted diseases: detection and management. Rev Infect Dis 1990;12:5682-5690.

Tilelli JA, Turek D, Jaffe AC. Sexual abuse of children. Clinical findings and implications for management. N Engl J Med 1980;302:319-323.

White ST, Coda FA, Ingram DA, et al. Sexually transmitted diseases in sexually abused children. Pediatrics 1983; 72:16-21.

Gonorrhea

Amstey MS, Steadman KT. Asymptomatic gonorrhea and pregnancy. J Am Vener Dis Assoc 1976;3:14.

Apicella MA. Serogrouping the *Neisseria gonorrhoeae:* identification of four immunologically distinct acidic polysaccharides. J Infect Dis 1976;134:377.

Armstrong JH, Zacarias F, Rein MF. Ophthalmia neonatorum: a chart review. Pediatrics 1976;57:884-892.

Bernstein GA, Davis JP, Katcher ML. Prophylaxis of neonatal conjunctivitis. An analytic review. Clin Pediatr 1983;21:545-550.

Branch G, Paxton R. A study of gonococcal infection among infants and children. Public Health Rep 1965;80:347-352.

Britigan BE, Cohen MS, Sparling PF. Gonococcal infections: a model of molecular pathogenesis. N Engl J Med 1985;312:1683-1694.

Catlin BW. Nutritional profiles of *Neisseria gonorrhoeae, Neisseria meningitis* and *Neisseria lactamica* in chemically defined media and the use of growth requirements for gonococcal typing. J Infect Dis 1973;128:178-194.

Edwards LE, et al. Gonorrhea in pregnancy. Am J Obstet Gynecol 1978;132:637.

Fransen L, Naanze H, Klauss V, et al. Ophthalmia neonatorum in Nairobi, Kenya: the roles of *Neisseria gonorrhoeae* and *Chlamydia trachomatis*. J Infect Dis 1986; 153:862-869.

Groothius J, Bischoff MC, Javrequi LE. Pharyngeal gonorrhea in young children. Pediatr Infect Dis 1983;2:99-101.

Handsfield HH, Hodson EA, Holmes KK. Neonatal gonococcal infection. JAMA 1973;225:697.

Hein K, Marks A, Cohen MI. Asymptomatic gonorrhea: prevalence in a population of urban adolescents. J Pediatr 1977;90:634-635.

Holmes KK, Counts GW, Beaty HN. Disseminated gonococcal infection. Ann Intern Med 1971;74:979.

Hook EW III, Holmes KK. Gonococcal infections. Ann Intern Med 1985;102:229-243.

Hook EW III, Judson FN, Handsfield HH. Auxotype/serovar diversity and antimicrobial resistance of *Neisseria gonorrhoeae* in two mid-sized American cities. Sex Transm Dis 1987;14:141-146.

Ingram DL, White ST, Durfee MR et al. Sexual contact in children with gonorrhea. Am J Dis Child 1982;136:994-996.

Judson FN, Ehret JM, Handsfield HH. Comparative study of ceftriaxone and spectinomycin for treatment of pharyngeal and anorectal gonorrhea. JAMA 1985;253:1417-1419.

Knapp JS, Holmes KK. Disseminated gonococcal infections caused by *Neisseria gonorrhoeae* with unique nutritional requirements. J Infect Dis 1975;132:204.

Laga M, Naamara W, Brunham RC, et al. Single dose therapy of gonococcal ophthalmia neonatorum. N Engl J Med 1986;315:1382-1385.

Laga M, Plummer FA, Piot P, et al. Prophylaxis of gonococcal and chlamydial ophthalmia neonatorum. N Engl J Med 1988;318:653-657.

McClure EM, Stack MR, Tanner T, et al. Pharyngeal culturing and reporting of pediatric gonorrhea in Connecticut. Pediatrics 1986;78:509-510.

Nelson JD. The bacterial etiology and antibiotic management of septic arthritis in infants and children. Pediatrics 1972;50:437-440.

Nelson JD, Mohs E, Dajani AS, Plotkin SA. Gonorrhea in preschool and school aged children. A report of the prepubertal gonorrhea cooperative study group. JAMA 1976;236:1359.

Petersen BH, Lee TJ, Synderman R, et al. *Neisseria meningitis* and *Neisseria gonorrhoeae* bacteremia associated with C6, C7, or C8 deficiency. Am Intern Med 1979; 90:917-920.

Potterat JJ, Markewich GS, Rothenberg R. Prepubertal infections with *Neisseria gonorrhoeae:* clinical and epidemiologic significance. Sex Transm Dis 1978;5:1-3.

Potterat JJ, Markewich GS, King RD, et al. Child-to-child transmission of gonorrhea. Report of asymptomatic genital infection in a boy. Pediatrics 1986;78:711-712.

Rawstron SA, Hammerschlag MR, Gullans C, et al. Ceftriaxone treatment of penicillinase-producing *Neisseria gonorrhoeae* infections in children. Pediatr Infect Dis 1989;8:445-448.

Rettig PJ, Nelson JD, Kusmiess H. Spectinomycin therapy for gonorrhea in prepubertal children. Am J Dis Child 1980;134:559-563.

Rothenberg R. Ophthalmia neonatorum due to *Neisseria gonorrhoeae:* prevention and treatment. Sex Transm Dis 1979;6:187-191.

Schwarz SK, Zenilman JM, Schnell D, et al. National surveillance of antimicrobial resistance in *Neisseria gonorrhoeae*. JAMA 1990;264:1413-1417.

Stamm WE, Guinan ME, Johnson C, et al. Effect of treatment regimens for *Neisseria gonorrhoeae* on simultaneous infection with *Chlamydia trachomatis*. N Engl J Med 1984;310:545-549.

Whittington WL, Rice RJ, Biddle JW, Knapp JS. Incorrect identification of *Neisseria gonorrhoeae* from infants and children. Pediatr Infect Dis 1988;7:3-10.

Weisner PJ, Tranca E, Bonin P, et al. Clinical spectrum of pharyngeal gonococcal infection. N Engl J Med 1973; 288:181-185.

Pelvic inflammatory disease

Bowie WR, Jones H. Acute pelvic inflammatory disease in outpatients: association with *Chlamydia trachomatis* and *Neisseria gonorrhoeae*. Ann Intern Med 1981;95:685-688.

Gates W. Sexually transmitted organisms and infertility: the proof of the pudding. Sex Transm Dis 1984;11:113-116.

Cromer BA, Heald FP. Pelvic inflammatory disease associated with *Neisseria gonorrhoeae* and *Chlamydia trachomatis:* clinical correlates. Sex Transm Dis 1987; 14:125-129.

Eschenbach DA, Buchanan TM, Pollock HM, et al. Polymicrobial etiology of acute pelvic inflammatory disease. N Engl J Med 1975;293:166-171.

Mardh PA. An overview of infectious agents of salpingitis, their biology and recent methods of detection. Am J Obstet Gynecol 1980;138:933-951.

Patton DL. Immunopathology and histopathology of experimental chlamydial salpingitis. Rev Infect Dis 1985; 7:746-753.

Shafer M-A, Irwin CE, Sweet RL. Acute salpingitis in the adolescent female. J Pediatr 1982;100:339-350.

Walters MD, Gibbs RS. A randomized comparison of gentamicin-clindamycin and cefoxitin-doxycycline in the treatment of acute pelvic inflammatory disease. Obstet Gynecol 1990;75:867-872.

Wasserheit JN, Bell TA, Kiviat NB, et al. Microbial causes

SEXUALLY TRANSMITTED DISEASES **453**

of proven pelvic inflammatory disease and efficacy of clindamycin and tobramycin. Ann Intern Med 1986; 104:187-193.

Westrom L. Incidence, prevalence and trends of acute pelvic inflammatory disease and its consequences in industrialized countries. Am J Obstet Gynecol 1980;138:880-892.

Wolner-Hanssen P, Eschenbach D, Paavonen J, et al. Treatment of pelvic inflammatory disease: use of doxycycline with an appropriate B-lactam while we wait for better data. JAMA 1986;256:3262-3263.

Syphilis

Ackerman AB, Goldfaden G, Cosmides JC. Acquired syphilis in early childhood. Arch Dermatol 1972;106:92-93.

Alderete JF, Baseman JB. Surface-associated host proteins on virulent *Treponema pallidum*. Infect Immunol 1979; 26:1048.

Baker-Zander S, Sell S. A histopathologic and immunologic study of the course of syphilis in the experimentally infected rabbit: demonstration of long-lasting cellular immunity. Am J Pathol 1980;101:387.

Beck-Sague C, Alexander ER. Failures of benzathine penicillin G therapy in early congenital syphilis. Pediatr Infect Dis 1987;6:1061-1064.

Centers for Disease Control. Guidelines for the prevention and control of congenital syphilis. MMWR 1988a;37:1-13.

Centers for Disease Control. Continuing increase in infectious syphilis—United States. MMWR 1988b;37:35-37.

Centers for Disease Control. Summary of notifiable diseases, United States 1989. MMWR 1989;38:3.

Centers for Disease Control. Congenital syphilis—New York City, 1986-1988. MMWR 1989;38:825-829.

Cohen DA, Boyd D, Pabhudas I, Mascola L. The effects of case definition, maternal screening, and reporting criteria on rates of congenital syphilis. Am J Public Health 1990;80:316-317.

Deacon WE, Lucas JB, Price EV. Fluorescent treponemal antibody-absorption (FTA-ABS) test for syphilis. JAMA 1966;198:624.

Duncan WC, Knox JM, Wende RD. The FTA-ABS test in Dark-field-positive primary syphilis. JAMA 1974;228:859-860.

Dunlop EMC, Al-Egaily MB, Houang ET. Penicillin levels in blood and CSF achieved by treatment of syphilis. JAMA 1979;241:2538.

Eagle H, Fleischman R, Muselman AD. The effective concentration of penicillin in vitro and in vivo for streptococci, pneumococci, and *Treponema pallidum*. J Bacteriol 1950;59:625-643.

Fiumara NJ, Lessell S. The stigmata of late congenital syphilis: an analysis of 100 patients. Sex Transm Dis 1983;10:126-129.

Fiumara NJ, Fleming WL, Downing JG, Good FL. The incidence of prenatal syphilis at the Boston City Hospital. N Engl J Med 1952;247:48-52.

Fiumara NJ. Syphilis in newborn children. Clin Obstet Gynecol 1975;18:183-189.

Fiumara NJ. Treatment of primary and secondary syphilis. Serological response. JAMA 1980;243:2500-2502.

Fojaco RM, Hensley GT, Moskowitz L. Congenital syphilis and necrotizing funisitis. JAMA 1989;261:1788-1790.

Frenz G, Hideon PB, Esperson F, et al. Pencillin concentrations in blood and spinal fluid after a single intramuscular injection of penicillin G benzathine. Eur J Clin Microbiol 1984;3:147.

Ginsberg CM. Acquired syphilis in prepubertal children. Pediatr Infect Dis 1983;2:232-234.

Harter CA, Benirschke K. Fetal syphilis in the first trimester. Am J Obstet Gynecol 1976;124:705.

Hovind-Hougen K. Morphology. In Shell RF, Musher DM (eds). Pathogenesis and immunology of treponemal infection. New York: Marcel Dekker, 1983.

Hira SK, Bhat GJ, Patel JB, et al. Early congenital syphilis: clinico-radiologic features in 202 patients. Sex Transm Dis 1985;12:177-183.

Idsoe O, Guthie T, Willcox RR. Penicillin in the treatment of syphilis. Bull WHO 1972;47 (suppl):1-68.

Jenkin HW, Sander PL. In vitro cultivation of *Treponema pallidum*. In Shell RF, Musher DM (eds). Pathogenesis and immunology of treponemal infection. New York: Marcel Dekker, 1983.

Kaufman RE, Olansky DC, Wiesner PJ. The FTA-ABS (IgM) test for neonatal congenital syphilis: a critical review. J Am Venereol Dis Assoc 1974;1:79-84.

Lukehart SA, Hook EW III, Baker-Zander SA, et al. Invasion of the central nervous system by *Treponema pallidum:* implications for diagnosis and treatment. Ann Intern Med 1988;109:855-862.

Mascola L, Pelosi R, Blount JH, et al. Congenital syphilis: why is it still occurring? JAMA 1984;252:1719-1722.

Mascola L, Pelosi R, Alexander CE. Inadequate treatment of syphilis in pregnancy. Am J Obstet Gynecol 1984;150:945-947.

McCracken GH Jr, Kaplan JM. Pencillin treatment for congenital syphilis. JAMA 1974;228:855.

Miller JL, Meyer PG, Parrott NA, Hill JH. A study of the biologic falsely positive reactions for syphilis in children. J Pediatr 1960;57:548-552.

Musher DM, et al. The interaction between *Treponema pallidum* and human polymorphonuclear leucocytes. J Infect Dis 1983;147:77.

Musher DM. Biology of *Treponema pallidum*. In Holmes KK, Mardh PA, Sparling PF, Wiesner PJ (eds). Sexually transmitted diseases. New York: McGraw-Hill, 1984.

Musher DM, Hamill RJ, Baughn RE. Effect of human immunodeficiency virus (HIV) infection on the course of syphilis and on the response to treatment. Ann Intern Med 1990;113:872-881.

Rathbun KC. Congenital syphilis. Sex Transm Dis 1983;10:93-99.

Sparling PF. Diagnosis and treatment of syphilis. N Engl J Med 1971;284:642.

Russell P, Altshuler G. Placental abnormalities of congenital syphilis. Am J Dis Child 1974;128:160-163.

Sanchez PS, Wendel GD, Grimpel E, et al. Diagnosis of congenital neurosyphilis by the rabbit infectivity test (RIT), and polymerase chain reaction (PCR). Pediatr Res 1991;29:286A.

Sanchez PJ, McCracken GH Jr, Wendel GS, et al. Molecular analysis of the fetal IgM response to *Treponema pallidum* antigens: implications for improved serodiagnosis of congenital infection. J Infect Dis 1989;508-517.

Scotti AT, Logan LL. A specific IgM antibody test in neonatal congenital syphilis. J Pediatr 1968;73:242-243.

Speer ME, Taber LH, Clark DB, Rudolph AJ. Cerebrospinal fluid levels of benzathine penicillin G in the neonate. J Pediatr 1977;9:996.

Srinivasan G, Ramamurthy RS, Bharathi A, et al. Congenital syphilis: a diagnostic and therapeutic dilemma. Pediatr Infect Dis 1983;2:436-441.

Taber LH, Huber TW. Congenital syphilis. Prog Clin Biol Res 1975;3:183.

Wendel GD. Gestational and congenital syphilis. Clin Perinatol 1988;15:287-303.

Yobs AR, Brown L, Hunter EF. Fluorescent antibody technique in early syphillis. Arch Pathol 1964;77:220-225.

Zenker PN, Rolfs RT. Treatment of syphilis, 1989. Rev Infect Dis 1990;12(suppl 6):S590.

Chlamydia trachomatis infections

Alexander ER, Harrison HR. Role of Chlamydia trachomatis in perinatal infection. Rev Infect Dis 1983;5:713-719.

Beem MO, Saxon EM. Respiratory tract colonization and a distinctive pneumonia syndrome in infants infected with Chlamydia trachomatis. N Engl J Med 1977;296:306-310.

Bell TA, Sandstrom KI, Gravett MG, et al. Comparison of ophthalmic silver nitrate solution and erythromycin ointment for prevention of natally acquired Chlamydia trachomatis. Sex Transm Dis 1987;14:195-200.

Blythe MJ, Katz BP, Caine VA. Historical and clinical factors associated with Chlamydia trachomatis genitourinary tract infection in female adolescents. J Pediatr 1988;112:1000-1004.

Brunham RC, Binns B, McDowell J, Paraskevas M. Chlamydia trachomatis infection in women with ectopic pregnancy. Obstet Gynecol 1986;67:722-726.

Chacko MR, Lovchik JC. Chlamydia trachomatis infection in sexually active adolescents: prevalence and risk factors. Pediatrics 1984;73:836-840.

Chambers CV, Shafer MA, Adger H, et al. Microflora of the urethra in adolescent boys: relationship to sexual activity and nongonococcal urethritis. J Pediatr 1987;110:314-321.

Chernesky MA, Mahony JB, Castriciano S, et al. Detection of Chlamydia trachomatis antigens by enzyme immunoassay and immunofluorescence in genital specimens from symptomatic and asymptomatic men and women. J Infect Dis 1986;154:141-148.

Eagar RM, Beach RK, Davidson AJ. Epidemiologic and clinical factors of Chlamydia trachomatis in Black, Hispanic and White female adolescents. West J Med 1985;143:3-41.

Fisher M, Swenson PD, Risucci D, Kaplan MH. Chlamydia trachomatis in suburban adolescents. J Pediatr 1987;111:617-620.

Fraser JJ, Rettig PJ, Kaplan DW. Prevalence of cervical Chlamydia trachomatis and Neisseria gonorrhoeae in female adolescents. Pediatrics 1982;71:333-336.

Golden N, Hammerschlag M, Neuhoff S, Gleyzer A. Prevalence of Chlamydia trachomatis cervical infection in female adolescents. Am J Dis Child 1984;138:562-564.

Hammerschlag MR. Chlamydial infections. J Pediatr 1989;114:727-734.

Hammerschlag MR, Cummings C, Roblin P, et al. Efficacy of neonatal ocular prophylaxis for the prevention of chlamydial and gonococcal conjunctivitis. N Engl J Med 1989;320:769-772.

Hammerschlag MR, Doraiswamy B, Alexander ER, et al. Are rectogenital chlamydial infections a marker of sexual abuse in children? Pediatr Infect Dis 1984;3:100-104.

Hammerschlag MR, Rettig PJ, Shields ME. False positive results with the use of chlamydial antigen detection tests in the evaluation of suspected sexual abuse in children. Pediatr Infect Dis 1988;7:11-14.

Hammerschlag MR, Roblin PM, Cummings C, et al. Comparison of enzyme immunoassay and culture for diagnosis of chlamydial conjunctivitis and respiratory infections in infants. J Clin Microbiol 1987;25:2306-2308.

Harrison HR, Alexander ER, Weinstein L, et al. Cervical Chlamydia trachomatis and mycoplasmal infections in pregnancy: epidemiology and outcomes. JAMA 1983;250:1721-1727.

Harrison HR, English MG, Lee CK, Alexander ER. Chlamydia trachomatis infant pneumonia. N Engl J Med 1978;298:702-708.

Hauger SB, Brown J, Agre F, et al. Failure of MicroTrak to detect C. trachomatis from genital tract sites of prepubertal children at risk for sexual abuse. Pediatr Infect Dis 1988;7:660-661.

Heggie AD, Lumicao GG, Stuart LA, et al. Chlamydia trachomatis infection in mothers and infants. Am J Dis Child 1981;135:507-511.

Heggie AD, Jaffe AC, Stuart LA, et al. Topical sulfacetamide vs oral erythromycin for neonatal chlamydial conjunctivitis. Am J Dis Child 1985;139:564-566.

Ingram DL, Runyan DK, Collins AD, et al. Vaginal Chlamydia trachomatis infection in children with sexual contact. Pediatr Infect Dis 1984;3:97-99.

Porder K, Sanchez N, Roblin PM, et al. Lack of specificity of Chlamydiazyme for detection of vaginal chlamydial infection in prepubertal girls. Pediatr Infect Dis 1989;8:358-360.

Radkowski MA, Kranzler JK, Beem MO, Tippk MA. Chlamydia pneumonia in infants: radiography in 125 cases. AJR 1981;137:703-706.

Rettig PJ, Nelson JD. Genital tract infection with Chlamydia trachomatis in prepubertal children. J Pediatr 1981;99:206-210.

Roblin PM, Hammerschlag MR, Cummings C, et al. Comparison of two rapid microscopic methods and culture for detection of Chlamydia trachomatis in ocular and nasopharyngeal specimens from infants. J Clin Microbiol 1989;27:968-970.

Saltz GR, Linnemann CC, Brookman RR, et al. Chlamydia trachomatis cervical infections in female adolescents. J Pediatr 1981;98:981-985.

Shafer MA, Vaughan E, Lipkin ES, et al. Evaluation fluorescein-conjugated monoclonal antibody test to detect Chlamydia trachomatis endocervical infections in adolescent girls. J Pediatr 1986;108:779-783.

Schachter J, Grossman M, Sweet RL, et al. Prospective study of perinatal transmission of Chlamydia trachomatis. JAMA 1986a;255:3374-3377.

Schachter J, Sweet RL, Grossman M, et al. Experience with the routine use of erythromycin in pregnancy. N Engl J Med 1986b;314:276-279.

Weiss SG, Newcomb RW, Beem MO. Pulmonary assessment of children after chlamydial pneumonia of infancy. J Pediatr 1986;108:661-664.

Bacterial vaginosis

Amsel R, Tolter PA, Spiegel CA, et al. Nonspecific vaginitis: diagnostic criteria and microbial and epidemiologic assocations. Am J Med 1983;74:14-22.

Bartley DL, Morgan L, Rimsza MA: *Gardnerella vaginalis* in prepubertal girls. Am J Dis Child 1987;141:1014-1017.

Hammerschlag MR, Cummings M, Doraiswamy B, et al. Nonspecific vaginitis following sexual abuse in children. Pediatrics 1985;75:1028-1031.

Samuels P, Hammerschlag MR, Cummings M, et al. Nonspecific vaginitis is an important cause of vaginitis in children. Presented at the 25th Interscience Conference on Antimicrobial Agents and Chemotherapy, 1985, Minneapolis, abstract #391.

Shafer M-A, Sweet RL, Ohm-Smith MJ, et al. Microbiology of the lower genital tract in post menarcheal adolescent girls, differences by sexual activity, contraception and presence of nonspecific vaginitis. J Pediatr 1985;107:974-981.

Spiegel CA, Amsel R, Holmes KK. Diagnosis of bacterial vaginosis by direct Gram stain of vaginal fluid. J Clin Microbiol 1983;18:170-177.

Thomason JL, Velbart SM, Anderson RJ, et al. Statistical evaluation of diagnostic criteria for bacterial vaginosis. Am J Obstet Gynecol 1990;162:155-160.

Trichomoniasis

Al-Salihi FL, Curram JP, Wang JS. Neonatal *trichomonas vaginalis:* report of three cases and review of the literature. Pediatrics 1974;53:196-200.

Fouts AC, Kraus SJ. *Trichomonas vaginalis:* Reevaluation of its clinical presentation and laboratory diagnosis. J Infect Dis 1980;141:137-143.

Jones JG, Yamauchi T, Lambert B: *Trichomonas vaginalis* infestation in sexually abused girls. Am J Dis Child 1985;139:846-847.

Kruger JN, Tam MR, Stevens CE, et al. Diagnosis of trichomoniasis. Comparison of conventional wet-mount examination with cytologic studies, cultures and monoclonal antibody staining of direct specimens. JAMA 1988;259:1223-1227.

Wolner-Hanssen P, Krieger JN, Stevens CE, et al. Clinical manifestations of vaginal trichomoniasis. JAMA 1989;261:571-576.

Human papilloma virus infection (condylomata acuminata)

Bauer HM, Greer CE, Chambers JC, et al. Genital human papilloma virus infection in female university students as determined by a PCR-based method. JAMA 1991;265:472-477.

Bender ME. New concepts of condyloma acuminata in children. Arch Dermatol 1986;122:1121-1124.

Boyd AS. Condylomata acuminata in the pediatric population. Am J Dis Child 1990;144:817-824.

Davis AJ, Emans SJ. Human papilloma virus infection in the pediatric and adolescent patient. J Pediatr 1989;115:1-9.

DeJong AR, Weiss JC, Brent RL. Condyloma acuminata in children. Am J Dis Child 1982;136:704-706.

Moscicki A-B, Palefsky J, Gonzales J, et al. Human papilloma virus infection in sexually active adolescent females: prevalence and risk factors. Pediatr Res 1990;28:507-513.

Rock B, Noghashfar Z, Barnett N, et al. Genital tract papilloma virus infection in children. Arch Dermatol 1986;122:1129-1132.

Seidel J, Zonana J, Tolten E. Condylomata acuminata as a sign of sexual abuse in children. J Pediatr 1979;95:553-554.

Other sexually transmitted diseases

Gellert GA, DurFee MJ, Berkowitz CD. Developing guidelines for HIV antibody testing among victims of pediatric sexual abuse. Child Abuse Neglect 1990;14:9-17.

Gutman LT, St Claire KK, Weedy C, et al. Human immunodeficiency virus transmission by child sexual abuse. Am J Dis Child 1991;145:137-141.

Leiderman BA, Grimm KT. A child with HIV infection. JAMA 1986;256:3094.

Schmid GP. Treatment of chancroid 1989. Rev Infect Dis 1990;12:80:S580-S589.

Szmuness W, Much MI, Prince AM, et al. On the role of sexual behavior in the spread of hepatitis B infection. Ann Intern Med 1975;83:489-495.

26

SMALLPOX (VARIOLA) AND VACCINIA

A full discussion of smallpox (variola) and vaccinia was included in Chapter 28 of the seventh (1981) edition of this book. Because the disease has been successfully eradicated and the requirement for vaccination has been abolished, the authors have chosen to restrict this chapter to brief general sections, comments on contemporary issues, remarks on related viruses and illnesses, and a list of significant references for those readers who choose to explore further this fascinating example of human conquest of a disease.

For more than 3,000 years smallpox was a widespread illness with serious morbidity and mortality. Nations in Africa and the Asian subcontinent reported hundreds of thousands of cases annually as recently as 1967. In that year the World Health Organization (WHO) began its 10-year program of smallpox eradication. On October 26, 1977, Ali Maow Maalin, a cook in the district hospital at Merka, Somalia, had the onset of his smallpox rash. He has gone down in history as the last known patient with endemic smallpox. In the years after Maalin's recovery the only known smallpox victims acquired their infection as the result of a laboratory contamination in Birmingham, England.

Several hundred episodes of suspected endemic smallpox have been reported to WHO since the case of Ali Maow Maalin, but none has been verified. Instead, they were chickenpox, herpes simplex, monkeypox, drug eruptions, or other skin disorders. Of special note is monkeypox, which has been reported with regularity from West and Central Africa. Originally recovered from monkeys who became ill in captivity, the virus has been responsible for human illness closely resembling smallpox, usually in children with no history of previous smallpox vaccination. Secondary spread among humans is quite unusual, but several cases have been documented. Serological assays can differentiate variola, vaccinia, and monkeypox infections (Walls et al., 1981).

The WHO Assembly on May 8, 1980, certified the final global eradication of smallpox (WHO, 1980). This is an achievement unique in the history of mankind's interaction with the microorganisms of the environment (Fenner et al., 1988). Smallpox virus exists today only in the deep freezers of two selected laboratories.

The two laboratories that maintain stocks of variola virus are at the Centers for Disease Control in Atlanta, Georgia, and the Research Institute for Viral Preparations in Moscow, Russia. They participate in the smallpox eradication surveillance and research program of the World Health Organization. Current plans call for destruction of the remaining stocks of smallpox virus in 1993, by which time complete genomic sequencing of the virus will have been achieved, permitting integration of this information with comparable studies of other members of the *Orthopox genus*.

SMALLPOX (VARIOLA MAJOR; VARIOLA MINOR OR ALASTRIM; VARIOLOID)

Smallpox was an acute, highly contagious, preventable disease caused by the variola virus, family Poxviridae, genus *Orthopoxvirus*. Other members of the genus include vaccinia, monkeypox, cowpox, camelpox, and ectromelia (mousepox). Smallpox was characterized by a 3- to 4-day prodromal period of chills, high fever, headache, backache, vomiting, and prostration. The temperature began to subside as the eruptive stage commenced on the third or fourth day. The eruption progressed from macular to papular to vesicular to pustular and finally to crusting during an 8- to 14-day period. The temperature rose again, and the constitutional symptoms intensified during the pustular stage. The rash had a characteristic peripheral or centrifugal distribution, with lesions at the same stage in any one regional area.

Variola major, variola minor or alastrim, and varioloid were the three chief forms of the disease. *Variola major* was classic smallpox. It had a high mortality rate that varied with the type of lesions as follows: ordinary-discrete, less than 10%; ordinary-semiconfluent, 25% to 50%; ordinary-confluent, 50% to 75%, flat, greater than 90%; hemorrhagic, nearly 100% (Koplan and Foster, 1979). In general, infants, pregnant women, and elderly patients had higher fatality rates. *Variola minor*, or alastrim, was a mild type of smallpox occurring in nonvaccinated persons. It was caused by a less virulent strain of the virus that bred true. The mortality rate was usually less than 1% except in rare instances when the rash became confluent or hemorrhagic. *Varioloid* was a mild form of smallpox occurring in previously vaccinated persons who had partial immunity. This mild disease was caused by a virulent strain of the virus capable of causing variola major in a nonimmunized contact (Koplan and Foster, 1979; Mazumder et al., 1975).

Etiology

The poxviruses are a family of large, ellipsoid, complex DNA viruses. They include more than 20 mammalian viruses plus groups of bird (avipox) and insect (entomopox) viruses. A number of the group can initiate human infection but only variola (smallpox) has been of worldwide significance. Humans are the only host for variola virus so that eradication of human infection left no sylvan or other occult reservoir from which virus could be re-introduced.

Smallpox and vaccinia viruses are morphologically indistinguishable and closely related immunologically. The elementary bodies can be identified in smears of vesicular fluid stained by the Paschen, Giemsa, or Gutstein method. As viewed with an electron microscope, they are brick shaped or ovoid and approximately 200 × 400 nm in size. Aggregates of these bodies in infected host cells form the so-called Guarnieri bodies, which are intracytoplasmic inclusions measuring approximately 10 μm in diameter. The viral genome is a single molecule of double-stranded DNA contained within a central core that in turn is enclosed by an external coat of lipid and protein surrounding two lateral bodies as well. Research continues on the classification and genetic relatedness of the many poxviruses and their interrelationships. All poxviruses apparently share a common inner core nucleoprotein antigen.

Infection with smallpox and vaccinia viruses stimulates the production of at least four types of antibody: antihemagglutinin, complement-fixing antibodies, neutralizing antibodies, and antibodies that inhibit agar gel precipitation. Levels of antihemagglutinin and complement-fixing antibodies rise significantly by the end of the second week of illness or vaccination; they persist for several months. Neutralizing antibodies develop later but persist for years.

Pathogenesis, pathology, clinical manifestations, diagnosis, differential diagnosis, complications, prognosis, immunity, epidemiological factors, treatment, preventive measures, isolation, quarantine, and control are discussed in Chapter 28 of the seventh edition and in references listed at the end of this chapter (Behbehani, 1983; Fenner et al., 1988).

VACCINIA

Nearly 200 years ago Edward Jenner reported his successful use of vaccinia virus inoculation to prevent smallpox (1798, reprinted 1896). Although the pedigree of later vaccinia strains became confused by their mixture with variola and an equine virus, standard vaccines since the last of the nineteenth century have been labeled *vaccinia*.

Vaccinia is an acute infectious disease induced by deliberate smallpox vaccination or by the accidental contact of abraded skin with infective material. It is characterized by the development of a localized lesion that progresses in sequence from papule to vesicle to pustule to crust. Fever and regional lymphadenitis may develop during the vesicular or pustular stage. The infection stimulates the production of antibodies that are protective against smallpox.

Clinical manifestations

The clinical manifestations of vaccinia are dependent for the most part on the immune status of the individual. Two types of reactions may result from a successful vaccination: a "major" response (pustular lesion or an area of definite induration or congestion surrounding a central lesion, scab, or ulcer 6 to 8 days after vaccination) or an "equivocal" response.

Major response. Three days after vaccination, the inoculated site becomes reddened and pruritic. It becomes papular on the fourth day and vesicular by the fifth or sixth day. A red areola surrounds the vesicle, which becomes umbilicated and then pustular by the eighth to the eleventh day. By this time the red areola has enlarged markedly. The pustule begins to dry, the redness subsides, and the lesion becomes crusted between the second and third week. By the end of the third week, the scab falls off, leaving a permanent scar that at first is pink in color but eventually becomes white.

At the end of the first week, between the vesicular and pustular phases, there may be a variable amount of fever, malaise, and regional lymphadenitis. These symptoms usually subside within 1 to 2 days and are more likely to occur in older children and adults than in infants.

Accelerated, modified, or vaccinoid reaction. Revaccination of a partially immune person is followed by an attenuated form of vaccinia with the following characteristics: (1) usually there is no fever or constitutional symptoms; (2) a papule appears by the third day, becomes vesicular by the fifth to seventh day, and dries shortly thereafter; (3) the vesicle and its red areola are relatively small; and (4) the scar, if present, is usually insignificant and disappears within 1 or 2 years.

Accelerated reactions may also result from scratching and autoinoculation with the vesicular fluid of a primary vaccinia pox. The accelerated lesions mature simultaneously with the initial primary lesion and heal without scarring as a rule.

• • •

The absence of a reaction does *not* mean that the person is immune. In most instances either the vaccine is not potent or the technique is at fault. Occasionally, a papule may result from needle trauma. To evaluate a vaccination, it would be ideal to inspect the lesion daily. When this is not practical, the optimal times of inspection are the third, seventh, and fourteenth days.

Vaccination procedures

Methods. The most commonly used method of vaccination is the multiple pressure method.

Precautions. Since vaccination is generally an elective procedure, it should be postponed in instances of intercurrent infection. Primary vaccination of individuals with eczema or other types of exfoliative dermatitis may be complicated by eczema vaccinatum, a severe and potentially fatal disease. Vaccination should be deferred until the skin lesions clear.

It is recommended that vaccination, in those few instances when indicated, be given as *one* inoculation over the *deltoid area*, with the *multiple pressure* or *multiple puncture technique* and a fully potent vaccine.

Immunity

Immunity develops between the eighth and eleventh days after vaccination. Antihemagglutinin, complement-fixing, and virus-neutralizing antibodies are demonstrable between the tenth and thirteenth days. Duration of immunity is extremely variable; it may range between 2 and 10 years. Revaccination at 3-year intervals is generally adequate to maintain optimal immunity (El-Ad et al., 1990).

Complications

Until May 1983 when it was withdrawn by Wyeth Laboratories (the sole U.S. producer) from general availability, smallpox vaccine occasionally was administered to patients with recurrent herpes simplex or papillomas in the mistaken expectation that doing so would interfere with development of new lesions or would accelerate the resolution of older ones. Because some of these patients suffered from underlying immunodeficiency disorders, they acquired life-threatening progressive vaccinia caused by unarrested local replication of vaccinia virus.

Currently, smallpox vaccine is available only from the Centers for Disease Control, Atlanta, Georgia, and is recommended only for laboratory workers who may be engaged in surveillance or research involving nonvariola orthopoxviruses. It seems appropriate and prudent to retain the following paragraphs on the possible complications of vaccination.

Secondary bacterial infection. The local lesion may become secondarily infected with staphylococci or streptococci, causing cellulitis.

Accidental infection. Autoinoculation by means of scratching an active lesion may produce secondary pocks over various parts of the body. The severity of this complication is governed by the site of inoculation. For example, a lesion of the eye with corneal involvement can result in ulceration, scarring, and blindness.

Toxic eruptions. An erythema multiforme type of eruption occasionally occurs between the seventh and tenth days at the height of the vaccinia reaction. The rash may be generalized or localized to a particular area. It usually clears within 3 to 5 days. It is considered a sensitivity reaction (Plate 6). This rash was most often seen in infants vaccinated before their first birthday.

Generalized vaccinia. This potentially serious complication arose between the seventh and fourteenth days after vaccination. A generalized eruption develops, with crops of lesions simulating a primary vaccination. Healing without scars takes place rapidly, being completed at the same time as the healing of the primary vaccinia lesion.

The possibility of serious consequences from the administration of recombinant vaccinia viruses or conventional vaccinia to human immunodeficiency virus (HIV)-infected individuals has been exemplified in recent case reports (Guillaume et al., 1991; Redfield et al., 1987).

Eczema vaccinatum. This potentially fatal complication of vaccinia develops in patients with eczema or other forms of exfoliative dermatitis who have been either vaccinated or exposed to an active case of vaccinia. The disease is characterized by high fever, severe toxicity, and an extensive vesicular and pustular eruption chiefly confined to the area of dermatitis (Plate 7 and Fig. 26-1). Healthy areas of skin also may become involved. The mortality may be significant.

Progressive vaccinia (vaccinia necrosum; prolonged vaccinia; vaccinia gangrenosa). Progressive vaccinia, a highly fatal complication, is fortunately rare. The initial vaccinal lesion fails to

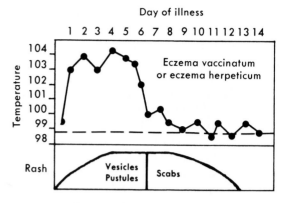

Fig. 26-1. Schematic diagram of the clinical course of eczema herpeticum or eczema vaccinatum.

heal and progresses to involve more and more areas of adjacent skin. The necrosis of the tissues continues to extend, often over a period of months. Metastatic lesions may develop in other parts of the skin, bones, and viscera. This complication has been observed in patients with immunological disorders. The common denominator has been depression of T-lymphocyte function, either congenital or acquired. Progressive vaccinia is also likely to occur in patients with immunological deficits caused by malignant disease of the lymphatic system (leukemia or lymphomas) and/or their therapy. Treatment has been attempted with vaccinia-immune globulin (VIG), N-methylisatin-β-thiosemicarbazone (methisazone, marboran), interferon, transfer factor, acyclovir, and rifampin. Cases have been too infrequent to evaluate therapy in an acceptable fashion.

Postvaccinal encephalitis. Postvaccinal encephalitis is a serious but rare complication. The incidence of postvaccinal encephalitis in Sweden from 1947 to 1954 was 1.9 per 100,000. Surveillance of complications of smallpox vaccination in the United States in 1968 revealed 2.9 cases of encephalitis per 1 million primary vaccinations; the highest incidence, 6.5 per 1 million, was observed in infants less than 12 months old (Goldstein et al., 1975; Lane et al., 1969).

The clinical picture is the same as that in other postinfectious encephalitides. The usual manifestations include fever, headache, vomiting, meningeal signs, paralysis, drowsiness, coma, and convulsions. The spinal fluid may contain an increase in number of mononuclear cells and amount of protein. Pathologically, the brain shows the same type of perivascular infiltration and demyelination as occur in encephalitis complicating measles and chickenpox. The mortality rate may be as high as 30% to 40%.

Treatment

Primary vaccinia requires no treatment. Dressings are unnecessary except to prevent the possible transmission of virus to susceptible contacts. Fever and pain in the arm may be treated with appropriate doses of acetaminophen. Superimposed pyogenic infections may require hot compresses and appropriate antimicrobial therapy. Patients with eczema vaccinatum need intensive supportive therapy; they should receive VIG, 0.6 ml per kilogram of body weight intramuscularly. The same dose would be indicated for patients with vaccinia necrosum. In general, the treatment of encephalitis is the same as that of any infectious or postinfectious encephalitis.

Preventive measures

Most complications of vaccinia are preventable. Vaccination is contraindicated under the following circumstances: evidence of eczema or other chronic forms of dermatitis in the vaccinated person or a close contact; or altered immune status from disease or immunosuppressive therapy.

In 1971 the United States Public Health Service accepted the recommendation of its Advisory Committee on Immunization Practices that *routine* smallpox vaccinations in the United States be discontinued. In 1976 the former recommendations of routine smallpox vaccination for hospital employees was also rescinded. Since that time the sole civilian group for whom vaccine has been indicated is laboratory workers directly involved with orthopoxviruses.

It is worth noting a renaissance of interest in widespread vaccinia administration. Smith et al. (1983) reported the successful incorporation into the vaccinia virus genome of coding sequences for the hepatitis B surface antigen. Gene portions from many other human viral pathogens have similarly been exploited to provide a vaccinia vector that could serve to induce immunity to a number of viral infections (Moss, 1991). The most active research with recombinant vaccinia viruses has focused on preparations expressing

HIV envelope glycoproteins (Cooney et al., 1991), which have already been used in human clinical trials. This promises to be an active area of investigation in the coming years.

REFERENCES

Smallpox

Bauer DJ, St Vincent L, Kempe CH, Downie AW. Prophylactic treatment of smallpox contacts with N-methylisatin-β-thiosemicarbazone (compound 33T57). Lancet 1963; 2:494.

Bauer DJ, et al. Prophylaxis of smallpox with methisazone. Am J Epidemiol 1970;90:130.

Baxby D. The origins of vaccinia virus. J Infect Dis 1977;136:453.

Behbehani AB. The smallpox story: life and death of an old disease. Microbiol Rev 1983;47:455-509.

Breman JG, Arita I. The confirmation and maintenance of smallpox eradication. N Engl J Med 1980;303:1263-1273.

Cho CT, Wenner HA. Monkeypox virus. Bacteriol Rev 1973;37:1.

Fenner F, Henderson DA, Arita I, et al (eds). Smallpox and its eradication. Geneva, Switzerland: World Health Organization, 1988;581-583.

Fenner F, Wittek R, Dumbell DR. The orthopoxviruses. San Diego: Academic Press, 1989, pp 10-13.

Henderson DA. The eradication of smallpox. Sci Am 1976;235:25.

Koplan JP, Foster SO. Smallpox: clinical types, causes of death, and treatment. J Infect Dis 1979;140:440.

Mazumder DNG, De S, Mitra AC, Mukherjee MK. Clinical observations on smallpox: a study of 1233 patients admitted to the Infectious Diseases Hospital, Calcutta, during 1973. Bull WHO 1975;52:301.

Ricketts TF, Byles JB. The diagnosis of smallpox, vols I and II. Reprinted from the 1908 London edition. U.S. Department of Health, Education, and Welfare, Bureau of Disease, Prevention and Environmental control, Division of Foreign Quarantine, 1966.

Walls HH, Ziegler DW, Nakano JM. Characterization of antibodies to orthopoxviruses in human sera by radioimmunoassay. Bull WHO 1981;59:253-262.

World Health Organization. Declaration of global eradication of smallpox. Weekly Epidemiol Rec 1980;55:145-152.

Vaccinia

Centers for Disease Control. Contact spread of vaccinia from a recently vaccinated Marine—Louisiana. MMWR 1984;33:37-38.

Centers for Disease Control. Contact spread of vaccinia from a National Guard vaccinee—Wisconsin. MMWR 1985; 34:182-183.

Cooney EL, Collier AC, Greenberg PD, et al. Safety of and immunological response to a recombinant vaccinia virus vaccine expressing HIV envelope glycoprotein. Lancet 1991;337:567-572.

El-Ad B, Roth Y, Winder A, et al. The persistence of neutralizing antibodies after revaccination against smallpox. J Infect Dis 1990;161:446-448.

Goldstein JA, Neff JM, Lane JM, Koplan JP. Smallpox vaccination reactions, prophylaxis, and therapy of complications. Pediatrics 1975;55:342.

Guillaume JC, Saiag P, Wechsler J, et al. Vaccinia from recombinant virus expressing HIV genes (letter). Lancet 1991;377:1034-1035.

Jenner E. An inquiry into the causes and effects of the variolae vacciniae, a disease discovered in some of the western counties of England, particularly Gloucestershire, and known by the name of cowpox. Reprinted by Cassell and Co, Ltd, 1896. Available in Pamphlet vol 4232, Army Medical Library, Washington, DC.

Kempe CH. Studies on smallpox and complications of smallpox vaccination. Pediatrics 1960;26:176.

Lane JM, Ruben FL, Neff JM, Millar JD. Complications of smallpox vaccination, 1968. N Engl J Med 1969;281:1201.

Moss B. Vaccinia virus: a tool for research and development. Science 1991;252:1662-1667.

Neff JM, et al. Complications of smallpox vaccination. National survey in the United States, 1963. N Engl J Med 1967;276:125.

Redfield RR, Wright DC, James WD, et al. Disseminated vaccinia in a military recruit with human immunodeficiency virus (HIV) disease. N Engl J Med 1987;316:673-676.

Smith GL, Mackett M, Moss B. Infectious vaccinia virus recombinants that express hepatitis B virus surface antigens. Nature 1983;302:490-495.

Tyzzer EE. The etiology and pathology of vaccinia. J Med Res 1904;11:180.

Zagury D, Leonard R. Fouchard M, et al. Immunization against AIDS in humans. Nature 1987;326:249-250.

27

STAPHYLOCOCCAL INFECTIONS

ALICE PRINCE

Staphylococcus aureus is an important cause of illness in infants, children, and adolescents. In addition to the common *S. aureus* infections of the skin and soft tissue such as impetigo, furuncles, and wound infections, life-threatening infections caused by *S. aureus* such as sepsis, endocarditis, and pneumonia also occur. Several diseases such as scalded skin syndrome and toxic shock syndrome are caused by endotoxins produced by staphylococci. These organisms may colonize mucous membranes or skin without producing generalized evidence of infection. The common use of indwelling central venous catheters has made infection caused by coagulase-negative staphylococci a very common clinical problem, both in neonates and in children who are immunologically compromised.

ETIOLOGY
Microbiology

Staphylococci are gram-positive organisms that can occur singly or in pairs, short chains, or clusters (the term *staphylococci* is derived from the Greek word meaning a bunch of grapes). Staphylococci grow well on artificial media and are very hardy organisms that can persist on nonphysiological surfaces for long periods of time. Colonies of *S. aureus* grow well under aerobic and anaerobic conditions, producing a golden pigmentation under some conditions. *S. aureus* ferments a variety of sugars, including mannitol under anaerobic conditions and tolerates media with high concentrations of sodium chloride.

The cell wall of a staphylococcus is composed primarily of peptidoglycan, teichoic acid, and protein A. The peptidoglycan comprises approximately 50% of the cell wall and consists of repeating subunits of N-acetylmuramic acid and N-acetylglucosamine. The peptidoglycan component of *S. aureus* is involved in the host immune response to staphylococci; it elicits the production of interleukin-1 (IL-1) from human monocytes, which is important in the production of the febrile response. Peptidoglycan can activate complement and stimulate antibody production.

Teichoic acid, the second major component of the cell wall, is composed of repeating units of glycerol phosphate and can be important in the immunological response to the organism.

The protein A component is also important in the immune response to staphylococci. Protein A has high affinity for the Fc fragment of immunoglobulins. It binds IgG and fixes complement. Another cell-wall component is coagulase, which binds fibrinogen and causes aggregation of the organisms.

Exoproducts

Much of the virulence of *S. aureus* is due to the production of exoproducts, enzymes and toxins important in the pathogenesis of staphylococcal infections and their relative virulence (Hodes and Barzilai, 1990). The toxins produced, in general, act on membranes. The exfoliatins (ETA and ETB), or epidermolytic toxins, are responsible for dermatological lesions characterized by erythema and desquamation resulting from the splitting of the desmosomes that link the epidermal cells. ETB is responsible for staphylococcal scalded skin syndrome, which occurs in newborns and young children. ETB usually is produced by organisms of phage group II and is plasmid encoded. ETA is a chromosomal enzyme and is found in several different phage groups. Exfoliatins produce characteristic changes in the epidermis of infants. Another toxin, leukocidin, is toxic to phagocytes, causing pores in their membranes. At least four other staphylococcal toxins are hemolysins (alpha, beta, gamma, delta) with distinct properties. Several of them (alpha, beta, gamma) cause hemolytic effects, whereas the delta toxin disrupts membranes by a detergent-like action.

Two other exotoxins, TSST-1 and TSST-2, are responsible for the production of toxic shock syndrome, which is characterized by hypotension, fever, a desquamative rash, and multisystem involvement (Davis et al., 1980). These toxins have profound effects on the immune system, including the induction of IL-1 production (Parsonnet, 1989; Schlievert et al., 1981).

Other exotoxins characteristically produced by staphylococci include catalase, coagulase, and hyaluronidase. Catalase is produced by all staphylococci. It is required for the conversion of hydrogen peroxide, which is generated by the organisms, to water and oxygen. This enzyme can also metabolize the hydrogen peroxide generated by phagocytes in the process of trying to kill the organism. Thus catalase is important in the pathogenicity of staphylococci. Coagulase is used to differentiate S. *aureus* from other staphylococcal species. It triggers the final steps in the clotting cascade, resulting in clot formation. Hyaluronidase destroys the hyaluronic acid that comprises much of the extracellular matrix of connective tissue. It is believed important in facilitating the spread of organisms through tissues.

Staphylococci can also produce several different **enterotoxins**, which are associated with gastrointestinal symptoms, particularly vomiting and diarrhea. They are heat-stable proteins (100° C, 212° F, for 30 minutes) typically produced by organisms contaminating milk-containing foodstuffs that were not refrigerated properly.

Antimicrobial susceptibility

The vast majority of S. *aureus* isolates are resistant to penicillin by virtue of β-lactamase production, generally attributed to the presence of a plasmid-associated β-lactamase. The few strains that do not harbor these plasmids are highly susceptible to penicillin G (minimal inhibitory concentration [MIC], 0.02 or less), which remains the drug of choice for infections caused by these rare, susceptible strains. More than 80% of clinical isolates of S. *aureus* are penicillinase positive. These enzymes recently have been differentiated into several groups based on differences in the β-lactamase produced. The staphylococcal β-lactamases can be chromosomal and inducible or can be constitutively produced. Their activity against "β-lactamase–stable" penicillins such as oxacillin, methicillin, and nafcillin also varies, as does their activity against first-generation cephalosporins such as cephalothin or cefazolin, which are extremely stable to these enzymes (Neu, 1985). The β-lactamase inhibitors clavulanic acid and sulbactam have excellent affinity for the staphylococcal β-lactamases and, when used in combination with amoxicillin or ampicillin, provide excellent coverage against these organisms. The plasmids encoding the staphylococcal β-lactamases can also express resistance to macrolide antibiotics, aminoglycosides, the lincosamides, and heavy metals.

Development of resistance to the β-lactamase–stable penicillins and to the cephalosporins has become an increasing problem (Kline and Mason, 1988). These organisms, collectively labeled methicillin-resistant S. *aureus* (MRSA), are associated with up to 30% of the clinical isolates at some medical centers. The molecular basis for MRSA is complex and not well understood. All MRSA contain a *mec* gene associated with an altered penicillin-binding protein (PBP2A) that has very low affinity for β-lactam antibiotics (Hartmann and Tomasz, 1984; de Lencastre et al., 1991). Expression of this gene is highly variable. High-level methicillin resistance can be associated with the induction of *mec*. In addition, the production of very high levels of β-lactamase is associated with failure of β-lactam antibiotic therapy against certain strains. Both β-lactamase production and the expression of *mec* can be induced at the same

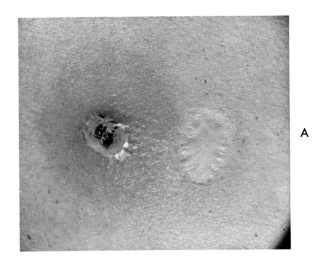

A

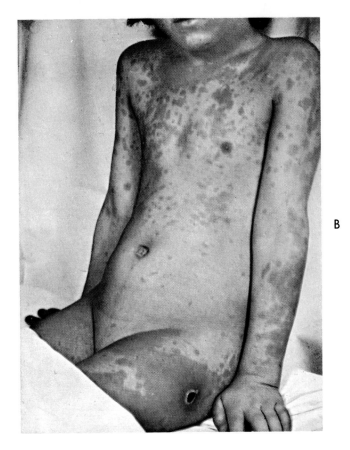

B

Plate 6
A, Primary take in a previously vaccinated person. **B,** Toxic eruption complicating vaccinia.
(From Top FH, Wehrle PF, eds. Communicable and infectious diseases, ed 8. St. Louis. The
CV Mosby Co., 1976.)

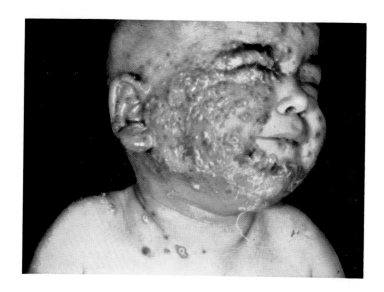

Plate 7
Eczema vaccinatum. (Courtesy Dr. Otto E. Billo; from Stimson PM, Hodes HLA. Manual of the common contagious diseases. Philadelphia. Lea & Febiger, 1956.)

time by common regulatory elements. Identification of MRSA in clinical laboratories is done by identifying organisms with an oxacillin MIC greater than 4 μg/ml after incubation at 35° C (95° F). Organisms that are high β-lactamase producers may be oxacillin resistant but are susceptible to amoxicillin plus clavulanic acid (Augmentin); strains with high-level expression of *mec* (altered PBPs) also are clavulanic acid resistant.

Staphylococci can also produce aminoglycoside-modifying enzymes that provide resistance to the aminoglycosides gentamicin, tobramycin, and amikacin. These enzymes are frequently plasmid associated and may be transferrable from strain to strain along with the antibiotic-resistance determinants for other clinically used drugs such as erythromycin or clindamycin.

HOST FACTORS

The normal host is usually quite resistant to infection by *S. aureus*. However, in the presence of a foreign body (Falcieri et al., 1987) or if there are predisposing conditions, staphylococci in the environment provide a common cause of infection. The hallmark of staphylococcal infection is suppuration—the organism elicits a brisk phagocytic response; however, several host factors determine susceptibility to staphylococcal infection. Staphylococci generally are opsonized, phagocytosed, and killed within the phagolysosome, with phagocytic function particularly important in the defense against staphylococci. In patients with chronic granulomatous disease of childhood, recurrent staphylococcal infections occur because of the inability to generate the superoxide required for intracellular killing of *S. aureus*. The catalase produced by staphylococci destroys the hydrogen peroxide involved in bacterial killing. Other immunological defects such as those present in patients with Job syndrome, Chédiak-Higashi syndrome, or Wiskott-Aldrich syndrome predispose the patients to staphylococcal and other common infections.

Opsonization of *S. aureus* occurs readily because the Fc fragment of immunoglobulin recognizes protein A, and the presence of receptors for complement, including C3b, facilitates phagocytosis. Thus the organisms can be opsonized by antibody, chiefly IgG, or, in nonimmune patients, by complement, by either the classic or alternate pathways.

CLINICAL MANIFESTATIONS AND MANAGEMENT
Skin and soft-tissue infections

One of the most common presentations of *S. aureus* infection is localized infection of the skin, which may range from small localized processes, including impetigo, paronychia, or small furuncles, to extensive areas of cellulitis. The organisms gain access to the integument after nasal colonization or through small breaks in the skin. Staphylococci multiply locally, producing the exoproducts and toxins outlined previously that facilitate spread throughout the surrounding connective tissue. A brisk polymorphonuclear leukocyte response and ensuing phagocytosis and bacterial killing follow. Thrombosis of surrounding small blood vessels occurs, with the deposition of fibrin. As this process continues, a central area of necrosis develops consisting of dead and dying tissue, phagocytes, and bacteria, surrounded by a fibrinous capsule. Thus a small localized skin infection such as impetigo may progress to cellulitis involving the underlying soft tissues and then result in frank abscess formation. Treatment of staphylococcal skin infections depends on the extent of disease; abscesses, in which there is poor penetration of antibiotics into the necrotic center of the lesion, require drainage; superficial cellulitis can be treated with oral or topical antimicrobials.

Impetigo, particularly bullous impetigo, is most often caused by *S. aureus* (Albert et al., 1970). The infection usually begins with a small area of erythema that progresses into bullae filled with cloudy fluid. These bullae are found most commonly on the extremities. The bullae rupture and heal with crust formation. Impetigo is most common in the summer months. Clinically, impetigo may be confused with the early stages of varicella and with insect bites. Treatment of impetigo traditionally has included systemic antistaphylococcal antibiotics (Demidovish et al., 1990), particularly if there are systemic signs such as fever, although topical therapy with agents such as mupirocin also is highly effective for treating localized infections (McLinn, 1988).

Staphylococcal lymphadenitis is a common infection in children, usually seen initially as a tender, erythematous mass in the cervical chain of lymph nodes, with accompanying fever (Hieber and Davis, 1976). Traditionally, cervical adenitis was considered a complication of streptococcal pharyngitis; however, staphylococci now are frequently the cause of these infections, although the possibility of mycobacterial infection should be considered. Surgical drainage of areas of staphylococcal lymphadenitis is preferable if the lesions are fluctuant. More often the area is indurated and not amenable to drainage. In these cases treatment of staphylococcal cervical adenitis with antistaphylococcal β-lactam antibiotics (oxacillin, methicillin, nafcillin) is usually successful, although resolution of all swelling may take weeks.

Mastitis caused by *S. aureus* is a common clinical problem, in both nursing mothers and neonates. The production of lipase by staphylococci is thought to contribute to their ability to cause this infection in a lipid-rich environment. The infection may begin as a localized cellulitis but can progress to frank abscess formation requiring drainage.

Diseases caused by staphylococcal toxins

Staphylococcal scalded skin syndrome originally was described as an exfoliative dermatitis of infants by Ritter von Rittershain. The disease is caused by staphylococci of phage group II producing exfoliative toxins (Melish and Glasgow, 1970) (Figs. 27-1 and 27-2). Specifically, phage type 71, which produces exfoliative toxins, is most often associated with this disease. The patient usually presents with generalized erythema, which progresses to bullae formation followed by generalized desquamation (Gooch and Britt, 1978). The skin is painful to the touch and becomes extremely friable; and even gentle stroking leads to peeling (Nikolsky's sign). Histopathologically, the skin separates intradermally at the stratum granulosum layer. Cultures

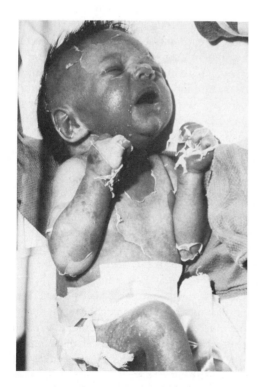

Fig. 27-1. Newborn infant with scalded skin syndrome in exfoliative stage. (From Melish ME, Glasgow LA. Reprinted by permission of New England Journal of Medicine 1970;282:1114.)

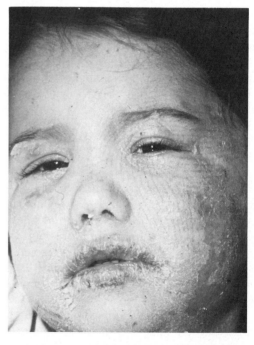

Fig. 27-2. Two-year-old girl in the resolving phase of the scalded skin syndrome undergoing secondary desquamation. Large, thick flakes of dried skin are concentrated particularly about the mouth. (From Melish ME and Glasgow LA. Reprinted by permission of the New England Journal of Medicine 282:1114, 1970.)

of the skin or nasopharynx are usually positive for *S. aureus*. Blood cultures are generally negative. Systemic treatment with antistaphylococcal antibiotics is indicated. This syndrome classically is found in infants but also occurs in older children. It can be reproduced in infant but not adult mice (Melish and Glasgow, 1970). A similar clinical syndrome in older patients, toxic epidermal necrolysis or Lyell's disease, is differentiated from scalded skin syndrome by intraepithelial splitting at the dermoepidermal junction and usually is caused by hypersensitivity to drugs such as sulfonamides or barbiturates. A skin biopsy may be a helpful diagnostic test in confusing situations.

Toxic shock syndrome is another disease caused by toxin-producing staphylococci (Davis et al., 1980). This syndrome was described by Todd, who observed seven children with a severe multisystem illness characterized by high fever, scarlatiniform rash, vomiting, diarrhea, renal and hepatic dysfunction, disseminated intravascular coagulation (DIC), and shock (Wiesenthal and Todd, 1984). This syndrome is similar to staphylococcal scarlet fever syndrome. A large increase in cases noted in young women was associated with the use of hyperabsorbent tampons (Parsonnet, 1989). The women were initially seen during their menses while using tampons; they had fever, vomiting, diarrhea, myalgias, and a characteristic "sunburn" type rash. *S. aureus* has been isolated from the tampon or from another focus of infection in patients with nonmenstrual toxic shock syndrome as it was in the cases originally described by Todd. The rash progresses to generalized desquamation, usually involving the palms and soles. Analysis of the staphylococci isolated from these cases, using gene probes, has demonstrated the presence of DNA associated with the production of TSST-1 (in the majority of menstrual-related cases) or TSST-2. Antibodies to these toxins appear to be protective. Treatment of toxic shock syndrome focuses primarily on reversing shock and hypotension, removing the focus of the staphylococcal infection, and providing treatment with antistaphylococcal antibiotics.

Staphylococcal gastrointestinal disease is produced by organisms expressing the heat-stable enterotoxin B. The disease usually occurs in outbreaks in which a common food source is contaminated by an individual carrying staphylococci (Holmberg and Blake, 1984). The toxin-producing organisms proliferate in food that is uncooked or only partially cooked (custards, potato salad) and not properly refrigerated. Patients develop an acute onset of vomiting and watery diarrhea 2 to 6 hours after ingestion. Symptoms are self-limited, and providing supportive therapy consisting of fluid replacement is sufficient. The use of antimicrobial agents is not necessary.

Illnesses caused by *S. aureus* bacteremia

Septicemia caused by *S. aureus* can occur in both normal (Hieber and Davis, 1976; Hodes and Barzilai, 1990, Musher and McKenzie, 1977; Sheagren, 1984) and immunocompromised hosts (Ladisch and Pizzo, 1978). As ubiquitous organisms, staphylococci gain access to the blood after colonization of the nasopharynx, through breaks in the skin, or from colonization of indwelling plastic catheters or other foreign bodies. High-grade bacteremia follows, with the usual signs of fever and tachycardia in an acutely ill patient. Although uncomplicated staphylococcal bacteremia can occur in previously well patients, including adolescents (Shulman and Ayoub, 1976), the organism can also seed other sites, causing local complications.

Endocarditis is a major complication of staphylococcal septicemia (Bayer, 1982). Although this was historically a disease of intravenous drug abusers, staphylococcal endocarditis is also a complication of congenital heart disease. This entity may present in a previously well child with asymptomatic cardiac pathology such as mitral valve prolapse or with an asymptomatic ventricular septal defect (Fig. 27-3). These lesions produce turbulent blood flow, causing a reactive focus on the cardiac endothelium that presents a nidus for fibrin and platelet deposition and exposes fibronectin (Hamill, 1987). During transient bacteremia, staphylococci can lodge in these fibrinous lesions, bind to fibronectin, and proliferate. These patients are acutely ill, often with septic shock, with petechiae on the palms and soles, and have repeated blood culture results positive for *S. aureus*. Embolic phenomena are common with this disease and may include pulmonary emboli, renal emboli, or central nervous system (CNS) involvement with significant sequelae, including stroke (Saiman and Prince, 1989). Management of these patients includes detailed hemodynamic assessment and echocardiography, which may help document the nature

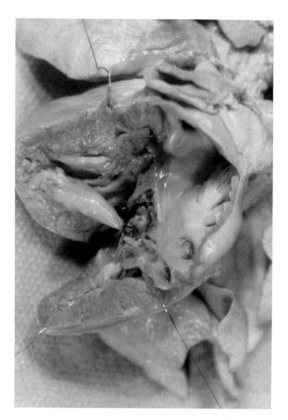

Fig. 27-3. Vegetation on the systemic (tricuspid) valve of a 15-month-old patient with hypoplastic left-heart syndrome. The cause of death was a cerebral vascular accident caused by septic emboli and a mycotic aneurysm.

and size of vegetations. Because *S. aureus* endocarditis can be a fulminant disease resulting in destruction of the infected valve, open heart surgery can be an important therapeutic option. For hemodynamically stable patients who are not embolizing from their infection, treatment with adequate levels of antistaphylococcal antibiotics can be curative.

Another group of patients at risk for staphylococcal endocarditis are patients with indwelling central venous catheters (Decker and Edwards, 1988; Saiman and Prince, 1989). Premature neonates dependent on parenteral nutrition, oncology patients, and patients with immunodeficiencies who have permanent central catheters are particularly at risk for seeding the catheter and adjacent endothelial tissue with *S. aureus*. Some of these infections can be managed without removal of the catheter, although,

when feasible, removal of the infected line and treatment with intravenous antibiotics are preferred.

Pulmonary infections caused by *S. aureus* can also be a complication of septicemia or can be due to aspiration of these organisms. Young infants with staphylococcal pneumonia usually present with high fever, respiratory distress, and pulmonary infiltrates (Fig. 27-4). The roentgenographic findings progress to dense consolidation, followed by pneumatocele (multiple, thin-walled abscesses with air-fluid levels) formation (Chartrand and McCracken, 1982). The areas of consolidation can extend to the pleura, resulting in empyema. Management of the patient with staphylococcal pneumonia is complex; both medical and surgical approaches have historical precedent (Pont and Rountree, 1963). Although the mainstay of therapy is antistaphylococcal antibiotics, the question of drainage of staphylococcal empyema is difficult to resolve. Diagnostic pleurocentesis and drainage with a chest tube are frequently done. Because blood cultures may be negative in patients with staphylococcal pneumonia, diagnosis by bronchoscopy or by pleural tap may be necessary to confirm the cause of the pneumonia. This procedure can be guided by either ultrasonography or computed tomography to facilitate drainage of loculated fluid. Resolution of fever and pleural fluid may take weeks. Open thoracotomy is another therapeutic option, which often is unnecessary if appropriate treatment and drainage can be accomplished with less invasive procedures.

Bone and joint infections are often a consequence of staphylococcal bacteremia in children, with 90% of cases occurring in children under the age of 15 years (Faden and Grossi, 1991; Waldvogel et al., 1970). These infections are most common in the metaphyseal portions of the long bones. The children present with fever and bony tenderness or, in infants, with irritability or refusal to walk. Laboratory findings are rarely diagnostic; the white blood cell (WBC) count may or may not be elevated, although the erythrocyte sedimentation rate usually is high. The diagnosis of acute hematogenous osteomyelitis can be made frequently by a radionuclide scan using technetium 99m phosphonate, for plain radiographs of the involved areas do not show the classic changes of periosteal new bone formation until the infection has been present for

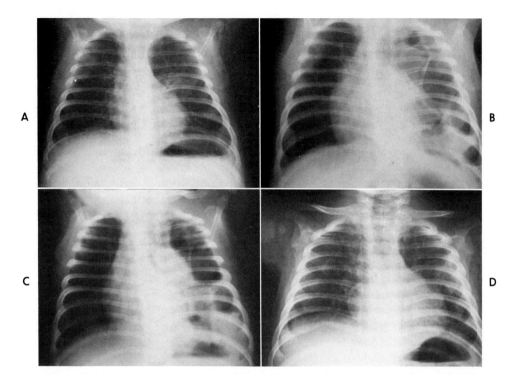

Fig. 27-4. Roentgenograms of a 3-month-old infant with acute staphylococcal pneumonia, showing the typical progression from consolidation to pneumatocele formation and pyopneumothorax to final resolution. **A,** Roentgenogram taken at admission, February 6, 1958 (third day of illness), showing an area of consolidation in the left midlung field. **B,** Roentgenogram taken February 10, 1958 (seventh day of illness), showing pneumatocele formation and pyopneumothorax. The heart and mediastinum are displaced to the opposite side. **C,** Roentgenogram taken February 28, 1958 (twenty-fifth day of illness), showing pneumatoceles, pyopneumothorax, and shift of mediastinum still present. **D,** Roentgenogram taken March 28, 1958 (fifty-third day of illness), showing considerable clearing.

10 to 14 days (Ledesma-Medina and Newman, 1989).

Depending on the site of osteomyelitis, adjacent septic arthritis can also result. This occurs when osteomyelitis is present within the portion of the bone enclosed by the joint capsule such as in the hip or shoulder. In these patients there is limited range of movement of the affected joint, and soft-tissue swelling may be evident either clinically or by x-ray examination. Diagnosis can be confirmed by aspiration of the joint and drainage as necessary. Because of the virulence of *S. aureus* with its associated toxins, *S. aureus* septic arthritis of the hip usually requires surgical drainage to prevent destruction of the joint (Bray and Schmid, 1986).

Hematogenous septic arthritis can also occur without underlying osteomyelitis. This is confirmed by finding purulent joint fluid, with poly-morphonuclear leukocytes, a high protein content, and gram-positive cocci, on a smear but finding negative results on films of the bone and on ^{99m}Tc scans of the surrounding bones. Prompt antibiotic treatment and appropriate drainage usually result in excellent cure rates. Particularly if the infecting organism has been isolated, oral antimicrobial agents are effective in curing staphylococcal bone and joint infections if patients comply with therapy (Tetzlaff et al., 1978). Detailed discussions of bone and joint infections are found in Chapter 16.

ANTIMICROBIAL AGENTS TO TREAT *S. AUREUS* INFECTIONS

A large number of antimicrobial agents are highly active against *S. aureus*, including parenteral drugs, oral drugs, fixed combinations, synergistic combinations, and antimicrobials with activity against MRSA and the coagulase-negative staphylococci.

Oral antistaphylococcal antimicrobials include dicloxacillin, cloxacillin, amoxicillin plus clavulanic acid (Augmentin), cephalexin, cefaclor, erythromycin, clindamycin, and ciprofloxacin. These antimicrobials could be used for treating skin and soft-tissue infections in ambulatory patients in whom *S. aureus* is a likely pathogen. In older patients oral fluoroquinolone antibiotics have been effective against bone and soft-tissue infections caused by staphylococci (Greenberg et al., 1987).

For severe life-threatening infections in areas in which methicillin-resistant organisms are common, vancomycin would be the drug of choice until a causative agent has been identified and its antimicrobial susceptibility established (Kline and Mason, 1988; Storch and Rajagpolan, 1986). Other parenteral agents for severe staphylococcal infections include oxacillin, nafcillin, methicillin, ticarcillin and clavulanate (Timentin), cephalothin, cefazolin, cefuroxime, imipenem, and clindamycin (Neu, 1985). Although the β-lactamase stable penicillins have been considered the "drugs of choice" for staphylococcal infections, the increased numbers of strains with altered penicillin-binding proteins and hyperproduction of β-lactamase have resulted in an increase in the use of vancomycin for staphylococcal infections. For the treatment of endocarditis or other infections with persistent bacteremia, combination therapy, combining rifampin, which can be accumulated within the phagocyte, with vancomycin or a β-lactam agent, may be useful. Aminoglycosides also can be added to vancomycin or β-lactam agents; however, nephrotoxicity increases when vancomycin and aminoglycosides are used at the same time.

EPIDEMIOLOGY

The usual source of staphylococcal infection is nasal colonization. The organism colonizes the anterior nares and can then be aerosolized in droplets or, more commonly, can be spread by intrapersonal contact. Small breaks in the skin can become infected, or the organism can disseminate in a nosocomial setting from hospital personnel to patients. Careful handwashing is of utmost importance in preventing spread of the organism.

Analysis of the epidemiology of staphylococcal infections, particularly in neonatal nurseries or after nosocomial outbreaks, has been performed using a variety of techniques. Historically, phage typing has been extremely useful. However, because staphylococci have numerous transferrable genetic elements such as plasmids, transposons, and prophages, more recent studies have used molecular biological techniques to trace the lineage of a particular strain. Either plasmid analysis, Western hybridization, or DNA-DNA hybridization using gene probes for a specific virulence determinant (e.g., TSST-1) can be used.

INFECTIONS CAUSED BY COAGULASE-NEGATIVE STAPHYLOCOCCI
Microbiology

Coagulase-negative staphylococci such as those belonging to the *S. epidermidis* group are considered "normal flora," commensal organisms that colonize the skin. Because these staphylococci do not ordinarily possess the virulence factors common to *S. aureus*, they rarely produce fulminant infections. The coagulase-negative staphylococci are differentiated from *S. aureus* on the basis of their lack of coagulase, lack of β-hemolysis on blood agar plates, and inability to ferment mannitol. The coagulase-negative staphylococci frequently contain plasmids that can be transferred to *S. aureus*. In addition, the majority of strains possess the *mec* gene, conferring resistance to most β-lactam antibiotics on the basis of penicillin-binding proteins with reduced affinity for β-lactams.

Catheter sepsis. These ubiquitous coagulase-negative staphylococci readily colonize plastic catheters and are associated with many infections both in neonates (Noel and Edelson, 1984) and in immunocompromised patients with indwelling venous access lines (Decker and Edwards, 1988; Quie and Belani, 1987; Wade et al., 1982). Coagulase-negative staphylococci frequently produce an extracellular "slime" layer that facilitates their attachment to plastic lines and other implanted foreign bodies (Diaz-Mitoma et al., 1987). Virtually all indwelling catheters do become colonized by these organisms, but symptomatic infections are infrequent. When large numbers of organisms are present, transient bacteremia may occur. It may be accompanied by clinical signs, which are most significant in premature neonates. In this patient population coagulase-negative staphylococcal bacteremia may be associated with fever or hypothermia, cardiovascular instability, or glucose intolerance. Older patients with bacteremia resulting from these organisms may have transient fever but generally have few clinical signs to indicate a systemic infection. Treatment of sepsis caused by coagulase-negative staphylococci may be attempted without removing the infected line in such patients. Because these organisms invariably have penicillin-binding proteins (PBP2A) with low affinity for β-lactam compounds, these infections require treatment with vancomycin (Archer, 1988).

Endocarditis. As increasing numbers of pediatric patients with congenital heart disease undergo open heart surgery with the placement of prosthetic valves, endocarditis caused by coagulase-negative staphylococci has increased correspondingly. Unlike endocarditis caused by S. *aureus*, these infections are more indolent in nature and may be difficult to diagnose as a result of the use of intermittent courses of antimicrobial agents for "fever" in these patients. In addition, a single positive value for coagulase-negative staphylococci in a blood culture is often considered the result of contaminants if endocarditis is not part of the differential diagnosis.

Central nervous system infections. The coagulase-negative staphylococci can also colonize the plastic tubing used to shunt cerebrospinal fluid (CSF) in premature neonates after intraventricular hemorrhages or in older patients with shunts for hydrocephalus and other indications. These organisms gain access to the CNS either through suture sites in the skin or at the time of the operation. Again, the organisms have a great affinity for plastic catheters (Slight et al., 1985). S. *epidermidis* species in the CNS cause a relatively indolent infection characterized by fever but relatively minimal systemic findings. Examination of the CSF, however, can reveal the high protein and low glucose values expected with bacterial infection of the CNS, a polymorphonuclear leukocyte response, and bacteria on Gram stain. These infections are rarely cured without replacement of the infected hardware.

Urinary tract infections. Another group of coagulase-negative staphylococci, S. *saprophy-* *ticus*, is associated with urinary tract infections in adolescent girls (Jordan et al., 1980). This organism should not be considered "commensal flora" in this setting.

Treatment

The resistance of the coagulase-negative staphylococci to β-lactam antibiotics, the presence of foreign bodies, and, in patients with CNS shunt infections, the lack of meningeal inflammation that facilitates transport of antimicrobial agents into the CSF are all major factors to consider in the treatment of these infections. Vancomycin has been the treatment of choice for infections caused by coagulase-negative staphylococci. Rifampin, with its increased penetration into CSF in the absence of inflammation, can be added to the vancomycin (Gombert et al., 1981). Treatment of all of these infections is likely to remain a problem because vancomycin-resistant organisms have been identified.

PREVENTIVE MEASURES

The ubiquity of staphylococci, their ready adaptability, and the nature of the parasite-host relationship make it difficult to control human staphylococcal infections.

Measures in hospitals

Careful handwashing with a detergent before and after handling patients is the mainstay of the prevention of infection.

It is most important to exclude from hospitals all persons with acute staphylococcal infections of the skin or mucous membranes, who may be shedding particularly virulent staphylococci. The topical application of antistaphylococcal creams and ointments for the control of organisms carried in the nose or skin is not advisable.

Prevention of food poisoning

Persons with obvious staphylococcal infections of the skin, especially of the hands, should be excluded temporarily from the preparation or handling of food. Sliced and chopped meats, custards, and cream fillings should be refrigerated promptly to avoid multiplication of staphylococci accidentally introduced. Pastries should be filled with custard immediately before sale, or there should be adequate heating of the finished product. All leftover foods should be refrigerated promptly.

Antimicrobial prophylaxis

One dose of vancomycin or a second-generation cephalosporin such as cefazolin are administered to patients just before surgery of the abdomen, pelvis, or head and neck and in patients with prosthetic heart valves or patches and may be continued for 24 to 48 hours postoperatively, to prevent wound infection and/or endocarditis. The potential risks of allergic reactions, emergence of resistant bacterial strains, and superinfection must be weighed against potential benefits to the patient (Hirschmann and Inui, 1980; Medical Letter, 1992).

REFERENCES

Albert SR, Baldwin S, Czekajewski A, et al. Bullous impetigo due to group II *Staphylococcus aureus*. Am J Dis Child 1970;120:10-13.

Antimicrobial prophylaxis in surgery, Med Lett 1987; 29:91-94.

Archer GL. Molecular epidemiology of multiresistant *Staphylococcus epidermidis*. J Antimicrob Chemother 1988; 21(Suppl):133-138.

Bayer AS. Staphylococcal bacteremia and endocarditis: state of the art. Arch Intern Med 1982;142:1169-1177.

Bray SB, Schmid FR. A comparison of medical drainage (needle aspiration and surgical drainage (arthrotomy or arthroscopy) in the initial treatment of infected joints. Clin Rheum Dis 1986;12:501-522.

Chartrand SA, McCracken GH. Staphylococcal pneumonia in infants and children. Pediatr Infect Dis 1982;1:19-23.

Davis JP, Chesney PJ, Wand PJ, LaVenture M. Toxic-shock syndrome: epidemiologic features, recurrence, risk factors, and prevention. N Engl J Med 1980;303:1429-1435.

Decker MD, Edwards KM. Central venous catheter infections. Pediatr Clin North Am 1988;35:579-612.

de Lencastre H, Sa Figueiredo AM, Urban C, et al. Multiple mechanisms of methicillin resistance and improved methods for detection in clinical isolates of *Staphylococcus aureus*. Antimicrob Agents Chemother 1991;35:632-639.

Demidovish CW, Wittler RR, Ruff ME, et al. Impetigo. Current etiology and comparison of penicillin, erythromycin and cephalexin therapies. Am J Dis Child 1990;144:1313-1315.

Diaz-Mitoma F, Harding GKM, Hoban DJ, et al. Clinical significance of a test for slime production in ventriculoperitoneal shunt infections caused by coagulase-negative staphylococci. J Infect Dis 1987;156:555-560.

Faden H, Grossi M. Acute osteomyelitis in children. Reassessment of etiologic agent and their clinical characteristics. Am J Dis Child 1991;145:65-69.

Falcieri E, Vaudauz P, Huggler E, et al. Role of bacterial exopolymers and host factors on adherence and phagocytosis of *Staphylococcus aureus* in foreign body infection. J Infect Dis 1987;155:524-531.

Gombert ME, Landesman SH, Corrado ML, et al. Vancomycin and rifampin therapy for *Staphylococcus epidermidis* meningitis associated with CSF shunts. Report of three cases. J Neurosurg 1981;55:633-636.

Gooch JJ, Britt EM. *Staphylococcus aureus* colonization and infection in newborn nursery patients. Am J Dis Child 1978;132:893-896.

Greenberg RN, Kennedy DJ, Reilly PM, et al. Treatment of bone, joint, and soft tissue infections with oral ciprofloxacin. Antimicrob Agents Chemother 1987;31:151-155.

Hamill RJ. Role of fibronectin in infective endocarditis. Rev Infect Dis 1987;9:S360-S371.

Hartman BM, Tomasz A. Low-affinity penicillin binding protein associated with beta-lactam resistance in *Staphylococcus aureus*. J Bacteriol 1984;158:513-518.

Hieber JP, Davis AT. Staphylococcal cervical adenitis in young infants. Pediatrics 1976;57:424.

Hieber JP, Nelson AJ, McCracken GH. Acute disseminated staphylococcal disease in childhood. Am J Dis Child 1977;131:181-185.

Hirschmann JV, Inui TS. Antimicrobial prophylaxis: a critique of recent trials. Rev Infect Dis 1980;2:1-23.

Hodes DS, Barzilai A. Invasive and toxin-mediated *Staphylococcus aureus* diseases in children. Adv Pediatr Infect Dis 1990;5:35-68.

Holmberg SD, Blake PD. Staphylococcal food poisoning in the United States. New facts and old misconceptions. JAMA 1984;251:487-489.

Jordan PA, Iravani A, Richard GA et al. Urinary tract infection caused by *Staphylococcus saprophyticus*. J Infect Dis 1980;142:510-515.

Kline MW, Mason EO Jr. Methicillin-resistant *Staphylococcus aureus*: pediatric perspective. Pediatr Clin North Am 1988;35:613-624.

Ladisch S, Pizzo PA. *Staphylococcus aureus* sepsis in children with cancer. Pediatrics 1978;61:231-234.

Ledesma-Medina J, Newman B. Use of imaging techniques in the diagnosis of infectious diseases of children. Adv Pediatr Infect Dis 1989;4:1-50.

McLinn S. Topical mupirocin vs. systemic erythromycin treatment for pyoderma. Pediatr Infect Dis J 1988; 7:785-790.

Melish ME, Glasgow LA. The staphylococcal scalded skin syndrome: development of an experimental model. N Engl J Med 1970;282:1114.

Musher DM, McKenzie SO. Infections due to *Staphylococcus aureus*. Medicine 1977;56:383.

Neu HC. Relations of structural properties of beta-lactam antibiotics to antibacterial activity. Am J Med 1985; 79:2-13.

Noel GJ, Edelson PJ. *Staphylococcus epidermidis* bacteremia in neonates. Further observations and the occurrence of focal infection. Pediatrics 1984;74:832-837.

Parsonnet J. Mediators in the pathogenesis of toxic shock syndrome: overview. Rev Infect Dis 1989;11(Suppl 1):S263-S269.

Peters G, Locci R, Pulverer G. Adherence and growth of coagulase-negative staphylococci on surfaces of intravenous catheters. J Infect Dis 1982;146:479.

Pont ME, Rountree WC. The medical and surgical treatment of staphylococcal pneumonia. Dis Chest 1963; 43:176-185.

Quie PG, Belani KK. Coagulase-negative staphylococcal adherence and persistence. J Infect Dis 1987;156:543-547.

Saiman L, Prince AS. Infections of the heart. Adv Pediatr Infect Dis 1989;4:139-155.

Schlievert PM, Shands KN, Dan BB, et al. Identification and characterization of an exotoxin from *Staphylococcus aureus* associated with toxic-shock syndrome. J Infect Dis 1981;143:509.

Sheagren JN. *Staphylococcus aureus:* the persistent pathogen. N Engl J Med 1984;310:1368-1374,1437-1440.

Shulman ST, and Ayoub EM. Severe staphylococcal sepsis in adolescents. Pediatrics 1976;58:59-66.

Slight PH, Gundling K, Plotkin SA, et al. A trial of vancomycin for prophylaxis of infections after neurosurgical shunts. N Engl J Med 1985;312:921.

Storch GA, Rajagpolan L. Methicillin-resistant *Staphylococcus aureus* bacteremia in children. Pediatr Infect Dis 1986;5:59-67.

Tetzlaff TR, McCracken GH, Nelson JD. Oral antibiotic therapy for skeletal infections of children. J Pediatr 1978;92:485.

Van Scoy RE, Welkowske CJ. Prophylactic use of antimicrobial agents. Mayo Clin Proc 1983;58:241-245.

Wade JC, Schimpff SC, Newman KA, et al. *Staphylococcus epidermidis:* an increasing cause of infection in patients with granulocytopenia. Ann Intern Med 1982;97:503-508.

Waldvogel FA, Medoff G, Swartz MN. Osteomyelitis: a review of clinical features, therapeutic considerations and unusual aspects. I. Hematogenous osteomyelitis. N Engl J Med 1970;282:198.

Wiesenthal AM, Todd JK. Toxic shock syndrome in children aged 10 years or less. Pediatrics 1984;74:112-117.

28

STREPTOCOCCAL INFECTIONS, GROUP A

EDWARD L. KAPLAN
SAUL KRUGMAN

Group A β-hemolytic streptococcal infections are among the most common bacterial infections in children. Although frequently causing no greater problem than uncomplicated tonsillitis or pharyngitis, they can result in serious and life-threatening suppurative and nonsuppurative complications. Scarlet fever, erysipelas, toxic shock-like syndrome, acute poststreptococcal glomerulonephritis, and acute rheumatic fever comprise only a partial list of the problems caused by the group A β-hemolytic streptococcus. These infections have become particularly important because during the latter part of the 1980s and early 1990s, complications of group A streptococcal infections appear to have become more common than in previous decades.

ETIOLOGY

Although other β-hemolytic streptococci such as those in groups B, C, and G can cause serious infections in humans, the group A hemolytic streptococci are most frequently responsible. These microorganisms are characterized by their tendency to grow in chains. The capsules are composed largely of hyaluronic acid. Loss of the capsule by desiccation is thought to account for lability of these organisms, explaining why transmission by fomites is rare. The optimal temperature for growth of the streptococcus is 37° C; it is inhibited at temperatures above 40° C.

The serological grouping of hemolytic streptococci is based on the presence of group-specific antigens. Lancefield (1933) identified 12 groups, A through L. Although group A streptococci are responsible for most human infections, other groups may be associated with disease in humans. Grouping of hemolytic streptococci is achieved by a precipitin technique (Lancefield, 1933) or by the fluorescent antibody (FA) technique. Group A streptococci may also be differentiated from other groups by a nonserological procedure described in 1953 by Maxted, who used bacitracin in a simple antibiotic plate method. The principle of this test is that group A strains are more sensitive to bacitracin than other groups of streptococci. Growth of most group A strains is inhibited by a special 0.04 unit bacitracin disk. In an analysis of 12,560 strains, the bacitracin test agreed with the precipitin test in 95.8% of cases (Moody, 1972). Serological grouping by the FA technique can be carried out with accuracy. However, the possibility for false-positive or false-negative results and the expense of the necessary laboratory equipment have resulted in an overall decrease in the use of this technique.

A major component of the bacterial cell wall is group A carbohydrate, which has antigenic components that cross-react with glycoprotein from human cardiac valves (Goldstein et al., 1968).

The most important surface protein is the M protein; it determines the type specificity of group A streptococci. More than 80 types have been identified. In addition, M proteins play an important role in virulence. They inhibit the phagocytosis of streptococci by host leukocytes by obscuring the C3b receptor. This antiphagocytic effect can be neutralized by specific antibody. Cross-protection between different types does not occur, and M proteins are also poorly antigenic in man. Two additional protein antigens, T and R, have no known role in the virulence of the organism or in eliciting protective type-specific antibody.

The inner layer of the cell wall is composed of mucopeptide, or peptidoglycan. Experimental injection of this material into rabbits has induced carditis (Rotta and Bednat, 1969), but whether it is involved in the pathogenesis of acute rheumatic fever remains unknown because no experimental animal model exactly mimics acute rheumatic fever in humans.

Group A hemolytic streptococci secrete a number of toxins and enzymes such as streptokinase, deoxyribonucleases, streptolysins S and O, hyaluronidase, and several erythrogenic toxins. Streptolysins cause beta hemolysis observed on blood agar cultures. Infection with streptococci that elaborate any of these substances is also followed by the production of specific antibodies for the substance such as antistreptokinase, antideoxyribonuclease, antistreptolysin O, hyaluronidase, and erythrogenic antitoxin. The measurement of these antibodies may be used as an aid to diagnosis of the sequelae of these infections. Antistreptolysin O, for example, is present in high titer in the serum of most patients recovering from a recent streptococcal infection. A test that purports to measure several different antibodies at the same time using an agglutination technique (the Streptozyme test) has been used since the early 1970s, but significant problems have been reported with this test. Batch-to-batch variation in the reagent and difficulty in reading the agglutination have led to concern about its accuracy.

The erythrogenic toxin is responsible for the rash of scarlet fever. The identification of three immunologically distinct rash-producing toxins explains the occasional occurrence of several episodes of scarlet fever in the same person (Zabriskie, 1964; Watson and Kim, 1970). Production of erythrogenic toxin is mediated by lysogeny (Zabriskie, 1964). A role for these toxins has also been proposed in the pathogenesis of the streptococcal toxic shock-like syndrome.

PATHOLOGY

The local lesions caused by the hemolytic streptococcus show the characteristic inflammatory reaction of hyperemia, edema, and polymorphonuclear cell infiltration. In scarlet fever the pathogenic changes are due to both the toxin and the microorganism. There is generalized lymphoid hyperplasia. Some cases reveal the characteristic findings of acute glomerulonephritis. During the height of the rash, the skin shows signs of hyperemia, edema, and polymorphonuclear cell infiltrates in the corium.

EPIDEMIOLOGICAL FACTORS

People of all ages, sexes, and races are susceptible to streptococcal infections. The incidence varies with age according to the clinical type of infection. In general, however, it is lowest in infancy, begins to rise gradually thereafter, and reaches a peak just before adolescence. In the pediatric age group, group A streptococcal infections of the throat are most common in children between 6 and 15 years of age. Although the incidence of group A streptococcal upper respiratory tract infection is lower among preschool-age children, outbreaks of group A streptococcal upper respiratory tract infections have been documented in day-care facilities (Smith et al., 1989). Streptococcal infections of the skin are more common in preschool-age children.

Although the incidence of streptococcal upper respiratory tract infection was believed greater in temperate zones, it is now recognized that group A streptococcal infections and their sequelae occur widely in the tropics. The geographical distribution of skin infections seems to favor warmer or tropical climates and to occur mainly in summer or early fall in temperate climates. However, streptococcal impetigo occurs even in winter months in temperate zones. In the United States streptococcal pharyngitis occurs most often during late winter and early spring.

Group A streptococci are spread primarily by the respiratory route. Individuals with acute streptococcal infection, especially those who harbor large numbers of organisms in their anterior nares, are especially likely to spread this organism to close contacts. In contrast, those individuals who harbor small numbers of organisms with the upper respiratory tract infection appear less likely to spread the organism. Contaminated foods (especially milk, ice cream, other dairy products, and eggs or egg products) have been responsible for a number of well-documented foodborne epidemics.

IMMUNITY

As indicated previously, group A hemolytic streptococci are composed of various antigenic constituents and elaborate extracellular antigenic material. Two of these antigens, type-specific M protein and erythrogenic toxin, stimulate the production of antibodies that provide a person with at least two types of resistance—antibacterial immunity and antitoxic immunity.

It has been postulated that the development of immunity and hypersensitivity may play a role in the changing pattern of streptococcal disease with advancing age. The nonspecific, nonlocalizing character of streptococcal disease in infants may represent the initial type of response to the microorganism.

Antibacterial immunity

Antibacterial immunity is related to the type-specific M component of group A hemolytic streptococci. A person who is infected with a given type of streptococcus develops antibodies against strains of the same type only. For example, infection with type 4 streptococcus is followed by development of antibodies against type 4 but not against heterologous types. These bacteriostatic antibodies have been demonstrated in patients' sera for several years after infection.

The current hypothesis of type-specific antibacterial immunity is supported by data obtained from many immunological and epidemiological studies. Theoretically, during a lifetime a person can develop at least 40 or more streptococcal infections, some apparent and others inapparent. Each infection in turn, would in all probability be caused by a different type of streptococcus. It has been demonstrated that the serum of infants and young children has a limited number of these type-specific bacteriostatic antibodies. As a person's age increases, a larger number of these type-specific antibodies develops as a result of repeated infections. However, second attacks of streptococcal infection with the same type have occurred. The capacity of early penicillin therapy to decrease the response to various streptococcal antigens may explain some of these second attacks. This reduced response has prompted controversy about whether early

treatment can be detrimental to the patient. Recent evidence suggests that this is not true (Gerber et al., 1990).

Antitoxic immunity

Antitoxic immunity is acquired either passively or actively. The antitoxic immunity of infancy is transplacental in origin and disappears before the end of the first year. Actively acquired antitoxin resulting from infection probably persists for life. Antitoxic immunity for the most part has group rather than type specificity, which is characteristic of antibacterial immunity.

• • •

In summary, the immune status of a person may affect the type of infection acquired after exposure to a particular pathogenic strain of streptococcus. The hypothetical example in Fig. 28-1, which assumes exposure to toxic group A hemolytic streptococcus type 4, illustrates this graphically. It may be noted that (1) type 4 antibacterial immunity prevents clinical disease regardless of the antitoxic status; (2) when type 4 antibacterial immunity is absent but antitoxic immunity is present, streptococcal pharyngitis or tonsillitis may develop, but scarlet fever will not occur; and (3) when neither type 4 antibacterial nor antitoxic immunity is present, scarlet fever may develop.

CLINICAL MANIFESTATIONS

The clinical manifestations of streptococcal disease are governed by many factors, the most important being the portal of entry, the variety of infecting streptococci, the patient's age, and the immune status of the host. The effect of type-specific immunity has been discussed. Powers and Boisvert (1944) emphasized the importance of the age factor in relation to the type of clinical response. They described the manifestations of streptococcal infections, or "streptococcosis," for three pediatric age groups: under 6 months, 6 months to 3 years, and 3 to 12 years.

Streptococcosis in infants under 6 months of age

Streptococcosis in infants under 6 months of age is characterized by nasopharyngitis associated with a thin mucopurulent nasal discharge and irregular rises in temperature. Frequently, there are excoriations around the nares. The

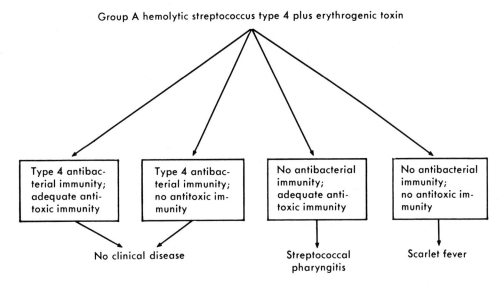

Group A hemolytic streptococcus type 4 plus erythrogenic toxin

| Type 4 antibac-terial immunity; adequate anti-toxic immunity | Type 4 antibac-terial immunity; no antitoxic im-munity | No antibacterial immunity; adequate anti-toxic immunity | No antibacterial immunity; no antitoxic im-munity |

No clinical disease   Streptococcal   Scarlet fever
                              pharyngitis

Fig. 28-1. Effect of immune status on streptococcal infections (see text).

acute symptoms last for approximately 1 week, but persistent nasal discharge and irritability may continue for 6 weeks. The disease may be clinically indistinguishable from the common cold. It can be confirmed only by means of a culture of the nasal discharge.

Streptococcosis in children 6 months to 3 years of age

In streptococcosis in children 6 months to 3 years of age there is an insidious onset of low-grade fever, mild constitutional symptoms, and mild nasopharyngitis. The nasal discharge can be clear, and the anterior cervical lymph nodes are usually enlarged and tender. It should be remembered, however, that the "classic" strep-tococcal upper respiratory tract infection can oc-cur in young children and should not be over-looked. Sinusitis and otitis media are frequent complications. The low-grade fever and symp-toms may persist for as long as 4 to 8 weeks. This type of infection is clinically similar to var-ious nonspecific respiratory tract infections. Di-agnosis can best be established by nasopharyn-geal culture.

Streptococcal infection in children 3 to 12 years of age

In children 3 to 12 years of age streptococcal infection usually is manifested as acute follicular tonsillitis, pharyngitis, or scarlet fever. Strep-tococcal tonsillitis is essentially scarlet fever without a rash. The clinical picture, complica-tions, prognosis, and treatment are identical to those of scarlet fever; consequently, they are considered in the discussion of scarlet fever.

Scarlet fever

The incubation period of scarlet fever is 2 to 4 days, with a range of 1 to 7 days. The disease is ushered in abruptly by fever, vomiting, sore throat, and constitutional symptoms such as headache, chills, and malaise. Within 12 to 48 hours after onset, the typical rash appears. In some cases abdominal pain is an early and prom-inent symptom. The association of this manifes-tation with vomiting may suggest the possibility of a surgical abdomen. The combination of vom-iting and abdominal pain in streptococcal ton-sillitis without rash is also frequently seen.

The significant findings are fever, enanthem, and exanthem.

Fever. In the typical case (Fig. 28-2) the tem-perature rises abruptly to 39.4° C (103° F) and reaches its peak by around the second day. It then gradually falls to normal by lysis within 5 or 6 days. A severe case has a higher and more protracted temperature course. Occasionally in mild scarlet fever the temperature may be low (under 38.3° C; 101° F) or normal. The pulse rate is frequently increased out of proportion to the fever. Today, a typical temperature course

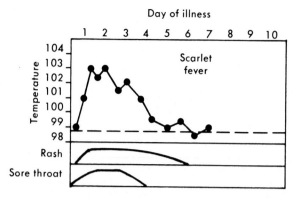

Fig. 28-2. Schematic diagram of a typical case of untreated uncomplicated scarlet fever. The rash usually appears within 24 hours of onset of fever and sore throat.

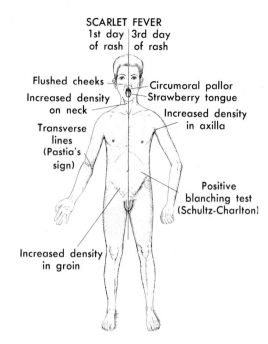

Fig. 28-3. Schematic drawing illustrating development and distribution of scarlet fever rash.

is rarely seen; it usually drops precipitously to normal within 24 hours after penicillin therapy is begun.

Enanthem. The enanthem includes lesions of the tonsils, pharynx, tongue, and palate. The tonsils are enlarged, edematous, reddened, and covered with patches of exudate. The pharynx also is edematous and beefy red in appearance. In mild cases the tonsils and pharynx show moderate erythema and little or no exudate. Severe cases may be characterized by membranous ulcerative tonsillitis clinically indistinguishable from diphtheria (Plate 8). The tongue changes in appearance as the disease progresses. During the first 1 or 2 days the dorsum has a white fur coat, and the tip and edges are reddened. As the papillae become reddened and edematous, they project through the coat, producing the so-called white strawberry tongue. By the fourth or fifth day the white coat has peeled off. The red, glistening tongue studded with prominent papillae presents the appearance of a red strawberry (Plate 9). The palate is usually covered with erythematous punctiform lesions and occasionally with scattered petechiae. The uvula and the free margin of the soft palate are reddened and edematous (Plate 8).

Exanthem. The rash usually appears within 12 hours after onset of the illness; occasionally, it may be delayed for 2 days. The rash is an erythematous punctiform eruption that blanches on pressure. The punctate lesions, pinhead in size, give the skin a rough sandpaper-like texture.

The rash of scarlet fever resembles a "sunburn with goose pimples" (Plate 9).

The exanthem (Fig. 28-3) has the following distinctive features:

1. It becomes generalized very rapidly, usually within 24 hours.
2. The punctiform lesions are usually not present on the face. The forehead and cheeks are red, smooth, and flushed, and the area around the mouth is pale (circumoral pallor).
3. It is more intense in skin folds such as the axillae and the groin and at sites of pressure such as the buttocks.
4. It has areas of hyperpigmentation, occasionally with tiny petechiae in the creases of the folds of the joints, particularly in the antecubital fossae. These lesions form transverse lines (Pastia's sign) that persist for a day or so after the rash has faded.
5. If the eruption is severe, minute vesicular lesions (miliary sudamina) may be scattered over the abdomen, hands, and feet.
6. It desquamates.

The rash, fever, sore throat, and other clinical manifestations clear up by the end of the first

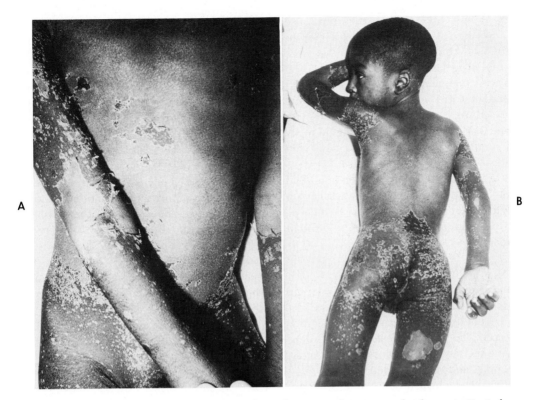

Fig. 28-4. Desquamation in a patient 16 days after onset of severe scarlet fever. **A,** Typical circular punched-out areas in groin and upper thighs. **B,** Sequence of spread from face to trunk and finally to extremities.

week. The period of desquamation follows shortly thereafter.

Desquamation. Desquamation is one of the most characteristic features of scarlet fever. The extent and duration of the desquamation are directly proportional to the intensity of the rash. It becomes apparent first on the face at the end of the first week as fine branny flakes. Then it spreads to the trunk and finally to the extremities, becoming generalized by the third week (Fig. 28-4). The desquamating skin of the trunk comes off in larger, thicker flakes. Frequently, circular areas of epidermis of variable size peel off, giving the skin a punched-out or pinhole appearance. The hands and feet usually are the last to desquamate, becoming involved between the second and third weeks. The tips of the fingers characteristically show splitting of the skin at the free margins of the nails. In severe cases an epidermal cast of the fingers, hands, or feet may be shed. In mild cases of scarlet fever the process of desquamation may be complete in 3 weeks; in severe cases it may persist for as long

as 8 weeks. Sometimes a retrospective diagnosis may be made on the basis of peeling skin and a history of a sore throat associated with a rash several weeks before. Occasionally, the eruption may be missed entirely. Rarely, the rash of scarlet fever is confused with mucocutaneous lymph node syndrome (Kawasaki disease).

Surgical scarlet fever

The portal of entry in classic scarlet fever is the nasopharynx. Occasionally, however, hemolytic streptococci may infect the site of a wound, a burn, or other type of skin lesion. Under these circumstances, so-called surgical scarlet fever may develop. The clinical manifestations are identical to those described earlier except that the pharyngeal and tonsillar involvement are absent. However, there may be local inflammatory signs at the wound or operative site.

Streptococcal sepsis

Although group A streptococci are most often considered in the context of surface infections of the respiratory tract or skin, they can cause serious invasive disease in normal children, newborns, and compromised hosts. These are usually fulminant bacteremic or septicemic infections with pneumonia, empyema, osteomyelitis, endometritis, meningitis, or soft-tissue abscesses (Burech et al., 1976). In the late 1980s and early 1990s an increasing number of cases of fulminant group A streptococcal bacteremia associated with a toxic shock-like syndrome were reported, occurring even in normal children. Such streptococcal infections have a very high mortality rate (reported as high as 30%). This condition can occur in association with varicella.

Streptococcal infections of the skin

Eczema streptococcum. Infants with weeping eczematoid lesions are prone to develop secondary infections, particularly with hemolytic streptococci. The resulting lesion shows extensive erythema, serosanguineous exudate, crusting, weeping, and regional adenopathy.

Impetigo. The characteristic superficial purulent crusting lesions may be caused by either hemolytic streptococci or staphylococci. The vesicular stage of streptococcal impetigo may be transient, and vesicles are small (1 to 2 mm in diameter). The typical lesion is a thick, adherent, amber-colored crust on an erythematous base; there can be an associated local lymphadenopathy (Wannamaker, 1970). Bullous impetigo is usually caused by staphylococci. These vesicular lesions are large (1 to 2 cm in diameter); they rupture and form thin crusts without accompanying lymphadenopathy.

Erysipelas. Erysipelas, formerly very common, is rarely seen today. It is characterized by a red, indurated thickening of the skin. It begins as a small lesion that spreads marginally for approximately 4 to 6 days. The margins have a raised, firm, tender, palpable border. On the face the rash may assume a butterfly distribution. The skin lesion is usually associated with fever and constitutional symptoms that subside when the rash stops progressing.

Histologically, there is evidence of an inflammatory reaction involving the superficial lymph vessels. The lymph channels are crammed with fibrin, leukocytes, and streptococci. The progressively diffuse lymphatic involvement accounts for the peculiar spread and evolution of the lesion.

DIAGNOSIS

The diagnosis of streptococcal infections, including scarlet fever, can be established by (1) characteristic clinical features, (2) isolation of the causative agent, (3) serological tests, and (4) other confirmatory tests (Wannamaker, 1972).

Characteristic clinical features

The triad of fever, vomiting, and sore throat associated with an exudative tonsillitis and an erythematous punctiform eruption suggests scarlet fever. The same symptoms and signs without a rash point to streptococcal tonsillitis.

Stillerman and Bernstein (1961) observed that groups of symptoms and signs are better indicators of streptococcal pharyngitis than single symptoms and signs. The following four syndromes were associated with positive cultures in more than 70% of the cases:

1. Moderate redness of the oropharynx, exudate over the tonsils, and cervical adenitis (75%)
2. Marked redness of the oropharynx with or without tonsillar exudate, and cervical adenitis (74%)
3. Moderate or marked redness of the oropharynx, no tonsillar exudate, and petechiae on the palate, with or without cervical adenitis (95%)
4. Moderate or marked redness of the oropharynx, tonsillar exudate, and petechiae on the palate, with or without cervical adenitis (100%)

Isolation of causative agent

The throat culture is the most useful and most important confirmatory test. Group A hemolytic streptococci may be isolated from the throat, the nasopharynx, or an infected wound. A positive throat culture is usually indicative of an acute streptococcal infection; it may also indicate the presence of a carrier state. A quantitative throat swab culture usually but not always reveals a correlation between the isolation of large numbers of streptococci and the presence of a streptococcal pharyngitis (Breese et al., 1972). Studies by Bell and Smith (1976) revealed a heavy growth of *Streptococcus pyogenes* in 71% of throat swabs taken from 1,054 children with pharyngitis, as compared with 1.7% of 462 normal children who were carriers.

Diagnosis of streptococcal impetigo is made by isolation of the organism from a skin lesion.

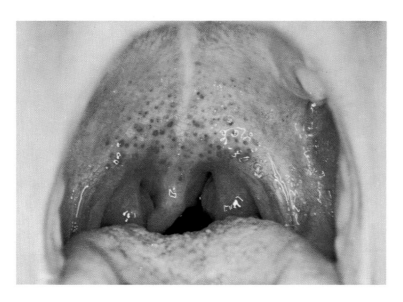

Plate 8
Marked petechial stippling of the soft palate in scarlet fever. (From Stillerman M, Bernstein SH. Am J Dis Child 1961;101:476.

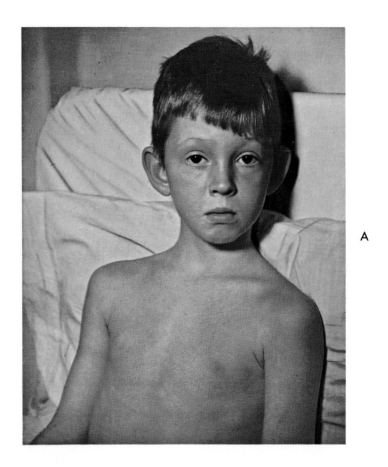

A

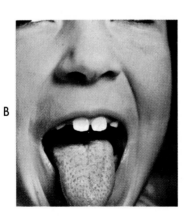

B

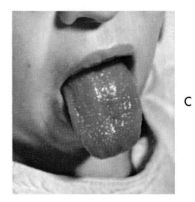

C

Plate 9
Scarlet fever, **A,** Punctate, erythematous rash (second day). **B,** White strawberry tongue (first day). **C,** Red strawberry tongue (third day). (Courtesy Dr. Franklin H. Top, Professor and Head of the Department of Hygiene and Preventive Medicine, State University of Iowa, College of Medicine, Iowa City, Iowa; and Parke, Davis & Company's *Therapeutic Notes.*)

Staphylococci may also be isolated simultaneously.

Rapid antigen detection and serological tests

Rapid antigen detection tests for confirming the presence of group A streptococci on throat swabs are commercially available (Kaplan, 1988). In general, the specificity of these tests is much better than their sensitivity. These tests are, however, helpful in the rapid diagnosis of streptococcal upper respiratory tract infections and of streptococcal pyoderma (Kaplan et al., 1989). Because of several reports of decreased sensitivity, most clinicians who receive a negative result from a rapid antigen detection test for group A streptococci in a patient who has symptoms compatible with this infection also obtain a conventional throat culture. The throat culture remains the "gold standard" for the confirmation of group A streptococcal upper respiratory tract infections.

Streptococcal antibody tests are used to confirm a previous group A streptococcal infection. There are few, if any, indications for the use of streptococcal antibody tests in patients with uncomplicated group A streptococcal upper respiratory tract infection. A number of antibody tests are commercially available. The antistreptolysin O test has been used most widely. In addition, the antideoxyribonuclease B test is available and has the advantage that, in contrast to the antistreptolysin test, its response is brisk, even after pyoderma. The antihyaluronidase test is also commercially available but is used less widely. The Streptozyme agglutination test has been used, but for reasons stated previously, it cannot be recommended.

Group A streptococcal antibody levels may vary with age, with season of the year, and with site of infection and also are dependent on the interval since the streptococcal infection. For example, the peak for the antistreptolysin O titer usually is reached 3 to 6 weeks after an infection, whereas the peak for the antideoxyribonuclease B titer occurs somewhat later at approximately 6 to 8 weeks after infection. The results of the laboratory test are influenced by when the serum is obtained. Early eradication of hemolytic streptococci by antimicrobial therapy may suppress the development of antibodies.

Following impetigo, it is rare for antibodies to antistreptolysin O to rise. Although all group A streptococci produce streptolysin O, cholesterol in the skin binds to the toxin and prevents development of the immune response after impetigo (Kaplan and Wannamaker, 1976).

Other confirmatory tests

The typical blood picture shows leukocytosis with a predominance of polymorphonuclear leukocytes. An increase in number of eosinophils to between 5% and 10% of the total white blood cell count is a common finding in patients with scarlet fever.

DIFFERENTIAL DIAGNOSIS

The differential diagnosis of scarlet fever is discussed in detail in Chapter 36. Some of the conditions that may be confused with this disease are rubella, measles, exanthem subitum, erythema infectiosum, Lyme disease, infectious mononucleosis, staphylococcal scalded skin syndrome, Kawasaki syndrome, and toxic shock syndrome. Sunburn in a child with nonspecific pharyngitis may be confused with scarlet fever; the absence of eruption in the bathing suit area clarifies the diagnosis. Heat rash (miliaria) also may simulate a scarlatiniform eruption.

The differential diagnosis of exudative and membranous tonsillitis is covered in the chapters on diphtheria (p. 50) and Epstein-Barr virus infections (infectious mononucleosis; p. 95).

Wannamaker in 1970 and Peter and Smith in 1977 described the comparative features of streptococcal infections of the throat and skin. The organisms causing disease in these two organ systems apparently are different. For example, nephritogenic types that cause pharyngitis are rarely isolated from the skin (Anthony et al., 1969). The various features of these infections are listed in Table 28-1.

COMPLICATIONS

Complications following streptococcal infections may occur early or late in the course of the disease.

Early complications

Early complications are generally the result of an extension of the streptococcal infection; they usually occur during the first week of illness. Thus spread of the infection to the regional lymph nodes results in cervical adenitis. Progression of the infection into the middle ear is followed by otitis media. Sinusitis also may be produced by invading hemolytic streptococci.

Table 28-1. General features of streptococcal infections at different sites

	Streptococcal pharyngitis and tonsillitis	Streptococcal impetigo and pyoderma
Clinical features		
Erythema	Usually present and generalized	Often minimal and localized to immediate area around lesion
Vesicular stage	Absent	Typical of early lesion but transient
Pustular stage	Patchy exudate; pustules sometimes confluent	Pustules usually discrete; flora often mixed
Crusted stage	Absent	Frequent and characteristic
Local pain	Common; may be intense	Usually absent
Systemic reaction	Fever, headache, and malaise common	Unusual
Regional adenitis	Common	Less common, but adenopathy frequently seen
Deep-seated cellulitis	May occur	Perhaps less common
Bacteremia	Rare	May be relatively more frequent
Scarlatiniform rash	Sometimes present	Rare
Course	Typically acute except in infants	Often chronic; lesions may become ecthymatous
Laboratory findings		
Leukocytosis	Usually present	Often absent
Bacterial agent	Group A streptococci	Group A streptococci; often also large numbers of staphylococci
Serologic types of group A streptococci	Many different types	Few types predominate
Antistreptolysin O response	Common	Uncommon
Epidemiological factors		
Seasonal occurrence	Winter and spring	Late summer and early fall
Common-source epidemics	May occur	Not described
Geographical distribution	More common in temperate or cold climates	Common in hot or tropical climates
Age	Young school-age children	Children of preschool age
Sex	Equal incidence	Equal incidence
Transmission	Direct spread from human reservoirs, particularly nasal carriers	Unknown; insects may be mechanical vectors
Carrier state	Common in pharynx of many populations	Unusual on skin except in certain situations
Preceding trauma	Not present	May predispose to natural or experimental infection
Preceding viral infection	Uncommon	Uncommon
Complications		
Acute nephritis	Occurs; partially preventable (50%)	Occurs; preventability unknown
Acute rheumatic fever	Occurs; preventable	Does not occur
Treatment		
Local	Not important	Removal of crusts and scrubbing with hexachlorophene soap
Systemic	Single intramuscular injection of benzathine penicillin G or oral administration of penicillin for 10 days	May not be necessary; extensive lesions may require intramuscular injection of benzathine penicillin G

From Wannamaker LW. N Engl J Med 1970; 282:23.

Bronchopneumonia is a rare early complication of streptococcal involvement of the upper respiratory tract. Early bacterial complications rarely occur in adequately treated patients. Other less common complications include mastoiditis, septicemia, and osteomyelitis. A toxic shock-like syndrome (not related to the staphylococcal toxic shock syndrome discussed in Chapter 27) is an uncommon, but often very severe infection with high morbidity and mortality (Stevens et al., 1989). The precise pathogenetic mechanisms responsible for the development of the group A streptococcal toxic shock-like syndrome have not been identified.

Late complications

The late or nonsuppurative sequelae of group A streptococcal infections are acute rheumatic fever and acute poststreptococcal glomerulonephritis. The pathogenetic mechanisms responsible for the development of these nonsuppurative sequelae also remain a mystery. Generally speaking, they are believed to result from an abnormal host immune response to one or more as yet undefined group A streptococcal extracellular or somatic antigens. Although numerous hypotheses describing various specific antigens have been described, confirmatory evidence is lacking. These nonsuppurative sequelae usually develop after a latent period of 1 to 3 weeks and may follow both abnormally evident and inapparent infections.

Rheumatic fever. Although very common in North America and in Europe before, during, and immediately after the Second World War, the incidence of acute rheumatic fever in these industrialized countries declined remarkably in the 1960s and 1970s. Rheumatic fever incidence figures of less than 1 case per 100,000 people per year were common in the United States by the late 1970s. In contrast, in developing countries of the world rheumatic fever and rheumatic heart disease remain very significant public health problems (World Health Organization Study Group, 1988). Very high prevalence rates of rheumatic heart disease have been described in schoolchildren in a number of developing countries around the world, making this nonsuppurative sequel of group A streptococcal infections a major cardiovascular problem in the world today.

In the mid-1980s an unexpected "resurgence" of acute rheumatic fever occurred in the United States, affecting not only schoolchildren but also military recruits (Markowitz and Kaplan, 1989). The exact reasons for this resurgence are not completely understood, but the increase likely was associated with the introduction and spread of specific serotypes of group A streptococci (M types 1, 3, 5, 6, and 18), many with a mucoid phenotype.

Rheumatic fever is a relatively uncommon but serious complication of streptococcal infections; its incidence is approximately 3% after exudative pharyngitis. Rheumatic fever has not been associated with streptococcal impetigo. With optimal penicillin therapy for the preceding streptococcal infection, the attack rate is reduced to almost zero. Recurrent attacks of rheumatic fever, on the other hand, are a frequent complication of streptococcal infection, but most can be prevented by prophylactic penicillin. The disease is rare in children under 3 years of age; it occurs most often in children 5 to 15 years of age. The clinical manifestations of fever, polyarthritis, and carditis occur 7 or more days after the onset of the streptococcal infection.

Nephritis. Nephritis is a more common complication than rheumatic fever, but its incidence is variable. Certain strains of group A hemolytic streptococci—for example, types 12, 49, 55, and 57—are nephritogenic, and infections with these microorganisms may be followed by a high incidence of nephritis. Nephritis, unlike rheumatic fever, can follow infection of either the throat or the skin, but the serotypes of group A streptococci known as "nephritogenic" and associated with these two sites differ. For example, type 12 is classic throat strain producing nephritis, whereas serotypes such as 49, 55, and 57 usually are associated with skin infections and also are nephritogenic. Nephritis is usually manifested by fever, bloody urine, moderate edema, and, occasionally, hypertension and azotemia. In contrast to rheumatic fever, only one attack usually occurs; recurrences are unlikely. The rarity of recurrences may be due to the limited number of nephritogenic types of streptococci. Although residua of acute poststreptococcal nephritis have been noted in adult patients, it is generally believed that the long-term prognosis for children with acute streptococcal nephritis is excellent, seldom leading to residual renal disease.

PROGNOSIS

The prognosis for patients with adequately treated streptococcal infections is excellent. Serious septic complications can be easily prevented and treated. Adequate therapy will also reduce the incidence of rheumatic fever, thereby improving the prognosis. Deaths caused by scarlet fever and other streptococcal infections, very common some decades ago, are rare in the late 1980s and 1990s. However, as mentioned previously, there has been an increase in the late 1980s and early 1990s of severe streptococcal suppurative infections with a high mortality rate.

TREATMENT
Antimicrobial therapy

The treatment of streptococcal infections, including scarlet fever, has been revolutionized by antimicrobial therapy. Penicillin remains the preferred drug. Strains of group A hemolytic streptococci are uniformly susceptible to penicillin. Penicillin therapy is consistently followed by a dramatic subsidence of fever and constitutional symptoms. Atlhough at one time it was believed that penicillin had little effect on the acute symptoms of streptococcal sore throat, this belief is erroneous. For years some investigators (Breese et al., 1972; Hall and Breese, 1984) have maintained that administering penicillin reduces the symptoms of streptococcal sore throat more rapidly than no treatment. Indeed, several recent studies have demonstrated that prompt therapy is associated with more prompt resolution of the symptoms, allowing children to return to school and parents to work at an earlier time. Nelson (1984), in a double-blind study, demonstrated this phenomenon. Thus not only does prompt penicillin therapy prevent the sequelae of streptococcal infection of the throat, but also it rapidly alleviates symptoms (Gerber et al., 1990). Optimal treatment eradicates the streptococci from the site of infection, prevents septic complications, and reduces the incidence of rheumatic fever. Early institution of therapy interferes with the development of antistreptolysin O antibodies. It is uncertain whether the incidence of nephritis is affected by early penicillin therapy.

Optimal penicillin therapy can be achieved by a variety of regimens. Because of the absence of documented resistance by group A streptococci to penicillin, it remains the therapy of choice. The goal in treating streptococcal upper respiratory tract infection is to eradicate the organism. This usually can be accomplished by either 10 days of oral therapy (250 μg of penicillin V three or four times a day for 10 days) or by a single injection of intramuscular benzathine penicillin G, a repository form of the antibiotic (American Heart Association, 1988). Oral therapy may not always be effective because of a lack of patient compliance. The use of intramuscular benzathine penicillin G (600,000 units for children weighing <60 pounds and 1,200,000 units for children weighing >60 pounds) eliminates the problem of compliance. Mixtures of benzathine penicillin G with either procaine penicillin or in some instances with aqueous penicillin G are available. However, the total penicillin dosage should be based on the amount of benzathine penicillin G in the mixture because the other forms are rapidly excreted.

Although penicillin remains the treatment of choice, treatment failures (failure to eradicate the organism from the upper respiratory tract) have been documented. There is some indication that these instances may have been increasing during the last two decades (Kaplan, 1985). An alternative drug for use in penicillin-allergic patients is erythromycin. It can be given at a dose of 40 mg/kg/day in three or four divided doses. A maximum dose is 1 g/24 hours.

Alternative antibiotics that can be used in place of penicillin or the macrolides include a number of the cephalosporins. Careful review of the literature suggests no significant superiority of any of these alternative antibiotics.

Impetigo is treated best with penicillin given parenterally plus bacitracin given topically. Although it is unclear whether antibiotic therapy can prevent the nephritis that may follow impetigo, therapy will decrease the spread of the organism to others.

Patients who are allergic to penicillin may be treated with erythromycin estolate (Ginsberg et al., 1984) or a cephalosporin. Sulfonamides are *not* effective for the treatment of an established streptococcal infection. Tetracyclines are *not* recommended because of the high incidence of strains resistant to this antibiotic.

Supportive therapy

Although bed rest is recommended during the febrile period of streptococcal pharyngitis, it is virtually impossible to keep most children in bed when they feel well. Acetaminophen is indicated for relieving sore throat and malaise. An adequate fluid intake should be encouraged during the febrile period. A regular diet should be offered when tolerated.

PREVENTIVE MEASURES

The widespread prophylactic use of penicillin to prevent streptococcal infections has been recommended in epidemic conditions. Furthermore, penicillin still is used for secondary prevention of recurrent attacks of rheumatic fever. Clear-cut indications for prophylaxis for entire populations have not been established, but generally speaking, in those situations in which there is a documented community-wide outbreak of severe streptococcal infections with sequelae, the use of broad prophylaxis has been successful in many instances. Ideally, the results of a throat culture should resolve the question of whether or not to treat a person. Examples of populations in which widespread prophylaxis has been administered include schools, military populations, or other populations living in close quarters.

To provide long-term secondary rheumatic fever prophylaxis for prevention of recurrent rheumatic fever, regular injections of intramuscular benzathine penicillin G have proven most effective. In the United States injections every 4 weeks are adequate. Recent data have suggested, however, that in high-risk patients or in those countries where the risk of recurrence is quite high, injections given every 3 weeks may be indicated. Although sulfadiazine can be used for secondary rheumatic fever prophylaxis, it cannot be used for treatment of group A streptococcal infections. In patients who can take neither sulfadiazine nor penicillin, erythromycin has been used successfully for secondary prevention.

ISOLATION AND QUARANTINE

Specific penicillin therapy that rapidly eradicates hemolytic streptococci has reduced the need for periods of isolation.

Quarantine measures usually are not indicated.

REFERENCES

American Heart Association, Committee on Rheumatic Fever, Endocarditis, and Kawasaki Disease. Prevention of rheumatic fever. Circulation 1988;78:1082-1088.

Anthony BF, Kaplan EL, Wannamaker LW, et al. Attack rates of acute nephritis after type 49 streptococcal infection of the skin and of the respiratory tract. J Clin Invest 1969;48:1697-1704.

Bell SM, Smith DD. Quantitative throat swab culture in the diagnosis of streptococcal pharyngitis in children. Lancet 1976;2:61.

Breese BB, et al. Beta-hemolytic streptococcal infection: the clinical and epidemiologic importance of the number of organisms found in culture. Am J Dis Child 1972;124:352.

Burech DL, Koranyi KI, Haynes RE. Serious group A streptococcal diseases in children. J Pediatr 1976;88:972.

Gerber MA, Randolph MF, DeMeo KK, Kaplan EL. Lack of impact of early antibiotic therapy for streptococcal pharyngitis on recurrence rates. J Pediatr 1990;117:853-858.

Ginsberg CM, McCracken GH, Steinberg JB, et al. Treatment of group A streptococcal pharyngitis in children. Clin Pediatr 1984;21:83-88.

Ginsberg CM, McCracken GH, Crow SD, et al. Erythromycin therapy for group A streptococcal pharyngitis. Results of a comparative study of the estolate and ethylsuccinate formulations. Am J Dis Child 1984;138:536-539.

Goldstein I, Rebeyotte P, Parlebas J, et al. Isolation from heart valves of glycopeptides which share immunological properties with *Streptococcus hemolyticus* group A polysaccharides. Nature 1968;219:866-868.

Hall CB, Breese BB. Does penicillin make Johnny's strep throat better? Pediatr Infect Dis 1984;3:7-9.

Kaplan EL. The group A streptococcal upper respiratory tract carrier state: an enigma. J Pediatr 1980;97:337-345.

Kaplan EL. Benzathine penicillin for treatment of group A streptococcal pharyngitis: a reappraisal in 1985. Pediatr Infect Dis 1985;4:592-596.

Kaplan EL. The rapid identification of group A β-hemolytic streptococci of the upper respiratory tract. Pediatr Clin North Am 1988;35:535-342.

Kaplan EL, Wannamaker LW. Suppression of the antistreptolysin O response by cholesterol and by lipid extracts of the rabbit skin. J Exp Med 1976;144:754-767.

Kaplan EL, Reid HFM, Johnson DR, Kunde CA. Rapid antigen detection in the diagnosis of group A pyoderma: influence of a "learning curve effect" on sensitivity and specificity. Pediatr Infect Dis 1989;8:591-593.

Lancefield RC. A serological differentiation of human and other groups of hemolytic streptococci. J Exp Med 1933;57:571.

Markowitz M, Kaplan EL. Reappearance of rheumatic fever. Adv Pediatr 1989;36:39-66.

Maxted WR. The use of bacitracin for identifying group A haemolytic streptococci. J Clin Pathol 1953;6:224.

Moody MD. Old and new techniques for rapid identification of group A streptococci. In Wannamaker LW, Matsen JM (eds). Streptococci and streptococcal diseases: recognition, understanding, management. New York: Academic Press, 1972, pp 177-188.

Nelson JD. The effect of penicillin therapy on the symptoms and signs of streptococcal pharyngitis. Pediatr Infect Dis 1984;3:10-13.

Supportive treatment

Good medical and nursing care must minimize stimuli that may precipitate a convulsion. Procedures such as catheterization or placement of indwelling lines should be carried out at a time when any sedative is exerting its maximal effect. Such procedures preferably are performed early in the course of clinical illness. In addition, care should be taken to anticipate and prevent complications such as aspiration pneumonia, lower bowel obstruction resulting from fecal impaction, urinary retention, and decubitus ulcers. Adequate sedation may prevent a compression fracture of the vertebra. Respiratory support is essential, and intubation or tracheostomy with respirator ventilation may be required.

Tracheostomy

The combination of heavy sedation, difficulty in swallowing, laryngospasm, and accumulation of secretions leads to obstruction of the airway. A relatively low mortality rate of 10% was reported by Edmondson and Flowers (1979), who treated 100 patients with tetanus on an intensive care unit. Intubation can be lifesaving.

PREVENTIVE MEASURES
Active immunization

Since many cases of tetanus follow minor abrasions and lacerations that are ignored, control of the disease can be achieved best by active immunization with toxoid before exposure. All infants should be immunized routinely with tetanus toxoid that is incorporated with diphtheria toxoid and pertussis vaccine. The usual basic series of the triple antigen is given at 8-week intervals for three doses beginning at 2 to 4 months of age. Booster doses are given approximately 1 and 4 years later and at 10-year intervals thereafter.

In the event of an injury, administration of an additional booster dose of tetanus toxoid may be indicated; a protective antitoxin level is usually achieved within 1 week. A booster dose can provoke an adequate response after a 10-year lapse since the last injection. In severe, crush, and heavily contaminated wounds, particularly compound skull fractures, human tetanus immunoglobulin (250 units) should be given intramuscularly in conjunction with the toxoid. This procedure should prevent a potential short-incubation-period disease. Patients recovering from tetanus *may not be immune;* therefore they should be actively immunized with tetanus toxoid.

Passive immunization

Persons who have not been actively immunized should be protected with human tetanus immunoglobulin in the event of an injury. Although the usual dose is 250 units given intramuscularly, patients with severe wounds may need 500 units.

Care of a wound

A wound should be cleansed thoroughly, foreign bodies and necrotic tissues should be removed, and the area should be débrided when indicated.

• • •

The guidelines for the use of currently licensed vaccine(s) as recommended by the Immunization Practices Advisory Committee (ACIP) are included in Chapter 4.

REFERENCES

Adams JM, Kenny JD, Rudolph AJ. Modern management of tetanus neonatum. Pediatrics 1979;64:472.

Armitage P, Clifford R. Prognosis in tetanus: use of data from therapeutic trials. J Infect Dis 1978;138:1-8.

Bagratuni L. Cephalic tetanus: with report of a case. Br Med J 1952;1:461.

Bizzini B. Tetanus toxin. Microbiol Rev 1979;43:224-240.

Brand DA, Acampora D, Gottlieb ZD, et al. Adequacy of antitetanus prophylaxis in six hospital emergency rooms. N Engl J Med 1983;309:636-640.

Brooks VB, Asanuma H. Action of tetanus toxin in the cerebral cortex. Science 1962;137:674.

Brooks VB, Curtis DR, Eccles JC. Mode of action of tetanus toxin. Nature 1955;175:120.

Christie AB. Infectious diseases: epidemiology and clinical practice. Baltimore: Williams & Wilkins, 1969.

Edmondson RS, Flowers MW. Intensive care in tetanus: management, complications and mortality in 100 cases. Br Med J 1979;1:1401.

Edsall G. Specific prophylaxis of tetanus. JAMA 1959; 171:417.

Edsall G. Passive immunization. Pediatrics 1963;32:599.

Eidels L, Proia RL, Hart DA. Membrane receptors for bacterial toxins. Microbiol Rev 1983;47:596-620.

Goyal RK, Neogy CN, Mathur GP. A controlled trial of antiserum in the treatment of tetanus. Lancet 1966; 2:1371.

Kaeser HE, Sauer A. Tetanus toxin: a neuromuscular blocking agent. Nature 1969;223:842.

Kerr JH, et al. Involvement of the sympathetic nervous system in tetanus: studies on 82 cases. Lancet 1968;2:236.

Kessimer JG, Habig WH, Hardegree MC. Monoclonal antibodies as probes of tetanus toxin structure and function. Infect Immun 1983;42:942-948.

Laird WJ, Aronson W, Silver RP, et al. Plasmid associated toxigenicity in *Clostridium tetani*. J Infect Dis 1980; 142:623.

Levine L, Edsall G. Tetanus toxoid: what determines reaction proneness? J Infect Dis 1981;144:376.

Looney JM, Edsall G, Ispen J Jr, Chasen WH. Persistence of antitoxin levels after tetanus toxoid inoculation in adults and effects of a booster dose after intervals. N Engl J Med 1956;254:6.

Marie A, Morax V. Recherches sur l'absorption de la toxine tetanique. Ann Inst Pasteur 1902;16:818.

McCracken GH Jr, Dowell DL, Marshall FN. Double-blind trial of equine antitoxin and human immune globulin in tetanus neonatorum. Lancet 1971;1:1146.

Meyer H, Ransome F. Untersuchungen uber den Tetanus. Arch Exp Pathol Pharmakol 1903;49:369.

Pratt EL. Clinical tetanus: a study of 56 cases, with special reference to methods of prevention and a plan for evaluating treatment. JAMA 1945;129:1243.

Rubbo SD, Suri JC. Passive immunization against tetanus with human immune globulin. Br Med J 1962;2:79.

Rubinstein HM. Studies on human tetanus antitoxin. Am J Hyg 1962;76:276.

Smolens J, Vogt A, Crawford MN, Stokes J Jr. The persistence in the human circulation of horse and human tetanus antitoxins. J Pediatr 1961;59:899.

Stanfield JP, Gall D, Braden PM. Single dose–antenatal tetanus immunization. Lancet 1973;1:215.

Veronesi R. Clinical observations on 712 cases of tetanus subject to four different methods of treatment: 18.2 percent mortality rate under a new method of treatment. Am J Med Sci 1956;232:629.

30

TICK-BORNE INFECTIONS

RICKETTSIA

Rickettsiae are obligate intracellular gram-negative bacteria that multiply in arthropod vectors; the blood-eating habits of these vectors have involved their vertebrate hosts in the complex life cycle of these microorganisms. Except for epidemic typhus, humans are the incidental hosts for most rickettsial infections, and the geographical distribution of rickettsiae reflects that of the vector. Diseases such as typhus have been recognized for centuries, but not until the early twentieth century was the causative group of agents recognized when Dr. Howard T. Ricketts produced disease by injecting blood from a patient with Rocky Mountain spotted fever into a guinea pig.

The taxonomy of the order Rickettsiales is shown in Fig. 30-1. The tribes Rickettsieae and Ehrlichieae have four genera with agents causing human disease. The *Rickettsia* genus is further divided into three groups—typhus, spotted fever, and scrub typhus—with 10 species of organisms in these groups causing human illness. All Rickettsiaceae are limited to intracellular growth except *R. quintana*, the causative agent of trench fever, which grows extracellularly in the lumen of its host, the body louse, and without cells on enriched medium. *Coxiella burnetti*, although similar to the other genera of rickettsiae in morphology and intracellular growth, differs in major ways. This organism produces a sporelike small cell, has dissimilar DNA base composition, and is transmitted by aerosol to humans.

The spectrum of clinical illnesses produced by four of the genera of the Rickettsiaceae family include vasculitis (Rocky Mountain spotted fever); pneumonia (Q fever); febrile illness with vesicular rash (trench fever); febrile illness with infection of white blood cells (WBC) (ehrlichiosis); recrudescent febrile infection (Brill-Zinsser disease); and endocarditis (Q fever) (Table 30-1). Endothelial damage and secondary inflammation are the hallmarks of these Rickettsiaceae infections.

Etiology

Rickettsiales are pleomorphic coccobacillary organisms ranging from 0.3 to 0.6 μm in width and from 0.8 to 2.0 μm in length. They are gram negative but stain poorly, and visualization is best accomplished using a Gimenez modification of the Macchiavello method, which stains organisms red. These bacteria have a three-layered cell wall, trilaminar plasma membrane, ribosome-like particles, and intracellular organelles. They possess both RNA and DNA, and they divide by binary fission. The genome is large, varying from 1.0 to 1.5 × 10⁹ daltons. Apparently a single chromosome is organized as are other bacteria and plasmids. They have developed carrier-mediated exchange transport systems for phosphorylated compounds (ADP and ATP) similar to those of mitochondria. The genome size, DNA-DNA hybridization, and guanosine-cytosine content are similar within species of a group, but significant differences

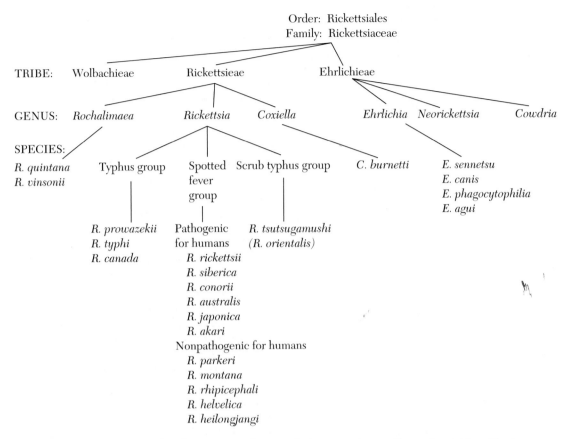

Order: Rickettsiales
Family: Rickettsiaceae

TRIBE: Wolbachieae   Rickettsieae   Ehrlichieae

GENUS: *Rochalimaea*   *Rickettsia*   *Coxiella*   *Ehrlichia*   *Neorickettsia*   *Cowdria*

SPECIES:

R. quintana   Typhus group   Spotted Scrub typhus group   *C. burnetti*   *E. sennetsu*
R. vinsonii   fever   *E. canis*
                                  group   *E. phagocytophilia*
                                                                                   E. agui

         R. prowazekii   Pathogenic   *R. tsutsugamushi*
         R. typhi   for humans   *(R. orientalis)*
         R. canada   *R. rickettsii*
                              R. siberica
                              R. conorii
                              R. australis
                              R. japonica
                              R. akari
                           Nonpathogenic for humans
                              R. parkeri
                              R. montana
                              R. rhipicephali
                              R. helvelica
                              R. heilongjangi

Rickettsieae: pathogenic or related to species pathogenic for humans who usually are the accidental host.
Ehrlichieae: pathogenic for vertebrate host but not known as pathogenic for human; two exceptions.
Wolbachia: confined to arthropods as pathogens or symbiotes.

Fig. 30-1. Taxonomy of Rickettsiales.

exist between groups (e.g., between *Coxiella* and *R. prowazekii*).

All members of the genus *Rickettsia* can obtain access to cytoplasm by traversing the host cell membrane and are unstable extracellularly, whereas *C. burnetti* (genus *Coxiella*) is very resistant to heat and dryness. Only *R. quintana* (of genus *Rochalimaea*) can multiply extracellularly. All members of the Rickettsiaceae family can be propagated in various tissue culture systems, embryonated eggs, laboratory animals, and certain arthropods. Generally, typhus group organisms grow in the cytoplasm, and spotted fever group organisms grow in the cytoplasm and nucleus.

Antigenic differences help classify these microorganisms. There is no common group antigen for all members of the Rickettsiaceae family

or of the tribe Rickettsieae. The antigens thought to induce a protective response to the typhus genus are species-specific for *R. prowazekii* or *R. typhi*, and a 155-kilodalton polypeptide and a 120-kilodalton polypeptide induce a protective humoral response.

The spotted fever group

Rickettsiae in the spotted fever group cause a diffuse infectious vasculitis involving the skin and produce a rash typically petechial or purpuric in character. Any of the viscera may be involved with the clinical disease, which encompasses a spectrum from unrecognized infection to fatal illness.

Rocky Mountain spotted fever (tick-borne typhus). This acute infectious disease, Rocky Mountain spotted fever (tick-borne typhus), is

Table 30-1. Rickettsial diseases

Causative agent	Diseases
R. prowazekii	Epidemic typhus, Brill-Zinsser disease
R. typhi	Endemic or murine typhus
R. canada	?—disease similar to Rocky Mountain spotted fever
R. rickettsii	Rocky Mountain spotted fever
R. akari	Rickettsial pox
R. sibirica	North Asian tick typhus
R. australis	Queensland tick typhus
R. japonica	Japanese spotted fever
R. conorii	Boutonneuse fever
R. tsutsugamushi	Scrub typhus (chigger-borne typhus, mite-borne typhus, Japanese River fever, rural fever, tropical typhus)
Rochalimaea quintana	Trench fever
Coxiella burnetti	Q fever
Ehrlichia sennetsu	Sennetsu rickettsiosis
E. canis (or related organism)	Ehrlichiosis

limited to the Western Hemisphere. The disease is most prevalent in the Piedmont region of the southeastern United States and in Oklahoma. Small numbers of cases have been recognized over the years in almost every state (Fig. 30-2). Approximately 650 cases of disease were reported to the Centers for Disease Control (CDC) in 1990. This disease is responsible for 95% of all reported rickettsial infections in the United States. Exposure to the vectors determines the epidemiological features of the disease. Thus the incidence is seasonal, with most cases coinciding with tick exposure between April and September (D'Angelo et al., 1978; Wilfert et al., 1984). Rural and suburban dwellers are more likely to acquire disease than urban residents. Similarly, very young infants (<2 years old) are rarely exposed, and illness in this age group is unusual. Persons who are outdoors in the typical oak, hickory, and pine forest habitat more likely will be exposed and acquire the disease.

Four species of *Ixodes* (hard) ticks indigenous in the United States harbor *R. rickettsii*. The wood tick, *Dermacentor andersoni*, is the western vector of *R. rickettsii*, and *D. variabilis*, or the dog tick, is the culprit in the Southeast. Ticks obtained from their habitat (not from dogs) harbor rickettsiae at varying frequencies (<1% to 10%); however, only one tick of 2,510 (0.03%) had *R. rickettsii* in one North Carolina study. The Lone Star tick (*Amblyomma americanum*) and the rabbit tick (*Haemaphysalis leporispalustris*) only occasionally transmit disease to humans, but they may be important in maintenance of infection in animals. The infected tick must ingest a blood meal to "activate" the rickettsia. This phenomenon probably is related to increasing the temperature of the organism, which microscopically correlates with the presence of a microcapsular slime layer (Hayes and Burgdorfer, 1982). Infection is transmitted to humans by a tick bite or by handling an infected tick that has had a blood meal. Infection is transmitted within the laboratory by aerosol (Oster et al., 1977), but aerosol transmission is not known to occur in nature. Very rarely, transmission from human to human has occurred through a blood transfusion from a patient incubating disease or through an accidental stick by a needle contaminated with infected blood.

Etiology and ecology. *R. rickettsii* are morphologically similar to other rickettsiae. *R. rickettsii* and *R. prowazekii* have a slime layer (glycocalix), probably composed of polysaccharide and external to the cell wall, which could be antigenically important and/or relate to cell attachment (Silverman et al., 1978). *R. rickettsii* are labile and are killed by drying at room temperature, by moist heat (50° C), and by formalin or phenol. *R. rickettsii* multiply in the nucleus and cytoplasm and produce demonstrable cytopathic effects. Scanning electron microscopic studies have shown *R. rickettsii* exiting from cells on long cytoplasmic projections without cell lysis. Large numbers of cells become infected relatively quickly. These microorganisms live within ticks, causing no disease, and are transovarially transmitted by tick progeny. The ticks pass through four stages in their life cycle, and they can acquire infection at any stage by feeding on a rickettsemic animal. The infection is passed by the vector through its sequential stages of

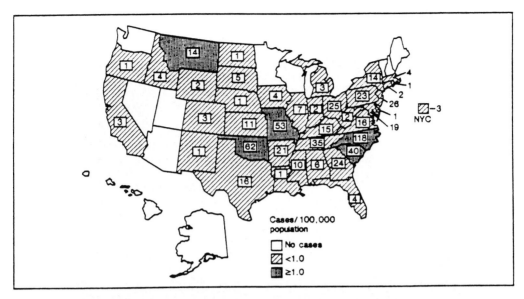

Fig. 30-2. Reported cases and rates of Rocky Mountain Spotted Fever, by state—United States, 1989. (From MMWR 1990; 39:281.)

development: egg to larvae to nymph to adult (i.e., transtadially). The arthropods are both reservoirs and vectors of infection. *R. rickettsii* shares antigens with *R. montana*, and in animals immunization with *R. montana* can protect against fatal *R. rickettsii* infection. It is theoretically possible that interrelationships of rickettsiae in nature may affect the clinical expression of human disease.

Pathogenesis and pathology. Rickettsiae gain entry in endothelial cells of small blood vessels (Silverman and Bond, 1979; Silverman, 1984). They are engulfed with host cell membrane. Phospholipase may aid in the escape from the phagosome and contribute to host cell membrane damage. In mammals organisms multiply in the vascular endothelium and smooth muscle, producing endothelial damage and small vessel occlusion, with extravasation of blood and fluid and attendant serum electrolyte changes. Typhus rickettsiae increase endothelial and macrophage secretion of arachidonate-derived autocoids. Activation of the kallikrein-kinin system has been documented in humans as has disseminated intravascular coagulation. The vasculitis is apparent in many tissues (Fig. 30-3), especially skin, that of the central nervous system (CNS), heart, lungs, liver, and kidney. Severe disease can cause occlusion of larger vessels and

gangrene. In animal models the rickettsiae themselves cause cellular damage. Cell-mediated immunity to *R. rickettsii* antigens has been demonstrated in vitro and may contribute to eradication of organisms in tissues, but the host immune response is not necessary or responsible for the tissue damage.

Clinical manifestations. The incubation period is usually 5 to 7 days, with a range of 3 to 12 days. Recognized illness is characterized by a short prodromal period of headache, malaise, and myalgias. The abrupt onset of fever may be accompanied by chills, and the severity of myalgias and headache may increase. Usually, the rash is noted 2 to 4 days after onset of illness. It begins as a maculopapular eruption with a peripheral distribution. The skin lesions appear first on the thenar eminence and the flexural surfaces of the wrist and ankle. The rash spreads to involve the arms, legs, chest, and, lastly the abdomen. The palms and soles are nearly always affected. The lesions are at first discrete, macular, and maculopapular, blanching on pressure. Within 1 to 3 days, the rash becomes hemorrhagic, and lesions may become confluent, with areas of necrosis at sites of maximal involvement. Gangrene of fingers, toes, genitalia, or nose may develop. During the period of convalescence, the rash becomes pigmented, and evidence of

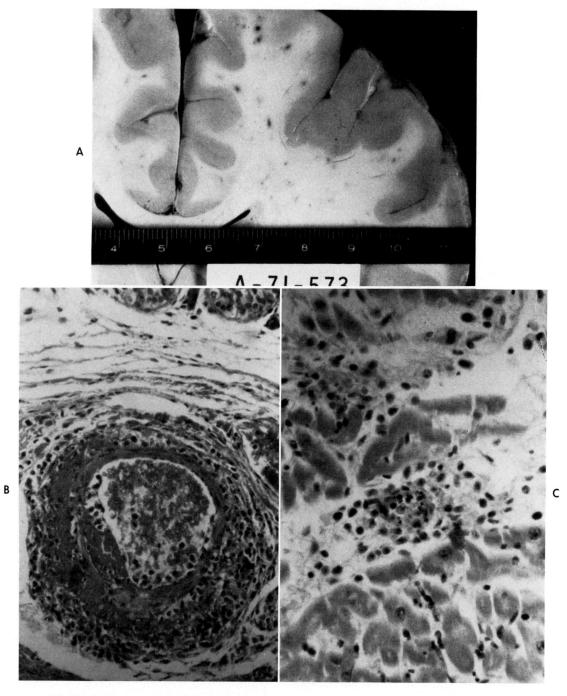

Fig. 30-3. Postmortem pathology of Rocky Mountain spotted fever. **A,** Brain with evidence of petechial hemorrhages. **B,** Tunica testes showing prominent vasculitis with endothelial thickening and fibrin deposition. **C,** Vasculitis of myocardium.

desquamation appears over the more severely affected areas.

The illness varies in severity even in the absence of specific antimicrobial therapy. Mortality rates are 5% to 10%, and factors associated with increased fatality include increased age and an increased length of time from onset to initiation of therapy (Hattwick et al., 1978). The diffuse organ involvement of this infection results in protean manifestations. Myalgia and associated elevations of muscle enzymes are common. Hepatic involvement is frequent and may produce mild to severe hepatocellular dysfunction and jaundice. The gastrointestinal tract manifestations include abdominal pain, vomiting, and diarrhea. The frequent myocardial involvement is evident microscopically, with apparent vasculitis and inflammation (see Fig. 30-3). The patient may have an altered sensorium or be comatose, and the cerebrospinal fluid (CSF) frequently contains an increased WBC count but usually fewer than 100 to 200 WBC/mm^3. The peripheral WBC count is often normal but with a shift to the left, with prominent vacuolization of polymorphonuclear cells. Hyponatremia and mild peripheral edema are frequent consequences of the vasculitis, and corrective supportive measures may include infusion of a colloid solution to increase intravascular volume. Increased antidiuretic hormone (ADH) levels have also been observed in patients with this disease.

Hospitalized patients represent the more severely ill; their course of illness may range from days to weeks. Prolonged fever of 10 days to several weeks or relapse after cessation of therapy has been observed. Some persons with measurable specific antibody titers have had no known illness consistent with Rocky Mountain spotted fever. It is likely that asymptomatic or mildly symptomatic infections occur.

Diagnosis. Clinical suspicion of Rocky Mountain spotted fever is all important in endemic areas, especially during the months of seasonal occurrence of tick exposure. A febrile illness, particularly with rash, often constitutes enough evidence for initiation of therapy. Additional features such as a known tick bite or attachment, myalgias, headache, and hyponatremia constitute a compelling clinical constellation. Laboratory diagnosis is dependent on the demonstration of antibodies, which are rarely present during the first 3 to 5 days of illness. Thus specific therapy should not await confirmation of the diagnosis by serological tests.

Laboratory diagnosis. Isolation of *R. rickettsii* from the blood is expensive and time consuming because it requires cell culture or animal inoculation and is done in only a few research laboratories. Recognition of positive cultures requires several days; therefore awaiting laboratory confirmation is not practical for early diagnosis.

Detection of intracellular *R. rickettsii* by fluorescein-conjugated antibody in skin biopsies obtained from an area of rash has yielded the earliest diagnosis (Woodward et al., 1976) (Fig. 30-4). Areas of normal skin do not demonstrate the presence of *R. rickettsii*. Antibiotic therapy given for more than 24 hours before obtaining test specimens may result in negative immunofluorescent stains of tissue from patients with known disease. Similarly, if specific antisera are available, it is possible to demonstrate the presence of intracellular organisms in tissues obtained at autopsy.

Polymerase chain reaction (PCR) testing has been reported to diagnose an acute rickettsial infection (typhus). The pair of oligonucleotide primers was based on a 434–base-pair DNA sequence from *R. rickettsii*. This primer pair resulted in successful amplification of DNA from

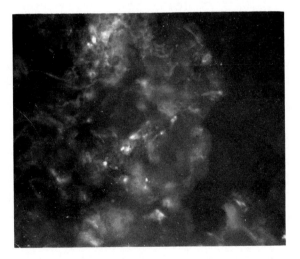

Fig. 30-4. Photomicrograph of a skin biopsy obtained from a 5-year-old child on the sixth day of illness. *R. rickettsii* are demonstrated by immunofluorescence. (×235.) (Courtesy Dr. David H. Walker, University of North Carolina at Chapel Hill.)

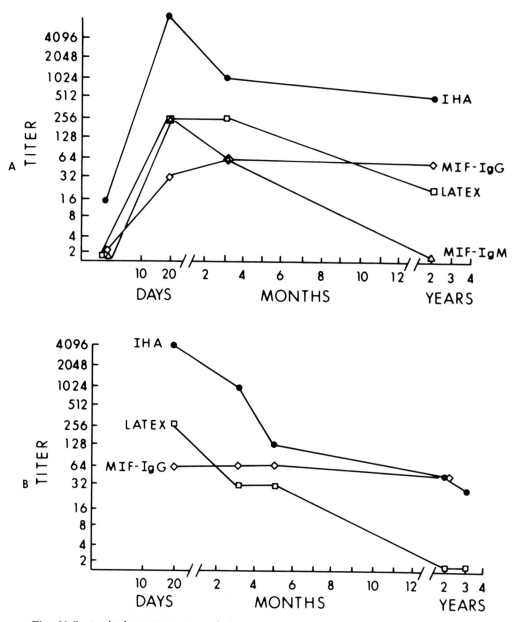

Fig. 30-5. Antibody titers to *R. rickettsii* measured by indirect hemagglutination *(IHA)*, microimmunofluorescence *(MIF)* for IgG and IgM, and latex agglutination. Titers are plotted by the time they were obtained in relation to onset of symptomatic illness. **A,** Titers obtained from serum of 62-year-old man with rash and fever hospitalized for 5 days and treated with tetracycline. **B,** Titers obtained from serum of 3-year-old boy who had a rash and fever; he was not hospitalized and did not receive specific therapy.

R. typhi, *R. prowazekii*, *R. rickettsii*, and *R. canada* and can be done in 48 hours. However, the sensitivity and general applicability have not been determined. In the near future this technology probably will provide a means of detecting those intravascular organisms during the acute illness.

Confirmation of disease generally is accomplished by serological demonstration of antibodies that appear during convalescence. Nonspecific testing traditionally has been accomplished with the Weil-Felix reaction. Because of their polysaccharide O antigens, several strains of proteus (OX-19, OX-2, OX-K) are agglutinated by antibodies formed in response to rickettsial infections. Antibodies are detected after the first week of illness, and a fourfold increase is suggestive of recent infection. The test is easy and inexpensive but lacks specificity and sensitivity.

Specific antibody to rickettsiae can be measured by indirect hemagglutination (IHA), microimmunofluorescence (micro-IF), latex agglutination, enzyme-linked immunosorbent assay (ELISA), and complement-fixation (CF) tests. The latter lacks sensitivity and is no longer in general use in the United States; antibodies detected by CF may be delayed in appearance, and their development has been aborted by specific antibiotic therapy. Neither the latex agglutination nor the ELISA test is commercially available. Some state health laboratories provide one or more of these tests. The sensitivity and specificity of IHA, micro-IF, and latex agglutination tests are comparable (Philip et al., 1977). An antibody rise of four-fold or greater in two sera is diagnostic of acute infection.

Demonstration of specific IgM antibody by immunofluorescence or ELISA suggests recent infection (Clements et al., 1983). A comparison of antibody measurements on two patients is depicted in Fig. 30-5.

Host defenses. It seems probable that a single infection with *R. rickettsii* confers immunity. This belief is substantiated by volunteer studies. Persons who have been sequentially challenged twice with *R. rickettsii* have disease only after the first exposure (DuPont et al., 1973). A spectrum of antibodies can be demonstrated in response to *R. rickettsii* (Anacker et al., 1983). Crossed immunoelectrophoresis demonstrates antibody responses to different antigens of the organism. It is currently unknown which antibody or antibodies confer protection against *R. rickettsii*. Antibody coating of *R. rickettsii* is necessary for phagocytosis and killing of the organism by guinea pig peritoneal macrophages in cell culture systems. Lymphocyte sensitization to *R. rickettsii* has been demonstrated in vitro from patients with prior infection and exposed to spotted fever group antigens. The relative roles of antibody and cell-mediated immunity in recovery from infection or protection against subsequent infection in human beings are unknown.

Differential diagnosis. In the absence of rash (e.g., in the early days of illness or in the unusual patient in whom no rash develops during the illness) it is difficult to make a specific diagnosis. The disease must be suspected in endemic areas. The differential diagnosis includes other rash diseases. Meningococcemia is difficult to distinguish from Rocky Mountain spotted fever. Atypical measles, which occurs in individuals previously vaccinated with inactivated (killed) measles virus vaccine, may also resemble Rocky Mountain spotted fever. Other species of rickettsiae that cause tick-borne disease and resemble Rocky Mountain spotted fever are found on several continents other than North America. Epidemic typhus is no longer present in the United States, but the clinical illness is similar to that of Rocky Mountain spotted fever. The skin rash classically appears as a patchy cutaneous erythema; it then progresses to the petechial form but usually spares the palms, soles, and face. Occasionally, recrudescent typhus, Brill-Zinsser disease, occurs in the United States, but primarily it occurs in immigrants from previously endemic areas. Murine typhus is usually a mild illness, and the rash tends to appear first on the trunk and spread to the extremities. Generally, the rash is macular or maculopapular and does not become petechial. This rickettsial infection is most likely to be confused with that of Rocky Mountain spotted fever within the United States.

Complications. Complications of Rocky Mountain spotted fever are more likely to occur in untreated patients or in patients whose specific therapy is initiated after more than 4 days of clinical illness (Hattwick et al., 1978). CNS sequelae have been observed after infection, but generally the prognosis is excellent for recovery. Occasionally, amputation of fingers and toes or other tissues may be necessitated by gangrene. Arrhythmias have been observed as a manifestation of the myocardial involvement.

Treatment. The only appropriate therapy is tetracycline or chloramphenicol, which alters the course of infection most significantly when instituted early in the course of illness. Rocky Mountain spotted fever is not transmitted from human to human except for the unusual circumstance of blood transfusion or needle puncture. Therefore isolation of patients is unnecessary.

Prevention. Nonspecific measures to diminish exposure to ticks should be taken but are not optimally successful. Individuals who are exposed to ticks and tick-infested environments should inspect themselves for ticks and carefully remove any they find. A period of time is necessary for activation of *R. rickettsii* in infected ticks; therefore early removal of ticks could in theory prevent infection. Attached ticks should be removed with forceps and gentle traction. Tick tissues and tick feces are highly infectious if the vector contains *R. rickettsii.*

There is no available vaccine for prevention of Rocky Mountain spotted fever. An early product made from egg-grown rickettsiae was used until it was shown conclusively that it failed to prevent infection. An experimental vaccine grown in cell-culture systems was subjected to experimental trials in animals and humans. Although humoral antibodies and lymphocyte sensitization could be demonstrated, people were not protected against challenge with *R. rickettsii*; therefore studies on this vaccine have been discontinued. Thus treating the disease is more effective than available preventive measures.

Rickettsialpox. Rickettsialpox is caused by *R. akari*, an organism of the spotted fever group that cross-reacts serologically with *R. rickettsii*. The disease is usually a mild febrile illness heralded by the development of a local eschar. Subsequently, a papulovesicular rash appears.

Etiology and ecology. The common house mouse in the United States is infested with a mite (formerly *Allodermanyssus sanguineus*, now *Lipryssoides sanguineus*) that may be infected with *R. akari*. This rickettsia has also been found in a wild Korean rodent *(Microtus fortis)*. This rickettsial infection may also be transmitted transovarially to the progeny of an infected mite. Humans enter the cycle of infection accidentally, often as the result of displacement of a rodent population by construction or during reduction of the rodent population by control programs. The mite attacks humans when its normal murine host is scarce. This rickettsia is infective for mice and guinea pigs but not for monkeys.

Epidemiology. All ages and both sexes are equally susceptible to rickettsialpox. The majority of cases have been reported in New York City where the disease was originally described in the Kew Gardens area of the borough of Queens in 1946 (Sussman, 1946; Greenberg, 1948). It has also been identified in West Hartford, Connecticut; Boston; Philadelphia; Arkansas; Delaware; and Russia.

Clinical manifestations and pathology. The estimated incubation period is 10 to 24 days. A triad of symptoms occur in sequence: the initial eschar, a febrile illness, and a generalized papulovesicular eruption.

The primary lesion at the site of the original mite bite is a local erythematous papule that evolves into a vesicle over a period of 2 days and then into an eschar. Most patients are not aware of either the bite or the lesion. The eschar resolves over a period of 3 to 4 weeks, and this lesion is usually associated with enlarged regional lymph nodes.

Approximately 3 to 7 days after the appearance of the eschar, fever with chills begins abruptly. Often there are headache, malaise, and myalgia. Within 72 hours of the onset of fever, the generalized rash develops. There is no characteristic distribution of this rash. It may occur on any part of the body, but it only rarely involves the palms or soles. The lesions are initially maculopapular and discrete, but small vesicles form on the summit of the papules. The lesions dry and may have tiny scabs that fall off without leaving scars. The entire course of illness is approximately 2 weeks. The WBC (2,400 to 4,000) usually shows leukopenia with relative lymphocytosis.

Because there have been no reported deaths from this disease, the available pathology consists of examination of the cutaneous manifestations (Dolgopol, 1948). The initial lesion is a firm nodule approximately 1 cm in diameter. It consists of a vesicle or pustule covered with dry epithelium or crust. Histologically, the vesicle is situated subepidermally and may arise from vacuolar changes of the basal layer. Mononuclear infiltration of the epidermis is seen, with a mixed polymorphonuclear mononuclear cell infiltrate in the dermis. The capillaries of the corium are dilated and surrounded by mononuclear cells. There is endothelial swelling in blood vessels.

Diagnosis. The diagnosis of rickettsialpox can be made clinically and confirmed by antibody determinations. Weil-Felix antibodies do not appear after infection with *R. akari*. However, more specific testing available at the CDC or research laboratories can demonstrate an antibody response 1 to 2 months after the onset of illness. Shared antigens of *R. rickettsii* and *R. akari* may result in detectable antibodies for Rocky Mountain spotted fever in patients with rickettsialpox.

R. akari has been isolated from both the blood and the vesicular fluid of infected persons. Using a research laboratory or one specifically interested in the diagnosis of this infection is necessary for obtaining diagnosis by culture because animals and embryonated eggs are used.

Differential diagnosis. Rickettsialpox has been confused with varicella (chickenpox) and is the only rickettsial disease characterized by the appearance of vesicular lesions. The presence of a primary eschar, however, should rule out varicella infection. The vesicular lesions in rickettsialpox are smaller than those in varicella and are usually situated on top of a papule. Rickettsialpox can affect all ages, but varicella is more likely to occur in children. The typical crusting of varicella lesions may not be observed in many of the rickettsialpox lesions. The diffuse nature of the vesicular lesions is in contrast to the characteristic sequential eruption and distribution of varicella vesicles. This difference should also help to distinguish this illness from primary herpes simplex infection. The demonstration of multinuclear giant cells and/or isolation of either herpes simplex or varicella-zoster virus will easily distinguish these infections. Hand, foot, and mouth disease does not have a primary eschar, and its scattered sparse lesions are usually tender and painful.

Prognosis. Untreated rickettsialpox is a benign, self-limited, nonfatal disease. No complications have been described.

Treatment and control measures. Tetracycline or chloramphenicol has been reported to modify the course of illness. Prevention is directed at control of the rodent host of the vector. No vaccines are available, and there is little stimulus to develop additional preventive measures because of the mild nature of this disease.

Other tick-borne diseases. An illness similar to Rocky Mountain spotted fever but generally milder has been ascribed to several tick-borne rickettsiae. North Asian tick typhus is caused by *R. sibirica* and occurs in Central Asia, Siberia and Mongolia. Queensland tick typhus is caused by *R. australis* and is found only in Australia. South African tick bite fever, Kenya tick typhus, Indian tick typhus, or boutonneuse fever (Mediterranean region) (different names for the same illness) is caused by *R. conorii*. *R. japonica* is the causative agent of Japanese spotted fever. All four of these rickettsiae infect species of *Ixodes* ticks and subsequently their wild animal host. Humans are only incidentally infected and are not important as reservoirs or for transmission of these illnesses. In contrast to Rocky

Mountain spotted fever, these rickettsial illnesses are characterized by a local skin lesion at the site of tick attachment and with the formation of an eschar as described for rickettsialpox. The illnesses are milder than Rocky Mountain spotted fever. Group-reactive complement-fixing antibodies have been demonstrated in response to infection with any of these four rickettsiae, but the Weil-Felix test is only inconsistently positive. The geographical distribution of the individual rickettsiae overlaps very little, so the diagnosis can be specific. These rickettsiae are also sensitive to chloramphenicol and tetracycline.

The typhus group

The typhus group of rickettsiae causes epidemic typhus (including recrudescent disease) and murine typhus. These organisms share a common group-specific antigen and are characterized by intracytoplasmic growth.

Epidemic typhus (louse-borne typhus). Epidemic typhus is an acute, potentially fatal infectious disease caused by *R. prowazekii* that has played an important role in history. For example, it has been estimated that in World War I more than 3 million Russians died as a result of this infection.

Etiology and ecology. *R. prowazekii* is similar to the previously described rickettsial species. The organisms multiply in cytoplasm much as do classic bacteria in liquid medium, and there are few cytopathic effects in the cells in which they grow. The organism is infectious for mice, guinea pigs, and embryonated eggs. Infectivity is preserved by lyophilization or storage at $-70°$ C. This organism can infect both the human body louse (*Pediculus humanus corporis*) and the head louse (*P. humanus capitis*). *P. humanus corporis* feeds only on humans, and all three stages of the life cycle of the louse (egg, nymph, and adult) can occur on the same host. The louse becomes infected by taking a blood meal from a person with rickettsemia. *R. prowazekii* multiplies in the epithelial cells of the intestine of the louse. After 3 to 7 days, large numbers of rickettsiae are excreted in the feces. Fortunately, lice do not transmit the rickettsiae to their progeny, and infected lice die within several weeks. An infected louse transmits disease by moving to another person and excreting feces during the blood meal. The abrasions induced by scratching provide a portal of entry for the rickettsiae deposited on the skin. Rarely, infections have been acquired by inhalation of dry infective feces of the louse. For practical purposes, humans are the only apparent reservoir of infection; however, the flying squirrel (*Glaucomys volans*) and its lice and fleas have been an occasional reservoir responsible for disease in Virginia, North Carolina, and West Virginia (Sonenshine et al., 1978).

Clinical manifestations and pathology. After an incubation period of 7 to 14 days, epidemic typhus begins abruptly with fever, chills, headache, malaise, and generalized aches and pains. The fever and constitutional symptoms increase in severity and are followed by a rash that erupts on the fourth to sixth day of illness. The maculopapular rash appears first on the trunk near the axillae and spreads to involve the extremities. The face, palms, and soles are usually not involved. Initially, the lesions are discrete pleomorphic macules that blanch on pressure. During the second week of illness, the skin lesions become petechial and purpuric and are followed by brownish pigmentation.

In the untreated patient fever lasts for 2 weeks and then falls by lysis over a period of 2 to 3 days. Severe illness is characterized by stupor, delirium, hallucinations or excitability, mental dullness, marked weakness, prostration, and temporary deafness. By the second and third weeks the patient either recovers or progresses to coma and death. The disease also is characterized by manifestations from the cardiovascular system. Early in the course of infection relative bradycardia may be present; later, tachycardia and gallop rhythm may reflect the myocardial damage. Spenomegaly, albuminuria, and elevated blood urea nitrogen (BUN) usually develop. The complete blood count (CBC) may reveal leukopenia and anemia.

The typical pathological lesion involves the endothelial cells of the small blood vessels. Multiplication of the rickettsiae causes edema, fibrin and platelet deposition, and obstruction of the vessels, which may be followed by thrombosis, hemorrhage, and perivascular accumulations of neutrophils, macrophages, and lymphocytes. The vascular lesions are widely disseminated, but they are most numerous in the skin, myocardium, skeletal muscle, kidneys, and CNS.

Diagnosis. The clinical picture should suggest the diagnosis of epidemic typhus, and appropriate therapy should not await laboratory confirmation of disease. Isolation of *R. prowazekii* can substantiate the clinical diagnosis, but doing so is potentially dangerous and is difficult and must be done by specifically trained personnel and special equipment. Primary isolations of *R. prowazekii* can be accomplished by inoculating blood into guinea pigs and adult white mice or into the yolk sac of embryonated eggs. Infection with *R. prowazekii* also induces the formation of antibodies that agglutinate *Proteus vulgaris* OX polysaccharide antigens. These agglutinins appear in the second week after onset of illness, and agglutination is usually maximal with OX-19 strains. A fourfold rise in agglutination titers is suggestive of recent infection; obtaining serial specimens often is necessary to document the antibody increment. Complement-fixing antibodies are demonstrable in the third week after onset of illness. However, as with Rocky Mountain spotted fever, immunofluorescent tests and microagglutination procedures are more sensitive and are specifically available in specialized laboratories (Ormsbee, 1977).

Differential diagnosis

Endemic typhus. Endemic typhus is clinically similar to but usually much milder than epidemic typhus. It is less likely its rash will be hemorrhagic. If the agent is isolated or injected into guinea pigs, scrotal edema is produced; this result does not occur after injection with *R. prowazekii.* Specific antibody measurements will establish the correct diagnosis.

Rocky Mountain spotted fever. The distribution of the rash of Rocky Mountain spotted fever should be different, with concentration of the face and extremities. A specific antibody test will help distinguish these two illnesses.

Scrub typhus. A primary lesion usually is present with this infection, which consists of a papule progressing to a vesicle and then to a scab with an ulcer. This severe febrile illness and rash could be confused with typhus. Antibody determinations distinguish epidemic typhus and scrub typhus.

Meningococcemia. Meningococcemia usually progresses more rapidly than typhus, a fact that may be helpful in making a clinical diagnosis. Isolation of the organism from the blood is diagnostic. This infection is commonly associated with meningitis.

Measles. The respiratory tract symptoms of coryza, conjunctivitis, and fever that precede the maculopapular eruption often provide a useful clinical distinction of measles from typhus. The distribution of the rash, with its initial appearance on the face and neck, is different from that of typhus. Hemorrhagic lesions are uncommon in patients with measles, and the fever usually subsides after the first week of illness.

Complications. Otitis media, parotitis, and bronchopneumonia may complicate epidemic typhus. Gangrene of portions of the extremities may also result from the vasculitis and thrombosis.

Prognosis. Untreated epidemic typhus fever is a severe and potentially fatal infection. The mortality rate ranges from 10% to 40%. The severe myocardial and CNS involvement is not usually followed by sequelae. The prognosis is considerably improved by specific antimicrobial therapy early in the course of disease. Case fatality rates increase with increasing age.

Epidemiology. Epidemic typhus is worldwide in distribution. All ages and both sexes are equally susceptible. It occurs chiefly in Asia, Africa, Europe, Central America, and South America. During World War II the disease was epidemic in Russia, Poland, Germany, Spain, and North Africa. Conditions that promote louse infestation, including crowding, lack of bathing, and conditions under which the same clothing is worn for prolonged periods, help propagate the disease. The conditions favorable for propagation of lice and disease are associated with war, poverty, and famine. Lice apparently seek locations where the temperature is approximately 20° C and will abandon the host when the body temperature rises to 40° C.

A few sporadic cases of epidemic typhus in the United States have been associated with the flying squirrel and have raised questions about whether this animal is a reservoir for this agent. The means of transmission of disease between these animals and man is not understood.

Brill-Zinsser disease. Recrudescent infection has occurred many years after an individual has had epidemic typhus. It was first suggested in 1934 that this recurrence was a relapse of a prior epidemic typhus infection. Thus the disease may occur in an individual living in the United States in a lousefree environment. Brill-Zinsser disease most frequently is observed in immigrants from endemic areas. An additional aspect of recrudescent disease is that lice feeding on such a patient can become infected and subsequently initiate another cycle of transmission. Thus latent human infection represents an interepidemic reservoir. Weil-Felix antibodies usually do not develop in patients with Brill-Zinsser disease. However, the demonstration of specific antibodies, which are IgG in immunoglobulin class, may occur earlier. The IgG and IgM determinations are usually performed using microimmunofluorescence.

Management and therapy. Patients with epidemic typhus must be deloused, which can be accomplished by bathing with soap and water and weekly dusting with 10% dichlorodiphenyltrichloroethane (DDT), 1% lindane, or another effective agent lethal to the lice.

Tetracycline or chloramphenicol is an appropriate specific antimicrobial therapy. A therapeutic response is ordinarily apparent within 48 hours, and earlier therapy is more likely to induce a prompt response.

After the patient and his clothing have been freed of lice, no isolation is necessary because the patient will not transmit disease to other persons. A susceptible contact who is known to have lice should be freed of infestation. After that, quarantine is not necessary.

Prevention. Current studies have refined and purified species-specific protein antigens of *R. prowazekii* and *R. typhi* that are essential for protection. These purified large polypeptides do not have significant endotoxin content. Both humoral and cellular immunity to these antigens does develop in humans after natural infection, and these "subunit vaccines" have been tested successfully for immunogenicity and efficacy in guinea pigs.

Murine typhus (endemic typhus, flea-borne typhus, rat typhus). Endemic typhus fever is an acute, relatively mild infection caused by *R. typhi*. It is characterized clinically by headache, fever, malaise, and a maculopapular eruption with a centripetal distribution. Essentially, it is a modified version of epidemic typhus fever.

Etiology and ecology. *R. typhi* is a natural infection of rodents that is spread to humans by the rat flea *(Xenopsylla cheopis)* and the rat louse *(Polyplax spinulosus)*. The vector, most frequently the rat flea, acquires *R. typhi* infection by feeding on a rickettsemic mouse or rat. The rickettsiae multiply in cells of the gut of the flea and in malpighian tubules. Thus infected, the flea may infect other susceptible rodents. Rickettsiae can be demonstrated in rodent brains for a period up to several months. Fleas do not transmit *R. typhi* transovarially, so the murine hosts constitute the reservoir for the microorganisms. The occasional transmission of *R. typhi* to humans occurs when the infected flea that is taking a blood meal incites scratching; the host then inoculates the infected feces into the excoriation. Infection is not transmitted by the flea bite. The flea feces are also infective if accidentally transmitted through a mucosal surface such as the conjunctiva. *R. typhi* is very similar to *R. prowazekii* and is also infective for rats, mice, guinea pigs, and the yolk sac of embryonated eggs.

Clinical manifestations. The incubation period of murine typhus ranges from 1 to 2 weeks. Clinically, endemic typhus is indistinguishable from a mild case of epidemic typhus fever. The onset of fever, headache, malaise, myalgias, and a maculopapular nonpruritic skin rash that becomes apparent on the third to fifth day of disease are typical features of the illness. The rash is typically sparse, discrete, and rarely hemmorrhagic. In the untreated patient the febrile course seldom persists for more than 2 weeks. The reported mortality rate is less than 2%. Cardiac, CNS, and renal manifestations occur less frequently than in patients with epidemic typhus.

Diagnosis. Weil-Felix agglutinins to *Proteus* OX-19 usually appear in the second week of infection. More sensitive and specific serological assessment includes antibodies measured by micro-IF. The CF assay is a standard method, generally available but less sensitive.

Epidemiology. Murine typhus fever has a worldwide distribution and is endemic in many countries, including the United States. In the United States the largest concentration of cases has occurred in the southern states along the Gulf of Mexico and the Atlantic seaboard. Over the past 10 years approximately three fourths of the reported cases in the United States have occurred in Texas. Clearly, the disease occurs in areas that are rat or mice infested, and these animals tend to accumulate in large numbers where grains and feeds are stored. The disease occurs most often during the summer months.

Immunity. Endemic typhus is usually followed by lasting immunity. There is cross-protection between this disease and epidemic typhus fever, although they are caused by different organisms.

Treatment. The treatment is the same as that for epidemic typhus. This disease does not spread from human to human but is dependent totally on an infected vector.

Diagnosis. The serological cross-reactions among members of the typhus group are common, but usually the response to the homologous antigen is the greatest. Inoculation of organisms or blood containing organisms into the peritoneal cavity of a guinea pig produces severe vesicular lesions and scrotal swelling. This is a much more severe disease for this animal than that induced by the inoculation of *R. prowazekii*.

Rickettsia canada infection. In 1967 a new species of rickettsia was isolated from rabbit ticks (*Haemaphysalis leporispalustris*) in Ontario, Canada. *R. canada* has been replaced in the typhus group on the basis of guanosine and cytosine content, DNA-DNA hybridization, and genome size. However, it grows in both the cytoplasm and nuclei of infected cells, a characteristic of the spotted fever group, and it has serological cross-reactivity with the spotted fever group organisms. This organism has not yet been isolated from a human source. Thus its role in human disease is unknown, although there is serological evidence that several patients with a Rocky Mountain spotted fever–type illness were infected with this rickettsia.

Scrub typhus. An additional scrub typhus group of rickettsiae is capable of producing a single clinical illness in humans. Demonstrably different surface antigens classify organisms as Karp, Gilliam, or Kato. The different antigenic types do not seem to influence the manifestations of infection, and persons can become infected and sustain clinical illness more than once by these rickettsiae.

Etiology. *R. tsutsugamushi* (or *R. orientalis*) is the causative agent. This rickettsia has been studied in cell culture systems and observed to form blebs from its outer membranes just as some other gram-negative organisms do. The organism infects several species of trombiculid mites. The mites have a four-stage life cycle (i.e., eggs, larvae, nymphs, and adults), and *R. tsutsugamushi* is transmitted transtadially. The larva, or chigger, is the only stage that feeds on vertebrates. After a blood meal the chigger detaches and matures into a nymph and then into an adult. The nymphs and adults are free-living arthropods in the soil. Therefore trombiculid mites are the vectors and the reservoirs of the rickettsial infections they transmit.

The natural cycle of infection involves chiggers in small mammals or ground-feeding birds. Humans accidentally enter the natural cycle of infection in areas of secondary or scrub vegetation but also beaches, deserts, and rain forests. The disease is endemic in a geographical area of approximately 5 million square miles that includes Australia, Japan, Korea, India, and Vietnam. Appreciable morbidity from scrub typhus was sustained during World War II by both American and Japanese soldiers. The disease usually occurs sporadically unless a group of people is brought into an endemic mite-infested area; then an outbreak may occur.

Clinical manifestations. The incubation period of scrub typhus ranges from 1 to 3 weeks, and the illness is very similar to other rickettsial infections, with abrupt onset of fever, headache, vomiting, myalgia, and abdominal pain. A local cutaneous lesion evolves from a small indurated or vesicular lesion into an ulcerated area that is present at the time of onset of symptoms. An eschar is usually present as is local lymphadenopathy. Approximately 1 week after the onset of fever, a macular or maculopapular rash appears and is apparent first on the trunk. Fatality rates in epidemics have varied from 0% to 50%. Appropriate therapy alters the disease and prevents fatal illness.

Variation in surface antigenicity of the causative organism permits reinfection and clinically apparent disease to occur in a single individual. Thus infection with one strain of *R. tsutsugamushi* does not confer protection against another strain.

Diagnosis. The serological diagnosis is somewhat complex because of the different antigens that do not cross-react. A series of antigens, usually three, must be used in a test such as the CF assay. As stated previously, the strains represented are the Karp, Gilliam, and Kato. A Weil-Felix reaction may be positive, with agglutinins to *Proteus* OX-K. The time course is similar to that of other rickettsial infections, with antibodies becoming detectable in the second week of illness. The agglutinins are less sensitive than measurement of antibody by immunofluorescence.

Treatment. Tetracycline and chloramphenicol are effective therapeutic agents that inhibit the growth of rickettsiae and usually produce prompt clinical improvement. Relapse or recrudescence of self-limited fever has been observed in patients whose therapy was initiated before 5 days of illness. If antibiotics are discontinued too early, relapse has also been observed.

TRENCH FEVER

The illness caused by *Rochalimaea quintana* originally was recognized during World War I and was not described again until epidemic occurrences during World War II. The illness has been reported primarily in Europe, although *R. quintana* has also been isolated from lice in Mexico. The louse-human-louse cycle is like that of epidemic typhus, with no known animal reservoirs. *R. quintana* multiplies in an extracellular environment in the lumen of the gut of the arthropod host. Once a louse is infected, it excretes rickettsiae in its feces for the duration of its life. Surprisingly, the DNA of this organism hybridizes with that of 25% to 33% of the typhus group of organisms, suggesting more homology than would have been expected between these genera. Transovarial transmission of infection does not occur.

The incubation period in volunteers is 8 to 18 days, and the clinical manifestations are variable. A mild, afebrile disease may occur along with other symptoms, including headache, malaise, myalgias, and bone pain. Rash is not prominent, but a macular eruption resembling the rose spots of typhoid fever may occur. This rickettsial species can be isolated in enriched blood agar media or grown in the yolk sacs of embryonated eggs. The usual laboratory animals— mice, rabbits, and guinea pigs—are not useful for isolation of *R. quintana*. Indirect immunofluorescence, complement fixation, and passive hemagglutination assays have been used to assess antibody status. *R. quintana* has been isolated from apparently healthy patients years after their original attack of disease.

In vitro sensitivity testing suggests that chloramphenicol and tetracycline would be effective therapy, although no data substantiate their efficacy in people.

Q FEVER

Coxiella burnetti was isolated simultaneously from infected persons in Australia and from wood ticks in Montana and was identified as a rickettsia in 1939 (Burnet and Freeman). The name of the disease, *Q fever*, is derived from the first initial of "query," which was the clinical designation for this unusual febrile illness.

Etiology. *C. burnetti* grows intracellularly in membrane-bound vesicles primarily in monocytes and macrophages. As an obligate intracellular organism, it parasitizes eukaryotic cells and goes through its developmental cycle in the phagolysosome. These organisms actively metabolize at a pH of 4.5, which is the intravacuolar pH, and not at a pH of 7.0. Thus this organism thrives in the usually hostile environment of the phagolysosome. Surface antigenic differences define phase I and phase II organisms, which are morphologically the same. Phase I organisms exist in nature, and phase II organisms emerge with passage in embryonated eggs. Reversion occurs after animal passage.

The ecology of this rickettsia is more complex than those previously described. One cycle involves arthropods, especially ticks, which infect a variety of vertebrates, including domestic animals but not humans. Another cycle is maintained among domestic animals. These animals may have inapparent infections and shed large quantities of infectious organisms in urine, milk, feces, and placental products. *C. burnetti* resists desiccation and exposure to light or ambient temperatures after it is shed by the infected animal; therefore aerosolization of infectious material occurs. Humans and animals may be infected by inhalation of such material. An alternative mode of acquisition of infection is ingestion of infected milk or the handling of contaminated wool or hides. *C. burnetti* also can penetrate the skin (e.g., through a minor abrasion) and mucous membranes. Rarely, human-to-human transmission has occurred. Q fever has been an occupational risk in abattoir workers, dairy and other farm workers, persons employed in tanneries, in wool and felt plants, and in the laboratory setting. Four outbreaks, involving as many as 100 persons, occurred recently in major university teaching hospitals. This occupational hazard is receiving increased attention.

Clinical manifestations. The incubation period of Q fever is 2 to 3 weeks, and illness usually begins abruptly with fever, chills, headache, malaise, and weakness. After 5 or 6 days of symptoms, cough and chest pain occur, and rales may be audible. X-ray studies reveal pneumonia that is usually apparent by the third day of illness.

The consolidation clears over a period of 1 to 2 weeks (Derrick, 1973). The reported pathology in the lungs consists of peribronchial and perivascular mononuclear infiltrates of lymphocytes, plasma cells, and monocytes. Fibrinous exudate fills the alveoli and bronchioles. Skin rash is not a part of the clinical syndrome, and its absence is unique among the rickettsial diseases. There is a spectrum of illness, and people have been proved infected without any obvious symptoms; in addition, asymptomatic recrudescence of infection has occurred during pregnancy. Prolonged fever, endocarditis, and hepatitis complete the clinical spectrum. Unfortunately, Q fever endocarditis can occur months or years after the acute attack. The diagnosis should be considered when a previous history of such illness is obtained from someone of the appropriate occupation or exposure with culture-negative illness. Organisms isolated from persons with chronic illness contain a large plasmid (QpRS), whereas a smaller plasmid (QpH1) is present in organisms isolated from persons with acute illness. There is interest in these differences because they may relate to the altered expression of disease.

Diagnosis. The compatible clinical picture, isolation of *C. burnetti* from the blood or sputum, and serological tests establish the diagnosis. Unfortunately, isolation of the organism requires inoculation of blood or sputum into an animal such as a guinea pig, mouse or hamster, or embryonated eggs or cell culture. Because of the possibility of transmission in the laboratory setting, this procedure is available only in research laboratories accustomed to dealing with the organism. Consequently, it is more reasonable to rely on serological confirmation of the diagnosis.

Purified antigens are used by several state health departments to perform the CF test. Since *C. burnetti* exists in two phases, reagents have been prepared using phase I and phase II antigens, which have been useful in distinguishing acute from chronic or past infection. Nevertheless, assessment by CF antibodies underestimates the prevalence of infection, and an intradermal skin test is more reliable. A microagglutination test has been a useful epidemiological tool. The use of ELISA for specific IgM antibody to *C. burnetti* may be helpful in diagnosing acute infection (Field et al., 1983).

There are no Weil-Felix agglutinins in response to infection with *C. burnetti*.

Differential diagnosis. The differential diagnosis includes illness that relates to the particular system that is most prominently affected. Thus influenza or mycoplasmal pneumoniae is considered when respiratory complaints are present. When CNS complaints are present, meningitis is considered. Abnormal liver function studies suggest hepatitis, and with gastrointestinal manifestations, typhoid fever is included in the diagnostic considerations.

Prognosis. The mortality rate of Q fever before antimicrobial therapy was available was approximately 1%. Fatalities are extraordinarily rare with specific therapy; the only exception is the unfortunate patient with endocarditis for whom the mortality rate is higher.

Treatment. Tetracycline or chloramphenicol is indicated and should be administered for several days after the patient with Q fever has become afebrile. Good clinical response is not as dramatic as that observed with some other rickettsial infections. Studies have suggested that replacement of an involved heart valve with a prosthetic valve and long-term therapy may improve the prognosis for patients with endocarditis caused by *C. burnetti*.

Preventive measures include pasteurization of milk; otherwise, it is difficult to interrupt the transmission of infection. A specific suggestion to protect laboratory personnel working with sheep or their tissues is for them to do their research in a setting distinct from other hospital research and away from patient care. Use of seronegative flocks may be considered as an alternative to containment procedures, and a skin test is the best assessment of status of at-risk personnel. Lymphocyte transformation studies and skin testing are better predictors of immunity than antibody because antibody-negative persons may be immune. Human beings rarely transmit disease to one another; thus isolation of the infected patient is not indicated. An early vaccine from phase II organisms was used effectively in Public Health Service and Army laboratories, but adverse reactions limited any general applicability of the vaccine. Recently, a formalin-inactivated phase I *C. burnetti* vaccine has undergone study. Phase I antigens increase the protective efficacy, and such a vaccine has provided protection in challenge studies. Thus a practical vaccine may become a reality in the foreseeable future.

EHRLICHIOSIS

Ehrlichieae is one of the three tribes of the family Rickettsiaceae (see Fig. 30-1). The genus *Ehrlichia* has six species, two of which, *E. sennetsu* and *E. canis*, apparently cause human illness—sennetsu fever and ehrlichiosis, respectively.

Etiology. Ehrlichieae are obligate intracellular bacteria nominally grouped with rickettsiae (see Fig. 30-1). These organisms replicate within the phagosome in the host cell and have a tropism for circulating leukocytes. All *Ehrlichia* presumably are tick borne. The presumed vector for *E. canis* is *Rhipicephalus sanguineus* of dogs. The vector for *E. sennetsu* is unknown. *E. sennetsu* grows readily in human and canine monocytes, in a variety of cell cultures, and in mice, whereas *E. canis* grows only in canine monocytes. *Ehrlichia*, like *Chlamydia*, go through developmental stages of elementary bodies, initial bodies, and morulae. The individual organisms, called *elementary bodies*, are small gram-negative rods measuring 0.5 μm in diameter. They are phagocytized by monocytes, and phagolysosomal fusion fails to occur. The elementary bodies grow and divide by binary fission within the phagosome and form initial bodies, which are composed of many elementary bodies and are apparent as inclusions in 3 to 5 days. These initial bodies grow further and divide during the next 7 to 12 days so that by light microscopy the configuration resembles a mulberry, or morula. Each infected monocyte can contain several of these inclusions. Rupture of the infected cells releases individual elementary bodies from the broken morulae. The data suggest that the agent causing the human illness ehrlichiosis is closely related to *E. canis*.

Clinical manifestations. In the 1950s sennetsu fever was described, manifested as fever, lymphadenopathy, and atypical lymphocytosis. A rickettsia-like agent was isolated from the blood, lymph nodes, and bone marrow of this patient. The provisional name associated with the organism was *Rickettsia sennetsu*; however, the organism has been reclassified as *E. sennetsu*.

The disease rarely has been reported outside of Japan. One serological survey from Malasia suggested that patients with febrile illnesses had antibodies to this organism. The mode of transmission of the organism is unknown, and the illness occurs predominately in the summer and fall. The incubation period is approximately 14 days, with sudden onset of illness and generalized adenopathy developing within the first week of illness. The untreated illness is benign, and no fatalities or serious complications have been described.

In 1987 the first case of human ehrlichiosis in the United States was reported (Maeda et al., 1987). Since 1986 more than 100 cases of human ehrlichiosis have been identified by the CDC. Fourteen states in the south central and south Atlantic regions have reported the illness, possibly resulting in part from considering the diagnosis of Rocky Mountain spotted fever. The epidemiology thus far is very similar to that of Rocky Mountain spotted fever, with a seasonal prevalence occurring from May to July and with more cases observed in rural areas. Patients report a tick bite or exposure to ticks in the 4 weeks before the onset of illness.

The clinical illness is similar to that of Rocky Mountain spotted fever except that only a minority of patients, perhaps 20%, have a rash. Leukopenia and thrombocytopenia are detected in most patients in the first weeks of illness. Fishbein et al. (1987, 1989) reported leukopenia in 57% of their patients and thrombocytopenia in 85% at the time of hospital admission. Over three quarters of the patients have elevated alanine or aspartate aminotransferase values during the course of their illness, and most abnormalities are noted in the first week.

During the acute illness inclusion bodies may be seen in atypical lymphocytes, neutrophils, and monocytes. These inclusions are dark blue, round, and approximately 2 to 5 μm in diameter. Electron microscopic examination shows aggregates of organisms in membrane-lined vacuoles. No ehrlichiae have been isolated from patients ill with disease. However, the antibody response of patients is measured by the *E. canis* fluorescent antibody test. Antibodies rise during the first 3 weeks of illness and peak approximately 6 weeks after the onset of illness.

Prognosis. Fatal infection with ehrlichiosis has occurred; however, serological surveys suggest that unrecognized infection occurs, too. Thus a broad spectrum of disease exists, with some patients having asymptomatic or totally unrecognized illness. The illness may be prolonged in some patients and may require considerable time to full recovery.

Differential diagnosis. Many of the patients with ehrlichiosis have been identified because the illness is similar to Rocky Mountain spotted fever. The differential diagnosis for ehrlichiosis includes Rocky Mountain spotted fever, leptospirosis, Lyme disease, and babesiosis.

Treatment. Chloramphenicol or tetracycline is the drug of choice. There is more reported experience with the use of tetracycline in management of this infection.

BABESIOSIS

Infection with members of the protozoan genus *Babesia* has caused identifiable illness in the United States and Europe. This febrile illness with associated hemolysis primarily affects middle-aged and older persons. *Babesia* are transmitted by ticks; therefore the illness, its epidemiology, and its relationship to the other tick-borne entities are considered within this chapter.

Etiology. Many species of *Babesia* can infect a variety of domestic and wild animals throughout the world. In the United States *B. microti* is the principal cause of human infection. In Europe *B. divergens*, a parasite of cattle, also infects people. *Ixodes* ticks transmit *Babesia* species. The nymphal stage of the deer tick, *Ixodes dammini*, is the principal vector of *B. microti* in the United States. To date, the principal endemic focus for babesiosis in the United States is coastal New England. Most of the cases have occurred in Nantucket and Martha's Vineyard, Massachusetts, and on Shelter Island off the coast of Long Island, New York. Other cases have been documented in Rhode Island and Washburn County, Wisconsin. As with the other tick-borne diseases, the majority of cases occur from June through September.

I. dammini requires three separate hosts during its maturation through larval, nymph, and adult stages. Many species of birds and mammals harbor the various stages of this tick. *B. microti* is transtadially transmitted from larvae to nymphs, not from the nymphal stage to the adult stage of the tick. Therefore transovarial transmission of this infection does not occur, and the reservoir of infection is probably in the larvae and nymphal forms of the vector. Female ticks lay their eggs on the ground, and the six-legged larvae emerge in late spring, with their blood meal obtained from a rodent host from July to September. Ordinarily, the larvae develop into nymphs in the fall; if they have acquired infection during their blood meal, it is carried over to the nymph stage. The nymphs do not attach to animals until the spring after their emergence as larvae. The nymphs become active in the early spring, and although they are the second stage of development, their feeding on animals occurs earlier in the year than that of the larvae. The nymphs infect rodents; thus the cycle is continued. The small rodents such as voles and white-footed deer mice (*Peromyscus* species) are the principal reservoirs for *B. microti*. Adult ticks are most active in the late summer and fall but are not infectious for humans because the babesiae are not transmitted from the nymph to the adult tick. The adult tick takes only a single meal; therefore if it acquired *Babesia* from an animal, it would not take a second meal and expose a human.

Babesia are intraerythrocytic protozoa (piroplasms). They have solid pyriform shapes and frequently are arranged in pairs. It is possible to infect a variety of animals experimentally, and removal of the spleen often augments the duration and severity of infection. A microscopic study of an extensively parasitized patient during illness has shown that usually one to four of the basophilic parasites are seen in infected red blood cells, but as many as five to 12 parasites per cell can be visualized. Varying developmental stages of the parasite, including ring, ameboid, and other forms, can be seen even within a single cell. Extracellular merozoites are present singly or in a syncytial structure. Free ribosomes, occasional endoplasmic reticulum, and small dense bodies may be seen in the cytoplasm of merozoites with a single large membrane-limited dense body (rhoptry). Trophozoites are surrounded by a single plasma membrane. Red blood cells viewed early in the course of illness show membrane changes, with protrusions and perforations. Spherical inclusions in red blood cells corresponding to the parasites have been seen through the scanning electron microscope.

Clinical manifestations. The incubation period apparently is 1½ to 3 weeks after a tick bite. Onset is heralded by the development of fatigue and malaise, followed by fever from 38° to 39° C. The patient may have shaking chills, arthralgia, myalgia, and depression. The disease is somewhat like malaria but without the periodicity. The patient may have mild jaundice and splenomegaly, and the most severe disease occurs in patients without a spleen. Jaundice, thrombocytopenia, and disseminated intravascular coagulation have been noted. Postmortem findings in the lungs are consistent with adult respiratory distress syndrome. In the bone marrow hemophagocytosis has been observed.

Most *B. microti* infections are self-limited. Serological surveys have confirmed the existence of antibodies in persons who did not have recognizable disease. Unfortunately, healthy individuals may be carrying the organism, for transfusion has resulted in transmission of infection to recipients, and a single instance of transplacental transmission to an infant has been described. Some studies of the hematological and immunological findings in acute babesiosis indicate the presence of lymphocytosis with some increase in the number of B-lymphocytes and null cells. There is a relative T-cell depletion. The level of circulating immune complexes, as determined by the C1q-binding assay, is increased.

Diagnosis. *B. microti* is visible in the peripheral blood smear, and the examination is conducted as for malaria. Patients will have hemolytic anemia, with elevated reticulocyte counts and visible parasites in their red blood cells. The principal differential diagnosis in endemic areas is malaria caused by *Plasmodium falciparum*. The ringlike structures are present in both entities, but the malarial parasite usually is associated with a brown granular pigment that is absent in babesiosis. Additionally, in patients with falciparum malaria other intraerythrocytic forms besides rings may be seen, and the banana-shaped gametocyte is the hallmark. Inoculation of blood into guinea pigs may result in small numbers of babesial organisms not seen in the peripheral smears.

Serological testing by indirect fluorescent antibody is available through the CDC. Titers greater than 1:64 are suggestive of recent infection, but two sera demonstrating a fourfold or greater rise are diagnostic.

Treatment. Babesiosis is treated with quinine and clindamycin. Patients who are extremely ill require exchange transfusion to diminish the load of parasites.

The *Babesia* are transmitted by the same vectors and therefore require the same animal hosts as those involved in transmission of Lyme disease. It has been suggested that a person with one of these infections should be evaluated for the other infection.

LYME DISEASE

Lyme disease was described in 1977 by Steere et al. The cutaneous manifestations, including erythema migrans, provided a link to other previously described illnesses in Europe, which included chronic lymphocytic meningitis (sometimes with cranial or peripheral neuritis) and chronic skin disease (acrodermatitis chronica atrophicans). These entities became associated when the causative organism, *Borrelia burgdorferi*, was identified in 1982 (Burgdorfer et al.).

Etiology. *Borrelia* species are in the Eubacterial phylum of spirochetes. Its DNA is 39% to 59% homologous with other *Borrelia*. *B. burgdorferi* measures 0.2 to 0.3 μm × 20 to 30 μm and has the characteristic cylindrical morphology of all spirochetes, with its protoplasm surrounded by a cell membrane, seven to 11 flagella, and an outer membrane. *Borrelia* grow in a complex liquid medium (Barbour/Stoenner-Kelly) and are microaerophilic. Isolation of organisms from patients is very difficult, and the bacteria grow slowly.

Movement of the outer membrane can occur so that the organism becomes capped by the membrane. At least 30 proteins are in *B. burgdorferi*, and the two major outer surface proteins have attracted considerable attention. Outer surface protein A (30 to 32 kilodaltons) and outer surface protein B (34 to 36 kilodaltons) are both encoded by a 49-kilodalton linear plasmid that always is present as one of four to nine plasmids. The plasmid-encoded proteins in the outer membrane may facilitate antigenic changes. The organism loses its pathogenicity in culture. Some of the plasmids may be lost during passage in vitro, and since a concurrent loss of infectivity occurs, it is speculated that virulence factors are encoded by these plasmids. There are differences between the outer-surface proteins of American and European isolates. This observation leads to concern about the possibility of protecting against this infection with a single protein. Although there are different immunotypes or subtypes of *B. burgdorferi*, there is no system of subclassification at present.

B. burgdorferi is transmitted by certain *Ixodes* ticks, including *I. dammini* in the northeastern and midwestern United States, *I. pacificus* in the western United States, *I. ricinus* in Europe, and *I. persulcatus* in Asia. The life cycle of the spirochete is dependent on horizontal transmission of infection. The preferred host for both the larval and nymphal stages of *I. dammini* is the white-footed mouse, *Peromyscus leucopus*. The infected nymphs must transmit infection to the mice in early summer during their single feeding. In late summer the asymptomatic infected mice who remain spirochetemic transmit the organism to larvae. The larvae that take their blood meal from an infected mouse become infected and harbor organisms in their midgut. The larvae molt to become nymphs the following year, attach to another host, and inject *B. burgdorferi* with saliva into the host, and the cycle is continued. Experimentally, the ticks must remain attached for 24 hours or more before transmission occurs. *B. burgdorferi* has been found in 10% to 35% of *I. dammini* ticks in Connecticut and in Shelter Island, New York. The white-tailed deer are not essential to the life cycle of the spirochetes but are important for the survival of the tick. There is no known illness in wild animals as a result of this infection.

Epidemiology. Lyme disease is the most commonly reported vector-borne infection in the United States (MMWR, 1988). Erratic cases have been identified in more than 40 states, but three areas of the country have the majority of disease: Massachusetts to Maryland in the Northeast; Wisconsin and Minnesota in the Midwest; and California and Oregon in the West. In Europe thousands of cases of Lyme borreliosis occur each summer and are reported from Germany, Austria, Switzerland, France, Sweden, and other countries. It has been postulated that the recent protection of deer, with the resulting increase in the population, has increased the contact of people with mice and ticks. However, on the West Coast where *I. pacificus* ticks are the vector, only sporadic cases of disease are observed, perhaps because the nymphal stage of the tick feeds primarily on lizards, which are not susceptible to infection with *B. burgdorferi*.

Clinical manifestations and pathogenesis. Infection with the spirochete produces a constellation of symptoms; characteristically, the disease occurs in stages as described by Asbrink and Hobmark (1988). Stage 1 may be asymptomatic or characterized by localized erythema migrans. In days or weeks disseminated infection, or stage 2, occurs. Within weeks or months intermittent symptoms occur. Persistent infection or late infection is referred to as stage 3 and usually begins a year or more after the original onset of disease. Any patient may have one or all of the stages.

Localized erythema migrans or early infection: stage 1. B. burgdorferi is injected by the tick into the host. The organism spreads in the skin in 60% to 80% of patients and produces erythema migrans. Systemic symptoms such as fever or regional adenopathy may accompany the skin disease. Organisms can be cultured from the skin or seen in a biopsy specimen. Specific antibody to the spirochete often is lacking. The erythema migrans lesions fade, even if the patient is untreated, and generally last 3 to 4 weeks. They may recur and have been reported for as long as 1 day to 14 months.

Disseminated infection or early infection: stage 2. The organism may be hematogeneously disseminated or spread through the lymph. It has been recovered from blood and visualized in tissues such as the retina, muscle, bone, synovium, myocardium, spleen, meninges, liver, and brain. The most common manifestations of disseminated infection include skin, CNS, or musculoskeletal involvement. In the skin annular skin lesions occur in approximately half of the patients and resemble the primary erythema migrans but are smaller and migrate less. Headache and mild stiffness of the neck are common but typically last only several hours. The CSF is normal. The musculoskeletal symptoms include migratory pain of joints, tendons, bone, or muscle, also lasting only a few hours or days. At this time the patient's mononuclear cells have demonstrable increased responsiveness to *B. burgdorferi* antigens. Specific IgM antigen response to a 41-kilodalton flagellar antigen reaches peak titers 3 to 6 weeks after infection. Polyclonal activation of cells may occur. IgG antibody develops, and the specific response to the antigens of the organism is primarily of the IgG1 and IgG3 subclasses. These antibodies are required for serum bactericidal activity by the classic complement pathway (Kochi and Johnson, 1988). Polymorphonuclear leukocytes and

monocytes phagocytize and kill the spirochete. There is some degree of vasculitis in multiple sites, and immune complexes are present in and around blood vessels.

The organism gains access to sites where it is sequestered and survives by unknown mechanisms. Approximately 15% to 20% of Lyme disease patients in the United States develop neurological involvement. The most common manifestation is meningitis with cranial or peripheral neuropathy superimposed. Radicular pain is characteristically described. The patients with meningitis may have lymphocytic pleocytosis, with approximately 100 cells, that is accompanied by an elevated protein level. The spirochete has been cultured from the CSF, and the intrathecal production of specific antibody has been demonstrated. It is also possible to demonstrate that mononuclear cells capable of responding to *B. burgdorferi* are present. T-cell clones from infected patients also may react with autoantigens.

Isolated facial palsy is the most common cranial nerve finding. Asymmetrical peripheral neuritis occurs and may involve motor and/or sensory components. Neurologically, axonal injury with perivascular infiltration of lymphocytes and plasma cells around epineural blood vessels can be seen. Axonal nerve involvement is suggested by electrophysiological studies. Neurological abnormalities last for weeks or months but may recur and/or become chronic.

Cardiac involvement occurs briefly in 4% to 8% of patients in the United States. Variable atrioventricular block is the most common manifestation, but some patients have myocarditis and/or pericarditis. Fortunately, heart blockage is rarely persistent.

From 2 weeks to 2 years after the onset of disease and most commonly at approximately 6 months, episodes of arthralgia or migratory musculoskeletal pain occur in as many as 60% of patients. This is usually oligoarticular arthritis that is asymmetrical and occurs primarily in the large joints. When joint fluid is examined in the presence of symptoms, WBC counts range from 500 to 110,000.

Persistent infection or late infection: stage 3. During the second or third years of illness, the episodes of arthritis become longer and may last for months. A biopsy reveals villous hypertrophy, fibrin deposition, and a mononuclear cell infiltrate. The expression of the human leukocyte antigen DR (HLA-DR) on many cell types has been noted, and spirochetes have been seen around blood vessels. Joint disability occurs, and in severe cases there may be erosion of cartilage and bone. Interleukin-1 is stimulated directly by *B. burgdorferi* and has been measured in joint fluid. This mediator may contribute to the synovial proliferation. The number of patients experiencing the chronic symptoms diminishes with each passing year, and it is unusual for a patient to experience more than several years of joint inflammation. Those patients with the most severe arthritis have HLA-DR2 or HLA-DR4 antigens (Steere et al., 1990). It is speculated that these genetically susceptible persons may have an autoimmune response triggered by this organism.

Recently, progressive encephalomyelitis has been reported in West Germany (Ackermann et al., 1988). Findings as diffuse as spastic paraparesis, bladder dysfunction, ataxia, and seventh or eighth cranial nerve deficits have been described. The intrathecal presence of antibody to *B. burgdorferi* was demonstrated. Those patients who have more subtle symptoms of CNS dysfunction without any classic symptoms of Lyme disease are diagnostic problems. The presence of CSF antibody to *B. burgdorferi* is unfortunately inconsistent.

Acrodermatitis chronica atrophicans has been described primarily in Europe. This skin lesion begins with blue-red discoloration and swollen skin, usually on an extremity. Ultimately, atrophy of the skin occurs. *B. burgdorferi* has been cultured from these lesions as long as 10 years after their onset. Pathologically, the rete ridges of the epidermis are lost, and there is a mononuclear cell infiltrate.

Congenital infection. Infants have been described who acquired *B. burgdorferi* transplacentally. Their mothers had Lyme disease during the first trimester of pregnancy. Spirochetes were visualized in fetal tissues, and both infants died—one with congenital cardiac malformation and one with encephalitis. The frequency and risk of congenital infection are unknown but are considered unusual.

Diagnosis. The direct visualization and the culture of *B. burgdorferi* are exceedingly difficult. Therefore diagnosis is made by the use of serological tests, which has been problematic. ELISA is in general use and is believed more sensitive than the immunofluorescent antibody tests. Most patients with Lyme disease will have elevated antibody titers to *B. burgdorferi* after several weeks of infection. Unfortunately, the serological testing is not yet standardized, and the results obtained from various laboratories differ significantly. Thus these serological values must be interpreted with caution, and the physician must be aware that there are false-positive and false-negative results.

As might be anticipated, false-negative antibody determinations occur primarily during the first weeks of infection. If it is possible to obtain an IgM ELISA assay, approximately 90% of patients will have demonstrable IgM antibodies to *B. burgdorferi*. False-positive IgM assays have been documented in healthy subjects and in patients with other illnesses, including syphilis and Rocky Mountain spotted fever. In the research laboratory, development of assays using specific proteins such as the 41-kilodalton flagellar antigen or outer surface proteins is being investigated. To complicate the diagnosis further, asymptomatic infection does occur; therefore the presence of antibodies in an individual who is having symptoms of an illness does not necessarily mean that the illness is Lyme disease.

Differential diagnosis. The spectrum of manifestations caused by this organism makes the differential diagnosis very large. The publicity attached to this infection has amplified the public awareness, and the infection may be overdiagnosed. The early symptoms of multiple sclerosis, amyotrophic lateral sclerosis, or Alzheimer's disease have not been described in association with *B. burgdorferi*. The acute skin rash is pathognomonic, but the later stages of disease may present problems in differential diagnosis.

Treatment. There is now agreement that *B. burgdorferi* is extremely sensitive to tetracycline and moderately sensitive to penicillin in vitro. Ampicillin, imipenem, and ceftriaxone are also antibiotics to which the organism is sensitive. Although the organism is sensitive to erythromycin in vitro, it is believed that it is not an effective therapy in vivo.

The recommended therapy for this infection may change as additional studies are done. The current recommendations include tetracycline therapy for early Lyme disease and for localized stage 1 or disseminated stage 2 infection. Doxycycline may be preferable because of the more sustained serum and tissue levels. Amoxicillin is the best alternative for children and is an acceptable alternative to doxycycline in adults. Clinical response determines the duration of therapy, which will fall between 10 and 30 days. Some patients may require repeat therapy with an oral or intravenous drug. Patients who are treated early in disease may lose specific antibodies in several months and may become reinfected.

Antibiotic therapy has been recommended for all patients with objective neurological abnormalities unless they have the isolated finding of a facial palsy without any CSF abnormalities. Ceftriaxone is recommended for treatment of the neurological abnormalities because it penetrates the blood-brain barrier better than penicillin. Doxycycline or chloramphenicol may be an acceptable alternative in the allergic patient.

Treatment of stage 3 disease does not result in rapid response. Failure apparently is similar with patients who receive oral doxycycline, amoxicillin and probenecid, or intravenous penicillin or ceftriaxone. Supplementary therapy with steroids may be indicated for patients with Lyme disease carditis if there is no response to antibiotic therapy.

REFERENCES

R. rickettsii

Abramson JS, Givner LB. Should tetracycline be contraindicated for therapy of presumed Rocky Mountain spotted fever in children less than 9 years of age? Pediatrics 1990;86:123-124.

Anacker RL, Lissh RH, Mann RE, et al. Antigenic heterogeneity in high and low virulence strains of Rickettsia rickettsii revealed by monoclonal antibodies. Infect Immun 1986;51:653.

Anacker RL, Philip RN, Casper E, et al. Biological properties of rabbit antibodies to a surface antigen of Rickettsia rickettsii. Infect Immun 1983;40:292.

Anderson BE, Tzianabosj I. Comparative sequence analysis of a genus common rickettsial antigen gene. J Bacteria 1989;171:5199.

Bradford WD, Croker BP, Tisher CC. Kidney lesions in Rocky Mountain spotted fever. Am J Pathol 1979;97:383.

Bradford WD, Hawkins HK. Rocky Mountain spotted fever in childhood. Am J Dis Child 1977;131:1228.

Clements ML, Dumler JS, Fiset P, et al. Serodiagnosis of Rocky Mountain spotted fever: comparison of IgM and IgG enzyme-linked immunosorbent assays and indirect fluorescent antibody test. J Infect Dis 1983;148:876.

D'Angelo LJ, Winkler WG, Bergman DJ. Rocky Mountain spotted fever in the United States, 1975-1977. J Infect Dis 1978;138:273.

DuPont HL, Hornick RB, Dawkins AT, et al. Rocky Mountain spotted fever: a comparative study of the active immunity induced by inactivated and viable pathogenic R. kettsii. J Infect Dis 1973;128:340.

Feng WC, Waner JL. Serological cross-reaction and cross-protection in Guinea pigs infected with Rickettsia rickettsii and Rickettsia montana. Infect Immun 1980;28:627.

Hattwick MAW, Retailliau H, O'Brien RJ, et al. Fatal Rocky Mountain spotted fever. JAMA 1978;240:1499.

Hayes SF, Burgdorfer W. Reactivation of Rickettsia rickettsii in Dermacentor andersoni ticks: an ultrastructural analysis. Infect Immun 1982;37:779.

Hechemy KE, Michaelson EE, Anacker RL, et al. Evaluation of latex Rickettsia rickettsii test for Rocky Mountain spotted fever in 11 laboratories. J Clin Microbiol 1983;18:938.

King WV. Experimental transmission of Rocky Mountain spotted fever by means of the tick. Public Health Rep 1986;21:863.

McDade JE, Newhouse VF. Natural history of Rickettsia rickettsii. Ann Rev Microbiol 1986;40:287.

McDonald GA, Anacker RL, Gargjian K. Cloned gene of Rickettsia rickettsii surface antigen: candidate vaccine for Rocky Mountain spotted fever. Science 1987;235:83.

Oster CN, Burke DS, Kenyon RH, et al. Laboratory-acquired Rocky Mountain spotted fever: the hazard of aerosol transmission. N Engl J Med 1977;297:859.

Philip RN, Casper EA, MacCormack JN, et al. A comparison of serologic methods for diagnosis of Rocky Mountain spotted fever. Am J Epidemiol 1977;105:56.

Silverman DJ. Rickettsia rickettsii-induced cellular injury of human vascular endothelium in vitro. Infect Immun 1984;44:545.

Silverman DJ, Bond SB. Infection of human vascular endothelial cells by Rickettsia rickettsii. J Infect Dis 1979;26:714.

Silverman DJ, Wisseman CL. In vitro studies of rickettsia-host cell interactions: ultrastructural changes induced by Rickettsia rickettsii infection of chicken embryo fibroblasts. Infect Immun 1984;149:201.

Silverman DJ, Wisseman CL Jr, Waddell AD, Jones M. External layers of Rickettsia prowazekii and Rickettsia rickettsii: occurrence of a slime layer. Infect Immun 1978;22:233.

Todd WJ, Burgdorfer W, Wray GP. Detection of fibrils associated with Rickettsia rickettsii. Infect Immun 1983;41:1252.

Walker DH, Firth WT, Edgell CJS. Human endothelial cell culture plaques induced by Rickettsia rickettsii. Infect Immun 1982;37:301.

Walker TS. Rickettsial interactions with human endothelial cells in vitro: adherence and entry. Infect Immun 1984;44:205.

Wells GM, Woodward TE, Fiset P, Hornick RB. Rocky Mountain spotted fever caused by blood transfusion. JAMA 1978;239:2763.

Wilfert CM, MacCormack JN, Kleeman K, et al. Epidemiology of Rocky Mountain spotted fever as determined by active surveillance. J Infect Dis 1984;150:469-479.

Woodward TE, Pedersen SE, Oster CN, et al. Prompt confirmation of Rocky Mountain spotted fever. Identification of rickettsiae in skin tissues. J Infect Dis 1976;134:297.

Spotted fever group

Burgdorfer A, Sexton DJ, Gerloff RK, et al. Rhipicephalus sanguineus: vector of a new spotted fever group rickettsia in the United States. Infect Immun 1975;12:205.

Hayes SF, Burgdorfer W. Ultrastructure of *Rickettsia rhipi-cephali*, a new member of the spotted fever group rickettsiae in tissues of the host vector Rhipicephalus sanguineus. J Bacteriol 1979;137:605.

Treadwell TL, Phillips SD, Jablonski WJ. Mediterranean spotted fever in children returning from France. Am J Dis Child 1990;144:1037-1038.

Uchida T, Yu X, Uchiyama T, Walker DH. Identification of a unique spotted fever group Rickettsia from human in Japan. J Infect Dis 1989;159:1122-1126.

Yagupsky P, Gross EM, Alkan M, Bearman JE. Comparison of two dosage schedules of Doxycycline in children with rickettsial spotted fever. J Infect Dis 1987;155:1215-1219.

Rickettsialpox

Brettman LR, Lewin S, Holzman RS, et al. Rickettsialpox: report of an outbreak and a contemporary review. Medicine 1981;60:363.

Dolgopol VB. Histologic changes in rickettsialpox. Am J Pathol 1948;24:119.

Greenberg M. Rickettsialpox in New York City. Am J Med 1948;4:866.

Huebner RJ, Jellison WL, Pomerantz C. Rickettsialpox—a newly recognized disease. IV. Isolation of a rickettsia apparently identical with the causative agent of rickettsialpox from Allodermanyssus sanguineus, a rodent mite. Public Health Rep 1946;61:1677.

Sussman LN. Kew Gardens' spotted fever. NY Med J 1946;2:27.

Wong B, Singer C, Armstrong D, Millian SJ. Rickettsialpox. Case report and epidemiologic review. JAMA 1979; 242:1998.

Typhus group

Berman SJ, Kundin WD. Scrub typhus in South Vietnam, a study of 87 cases. Ann Intern Med 1973;79:26.

Brown GW, Robinson DM, Huxsall DL, et al. Scrub typhus: a common cause of illness in indigenous populations. Trans R Soc Trop Med Hyg 1976;70:444.

Dasch GA, Samms JR, Weiss E. Biochemical characteristics of typhus group rickettsiae with special attention to the *Rickettsia prowazekii* strains isolated from flying squirrels. Infect Immun 1978;19:676.

Duma RJ, Sonenshine DE, Bozeman FM, et al. Epidemic typhus in the United States associated with flying squirrels. JAMA 1981;245:2318.

Ormsbee RA. Serologic diagnosis of epidemic typhus fever. Am J Epidemiol 1977;105:261.

Osterman JV, Eisemann CS. Surface proteins of typhus and spotted fever group rickettsiae. Infect Immun 1978; 21:866.

Samra Y, Shaked Y, Maier MK. Delayed neurologic display in murine typhus: report of two cases. Arch Intern Med 1989;149:949-951.

Silpapojakul K, Chupuppakarn S, Yuthasompob S, et al. Scrub and murine typhus in children with obscure fever in the tropics. Pediatr Infect Dis 1991;10:200-203.

Sonenshine DE, Bozeman M, Williams MS, et al. Epizo-otiology of epidemic typhus (R. prowazeki) in flying squirrels. Am J Trop Med Hyg 1978;27:339.

Traub R, Wisseman CL. The ecology of chigger-borne rickettsiosis (scrub typhus). J Med Entomol 1974;11:237.

Q fever

Amano KI, Williams JC. Sensitivity of *Coxiella burnetii* peptidoglycan to lysozyme hydrolysis and correlation of sacculus rigidity with peptidoglycan-associated proteins. J Bacteriol 1984;160:989.

Ascher MS, Berman MA, and Ruppanner R. Initial clinical and immunologic evaluation of a new phase I Q fever vaccine and skin test in humans. J Infect Dis 1983;148:214.

Baca OG, Paretsky D. Q fever and *Coxiella burnetii*: a model for host-parasite interactions. Microbiol Rev 1983;47:127.

Burnet FM, Freeman M. A comparative study of rickettsial strains from an infection of ticks in Montana (United States of America) and from Q fever. Med J Aust 1939;2:887.

Derrick EH. The course of infection with *Coxiella burnetii*. Med J Aust 1973;1:1051.

Field PR, Hunt JG, Murphy AM. Detection and persistence of specific IgM antibody to Coxiella burnetii by enzyme-linked immunosorbent assay: a comparison with immunofluorescence and complement fixation tests. J Infect Dis 1983;148:477.

Hart RJC. The epidemiology of Q fever. Postgrad Med J 1973;49:535.

Sawyer LA, Fishbein DB, McDade JE. Q fever: current concepts. 1987;9:935-946.

Williams JC, Peacock MG, McCaul TF. Immunological and biological characterization of *Coxiella burnetii*, phases I and II, separated from host components. Infect Immun 1981;32:840.

Babesiosis

Benach JL, Habicht GS, Hamburger MI. Immunoresponsiveness in acute babesiosis in humans. J Infect Dis 1982;146:369-380.

Esernio-Jenssen D, Scimeca PG, Benach JL, Tenenbaum MJ. Transplacental/perinatal babesiosis. J Pediatr 1987; 110:570-572.

Healy GR. Babesia infections in man. Hosp Pract 1979; June:107-116.

Steketee RW, Eckman MR, Burgess EC, et al. Babesiosis in Wisconsin: a new focus of disease transmission. JAMA 1985;253:2675-2678.

Sun T, Tenenbaum MJ, Greenspan J, et al. Morphologic and clinical observations in human infection with *Babesia microti*. J Infect Dis 1983;148:239-248.

Wolf RE, Gleason NN, Schoenbaum JC, et al. Intraerythrocytic parasitosis in humans with entopolypoides species (Family Babesiidae). Ann Intern Med 1978;88:769-773.

Ehrlichiosis

Barton LL, Dawson JE, Letson WG, et al. Simultaneous ehrlichiosis and lyme disease. Pediatr Infect Dis 1990;9:127-129.

Barton LL, Foy TM. Ehrlichia canis infection in a child. Pediatrics 1989;4:580-582.

Dawson JE, Fishbein DB, Eng TR, et al. Diagnosis of human ehrlichiosis with the indirect fluorescent antibody test: kinetics and specificity. J Infect Dis 1990;162:91-95.

Dawson JE, Rikihisa Y, Ewing SA, Fishbein DB. Serologic diagnosis of human ehrlichiosis using two *Ehrlichia canis* isolates. J Infect Dis 1991;163:564-567.

Edwards MS, Jones JE, Leass DL, et al. Childhood infection caused by *Ehrlichia canis* or a closely related organism. Pediatr Infect Dis 1988;7:651-654.

Eng TR, Harkess JR, Fishbein DB, et al. Epidemiologic, clinical, and laboratory findings of human ehrlichiosis in the United States. JAMA 1990;264:2251-2258.

Fishbein DB, Kemp A, Dawson JE, et al. Human ehrlichiosis: prospective active surveillance in febrile hospitalized patients. J Infect Dis 1989;160:803-809.

Fishbein DB, Sawyer LA, Holland CJ, et al. Unexplained febrile illnesses after exposure to ticks. JAMA 1987; 257:3100-3104.

Harkess JR, Ewing SA, Brumit T, Mettry CR. Ehrlichiosis in children. Pediatrics 1991;87:199-203.

Maeda K, Markowitz N, Hawley RC, et al. Human infection with *Ehrlichia canis*, a leukocytic rickettsia. N Engl J Med 1987;316:853-856.

McDade JE. Ehrlichiosis-A disease of animals and humans. J Infect Dis 1989;161:609-617.

Rohrback BW, Harkess JR, Ewing SA, et al. Epidemiology and clinical characteristics of persons with serologic evidence of *E. canis* infection. Am J Pub Health 1990;80:442.

Lyme disease

Ackermann R, Rehse-Kupper B, Gollmer E, Schmidt R. Chronic neurologic manifestations of erythema migrans, borreliosis. Ann NY Acad Sci 1988;539:16-23.

Asbrink E, Hobmark A. Early and late cutaneous manifestations of Ixodes born borreliosis (erythema migrans borreliosis, lyme borreliosis). Ann NY Acad Sci 1988; 539:4-15.

Benach JL, Bosler EM, Hanrahan JP, et al. Spirochetes isolated from the blood of two patients with lyme disease. N Engl J Med 1983;308:740-742.

Burgdorfer W, Barbour AG, Hayes SF, et al. Lyme disease/ a tick born spirochetosis? Science 1982;216:1317-1319.

Dattwyler RJ, Volkman DJ, Luft BJ, et al. Seronegative lyme disease: dissociation of specific T and B lymphocyte responses to *Borrelia burgdorferi*. N Engl J Med 1988;319:1441-1446.

Duray PH, Steere AC. Clinical and pathologic correlations of lyme disease by stage. Ann NY Acad Sci 1988; 539:65-79.

Eichenfield AH, Goldsmith DP, Benach JL, et al. Childhood lyme arthritis: experience in an endemic area. J Pediatr 1986;109:753-758.

Fikrig E, Barthold SW, Kantor FS, Flavell RA. Protection of mice against the lyme disease agent by immunizing with recombinant OspA. Science 1990;250:553-556.

Kochi SK, Johnson RC. Role of immunoglobulin G and killing of *Borrelia burgdorferi* by the classical complement pathway. Infect Immun 1988;56:314-321.

Lastavica CC, Wilson ML, Berardi VP, et al. Rapid emergence of a focal epidemic of lyme disease in coastal Massachusetts. N Engl J Med 1989;320:133-137.

Logigian EL, Kaplan RF, Steere AC. Chronic neurologic manifestations of lyme disease. N Engl J Med 1990;323:1438-1444.

Lyme disease—Connecticut. MMWR 1988;37:1-3.

Rosa PA, Schwan TG. A specific and sensitive assay for the lyme disease spirochete *Borrelia burdorferi* using the polymerase chain reaction. J Infect Dis 1989; 160:101829.

Steere C, Dwyer E, Winchester R. Association of chronic lyme arthritis with HLA-DR4 and HLA-DR2 Alleles. N Engl J Med 1990;323:219-223.

Steere AC, Malawista SE, Snydman DR, et al. Lyme arthritis: an epidemic of oligoarticular arthritis in children and adults in three Connecticut communities. Arthritis Rheum 1977;20:7-17.

Steere AC. Medical Progress-Lyme disease. N Engl J Med 1989;321:586-596.

Steere AC, Grodzicki RL, Kornblatt AN, et al. The spirochetal etiology of lyme disease. N Engl J Med 1983;308:733-740.

Szczepanski A, Benack JL. Lyme borreliosis: host responses to *Borrelia burgdorferi*. Microbiol Rev 1991;55:21-34.

Williams CL, Strobino B, Lee A, et al. Lyme disease in childhood: clinical and epidemiologic features of ninety cases. Pediatr Infect Dis 1990;9:10-14.

31

TOXOPLASMOSIS

RIMA McLEOD
JACQUELINE WISNER
KENNETH BOYER

Toxoplasmosis is disease caused by the ubiquitous, obligate intracellular protozoan *Toxoplasma gondii*. Infection is usually acquired orally or transplacentally, rarely by inoculation in a laboratory accident, by blood or leukocyte transfusion, or from a transplanted organ. Disease may also occur as the result of recrudescence of latent infection in immunocompromised individuals.

Clinical signs and symptoms depend in part on the host's immunological status. In the immunologically healthy older child the acute infection may be asymptomatic, cause self-limited lymphadenopathy with or without fatigue and malaise, or occasionally cause significant organ damage. In the child who is immunocompromised by acquired immunodeficiency syndrome (AIDS), organ transplantation, or cytotoxic therapy for malignancy or vasculitis, initial infection or recrudescence of latent infection may cause severe illness. The most common presentation in immunocompromised individuals is with neurological disease.

Congenitally acquired toxoplasmosis almost always causes morbidity and occasionally causes mortality. Most congenital infections are not recognized at birth but are manifested in later infancy, childhood, or adulthood. When infection is acquired by a mother early in gestation, transmission of the infection to her fetus occurs less frequently than when her infection is acquired later in gestation. When infection is transmitted, however, neurological and ophthalmological impairment is often severe. Involvement is less severe at birth in infants born to mothers who acquired the disease later in gestation. Nonetheless, although these infants usually appear normal in initial newborn examinations, 80% to 90% of them have ophthalmological lesions by adolescence. Because *T. gondii* is a major opportunistic pathogen for patients with AIDS, congenital transmission of human immunodeficiency virus (HIV) and *T. gondii* from such mothers is an emerging problem, often causing extensive, fulminant, disseminated toxoplasmosis in the newborn infant.

Toxoplasmosis not only causes substantial morbidity and mortality for affected individuals, but also major expenditures for health care. For example, in 1975 Wilson and Remington estimated that the average lifetime cost of special care for each child with congenital toxoplasmosis was $67,000. Since the estimated incidence of congenital toxoplasmosis is 1.1 per 1,000 births, an estimated 3,300 infants will be affected each year in the United States, resulting in a cost of $221,000,000 for lifetime care in 1975 dollars for infants born in just 1 year. Estimated productivity losses resulting from infection of children born in 1 year in the United States are $65 million to $1.6 billion, and estimated total preventable costs are $368 million to $8.7 billion dollars (Wilson and Remington, 1980; Roberts and Frenkel, 1990).

Congenital *Toxoplasma* infection in the fetus can be prevented by pregnant women if they avoid consumption of raw or undercooked meat and avoid accidental ingestion of material contaminated with cat feces. Serological testing and antimicrobial therapy are important for prevention and treatment. Antimicrobial therapy given to an acutely infected mother can block transmission to her fetus (Desmonts and Couvreur, 1979). Such therapy can also cure signs of infection caused by proliferating tachyzoites in congenitally infected fetuses (Daffos et al., 1988; Hohlfeld et al., 1989), infants (McLeod et al., in press), and immunocompromised individuals (McLeod et al., 1979). Vaccines to prevent oocyst shedding from cats (Frenkel et al., 1991) and vaccines that potentially could protect against initial infection or disease in humans (McLeod et al., 1988; Prince et al., 1989; Duquesne et al., 1990) are still experimental.

HISTORY

In 1908 Nicolle and Manceaux described tachyzoites in spleen and liver mononuclear cells from the North African rodent *Ctenodactylus gundi*. In 1923 *T. gondii* was implicated in human disease when Janku, an ophthalmologist in Prague, found cysts containing *T. gondii* in the retina of an 11-month-old child with congenital hydrocephalus. In 1937 Wolf and Cowen described an infant with granulomatous encephalitis. The protozoan parasite causing this infection was later identified by Sabin as *T. gondii*. In 1948 Sabin and Feldman developed the Sabin-Feldman dye test, which permitted serological testing and provided another means, in addition to histopathology, for detecting disease caused by *T. gondii*. In 1970 *T. gondii* was classified among the coccidia, and it was discovered that the domestic cat and other felines were the only hosts in which the sexual form develops. In the 1960s through the 1980s the full spectrum of clinical syndromes caused by *T. gondii* was defined, as were more rational approaches to antimicrobial therapy in different clinical settings.

Recent developments in immunology and molecular and cell biology and new developments in the care of pregnant women, children, and immunocompromised individuals have led to development of improved diagnostic tests and approaches to care for patients with toxoplasmosis. Recent studies also have further elucidated the pathogenesis of the infection, facilitated diagnostic testing, contributed to the development of effective antimicrobial agents, and

provided the groundwork for development of vaccines.

THE ORGANISM

T. gondii, a coccidian parasite, exists in a number of forms: tachyzoites (the rapidly proliferative form, formerly referred to as "trophozoites"); bradyzoites (which replicate more slowly than tachyzoites and exist within tissue cysts); and oocysts (which contain highly infectious sporozoites).

Tachyzoites

Tachyzoites (Fig. 31-1, *A*) are crescent or oval in shape and are approximately 2 to 4 μm wide and 4 to 8 μm long. They stain well with either Wright's or Giemsa stain. Tachyzoites can invade and multiply in all mammalian cells. Their reproduction is by endodyogeny, a process of internal budding in which two daughter cells are formed within the parent cell. Daughter cells are released when the host cell wall is disrupted or lysed. Tachyzoites are fastidious and do not survive freezing, thawing, desiccation, or exposure to normal gastric secretions.

Bradyzoites

Bradyzoites (Fig. 31-1, *B*) in tissue cysts are crescent-shaped organisms that appear similar to tachyzoites but replicate more slowly. They have unique epitopes that are not expressed by tachyzoites or sporozoites. Tissue cysts vary in size and contain a few to approximately 10,000 bradyzoites. Tissue cysts can be stained with periodic acid–Schiff (PAS) stain. Primary human infection can also occur by ingestion of bradyzoites within cysts in raw or undercooked meat. After ingestion, the cyst wall is disrupted by pepsin or trypsin. The liberated bradyzoites can remain viable for up to 2 hours in pepsin–hydrogen chloride or as long as 6 hours in trypsin. Bradyzoites then invade the digestive tract mucosa and can disseminate throughout the body. Tissue cysts have been found in virtually every organ but appear to have greatest predilection for the retina, brain, heart, and skeletal muscle. Cysts remain viable throughout the life of the host. These tissue cysts can be a source of local or disseminated infection if the host becomes immunocompromised. Freezing to −20° C (−4° F), heating to 60° C (140° F), desiccation, and irradiation destroy viability of encysted bradyzoites.

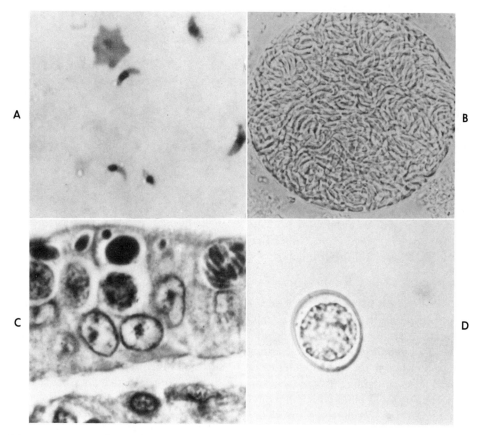

Fig. 31-1. Forms of *Toxoplasma gondii*. **A,** Tachyzoite. **B,** Bradyzoite in tissue cyst. **C,** Gametocytes in cat ileum. **D,** Unsporulated oocyst. (Adapted from Dubey JP, Beattie CP. Toxoplasmosis of animals and man. Boca Raton, Fla.: CRC Press, Inc., 1988, and Gardiner CH, Fayer R, Dubey JP. An atlas of protozoan parasites in animal tissues. Washington, D.C.: U.S. Department of Agriculture, Agriculture Handbook No. 651, 1988.)

Oocysts and sporozoites

Oocysts (Fig. 31-1, *C*) are oval in shape and are approximately 10 to 12 μm in diameter. They complete the life cycle of *T. gondii* within the intestine of its definitive host, cats. They are found in the cat intestine only during primary infection or, rarely, in a chronically infected cat that acquires another coccidian parasite, *Isospora*. Oocysts can remain infectious in warm, moist soil for 1 year or more and easily resist the gastric acid barrier after ingestion. They can be killed by exposure to nearly boiling water for 5 minutes, by burning, or by contact with strong ammonia (7%) for 3 hours. Oocysts sporulate 1 to 5 days after excretion, and the sporozoites become highly infectious if they are ingested.

Life cycle

There are two life cycles for *T. gondii*. The complete cycle, with schizogony (an asexual cy-cle) and gametogony (sporulating sexual cycle), which results in the formation of infectious oocysts, occurs only in members of the cat family. In all other animals only an incomplete cycle by schizogony occurs, forming tachyzoites or bradyzoites in tissue cysts. *Toxoplasma* are acquired by susceptible cats when they eat meat (e.g., mice) that contains tissue cysts or ingest oocysts excreted by other recently infected cats (Fig. 31-2). *T. gondii* then multiplies through both schizogonic and gametogonic cycles in the tips of villi in the cat's distal ileum. The time of the first appearance of oocysts in cat feces depends on the form of *Toxoplasma* ingested: 3 to 5 days after ingestion of tissue cysts; 7 to 10 days after ingestion of tachyzoites; and 20 to 24 days after the ingestion of oocysts. For a brief 1- to 3-week period, an acutely infected cat can excrete 10^7 to 10^9 oocysts per day.

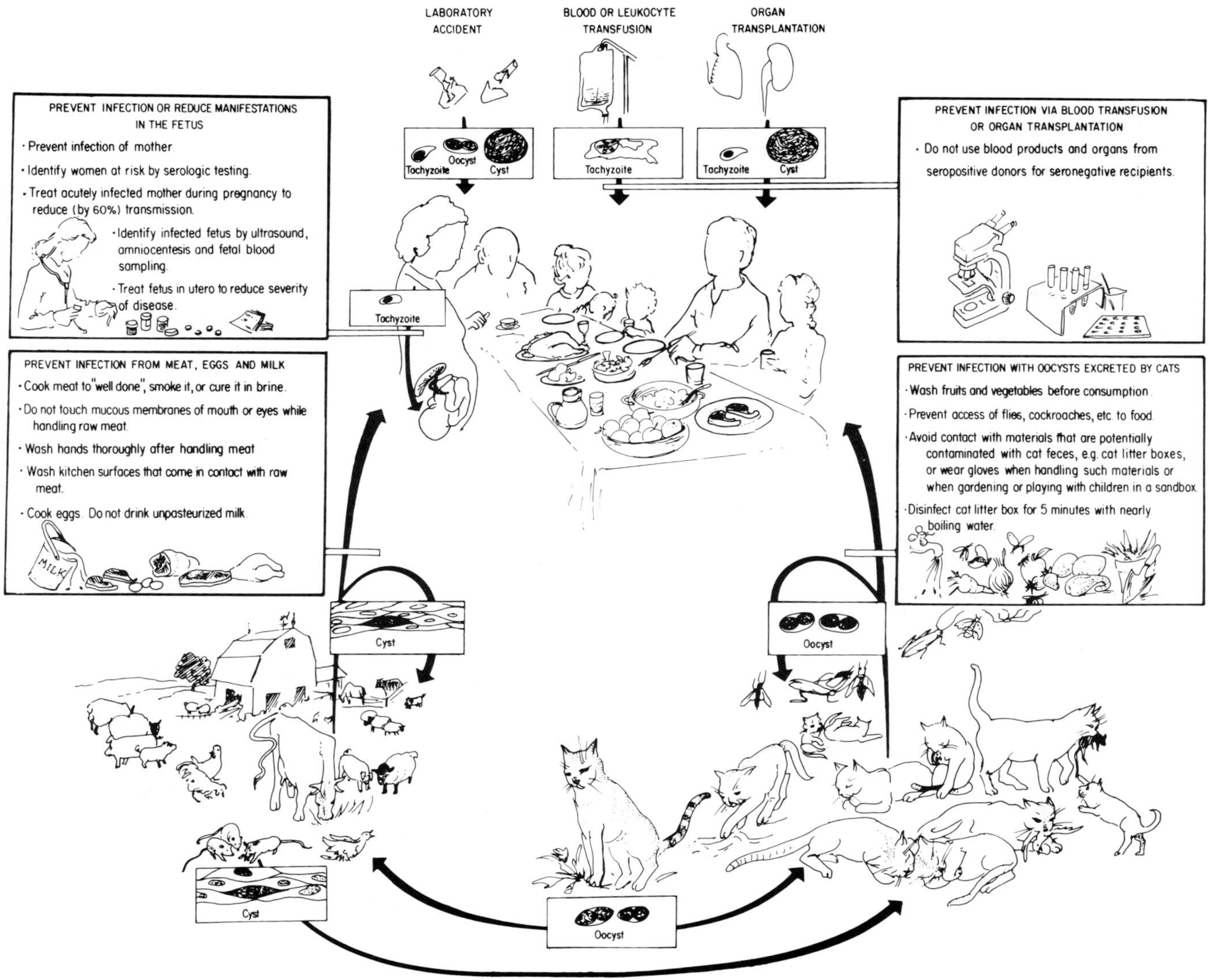

Fig. 31-2. Life cycle of *T. gondii* and prevention of acquisition by humans. Infection of older children and adults occurs primarily after ingestion of cysts in undercooked meat or oocysts excreted by cats or by the fetus transplacentally from an acutely infected mother. After ingestion, organisms invade the intestinal epithelium, either hematogenously or through lymphatics, are spread to other tissues, and when there is a normal immune response, they form cysts. Rarely, infection is acquired by blood or leukocyte transfusion, in a transplanted organ, or via a laboratory accident. (Adapted from McLeod and Remington. In Behrman RL, Vaughan VC III, Nelson WE [eds]. Nelson's textbook of pediatrics, ed 14. Philadelphia, WB Saunders, 1990.)

EPIDEMIOLOGY

The prevalence of *Toxoplasma* infection in cats and in tissue cysts in meat used for human consumption varies widely, depending in part on locale (Remington and Desmonts, 1990). In early studies in the United States 50% of domestic cats were seropositive. In a study in Costa Rica where the overall antibody prevalence in people was 60%, over 20% of 237 cats were shedding oocysts when examined, and 60% overall were infected as shown by either oocyst shedding or *T. gondii*–specific antibody (Ruiz and Frenkel, 1980). *T. gondii* has been isolated from the skeletal muscle of 23% of market and 42% of breeder pigs in the United States. The prevalence in Czechoslovakia ranged from 43% to 73%. Sheep used for human consumption had a prevalence rate of 4% to 22% in California. Cattle apparently are infected less commonly than sheep or pigs in the United States, Europe, and New Zealand. The combined prevalence rates range from 1% to 33%.

The prevalence of infection in humans is also highly variable, depending in part on locale and age. Highest rates of seropositivity occur in El Salvador, Tahiti, and France, where the prevalence of seropositivity is greater than 90% by the fourth decade of life. In the United Kingdom and in the United States approximately 10% of the population has IgG antibody at 10 years of age, 20% at 20 years, and 50% at 70 years. The prevalence of infection lessens in colder regions, in hot and arid climates, and at high elevations. There is no significant difference in prevalence between men and women.

There have been clusters of cases of toxoplasmosis and/or *T. gondii* infection caused by common exposures in a riding stable or to water, associated with eating similarly prepared meat, and in families. Data in experimental animals demonstrate significant immunogenetic differences in the manifestations of infection in mice (Brown and McLeod, 1990).

Congenital toxoplasmosis occurs when the mother acquires the infection for the first time during pregnancy. The risk of infection in an obstetrical population depends on two factors: (1) the incidence of primary infection in the population as a whole and (2) the proportion of women of childbearing age who have not been previously infected.

In the relatively few studies of prevalence of *Toxoplasma* antibodies in pregnant women,

Table 31-1. Inverse relationship between incidence of fetal infection and severity of fetal damage following acutely acquired maternal infection with *T. gondii* at different stages of gestation

Trimester of pregnancy	Fetuses infected (%)	Severity of illness
1	17	Most severe
2	25	Intermediate severity
3	65	Least severe or subclinical

Data from Remington JS, Desmonts G. In Remington JS, Klein JO (eds). Infectious diseases of the fetus and newborn infant, ed 3. Philadelphia: WB Saunders, 1990.

there is geographical variation. In the United States 39% of 23,000 pregnant women in the Collaborative Perinatal Project had *T. gondii*–specific serum antibody. Other studies indicate a varying incidence of seropositivity in women of childbearing age in the United States: Denver, 3%; Palo Alto, California, 10%; Chicago, 12%; Boston, 14%; and Birmingham, Alabama, 30% (Remington and Desmonts, 1990). Seroprevalence studies of women of childbearing age from other nations or cities outside the United States also demonstrate variability in rates of seropositivity: Thailand, 3%; Australia, 4%; Japan, 6%; Scotland, 13%; London, 20%; Poland, 36%; Belgium, 53%; and Paris, 73%. Published estimates for the incidence of congenital toxoplasmosis range from 0.1 to 10 per 1,000 live births. Approximations per 1,000 births for individual cities are as follows: Birmingham, Alabama, 0.12; London, 0.07 to 0.25; Glasgow, Scotland, 0.46 to 0.93; Basel, Switzerland, 1; Brussels, 2; Melbourne, 2; and Vienna, 6 to 7. Sera from 330,000 newborns in Massachusetts and New Hampshire were tested using the double-sandwich (DS) IgM enzyme-linked immunosorbent assay (ELISA) of Remington and Naot, and the incidence of seropositivity using this test was 1 per 10,000 live births.

Acute maternal infection is transmitted to the fetus in approximately 40% of cases. Incidence and severity of congenital infection depend in part on the time of acquisition of infection during pregnancy (Table 31-1). By the last weeks of gestation, the incidence of transmission to the fetus approaches 100%. The severity of manifestations of infection at birth decreases the later in gestation the infection is acquired. Approximately half of the infected infants detected in serological screening programs who were initially believed normal based on routine newborn evaluations had one or more signs of infection apparent with more complete evaluations. Almost all infected infants will have some evidence of infection (e.g., chorioretinitis) by adolescence if untreated or treated for only 1 month.

PATHOGENESIS

After acquisition by the older child or adult (usually through the gastrointestinal tract), organisms invade cells directly or are phagocytosed by leukocytes. Within these cells, organisms multiply, cause cell lysis, and are spread throughout the body hematogenously or through the lymphatics. Organisms can infect every mammalian cell. Proliferation of tachyzoites results in rupture of infected cells and eventually in areas of localized tissue necrosis surrounded by infiltrates of inflammatory cells. The eventual outcome of acute infection depends on the host's immune response. Cysts form in immunocompetent hosts in whom both cellular and humoral immunity is intact. Cyst formation can be demonstrated as early as the seventh day after infection. Cysts can persist in many organs and tissues after immunity is acquired; thus *T. gondii* remains in tissues for the life of the host.

In immunodeficient individuals and in some apparently immunologically normal individuals the acute infection is not contained by an effective immune response; it may cause marked destruction of the host's tissues, leading to, for example, pneumonitis, myocarditis, or necrotizing encephalitis. Encysted organisms may also cause recrudescent disease in previously immunocompetent patients. Such previously latent infection is the major source of disease caused by *T. gondii* in patients with AIDS, in transplant recipients, or in older children who develop new or recrudescent chorioretinitis as a sequela of congenital *T. gondii* infection.

When a mother acquires *T. gondii*, tachyzoites are hematogenously spread to the placenta. The organism then can be transmitted transplacentally directly to the fetus during gestation or at birth. Overall, in approximately 60% of cases, maternal acute infection does not result in fetal infection. However, as stated previously, almost all infected infants will have manifesta-

tions of infection (e.g., chorioretinitis) by adolescence if they are untreated. It has been suggested that the differences in rates of transmission during gestation depend on placental blood flow, virulence of the *T. gondii* strain, possibly genetic susceptibility of the patient, and the number of organisms hematogenously spread to the placenta. As in other congenital infections, the greater severity of toxoplasmic infection acquired early in gestation relates to the sensitivity of early fetal organs to damage by intracellular parasites, the placental barrier separating the fetus from the mother's humoral and cell-mediated immune responses, and the fetus' intrinsic immunological immaturity. The most profoundly affected babies frequently exhibit specific immunological tolerance in the perinatal period (McLeod et al., 1990).

PATHOLOGY

Information about pathological changes observed in toxoplasmosis in humans is largely derived from lymph node biopsies, from autopsy data described in fatal congenital infections, or from immunodeficient individuals. Limited information is available on the pathological changes in immunocompetent individuals since acute infection is usually asymptomatic or self-limited in such persons.

Tachyzoites and tissue cysts are only rarely observed in conventionally stained sections. Tachyzoites may be observed with Wright's or Giemsa stain but are best demonstrated with the immunoperoxidase technique. Tissue cysts stain well with PAS stain, silver impregnation stains, and immunoperoxidase techniques.

Lymph nodes

In acute acquired lymphadenopathic toxoplasmosis (Fig. 31-3) there is a characteristic triad of (1) reactive follicular hyperplasia, with (2) irregular clusters of epithelioid histiocytes, and (3) monocytoid cells that distend the subcapsular and trabecular lymph node sinuses (Dorfman and Remington, 1973). Tachyzoites and tissue cysts are only very rarely demonstrable in affected nodes.

Eye

Single and multiple foci of tissue necrosis in the retina and choroid are the earliest manifestations of *Toxoplasma* involvement of the eye. Secondary changes such as vitritis, iridocyclitis,

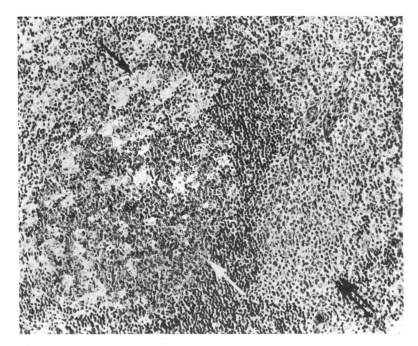

Fig. 31-3. Lymph node biopsy showing characteristic lymph node pathology in lymphadenitis caused by *Toxoplasma*. Epithelioid cells *(black arrow)* encroach upon and blur margins of germinal center *(white arrow)*. There is focal distension of subcapsular and trabecular sinuses by "monocytoid" cells *(double black arrows)*. Irregular clusters of epithelioid cells are scattered throughout paracortical lymphoid stroma. (Adapted from Dorfman RF, Remington JS: N Engl J Med 1973; 289-878.)

and cataracts are complications of the chorioretinitis. Organisms first lodge in the capillaries of the inner layer of the retina, invade the endothelium, and extend to adjacent tissues. An intense local inflammatory reaction develops, with edema, infiltration of polymorphonuclear neutrophils (PMNs), lymphocytes, plasma cells, mononuclear cells, and occasionally eosinophils. Both intracellular and extracellular tachyzoites and tissue cysts may be seen. Eventually, scarring of the choroid develops.

Central nervous system

Along with involvement of the eye, congenital toxoplasmosis most often involves the central nervous system (CNS). In the CNS there may be acute or focal diffuse meningoencephalitis, with cellular necrosis, microglial nodules, and perivascular mononuclear inflammation. In patients with congenital infection vascular thrombosis produces extensive areas of necrosis, often several centimeters in diameter. The basal ganglia are often heavily involved, and scattered cortical lesions are often seen as well. Large

areas of necrosis in congenital toxoplasmosis may lead to sloughing of periventricular tissue, which causes obstruction of the aqueduct of Sylvius or foramen of Monro and subsequent hydrocephalus. The protein count of such ventricular fluid is high (grams per deciliter) and contains large amounts of *Toxoplasma* antigen. Eventually, necrotic brain tissue may calcify, giving rise to the typical findings in conventional radiographs and computed tomographic (CT) scans.

In cases of acute CNS infection acquired postnatally or with immunocompromise, there is focal or diffuse meningoencephalitis with necrosis and microglial nodules. In immunocompromised patients such as infants and children with both congenital toxoplasmosis and AIDS, the major finding is necrotizing encephalitis in both acute and recrudescent disease.

Other sites

Rarely, *Toxoplasma* gives rise to interstitial pneumonitis. The myocardium is a frequent site for necrosis, inflammation, and encysted organisms. Acute and chronic pericarditis have also been described. Infection of kidney (and antigen-antibody complex glomerulonephritis), spleen, liver, adrenals, pancreas, stomach, intestine, thyroid, thymus, testes, ovaries, and skin also have been described (reviewed in Remington and Desmonts, 1990).

CLINICAL MANIFESTATIONS
Acute acquired toxoplasmosis in apparently immunologically normal older children and adults

Infection acquired after birth is generally asymptomatic in 80% to 90% of immunologically normal persons, including pregnant women. Those with clinically apparent disease generally have lymphadenopathy with or without a "mononucleosis-like" illness. Rarely, severe systemic disease or specific organ involvement (e.g., encephalitis or chorioretinitis) occurs.

Lymphadenopathy is the most commonly recognized clinical manifestation of acute, acquired toxoplasmosis (McCabe, et al, 1984). Lymphadenitis can be generalized, but in approximately two thirds of patients only one area is affected. Cervical lymph nodes are the most frequently involved. However, axillary, inguinal, retroperitoneal, and mesenteric lymph nodes may also be involved. Lymph nodes generally measure 0.5 to 3.0 cm and can be tender or nontender. They are often firm, discrete, smooth, and mobile, but they do not suppurate or ulcerate. Although self-limited, lymphadenopathy can persist or recur for up to 1 year. Retroperitoneal or mesenteric node involvement with fever may mimic appendicitis. Toxoplasmic lymphadenopathy often raises concern about lymphoma or other malignancy. Appropriate serological testing can differentiate this condition and avert the need for lymph node biopsy.

Occasionally, lymphadenopathy is accompanied by a constellation of symptoms suggestive of infectious mononucleosis, or these symptoms may occur alone. This infection also has a self-limited course; however, fatigue and lymphadenopathy may persist for months to a year. It usually ends with complete recovery.

Significant systemic disease can occur. Onset may be insidious, with weakness and malaise that persist for 6 to 10 days, followed by fever, rash, and symptoms of pneumonia or hepatitis. Temperature may be as high as 41° C (105.8° F). Abdominal pain may be present. A maculopapular, generalized rash may occur. It appears similar to that of Rocky Mountain spotted fever except that the palms of the hands and the soles of the feet are spared. These skin lesions are bright red to pale pink and may blanch with pressure. Signs of pneumonia may appear simultaneously with the rash or later. Roentgenographic examination of the chest may show irregular areas of increased density in the lower lobes or only accentuation of the hilar or lower lobe markings.

Systemic toxoplasmosis in immunologically normal individuals has also been manifested as hepatitis, polymyositis, pericarditis with effusion, myocarditis, or meningoencephalitis. Toxoplasmic meningoencephalitis has been characterized by headache, vomiting, seizures, focal neurological signs, and/or transitory confusion (Townsend et al., 1975). Temperature was not always elevated at the onset. Lymphadenopathy and splenomegaly were present in some cases. Cerebrospinal fluid (CSF) had increased numbers of white blood cells (WBCs), particularly mononuclear cells. Protein and glucose concentrations were normal or simulated bacterial meningitis. The patient's condition may steadily deteriorate, ending in death or survival with residual brain damage manifested by seizures or focal neurological deficits. Complete recovery without residua has also been described.

Infection in the immunocompromised individual

Immunocompromised patients such as those with AIDS, malignancy, autoimmune disease and its therapy, and solid organ or bone marrow transplants are at risk for severe toxoplasmosis. In most cases toxoplasmosis is the result of reactivation of latent rather than of primary infection.

Approximately 50% of patients with AIDS who are chronically infected with *T. gondii* will develop toxoplasmosis. Why the other 50% of such patients do not reactivate their infections is unknown. Pediatric AIDS and congenital *T. gondii* infections have been reported in the same infants. Such dual infections, including encephalitis and involvement of other organs (e.g., heart and lungs), usually have been fulminant and rapidly fatal. *T. gondii* infection has most often been diagnosed at postmortem examination. This infection is emerging as a particular problem in populations in whom the prevalence

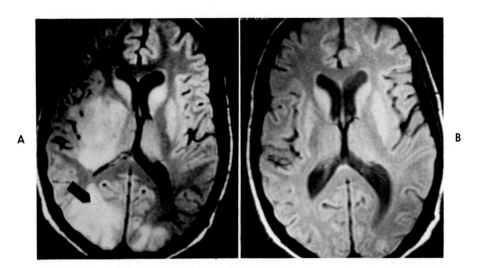

Fig. 31-4. MRI of the brain of a patient with AIDS and toxoplasmic encephalitis before (**A**) and after (**B**) antimicrobial therapy. Note that large areas of necrosis and inflammation in **A** *(arrow)* have resolved in **B**.

of both *T. gondii* and HIV infections is relatively high.

Typical signs and symptoms of toxoplasmic encephalitis in adult AIDS patients include headache, fever, and focal neurological deficits. Less commonly, meningitis, spinal cord involvement, or signs that reflect involvement of other organs are present. CNS lesions occur throughout the brain, with predilection for involvement of the basal ganglia and corticomedullary junction. Diffuse encephalitis diagnosed only at autopsy also has been reported (LePort, 1991), but most often there are focal lesions that enhance with contrast on brain CT scan or brain magnetic resonance imaging (MRI) scans. MRI scans almost always show multiple lesions (Fig. 31-4).

In a recent series of adult AIDS patients with toxoplasmosis (Leport, 1991), the most frequent clinical localization was in the brain, with focal abscesses (83%) and diffuse encephalitis (in the 17% with a normal CT scan). Fever occurred in 60% to 70%, 40% to 50% had headaches, 35% to 40% were confused, and 40% to 80% had focal neurological signs. Specific IgG antibodies are detectable in most (>95%) adult patients with AIDS and toxoplasmosis. Of affected patients with toxoplasmic chorioretinitis 65% had concomitant cerebral localization. With appropriate treatment, there is usually an initial improvement within a few weeks and complete resolution of lesions seen on brain CT scan in 1 to 6

months. Delayed or absent response to this treatment is an indication for brain biopsy. Rupture of thrombosed vessels (secondary to intimal and perivascular inflammatory cell infiltrates) has occurred. At autopsy, 40% to 70% of patients with AIDS and toxoplasmosis have involvement of the heart and lung, and involvement of pancreas, stomach, and intestine is remarkable.

In older immunocompromised children toxoplasmosis generally occurs as a result of reactivation of latent infection. However, *T. gondii* may actually be transmitted through organ transplantation and leukocyte transfusion (see Fig. 31-2). Symptomatic toxoplasmosis has occurred when *T. gondii*–infected hearts or kidneys have been transplanted into seronegative recipients. The diagnosis of reactivated or primary toxoplasmosis in recipients of bone marrow transplants may be particularly difficult because *T. gondii*–specific antibody may be absent or may not increase in titer. Increase in antibody titer without overt disease has occurred when *T. gondii*–infected hearts have been transplanted into seropositive recipients.

Congenital toxoplasmosis

Clinical manifestations. Approximately 40% of untreated women who acquire the infection during pregnancy transmit *Toxoplasma* to their fetus. In an otherwise healthy woman transmission to the fetus occurs only in the setting of

Table 31-2. Numbers and percentages of 300 patients with congenital toxoplasmosis with various clinical manifestations at presentation

Clinical manifestations	Age when first diagnosed								
	1-5 mo	6-11 mo	12-23 mo	2-3 yr	4-7 yr	8-14 yr	15-29 yr	30 yr	Total
Neurological disorders	42 (58)*	26 (81)	24 (57)	20 (42)	14 (42)	21 (54)	7 (29)	1	155 (52)
Hydrocephalus or microcephalus	40 (55)	12 (38)	14 (33)	6 (13)	—	4 (10)	1 (4)	1	78 (26)
Ocular disorders	52 (71)	27 (84)	32 (76)	26 (54)	31 (94)	35 (90)	24 (100)	1	228 (76)
Intracranial calcification	28 (38)	12 (38)	17 (40)	14 (29)	11 (33)	10 (26)	4 (17)	2	98 (33)
Jaundice	20 (27)	1 (32)	—	—	—	—	—	—	21
Hepatospleno-megaly	13 (18)	—	—	—	—	—	—	—	13
TOTALS	73	32	42	48	33	39	24	2	300

Modified from Couvreur J, Desmonts G. Dev Med Child Neurol 1962, 4:519-530.
*Figure outside parentheses, number; figure inside parentheses, percentage of patients diagnosed at that age with this manifestation.

primary (not recrudescent) infection. Only 10% to 40% of women giving birth to congenitally infected infants recall any signs or symptoms of acute infection. Rarely, cases of congenital transmission have been reported in women chronically infected with *T. gondii* and immunosuppressed from corticosteroid treatment or AIDS.

Manifestations of congenital infection are protean and vary from a mild or asymptomatic infection to a generalized infection dominated by signs of irreversible CNS damage. Disease may be seen initially in the neonatal period, in the first months of life, or at later ages—up to adulthood. Newborns and young infants are usually detected based on systemic, neurological, or ophthalmological signs (Table 31-2). Older children are seen with ophthalmological and, less frequently, neurological disease. Couvreur et al. (1984) reported data that indicate the spectrum and frequency of signs and symptoms noted in newborn infants born to mothers whose infections had been diagnosed in a systematic serological screening program. Only 10% had substantial CNS, ocular, or systemic involvement; 34% had normal clinical examinations with the exception of retinal scars or isolated calcifications; and 55% had no abnormalities detected. These French prospective data likely underestimate the true proportion of severe infection because the most severe cases were not referred, therapeutic abortion often eliminated the most severely involved fetuses, and gesta-

tional spiramycin therapy may have reduced the severity of infection. Between 33% and 50% of the infants initially thought to have subclinical infection had signs of infection (most commonly, abnormal CSF) with more detailed evaluation. At face value, however, these data imply that 90% of the infants with congenital toxoplasmosis would have been missed with a routine newborn physical examination.

In infants with generalized or primarily neurological disease and with no or brief treatment, substantial long-term morbidity can be expected (Table 31-3). For example, of infants with neurological disease who were reevaluated at 4 years of age (Eichenwald, 1960), 89% had IQs less than 70, 83% had convulsions, 76% had spasticity and palsies, 69% had severely impaired vision, 20% were deaf, and only 9% were normal. Only 16% of the children who initially presented with generalized disease were normal at follow-up. In a study by Wilson et al. (1980) the outcome for infants who had "subclinical" infection at birth and who were evaluated when they were 9 to 10 years old also revealed substantial sequelae (Table 31-4). Sixteen percent were mentally retarded, 17% had seizures, 27% had unilateral blindness and 20% had bilateral blindness, 25% had hearing impairment, and 86% had sequentially lower IQ scores when tested at 5-year intervals. With 1 year of treatment, outcome apparently is substantially better for most (but not all) such infants (McLeod et al., 1991).

Table 31-3. Signs and symptoms occurring before diagnosis or during the course of untreated acute congenital toxoplasmosis in 152 infants and 101 of these same children when they had been followed 4 years or more

	Frequency of occurrence (%) in patients with	
	*Neurological disease**	*Generalized disease†*
Signs and symptoms	*108 Patients*	*44 Patients*
Infants		
Chorioretinitis	102 (94)‡	29 (66)
Abnormal spinal fluid	59 (55)	37 (84)
Anemia	55 (51)	34 (77)
Jaundice	31 (29)	35 (80)
Splenomegaly	23 (21)	40 (90)
Convulsions	54 (50)	8 (18)
Fever	27 (25)	34 (77)
Intracranial calcification	54 (50)	2 (4)
Hepatomegaly	18 (17)	34 (77)
Lymphadenopathy	18 (17)	30 (68)
Vomiting	17 (16)	21 (48)
Hydrocephalus	30 (28)	0 (0)
Diarrhea	7 (6)	11 (25)
Pneumonitis	0 (0)	18 (41)
Microcephalus	14 (13)	0 (0)
Eosinophilia	6 (4)	8 (18)
Rash	1 (1)	11 (25)
Abnormal bleeding	3 (3)	8 (18)
Hypothermia	2 (2)	9 (20)
Cataracts	5 (5)	0 (0)
Glaucoma	2 (2)	0 (0)
Optic atrophy	2 (2)	0 (0)
Microphthalmia	2 (2)	0 (0)
	70 Patients	*31 Patients*
Children 4 years (or more) old		
Mental retardation	62 (89)	25 (81)
Convulsions	58 (83)	24 (77)
Spasticity and palsies	53 (76)	18 (58)
Severely impaired vision	48 (69)	13 (42)
Hydrocephalus or microcephalus	31 (44)	2 (6)
Deafness	12 (17)	3 (10)
Normal	6 (9)	5 (16)

Modified from Eichenwald H. In Siim JC (ed). Human toxoplasmosis. Copenhagen: Munksgaard, 1960, pp 41-49. Study was performed in 1947. The most severely involved institutionalized patients were not included in the later study of 101 children.

*Patients with central nervous system disease in the first year of life.

†Patients with nonneurological diseases during the first 2 months of life.

‡Figure outside parentheses, number; figure inside parentheses, percentage.

Table 31-4. Development of adverse sequelae in children born with subclinical congenital toxoplasma infection

	Group 1* (n = 13)	Group 2† (n = 11)
Ophthalmological finding		
No sequelae	2	0
Chorioretinitis		
Bilateral		
Bilateral blindness	0	5
Unilateral blindness	3	3
Moderate unilateral visual loss	0	1
Minimal or no visual loss	5	1
Unilateral		
Minimal or no visual loss	3	0
Mean age at onset (yr)	3.67	0.42
Range	0.08-9.33	0.25-1.00
Recurrences of active chorioretinitis	3	2
Neurological finding‡		
No sequelae	8	3
Major sequelae		
Hydrocephalus	0	1
Microcephaly	1	1
Seizures	1	3
Severe psychomotor retardation	1	2
Minor sequelae		
Mild cerebellar dysfunction	2	4
Transiently delayed psychomotor development	2	2
Other abnormality		
Sensorineural hearing loss		
Moderate unilateral	1 of 10	1 of 9
Mild unilateral	1 of 10	0 of 9
Mild bilateral	1 of 10	1 of 9
Precocious puberty	2	0
Premature thelarche	0	1
Miscellaneous	3	1

Modified from Wilson et al. Pediatrics 1980;66:767-774.

*No abnormalities found on an extensive newborn evaluation based on awareness of a diagnosis of congenital toxoplasmosis.

†No abnormalities found on a routine newborn physical examination.

‡Eighty-six percent of eight children who were tested had sequentially lower intelligence quotient scores.

Reported cutaneous manifestations in congenitally infected infants have included thrombocytopenia (e.g., petechiae, hemorrhage, ecchymoses) and rashes (fine punctate; diffuse maculopapular; lenticular deep blue-red; sharply defined and diffuse blue papules). The entire body, including palms and soles, has been involved with macular rashes. Jaundice, cyanosis, and edema secondary to hepatic, pulmonary, myocardial, and renal involvement have been reported.

General and systemic findings have included prematurity, low Apgar scores, intrauterine growth retardation, instability of temperature regulation with hypothermia, lymphadenopathy, hepatosplenomegaly, signs of myocarditis, pneumonitis, nephrotic syndrome, vomiting, diarrhea, and feeding problems. Endocrine abnormalities have also been reported and include hypothyroidism, diabetes insipidus, sexual precocity, and partial anterior hypopituitarism.

Neurological abnormalities have ranged from subtle findings to severe encephalitis. Hydrocephalus may be the only clinical manifestation of congenital toxoplasmosis and may be compensated or may require shunt placement. It may be seen in the perinatal period, later in infancy, or, rarely, up to adulthood. A variety of different seizure patterns may occur in the perinatal period and later in life. Central focal motor deficits have been noted as have signs of spinal or bulbar involvement. Microcephaly in untreated infants is generally associated with diminished cognitive functioning. Mild and severe sensorineural hearing loss has been reported in approximately 20% of children with no or brief treatment, but it was not found in a recent study of treated infants and children (McGhee et al., 1992).

CSF is abnormal in at least one third of congenitally infected infants. Abnormalities include CSF lymphocytic pleocytosis, hypoglycorrhachia, and elevated protein level. Remarkable elevations of CSF protein levels (with values of grams per deciliter when there is aqueductal obstruction and ventricular dilation) are characteristic of this congenital infection. Local production of *T. gondii*–specific antibodies may be present in CSF. Brain CT scan with contrast can determine ventricular size, detect calcifications, and define active inflammatory lesions and porencephalic cystic structures. Skull radiographs and ultrasonography are less sensitive than CT scan for detection of calcifications, but ultrasonography may be useful for following ventricular size. Brain MRI and radionuclide scans may be useful to detect active inflammation.

Case summaries that provide examples of infants with subclinical infection, generalized systemic, neurological, and ophthalmological disease, and severe neurological and ophthalmological disease follow:

CASE 1: PATIENT WITH SUBCLINICAL DISEASE. The patient's family lived in a rural area, and two stray cats lived nearby. Although they had no known contact with these cats or with feces from the cats, the family did have a sandbox where the pregnant mother played in the sand with her older children. The mother also prepared a large number of hamburgers for a picnic 2 to 3 weeks before delivery of her son, but she did not recall sampling raw hamburger or eating raw or undercooked meat during her infant's gestation. She had no history of consuming raw milk or raw eggs.

The mother's pregnancy, labor, and delivery were uncomplicated. Her infant was born appropriate for gestational age (AGA) with Apgar scores of 9 and 9 and a birth weight of 3.9 kg, and he had no medical problems in the perinatal period. On the day after delivery, the patient's mother noted that she had an enlarged posterior auricular lymph node. She had no other symptoms or signs and an otherwise normal physical examination, which included a retinal examination. The affected lymph node was excised, and microscopic studies of it revealed epithelioid histiocytes and monocytoid cells characteristic of toxoplasmic lymphadenopathy (similar to those shown in Fig. 31-3). Serological tests for the mother and the child were obtained: the infant's serum Sabin-Feldman dye test titer was 1:8000, his serum IgM ELISA level was 11, the IgM ISAGA level was 12, and the IgA ELISA level was 11 (see p. 548 for definitions of terms). His mother's serum Sabin-Feldman dye test titer was 1:1024 (300 IU), her IgM ELISA level was 11, and her AC/HS was 1600/>3200.

Results of general ophthalmological and neurological examinations, auditory brain stem response testing, and head CT scan with and without contrast were normal. CSF at 5 weeks of age had 30 WBCs/mm³, with 3% PMNs, 91% lymphocytes, 3% monocytes, a protein level of 68 mg/dl, and a glucose level of 39 mg/dl.

The patient is being treated with pyrimethamine, sulfadiazine, and leucovorin for 1 year and has had no clinical manifestations (other than slightly elevated

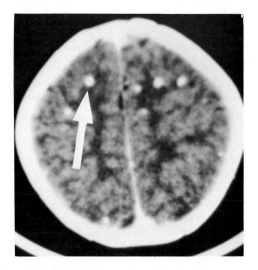

Fig. 31-5. Brain CT scan of an infant with congenital toxoplasmosis that demonstrates calcifications. This infant and other treated infants have developed normally in spite of calcifications *(arrow)* and even microcephaly.

CSF protein levels) of his third-trimester congenital infection.

CASE 2: PATIENT WITH GENERALIZED SYSTEMIC, NEUROLOGICAL, AND OPHTHALMOLOGICAL DISEASE. This boy was the product of a first pregnancy and unremarkable gestation. During pregnancy his mother occasionally sampled raw hamburger, gardened, and had a pet cat but did not change the litter box.

An emergency cesarean section was performed after 30 hours of labor because of fetal distress (decreased fetal heart rate). The infant's Apgar scores were 2 at 1 minute and 3 at 5 minutes, leading to intubation and mechanical ventilation for his first 24 hours of life. During those 24 hours he had one episode that was considered to be a seizure, and administration of phenobarbital was begun. His birth weight was 3,450 g (50th percentile); length, 19 inches (50th percentile); and head circumference, 36 cm (50th percentile). His platelet count on the first day of life was 44,000/mm³; thus a platelet transfusion was given and the platelet count subsequently returned to normal. Because of his asphyxial episode, a head CT scan was performed and revealed multiple discrete intracranial calcifications. Because of the presence of calcifications (similar to those in Fig. 31-5), the diagnosis of toxoplasmosis was suspected. An ophthalmological examination revealed bilateral chorioretinitis, which was more prominent on the right side than on the left and involved the right macula.

Hepatosplenomegaly was present, but the infant was considered normal otherwise. An examination of his CSF revealed 30 WBCs/mm³, with a predominance of lymphocytes, a protein level of 215 mg/dl, and a glucose level of 86 mg/dl. Serological test results included a serum dye test titer of 1:1024, an IgM ELISA level of 2.0, and an IgA ELISA level of 2.5. The mother's serum on the same dates had a dye test titer of 1:8000, DS IgM ELISA level of 0.2, IgA ELISA level of 0.2, and AC/HS of 400/3200. The infant was given pyrimethamine, sulfonamides, and leucovorin. His hepatosplenomegaly resolved. He is now 2 years old and has developed completely normally, with strabismus related to his macular scar as his only overt abnormality.

CASE 3: PATIENT WITH SEVERE NEURO-LOGICAL AND OPHTHALMOLOGICAL DIS-EASE.

This boy's mother was a 21-year-old woman of Laotian descent with known hepatitis B surface antigenemia. She had minimal exposure to cats during the third trimester (i.e., she had visited in a house in which cats were present). She did not own a cat, nor did she clean a litterpan or get scratched or bitten. She had no gardening or sandbox exposure. On one occasion she ate rare meat during the third trimester; however, she usually consumed well-cooked meat. She denied consumption of raw milk or raw eggs. In the eighth week of gestation a 1-week illness occurred, with swelling of her neck and face and with fever, lymphadenopathy, and night sweats. She was hospitalized, treated with antibiotics for presumed facial cellulitis, and had complete resolution of her symptoms. She also had intermittent headaches throughout her pregnancy. During the twenty-eighth week of gestation, at her request, a fetal ultrasound was performed that demonstrated a fetus with hydrocephalus. From that time on, she routinely underwent ultrasonography every 2 weeks until the thirty-fifth week of gestation.

A male infant was delivered at 35 weeks' gestation (34 weeks by Dubowitz) by cesarean section because of increasing ventriculomegaly. The infant's birth weight was 2,325 g (70%); head circumference, 34.5 cm (>90%); and length, 18 inches (70%). Apgar scores were 4 and 9 at 1 and 5 minutes of age, respectively. Hydrocephalus was prominent at birth as demonstrated by CT (similar to that in Fig. 31-6). The patient underwent ventriculoperitoneal shunting at 5 days of age, with resolution of increased intracranial pressure and appearance of thicker cortical mantle. Testing of ventricular fluid revealed 870 red blood cells, 43 WBCs, protein level of 1,155 mg/dl, and glucose level of 26 mg/dl. His serum Sabin-Feldman dye test titer was 1:4096, and DS IgM ELISA level was 4. His IgA ELISA level was 3. His mother's serum Sabin-Feld-

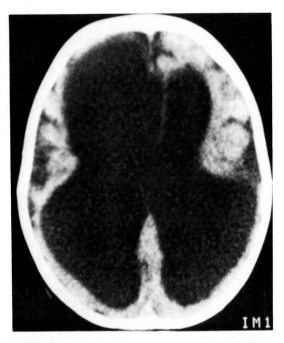

Fig. 31-6. Brain CT scan of an infant with congenital toxoplasmosis and hydrocephalus. Some (but not all) such treated infants with hydrocephalus from congenital toxoplasmosis have developed normally (with normal motor and cognitive function following prompt placement of ventriculoperitoneal shunts and with antimicrobial therapy). Poorer prognosis has been associated with delays in shunt placement or revisions or intercurrent complications such as prolonged hypoxia and/or hypoglycemia.

man dye test titer was 1:2048, IgM ELISA level was 4, IgA ELISA level was 12, and AC/HS was 800/3200.

Other complications noted during the infant's initial hospitalization included transient anemia, thrombocytopenia, transient hyperbilirubinemia, elevation of liver transaminases, and diabetes insipidus. His examination also documented severe chorioretinitis, microophthalmia, hepatosplenomegaly, an umbilical hernia, and a hydrocele with micropenis. Administration of pyrimethamine, sulfadiazine, and folinic acid was begun at 18 days of age. At 24 days of age prednisone was added and eventually tapered. He was started on vasopressin therapy.

A repeat CT scan showed worsening hydrocephalus. Four months later, another repeat CT scan was performed and showed increased cerebral atrophy without clear indication of increased intracranial pressure. The infant is blind and has substantial development delay.

Ophthalmological disease

Clinical manifestations. In the United States and in Western Europe, *T. gondii* is the most common cause of chorioretinitis, estimated to cause approximately 35% of cases. Toxoplasmic chorioretinitis is most frequently observed as an initial manifestation of or with reactivation of congenital infection. Almost all untreated congenitally infected individuals will develop chorioretinal lesions (Koppe et al., 1986). Chorioretinitis is estimated to occur in 1% of immunologically normal individuals with acute acquired toxoplasmosis.

Infants with active congenital ocular toxoplasmosis may have microophthalmia, impaired vision, cataracts, chorioretinal scars, chorioretinitis, iritis, leukocoria, anisometropia, nystagmus, optic atrophy, microcornea, or strabismus. Older children may complain of blurred vision, photophobia, epiphora, loss of central vision, or "floaters." Recurrent symptoms occur at irregular intervals. Data from Couvreur et al. (1984)

suggest that the appearance of recurrent or new retinal lesions during the first years of life may be prevented by therapy in alternate months with pyrimethamine and sulfadiazine and spiramycin. Longer follow-up is needed for definitive conclusions about whether such therapy reduces symptomatic, progressive ophthalmological disease.

During an ophthalmoscopic examination acute focal retinitis is seen as a fluffy white-yellow lesion with surrounding retinal edema and hyperemia (Fig. 31-7, *A*). Overlying vitritis may obscure the retina. Active lesions often are adjacent to old inactive lesions. Inactive lesions characteristically are atrophic, white to gray plaques, with distinct borders and choroidal black pigment (Fig. 31-7, *B*). The lesions may be single or multiple, large, small, unilateral, or bilateral. They are often found at the posterior pole of the retina but also occur in the periphery. Papillitis (most often unilateral), optic atrophy, retinal detachment, and cortical blindness have

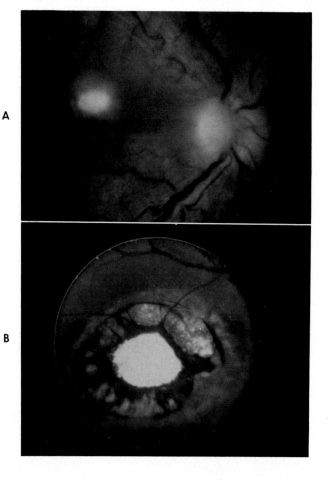

A

B

Fig. 31-7. Toxoplasmic chorioretinitis with acute lesion (**A**) and inactive macular scar (**B**). In **A**, there is focal necrotizing retinitis with cotton-like patch in the fundus. Acute lesions (**A**) appear soft and white, have indistinct borders and may have associated vitritis. Older lesions (**B**) are whitish gray and sharply demarcated and often have areas with choroidal pigment. (Adapted from McLeod R, Remington JS. In Behrman RL, Vaughan VC III, Nelson WE [eds]. Nelson's textbook of pediatrics, ed 14. Philadelphia: WB Saunders, 1990, and Remington JS, Desmonts G. In Remington JS, Klein JO [eds]: Infectious diseases of the fetus and newborn infant, ed 3. Philadelphia: WB Saunders, 1990.)

also been observed. Other ophthalmological findings include cells in the anterior chamber, neovascular formation on the iris' surface, sometimes with increased intraocular pressure, and glaucoma. The following case illustrates some of these findings.

CASE 4: PATIENT WITH TOXOPLASMIC CHORIORETINITIS. Her mother gardened and sampled uncooked hamburger during this child's gestation. The perinatal history was unremarkable except for the birth weight of 5 pounds, 9 ounces at a gestational age of 37 weeks. She had no medical problems identified in the newborn period and did not require hospitalization or treatment for any serious medical illness. Before entering nursery school when she was 4 years old, she had a routine ophthalmological examination, which revealed decreased vision in her right eye and bilateral macular scars. Her visual acuity was 20/125 OD and 20/25 OS. There were cells in the anterior vitreous of the right eye and a few cells in the anterior vitreous of the left eye. The right vitreous had 1 to 2+ haze caused by the cells. In the right eye there was a one-disc diameter foveal scar with a hyperpigmented center surrounded by a deeply pigmented area. A small, one-eighth disc-diameter area of active retinitis was present between the disc and the macular scar. The left fundus had a trace of vitreous haze with macular scarring. The child's serum *Toxoplasma* IgG indirect fluorescent antibody (IFA) titer was 1:4096, and her *Toxoplasma* IgM IFA titer was 0. The mother's serum contained *Toxoplasma*-specific IgG antibody. The child's active ocular toxoplasmosis was treated with prednisone, pyrimethamine, triple sulfonamides, and clindamycin. Signs of active retinal disease and vitritis resolved, and therapy was discontinued.

Three years later, her visual acuity was 20/50 OD and 20/30 OS. She had normal discs and vessels in both eyes, with bilateral macular scarring (similar to Fig. 31-7, *B*).

Holland et al. (1988) described eight patients with presumed toxoplasmic retinochoroiditis and AIDS. Their retinal lesions were frequently bilateral and multifocal. Hemorrhage was minimal, but prominent inflammatory reactions in the vitreous and anterior chamber were common. Preexisting retinal scars were rare. Occasionally, tachyzoites were visualized in inner retinal layers in pathological specimens.

DIAGNOSIS

Multiple serological tests may be needed to establish the diagnosis of acutely acquired or congenital *Toxoplasma* infection. Each laboratory must establish test values that are diagnostic of infection in particular clinical settings and must provide interpretation of the test results and appropriate quality control. If therapy is based on serological test results, these results should be confirmed in a reference laboratory (e.g., Palo Alto Research Institute, Palo Alto, California, 415-326-8120). Diagnosis may also be established by microscopic demonstration of tachyzoites in smears prepared from body fluids (e.g., CSF) or tissue sections (e.g., brain biopsy) or by actual isolation of the organism from tissues such as placenta, fetal blood, amniotic fluid, or body fluids that are inoculated into tissue culture or mice. Characteristic histopathology may also be noted in a lymph node biopsy.

Isolation

T. gondii can be isolated by inoculation of specimens (from body fluids, leukocytes, fetal blood clots, bone marrow, or homogenates of placenta) into the peritoneum of seronegative mice or into tissue culture. Ideally, material should be processed immediately, although *T. gondii* has been isolated from tissues and blood stored at 4° C overnight. Freezing or treatment of specimens with formalin kills the organism. Six to 10 days later, or earlier if the mice die, the peritoneal fluid of inoculated mice is examined microscopically for tachyzoites. If mice survive 4 to 6 weeks, their sera are then tested for IgG *Toxoplasma* antibody. If their sera contain specific antibody, definitive diagnosis is made by visualization of tissue cysts in the mouse brain. If no cysts are found, homogenates of mouse brain, liver, and spleen are subinoculated into other mice, and the process is repeated.

Tissue cultures (e.g., of fibroblasts) have also been used to isolate *T. gondii*. This apparently is a more convenient but less sensitive method than inoculation into mice. Tissue cultures are inoculated with clinical samples; and if the result is positive, plaques generally form as early as 4 days after inoculation. Cultures are stained with Wright's or Giemsa stain and examined for plaques that contain necrotic cells and replicating tachyzoites. Isolation of *T. gondii* from placenta, blood, or body fluids (e.g., CSF or amniotic fluid) is diagnostic for both acute and congenital toxoplasmosis. In contrast, in suspected cases of reactivated disease, isolation of *T. gondii* from tissue homogenates may only reflect the presence of tissue cysts in a chronic, latent infection.

Histology

Tissue sections, smears from brain biopsy, bone marrow aspirates, or cytocentrifuge specimens of body fluids that demonstrate free or intracellular tachyzoites confirm the diagnosis of acute infection. Because tachyzoites are often difficult to see in ordinary stains, immunofluorescent antibody and immunoperoxidase techniques may be useful (Conley et al., 1981). The finding of tissue cysts is diagnostic of infection with *Toxoplasma* but does not differentiate between acute and chronic infection. Tissue cysts in the placenta or any tissue samples from a newborn do, however, indicate congenital transmission. Toxoplasmic lymphadenitis has characteristic histological features (see "Pathology"), but tachyzoites are generally not demonstrable.

Serological testing

Clinical use of serological tests and representative results in specific clinical settings. Serological tests to detect *T. gondii*–specific IgG, IgM, or IgA antibodies include the Sabin-Feldman dye test, IFA tests, agglutination tests, and ELISAs. DNA probe methods (e.g., the polymerase chain reaction) have been described recently and appear promising for prenatal diagnosis of congenital infection by amniocentesis. Tables 31-5 and 31-6 list specific tests that may be useful in particular clinical settings. Representative serological test results from various clinical forms of infection are also listed in Table 31-6.

IgG antibodies. The following serological tests detect IgG antibodies to *T. gondii*: Sabin-Feldman dye test, IFA, IgG ELISA, direct agglutination, and complement fixation. The Sabin-Feldman dye test and the IgG IFA test measure the same antibodies, and titers are usually of approximately the same magnitude. The Sabin-Feldman dye test is both sensitive and specific. It is generally viewed as the "gold standard" for detection of *T. gondii*–specific IgG. In this test live tachyzoites incubated with serum that contains antibodies to *Toxoplasma* and an exogenous source of complement will change in shape and no longer take up the vital stain, alkaline methylene blue dye, indicating cell death. The dye test titer is the serum dilution at which half of the tachyzoites are killed. The IgG IFA test measures *Toxoplasma*-specific IgG antibodies, using formalin-fixed tachyzoites, the patient's serum, and antibody to human IgG that is fluorescein conjugated. In both the IgG IFA test and the dye test, antibodies usually appear 1 to 2 weeks after infection and reach high titers (>1:1000) after 6 to 8 weeks. Low titers of such IgG antibody usually persist for life.

Results that demonstrate *Toxoplasma*-specific IgG using IgG ELISA also correlate well with results of the Sabin-Feldman dye and IgG IFA tests. The complement-fixation test, however, detects IgG antibody that is generated less rapidly than antibody detected by the dye test, IgG IFA test, or IgG ELISA. Antibody detected with the complement-fixation test appears in the serum 3 to 8 weeks after infection, rises over the next 2 to 8 months, and then declines to low levels within a year. This test is not useful for detection of acute infection because of high false-negative rates.

Agglutination tests to detect IgG antibody are available commercially in Europe. Formalin-preserved whole parasites are used to detect IgG. Interference of nonspecific IgM antibodies is a problem that can be eliminated with the use of 2-mercaptoethanol. This test is accurate, simple, and relatively inexpensive.

IgM antibodies. Tests to detect IgM antibodies to *Toxoplasma* include the IgM IFA, double-sandwich enzyme-linked immunosorbent technique (DS IgM ELISA), and IgM ISAGA (an agglutination test). Since IgM antibodies usually appear within the first weeks of infection and disappear more rapidly than IgG antibodies, they are used to detect acute infection. IgM does not cross the placenta, so IgM antibodies detected in fetal or neonatal blood samples represent synthesis by an infected fetus or infant. IgM antibodies often are not present in sera of immunodeficient patients with active infection or in normal or immunodeficient patients during recrudescence in the eye. Specific IgM can be detected in sera of approximately 75% of newborns with congenital toxoplasmosis (when sera are tested using the DS IgM ELISA).

Although the IgM IFA is useful for the diagnosis of acute infection with *T. gondii* in the

Table 31-5. Approach to serological diagnosis of toxoplasmosis

Patient and specimen	T. gondii–specific IgG*				T. gondii–specific IgM†				T. gondii–specific IgA	Other tests		
	Dye test	IFA	IgG ELISA	Direct agglutination	DS-IgM ELISA	ISAGA	ELISA for IgM to P30	IFA	IgA ELISA	PCR	Isolation	AC/HS
Newborn congenital toxoplasmosis												
Serum	C	C	C	C	C	C	C Do not use	C	R		C	C
Cerebrospinal fluid (CSF)	C				C					R	C	
Peripheral blood clot or peripheral blood cells (WBC)											C	
Placenta										R	C	
Pregnant woman												
Maternal serum	C	C	C	C	C	C	C	C				
Amniotic fluid									C	R	C	C
Fetal serum					C	C			R		C	
Fetal WBCs/clot										R	C	
Immunologically normal child												
Serum	C	C	C	C	C	C	C	C				C
CSF	C	C	C		C							
Immunologically deficient child												
Serum	C	C	C	C	C‡	C‡	C‡	C‡		R	C	
CSF	C	C	C	C	C‡	C‡	C‡	C‡		R	C	

IFA, indirect fluorescent antibody; ELISA, enzyme-linked immunosorbent assay; ISAGA, immunosorbent test for IgM; PCR, polymerase chain reaction; AC/HS, differential agglutination test; C, commercially available; R, research test at present in reference laboratories.

*When properly standardized, any one of these tests is useful for demonstration of IgG antibody.

†ISAGA is usually most sensitive; IFA is least sensitive (do not use for congenital infection).

‡Rarely positive.

Table 31-6. Guidelines for interpretation of serological tests for toxoplasmosis

Test	Positive titer	Titer in acute infection	Titer in chronic infection	Duration of elevation of titer
IgG				
Sabin-Feldman dye test	Undiluted	1:4 to ≥1:1000 (usual)	1:4 to 1:2000	Years
Direct agglutination test	≥1:20	Rises slowly from negative to low titer to high titer (1:512)	Stable (≥1:1000) or slowly decreasing titer	≥1 yr
Indirect fluorescent IgG antibody (IgG IFA)	≥1:10	≥1:1000	1:8 to 1:2000	Years
Indirect hemagglutination test (IHA)	≥1:16	≥1:1000	1:16 to 1:256	Years
Complement fixation (CF)	≥1:4	Varies among laboratories	Negative to 1:8	Years
IgM				
Indirect fluorescent IgM antibody (IgM IFA)	≥1:2, infants ≥1:10, adults	≥1:80	Negative to 1:20	Weeks to months, occasionally years
Double-sandwich IgM ELISA	≥0.2, newborn infant, fetus ≥1.7, older children, adults	≥6	Negative to 1.7 (older children, adults)	Can be >1 yr
Immunosorbent test for IgM (ISAGA)	≥8, adult 1-7, indeterminate	≥8	Negative to 1	Unknown, can be ≥1 yr
IgA				
IgA, enzyme-linked immunosorbent assay (ELISA)	≥1.0 infants ≥1.3 adults	>1.0, infants >1.3, adults	Negative to <1.0 Negative to <1.3	Weeks to months, occasionally longer
Polymerase chain reaction	Positive	Positive	Negative	Only when *Toxoplasma* DNA present

Modified from McLeod R, Remington JS. Toxoplasmosis. In Braunwald E, et al. (eds). Harrison's principles of internal medicine, ed 11. New York: McGraw-Hill, 1987, pp 791-797.

*Values are those of one reference laboratory; each laboratory must provide its own standards and interpretation of results in each clinical setting.

older child and adult, it is relatively insensitive and therefore not reliable in detection of infection in infants. It detects only 25% of congenital *Toxoplasma* infections. Moreover, sera containing antinuclear antibodies or rheumatoid factor may yield false-positive reactions in the IgM IFA test.

The DS IgM ELISA is more specific and sensitive for detecting anti-*Toxoplasma* IgM antibodies than the IgM IFA (Naot and Remington, 1980). It is useful for detection of both congenital toxoplasmosis in the infant and acute toxoplasmosis in the older child. Values indicative of infection must be determined by each labora-

Table 31-7. Interpretation of the AC/HS test

HS result (IU/ml)	AC result (IU/ml)							
	<50	50	100	200	400	800	1600	>1600
<100	NA	NA	A	A	A	A	A	A
100	NA	NA	A	A	A	A	A	A
200	NA	NA	A	A	A	A	A	A
400	NA	NA	A	A	A	A	A	A
800	NA	NA	NA	A	A	A	A	A
1600	NA	NA	NA	NA	A	A	A	A
3200	NA	NA	NA	NA	NA	A	A	A
>3200	NA	NA	NA	NA	NA	NA	A	A

Modified from Thulliez P, Remington JS. J Clin Microbiol 1990;28(9):1928-1933.
NA, not acute; A, acute.

tory. In one reference laboratory, levels of 1.7 (ELISA units) or greater usually indicate recently acquired infection in an older child or adult, although presence of specific serum IgM antibody can persist for up to 2 years. In that laboratory a value in serum of greater than 0.2 suggests congenital infection in a fetus or neonate. The DS IgM ELISA detects 75% of infants with congenital *Toxoplasma* infection compared to detection of 25% of such infants using the IgM IFA. If a fluorescent antibody (FAB) is used, the DS IgM ELISA avoids false-positive test results caused by rheumatoid factor or antinuclear antibody.

The IgM ISAGA combines trapping of the patient's IgM to a solid surface and the use of formalin-fixed organisms or antigen-coated latex particles. It apparently is more sensitive than the DS IgM ELISA and, in the same manner, avoids false-positive results from rheumatoid factor or antinuclear antibodies.

IgA and IgE antibodies and AC/HS. Other tests to detect antibody to *T. gondii* include the IgA ELISA, the enzyme-linked immunofiltration assay (for IgA and IgE), and a differential agglutination test, AC/HS (Dannemann et al., 1990). The IgA ELISA apparently is even more sensitive than the IgM ELISA for detection of congenital infection (Decoster et al., 1988; Stepick-Biek et al., 1990). Both *T. gondii*–specific IgM and IgA antibodies demonstrated in ELISA or ISAGA may remain elevated for prolonged times (i.e., many months to years in older children and adults) but more commonly are present

only a short time. The AC/HS (Dannemann et al., 1990) is useful in differentiating recent from remote acquisition of infection in older children and adults (Table 31-7). In this test greater agglutination of acetone-fixed tachyzoites (relative to agglutination of formalin-fixed tachyzoites) is detected in patients with acute infection. This test may be particularly helpful in differentiating recent from remote infection in a pregnant woman.

Local antibody production. The amount of *T. gondii*–specific antibody produced locally in CSF or aqueous humor has also been used to establish the presence of *T. gondii* infection. An organism-specific antibody index (OSAI), previously called "antibody coefficient (C)" or "*Toxoplasma*-specific index," is calculated as follows:

$$OSAI = \frac{\text{Reciprocal titer in body fluid} \div \text{Concentration of IgG in body fluid}}{\text{Reciprocal titer in serum} \div \text{Concentration of IgG in serum}}$$

An OSAI greater than or equal to 8 (in aqueous humor for ophthalmological infection), greater than or equal to 4 (in CSF for congenital infection), or greater than or equal to 1 (in CSF for AIDS patients) indicates local antibody production. If the serum dye test titer is greater than or equal to 1,000, it is usually not possible to demonstrate local antibody production. IgM may also be present in CSF.

Antibody load. In patients with congenital

toxoplasmosis serum *T. gondii*–specific IgG antibody present at birth usually reflects the level of passively transferred maternal IgG antibody. Synthesis of specific antibody by the infected infant often can be detected by serial measurement of the ratio of *T. gondii*–specific IgG to total IgG and comparison to the expected linear decline in this ratio in an uninfected infant (Remington and Desmonts, 1990). However, antimicrobial therapy may delay detection of the baby's specific antibody synthesis by this means.

Polymerase chain reaction (PCR). This technique is promising for detection of *Toxoplasma* DNA in amniotic fluid and could potentially be useful for its detection in CSF or peripheral blood. PCR is used to amplify *T. gondii* DNA, which then is identified by hybridization with a labeled probe. In a recent study by Grover et al. (1990), amniotic fluid samples of 43 documented cases of acute maternal *Toxoplasma* infections were studied using PCR. PCR correctly identified 8 of 10 samples of amniotic fluid from four cases of congenital infection when other methods performed on fetal samples gave the following results: serum IgM ISAGA, 3 of 10; amniotic fluid inoculation into tissue culture, 4 of 10; amniotic fluid inoculation into mice, 7 of 10.

Diagnosis in utero

Fetal blood sampling (percutaneous umbilical blood sampling [PUBS]), in combination with amniocentesis and fetal ultrasound, has been very useful in the diagnosis and treatment of congenital toxoplasmosis (Daffos et al., 1988; Hohlfeld et al., 1989). These procedures should be performed only by physicians with considerable technical experience with the procedures and with the processing and interpretation of the data acquired. An example of the use of these techniques and of the need for experience and skill in interpretation of these results follows.

CASE 5. A 19-year-old woman had headaches, malaise, fatigue, and cervical lymphadenopathy 1 month before conception. She did not seek medical care, and her symptoms resolved over a 2-week period. She had cats and kittens that roamed outdoors, but she did not handle their litterbox. She denied ingesting any raw or rare meat. On her first prenatal visit at 12 weeks' gestation by dates, serological test

results were as follows: Sabin-Feldman dye test 1: 2048; IgA ELISA, 10; IgM ELISA, 6; and AC/HS, greater than 1600/1600. Results from a fetal ultrasound at 14 weeks' gestation were normal. Spiramycin (3 g/day orally) was begun.

A PUBS at 20 weeks' gestation revealed the following: Beta human chorionic gonadotropin (HCG) levels, indicative of fetal blood sample. *T. gondii*–specific IgM was 0 (by ISAGA). A clot from 4 ml of fetal blood and a cell pellet from 19 ml of amniotic fluid were inoculated into mice. Subinoculation studies were all negative.

Spiramycin therapy was continued until delivery. Fetal ultrasound examinations were repeated every 2 weeks and were normal. The patient tolerated spiramycin therapy without any ill effects. She delivered a normal, uninfected infant, who was evaluated as described in the box.

Evaluation of the infant at birth

Diagnostic tests (in addition to *T. gondii*–specific serological tests, attempts to isolate the organism, and histological tests) that may be useful in evaluation of fetuses and infants with congenital toxoplasmosis are listed in the box.

THERAPY

Pyrimethamine plus sulfadiazine or trisulfapyrimidines (triple sulfa) act synergistically against *T. gondii*. These antimicrobial agents (plus leucovorin) currently comprise the standard treatment for toxoplasmosis. In addition, spiramycin has been used extensively in France to prevent in utero transmission of infection to fetuses of acutely infected women (Desmonts and Couvreur, 1974) and has been included in treatment regimens for congenital toxoplasmosis after birth (Remington and Desmonts, 1990). Clindamycin has been used in conjunction with pyrimethamine to treat toxoplasmosis in AIDS patients who have been unable to tolerate therapy with sulfadiazine. New antimicrobial agents that apparently are effective against encysted bradyzoites are promising.

Pyrimethamine

Pyrimethamine (Daraprim) inhibits dihydrofolate reductase. The plasma half-life is 90 hours in adults and 60 hours in infants (McLeod et al., in press). Pyrimethamine has caused bone marrow suppression manifested by thrombocytopenia, granulocytopenia, and megaloblastic anemia. Reversible granulocytopenia is the most frequent adverse effect in treated infants. Seizures have also occurred with overdosage of pyrimethamine. Patients being treated with pyrimethamine should have their neutrophil counts monitored once weekly and their platelet counts and hematocrit level monitored once monthly. Folinic acid (leucovorin calcium) should always be administered with pyrimethamine to prevent bone marrow suppression. Folinic acid does not block the inhibitory effect of pyrimethamine and sulfadiazine on *Toxoplasma* replication at dosages used in the treatment of congenital toxoplasmosis.

Zidovudine, on the other hand, appears to antagonize the antitoxoplasmic effect of pyrimethamine and its synergy with sulfadiazine in vitro. Therapy with phenobarbital appears to reduce the half-life of pyrimethamine in infants (McLeod et al., in press) probably by induction of hepatic enzymes, which degrade pyrimethamine. Pyrimethamine levels in fetal serum when mothers receive 50 mg pyrimethamine daily are in a relatively low but are in a potentially therapeutic, range (Dorangeon et al., 1990).

Sulfonamides

Sulfadiazine or trisulfapyrimidines (sulfadiazine, sulfamerazine, and sulfamethazine) should be used in combination with pyrimethamine for the treatment of toxoplasmosis. Other sulfonamides are less effective. Sulfadiazine and trisulfapyrimidines antagonize folic acid synthesis by inhibition of dihydrofolate synthetase. Sulfadiazine is rapidly absorbed from the gastrointestinal tract, and peak plasma concentrations are reached within 3 to 6 hours after ingestion of a single dose. Equilibration between maternal and fetal circulation is also established in this time. Sulfonamides readily pass through the placenta and reach the fetus in concentrations sufficient to exhibit both antimicrobial and toxic effects.

The side effects of sulfadiazine or trisulfapyrimidines include bone marrow suppression, diarrhea, rash, crystalluria with possible stone formation, and acute reversible renal failure. An increase in fluid intake, with maintenance of high urinary flow, is important in patients treated with sulfonamides. Hypersensitivity reactions can also occur, especially in patients with AIDS. Sulfadiazine interferes with the metabolism of hepatic microsomal enzymes and may inhibit metabolism of phenytoin, causing higher serum levels of this antiepileptic agent. Sulfonamides may also potentiate coumarin anticoagulants by displacing them from binding sites.

Spiramycin

Spiramycin is a macrolide and is available to physicians in the United States with individual permission of the Food and Drug Administration (telephone number, 301-443-5680) and can be obtained from the drug manufacturer, Rhone Poulenc (telephone number, 609-520-0880). It appears to reduce transmission of *T. gondii* from acutely infected pregnant women to their fetuses in utero by 60% (Desmonts and Couvreur, 1979). It is absorbed best without food. Side effects are usually minimal but have included gastrointestinal distress, local vasospasm, dysesthesias, dizziness, flushing, nausea, vomiting, tearing, diarrhea, anorexia, and allergy. There are no known deleterious effects on the fetus.

Clindamycin

Clindamycin is effective against murine toxoplasmosis. However, its effect in human infection is controversial. Despite its absent penetration into CSF and absent in vitro activity against *T. gondii* (presumably a metabolite is active in vivo), clindamycin has been used in combination with high dosages of pyrimethamine to treat successfully toxoplasmic encephalitis in patients with AIDS (with efficacy equal to treatment with pyrimethamine and sulfadiazine). It is recommended as an alternative therapy in conjunction with pyrimethamine if sulfonamide therapy cannot be tolerated. Uncontrolled studies have reported use of clindamycin to treat ocular toxoplasmosis.

Other antimicrobial agents

Because of the adverse effects of current antimicrobial agents effective against *T. gondii* and the great need for antimicrobial agents effective against encysted organisms, active research continues to develop new therapies for toxoplasmosis. Several new antimicrobial agents are in animal experimental or clinical trials. They include napthoquinone (566C80), which appears to inhibit protozoan mitochondrial electron transport, new macrolides (roxithromycin, clarithromycin, and azithromycin), folic acid antagonists (piritrexim), purine antagonists (aprinocid), 1,2,4-trioxanes (pentatrioxane and hexatrioxane), and immunomodulators (recombinant interleukin-2 and γ-interferon). Napthoquinone, azithromycin, and aprinocid are of particular interest because of their antimicrobial effect against encysted organisms (Huskinson-Mark et al., 1991), an effect not exhibited by pyrimethamine and sulfadiazine.

Therapy in specific clinical settings

Summaries of currently used therapies for toxoplasmosis in specific clinical settings are in Tables 31-8 and 31-9.

Table 31-8. Management of pregnancies at risk for fetal infection according to time of maternal infection

Time of maternal infection	Pregnancies with fetal infection (%)	Prenatal diagnostic tests	Management
Periconception	1 with treatment	Ultrasound every 2 wk; fetal blood sampling plus amniocentesis	Spiramycin; if fetal infection, termination or possibly antiparasitic treatment
5 to 16 wk	4 with treatment; 12 without treatment	Ultrasound every 2 wk; fetal blood sampling plus amniocentesis	Spiramycin; if fetal infection, termination or possibly antiparasitic treatment
16 to 28 wk	20 with treatment	Ultrasound every 2 wk; fetal blood sampling plus amniocentesis	Spiramycin; if fetal infection, antiparasitic treatment or possibly termination
28 wk to term	20 to 30 with treatment	Ultrasound every 2 wk*	Spiramycin; neonatal diagnosis; postnatal treatment*

Modified from Daffos F, et al.: N Engl J Med 1988;318:271.

*An alternative approach is prenatal diagnosis and antiparasitic treatment as specified for maternal acquisition at 16 to 28 weeks or with pyrimethamine, sulfadiazine, and folinic acid without spiramycin.

Table 31-9. Treatment of toxoplasmosis

Manifestation of disease	Therapy	Dosage (oral unless specified)	Duration
Congenital toxoplasmosis*	Pyrimethamine*	Loading dose: 2 mg/kg per day for 2 days, then 1 mg/kg/day for 2 or 6 months, then this dose on each Monday, Wednesday, and Friday	1 yr
	and Sulfadiazine*	100 mg/kg/day in two daily divided doses	1 yr
	and Leucovorin (folinic acid)*	5-10 mg three times weekly†	1 yr
	Spiramycin‡	100 mg/kg/day in divided doses used in alternate months in place of pyrimethamine/sulfadiazine/leucovorin in France	1 yr
	Corticosteroids (prednisone)§	1 mg/kg/day in two daily divided doses	Until resolution of elevated (≥1 g/dl) cerebrospinal fluid protein level or active chorioretinitis that threatens vision
In immunologically normal children			
Lymphadenopathy	No therapy	—	—
Significant organ damage that is life threatening	Pyrimethamine	A = Loading dose: 2 mg/kg/day (maximum, 50 mg) for 2 days, then maintenance, 1 mg/kg/day (maximum, 25 mg)	D = Usually 4-6 wk or 2 wk beyond time that signs and symptoms have resolved
	and Sulfadiazine	B = Loading dose: 75 mg/kg, then maintenance, 50 mg/kg q 12 hr	Same as D
	Leucovorin	C = 5-20 mg three times weekly†	Same as D
Active chorioretinitis in older children	Pyrimethamine and	Same as A	Same as D
	Sulfadiazine and	Same as B	
	Leucovorin	Same as C	
	Corticosteroid§	Same as for congenital toxoplasmosis	Same as for congenital toxoplasmosis

*Optimal dosage, feasibility, toxicity currently being evaluated or planned in ongoing National Collaborative Treatment Trial (312-791-4152).

†Adjusted for megaloblastic anemia, granulocytopenia, or thrombocytopenia; blood counts, including platelets, should be monitored as described in text.

‡Available only on request from the Food and Drug Administration (301-443-5680).

§Corticosteroids should be continued until signs of inflammation (high CSF protein ≥1 g.dl) or active chorioretinitis that threatens vision have subsided, dosage then can be tapered and discontinued; use only in conjunction with pyrimethamine, sulfadiazine, and leucovorin.

Continued.

Table 31-9. Treatment of toxoplasmosis—cont'd

Manifestation of disease	Therapy	Dosage (oral unless specified)	Duration
In immunocompromised children			
Non-AIDS	Pyrimethamine	Same as A	E = 4-6 wk beyond complete resolution of symptoms and signs
	and		
	Sulfadiazine	Same as B	Same as E
	and		
	Leucovorin	Same as C	Same as E
AIDS	Pyrimethamine	Same as A	Lifetime
	and		
	Sulfadiazine	Same as B	Lifetime
	and		
	Leucovorin	Same as C	Lifetime
	Clindamycin may be used instead of sulfadiazine	Reported trials for adults but not infants and children	Lifetime
	Experimental 566C80#	Experimental#	Lifetime
In pregnant women with acute toxoplasmosis			
First 21 wk of gestation or until term if fetus not infected	Spiramycin‡	1.5 g q 12 hr without food	F = Until fetal infection documented or excluded at 21 weeks; if documented, in alternate months with pyrimethamine, leucovorin, and sulfadiazine
If fetal infection confirmed after 17th wk of gestation or if infection acquired in last few weeks of gestation	Pyrimethamine	Loading dose: 100 mg/day in divided doses for 2 days followed by 50 mg daily	Same as F
	and		
	Sulfadiazine	Loading dose: 75 mg/kg/day in two divided doses (maximum, 4 g/day) for 2 days, then 100 mg/kg/day in two divided doses (maximum, 4 g/day)	Same as F
	and		
	Leucovorin†	5-20 mg qd	Same as F

Available as compassionate protocol when other medications cannot be tolerated.

Congenital toxoplasmosis. Infected newborns should be treated whether or not they have overt clinical signs of infection.

In a study in France mothers received pyrimethamine and sulfonamide therapy to treat their infected fetuses in utero as outlined in Tables 31-8 and 31-9 (Daffos et al., 1988; Hohlfeld et al., 1989). Outcome was considerably better than was found for comparable historical controls who did not receive such treatment in utero. Forty-one treated children had subclinical infection, and 12 had only isolated asymp-

WEIGH BABY <u>EACH</u> WEEK.
INCREASE MEDICATIONS ACCORDINGLY.

Medication syringe marked with number of ml
to be given in each dose during that week.

Dispensing caps

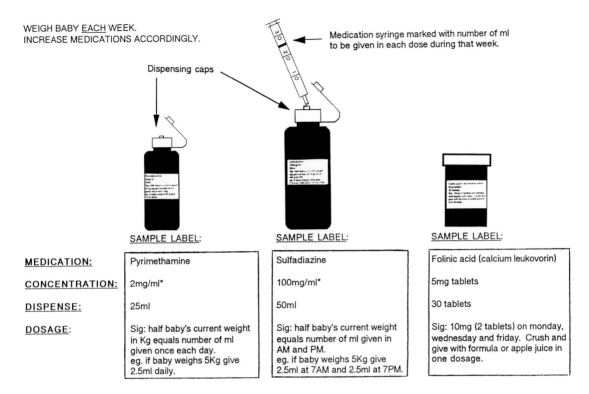

	SAMPLE LABEL:	SAMPLE LABEL:	SAMPLE LABEL:
MEDICATION:	Pyrimethamine	Sulfadiazine	Folinic acid (calcium leukovorin)
CONCENTRATION:	2mg/ml*	100mg/ml*	5mg tablets
DISPENSE:	25ml	50ml	30 tablets
DOSAGE:	Sig: half baby's current weight in Kg equals number of ml given once each day. eg. if baby weighs 5Kg give 2.5ml daily.	Sig: half baby's current weight equals number of ml given in AM and PM. eg. if baby weighs 5Kg give 2.5ml at 7AM and 2.5ml at 7PM.	Sig: 10mg (2 tablets) on monday, wednesday and friday. Crush and give with formula or apple juice in one dosage.

*Suspended in sugar solution. Suspension at usual concentration must be made up each week. Store refrigerated.

Fig. 31-8. Preparation and administration of medications used to treat congenital toxoplasmosis in a National Collaborative Study. (Adapted from McAuley et al, in preparation.)

tomatic signs (retinal scar with normal vision or cerebral calcifications with normal neurological status). Only one had signs of severe congenital infection.

The most extensive experience in treatment of congenital toxoplasmosis after birth has been with the regimen of Dr. Jacques Couvreur. It uses alternate courses of pyrimethamine, sulfadiazine, and spiramycin (see Table 31-9). Couvreur et al. (1984) reported a reduction in early ophthalmological sequelae with this treatment.

In addition, a U.S. National Collaborative prospective, controlled treatment study with long-term follow-up to determine feasibility, safety, efficacy, and optimal dosage for treatment with pyrimethamine and sulfadiazine is on-going (McGhee et al., 1992; McLeod et al., 1991; Roizen et al., 1992; Mets et al., 1992). Preliminary results from this trial indicate that signs of active disease resolve with therapy and suggest that early outcome for most (but not all) treated infants is substantially better than out-

come reported for untreated infants or those treated for only 1 month as described in the earlier literature (Eichenwald, 1960; Wilson et al., 1980). Neurological, developmental, auditory, and ophthalmological outcomes are evaluated. Study of the effect of newer antimicrobial agents that eliminate encysted organisms on ophthalmological and neurological sequalae is also planned. Infants can be referred to this National Collaborative study by telephoning 312-791-4152.

A method for preparation of pyrimethamine and sulfadiazine to facilitate their administration to infants, which currently is being used in this National Collaborative study, is shown in Fig. 31-8. Dosages of medications being evaluated are outlined in Table 31-9. Therapy with corticosteroids (prednisone, 1 mg/kg/day, divided into two doses) has been recommended when there is elevated CSF protein (≥ 1 g/dl) and/or active chorioretinitis that threatens vision (Remington and Desmonts, 1990).

Immunologically normal children with lymphadenopathy, severe symptoms, or damage to vital organs. Children with lymphadenopathy alone do not need specific treatment. If severe or persistent symptoms occur or there is evidence of organ damage, therapy with a combination of pyrimethamine, sulfadiazine, and leucovorin is indicated. Patients who are immunologically normal but have severe symptoms or damage to vital organs (e.g., chorioretinitis, myocarditis, or pneumonitis) should be treated until all symptoms and signs resolve, followed by an additional 2 weeks of therapy. The usual course of therapy is approximately 4 to 6 weeks; dosages of medications are in Table 31-9. A loading dose of pyrimethamine (2 mg/kg body weight, maximum of 50 mg) is given daily for 2 days, followed by a maintenance dose (1 mg/kg body weight, maximum of 25 mg) daily. The loading dose of sulfadiazine is 75 mg/kg body weight, followed by a maintenance dose of 50 mg/kg body weight every 12 hours. Folinic acid (calcium leucovorin) is administered orally whenever pyrimethamine is given. Dosage is 5 to 20 mg given three to seven times weekly, depending on the results of blood and platelet counts.

Active chorioretinitis in older children. Chorioretinitis is the most frequent manifestation of congenital disease, and relapse may occur throughout childhood and adult life. Although active chorioretinitis may remit spontaneously without specific therapy, treatment with pyrimethamine, sulfadiazine, and leucovorin appears to reduce signs and symptoms. Therapy for active chorioretinitis is outlined in Table 31-9. Therapy should be given in conjunction with care by an ophthalmologist. With treatment, borders of retinal lesions sharpen, and vitreous haze should disappear within approximately 10 days. Corticosteroids should be added if lesions involve the macula, optic nerve head, or papillomacular bundle. Use of clindamycin has been described extensively in the ophthalmological literature and has been recommended as an alternative to the sulfonamide-pyrimethamine combination. However, definitive studies demonstrating efficacy have not been performed. In some severe cases, vitrectomy and/or removal of the lens has been used to improve visual acuity. Retinal detachment (which is potentially surgically correctable) has been reported.

Immunocompromised patients. Toxoplasmosis in patients who are immunocompromised by underlying disease (e.g., lymphoma, AIDS) or by therapy (e.g., corticosteroids, cytotoxic drugs) should be treated. Serological evidence of active infection in an immunocompromised patient, regardless of clinical signs and symptoms, or documentation of the presence of tachyzoites in tissue is an indication for treatment. In patients with AIDS clinical symptoms with radiological findings (CT or MRI) that are suggestive of infection may in themselves be indications for treatment. If there is no response to a therapeutic trial of pyrimethamine and sulfadiazine within approximately 10 to 14 days, brain biopsy to exclude other diagnoses should be considered. In 80% of patients with AIDS in whom the diagnosis was made antemortem, there was clear and rapid (<1 month) improvement with antimicrobial treatment. In the same group of patients more than half of those responding showed complete resolution of clinical and brain CT scan abnormalities. For immunosuppressed individuals, it is imperative to suspect and establish the diagnosis quickly and to begin treatment as soon as possible.

For children whose immunosuppression can be reduced (by discontinuation of chemotherapy or corticosteroids), treatment with sulfadiazine, pyrimethamine, and leucovorin should be continued for 4 to 6 weeks beyond complete resolution of all signs and symptoms of active disease.

In immunocompromised adults with AIDS relapse is frequent if therapy is discontinued. Until agents that can eliminate encysted organisms have demonstrated efficacy in humans, suppressive therapy with pyrimethamine and sulfadiazine should be continued for the remainder of such patients' lives. There are no reported results from studies to examine relative effects of different suppressive regimens, but some that have been recommended are included in Table 31-9. Recently, in a controlled study the combination of pyrimethamine and sulfadoxine, one tablet biweekly, was reported to reduce the occurrence of toxoplasmic encephalitis (Ruf et al., 1991). In this study the incidence of subsequent encephalitis was reduced to 4 (11%) out of 37 with prophylaxis and from 8 (67%) out of 12 without prophylaxis. When used as primary prophylaxis in seropositive individuals without overt disease, the incidence of subsequent encephalitis was reduced to 2 (5%) out of 38 with sulfadoxine and pyrimethamine (Fansidar) and 7 out of 28 (25%) without it. It is not known whether suppressive doses of pyrimethamine and sulfonamides are either necessary or effective in preventing relapse in infants with congenital or acute acquired toxoplasmosis and AIDS. Based on data in adults, it is reasonable to treat children with AIDS and toxoplasmic encephalitis with pyrimethamine and sulfadiazine for the remainder of their lives.

Pregnant women with acute acquired T. gondii *infection or chronic* T. gondii *infection and immunocompromise.* In general, if *Toxoplasma* infection is acquired by an immunologically normal mother before conception, the fetus is not at risk for congenital toxoplasmosis. There has been only one report of a normal woman who acquired *T. gondii* 2 months before conception who transmitted the infection to her fetus in utero. Treatment with spiramycin of an immunologically normal pregnant woman who acquires an acute infection during pregnancy reduces the chance of congenital infection in her infant by 60% (Desmonts and Couvreur, 1974). Spiramycin (1.5 g every 12 hours without food) is continued throughout pregnancy unless fetal infection is demonstrated by ultrasound and/or analysis of percutaneous fetal blood and amniotic fluid (see Table 31-8). If evidence of infection is present in the fetus, pyrimethamine, sulfadiazine, and leucovorin therapy (dosages are listed in Table 31-9) have been substituted in alternate months for spiramycin. If no fetal involvement is found, spiramycin alone is continued until term. Such treatment reduces the ability to isolate *T. gondii* from the placenta. *T. gondii* was isolated from placentas of untreated infected infants 95% of the time but only 80% of the time from placentas of infected infants whose mothers were treated with spiramycin and only 50% of the time from placentas of infants whose mothers were treated with pyrimethamine and sulfadiazine and spiramycin in alternate months (Couvreur et al., 1988).

Chronically infected women who become immunosuppressed by cytotoxic drugs, corticosteroids, or HIV infection have also transmitted *T. gondii* to the fetus. Most of these women develop toxoplasmosis by recrudescence of latent *T. gondii* rather than from newly acquired infection. Such women, who do not have overt toxoplasmosis, should at least receive spiramycin throughout pregnancy.

PROGNOSIS

Toxoplasmic lymphadenopathy in the immunologically normal individual is self-limited and resolves without antimicrobial therapy. Treatment with pyrimethamine, sulfadiazine, and leucovorin results in resolution of active signs of *T. gondii* infection in most immunologically normal, immunocompromised, and congenitally infected individuals (McLeod et al., 1979; McAuley et al., in preparation). The prognosis for infants with congenital toxoplasmosis that was untreated or was treated with 1 month of pyrimethamine and sulfadiazine was poor for those who had neurological or generalized infection at presentation in their first year of life (see Table 31-3). The prognosis also was guarded for those with subclinical infection at birth (see Table 31-4). The outcome is substantially better for most (but not all) infants who are treated in utero and/or for 1 year with pyrimethamine and sulfadiazine (Tables 31-10 and 31-11). Favorable outcomes have been associated with prompt diagnosis and initiation of antimicrobial therapy and with prompt attention to the need for shunting of patients with hydrocephalus and/or revision of malfunctioning ventriculoperitoneal shunts (McAuley et al., in press).

PREVENTION

At present, the major component of primary prevention is educating susceptible patients, especially seronegative pregnant or immunodeficient individuals. Given the morbidity, mortality, and expense of the disease in terms of care of affected patients, major attempts to define and initiate better forms of prevention are needed. All physicians responsible for the care of pregnant women, those attempting to conceive, or immunosuppressed patients should inform them of simple measures for prevention. Provision of informational material to pregnant women in France reduced the incidence of congenital infection by 50%. An educational pamphlet and videotape are also available (phone number, 800-323-9100).

The goal of primary prevention is to avoid ingestion of cysts or contact with sporulated oocysts. Methods of prevention are outlined in

Table 31-10. Comparison of ophthalmological, developmental, and audiological outcomes with postnatal treatment

Authors (year of publication)	Treatment	Number studied	Present age in years — mean (range)	Percent with impairment					
				Ophthalmological			Cognitive	Motor or seizures	Audiological
				Lesions	Vision	New			
Eichenwald (1960)	0 or 1 mo, P, S	104	4 (minimum)	NA	0, 42, 67*	NA	50, 81, 89	0, 58, 76	0, 10, 17
Wilson et al. (1980)	0 or 1 mo, P, S	23	8.5 (1-17)	93	47	22	55 (20 severe)	20	22, 30
Labadie and Hazemann (1984)	0	17	1 (NA)	28	NA	NA	NA	NA	NA
Couvreur et al. (1984)	1 yr, P, S, Sp	172	NA (2-11)	NA	NA	8	NA	NA	NA
Koppe et al. (1986)	0 or 1 mo, P, S	12	20 (NA)	80	NA	NA	0	0	NA
Hohlfeld et al. (1989)	Prenatal, 1 yr, P, S, Sp	43	NA (0.5-4)	12	NA	NA	0	0	NA
National Collaborative Study (historical control)	0	7	5.6 (2-10)	100	86	29	25	25	14
National Collaborative Study (treated)	Most for 1 yr, P, S	37	3.4 (0.3-10)	81	81	8	0, 24†	0, 24	0

From McLeod R et al. Exp Parasitol 1991;72:109-121.

P, pyrimethamine; S, sulfonamides; Sp, spiramycin; NA, data not available; lesions, any chorioretinal lesions; vision, vision impaired; new, new lesions.

*Subclinical, generalized, neurological.

Table 31-11. Fetal toxoplasmosis: outcome of pregnancy and infant follow-up after in utero treatment*

	Trimester										
	First				Second				Third		
	1972-1981		1982-1988		1972-1981		1982-1988		1972-1981		1982-1988
Outcome	Number	%	Number	%	Number	%	Number	%	Number	%	Number
Subclinical	1	10	6	67	23	37	33	77	74	68	2
Benign	5	50	2	22	28	45	10	23	31	29	0
Severe	4	40	1	11	11	18	0		3	3	0
TOTAL	10		9		62		43		108		2

Modified from Hohlfeld P, et al. J Pediatr 1989;115:765.

*Infants were not treated in utero 1972-1981 and were treated in utero 1982-1988. Trimester indicates time of acquisition of acute infection by the mother. Note in utero treatment was associated with marked diminution of clinical signs or severity of infection.

Fig. 31-2. Tissue cysts can be rendered noninfectious by heating meat or eggs to 66° C (150.8° F) or by smoking, curing, or freezing meat to $-22°$ C ($-7.6°$ F). Most home freezers do not become this cold. Hands should be washed thoroughly after handling raw meat and vegetables. Steak tartare or other foods featuring uncooked meat should be avoided. Eggs should not be ingested raw, and unpasteurized milk (particularly from goats) should not be consumed. Any kitchen surfaces that come in contact with raw meat or vegetables should be washed thoroughly. Patients should also be warned not to touch mucous membranes or eyes while handling raw meat.

To prevent infection with the oocyst, cat feces should be avoided. Cat feces should be disposed of daily (because sporulation occurs 1 to 5 days after excretion) either by incineration or by flushing down the toilet. Cat litter pans should be used with liners and changed by someone other than the pregnant or immunosuppressed individual. The pan can then be rendered free of viable oocysts by pouring boiling water into the pans and letting the water remain for at least 5 minutes before rinsing. Ammonia (7%) can also kill oocysts but requires 3 hours of exposure. Chlorine bleach, dilute ammonia, quaternary ammonia compounds, or other household detergents are not sufficient to destroy oocysts. When working in sand or soil possibly contaminated with cat feces, gloves should be worn. Hands should be thoroughly washed before handling any items that would be ingested or come in contact with mucous membranes. Since the cat is the only animal that is known to produce oocysts, efforts should also be directed toward preventing infection in cats. Feeding cats commercially dried, canned, or cooked food rather than allowing them to hunt possibly infected prey will reduce the likelihood of their infection. These general precautionary measures rather than serological testing of cats are recommended.

Although primary prevention theoretically can be achieved by education about hygienic measures as described previously, secondary prevention consists of identification of acutely infected individuals in high-risk populations and the early institution of specific therapy to prevent or minimize complications. Since approximately 90% of women infected during pregnancy have no clinical illness, sequential serological testing of seronegative pregnant women is the only way to identify the fetus at risk of congenital infection. Standardized screening, followed by sequential testing, is routinely performed in areas of high incidence such as France and Austria. However, there is no universally adopted policy for screening or sequential testing of pregnant women for congenital toxoplasmosis in the United States. Cost effectiveness has been suggested but not proven (McCabe and Remington, 1988). Problems with the reliability of some commercially available serological tests have in the past dissuaded certain authors from recommending widespread serological screening. Before the initiation of therapy in any setting, positive serological test results should be confirmed in a reference laboratory (e.g., Palo Alto Research Institute; phone number, 415-326-8120). Some serological screening programs have involved all women in their childbearing years before and during pregnancy to determine prior exposure (e.g., France), and some have involved screening of all newborns (e.g., the model of the Massachusetts State Screening Program). If women are seronegative, systematic serological screening at specific intervals during pregnancy is used. This is a reasonable approach because it is possible to prevent or modify illness caused by congenital *T. gondii* infection by treatment during gestation and because reliable serological tests are now commercially available in the United States. The individual suffering and the cost to families and society of caring for children born with congenital toxoplasmosis make increased use of screening tests potentially important (Featherstone, 1981).

THE FUTURE

Major future advances in prevention and treatment of toxoplasmosis are likely. Development of a vaccine to prevent infection in humans and cats or animals used for meat remains at an experimental stage, but a number of lines of investigation are promising. Use of educational programs for pregnant and immunocompromised individuals should further reduce infection rates. Paradigms for prevention of congenital infection or its sequelae are being developed and tested. More sensitive and specific serological and direct (e.g., PCR) tests are being evaluated. Additional reference laboratories to perform serological testing reliably are needed. Studies to determine optimal means to treat congenital toxoplasmosis and toxoplasmosis in patients with AIDS are in progress. Development and testing of new antimicrobial agents that eliminate encysted organisms that are the source of recrudescent disease in congenital, ophthalmological, and disseminated or neurological toxoplasmosis in immunocompromised individuals are promising and in progress.

GLOSSARY

AC/HS Differential agglutination test using acetone- (AC) and formalin- (HS) fixed tachyzoites; useful in determining whether infection was acquired in the 6 months before the serum sample was obtained.

Chronic infection with *T. gondii* Condition of asymptomatic parasite latency that follows primary infection or successful treatment of recrudescence.

Cyst Contains bradyzoites and is present in chronic infection.

Double sandwich (DS) IgA ELISA Measures *T. gondii*–specific IgA; possibly more sensitive than the DS IgM ELISA for diagnosis of congenital infection.

Double sandwich (DS) IgM ELISA Measures *T. gondii*–specific IgM; positive at birth in approximately 75% of congenitally infected infants.

IgM ISAGA Measures *T. gondii*–specific IgM; usually more sensitive than the DS IgM ELISA.

Mouse inoculation Inoculation of body fluid or placental tissue intraperitoneally into mice; mice then are observed for proliferating tachyzoites in their ascitic fluid, brain cyst development, and *T. gondii*–specific serum antibodies.

Oocyst Contains sporozoites and is excreted by cats.

Sabin-Feldman dye test "Gold standard" test for measurement of IgG antibody that damages the surface membrane of live tachyzoites in the presence of complement, rendering the tachyzoite unstained by the vital dye methylene blue; performed by reference laboratories.

***Toxoplasma gondii* bradyzoite** Slowly proliferative form present within tissue cysts in chronic, latent infection; source of infection ingested in undercooked meat.

***Toxoplasma gondii* sporozoite** Highly infectious form in oocyst, which sporulates after fecal excretion by cats.

***Toxoplasma gondii* tachyzoite** Rapidly proliferative form present in acute and/or active infection.

Toxoplasmosis Disease caused by *T. gondii*; may be primary or recrudescent.

REFERENCES

Aspock P. Prevention of congenital toxoplasmosis by serological surveillance during pregnancy: current strategies and future perspectives. In Marget W, Lang W, Gabler-Sandberger E (eds). Parasitic infections, immunology, mycotic infections, general topics, Vol. 3. Munich: MMV Medizin Verlag, 1986, pp 69-72.

Brown C, McLeod R. Class I MHC genes and CD8[+] T cells determine cyst number in *Toxoplasma gondii* infection. J Immunol 1990;145:3438-3441.

Burg JL, Grover CM, Pouletty P, Boothroyd JC. Direct and sensitive detection of a pathogenic protozoan, *Toxoplasma gondii*, by polymerase chain reaction. J Clin Microbiol 1989;27:1787.

Conley JK, Jenkins KA, Remington JS. *Toxoplasma gondii* infection of the central nervous system. Use of the peroxidase-antiperoxidase method to demonstrate *Toxo-*

plasma in formalin-fixed, paraffin-embedded tissue sections. Hum Pathol 1981;12:690.

Couvreur J, Desmonts G. Congenital and maternal toxoplasmosis. A review of 300 congenital cases. Dev Med Child Neurol 1962;4:519-530.

Couvreur J, Desmonts G, Aron-Rosa D. Le pronostic oculaire de la toxoplasmose congenitale: role du traitement. Ann Pediatr 1984;31:855-858.

Couvreur J, Desmonts G, Thulliez P. Prophylaxis of congenital toxoplasmosis. Effect of spiramycin on placental infection. J Antimicrob Chemother 1988;22:193-200.

Daffos F, Forestier F, Capella-Pavlovsky M, et al. Prenatal management of 746 pregnancies at risk for congenital toxoplasmosis. N Engl J Med 1988;318:271.

Dannemann BR, Vaughan WC, Thulliez P, et al. The differential agglutination test for diagnosis of recently acquired infection with *Toxoplasma gondii*. J Clin Microbiol 1990;28:1928.

Decoster A, Darcy F, Caron A, et al. IgA antibodies against P30 as markers of congenital and acute toxoplasmosis. Lancet 1988;2:1104.

Desmonts G, Couvreur J. Congenital toxoplasmosis. A prospective study of 378 pregnancies. N Engl J Med 1974;290:1110-1116.

Desmonts G, Couvreur J. Congenital toxoplasmosis: a prospective study of the offspring of 542 women who acquired toxoplasmosis during pregnancy. Pathophysiology of congenital disease. In Thalhammer O, Baumgarten K, Pollak A (eds). Perinatal medicine. Sixth European Congress. Stuttgart: Georg Thieme, 1979, p 51.

Desmonts G, Couvreur J. Natural history of congenital toxoplasmosis. Ann Pediatr 1984;31:799.

Desmonts G, Remington JS. Direct agglutination test for diagnosis of *Toxoplasma* infection. Method for increasing sensitivity and specificity. J Clin Microbiol 1980;11:562.

Dorangeon PH, Fay R, Marx-Chemla C, et al. Passage transplacentaire de l'association pyrimethamine-sulfadoxine hors du traitement antenatal de la toxoplasmose congenital. Presse Med 1990;2036:22-29.

Dorfman RF, Remington JS. Value of lymph node biopsy in the diagnosis of acute acquired toxoplasmosis. N Engl J Med 1973;289:878.

Duquesne V, Auriault C, Darey F, et al. Protection of nude rats against *Toxoplasma* infection by excreted-secreted antigen-specific helper T cells. Infect Immunol 1990;58:2120.

Eichenwald HF. A study of congenital toxoplasmosis, with particular emphasis on clinical manifestations, sequelae, and therapy. In Siim JC (ed). Human toxoplasmosis. Copenhagen: Munksgaard, 1960, p 41.

Featherstone H. A difference in the family. New York: Penguin, 1981.

Forestier F, Daffos F, Rainant M, Cox WC. The assessment of fetal blood samples. Am J Obstet Gynecol 1988;158:1184-1188.

Frenkel JK, Pfefferkorn ER, Smith DD, Fishback JL. Prospective vaccine prepared from a new mutant of *Toxoplasma gondii* for use in cats. Am J Vet Res 1991;52:759-763.

Grover CM, Thulliez P, Remington JS, et al. Rapid prenatal diagnosis of congenital *Toxoplasma* infection by using polymerase chain reaction and amniotic fluid. J Clin Microbiol 1990;28:2297.

Hoff R, Weiblen BJ, Reardon LA, Maguire JH. Screening for congenital toxoplasma infection. In Transplacental disorders: perinatal detection, treatment and management (including pediatric AIDS). New York: Alan R Liss, 1990, p 169.

Hohlfeld P, Daffos F, Thulliez P, et al. Fetal toxoplasmosis: outcome of pregnancy and infant follow-up after in utero treatment. J Pediatr 1989;115:765-769.

Holland GN, Engstrom RE Jr, Glasgow BJ, et al. Ocular toxoplasmosis in patients with the acquired immunodeficiency syndrome. Am J Ophthalmol 1988;106:653-667.

Huskinson-Mark J, Araujo FG, Remington JS. Evaluation of the effect of drugs on the cyst form of *Toxoplasma gondii*. J Infect Dis 1991;164:170.

Israelski DM, Remington JS. Toxoplasmic encephalitis in patients with AIDS. In Sande MA, Volberding PA (eds). The medical management of AIDS. Philadelphia: WB Saunders, 1988, pp 193-211.

Israelski DM, Tom C, Remington JS. Zidovudine antagonizes the action of pyrimethamine in experimental infection with *Toxoplasma gondii*. Antimicrob Agents Chemother 1989;33:30.

Khan A, Ely K, Kasper L. A purified parasite antigen (p30) mediates CD8 T cell immunity against fatal *Toxoplasma gondii* infection in mice. J Immunol 1991;147:3501-3506.

Koppe JG, Kloosterman GJ, deRoever-Bonnet H, et al. Toxoplasmosis and pregnancy, with a long-term follow-up of the children. Europ J Obstet Gynecol Reprod Biol 1974;413:101-110.

Koppe JG, Loewer-Sieger DH, DeRoever-Bonnet H. Results of 20-year follow-up of congenital toxoplasmosis. Lancet 1986;I:254-256.

Labadie MD, Hazeman JJ. Apport des bilans de sante de l'efant pour le depistage et l'etude epidemiologiquede la toxoplasmose congenitale. Ann Pediatr 1984;31:823-828.

Leport C. Toxoplasmosis in AIDS. 17th International Congress of Chemotherapy, June 28, 1991, Berlin, Germany.

Luft BJ, Naot Y, Araujo FG, et al. Primary and reactivated *Toxoplasma* infection in patients with cardiac transplants. Clinical spectrum and problems in diagnosis of a defined population. Ann Intern Med 1983;99:27.

Luft BJ, Remington JS. Acute *Toxoplasma* infection among family members of patients with acute lymphadenopathic toxoplasmosis. Arch Intern Med 1984;144:53.

McAuley J, Roizen N, Beckman J, et al. Early evaluations and treatment of 43 infants and children with congenital toxoplasmosis. (In preparation.)

McCabe RE, Brooks RG, Dorfman RF, Remington JS. Clinical spectrum in 107 cases of toxoplasmic lymphadenopathy. Rev Infect Dis 1987;9:754.

McCabe RE, Remington JS. Toxoplasmosis: the time has come. N Engl J Med 1988;318:313.

McGhee T, Wolters C, Stein L, et al. Absence of sensorineural hearing loss in treated infants and children with congenital toxoplasmosis. Otolaryngol Head Neck Surg. (In press.)

McLeod R, Berry PF, Marshall WH, et al. Toxoplasmosis presenting as brain abscesses. Diagnosis by computerized tomography and cytology of aspirated purulent material. Am J Med 1979;67:711-714.

McLeod R, Boyer K, Roizen N, et al. Treatment of congenital toxoplasmosis. 17th International Congress of Chemotherapy, June 18, 1991, Berlin, Germany.

McLeod R, Frenkel JK, Estes RG, et al. Subcutaneous and intestinal vaccination with tachyzoites of *Toxoplasma gondii* and acquisition of immunity to peroral and congenital *Toxoplasma* challenge. J Immunol 1988;140:1632-1637.

McLeod R, Hubbel J, Foss R, et al. Serum, cerebrospinal, and ventricular fluid levels of pyrimethamine in infants treated for congenital toxoplasmosis. Antimicrob Agents Chemother 1992 (in press).

McLeod R, Mack DG, Boyer KM, et al. Phenotypes and functions of lymphocytes in congenital toxoplasmosis. J Lab Clin Med 1990;116:623-635.

McLeod R, Mack D, Brown C. *Toxoplasma gondii*—new advances in cellular and molecular biology. Exp Parasitol 1991;72:109-121.

McLeod R, Remington JS. Toxoplasmosis. In Behrman RL, Vaughan VC III, Nelson WE (eds). Nelson's textbook of pediatrics, ed 14. Philadelphia: WB Saunders, 1990.

Mets M, et al. Ophthalmic findings in congenital toxoplasmosis. Sarasota, FL: Association for Research and Vision in Ophthalmology, 1992.

Mitchell CD, Erlich SS, Mastrucci MT, et al. Congenital toxoplasmosis occurring in infants perinatally infected with human immunodeficiency virus 1. Pediatr Infect Dis 1990;9:512.

Naot Y, Remington JS. An enzyme-linked immunosorbent assay for detection of IgM antibodies to *Toxoplasma gondii*: use for diagnosis of acute acquired toxoplasmosis. J Infect Dis 1980;142:757.

O'Connor GR. Manifestations and management of ocular toxoplasmosis. Bull NY Acad Med 1974;30:192.

Prince JB, Araujo FG, Remington JS, et al. Cloning of cDNAs encoding a 28 kilodalton antigen of *Toxoplasma gondii*. Mole Biochem Parasitol 1989;34:3-14.

Remington JS, Desmonts G. Toxoplasmosis. In Remington JS, Klein JO (eds). Infectious diseases of the fetus and newborn infant, ed 3. Philadelphia: WB Saunders, 1990, p 89.

Roberts T, Frenkel JK. Estimating income losses and other preventable costs caused by congenital toxoplasmosis in people in the United States. J Am Vet Med Assoc, 1990.

Roizen N, et al. Developmental and neurologic function in treated congenital toxoplasmosis. Baltimore: Society for Pediatric Research, May 1992.

Roux C, Desmonts G, Molliez N, et al. Toxoplasmose et grossesse. Bilan deux ans de prophylaxie de la toxoplasmose congenitale a la maternite de l'Hopital Saint Antoine (1973-1974). J Gynecol Obst Biol Repr 1976;5(2):249-264.

Ruf B, Schurmann D, Pohle HD. The efficacy of Fansidar® in preventing AIDS associated neurotoxoplasmosis and pneumocystis carinii pneumonia. Berlin: International Congress of Chemotherapy, 1991.

Ruiz A, Frenkel JK. *Toxoplasma gondii* in Costa Rican cats. Am J Trop Med Hyg 1980;29:1150.

Stepick-Biek P, Thulliez P, Araujo FG, Remington JS. IgA antibodies for diagnosis of acute congenital and acquired toxoplasmosis. J Infect Dis 1990;162:270-273.

Townsend JJ, et al. Acquired toxoplasmosis. Arch Neurol 1975;32:335.

Wilson CB, Remington JS. What can be done to prevent congenital toxoplasmosis? Am J Obstet Gynecol 1980;138:357-363.

Wilson CB, Remington JS, Stagno S, Reynolds DW. Development of adverse sequelae in children born with subclinical congenital *Toxoplasma* infection. Pediatrics 1980;66:767-774.

32

TUBERCULOSIS

DAVID P. SPEERT

Tuberculosis is an ancient disease that is known to have existed in prehistoric times. It is worldwide in distribution, affecting not only human beings but also many species of wild and domestic animals. In the early nineteenth century tuberculosis was the cause of death in more than one third of the autopsies performed in Paris. Tuberculosis was not considered an infectious disease until 1882, when Koch reported the discovery of the tubercle bacillus (Tb). The spread of tuberculosis became a concern of public health authorities, and measures directed toward its control were established. In the 1830s the death rate from tuberculosis in large cities in the United States was approximately 400 per 100,000 of the population. By 1900 the death rate had already fallen to 200 per 100,000. The downward trend accelerated after antimicrobial therapy became available, and in 1983 there were only approximately 2,000 deaths in the United States caused by tuberculosis.

The rate of decline of tuberculosis in the United States has slowed lately. Recent evidence suggests that the incidence is increasing. The first year in which there was an increase in reported cases of tuberculosis was 1986 (Rieder et al., 1989). This change has been attributed to the enhanced risk in individuals with the acquired immunodeficiency syndrome (AIDS) (Chapter 1). The increased number of new cases of tuberculosis is particularly evident in areas in which AIDS is most prevalent such as New York City, Florida, and California (Chaisson and Slutkin, 1989). In 1987 there were 22,517 reported cases of tuberculosis in the United States, a rate of 9.3 per 100,000.

Surveys using the tuberculin test have provided additional information about the prevalence of infection. In 1907 infection was almost universal in large cities. Surveys in St. Louis and Philadelphia in the following years showed that more than 50% of the general population reacted to tuberculin. By 1937 the rate of reactivity to purified protein derivative (PPD) of tuberculin of United States naval recruits 15 to 19 years old was 31.9%. Thirty years later, in the period from 1965 to 1969, 3% of naval recruits 17 to 21 years old showed reactions measuring 10 mm or more to tuberculin, and in 1973 only 2% reacted. In the United States in 1973 only 0.2% of children entering school at age 6 years reacted to tuberculin.

ETIOLOGY

Mycobacterium tuberculosis organisms are usually referred to as acid-fast bacilli. They do not stain with Gram stain, but when heated, they do absorb a carbolfuchsin stain; once stained, they resist decolorization by strong acids and alcohol. They also absorb the fluorescent auramine-rhodamine dye. The stain is not specific for *M. tuberculosis* and is also reactive with other Mycobacteriaceae.

Both *M. tuberculosis* and *M. bovis* are pathogenic for man. Children are equally susceptible to infection with either, but in the United States the campaign for the eradication of tuberculosis in cattle has made infection with *M. bovis* very rare. In addition, asymptomatic infection with atypical bacilli is found in all parts of the world. Such infections may result in skin sensitivity to tuberculin (Palmer et al., 1959) and occasionally in disease, especially cervical adenitis.

Atypical mycobacterial infections have gained new notoriety lately; they are a particular problem for individuals with impaired cell-mediated immunity such as those with AIDS (Horsburgh, 1991). These mycobacteria have introduced a new set of therapeutic challenges because they are resistant to a wide range of antituberculous agents and are capable of establishing a refractory state of intracellular parasitism. Infections with *M. avium* and *M. intracellulare* have become increasingly common in patients with AIDS and may be incurable.

PATHOGENESIS
Initial infection

The lung is the most common portal of entry of tubercle bacilli. If the bacilli are ingested, infection in the upper respiratory or intestinal tract may result (Lincoln, 1950). The initial infection produces a complex consisting of the local disease at the portal of entry and in the regional lymph nodes that drain that area, the Ghon complex. The term *primary tuberculosis* includes the primary complex and the local progression of disease; however, this term is no longer used under the modern classification of tuberculosis developed by the American Thoracic Society, but the concept of a special response of the body to the first infection with tubercle bacilli is still valid and is basic to an understanding of tuberculosis in children.

At the site of entry, the bacilli multiply and create an area of inflammatory exudate. Almost as soon as infection occurs, bacilli are carried through the lymphatic system to the nearest group of lymph nodes that drain the area in which the focus is situated. When the portal of entry is in the lung, the bronchopulmonary nodes usually form the complex. Until delayed hypersensitivity develops, the area of infection may expand and remains unencapsulated. With the onset of delayed hypersensitivity, the perifocal infiltration generally increases very rapidly, regional lymph nodes enlarge, and the initial lesion may become caseous and may become walled off. Caseous lesions may eventually calcify. Living tubercle bacilli may persist within these foci for years (Lincoln, 1950).

Progression of tuberculous disease usually involves the bronchi, the blood vessels, and the lymphatic channels supplying and draining the lung, all of which converge in the hilar area. Enlargement of hilar nodes may encroach on any of these structures. The ones most commonly affected are the bronchi, especially in infants, who often develop tuberculous endobronchitis. The infection may erode the bronchial wall to cause a fistula between the node and the bronchial lumen, with dissemination of the infection through the bronchi. The swelling of the bronchial mucosa may interfere with aeration and drainage of segments or of an entire lobe of the lung. Sequelae in the involved portion of lung are fibrosis, bronchiectasis, distortion of the bronchi, and pneumonia. Tuberculous lymph nodes sometimes compress or invade other adjacent structures such as the pericardium, esophagus, or blood vessels. During resolution of infection, the nodal component of the primary complex resolves less rapidly than does the parenchymal focus.

Hematogenous tuberculosis

During the early stage of disease small numbers of tubercle bacilli reach the bloodstream either directly from the initial focus or by way of the regional nodes and the thoracic duct. This sporadic dissemination (occult hematogenous tuberculosis) ceases after delayed hypersensitivity develops. Some disseminated tubercle bacilli progress at varying rates into foci of active disease. Such lesions may regress and heal completely, may progress immediately, or may remain quiescent but contain viable tubercle bacilli. These latent foci may become active again years after the initial infection.

Most complications resulting from hematogenous dissemination are caused by the invasion of an adjoining viscus or space by a tubercle or group of tubercles. For example, caseous tubercles in the cerebral cortex or on the meninges cause meningitis by the discharge of tubercle bacilli into the subarachnoid space. Acute generalized miliary tuberculosis usually results from the invasion of a blood vessel by a caseating focus of tuberculosis or by dissemination from a tubercle within the lumen of a blood vessel originally seeded during the early lymphohematogenous spread.

Although most complications result from hematogenous dissemination, a few do not. The frequent association of spondylitis with pleurisy or with renal tuberculosis is often due to involvement of adjacent paravertebral nodes. Most complications of primary tuberculosis develop during the first year after onset of the disease. In the Bellevue Hospital experience with untreated children, only approximately 5% of the survivors developed complications more than 1 year after the first infection (Lincoln, 1950). Chronic pulmonary tuberculosis of the type usually seen in adults rarely developed in children before adolescence; it occurred twice as often in girls as boys. Twenty percent of the cases in girls were diagnosed within 2 years of the date of menarche (Lincoln, 1950).

IMMUNITY
Host defense

M. tuberculosis evades host defenses and persists by mechanisms that are poorly understood. It appears that a state of intracellular parasitism is established in which the bacilli survive and grow within human cells. Macrophages form the first line of defense against inhaled mycobacteria, and it is within these cells that the initial infection may be established. The means by which *M. tuberculosis* resists killing by macrophages has been studied extensively but explained incompletely. Viable mycobacteria appear to prevent fusion of phagosomes (within which the bacteria are engulfed by the macrophage) with lysosomes, which contain the toxic substances for killing ingested microbes (Armstrong and D'Arcy Hart, 1975). The means by which normal macrophages kill mycobacteria and factors capable of enhancing this bactericidal activity are currently under investigation.

Cell-mediated immunity plays a critical role in the control of mycobacterial infections (Kaufmann, 1989). T cells elaborate an array of cytokines capable of activating macrophage bactericidal activities. It is this cell-mediated response to infection with *M. tuberculosis* that apparently controls the spread of primary infection. Cell-mediated immune mechanisms also enhance the tissue damage (caseous necrosis) that is characteristic of tuberculosis. Factors that compromise this cell-mediated immunity such as AIDS or therapy with corticosteroids may permit the infection to spread and cause symptomatic disease. Suppression of cell-mediated immunity by products of *M. tuberculosis* may also interfere with host defenses and permit persistence of the infection (Ellner and Wallis, 1989).

Gender

In the children studied in Bellevue Hospital, before the use of chemotherapy there were equal numbers of boys and girls. The mortality and incidence of meningitis were equal in both sexes. However, among tuberculin-reactive teenagers, active disease occurred more frequently in adolescent girls than in adolescent boys (Lincoln, 1950). Before chemotherapy was available, there was a higher death rate from tuberculosis in girls 15 to 18 years old than in boys of the same age group. At the present time the case rate and the death rate in most countries are highest among elderly men.

Genetic factors

Genetically determined susceptibility to tuberculosis has been demonstrated in laboratory animals (Schurr et al., 1990), and in humans there is evidence that the degree of resistance to tuberculosis may vary in different ethnic groups (Stead et al., 1990).

Age

Infants who are exposed to *M. tuberculosis* have a very high incidence of active and disseminated disease, which has been estimated as at least 35% of infected cases. It is probable that the infective dose for infants is less than 10 organisms. The majority of untreated infants who develop disease die. This extreme susceptibility of the very young decreases during early childhood until adolescence, when there again occurs an enhanced susceptibility to disease (Lincoln, 1950). After their early twenties humans are relatively resistant, and probably only approximately 1% of untreated and otherwise healthy young adults exposed to *M. tuberculosis* develop clinically apparent disease (Fig. 32-1).

Nutrition

It is difficult to separate the effects of poor nutrition on resistance to tuberculosis from those of other socioeconomic factors. Active disease, however, is inversely proportional to the degree of nutrition, and excellent nutrition is essential to the recovery of young children with tuberculosis. Recent evidence indicates that vitamin D enhances the ability of macrophages to inhibit growth of *M. tuberculosis* (Rook, 1988).

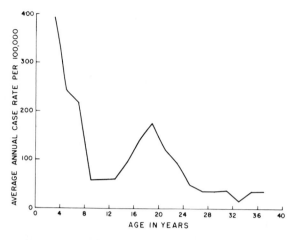

Fig. 32-1. Incidence of tuberculosis among PPD-reactive individuals by age when tuberculous disease was first diagnosed. Reprinted with permission of GW Comstock. (From Comstock GW, et al. Am J Epidemiol 1974;99:141.)

Intercurrent infections

Measles has the closest association with activation of latent disease, but other infectious diseases, especially pertussis, have also been incriminated. The skin reactivity to tuberculin disappears in the preeruptive stage of measles and does not reappear for 2 or 3 weeks, and disease may worsen during this time. There is abundant evidence that corticosteroid therapy without concurrent antituberculous therapy may precipitate disease.

EPIDEMIOLOGICAL FACTORS
Mode of spread

The source of infection in children is usually an adult or occasionally an adolescent who is usually a member of the household. When a person with contagious pulmonary tuberculosis coughs or sneezes, droplets of varying sizes containing tubercle bacilli are dispersed into the air. The particle must be of a particular size to gain access to an alveolus where infection begins. The number of tubercle bacilli discharged into the atmosphere by a patient depends on the number of organisms in the sputum, and the type and frequency of cough. Almost all initial infections occur in the lungs. Occasionally ingested bacilli find a portal of entry in the intestinal tract and, more rarely, in a tonsil or in the mucous membranes of the mouth. Other extrapulmonary sites of infection such as those in the skin or con-

junctiva are due to local contact with tubercle bacilli.

Although children most often acquire tuberculosis from another family member, the disease may also be contracted from any adult with inapparent (quiescent) disease or from someone with an undiagnosed chronic cough (Lincoln, 1967). Vertical transmission may on rare occasion give rise to congenital tuberculosis (Hageman et al., 1980).

Epidemic spread is possible whenever a large proportion of a population has never been exposed to tubercle bacilli, a situation that now exists in most schools. Epidemics are characterized by the finding of a number of newly infected children within a short period of time. The index case is often a teacher, other school personnel, or another student with active pulmonary disease (Lincoln, 1967; Steiner et al., 1976; Rideout and Hiltz, 1969).

Contagion of childhood tuberculosis

In general, primary pulmonary tuberculosis in young children is noninfectious for older children or adults. Bacilli are rarely recovered by culture, even from children with recent infections, unless gastric lavage is performed early in the morning. The number of colonies is usually very small, rarely over 10 and often only one or two. The contagiousness of chronic pulmonary tuberculosis in older children and adolescents is comparable to that of similar pulmonary disease in adults. Cavitation at the site of the initial focus is also an especially contagious form of tuberculosis. Fortunately, these forms of disease are uncommon in children, and when they occur, drug therapy usually causes a rapid decrease in the number of bacilli. Probably of greater concern in the prevention of spread of disease is the possibility that other infected members of a child's family will visit the hospital. For that reason, the child and all visitors probably should be restricted to the child's room pending investigation of the family.

DIAGNOSTIC CRITERIA
Tuberculin tests

The tuberculin skin test is the primary method of identifying persons who have been infected with tubercle bacilli (Lunn and Johnson, 1978; Thompson et al., 1979). PPD, used for intradermal testing in the United States, is prepared by heating tubercle bacilli; it was developed by Seibert and designated by the World Health Organization as the international PPD-tuberculin, usually called *PPD-S*. The potency of tuberculin is expressed in terms of international tuberculin units (TU): 1 TU is equivalent to approximately 0.00002 mg of PPD; 5 TU is the standard dose for intradermal testing. PPD is available commercially in a buffered diluent. Tuberculin is adsorbed to glass or plastic. To avoid reduction in potency by such adsorption, manufacturers add polysorbate 80 (Tween 80) to the diluent. This stabilized PPD will expire in 1 year. Transfer of tuberculin from one container to another should be avoided, and skin tests should be administered within 24 hours after the syringe has been filled.

The Mantoux test (intradermal test) is the most accurate and reliable method of testing for tuberculosis. To ensure reliability, the test must be applied properly. A tuberculin syringe should be used. The best site for testing is the central part of the volar surface of the forearm. The skin should be washed with alcohol and allowed to dry. The needle is inserted transversely into, but not beneath, the skin, and exactly 0.1 ml of test material is injected. A wheal at least 5 mm in diameter should be formed. The operator must ensure that the needle is within the dermal layers since a false-negative result may be obtained if the tuberculin is injected subcutaneously. For mass tuberculin surveys the Mantoux test may be administered with a jet injector using a specially adapted head for intracutaneous injection.

Tests should be read between 48 and 72 hours after the injection. If there is erythema without induration, the reaction should be considered negative. When there is an area of induration, it should be carefully palpated, and its maximal transverse diameter should be measured with a millimeter rule. Induration of less than 5 mm is considered a negative reaction. The test should be considered doubtful if the induration is more than 5 mm but less than 10 mm in diameter. The test should be repeated at a different site; a second test may give a decisive result. A test with 5 TU that results in 10 mm or more of induration is positive. Local reactions that may occur at the site of injection include marked swelling, erythema, vesiculation, and ulceration. In the case of such reactions, there may be lymphangitis and swelling of the regional lymph nodes. Application of topical steroids will help to control a severe local reaction.

The use of greater concentrations of PPD such as 250 TU is valuable only in excluding the diagnosis of generalized anergy. In testing as part of a physical examination or in surveys, it is not necessary to start with 1 TU.

Tests for skin reaction to tuberculin may also be done with multiple puncture devices. These tests should be considered screening tests rather than diagnostic tests. Reactions of 2 mm or less at each prong should be considered negative. Reactions larger than 2 mm are considered doubtful unless vesiculation has occurred. Doubtful screening reactions should be confirmed by means of a diagnostic Mantoux test with 5 TU of PPD. A Mantoux test should always be used if the physician suspects tuberculosis in an ill child.

When potent testing material is properly administered, a tuberculin skin test should produce positive results in the majority of tuberculous persons. Among the exceptions are severely dehydrated or moribund patients and those receiving treatment with corticosteroids. In addition, anergy to tuberculin is often present for 2 or 3 weeks after the onset of measles and during the incubation period of primary tuberculous infection. If the physician suspects tuberculosis and the PPD is nonreactive, the test may be repeated weekly until the uncertainty is resolved. In addition, an intradermal application of 0.1 ml tetanus toxoid or *Candida* 1:1,000 will help determine whether the patient is anergic.

History of exposure

One of the most helpful, and sometimes the most crucial, aspects of the diagnosis of tuberculosis in children is the elicitation of a history of exposure to a patient with active pulmonary disease. If tuberculosis is suspected, members of the family should be asked on more than one occasion if persons within the extended household have had compatible pulmonary disease, weight loss, or sweating. Visitors to the home in the prior 3 months should be assessed since a transient exposure to an alcoholic relative is a fairly common contact. In extended households, close friends of older household members should be included in the discussion of the health of persons to whom the child has been exposed.

Many extended families live in several adjacent homes, and all members of these homes should be considered as potential contacts. If the diagnosis remains uncertain, tuberculin testing of all household members will help to determine if the child is living in an environment in which there has been tuberculous exposure.

Roentgenological examination

Roentgenological examination of the chest should be done if tuberculosis is suspected and should include a lateral view.

Recovery of tubercle bacilli

The diagnosis of tuberculosis is established when *M. tuberculosis* is grown from infected material. Since other mycobacterial species look identical to *M. tuberculosis* on a smear, the diagnosis of tuberculosis by direct examination should be made with caution; however, the examination is helpful in suggesting a diagnosis. Mycobacteria are impervious to Gram stain and usually do not show on a specimen stained with Gram's method alone. Auramine-rhodamine stain allows a more sensitive and rapid identification of the presence of acid-fast organisms in a clinical sample than do the traditional acid-fast stains such as Kinyoun carbolfuchsin. Direct stains are of great value in the examination of cerebrospinal fluid (CSF) since meningitis caused by acid-fast bacilli other than tubercle bacilli is rare. Diagnostic specimens from suspected cases should be cultured for identification of *M. tuberculosis* and other mycobacteria and for determination of susceptibility of the organisms to antituberculous drugs. Cultures of tubercle bacilli usually display some growth in 3 to 4 weeks; however, they should be observed for at least 2 months.

In adults expectorated sputum is the most common source of pulmonary secretions for culture or animal inoculation. In children sputum is usually swallowed, and gastric lavage is a method for attempting recovery of tubercle bacilli that will yield organisms in approximately 35% of children with pulmonary tuberculosis. The number of bacilli recovered from the gastric lavage is usually very small in children, and the yield is increased when washings obtained on 3 successive days are pooled. Cultures obtained during the early phase of primary pulmonary tuberculosis are most likely to yield tubercle bacilli. Bronchoscopy provides a better yield. For adults and children old enough to cooperate, an effective method of inducing sputum is the inhalation of nebulized, warmed, hypertonic saline solution. This method is more acceptable to patients than gastric lavage, and the yield of positive cultures from it has been reported as good. Guinea pig inoculation of CSF or pleural fluid was an important method of diagnosis in the past, but it is now seldom used.

Histopathological examinations

Biopsies from diseased areas of the skeletal system, pleura, superficial lymph nodes, and liver may yield a diagnosis. Histopathological findings include noncaseating granulomas, caseating granulomas, and presence or absence of mycobacteria or acid-fast stains of the tissue.

Hematological examinations

Hematological examinations usually offer little help in making a diagnosis or prognosis. Mild secondary anemia is often present. The total white blood cell (WBC) count is often within normal limits. During some active phases of tuberculosis, there may be an elevation in the total count with an increase in number of polymorphonuclear leukocytes. The erythrocyte sedimentation rate is moderately elevated in most patients and decreases as the disease becomes inactive. No serological tests have as yet been devised that are of significant help in making a diagnosis or prognosis.

TREATMENT

The general care and supervision of a child with tuberculosis require careful planning. Close liaison should be maintained between the physicians caring for adults and those caring for children in the same family. The pediatrician should work closely with members of the local department of health, including the public health nurses and social workers. To function properly, social investigation should be organized on a family basis.

Most children with asymptomatic or early initial infection do not require hospital or sanatorium care. They may lead an essentially unrestricted life. Asymptomatic children remaining at home should be shielded against the anxiety of parents. The usual immunizations are indicated, including measles vaccine after therapy has begun.

Antituberculous drugs

In the child whose contact is known, it is almost certain that the sensitivity pattern of the contact's isolate will be the same as that of the child. Therefore determining the sensitivity of the contact's isolate may guide therapy for the ~hild.

A combination of bactericidal drugs for initial therapy is usually used to prevent treatment failures and to prevent the emergence of resistant *M. tuberculosis*. The possibility that resistant organisms may be included in the population increases with the size of the population of infecting organisms. The number of bacilli present in a cavity is vastly greater than the number in a nodular lesion, and numbers of organisms in asymptomatic persons who are PPD reactive are fewer still. When the estimated number of organisms is very large, the use of three drugs is advisable. For other forms of symptomatic disease, two are usually sufficient unless there is reason to expect an increased chance that the child has acquired a drug-resistant infection (primary resistance) (Kopanoff et al., 1978).

Chemotherapy for childhood tuberculosis

The therapy for childhood tuberculosis has included a number of standard regimens that appear to have had a high degree of success. Many of these regimens reflect adult experience and have been only moderately well studied in children. There are drug regimens that are highly recommended for adults for which there have been virtually no reported trials involving children. The following comments and suggested regimens are based on a number of years of successful experience in children. Improved understanding of the use of newer drugs in children will undoubtedly lead to changes in accepted courses of therapy (Table 32-1).

The three bactericidal antituberculous drugs that are used in children and are considered *first line* are isoniazid (INH), rifampin, and streptomycin. Pyrazinamide has recently gained favor as therapy of severe disease in children and is considered the drug of first choice by some experts. Most courses of childhood tuberculosis, in which drug resistance is not proven or highly likely, are well managed by a combination of these drugs.

Isoniazid. Isoniazid remains the single most valued form of therapy and has been available for 40 years (Hsu, 1984). It is mycobactericidal and may be given orally, intravenously, or intramuscularly. It is inexpensive and may be administered as a single daily dose. It is distributed to all areas of the body. There are genetically determined racial differences in the rate of acetylation of isoniazid that may influence rates of adverse reaction to some extent but do not appear to influence the efficacy of therapy.

There is competitive inhibition by isoniazid of pyridoxine utilization, which leads to peripheral neuritis. Although this is most common in older adults, it may also occur in children who have deficient nutrition. Supplementation of the diet with pyridoxine will prevent the reaction, and the usual dose is approximately 1 mg pyridoxine for every 10 mg isoniazid prescribed.

The other major adverse reaction to isoniazid

Table 32-1. Preferred therapy of tuberculosis in children

Drug	Daily dose	Route of administration	Notes on adverse reactions
Isoniazid	10 to 20 mg/kg; 300 mg maximum may be given in one dose	PO IM IV	Peripheral neuritis, prevented by pyridoxine; hepatotoxicity; use with caution when combined with rifampin
Rifampin	15 to 20 mg/kg, 600 mg maximum	PO	Hepatotoxicity; orange staining of secretions; use with caution with isoniazid; gastric irritation
Streptomycin	20 to 30 mg/kg, 1 g maximum	IM	Eighth nerve damage; assay serum concentration if renal impairment present
Pyrazinamide	20 to 40 mg/kg, 2 g maximum	PO	Hepatotoxicity; hyperuricemia
Ethambutol	15 to 20 mg/kg	PO	Optic neuritis; for this reason, avoid in children less than 12 years old
Ethionamide	15 to 20 mg/kg	PO	Hepatotoxicity; gastric irritation

is hepatotoxicity (Spyridis et al., 1979). It is very rarely of clinical significance in children. Conditions that appear to enhance the hepatotoxicity of isoniazid include concomitant use of phenytoin and rifampin. The great majority of hepatotoxic isoniazid reactions are asymptomatic, involve minor degrees of hepatic enzyme elevations, and resolve with continued therapy. Rare but serious reactions, which may be life threatening, are associated with continued use of isoniazid (and/or rifampin) after the onset of symptomatic disease. For this reason, it is good practice to warn the parents of signs and symptoms of early isoniazid hepatotoxicity and instruct them to discontinue the use of isoniazid if these signs occur and to return to the clinic for evaluation.

Signs of isoniazid toxicity that are recognizable to a layman include the following:
1. Right upper abdominal aching or pain
2. Dark urine
3. Poor appetite or vomiting
4. Yellow sclera
5. Fever of 38.3° C (101° F) for 2 days or more

One of the purposes of monthly follow-up visits during therapy is to ensure that the parent understands the indications for discontinuing therapy and the reasons for ensuring compliance with medication. Routine monitoring of liver function is not recommended.

If isoniazid is prescribed alone, doses of 10 to 20 mg per kilogram of body weight per day are usual. Tablets of 100 and 300 mg are readily available; the tablet may be crushed and mixed with a tasty food. If isoniazid is given in a regimen also containing rifampin, the isoniazid dose should not exceed 10 mg per kilogram of body weight per day.

Rifampin. Rifampin is an orally absorbed, bactericidal antituberculous drug that is widely distributed throughout the body, including the CSF. It is highly effective against *M. tuberculosis*, especially when combined with isoniazid. It is relatively safe but rarely may cause hepatotoxicity. Rifampin may be administered to young children as a suspension in syrup or sprinkled over food such as applesauce. The drug is excreted in urine and bile and causes an orange discoloration of urine and tears. Rifampin causes staining of soft contact lenses and may render oral contraceptives ineffective.

Rifampin should be administered with another antituberculous drug for persons with clinically apparent disease. Particular alertness to hepatic toxicity when it is combined with isoniazid is important, and the dose of each when used in combination should not exceed 10 mg/kg/day isoniazid and 15 mg/kg/day rifampin.

Pyrazinamide. Experience with pyrazinamide is limited in children, but it lately has gained favor because of its attractive pharmacokinetic properties. Pyrazinamide is given orally at a dose of 20 to 40 mg/kg/day; although it is quite toxic at the higher doses used previously, hepatotoxicity rarely occurs in adults treated with this dose. The drug is widely distributed in the body, attaining therapeutic levels within CSF. It is concentrated within macrophages, thereby permitting accumulation of the drug at one potential site of bacterial intracellular survival. Pyrazinamide is one of the drugs of first choice for therapy of serious tuberculous infections in children. When pyrazinamide is combined with other bactericidal drugs, the duration of therapy can be shortened substantially.

Streptomycin. Streptomycin remains a first-line drug in the treatment of advanced cases of tuberculosis in children. It is bactericidal and is given intramuscularly. It is frequently used for 3 to 12 weeks to initiate therapy and is discontinued after the disease is fully controlled. The main adverse reaction is eighth nerve deafness. Monitoring of serum concentrations of streptomycin probably assists in preventing this complication. Peak serum concentrations of 20 to 30 μg/ml are the goal.

Other agents. Other antituberculous agents are far less frequently used. Para-aminosalicylic acid (PAS) is administered orally, is inexpensive, and is well tolerated by children. However, it is marginally effective, and large doses are required; therefore it is often bypassed. Ethambutol is a mainstay of adult regimens. However, the main complication, optic neuritis, is difficult to diagnose in children in early stages; thus many pediatricians refrain from its use unless the patient is a teenager or an older adolescent. Finally, ethionamide is an isoniazid congener and, like isoniazid, is bactericidal and widely distributed throughout the body. Isoniazid-resistant strains are usually ethionamide sensitive. It is well tolerated by children; the main form of adverse reaction is hepatotoxicity. It may be useful when isoniazid resistance is known or suspected. The remaining antituberculous agents that are available are used rarely in children.

Corticosteroids. The use of steroid hormones in persons with tuberculosis is contraindicated unless antituberculous drugs are given at the same time. Used judiciously in conjunction with antituberculous drugs, steroids can improve the prognosis in conditions in which inflammation adversely affects outcome. Some experts recommend the routine use of steroids in all cases of tuberculous meningitis; recent evidence suggests that their use decreases both morbidity and mortality (Girgis et al., 1991). Other conditions in which steroid therapy should be considered include severe miliary disease, endobronchial disease with obstruction, and when there is evidence of pleural or pericardial effusions.

Therapy of specific manifestations of tuberculosis. Recommendations for therapy of pulmonary and extrapulmonary tuberculosis in children have changed substantially over the past decade. Whereas a minimum of 12 months of therapy for uncomplicated pulmonary disease was recommended in the past, impressive results with "short-course" therapy in adults (Cohn et al., 1990) have encouraged an appraisal of its use in children (Abernathy et al., 1983; Snider et al., 1988; Starke, 1988). With the institution of therapy with three bactericidal drugs (isoniazid, rifampin, and pyrazinamide) for the first phase, the total duration of therapy often can be reduced to 6 months. This regimen has proven efficacious for therapy of pulmonary disease, hilar adenopathy, and extrapulmonary disease other than meningitis or miliary disease. For the latter, more severe manifestations of tuberculosis, a minimum of 12 months of therapy is mandated, with four bactericidal drugs (isoniazid, rifampin, pyrazinamide, and streptomycin) given for the initial 2 months.

Recommendations for therapy of tuberculosis in children are evolving rapidly as more information accumulates about the efficacy of the newer short-course regimens. The reader is encouraged to consult the latest edition of the "Report of the Committee on Infectious Diseases of the American Academy of Pediatrics" (the "Red Book") when initiating therapy.

PREVENTION

Tuberculosis occurs more frequently in urban than in rural populations. The new active case rate in the District of Columbia is 11 times that in Iowa. Within cities the death rate and the rate of newly reported cases are still highest in persons at the low end of the socioeconomic scale. Philadelphia had an overall new case rate of 49 per 100,000 population in 1973; in the extreme northeastern portion of the city, a middle-class area, the rate was 14 per 100,000, whereas West Philadelphia had a rate of 131 per 100,000.

Case finding surveys are most fruitful in groups with a high probability of tuberculous infection such as contacts of newly diagnosed cases of tuberculosis, residents of economically depressed areas of large cities, and indigent patients suffering from diseases such as silicosis and alcoholism that predispose them to tuberculosis. As the rate of infection has decreased, the use of tuberculin surveys with roentgenographic examination of the reactors has become the method of case finding. The object of discovering persons with active tuberculosis is not only to cure the patient by specific therapy but also to prevent spread to other individuals, especially children. Studies have shown that treated patients rarely infect their contacts, even in the home. The major risk of infection occurs before the index case is diagnosed.

Schedules for routine screening with tuberculin have changed over the past few decades. Currently, most children receive a PPD test at 1 year of age. Thereafter some children continue to receive yearly examinations, whereas others will not receive another unless they are being examined as part of a diagnostic workup. It is prudent to plan a schedule that takes account of the extent of tuberculous disease in the patient's environment. If the disease is rare, a PPD test at 1 year, at entrance to school, and during high school would be a satisfactory schedule. However, for many populations, it should remain a part of the yearly examination during early childhood.

Any plan for prevention of tuberculosis should be concerned particularly with children. In areas with a low rate of infection much of the active tuberculosis found in adults is due to reactivation of disease originally acquired in early life. The identification of children who are PPD reactive may furnish clues to previously unknown cases of active tuberculosis in adults.

Preventive therapy

Soon after isoniazid was introduced, it was noticed that meningitis did not develop in infected children who were receiving this therapy, even when they had miliary tuberculosis. In 1955, 2,750 children with positive tuberculin tests were randomly assigned to receive either isoniazid or placebo for 1 year. During a follow-up period of 10 years, the rate of complications in the group that received placebo was 30.2 per 1,000 children as compared with 3.6 per 1,000 children who received isoniazid. Thirty-one of the 41 complications in the placebo group occurred within the first year, including six cases of meningitis and one of miliary tuberculosis. There were no instances of meningitis or miliary tuberculosis in the group that received isoniazid.

Since that time the concept of *preventive therapy* has developed. Preventive therapy is applied to the prevention of tuberculosis in two primary settings.

The first primary setting involves the patient who has been exposed within a household or other close setting to a person with active pulmonary tuberculosis but is nonreactive to PPD. In this circumstance the physician cannot determine if the patient has not acquired the infection or if the patient is infected but has not yet manifested delayed hypersensitivity to tuberculin. Since some patients, especially children, may progress rapidly during the first weeks after infection, it is not safe merely to observe such a patient. Therefore persons at significant risk of having recently been infected but who are PPD nonreactive should receive preventive therapy. The usual choice of therapy is isoniazid, and the duration is 2 to 3 months. At the end of that time the patient may be retested with PPD. If he has remained PPD nonreactive and is no longer exposed to an active case, therapy may cease. If he has become PPD reactive, he should complete a full course of preventive therapy, which is 1 year in duration.

Preventive therapy with isoniazid is not efficacious if the strain is resistant to isoniazid. If that is the case, rifampin is usually used in a similar regimen, but clinical studies concerning the efficacy of rifampin for prophylaxis have not been conducted.

Some health departments exclude children from their protocols for administration of preventive therapy. However, the precepts of preventive therapy apply with particular urgency to children, who are at increased risk of progressive tuberculosis compared to adults. The pediatrician should ensure that the children who are in contact with an infected adult receive adequate prophylaxis.

Other settings in which preventive therapy of PPD-nonreactive persons may be indicated include institutional outbreaks of tuberculosis and any closed setting in which it has been found that the development of disease or delayed hypersensitivity is occurring in several persons.

The other common setting in which preventive therapy is indicated is for the patient who is clinically well, has normal or minimal changes in the chest roentgenogram, and is PPD reactive. In this instance, if the patient is a child, a full course of preventive therapy should be planned, which would usually be isoniazid, 10 mg per kilogram of body weight per day, for 1 year. Persons who are particularly likely to progress to active disease include those who are very young, who have become infected within the past year, and who become immunosuppressed as a result of malignant disease, use of adrenocorticosteroids, or other illnesses such as measles.

When a positive tuberculin test is associated with tuberculous disease, delayed hypersensitivity ordinarily persists for many years, even if the disease has responded well to specific therapy. In contrast are those children whose only evidence of tuberculosis is delayed hypersensitivity to tuberculin. When they are retested a few years after the original reaction, it is not uncommon to find reversion of the tuberculin test to negative.

Bacille Calmette-Guérin vaccination

Bacille Calmette-Guérin (BCG), live attenuated strains of a related mycobacterium, has been used as a vaccine for over 50 years (Centers for Disease Control, 1979). It produces a varying degree of immunity to infection with virulent tubercle bacilli. Although the immunity is not complete and superinfections with human *M. tuberculosis* can occur, the illness is moderated and rarely progressive. The most important benefit of BCG vaccination is that the risk of disseminated disease is markedly diminished; both miliary tuberculosis and meningitis usually can be prevented by vaccination.

In the United States Rosenthal et al. (1961) reported a 74% reduction of morbidity in BCG-vaccinated children. Trials in Puerto Rico and in Georgia demonstrated that BCG was only approximately 30% effective in these populations.

A study very similar in design and execution, conducted by the British Medical Research Council among adolescents, reported that the vaccine was more than 80% effective. The discrepancies in results may be due to variations in the vaccine strains but are probably also related to prior subclinical infections with atypical acid-fast bacilli. In experimental animals atypical mycobacteria have the capacity to modify the course of subsequent infection with tubercle bacilli.

In the United States there are families in which tuberculosis is uncontrolled and active, and BCG vaccination may provide the wisest form of protection for some children (Kendig, 1969). The majority of PPD reactions within 1 year or more after BCG vaccination are less than 10 mm in diameter. Reactions larger than that are likely to represent infection with *M. tuberculosis*, and the child should be assessed accordingly. A very small number of deaths caused by BCG vaccination have been reported. They have mainly occurred in patients with immunodeficiency disorders. Since millions of children have been vaccinated, the procedure may be regarded as relatively safe.

CLINICAL SPECTRUM OF TUBERCULOSIS
Classification

The classification of tuberculous disease has undergone many revisions, and the literature is burdened with terms that have changed meaning with changing understanding of the disease process. In the 1970s the American Thoracic Society proposed a classification that is compatible with the disease in both children and adults. This classification is based on the patient's history of exposure, tuberculin reaction, symptomatic state, location of apparent disease, and treatment, and is as follows:

0. No tuberculosis exposure, not infected (no history of exposure, negative tuberculin skin test)
I. Tuberculosis exposure, no evidence of infection (history of exposure, negative tuberculin skin test)
II. Tuberculous infection, without disease (positive tuberculin skin test, negative bacteriological studies, no roentgenographic findings compatible with tuberculosis, no symptom caused by tuberculosis)

Chemotherapy status (preventive therapy)
A. None
B. On chemotherapy since (date)
C. Chemotherapy terminated (date)
   1. Complete (prescribed course of therapy)
   2. Incomplete
III. Tuberculosis: infected, with disease. The current status of the patient's tuberculosis shall be described by the following characteristics:
A. Location of disease
   1. Pulmonary
   2. Pleural
   3. Lymphatic
   4. Bone or joint
   5. Genitourinary
   6. Miliary
   7. Meningeal
   8. Peritoneal
   9. Other
   The predominant site shall be listed for each patient. Other sites may also be listed if significant. More precise anatomical sites may be specified.
B. Bacteriological status
   1. Positive by
      a. Microscopy only (date)
      b. Culture only (date)
      c. Microscopy and culture (date)
   2. Negative (date)
   3. Pending
   4. Not done
C. Chemotherapy status
   1. None
   2. On chemotherapy since (date)
   3. Chemotherapy terminated (date)
      a. Complete (prescribed course of therapy)
      b. Incomplete
D. Roentgenographic findings
   1. Normal
   2. Abnormal
      a. Cavitary or noncavitary
      b. Stable or worsening or improving
E. Tuberculin skin test
   1. Positive reaction
   2. Doubtful reaction
   3. Negative reaction
   4. Not done

Tuberculosis suspect: patients may be so classified until diagnostic procedures are complete. This classification should not be used for more than 3 months.

Tuberculous infection without disease

Asymptomatic primary infection is tuberculous infection in which the child is tuberculin reactive but has no apparent clinical illness and a normal or minimally abnormal roentgenogram of the chest. This condition may occur very early in an illness in which the child will progress to active disease or may remain quiescent and heal. Infants are most likely to have progressive disease, but over 80% of children who are more than 4 years of age and have not reached puberty will not progress. Adolescence is another period in which progression of primary disease is likely to occur. In any event, preventive therapy should be instituted.

Tuberculous infection with disease

Almost all cases of tuberculous disease in children are first (primary) infections. The incubation period of primary tuberculosis varies from 2 to 8 weeks. During this period the skin test is nonreactive. Tubercle bacilli may be cultured from material obtained by gastric lavage during the prereactive period before any changes appear on a chest roentgenogram. The usual mode of onset of the initial tuberculous infection is insidious. The patient, especially an infant, often has signs or symptoms of an infection of the upper respiratory tract that appear at the same time as the fever. Except for the anorexia and lassitude that can accompany any fever, there are no other symptoms associated with the onset of primary tuberculosis. Erythema nodosum can appear concomitantly with the fever of onset, but today this finding is infrequent. Abnormal physical findings from the pulmonary examination are rare even when an extensive lesion is seen on the roentgenogram.

Occasionally the onset of the initial pulmonary infection may be pneumonic, resembling lobar pneumonia, with fever, rapid respiratory rate, signs of dullness, bronchial breath sounds, and moist rales. These signs and symptoms often subside in a few days to 2 weeks. The WBC count, if it has been elevated, returns to a normal range, the abnormal physical signs disappear, and the child seems to have recovered from the acute illness. The roentgenogram, however, continues to show parenchymal infiltrates and enlargement of mediastinal nodes (Fig. 32-2). This type of onset, if associated with a nontuberculous pneumonia, may respond initially to antimicrobial therapy.

Course. There is nothing diagnostic about the appearance of a child with initial tuberculous infection. If the pulmonary lesion progresses locally or if there is marked progression by the lymphohematogenous route, the child will experience a period of illness that usually resolves. In a few weeks, if treatment has not begun, afternoon fevers ensue. In a large percentage of older children with primary pulmonary tuberculosis, the initial lesion remains localized and causes no major symptoms or signs, and even without specific therapy the fever is unlikely to continue more than 2 to 3 months. Alternately, the pulmonary component of the primary complex may progress locally, in which case extension into the bronchi produces disseminated areas of tuberculous pneumonia.

In the early stage of bronchial involvement infants often have a harsh expiratory cough. Older children usually have no cough, even when extensive disease is present. Small infants may have respiratory distress, especially during an intercurrent infection. Occasionally the clinical picture may be indistinguishable from nonspecific laryngotracheobronchitis. Transient wheezes or rhonchi are often heard, especially in infants. Bronchoscopic studies have shown that tuberculous bronchitis may persist for months or years, even in patients receiving specific therapy, and bronchiectasis has been a sequel of tuberculous bronchitis in many patients.

Roentgenographic appearance. The initial complex may appear on the roentgenogram at the time of onset or it may be inapparent. Parenchymal infiltrates that appear weeks or months after onset usually represent segmental obstruction or nontuberculous infection. In the adolescent or adult, new infiltrates may be due to chronic pulmonary tuberculosis. The appearance of the initial focus may vary from a round area less than 2 cm in diameter to one that occupies an entire lobe. Regardless of its size at onset there is usually little change for at least 3 months, after which the area of involvement may begin to diminish gradually. Infiltrates persisting for 2 years or longer are not rare.

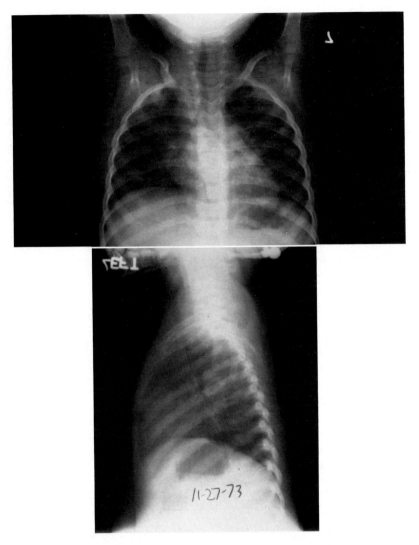

Fig. 32-2. Roentgenographic findings from a child with asymptomatic recent onset of pulmonary tuberculosis, demonstrating hilar and paratracheal adenopathy.

A primary focus without enlarged regional lymph nodes is rare, but enlarged lymph nodes without apparent parenchymal infiltrates are common. Hilar adenopathy may be the only roentgenographic evidence of tuberculosis and is best identified in a lateral view in which the nodes may form a rounded mass obscuring the bronchial bifurcation. Enlarged carinal nodes, often associated with foci in the lower lobes, are seen most easily in an oblique or a lateral view. The mass of nodes around the bifurcation may be so large that it displaces the heart and mediastinum.

In patients who have received antimicrobial therapy, calcification rarely is seen in the area of the parenchymal focus unless treatment was begun after the occurrence of extensive caseation necrosis. Calcification occurs more often in lymph nodes than in pulmonary foci. The usual minimal interval between infection and calcification in an older child is 1 year and in an adolescent or young adult may be longer than 5 years.

Differential diagnosis. The differential diagnosis of tuberculosis includes mycotic infections such as histoplasmosis and blastomycosis. Local epidemiological patterns may be helpful. The clinical and roentgenographic picture of locally progressive pulmonary tuberculosis may be confused with that of staphylococcal pneumonia in the infant or lung abscess in the older child. Biopsy or bronchoscopic examination may be required for causative diagnosis. The results of a tuberculin test also help distinguish between enlargement of the hilar nodes caused by tuberculosis and similar findings in sarcoidosis, Hodgkin's disease, or chronic pneumonia.

Hematogenous tuberculosis

Generalized tuberculosis in children may be caused by three types of hematogenous spread: (1) an occult dissemination in which clinical manifestations may or may not occur; (2) a single generalized dissemination that usually causes acute disease; and (3) repeated or protracted dissemination.

Occult hematogenous tuberculosis. The dissemination of a small number of tubercle bacilli through the blood early in the course of the first infection with tuberculosis has been termed *occult hematogenous tuberculosis*. Most of the dissemination takes place during the incubation period and for a short time after onset of disease, and it is unlikely to continue after hypersensitivity to tuberculin has been established. The bacilli are most commonly seeded to the apices of the lungs, the liver and spleen, and the superficial lymph nodes. Clinical manifestations during this episode usually last only a few days and are mild.

Acute miliary tuberculosis. Miliary tuberculosis is a complication of tuberculous infection that usually occurs within the first 6 months after onset of infection. All tubercles resulting from an acute generalized hematogenous spread are approximately the same size and are often the size of millet seed. The pulmonary infiltrates seen on the roentgenogram may be so small that they are barely visible.

An abrupt rise in temperature usually heralds the onset of miliary tuberculosis. Infiltrates become visible on the roentgenogram approximately 1 to 3 weeks after onset of fever. At this time there usually are no respiratory symptoms and no abnormal physical signs in the lungs. If diagnosis and treatment are delayed, fine rales may be heard, and dyspnea and cyanosis may develop. Enlargement of the liver, spleen, and superficial lymph nodes has occurred in approximately half of the children at the time of diagnosis. Choroid tubercles may occur but, in

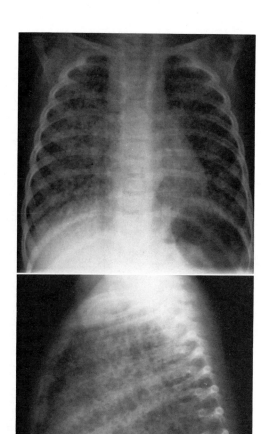

Fig. 32-3. Roentgenographic findings from a 6-month-old child with miliary tuberculosis. Note the nodular appearance and uniform size of the lesions. (Courtesy Drs. G. Gaisie and W. Clyde, University of North Carolina, Chapel Hill, N.C.)

spite of an intensive search, are found in only approximately 13% of tuberculous children. Specific therapy for miliary tuberculosis may prevent meningitis, but many patients are initially seen with both conditions.

Roentgenographic appearance. The even distribution of infiltrates throughout both lung fields is the most characteristic feature of the roentgenogram. Segmental obstruction, if present, produces the appearance of discrete areas of pneumonia. Examination of lateral views will usually reveal an equal distribution of tubercles over the entire lung fields. The lesions may resemble multiple nodules (Fig. 32-3).

Diagnosis. The PPD is nonreactive in many children who have miliary tuberculosis. If the tuberculin test is positive and if there is no roentgenographic evidence of miliary tuberculosis, the roentgenogram should be repeated frequently. Choroidal tubercles, if present, may be of great diagnostic importance (Olazábal, 1967). When they occur, however, they often do not appear until several weeks after the onset of miliary tuberculosis.

Culture of blood, bone marrow, or other tissue may confirm the diagnosis eventually, but these positive findings are obtained too late to help establish the initial diagnosis. Biopsy of the liver or bone marrow may be of greater value in achieving a rapid diagnosis.

Prognosis. In the preantibiotic era miliary tuberculosis was usually fatal within 3 months; most untreated children developed meningitis. The use of antituberculous therapy has improved the prognosis. Most treated patients recover if they are not moribund when first diagnosed.

COMPLICATIONS
Chronic pulmonary tuberculosis

Chronic tuberculosis is very uncommon in children; less than 5% of patients younger than 15 years old develop this form of pulmonary tuberculosis. Most cases of pulmonary tuberculosis of the adult type (chronic pulmonary tuberculosis) are caused by endogenous pulmonary reinfection or extension from a focus that was established during the initial bacteremic phase of primary disease and differs markedly from primary tuberculosis. Chronic pulmonary tuberculosis usually remains confined to the lung; unlike the initial infection, it does not represent the onset of a systemic disease.

The risk of developing chronic pulmonary tuberculosis increases during adolescence and develops generally within 1 or 2 years after the initial infection. When the date of conversion of the tuberculin test is known, the relatively short interval between initial infection and chronic pulmonary tuberculosis that can often be demonstrated suggests that many instances of chronic pulmonary tuberculosis, especially in young adults, represent local progression of initial disease. Evidence of early chronic pulmonary tuberculosis is most commonly seen roentgenographically above or below the clavicle in one or both lungs. Most small lesions in children and adolescents are unstable and tend to progress. Oblique and lordotic views may be valuable, and films made in expiration may help to uncover an apical focus. Frank hemoptysis is practically never seen in children and adolescents.

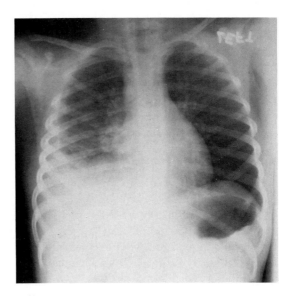

Fig. 32-4. Roentgenographic findings from a child with recent onset of pulmonary tuberculosis complicated by pleural effusion.

Pleural effusion

Pleural effusion is diagnosed in approximately 8% of children with initial pulmonary tuberculosis; two thirds of the cases of pleural effusion develop within 6 months of the onset of the primary disease. The complication occurs twice as frequently in boys as in girls and more often in children of school age than in younger children. Pleural effusion in children may occur as an extension from a subpleural primary focus, or the pleural lesion may result from hematogenous seeding to the pleura (Fig. 32-4). The onset of disease is occasionally insidious but more often is accompanied by fever and chest pain that is increased by deep breathing. The patient remains febrile for 1 to 2 weeks, followed by a gradual defervescence. By the end of the third week the temperature is usually normal, and most of the fluid has been absorbed.

The diagnosis of tuberculous pleural effusion is suggested by a positive tuberculin test, examination of the pleural fluid, or history. The diagnosis is confirmed by recovery of tubercle bacilli on culture from pleural fluid or from material obtained by pleural biopsy or by histological examination of biopsy material. Most often the fluid is clear, but occasionally it is slightly cloudy, and rarely it is frankly hemorrhagic. The albumin content is increased, and the WBC count is highly variable with a predominance of lymphocytes. Tubercle bacilli are recovered by culture in approximately 50% of cases. Needle biopsies of the parietal pleura show typical tubercles in approximately 60% of cases, and cultures of tissues obtained by this method also yield tubercle bacilli in most cases.

The immediate and long-term outlook for children with tuberculous pleural effusion has always been good. In untreated children the incidence of chronic pulmonary tuberculosis in later life was no greater than in those who never had this complication. Moderate to severe scoliosis developed in 5% of children with untreated tuberculous pleurisy, but few instances have been seen since the advent of chemotherapy. Thoracenteses that remove large amounts of fluid at one time or repeated thoracenteses for drainage of pleural fluid are not advised because the fluid will resolve during therapy. Arm and shoulder exercises designed to prevent scoliosis should be started.

Tuberculous meningitis

Meningitis is the most serious complication of tuberculosis (Lincoln et al., 1960; Sumaya et al., 1975); it is the most common cause of death from tuberculosis in childhood. Tuberculous meningitis was almost always fatal before effective therapy was available. Today it can be cured in at least 9 out of 10 patients, but complete neurological recovery in children depends to a large extent on early diagnosis followed by prompt and prolonged therapy. During the preantibiotic era the average course of meningitis from first symptom to death was only 19 days. Knowledge of the pathogenesis of meningitis helps in diagnosis and interpretation of the early physical signs and early changes in the CSF.

Pathogenesis. Tubercle bacilli that lodge in the cerebral cortex behave as metastatic foci; a caseous lesion forms that increases in size until it reaches the overlying meninges and infects

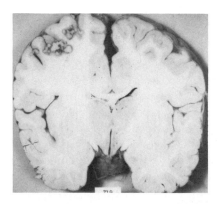

Fig. 32-5. Cerebral granulomas found at autopsy in a patient with tuberculous meningitis. Extension of the intracerebral focus to the CSF probably occurred first and developed into meningeal disease.

the subarachnoid space (Fig. 32-5). Sometimes the tuberculous focus may discharge caseous material and bacilli into the ventricular fluid, causing fulminating meningitis. Usually the infection of the meninges is gradual. Even in this early stage of meningeal involvement, examination of the CSF usually shows some deviations from normal.

A caseous focus may form, become encapsulated, and form a tuberculoma to produce symptoms simulating a brain tumor. A quiescent lesion may be activated by trauma or by an intercurrent systemic infection such as measles. The caseous focus that drains into the subarachnoid space may originate not only in the cortex, meninges, or choroid plexus but also in the bones enclosing the central nervous system (CNS). Thus tuberculous meningitis may also be due to direct extension from tuberculous mastoiditis or spondylitis.

Meningitis is an early complication of primary or miliary tuberculosis, usually developing within 6 months of the onset of infection. The first symptoms appear within 4 months of the estimated date of onset of tuberculosis in 40% of the cases. Fig. 32-6 demonstrates a tuberculous focus in a patient with miliary tuberculosis, shown by contrast-enhanced, computer-assisted tomographic scan.

The greatest involvement of the meninges is that surrounding the brain stem. The exudate at the base of the brain may cause obstruction of the basal cisterns, leading to hydrocephalus. Involvement of cerebral arteries and veins is

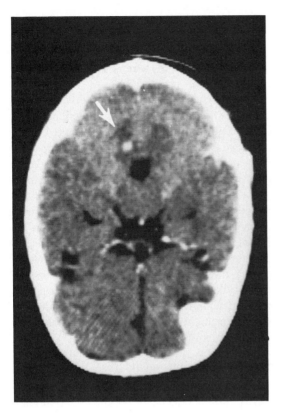

Fig. 32-6. Contrast-enhanced, computer-assisted tomographic identification of focal cerebral granuloma in a child with miliary tuberculosis and minimal abnormalities in cerebrospinal fluid examination.

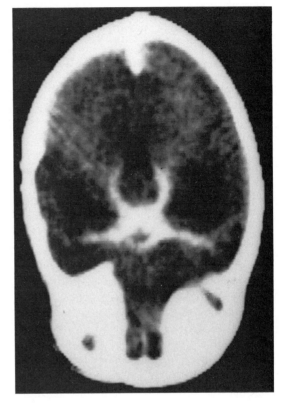

Fig. 32-7. Contrast-enhanced, computer-assisted tomographic visualization of the basilar view of the head, recording the extent of inflammatory activity in a child with advanced tuberculous meningitis.

common, and acute tuberculous arteritis may cause occlusion of the vessels with resulting severe neurological sequelae such as hemiparesis and seizure disorders.

The signs and symptoms of tuberculous meningitis often can be related to pathological changes in the CNS. The involvement of the cranial nerves is due to the exudate at the base of the brain (Fig. 32-7). Exudate or edema around the optic nerve causes visual disturbances in which changes in the optic discs are usually found. Impairment of extraocular muscles is common. Hemipareses usually result from cerebral involvement secondary to vascular changes. Neurological signs may be transient if they are due to cerebral edema or if the vascular lesion causing them can be reversed by therapy. If the area of infarction is large, the deficits may be permanent.

The onset of tuberculous meningitis is usually insidious. Fever, vomiting, and apathy are the most striking symptoms. Approximately 20% of

patients have infections of the upper respiratory tract at the time of onset of the meningitis, many with evidence of otitis media. Children over 4 years of age often complain of headache and abdominal pain.

The course of meningitis is classically divided into three stages. The initial stage of general symptoms lasts approximately a week. The second stage of neurological involvement may start abruptly with drowsiness, some resistance to neck flexion, sluggish pupillary reactions, strabismus, ptosis, positive Kernig's or Brudzinski's sign, absent abdominal reflexes, or increased deep tendon reflexes. In spite of drowsiness, patients usually respond to stimuli. Occasionally patients in the second stage have no evidence of meningeal irritation, but they develop signs or symptoms of encephalitis such as confusion, disorientation, slurred speech, grimacing, chewing, athetoid movements of the extremities, or peripheral tremors. Funduscopic examination is usually normal. Patients in the third

Table 32-2. Diagnostic findings in recent studies of tuberculous meningitis in children

Finding	Cases (%)
History of exposure to case with active tuberculosis	40-69
Abnormal roentgenogram of chest	44-88
Reaction to intermediate PPD <10 mm	6-48
CSF cell predominance of polymorphonuclear leukocytes	14-27
Papilledema	9-33
Cranial nerve palsies	12-13
Normal CSF glucose	13-22

stage of meningitis are usually unresponsive and exhibit neurological signs such as opisthotonos, decerebrate rigidity, marked irregular respirations, hemipareses, and cranial nerve palsies. Obstructive hydrocephalus may develop even during optimal therapy. The CSF is frequently xanthochromic, and the protein content is usually greater than 300 mg/dl of spinal fluid.

Diagnosis. Tuberculous meningitis usually is seen in children who have not previously been diagnosed as having tuberculosis. Diagnosis during the first stage depends largely on the family or social history indicating the possibility of tuberculosis, appreciation of the importance of a history of marked apathy or drowsiness, and administration of a tuberculin test. Many children with tuberculous meningitis react to tuberculin, and many children who develop meningitis have evidence of tuberculosis on chest roentgenogram. However, both of these findings may be absent (Table 32-2).

The characteristic CSF is clear with WBC counts ranging from 10 to 350 cells/mm³, predominantly lymphocytes or monocytes. Occasionally the initial count may be as high as 1,000 cells/mm³, predominantly polymorphonuclear leukocytes, and the glucose concentration may be decreased (<40 mg/dl), particularly in disease of longer duration. The protein content of the spinal fluid is usually above normal and increases on successive examinations. The chloride content of the fluid is frequently below normal in the second or third stage of meningitis but may be normal in the first stage. Tubercle bacilli often can be found on direct smear of CSF sediment but usually only after a meticulous search. In most patients tubercle bacilli can be recovered on culture. Confirmation of the diagnosis by this means is always desirable, but treatment should never be deferred pending the results of culture if there is reason to suspect this diagnosis.

Early in the second stage of tuberculous meningitis, differentiation from other infections by evaluation of the CSF may be difficult, but the decreasing glucose and increasing protein content may help distinguish tuberculous meningitis from viral encephalomyelitis, lead encephalopathy and brain tumors. Treatment may occasionally be begun while the diagnosis is being pursued since there is a close correlation between the prognosis and the stage of the disease at which treatment is initiated. Children treated during the first stage of meningitis almost invariably survive, often without significant sequelae, whereas children first treated after severe neurological changes have occurred are at great risk of a poor or fatal outcome.

Serous tuberculous meningitis

Serous meningitis is a clinical entity that resolves spontaneously; it occurs in tuberculous children who develop signs or symptoms that suggest tuberculous meningitis. This diagnosis was of great importance before specific therapy was available because the favorable prognosis was in marked contrast to that of true tuberculous meningitis. The differential diagnosis is less important today because all forms of active tuberculosis receive specific therapy.

Tuberculoma

Tuberculomas of the brain or spinal cord are isolated foci of active tuberculosis. Like other foci they may produce symptoms within a short period after initial infection, or they may remain silent for a time and later cause caseous meningitis or serous meningitis. Many tuberculomas are diagnosed as intracranial neoplasms.

Tuberculosis of the skeletal system

In most instances complications in the bones or joints appear early in infection and afflict approximately 4% of children with tuberculosis. In children who receive antituberculous therapy the risk of late skeletal complications has all but vanished. As with other complications, tuberculosis of the skeletal system usually results from early hematogenous dissemination of tubercle bacilli. Spondylitis may be due to lymphatic drainage from another area of tuberculosis such as pleura or kidney. Spondylitis is rare in infants, and dactylitis occurs almost exclusively in infants.

Skeletal infection usually begins in the metaphyseal portions of the epiphyses, and the necrotic process may invade the surrounding tissue to form cold abscesses that often appear at points far from their sources. The destruction may involve only the bone, but often it extends through the epiphysis into the capsule of the joint. The spine is the most common site of tuberculous bone involvement, followed, in order of frequency, by the hip and the knee. Dactylitis of the hands and feet is now uncommon. Multiple bony lesions are seen in disseminated forms of tuberculosis, especially in protracted hematogenous tuberculosis. Occasionally biopsy for culture or pathological examination may be indicated to confirm the diagnosis.

In tuberculosis of the spine (Pott's disease) the infection usually begins in the vertebral body. Destruction of the vertebral bodies may result in collapse, producing a kyphotic deformity (gibbus) and narrowing of the intervertebral space. Rigidity of the spine is due to muscular spasm from the resulting pain. Pain is a more prominent symptom of tuberculosis of the joints. It is usually localized to the involved joint and is increased by motion.

Local disability and referred pain often respond rapidly to therapy. Until pain on motion in the affected area is no longer present, some degree of rest is indicated. When treatment is given early, relatively little destruction of bone occurs. The need for surgical fusion in spondylitis has almost been eliminated by antituberculous drug therapy.

Tuberculosis of the superficial lymph nodes

Infection of the superficial lymph nodes was formerly the most common complication of tuberculosis in children. Cervical adenitis was believed to represent the regional adenopathy of tuberculosis of the tonsils, but this portal of entry is now very rare. In most instances generalized adenitis is an early hematogenous complication of tuberculosis. Excluding the patients with extrapulmonary primary tuberculosis, most persons with superficial adenitis of tuberculous origin also have pulmonary roentgenographic evidence of tuberculosis. If the diagnosis is otherwise in doubt, a biopsy may be done.

At the present time in the United States, adenitis of the superficial cervical nodes is far more likely caused by atypical acid-fast bacilli than to *M. tuberculosis*. The main findings differentiating between atypical mycobacterial infection and tuberculosis of the lymph nodes are tuberculin reactivity, history of contact with tuberculous persons, chest roentgenogram, response to antituberculous therapy, and results of cultures.

In patients with atypical mycobacteriosis the tuberculin test is usually indeterminate (5 to 9 mm) or weakly positive (10 to 12 mm). This is especially true in the southeastern portion of the United States where atypical mycobacterial colonization and disease are very prevalent. The chest roentgenogram is normal, whereas most children with tuberculous adenitis show evidence of pulmonary infection. In cervical adenitis caused by atypical bacilli, the nodes that are most often involved are those at the angle of the jaw, the submental group, and those in the preauricular area. The recovery of bacilli by culture from a specimen obtained by a needle biopsy or from material obtained from surgical resection is desirable to confirm the diagnosis. Pathological examination of biopsy material from both conditions shows findings that are identical. Although atypical mycobacteria seldom are sensitive to isoniazid, a course of therapy with isoniazid and rifampin for several months may be tried.

Antibiotic therapy directed toward possible pyogenic infection may be initiated for treatment of cervical adenitis. A favorable response within 1 to 2 weeks is consistent with the diagnosis of a nontuberculous infection. If the lymph nodes remain unchanged or increase in size, an aspirate or excision may be indicated. If nodal excision is done before the overlying skin has become involved, there should be no difficulty with wound healing. The biopsy provides material for pathological examination and culture.

Tuberculosis of the tonsils and adenoids, larynx, middle ear, and mastoids. Tuberculosis of a tonsil can result from infection caused by contact with material containing tubercle bacilli. This route of infection was important when the incidence of bovine tuberculosis was high and milk was not pasteurized, but it is now extremely rare in the United States. Tuberculous infection of the larynx is usually caused by infectious sputum in adolescents and adults who have chronic pulmonary tuberculosis.

The onset of tuberculous middle ear and mastoid disease is without pain or fever. Discharge from the ear canal and deafness are early symptoms (Skolnik et al., 1986). Facial paralysis develops more often in tuberculous otitis media than in other chronic infections of the middle ear. Infection of the labyrinth is also more common than in purulent infections, but it develops so gradually that symptoms are uncommon, even when function is destroyed.

Tuberculosis of the abdomen. Peritonitis may be localized, in which case it is called *plastic peritonitis* (Jakubowski et al., 1988). This most often results from direct extension of infection from lymph nodes or may originate from tuberculous salpingitis. In early cases there may be a small amount of loculated fluid. If the disease process is unchecked, the omentum becomes attached by adhesions and forms a mass in the epigastrium. The onset of peritonitis may be insidious, with low-grade fever as the only symptom. Occasionally the first symptoms are those of partial intestinal obstruction, vomiting, and pain. The lymph nodes and the surrounding exudate often can be palpated as irregular tender masses with a characteristic doughy feeling. Efforts to confirm the diagnosis by paracentesis incur the risk of perforating the intestine if it has adhered to the abdominal wall.

Generalized peritonitis with effusion may be due to direct extension from an initial infection in the gastrointestinal tract, but such instances are rare in the United States. The ascites also may result from hematogenous spread of the bacilli. The fluid increases rapidly, and a patient with a scaphoid abdomen may develop a tense, rounded abdomen within 48 hours. In children ascites apparently is an early complication.

Tuberculous enteritis was formerly a sequela of advanced pulmonary tuberculous disease in adults and adolescents. Its usual location is the lower half of the jejunum, the ileum, and the cecum. The disease apparently is acquired by superinfection of the mucosa with tubercle bacilli from swallowed sputum. Shallow ulcers produce pain and diarrhea alternating with constipation. Fistulas from the gastrointestinal tract may develop if therapy is neglected.

Tuberculosis of the skin

Extensive tuberculous disease of the skin such as progressive lupus vulgaris has always been rare in the United States. Cutaneous manifestations fall into two groups. The disease may be either localized, resulting from direct contact with tubercle bacilli, or have scattered lesions caused by dissemination through the bloodstream or lymphatics. In addition to tuberculous infection of the skin, other nonspecific skin conditions such as erythema nodosum are manifestations of tuberculosis as well as of other diseases.

Tuberculosis of the eye

The conjunctiva and cornea are the usual sites of tuberculous eye disease in children. Most often the organisms reach the eye by bacteremic spread. However, inoculation of *M. tuberculosis* into the conjunctiva can be caused by a cough or sneeze from a tuberculous individual or by inoculation of the bacilli on contaminated hands. A few yellowish gray nodules that resemble the early nodular lesions of trachoma may be found on the palpebral conjunctiva. When the nodules coalesce, a small ulcer is formed.

The lesions of phlyctenular conjunctivitis are small, grayish, jellylike nodules usually seen on the limbus and accompanied by injection of the blood vessels of the adjacent conjunctiva. They do not contain tubercle bacilli and are considered phenomena of hypersensitivity to tuberculin that occur in the initial stage of tuberculosis.

Tuberculosis of the endocrine and exocrine glands

Isolated instances of tuberculosis of the thyroid, parotid, pineal, and pituitary glands and of the thymus, pancreas, ovary, and testis have been observed. The adrenal is the gland in which tuberculosis has been diagnosed most frequently antemortem. Approximately 100 proved cases have been reported in children and many more in adults. The peak age incidence of Addison's disease is at approximately 30 years. Formerly it usually was caused by tuberculosis, but at present tuberculosis of the adrenal glands is rarely encountered.

Tuberculosis of the genital tract

The genital tract may be the portal of entry of tuberculous infection, but seeding through the blood or from a contiguous focus of active disease may also occur. The most common ev-

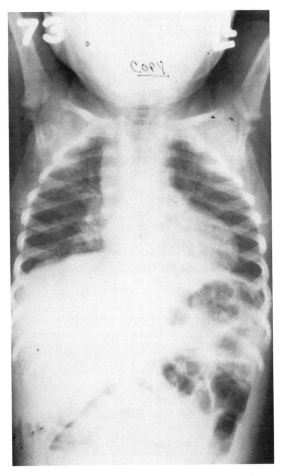

Fig. 32-8. Roentgenographic findings from a child with pulmonary tuberculosis complicated by pericardial effusion. Pericardiocentesis revealed serosanguineous fluid from which *M. tuberculosis* was not isolated.

idence of genital tuberculosis in boys is epididymitis (Gorse and Belshe, 1985). The nodular and painless or slightly painful enlargement is usually discovered in the course of a physical examination (Cabral et al., 1985). Tuberculosis of the fallopian tubes is the most common form of genital involvement in females and is often associated with some degree of endometritis, especially in women.

Tuberculosis of the urinary tract

Renal tuberculosis can occur at any age but is mainly a disease of young adults. Tuberculous disease of the kidney usually stems from hematogenous dissemination of bacilli to the cortex of the kidney, very often during the initial infection. Tubercle bacilli have been recovered

from the urine of children during occult hematogenous dissemination and from the urine of persons with miliary tuberculosis. Bacilluria indicates a focus of active disease, although it may originate in a single caseous tubercle. When renal tuberculosis progresses, the necrosis usually results in fistulous tracts leading into the pelvis of the kidney. The infection may spread through the ureter into the bladder. In males the prostate and epididymis may be involved.

In children who are not known to have tuberculosis, renal disease is usually first suggested by persistent pyuria from which no organisms can be cultured by routine methods. Common additional findings are albuminuria and hematuria. A urological examination is necessary to define the site and extent of renal and ureteral involvement. The earliest changes are usually in the upper or lower calyces in which there may be an irregularity caused by the erosion of the parenchyma. Cavities may be seen in patients with more advanced disease (Smith and Lattimer, 1973).

Tuberculous pericarditis

This complication is also usually the result of hematogenous dissemination to the pericardium, is most common in older children, and, if advanced, may lead to restrictive compromise of cardiac function (Fig. 32-8).

REFERENCES

Abernathy RS, Dutt AK, Stead WW, et al. Short-course chemotherapy for tuberculosis in children. Pediatrics 1983;72:801.

American Lung Association. Diagnostic standards and classification of tuberculosis and other mycobacterial diseases. New York: The Association, 1974.

American Thoracic Society. Preventive therapy of tuberculous infection. Am Rev Respir Dis 1974;110:371.

Armstrong JA, D'Arcy Hart P. Phagosome-lysosome interactions in cultured macrophages infected with virulent tubercle bacilli. Reversal of the usual nonfusion pattern and observations on bacterial survival. J Exp Med 1975;142:1.

Barksdale L, Kimm KS. Mycobacterium. Bacteriol Rev 1977;41:217.

Brickman HF, Beaudry PH, Marks MI. The timing of tuberculin tests in relation to immunization with live viral vaccines. Pediatrics 1975;55:392.

Brooks SM, Lassiter NL, Young EC. A pilot study concerning the infection risk of sputum positive tuberculous patients on chemotherapy. Am Rev Respir Dis 1973;108:799.

Cabral DA, Johnson HW, Coleman GU, et al. Tuberculous epididymitis as a cause of testicular pseudomalignancy in two young children. Pediatr Infect Dis 1985;4:59.

Centers for Disease Control. BCG vaccines. MMWR 1979;28:241.

Chaisson RE, Slutkin G. Tuberculosis and human immunodeficiency virus infection. J Infect Dis 1989;159:96.

Christensen WI. Genitourinary tuberculosis: review of 102 cases. Medicine 1974;53:377.

Cohn DL, Catlin BJ, Peterson KL, et al. A 62-dose, 6-month therapy for pulmonary and extrapulmonary tuberculosis. Ann Intern Med 1990;112:407.

Comstock GW. Frost revisited: the modern epidemiology of tuberculosis. Am J Epidemiol 1975;101:363.

Comstock GW, Livesay VT, Woolpert SF. The prognosis of a positive tuberculin reaction in childhood and adolescence. Am J Epidemiol 1974;99:141.

Dahlstrom G, Sjogren I. Side-effects of BCG vaccination. J Biol Stand 1977;5:147.

Edwards PQ. Screening for tuberculosis. Chest 1975;68:451.

Ellner JJ, Wallis RS. Immunologic aspects of mycobacterial infections. Rev Infect Dis 1989;11(Suppl):S455.

Farer LS, Lowell AM, Meador MP. Extrapulmonary tuberculosis in the United States. Am J Epidemiol 1979;109:205.

Ferebee SH. Controlled chemoprophylaxis trials in tuberculosis. A general review. Adv Tuberc Res 1970;17:28.

Girgis NI, Zoheir F, Kilpatrick ME, et al. Dexamethasone adjunctive treatment for tuberculous meningitis. Pediatr Infect Dis 1991;10:179.

Gorse GJ, Belshe RM. Male genital tuberculosis: a review of the literature with instructive case reports. Rev Infect Dis 1985;7:511.

Hageman J, Shulman S, Schreiber M, et al. Congenital tuberculosis: critical reappraisal of clinical findings and diagnostic procedures. Pediatrics 1980;66:980.

Horsburgh CR Jr. *Mycobacterium avium* complex infection in the acquired immunodeficiency syndrome. N Engl J Med 1991;324:1332.

Hsu KHK. Thirty years after isoniazid. Its impact on tuberculosis in children and adolescents. JAMA 1984;251:1283.

Jakubowski A, Elwood RK, Enarson DA. Clinical features of abdominal tuberculosis. J Infect Dis 1988;158:687.

Kaufmann SHE. In vitro analysis of the cellular mechanisms involved in immunity to tuberculosis. Rev Infect Dis 1989;11(Suppl):S448.

Kendig EL Jr. The place of BCG vaccine in the management of infants born of tuberculous mothers. N Engl J Med 1969;281:520.

Koch R. Die aetiologie der tuberculose. Berlin Klin Wochenschr 1882;xix:221.

Kopanoff DE, et al. A continuing survey of tuberculosis primary drug resistance in the United States: March 1975 to November 1977. A U.S. Public Health Service cooperative study. Am Rev Respir Dis 1978;118:835.

Lincoln EM. Course and prognosis of tuberculosis in children. Am J Med 1950;9:623.

Lincoln EM. Epidemics of tuberculosis. Arch Environ Health 1967;14:473.

Lincoln EM, Sewell EM. Tuberculosis in children. New York: McGraw-Hill, 1963.

Lincoln EM, Sordillo SVR, Davies PA. Tuberculosis meningitis in children: a review of 167 untreated and 74 treated patients with special reference to early diagnosis. J Pediatr 1960;57:807.

Lunn JA, Johnson AJ. Comparison of the Tine and Mantoux tuberculin tests. Report of the Tuberculin Subcommittee of the Research Committee of the British Thoracic Association. Br Med J 1978;1:1451.

Olazabal F Jr. Choroidal tubercles. JAMA 1967;200:374.

Palmer CE, Edwards LB, Hopwood L, Edwards PQ. Experimental and epidemiologic basis for the interpretation of tuberculin sensitivity. J Pediatr 1959;55:413.

Palmer CE, Shaw LW, Comstock GW. Community trials of BCG vaccination. Am Rev Tuberc 1958;77:877.

Porter JM, Snowe RJ, Silver D. Tuberculous enteritis with perforation and abscess formation in childhood. Surgery 1972;71:254.

Powell KE, Meador MP, Farer LS. Recent trends in tuberculosis in children. JAMA 1984;251:1289.

Rideout VK, Hiltz JE. An epidemic of tuberculosis in a rural high school in 1967. Can J Public Health 1969;60:22.

Rieder JL, Cauthen GM, Kelly GD, et al. Tuberculosis in the United States. JAMA 1989;262:385.

Rook GAW. The role of vitamin D in tuberculosis. Am Rev Respir Dis 1988;138:768-770.

Rose CE Jr, Zerbe GO, Lantz SO, Bailey WC. Establishing priority during investigation of tuberculosis contacts. Am Rev Respir Dis 1979;119:603.

Rosenthal SR, et al. BCG vaccination against tuberculosis in Chicago: a twenty-year study statistically analyzed. Pediatrics 1961;28:622.

Schurr E, Buschman E, Malo D, et al. E. Immunogenetics of mycobacterial infections; mouse-human homologies. J Infect Dis 1990;161:634.

Sifontes JE. Rifampin in tuberculosis meningitis. J Pediatr 1975;87:1015.

Skolnik PR, Nadol JB Jr, Baker AS. Tuberculosis of the middle ear: review of the literature with an instructive case. Rev Infect Dis 1986;8:403.

Small PM, Schecter GF, Goodman PC, et al. Treatment of tuberculosis in patients with advanced human immunodeficiency virus infection. N Engl J Med 1991;324:289.

Smith AM, Lattimer JK. Genitourinary tract involvement in children with tuberculosis. NY State J Med 1973;73:2325.

Snider DE Jr. TB in children: time for short-course chemotherapy. J Respir Dis 1987;8:70.

Snider DE Jr, Rieder HL, Combs D, et al. Tuberculosis in children. Pediatr Infect Dis 1988;7:271.

Spyridis P, et al. Isoniazid liver injury during chemoprophylaxis in children. Arch Dis Child 1973;54:65-67.

Starke JR. Modern approach to the diagnosis and treatment of tuberculosis in children. Pediatr Clin N Am 1988;35:441.

Stead WW, Senner JW, Reddick WT, Lofgren JP. Racial differences in susceptibility to infection by *Mycobacterium tuberculosis*. N Engl J Med 1990;322:422.

Steiner P, et al. Miliary tuberculosis in two infants after nursery exposure: epidemiologic, clinical and laboratory findings. Am Rev Respir Dis 1976;113:267.

Sumaya CV, et al. Tuberculosis in children during the isoniazid era. J Pediatr 1975;87:43.

Thompson NH, Glassroth JL, Snider DE Jr, Farer LS. The booster phenomenon in serial tuberculin testing. Am Rev Respir Dis 1979;119:587.

Wallgren A. The time-table of tuberculosis. Tubercle 1945;29:245.

33

URINARY TRACT INFECTIONS

KEITH M. KRASINSKI

The term *urinary tract infection* (UTI) refers to a clinical entity that may involve the urethra, bladder (lower urinary tract), and/or the ureters, renal pelvis, calyces, and renal parenchyma (upper urinary tract). Urethritis as a clinical entity is discussed in Chapter 25.

UTI is a convenient designation because it is often impossible to localize the infection to either the lower tract or the upper tract. Most bacterial UTIs are characterized by the presence of significant numbers of bacteria in the urine.

The designation *significant bacteriuria* refers to the number of bacteria in excess of the usual bacterial contamination of the anterior urethra. The presence of more than 100,000 bacteria per milliliter of urine in a clean voided specimen probably is the result of infection, not contamination at the time of voiding. *Asymptomatic bacteriuria* is defined as significant bacteriuria in a patient who has no clinical evidence of active infection.

Lower UTI is usually characterized by dysuria, frequency, urgency, and possibly suprapubic tenderness. The clinical manifestations of acute pyelonephritis may include fever, lumbar pain and tenderness, dysuria, urgency, and frequency associated with significant bacteriuria.

Recurrence of a UTI may be caused by a relapse or a reinfection. A relapse is a recurrence of the infection with the *same* infecting microorganism, perhaps indicating inadequate therapy. A reinfection is a new infection caused by a bacterium that is different from the one responsible for the previous episode. Specific identification

may require serotyping, pyocin typing, phage typing, or antibiotic typing of the bacterium (e.g., *Escherichia coli*), procedures that are not uniformly available to the clinician. These identification techniques may also be useful for associating individual incidents with hospital outbreaks of infection. Persistence of the UTI associated with the same organism for many months or years or frequent recurrences over many months or years are sometimes termed *chronic infection*.

ETIOLOGY

The microorganisms that cause UTIs include the following:

Gram-Negative Bacteria

E. coli
Klebsiella pneumoniae
Proteus mirabilis
Enterobacter aerogenes
Pseudomonas aeruginosa
Serratia marcescens
Salmonella species
Haemophilus influenzae
Gardnerella vaginalis

Gram-Positive Bacteria

Staphylococcus epidermidis
Enterococcus
Staphylococcus aureus
Staphylococcus saprophyticus
Streptococcus pneumoniae

Other Agents

Adenovirus types 11 and 21
BK virus

Candida albicans
Mycoplasma hominis
Ureaplasma urealyticum
Mycobacterium tuberculosis
Toxocara
Microfilariae
Enterobius vermicularis

The most common pathogens are the gram-negative bacilli. Of this group, *E. coli* is responsible for most acute infections. The other gram-negative bacteria such as *Proteus, Pseudomonas,* and *Klebsiella-Enterobacter* species more likely will be associated with chronic or recurrent infections. Salmonella bacteriuria is usually associated with Salmonella sepsis.

Gram-positive bacteria such as *S. epidermidis, S. saprophyticus,* and *S. aureus* have been identified as causes of UTIs. Coagulase-negative staphylococci have been detected as urinary tract pathogens in sexually active young women (Bailey, 1973; Vosti, 1975) and newborns (Khan et al., 1975). Coagulase-positive staphylococci may invade the urinary tract through the hematogenous route.

Adenovirus types 11 and 21 and the human papovavirus BK have been reported as causes of acute hemorrhagic cystitis (Mufson and Belshe, 1976; Padgett et al., 1987; Hashida et al., 1976; Rice et al., 1985). Symptomatic and asymptomatic BK viruria is associated with bone marrow transplantation. Fungi such as *C. albicans* may be responsible for UTIs in patients with indwelling catheters during the course of their treatment with antibiotics, in patients immunocompromised as a result of disease, steroids, or cytotoxic chemotherapy, and as a result of renal seeding during fungemia.

PATHOGENESIS

Bacterial invasion of the urinary tract may occur by direct extension, by ascending through the urethra, or by the hematogenous route. Lymphatic spread has been suggested, but it has not been proved (Murphy et al., 1960).

The ascending route is the most common pathway of infection. Bacteria that colonize the distal urethra may eventually spread to the bladder. Massage of the urethra such as occurs during masturbation and sexual intercourse forces bacteria into the bladder (Bran et al., 1972; Buckley et al., 1978). Hematogenous spread

may occur during the course of neonatal sepsis. In older children and adolescents with staphylococcal sepsis and/or endocarditis hematogenous spread to the kidney may result in abscess formation.

Abscesses also result from ascending infection from the collecting system, followed by renal seeding and localized liquefaction. This condition recently has been termed *lobar nephronia*. Intrarenal suppurative necrosis is most evident in the cortex when it occurs; however, abscesses also occur in the medulla. The natural methods of extension include rupture into the renal pelvis and extension through the renal capsule, producing a perinephric (perirenal) abscess.

The pathogenesis of a UTI is dependent in great part on factors associated with both the microorganism and the host. The following virulence factors of microorganisms are associated with UTIs:

1. Size of inoculum
2. Pili (mucosal cell adherence)
   a. Mannose sensitive type 1, common
   b. P pili
   c. X pili
3. Motility
4. Urease production
5. Surface antigens

Microorganism

Experimental studies in mice have revealed that the greater the number of organisms delivered to the kidney, the greater the chance of inducing pyelonephritis (Gorrill and De Navasquez, 1964). Thus the size of the inoculum is an important factor. Evidence accumulated during the course of studies by Gruneberg et al. (1968) and by Kaijser (1973) indicates that certain organisms apparently are particularly virulent for the urinary tract. Of the 150 or more *E. coli* O serogroups, only a few (01, 02, 04, 06, 07, 075) have been responsible for most UTIs, and these especially include those that possess large quantities of K antigen. *E. coli* K antigen types 11, 24, 36, and 37 account for the majority of isolates from children with pyelonephritis (Kaijser et al., 1977).

E. coli O antigens are cell-wall lipopolysaccharides that are immunogenic and induce local and systemic antibody responses in patients with pyelonephritis. Strains most often associated with pyelonephritis are representatives of 80 antigen groups. The specific O antigens appear to confer the ability to resist agglutination and bactericidal effects of serum in contrast to the O serotypes of organisms causing cystitis (Lindberg et al., 1975; Smith et al., 1977).

A primary pathogenic factor is the presence of pili. Pili are important for the attachment of E. coli and P. mirabilis to the urinary tract epithelium (Silverblatt, 1974). Almost all E. coli contain type 1 common pili that bind to mannose (Ofek et al., 1977). Attachment to mannose-containing receptors on epithelial cells of the urethra and vagina is thought of primary importance in colonizing the lower urinary tract (Iwahi et al., 1983; Svanborg-Eden et al., 1983). E. coli isolates from patients with cystitis have a greater avidity and adhere in higher numbers to uroepithelial cells than do E. coli fecal isolates (Svanborg-Eden et al., 1976, 1981). Uropathogenic E. coli and P. mirabilis are capable of altering their surface composition (phase variation) and tend to lose their type 1 pili on arrival in the kidney (Silverblatt, 1974; Ofek, et al., 1981). This ability to vary phase characteristics constitutes a selective advantage by promoting renal cell attachment and especially because variation of mannose receptors of type 1 pili allows escape from phagocytosis by polymorphonuclear leukocytes (Perry et al., 1983).

P pili cause mannose-resistant hemagglutination and bind to specific glycolipid receptor sites on human epithelial cells (Kallenius et al., 1981; Leffler and Svanborg-Eden, 1981; Svanborg-Eden et al., 1981, 1983). E. coli with P pili have their favored site of attachment on the uroepithelium of the kidneys where receptors are distributed with greatest density (Svanborg-Eden et al., 1976, 1983). UTIs are more likely to occur in persons who express the P blood group antigen (Lindberg et al., 1983).

A third type of pili, X pili, are also capable of binding to uroepithelium. Their receptor sites have not been identified; however, they also have an affinity for the upper urinary tract.

Motility probably also is an important pathogenic factor. Weyrauch and Bassett (1951) have shown that motile bacteria can ascend in the ureter against the flow of the urine. Moreover, the ascent of these bacteria may be facilitated by the decreased ureteral peristalsis attributed to the endotoxin of gram-negative bacilli.

The production of urease by the infecting bacteria may affect their capacity to cause pyelonephritis. When UTI was induced in experimental animals by the retrograde administration of P. mirabilis, a urease-producing organism, there was a high degree of correlation between the number of bacteria in the kidney and the extent of renal damage. However, treatment with a urease inhibitor reduced the extent of renal damage and the number of bacteria in the kidney without a significant decrease in the number of bacteria in the urine (Musher et al., 1975).

Host

The known host defense mechanisms of the urinary tract are as follows:

  Antibacterial activity of urine
  Prostatic secretions of postpubescent males
  Flushing mechanisms of the bladder
  Low vaginal pH
  Estrogen
  Antiadherence effect of uromucoid
  Antiadherence effect of mucopolysaccharide
  Humoral immunity
  Local secretory immunity, IgA
  Lack of P blood group antigen
  Normal flora

The long male urethra, in contrast to the short female urethra, has been implicated as a reason for the disproportionately high female-gender predilection for UTI.

Antibacterial activity of urine against certain bacteria has been described. Kaye (1968) has reported that extremes of osmolality, high urea concentration, low pH, and high concentration of organic acids may inhibit the growth of some bacteria that cause UTIs. However, with the usual range of pH (5.5 to 7.0) and osmolality (300 to 1,200), the rate of growth of E. coli has been reported as unaffected (Asscher et al., 1966).

The flushing mechanism of the bladder enhances the spontaneous clearance of bacteria. Voiding and dilution probably play an important role. However, when considering antimicrobial therapy, overhydration can have the negative effect of diluting and washing out the active antimicrobial.

In adolescents and adults prostatic fluid may inhibit bacterial growth (Stamey et al., 1968). The role of prostatic secretions in prepubescent males is unknown. The presence of estrogen may enhance the growth of some strains of *E. coli* (Harles et al., 1975). Glucose makes urine a better culture medium, and it inhibits the migrating, adhering, aggregating, and killing functions of polymorphonuclear leukocytes. In addition, the intact mucosal surfaces of animal bladders are resistant to bacterial invasion (Cobbs and Kaye, 1967).

Low vaginal pH apparently is an important factor responsible for lack of colonization (Stamey and Timothy, 1975). For example, serogroups of *E. coli* that usually cause UTIs are more resistant to low pH than serogroups that are less common causes of infection (Stamey and Kaufman, 1975). Similarly, low pH has an inhibitory effect on *P. mirabilis* and *P. aeruginosa* (Stamey and Mihara, 1976). This phenomenon may possibly account for the higher incidence of *E. coli* infection.

Tamm-Horsfall protein is secreted by renal tubular cells and is present in the urine as uromucoid (Orskov et al., 1980). Since uromucoid is rich in mannose residues, it may bind, prevent attachment, and allow adequate flushing out of bacteria. This hypothesis has been supported by an animal model in which mannose can prevent colonization (Aronson et al., 1979). Parsons et al. (1975) have demonstrated that an anti-adherence mechanism of the bladder (in rabbits) exists by pretreatment of the bladder with dilute hydrochloric acid. Acid-treated bladders had twentyfold to fiftyfold increases of bacterial adherence over controls. Adherence was enhanced by ablation of mucopolysaccharide and glycosaminoglycan from the surface of bladder epithelium (Parsons et al., 1978, 1979). This could result from exposure of additional binding sites. The rapid recovery of protection suggests a secretory component that inhibits binding. Increased adherence apparently is species specific (Sobel and Vardi, 1982).

It is possible that antibacterial mechanisms are responsible for the rapid disappearance of bacteria applied to bladder mucosa in an experimental model (Vivaldi et al., 1965; Cobbs and Kaye, 1967; Norden et al., 1968); however, the nature of these mechanisms has not been established. Secretory IgA does decrease adherence and colonization of perineal cells by *E. coli* (Stamey et al., 1978) and is increased in children with UTIs (Uehling and Stiehm, 1971).

The role of humoral immunity as a mechanism of the host's defense against UTI has not been satisfactorily clarified. Hanson et al. (1977) reported that *E. coli* acute pyelonephritis induced serum antibodies to O antigens but rarely to K antigens. In contrast, increased levels of O antibodies were not detected in sera from patients with cystitis or asymptomatic bacteriuria. Using the sensitive enzyme-linked immunosorbent assay (ELISA), Hanson et al. (1977) found high levels of *E. coli* O antibody in the urine of most patients with acute pyelonephritis, lower levels in those with asymptomatic bacteriuria and cystitis, and minimal or no detectable levels in the urine of healthy children. Serum antibodies to O antigen, K antigen, and type 1 pili have been found in patients with pyelonephritis (Hanson et al., 1977, 1981; Mattsby-Baltzer et al., 1982; Rene and Silverblatt, 1982), and IgM is the predominant species detected during acute infections. IgG antibody to the lipid A component of gram-negative rods is also detectable and may be a measure of the severity of renal disease and tissue destruction (Mattsby-Baltzer et al., 1981). A secretory IgA response can also be detected in the urine, apparently in both upper and lower tract disease (Hopkins et al., 1987).

Animal studies suggest that humoral antibody is protective against ascending infection because of organisms with P pili and O and K antigens (Mattsby-Baltzer et al., 1982; Kaijser et al., 1983; O'Hanley et al., 1983). The protective effect apparently is mediated by blocking of attachment to the uroepithelium of the upper urinary tract (Svanborg-Eden and Svennerholm, 1978). The role of the host's normal perineal flora—lactobacilli, *Staphylococcus epidermidis*, corynebacteria, streptococci, and anaerobes—in preventing colonization with uropathogens is not understood.

A number of factors intrinsic and extrinsic to the host combine to predispose to UTI. They include the following:

Intrinsic

    Obstruction
    Stasis
    Reflux
    Pregnancy
    Sexual intercourse (in females)

Hyperosmolality of renal medulla
Host cell receptor sites for attachment
Immunological cross reactivity of bacterial
    antigen and human protein
Chronic prostatitis
B or AB blood type
Genetic predisposition (?)
Immunodeficiency

Extrinsic

Instrumentation (catheters)
Antimicrobial agents

Probably the single most important host factor affecting the occurrence of UTIs is urinary stasis resulting from obstruction of urinary flow or bladder dysfunction. This predisposing host condition is more frequently observed in the younger patient and should prompt a more timely roentgenographic investigation of the urinary system. The most common causes of stasis are as follows:

Congenital anomalies of ureter or urethra
    (valves, stenosis, bands)
Calculi
Dysfunctional voiding
Extrinsic ureteral or bladder compression
Neurogenic bladder (functional obstruction)

The stasis resulting from these factors is associated with increased susceptibility to infection.

There is a striking correlation between vesicoureteral reflux and the occurrence of UTIs. Reflux, the retrograde flow of urine into the ureter and kidney, is caused by the incompetence of the normal valvular action of the ureterovesicular junction. It may occur when this area is affected by congenital anatomical defects, disease, or distal obstruction. Reflux tends to perpetuate infection by maintaining a residual pool of infected urine in the bladder after voiding. Children with reflux may develop upper UTIs and renal scarring. Smellie and Normand (1975) have reported that reflux can be detected in 30% to 50% of children with symptomatic or asymptomatic bacteriuria and that the scarred kidney associated with reflux is more susceptible to reinfection.

Physiological alterations of the urinary tract that increase the likelihood of UTI occur as a result of pregnancy. These changes include decreased bladder and ureteral tone, decreased ureteral peristalsis, hydroureter, and increased residual bladder urine, all of which serve to cause or aggravate obstruction, stasis, and reflux.

Sexual intercourse in females produces transient bacteriuria and is associated with an increased risk of UTI. This is substantiated by the studies of Nicolle et al. (1982) and Pfau et al. (1983), showing that 80% of UTIs begin within 24 hours of intercourse in sexually active women.

Hyperosmolality of the renal medulla inhibits the migration of polymorphonuclear leukocytes to damaged medullary tissue and decreases phagocytosis of bacteria (Rocha and Fekety, 1964).

Several facts suggest a genetic predisposition to UTI, including the association of blood group P antigen (Lindberg et al., 1983) with blood groups B and AB, that is, those lacking anti-B isohemagglutinin (Kinane et al., 1982). Studies on the occurrence of periurethral or vaginal defects in host defenses have been inconclusive. The finding of Stamey (1973) that persons subject to recurrences have a propensity to more frequent and prolonged colonization has not been supported by the work of others (Parsons et al., 1979; Kunin et al., 1980).

Adult males with chronic prostatitis are at risk for recurrent urinary tract infections because of intermittent seeding of their urinary bladders.

Finally, there is evidence that chronic interactions of the host's immune system with retained bacterial antigens or mimicking host antigens is responsible for chronic progressive renal damage. Bacterial antigen may not be eradicated and may trigger formation of antigen-antibody complexes (Hanson et al., 1977). Tamm-Horsfall protein antigen can permeate the renal interstitial spaces and evoke an aggressive humoral and cellular immune response (Work and Andriole, 1980; Mayrer et al., 1983). The most aggressive response occurs in persons with vesicoureteral reflux independent of bacteriuria. Furthermore, Tamm-Horsfall protein cross reacts with gram-negative bacilli (Fasth et al., 1980).

Two important extrinsic host factors, instrumentation and antimicrobial agents, predispose to UTI. This is particularly true in hospitalized patients with indwelling catheters and patients with chronic bladder dysfunction. Catheters produce their damage by eroding the slime layer of the urethra and bladder and by serving as a nidus for intraluminal concretions and bacterial colonization (Rubin, 1980). The pericannular space is not subject to mechanical washing out of bacteria as is the uncatheterized urethra. Suction ulcers of the bladder mucosa develop at the site of the bladder portal when urinary drainage systems are not properly vented (Monson et al., 1977). Antimicrobial agents apparently have the effect of altering the host's normal perineal flora, allowing easier colonization with uropathogens. In patients with urinary catheters antibiotics have the effect of shifting colonization to antibiotic-resistant strains (Britt et al., 1977; Butler and Kunin, 1968; Warren et al., 1982, 1983).

PATHOLOGY

Mucosal and submucosal edema and infiltration of the tissue with leukocytes are the prominent histopathological changes of cystitis.

In patients with acute pyelonephritis and upper UTIs the kidney is usually enlarged; its capsular surface is smooth, and the pelvic mucosa may also be involved. The microscopic findings include edema, congestion, polymorphonuclear infiltration of the interstitium, and abscess formation. Tubules may be distended by exudate consisting of leukocytes, bacteria, and debris, occasionally causing necrosis. The medulla is involved to a greater degree than the cortex.

In patients with chronic pyelonephritis the kidney is usually contracted; its surface is scarred, and its capsule is thickened. The calyces and pelvis are fibrotic, and the thickness of the parenchyma is decreased. The glomeruli show evidence of proliferation, crescents, and hyalinization, and they are surrounded by pericapsular fibrosis. The renal architecture is disrupted by fibrotic bands and collections of lymphocytes, eosinophils, and plasma cells. Tubules are atrophied and dilated.

CLINICAL MANIFESTATIONS

The clinical manifestations of UTIs are dependent on the age of the patient. The following symptoms in newborn infants and in those less than 2 years of age are characteristically nonspecific and apparently are related to the gastrointestinal tract rather than the urinary tract: failure to thrive, feeding problems, vomiting, diarrhea, abdominal distention, and jaundice. Infants may have signs of balanitis, prostatitis, and orchitis or manifestations of overt sepsis.

The infection in children more than 2 years of age may be characterized by fever, frequency, dysuria, abdominal pain, flank pain, and hematuria. The occurrence of enuresis in a child who has been toilet trained could be a manifestation of a UTI. Young infants and boys may have an obstructive uropathy characterized by dribbling of urine, straining with urination, or a decrease in the force and size of the urinary stream. These findings of obstruction can be aggravated by infection.

The manifestations of UTIs in adolescents and adults are fairly specific. Lower urinary tract symptoms include frequency and painful urination of a small amount of turbid urine that occasionally may be grossly bloody. Fever is usually absent. In contrast, upper UTI may be characterized by fever, chills, flank pain, and lower tract symptoms such as frequency, urgency, and dysuria. Occasionally the lower tract symptoms may appear 1 to 2 days before the upper tract symptoms. The clinical manifestations in some patients may be so atypical that they resemble gallbladder disease or acute appendicitis.

Given the appropriate clinical setting, the diagnosis is suggested by the detection of white blood cells (WBCs) and bacteria in the urine. The diagnosis of UTI requires confirmation by quantitative culture of urine and localization of the site of infection.

Presumptive tests

Pyuria. Pyuria is usually defined as the presence of more than five to eight WBCs per cubic millimeter of *uncentrifuged* urine. This usually represents more than one WBC per high-power field; it would be 50 to 100 WBCs/mm^3, that is, more than five WBCs per high-power field in *centrifuged* urine.

A standardized approach to urinalysis is valuable. Generally 5 ml of urine is centrifuged at 3,000 rpm for 3 minutes, followed by resuspension of the sediment. The occurrence of more than 20 WBCs per high-power field usually correlates with significant bacteriuria of 100,000 colonies in a clean-catch sample. However, pyuria does not necessarily indicate the presence of a UTI. Patients with or without pyuria may or may not have an infection. Unfortunately, false-positive results of approximately 30% have been reported (Brumfitt, 1965). It is likely that most patients with symptomatic UTIs will have pyuria.

Microscopic examination of urine for bacteria. A Gram stain of uncentrifuged urine is a useful test for the presumptive diagnosis of UTI. Infection is suggested by the presence of at least one bacterium per oil-immersion field in a midstream, clean-catch urine specimen, equivalent to approximately 100,000 bacteria per milliliter. On examination of centrifuged sediment, approximately 10 to 100 bacteria per high-power field correlate with significant bacteriuria.

Bioluminescence. The quantitative detection of bacterial production of ATP is another sensitive and specific screening test for UTI and detects both gram-positive and gram-negative organisms (Hanna, 1986).

Molecular detection of nucleic acids of prokaryotic cells in urine is being developed as a screening test for UTI. Although this strategy probably will be highly sensitive, it is also relatively expensive and labor intensive; thus its role in clinical-laboratory diagnosis of UTI remains to be determined.

Specific tests

Quantitative culture of urine. Urine for culture may be obtained as a midstream clean-catch specimen, by catheterization, or by suprapubic aspiration. A negative culture of a clean-catch specimen would obviate the need for catheterization or suprapubic aspiration. Urine collected as a bag specimen should not be submitted for bacterial culture.

Organisms, in any number, are considered significant when obtained by suprapubic aspiration. If the quantitative culture from a midstream sample reveals 100,000 bacteria or more per milliliter of urine, it indicates the presence of significant bacteriuria. A count of less than 10,000 bacteria per milliliter suggests probable contamination. The specificity of this technique is enhanced from 80% to 95% if significant bacteriuria is demonstrated on repeat testing.

A false-positive test may be due to contamination or prolonged incubation of urine before culture. False-negative results may reflect the following: prior antimicrobial therapy, the presence of a fastidious organism that grows slowly or is difficult to culture, rapid flow of urine, inactivation of bacteria by an extremely acid pH, or a break in technique such as spilling soap or

other cleansing agents into the urine. Therefore there are clinical situations in which colony counts of less than 100,000 may indicate significant bacteriuria.

Convenient, accurate, inexpensive culture techniques have become available for clinic or office practice and are most useful for screening for asymptomatic bacteriuria. They include the filter-strip, dip-slide, dip-strip, pad culture, and roll tube techniques. Of these techniques, the dip-slide apparently is the most sensitive and specific (Eichenwald, 1986). The filter-strip technique does not differentiate gram-negative and gram-positive bacteria. The dip-slide and dip-strip techniques do use discriminating agars that allow differentiation of gram-negative and gram-positive organisms.

The specific bacterium recovered by culture should be identified as a guide to appropriate therapy. Quantitative urine cultures should be performed. Commonly this is done using a 0.001 ml calibrated loop inoculated onto blood agar and MacConkey agar for gram-negative rods and onto chocolate agar for *H. influenzae*. The culture is incubated overnight, counted, and multiplied by 1,000. In special circumstances special media (e.g., Sabouraud dextrose agar for fungi and human embryonic kidney, HeLa, or Hep-2 tissue culture for viral isolation) are required. When suprapubic aspiration is performed, 0.1 ml of urine should be spread over the plate and incubated as above.

In uncomplicated disease the best test of antibiotic susceptibility is the test of cure. Successful treatment is followed by negative culture results within 24 to 72 hours after institution of therapy. If positive cultures are obtained, susceptibility results should be sought so that treatment can be tailored to the specific pathogen. Laboratory evaluation of response to therapy in children is required. For complicated disease, renal parenchymal disease, and nosocomially acquired organisms, antibiotic susceptibilities on the diagnostic urine specimen are useful in guiding therapy.

Localization of site of infection. It is important to determine if the infection involves the lower tract (probably cystitis) or the upper tract (probably pyelonephritis). Although pyelonephritis is classically associated with fever, flank pain or tenderness, decreased renal concentrating ability, and an elevated erythrocyte sedimentation rate (ESR), the absence of these findings does not reliably exclude upper tract disease. Collection of urine by ureteral catheterization for quantitative culture is the most reliable method of localizing the site of infection; however, it is an invasive test and may require general anesthesia; therefore its role in children is limited to research applications. Stamey et al. (1965) evaluated 95 females and 26 males by this method. Their observation that the site of infection was limited to the bladder in 50% of this group could not be predicted by history and physical examination. Localization by bladder washout (Fairley technique) is less invasive and does not require anesthesia; however, this is a cumbersome test and is not routinely performed.

The detection of antibody coating of bacteria is a sensitive, reliable, *noninvasive* indicator of renal bacteriuria in adults (Jones et al., 1974; Thomas et al., 1974). After addition of fluorescein-conjugated anti-human globulin to urine, the demonstration of fluorescence of the antibody-coated bacteria indicates upper tract involvement. Unfortunately, when this immunofluorescence technique has been applied to children with bacteriuria, it has been neither sensitive nor specific (Hellerstein et al., 1978; McCracken et al., 1981). Urinary lactic dehydrogenase (LDH) isoenzyme 5 is more accurate for localizing the site of infection in infants and children. Lorentz and Resnick (1979) have reported that elevations of urinary LDH greater than 150 and elevations of fractions 4 and 5 are good indicators of acute pyelonephritis.

C-reactive protein (CRP) is also useful for distinguishing upper from lower UTI and has a sensitivity and specificity of approximately 90% when compared to bladder washout (McCracken et al., 1981). A CRP value greater than 30 μg/ml suggests upper tract disease.

Finally, response to therapy is a clinical indication of the site of infection in adults. Studies in women indicate that more than 90% of patients with lower UTI but less than 50% of those with upper UTI are cured by a single dose of antibiotic if the organism is susceptible (Ronald et al., 1976; Fang et al., 1978). In children, however, recurrences of infection after short-duration therapy occur in approximately 30% of those treated (McCracken, 1982). This does not differ from the frequency of recurrences following conventional therapy.

DIFFERENTIAL DIAGNOSIS

The differential diagnosis of UTI is dependent in great part on the age of the patient. The clinical manifestations in newborn infants and in infants under 2 years of age are nonspecific. The findings of irritability, failure to thrive, vomiting, diarrhea, and jaundice suggest the possibility of *bacterial sepsis, acute gastroenteritis,* or *hepatitis*. The appropriate blood, stool, and urine cultures should provide a clue to the correct diagnosis.

In older children and adults the various conditions that may simulate cystitis or pyelonephritis should be considered. For example, the symptoms of gonorrheal or chlamydial urethritis may suggest a lower UTI. A right-sided pyelonephritis could be confused with acute appendicitis, gallbladder disease, or hepatitis. When the presenting complaint is hematuria and bacterial cultures are negative, viral cultures may reveal the diagnosis. Again, the appropriate cultures and serological tests should help identify the true diagnosis.

COMPLICATIONS

Failure to recognize and to treat acute UTIs may result in recurrent infections and progression to chronic pyelonephritis. Children with chronic pyelonephritis associated with ureteral reflux and obstructive uropathy may develop consequences of chronic renal failure such as anemia, hypertension, growth failure, and metabolic abnormalities. Nephrolithiasis and stricture formation may also develop and further complicate management. A rare complication is that of renal abscess, which may rupture into the perirenal space.

PROGNOSIS

The prognosis depends on the site of involvement, the presence or absence of obstructive uropathy, and vesicoureteral reflux and therefore is related to the age of the patient. Young patients with obstructive uropathy and infection are much more likely to have serious long-term sequelae. Most single, uncomplicated episodes of infection respond to specific antimicrobial therapy. However, approximately one third of these patients may relapse within 1 year. Relapses decrease in frequency beyond this time; however, 1% of patients may relapse up to 6 years after initial infection. The prognosis is less favorable for patients with obstructive lesions and for those with chronic pyelonephritis. In spite of specific antimicrobial therapy, most of these patients have repeated recurrences, and those with bilateral renal involvement may progress to chronic renal insufficiency.

Reflux can be detected in up to 50% of children with bacteriuria (Boineau and Lewy, 1975; Smellie and Normand, 1975). The confluence of infection and reflux is associated with renal scarring in a subset of these children (McCracken and Eichenwald, 1978; Huland and Busch, 1984; Smellie and Normand, 1975).

EPIDEMIOLOGY

UTIs involve all age groups from neonates to geriatric patients. Studies involving routine suprapubic puncture in over 1,000 infants revealed the presence of bacteriuria in 0.1% to more than 1% (Wiswell and Geschke, 1989; Wiswell et al., 1987; Wiswell and Roscelli, 1986). UTI was more common in males, with the majority of these infections occurring in uncircumcised infants. However, circumcision to prevent UTI is not warranted by the low frequency and usually mild nature of the disease. Premature infants have two to three times this rate of UTI. During preschool years, UTI is more common in girls (4.5%) than in boys (0.5%).

Long-term surveillance studies by Kunin et al. (1962) and Kunin (1970, 1976) of schoolchildren revealed persistent bacteriuria in 1.2% of girls and in 0.4% of boys. Each year an additional 0.4% of girls developed bacteriuria. Thus the overall prevalence in school girls was 5%. These studies indicated that the peak incidence of UTI in children occurred between 2 and 6 years of age. White girls tended to have more frequent reinfections than black girls. The incidence of UTI in females of high school and college age is approximately 2%.

TREATMENT

The objectives of treatment of children with UTIs are fourfold: (1) to eliminate the infection, (2) to detect and correct functional or anatomical abnormalities, (3) to prevent recurrences, and (4) to preserve renal function. The achievement of these goals requires successful identification of the causative microorganism, selection of optimal antimicrobial drugs and patient compliance in their use, roentgenographic evaluation of the urinary tract, screening for recurrent infections with periodic urine cultures, and use of general hygienic measures to prevent reinfections. Surgery may be required to correct severe reflux in children with UTIs and especially to correct obstructive lesions.

Antimicrobial therapy

Newborn infants with UTIs and children suspected of having pyelonephritis should be treated empirically at the time of diagnosis because of the frequency of associated bacteremia. Empiric therapy for newborn infants with UTI and suspected sepsis should include ampicillin (100 to 200 mg/kg/day) and gentamicin (5 mg/kg/day for infants <1 week of age and 7.5 mg/kg/day for infants >1 week of age) or another aminoglycoside. Table 33-1 provides recommendations for initial therapy of newborn infants *without sepsis or meningitis* when a specific organism can be predicted or when an organism has been isolated and susceptibilities are not yet available.

Older children with suspected pyelonephritis should be treated empirically with gentamicin (5 to 7.5 mg per kilogram of body weight per day), possibly with the addition of ampicillin. Table 33-2 contains recommendations for initial therapy of older children when a specific organism can be predicted or when an organism has been isolated and susceptibilities are not yet available. Children with mild symptoms and those with lower UTIs may not require antimicrobial therapy until the results of urine culture are available. If therapy is indicated before the results of culture become available, oral sulfisoxazole or triple sulfonamides are suggested because *E. coli* and other gram-negative bacilli are the most common pathogens. Ampicillin or amoxicillin (30 mg per kilogram of body weight per day in three doses) may be used as an alternative to sulfonamides. When the results of urine culture and antibiotic sensitivities are known, the antimicrobial therapy can be changed if necessary. If a repeat urine culture 48 hours after initiation of therapy is negative, the treatment should be continued, regardless of the results of in vitro sensitivity studies. If the repeat culture is still positive and the colony count has not decreased, the results of the sensitivity tests should be used as a basis for changing the antimicrobial therapy.

In adolescents with acute obstructive, persistent, or frequently recurrent UTIs and for those with nosocomially acquired organisms, fluoro-

Table 33-1. Initial therapy for predicted cause of acute urinary tract infections in newborn infants while awaiting susceptibility results

Gram stain	Cause	Initial therapy
Gram-negative rods	Coliforms (*Escherichia coli, Klebsiella pneumoniae, Enterobacter aerogenes*)	Gentamicin 3 mg/kg/day or amikacin 10 mg/kg/day
	Proteus mirabilis	Ampicillin 50 to 75 mg/kg/day
	Pseudomonas aeruginosa	Mezlocillin or ticarcillin 75 to 100 mg/kg/day or ceftazidime 100-150 mg/kg/day
Gram-positive cocci in chains	*Streptococcus faecalis*	Ampicillin 30 mg/kg/day IM or 50 mg/kg/day PO; add an aminoglycoside if synergy is needed
Gram-positive cocci in clusters	*Staphylococcus aureus*	Methicillin or oxacillin 50 to 75 mg/kg/day
	Staphylococcus aureus, methicillin resistant (MRSA)	Vancomycin 30 mg/kg/day
	Staphylococcus epidermidis	As for *S. aureus*

quinolones, imipenem-cilastatin, ticarcillin-cla-vulanate, or third-generation cephalosporins are acceptable alternative drugs.

For children in whom clinical and laboratory parameters indicate lower tract infection, the use of single-dose or short-term regimens should be restricted to those beyond the newborn period with their first UTI. Reexamination of the patient and reculture of the urine after short-term therapy is mandatory. Amoxicillin, cefad-roxil, nitrofurantoin, and trimethoprim-sulfa-methoxazole have all been used as short-term regimens.

McCracken and Eichenwald (1978) recommend that treatment be continued for 10 to 14 days. A "cure" is determined by the demonstration of several negative cultures after cessation of therapy. Therapeutic failures after short-course or conventional antibiotic treatment of susceptible organisms suggest upper tract disease. Consideration should be given to a 6-week regimen in patients who do not respond to conventional therapy. Follow-up should continue for at least 2 years with a routine culture schema such as monthly urine culture for the first 3 months followed by three cultures 3 months apart and two semiannual cultures. If reinfection occurs, the susceptibility of the organism should be determined, and the appropriate therapy should be instituted. Reinfection is differentiated from recurrence by typing the causative agent.

Radiological evaluation

After initial infection in all infants, in boys of any age, and, possibly, girls less than 3 years radiological evaluation is indicated. In girls more than 3 years of age imaging is also indicated in the presence of physical examination findings suggestive of possible renal or collecting system abnormalities, abnormal voiding, hypertension, or poor physical development (Eichenwald, 1986).

Information developed by these radiographic studies affects management. Children with no reflux or grade 1 reflux require only follow-up examination. Children with grade II or III reflux are candidates for suppressive therapy. Children with grade IV reflux are also candidates for suppressive therapy, and urological consultation should be obtained.

If radiographic studies are not performed in older girls after the primary infection, they are indicated if there is a recurrence. Radiographic studies are usually performed 6 weeks or longer after acute infection to avoid detection of grade I or II reflux caused by irritation of the vesicoureteral junction. Children with clinical signs of upper tract disease who fail to respond promptly to antibiotic therapy warrant evaluation with ultrasound or intravenous pyelography during their acute infection to investigate the role of obstruction. If grade III or IV reflux is detected, it probably will be persistent and not be the result of acute infection.

Table 33-2. Initial therapy for predicted cause of urinary tract infection in older children while awaiting susceptibility results

Clinical condition	Cause	Initial therapy*
Acute nonobstructive Gram-negative rods	Coliforms	Trisulfapyrimidines 120 to 150 mg/kg/day or sulfisoxazole 120 to 150 mg/kg/day or amoxicillin 30 mg/kg/day or trimethoprim (TMP) sulfamethoxazole (SMX), TMP 6 mg/kg/day, SMX 30 mg/kg/day
	Pseudomonas species	Carbenicillin 30 to 50 mg/kg/day PO or parenteral carbenicillin or mezlocillin 100 mg/kg/day
Gram-positive cocci in chains	Streptococcus faecalis	Ampicillin 50 to 100 mg/kg/day; add aminoglycoside if necessary for synergy
Gram-positive cocci in clusters	Staphylococcus aureus, Staphylococcus epidermidis	Nafcillin 100 mg/kg/day or vancomycin 40 mg/kg/day or cephalexin 25-50 mg/kg/day
	Staphylococcus aureus, methicillin resistant (MRSA)	Vancomycin 40 mg/kg/day
Acute nonobstructive with suspected sepsis	Coliforms	Gentamicin 5 to 7.5 mg/day
Acute obstructive	Coliforms	TMP 6 mg with SMX 30 mg/kg/day or nitrofurantoin 5 to 7 mg/kg/day × 3 weeks or gentamicin 3 mg/kg/day
Persistent, recurrent, or hospital acquired (acute therapy)	Coliforms	Amikacin 15 to 22 mg/kg/day or carbenicillin indanyl 10 to 30 mg/kg/day or TMP 30 mg with SMX, 6 mg/kg/day
Persistent, recurrent, or hospital acquired with sepsis	Coliforms	Amikacin 15 to 22 mg/kg/day or cefuroxime 75 to 150 mg/kg/day or moxalactam 150 to 200 mg/kg/day or mezlocillin 200 to 300 mg/kg/day or piperacillin 200 to 300 mg/kg/day or ceftriaxone 50-100 mg/kg/day or ceftazidime 100-150 mg/kg/day
Prophylaxis for chronic or recurrent infection		TMP 2 mg with SMX 10 mg/kg/day

*Alterations and subsequent therapy should be based on culture and sensitivity reports. The usual duration of therapy for acute infection is 10 days (Nelson, 1985).

Levitt et al. (1977) found that cystograms frequently revealed abnormalities in girls with dysuria and frequency (41%) but pyelograms rarely did (2%). However, if upper tract disease was suspected, pyelograms detected abnormalities in 40%, and findings included obstruction and hydronephrosis. This usually was true even if a first episode of UTI was being studied. In cases diagnosed as upper tract disease based on elevations of CRP and ESR and abnormal renal concentrating ability, 7% of children studied by intravenous pyelogram developed renal scarring (Pylkkanen et al., 1981). When diagnostic findings were expanded to include reflux and fever, in children less than 5 years, fever alone had a positive predictive value of 45%, and reflux had a positive predictive value of 40% for children likely to have radiographically demonstrable abnormalities (Johnson et al., 1985).

Ultrasonography is a rapid, noninvasive method for evaluating the renal parenchyma and renal collecting system and is capable of imaging the surrounding retroperitoneum without radiation exposure. In the hands of experienced individuals ultrasound has supplanted the intravenous pyelogram and voiding cystourethrogram. However, ultrasound may not be able to determine reliably the degree of renal scarring.

When detailed anatomical information is required, computerized tomography or magnetic resonance imaging should be performed. Radionuclide scanning is of limited value in its ability to define structural abnormalities. When imaging studies reveal reflux, they should be repeated in 6 months to follow the course of the finding. When no abnormality is detected, they ordinarily need not be repeated.

PROPHYLAXIS

Patients with frequent recurrences and those with persistent infections may require suppressive therapy for many years. As indicated in Table 33-2, the use of trimethoprim-sulfamethoxazole should be considered. No therapy with any prophylactic agent is completely safe because drug-related toxicities can occur.

Several regimens are available when breakthrough infections occur. Although low-dose ampicillin interferes with adherence of *E. coli* to bladder mucosa (Redjeb et al., 1982), the clinical relevance of this finding has not been determined.

Various nonspecific general measures may be helpful in preventing recurrences of UTIs. They include adequate fluid intake; frequent voiding, especially before bedtime; proper perineal hygiene, particularly after defecation; and avoidance of chronic constipation, which could produce rectal distention that might distort the bladder. Persons with functional abnormalities of the bladder benefit from intermittent catheterization programs. Acidification programs and long-term treatment with methenamine are occasionally effective; however, they are difficult to maintain.

REFERENCES

Aronson M, Medalia O, Schori L, et al. Prevention of colonization of the urinary tract of mice with *Escherichia coli* by blocking of bacterial adherence with methyl-a-D-mannopyanoside. J Infect Dis 1979;139:329-332.

Asscher AW, et al. Urine as a medium for bacterial growth. Lancet 1966;2:1037.

Bailey RR. Significance of coagulase-negative *Staphylococcus* in urine. J Infect Dis 1973;127:179.

Boineau FG, Lewy JE. Urinary tract infections in children: an overview. Pediatr Ann 1975;4:515-526.

Bran JL, Levison ME, Kaye D. Entrance of bacteria into the female urinary bladder. N Engl J Med 1972;286:626.

Britt MR, Garibaldi RA, Miller WA, et al. Antimicrobial prophylaxis for catheter-associated bacteriuria. Antimicrob Agents Chemother 1977;11:240-243.

Brumfitt W. Urinary cell counts and their value. J Clin Pathol 1965;18:550.

Buckley RM, McGuckin M, MacGregor RR. Urine bacterial counts following sexual intercourse. N Engl J Med 1978;298:321.

Butler HK, Kunin CM. Evaluation of specific systemic antimicrobial therapy in patients while on closed catheter drainage. J Urol 1968;100:567-572.

Cobbs CG, Kaye D. Antibacterial mechanisms in the urinary bladder. Yale J Biol Med 1967;40:93.

Eichenwald HF. Some aspects of the diagnosis and management of urinary tract infection in children and adolescents. Pediatr Infect Dis J 1986;5:760-765.

Fang LST, Tolkoff-Rubin NE, Rubin R. Efficacy of single-dose and conventional amoxicillin therapy in urinary tract infection localized by the antibody-coated bacteria technique. N Engl J Med 1978;298:413-416.

Fasth A, Ahlstedt S, Hanson LA, et al. Cross-reaction between Tamm-Horsfall glycoprotein and *Escherichia coli*. Int Arch Allergy Appl Immunol 1980;63:303-311.

Gorrill RH, De Navasquez SJ. Experimental pyelonephritis in the mouse produced by *Escherichia coli*, *Pseudomonas aeruginosa* and *Proteus mirabilis*. J Pathol Bacteriol 1964;87:79.

Gruneberg RN, Leigh DA, Brumfitt W. *Escherichia coli* serotypes in urinary tract infection: studies in domiciliary, antenatal and hospital practice. In O'Grady F, Brumfitt W. ed. Urinary tract infection. London: Oxford University Press, 1968, pp 68-70.

Hanna BA. The detection of bacteriuria by bioluminescence. Methods Enzymol 1986;311:22-27.

Hanson LA, et al. Antigens of *Escherichia coli*, human immune response, and the pathogenesis of urinary tract infections. J Infect Dis 1977;136:S144.

Hanson LA, Fasth A, Jodal U, et al. Biology and pathology of urinary tract infection. J Clin Pathol 1981;34:695-700.

Harles EMJ, Bullen JJ, Thompson DA. Influence of estrogen on experimental pyelonephritis caused by *Escherichia coli*. Lancet 1975;2:283-286.

Hashida Y, Gaffney PC, Yunis EJ. Acute hemorrhagic cystitis of childhood and papovavirus-like particles. J Pediatr 1976;89:85-87.

Hellerstein S, Kennedy E, Nussbaum L, et al. Localization of the site of urinary tract infections by means of antibody-coated bacteria in the urinary sediments. J Pediatr 1978;92:188-193.

Hopkins WJ, Uehling DT, Balish E. Local and systemic antibody responses accompanying spontaneous resolution of experimental cystitis in cynomolgus monkeys. Infect Immunol 1987;55:1951-1956.

Huland H, Busch R. Pyelonephritic scarring in 213 patients with upper and lower urinary tract infections: long term follow up. J Urol 1984;132:936-939.

Iwahi T, Abe Y, Nakao M, et al. Role of type I fimbriae in

the pathogenesis of ascending urinary tract infection induced by *Escherichia coli* in mice. Infect Immun 1983;39:1307-1315.

Johnson CE, Shurin P, Marchant C, et al. Identification of children requiring radiologic evaluation for urinary infection. Pediatr Infect Dis 1985;4:656-663.

Jones SR, Smith JW, Sanford JP. Localization of urinary tract infections by detection of antibody-coated bacteria in urine sediment. N Engl J Med 1974;290:591.

Kaijser B. Immunology of *Escherichia coli*: K. antigen and its relation to urinary-tract infection. J Infect Dis 1973;127:670.

Kaijser B, Olling S. Experimental hematogenous pyelonephritis due to *Escherichia coli* in rabbits: the antibody response and its protective capacity. J Infect Dis 1973;128:41.

Kaijser B, Hanson LA, Jodal U, et al. Frequency of *E. coli* K antigens in urinary tract infections in children. Lancet 1977;1:663-666.

Kaijser B, Larsson P, Olling S, et al. Protection against acute ascending pyelonephritis caused by *Escherichia coli* in rats, using isolated capsular antigen conjugated to bovine serum albumin. Infect Immunol 1983;39:142-146.

Kallenius G, Mollby R, Svensson SB, et al. Occurrence of P-fimbriated *Escherichia coli* in urinary tract infection. Lancet 1981;2:1369-1372.

Kaye D. Antibacterial activity of human urine. J Clin Invest 1968;47:2374.

Khan AJ, Evans HE, Bombeck E, et al. Coagulase negative-staphylococcal bacteriuria—a rarity in infants and children. J Pediatr 1975;86:309-313.

Kinane DF, Blackwell CC, Brettle RP, et al. ABO blood group, secretor state and susceptibility to recurrent urinary tract infection in women. Br Med J 1982;285:7-9.

Kunin CM. The natural history of recurrent bacteriuria in school girls. N Engl J Med 1970;282:1443.

Kunin CM. Urinary tract infections in children. Hosp Pract 1976;113:91.

Kunin CM, Polyak R, Postel E. Periurethral bacterial flora in women. Prolonged intermittent colonization with *Escherichia coli*. JAMA 1980;243:134-139.

Kunin CM, Zacha E, Paquin AJ. Urinary tract infections in school children. I. Prevalence of bacteriuria and associated urologic findings. N Engl J Med 1962;206:1287.

Leffler H, Svanborg-Eden C. Glycolipid receptors for uropathogenic *Escherichia coli* on human erythrocytes and uroepithelial cells. Infect Immunol 1981;34:920-929.

Levitt SB, Bekirov HM, Kogan SJ, et al. Proposed selective approach to radiographic evaluation of children with urinary tract infections. In Birth defects: Original article series, Vol 13, No. 5. New York: The National Foundation—March of Dimes, 1977, pp 433-438.

Lindberg H, Hanson LA, Jacobsson B, et al. Correlation of P blood group, vesiculoureteral reflux, and bacterial attachment in patients with recurrent pyelonephritis. N Engl J Med 1983;308:1189-1192.

Lindberg U, Hanson LA, Jodal U, et al. Asymptomatic bacteriuria in school girls. II. Differences in *E. coli* causing symptomatic and asymptomatic bacteriuria. Acta Pediatr Scand 1975;64:432-436.

Lorentz WB, Resnick MI. Comparison of urinary lactic de-

hydrogenase with antibody-coated bacteria in the urine sediment as a means of localizing the site of urinary tract infection. Pediatrics 1979;64:672.

Mattsby-Baltzer I, Claesson I, Hanson LA, et al. Antibodies to lipid A during urinary tract infection. J Infect Dis 1981;144:319-328.

Mattsby-Baltzer I, Hanson LA, Kaijser B, et al. Experimental *Escherichia coli* ascending pyelonephritis in rats: changes in bacterial properties and the immune response to surface antigens. Infect Immunol 1982;35:639-646.

Maybeck CE. Significance of coagulase negative staphylococcal bacteriuria. Lancet 1969;2:1150-1152.

Mayrer AR, Miniter P, Andriole VT. Immunopathogenesis of chronic pyelonephritis. Am J Med 1983;75:59-70.

McCracken GH Jr. Management of urinary tract infections in children. Pediatr Infect Dis 1982;1(suppl):52-56.

McCracken G, Eichenwald H. Antimicrobial therapy: therapeutic recommendations and a review of new drugs. J Pediatr 1978;93:366.

McCracken GH Jr, Ginsburg CM, Namasanthi V, et al. Evaluation of short-term antibiotic therapy in children with uncomplicated urinary tract infections. Pediatrics 1981;67:796-801.

Miller TE, North JD. Host response in urinary tract infections. Kidney Int 1974;5:179.

Monson TP, Macalalad FV, Hamman JW, et al. Evaluation of a vented drainage system in prevention of bacteriuria. J Urol 1977;177:216-219.

Mufson MA, Belshe RB. A review of adenoviruses in the etiology of acute hemorrhagic cystitis. J Urol 1976; 115:191.

Murphy JJ, et al. The role of the lymphatic system in pyelonephritis. Surg Forum 1960;10:880.

Musher DM, et al. Role of urease in pyelonephritis resulting from urinary tract infection with *Proteus*. J Infect Dis 1975;131:177.

Nelson JD. Pocketbook of pediatric antimicrobial therapy, ed 6. Dallas: Jodone Publishing Co. 1985.

Nicolle L, Harding GKM, Preiksaitis J, et al. The association of urinary tract infection with sexual intercourse. J Infect Dis 1982;278:635-642.

Norden CW, Green GM, Kass EH. Antibacterial mechanisms of the urinary bladder. J Clin Invest 1968;47:2689-2700.

Ofek I, Mirelman D, Sharon N. Adherence of *Escherichia coli* to human mucosal cells mediated by mannose receptors. Nature 1977;265:623-625.

Ofek I, Mosek A, Sharon N. Mannose-specific adherence of *Escherichia coli* freshly extracted in the urine of patients with urinary tract infections and of isolates subcultured from the infected urine. Infect Immunol 1981;34:708-711.

O'Hanley PD, Lark D, Falkow S, et al. A globaside binding *Escherichia coli* pilus vaccine prevents pyelonephritis (abstract). Clin Res 1983;31:372A.

Orskov I, Ferenez A, Orskov F. Tamm-Horsfall protein or uromucoid is the normal urinary slime that traps type I fimbriated *Escherichia coli*. Lancet 1980;1:887.

Padgett BL, Walker DL, Desquitado MM, et al. BK virus and non-hemorrhagic cystitis in a child. Lancet 1987; 1:770.

Parsons CL, Greenspan C, Mulholland SG. The primary

antibacterial defense mechanism of the bladder. Invest Urol 1975;13:72-76.

Parsons CL, Schrom SH, Hanno P, et al. Bladder surface mucin: examination of possible mechanisms for its antibacterial effect. Invest Urol 1978;6:196-200.

Parsons CL, Anwar H, Stauffer C, et al. *In vitro* adherence of radioactively labelled *Escherichia coli* in normal and cystitis prone women. Infect Immunol 1979;26:453-457.

Perry A, Ofek I, Silverblatt JF. Enhancement of mannose-mediated stimulation of human granulocytes by type I fimbriae aggregated with antibodies on *Escherichia coli* surfaces. Infect Immunol 1983;39:1334-1335.

Pfau A, Sacks T, Engtestein D. Recurrent urinary tract infections in premenopausal women: prophylaxis based on an understanding of the pathogenesis. J Urol 1983; 129:1152-1157.

Pylkkanen J, Vilska J, Koskimies O. The value of level diagnosis of childhood urinary tract infection in predicting renal injury. Acta Paediatr Scand 1981;70:879-883.

Redjeb SB, Slim A, Horchani A, et al. Effects of ten milligrams of ampicillin per day on urinary tract infections. Antimicrob Agents Chemother 1982;22:1084-1086.

Rene P, Silverblatt FJ. Serological response to *Escherichia coli* pili in pyelonephritis. Infect Immunol 1982; 37:749-754.

Rice SJ, Bishop JA, Apperly J, et al. BK virus as a case of haemorrhagic cystitis after bone marrow transplant. Lancet 1985;2:844-845.

Rocha H, Fekety FR. Acute inflammation in the renal cortex and medulla following thermal injury. J Exp Med 1964;119:131-138.

Ronald AR, Boutros P, Mourtada H. Bacteriuria localization and response to single-dose therapy in women. JAMA 1976;235:1854-1856.

Rubin M. Effect of catheter replacement on bacterial counts in urine aspirated from indwelling catheters. J Infect Dis 1980;142:291.

Silverblatt FS. Host-parasite interaction in the rat renal pelvis: a possible role of pili in the pathogenesis of pyelonephritis. J Exp Med 1974;140:1696-1711.

Smellie JM, Normand ICS. Bacteriuria, reflux and renal scarring. Arch Dis Child 1975;50:581.

Smith JW, Jones SR, Kaijser B. Significance of antibody-coated bacteria in urinary sediment in experimental pyelonephritis. J Infect Dis 1977;135:577-581.

Sobel JD, Vardi Y. Scanning electron microscopy study of *Pseudomonas aeruginosa in vivo* adherence to rat bladder epithelium. J Urol 1982;128:414-417.

Stamey TA. The role of introital enterobacteria in recurrent urinary infections. J Urol 1973;109:467-472.

Stamey TA, Govan DE, Palmer JM. The localization and treatment of urinary tract infections: the role of bactericidal urine levels as opposed to serum levels. Medicine 1965;44:1.

Stamey TA, Kaufman MF. Studies of introital colonization in women with recurrent urinary infections. II. A comparison of growth in normal vaginal fluid of common versus uncommon serogroups of *E. coli*. J Urol 1975;114:264.

Stamey TA, Mihara G. Studies of introital colonization in women with recurrent urinary infections. V. The inhibitory activity of normal vaginal fluid on *Proteus mirabilis* and *Pseudomonas aeruginosa*. J Urol 1976;115:416.

Stamey TA, Timothy MM. Studies of introital colonization in women with recurrent urinary infections. I. The role of vaginal pH. J Urol 1975;114:261.

Stamey TA, et al. Antibacterial nature of prostatic fluid. Nature 1968;218:444.

Stamey TA, Wehner N, Mihara G, et al. The immunologic basis of recurrent bacteriuria: role of cervicovaginal antibody in enterobacterial colonization of the introital mucosa. Medicine 1978;57:47-56.

Svanborg-Eden C, Svennerholm AM. Secretory immunoglobulin A and G antibodies prevent adhesion of *Escherichia coli* to human urinary tract epithelial cells. Infect Immun 1978;22:790-797.

Svanborg-Eden C, Hanson LA, Jodol U, et al. Variable adherence to normal human urinary tract epithelial cells of *Escherichia coli* strains associated with various forms of urinary tract infection. Lancet 1976;2:490-492.

Svanborg-Eden C, Hagberg L, Hanson LA, et al. Adhesion of *Escherichia coli* in urinary tract infection. CIBA Found Symp 1981;80:161-187.

Svanborg-Eden C, Gotschlich EC, Korhonan TK, et al. Aspects of structure and function of pili of uropathogenic *E. coli*. Prog Allergy 1983;33:189-202.

Thomas V, Shelokov A, Forland M. Antibody-coated bacteria in the urine and the site of urinary tract infection. N Engl J Med 1974;290:588.

Uehling DT, Stiehm ER. Elevated urinary secretory IgA in children with urinary tract infection. Pediatrics 1971; 47:40-46.

Vivaldi E, Munoz J, Cotran R, et al. Factors affecting the clearance of bacteria within the urinary tract. In Kass EH (ed). Progress in pyelonephritis. Philadelphia: FA Davis, 1965, pp 531-535.

Vosti CL. Recurrent urinary tract infections. Prevention by prophylactic antibiotics after sexual intercourse. JAMA 1975;231-934.

Warren JW, Anthony WC, Hoopes JM, et al. Cephalexin for susceptible bacteriuria in afebrile, long-term catheterized patients. JAMA 1982;248:454-458.

Warren JW, Hoopes JM, Muncie HL, et al. Ineffectiveness of cephalexin in treatment of cephalexin-resistant bacteriuria in patients with chronic indwelling urethral catheters. J Urol 1983;129:71-73.

Weyrauch HM, Bassett JB. Ascending infection in an artificial urinary tract. An experimental study. Stanford Med Bull 1951;9:25.

Wiswell TE, Geschke DW. Risks from circumcision during the first month of life compared with those for uncircumcised boys. Pediatrics 1989;83:1011-1015.

Wiswell TE, Roscelli JD. Corroborative evidence for the decreased incidence of urinary tract infections in circumcised male infants. Pediatrics 1986;78:96-99.

Wiswell TE, Enzenauer RW, Holton ME, et al. Declining frequency of circumcision: implications for changes in the absolute incidence and male to female sex ratio of urinary tract infections in early infancy. Pediatrics 1987; 79:338-342.

Work J, Andriole VT. Tamm-Horsfall protein antibody in patients with end-stage kidney disease. Yale J Biol Med 1980;53:133-148.

34

VARICELLA-ZOSTER VIRUS INFECTIONS

ANNE A. GERSHON
PHILIP LaRUSSA

Varicella is a common contagious disease of childhood that is caused by primary infection with varicella-zoster virus (VZV). It is characterized by a short or absent prodromal period and by a pruritic rash consisting of crops of papules, vesicles, pustules, and eventual crusting of nearly all the lesions. In normal children the systemic symptoms are usually mild, and serious complications are unusual. In adults, and in children with deficiencies in cell-mediated immunity, the disease may be manifested by an extensive eruption, severe constitutional symptoms, and pneumonia, with a fatal outcome if no therapy is given.

Zoster, which is caused by reactivation of latent VZV, is characterized by a localized unilateral rash consisting of varicella-like lesions in the distribution of a sensory nerve. Occasionally more than one nerve is involved, and in some patients hematogenous dissemination of virus occurs, leading to a generalized rash after the localized eruption. Zoster occurs most often in immunocompromised individuals; it is also more common in the elderly than in the young, and it is more likely to be accompanied by dermatomal pain in adults than in children.

ETIOLOGY

VZV, a member of the herpesvirus group, is composed of an inner core containing protein and DNA, an icosahedral capsid surrounded by a tegument, and an outer lipid-containing envelope. Enveloped VZV particles range in size from 150 to 200 nm (Fig. 34-1).

Weller et al., using tissue cultures of human embryonic cells and vesicular fluid from patients with chickenpox and zoster, was the first to propagate VZV in vitro (Weller and Witton, 1958). Weller demonstrated the presence of eosinophilic intranuclear inclusion bodies and multinucleated cells typical of varicella in culture, and he successfully passaged the agent in series, using the cellular components of infected tissue cultures. Using these cultures as the antigen, he demonstrated a rise in antibody titer in convalescent-phase serum from patients with varicella and patients with zoster.

The following body of evidence indicates that

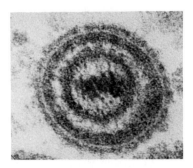

Fig. 34-1. Electron micrograph of varicella-zoster virus. This specimen was obtained from vesicular fluid of a child 1 day after the onset of varicella. The structural elements of the virion are the central DNA core, the protein capsid, the tegument, and the envelope. The last structure contains glycoproteins and is important for infectivity of the virion. ($\times$175,000.) (Courtesy Michael D. Gershon, M.D.)

the agents that cause varicella and zoster are identical:

1. Varicella has been transmitted to susceptible children by inoculating them with vesicular fluid from patients with zoster. The experimental disease was contagious, and it produced chickenpox in other children (Bruusgaard, 1932; Kundratitz, 1925).
2. The cytopathic effect of varicella virus in tissue cultures is neutralized not only by varicella immune serum but also by zoster immune serum. Both sera also neutralize virus obtained from patients with zoster (Weller and Coons, 1954).
3. Morphologically identical particles are seen in electron microscopic studies of vesicular fluid from patients with varicella and patients with zoster. Biopsies of skin lesions in both diseases reveal the same type of eosinophilic inclusion bodies, and smears of varicella and zoster lesions show the same type of multinucleated giant cells. Viruses from both clinical entities are indistinguishable by immunofluorescence assays (Weller and Witton, 1958).
4. Virus obtained from varicella and zoster lesions have the same DNA structure (Straus et al., 1984; Hayakawa et al., 1984; Williams et al., 1985; Gelb et al., 1987).

Glycoproteins specified by VZV are present both on the membranes of infected cells and on the envelope of the virus itself. At least five glycoproteins, designated I to V, have been identified for VZV. These glycoproteins play important roles in viral pathogenesis and in the generation of cellular and humoral immunity in the infected host. For example, some of the glycoproteins are required to facilitate transmission of VZV from one cell to another (Edson et al., 1985). In addition to glycoprotein antigens, VZV also synthesizes other structural and nonstructural proteins and polypeptides and viral enzymes and proteins that regulate viral development (Grose, 1987; Straus et al., 1988).

The linear double-stranded DNA genome of VZV has been fully sequenced (Davison and Scott, 1986). The genome is quite stable, as evidenced by the comparison of viral isolates obtained from patients during primary infection and during subsequent reactivation infection (Gelb et al., 1987; Hayakawa et al., 1984; Straus et al., 1984; Williams et al., 1985). Genome differences do exist, however, enabling differentiation of vaccine strains of VZV from wild-type

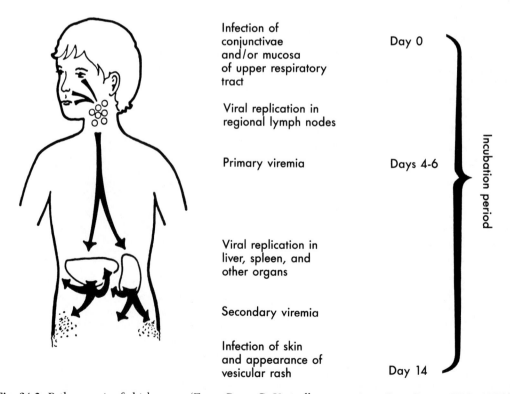

Infection of conjunctivae and/or mucosa of upper respiratory tract — Day 0

Viral replication in regional lymph nodes

Primary viremia — Days 4-6

Viral replication in liver, spleen, and other organs

Secondary viremia

Infection of skin and appearance of vesicular rash — Day 14

Incubation period

Fig. 34-2. Pathogenesis of chickenpox. (From Grose C. Varicella-zoster virus. Boca Raton: CRC, 1987.)

strains (Gelb et al., 1987; Martin et al., 1982).

VZV does not cause clinical disease in common laboratory animals, although simian forms of varicella have been described. Guinea pigs may be infected with VZV that has been adapted in vitro to guinea pig tissue; a high proportion of newborn and hairless animals so infected exhibit a papular rash (Myers et al., 1980; Myers et al., 1985; Myers et al., 1991).

PATHOLOGY

The following sequence of events is believed to occur when a varicella-susceptible person is infected (Fig. 34-2). The virus gains entry at the respiratory mucosa and presumably multiplies in the regional lymphatic tissue. Four to 6 days after infection a low-level primary viremia is believed to occur, allowing the virus to infect and multiply in the liver, spleen, and possibly other organs. Approximately 10 to 12 days after infection a secondary viremia of greater magnitude occurs, at which time the virus reaches the skin (Grose, 1981). The rash results, on the average, 14 days after infection. Viremia, which has been demonstrated during the early stage of clinical varicella, is more difficult to demonstrate in normal than in immunocompromised children (Asano et al., 1985a; Asano et al., 1990; Feldman and Epp, 1976; Feldman and Epp, 1979; Myers, 1979; Ozaki et al., 1986). Viremia has also been reported in some patients with zoster (Feldman et al., 1977; Gershon et al., 1978).

The skin lesions of varicella begin as macules, the majority of which progress to papules, vesicles, pustules, and crusts over a few days. Some lesions regress after the macular and papular stages. Vesicles are located primarily in the epidermis; the roof is formed by the strata corneum and lucidum and the floor by the deeper prickle cell layer. Ballooning degeneration of epidermal cells is followed by formation of multinucleated giant cells, many of which contain typical type A intranuclear inclusion bodies. Inclusion bodies are also present in endothelial cells. Vesicles are formed by accumulation of fluid derived from dermal capillaries, which fills in the space created by degenerating epidermal cells.

As the lesions progress, polymorphonuclear leukocytes invade the corium and vesicular fluid (Stevens et al., 1975), and the fluid changes from clear to cloudy. Interferon has been demonstrated in vesicular fluid and is believed to reflect the cell-mediated immune response to the

virus by the host (Merigan et al., 1978). The resolution of vesicular fluid is followed by the formation of a scab, which is at first adherent but later becomes detached. Mucous membrane lesions develop in the same way but do not progress to scab formation. The vesicles usually rupture and form shallow ulcers, which heal rapidly.

Although the most obvious target organ of the virus is the skin, children with benign cases of varicella and transiently elevated aspartate aminotransferase (AST) levels (>50 IU/l) have been described (Myers, 1982; Pitel et al., 1980). Postmortem examination of infants and adults who died of varicella reveals evidence of involvement of many organs. Areas of focal necrosis and acidophilic inclusion bodies may be present in the esophagus, liver, pancreas, kidney, ureter, bladder, uterus, and adrenal glands. The lungs show evidence of widely disseminated interstitial pneumonia, with numerous hemorrhagic areas of nodular consolidation. Histologically, the exudate consists chiefly of red blood cells, fibrin, and many mononuclear cells, some containing intranuclear inclusion bodies (Fig. 34-3). Encephalitis complicating varicella is pathologically similar to that with measles and to other types of postinfection encephalitis showing perivascular demyelination in the white matter.

Latent infection with VZV is believed to develop when sensory nerve endings in the epidermis are invaded by the virus during varicella when the virus is present on the skin. Virions presumably are transported up the sensory nerves to the ganglia where latency is established. During latency only a few viral genes are expressed, and infectious particles are not formed or released (Croen et al., 1988; Straus et al., 1988). As shown in Fig. 34-4, when viral reactivation occurs, infectious virions are produced once more, and virions are transported down the sensory nerve to the skin where vesicles appear (Hope-Simpson, 1965).

Patients with impaired cellular immunity have the highest rate of zoster; therefore it is believed that at least some aspects of VZV latency are under immunological control (Arvin et al., 1978, 1980). The incidence of zoster probably increases in the elderly because cell-mediated immune responses to VZV diminish with advancing age (Burke et al., 1982; Miller, 1980). An increased incidence of zoster with a short latency period has also been observed in children who experienced varicella in prenatal life or early

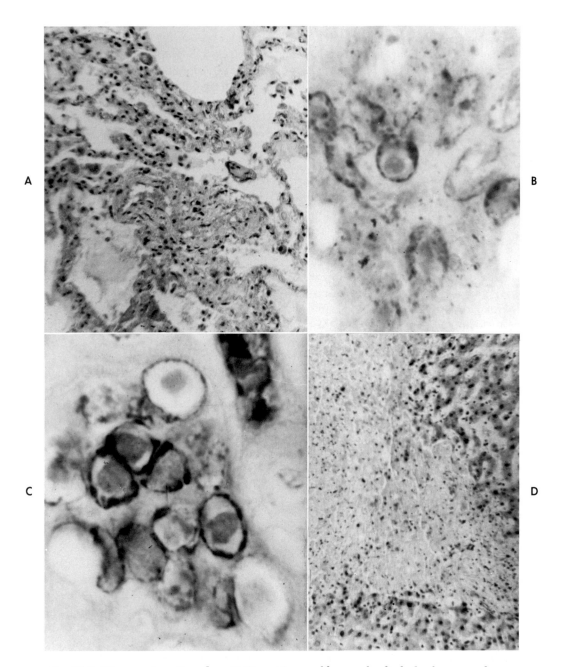

Fig. 34-3. Microscopic sections from E.W., a 44-year-old man who died of pulmonary edema after 5 days of hemorrhagic varicella associated with severe right upper quadrant abdominal pain, cough, dyspnea, tachypnea, cyanosis, and hemoptysis. **A,** Interstitial mononuclear cell infiltration and fibrinous exudate in the alveoli of the lung. **B,** Intranuclear inclusion bodies in the lung. **C,** Multinucleated cell with intranuclear inclusions in the skin. **D,** Typical focus of necrosis in the liver. (From Krugman S, et al. N Engl J Med 1957;257:843.)

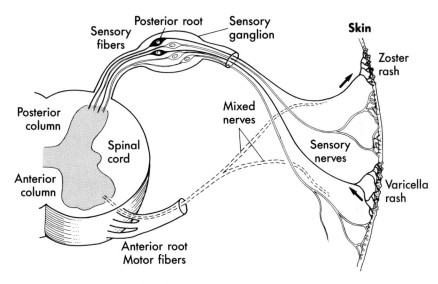

Fig. 34-4. Diagram of proposed pathogenesis of zoster. Latent VZV infection in dorsal root ganglia develops during the rash of varicella. Reactivation of VZV in ganglia may subsequently occur, resulting in zoster. Affected neurons and affected sensory nerves are in black. (Modified from Hope-Simpson RE. Proc R Soc Med 1965;58:9-20.)

infancy, presumably because of immaturity of the cell-mediated immune response to VZV during the primary infection (Baba et al., 1986; Brunell and Kotchmar, 1981; Dworsky et al., 1980; Guess et al., 1985). Brunell and Kotchmar (1981) described five infants with zoster, all of whose mothers had varicella between 3 and 7 months' gestation. These infants had no evidence of varicella after birth. Presumably all had varicella in utero since they developed zoster after an average latent period of only 21 months (range, 3 to 41 months). Usually the latent period between varicella and zoster lasts for decades.

Using in situ hybridization and polymerase chain reaction (PCR), VZV DNA and RNA and viral proteins have been demonstrated in human sensory ganglia obtained from autopsy material (Croen et al., 1988; Gilden et al., 1987; Hyman et al., 1983; Mahalingham et al., 1990; Vafai et al., 1988). These data prove that the site of VZV latency is sensory ganglia, although efforts to culture infectious virus from such ganglia have been unsuccessful. VZV DNA, RNA, and some proteins have also been found in the circulating peripheral white blood cells in elderly patients with postherpetic neuralgia (Vafai et al., 1988).

CLINICAL MANIFESTATIONS OF VARICELLA

After an incubation period of 14 to 16 days, with outside limits of 10 to 21 days, the disease

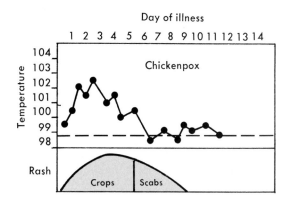

Fig. 34-5. Schematic diagram illustrating clinical course of typical case of chickenpox. Crops of lesions appear, with rapid progression from macules to papules to vesicles to scabs.

begins with low-grade fever, malaise, and the appearance of rash. In children the exanthem and constitutional symptoms usually occur simultaneously. In adolescents and adults the rash may be preceded by a 1- to 2-day prodromal period of fever, headache, malaise, and anorexia. The typical clinical course of varicella is illustrated in Fig. 34-5.

Rash

The typical vesicle of chickenpox is superficially located in the skin. It has thin, fragile walls

CHICKENPOX

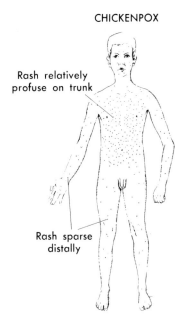

Rash relatively
profuse on trunk

Rash sparse
distally

Fig. 34-6. Schematic drawing illustrating typical distribution of rash of chickenpox.

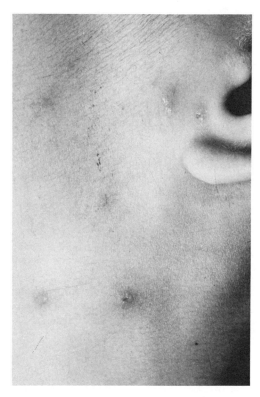

Fig. 34-7. Chickenpox lesions in various stages.

that rupture easily. In appearance it resembles a dewdrop, usually elliptical in shape, 2 to 3 mm in diameter, and surrounded by an erythematous area. This red areola is most distinct when the vesicle is fully formed and becomes pustular, and it fades as the lesion begins to dry. The drying process, which begins in the center of the vesicle or pustule, produces an umbilicated appearance and eventually a crust. After a variable interval of 5 to 20 days, depending on the depth of skin involvement, the scab falls off, leaving a shallow pink depression. The site of the lesion becomes white, with no evidence of scar formation. Secondarily infected lesions and prematurely removed scabs may be followed by scarring.

The lesions appear in crops that generally involve the trunk, scalp, face, and extremities. The distribution is typically central, with the greatest concentration of lesions on the trunk and face (Fig. 34-6). The rash is more profuse on the proximal parts of the extremities (upper arms and thighs) than on the distal parts (forearms and legs). A distinctive manifestation of the eruption is the presence of lesions in all stages in any one general anatomical area; macules, papules, vesicles, pustules, and crusts are usually located in proximity to each other (Fig. 34-7).

In the typical case of chickenpox three suc-

cessive crops of lesions appear over a 3-day period in the characteristic central distribution just described. The extremes of this picture may range from (1) a single crop of a few scattered lesions to (2) a series of five or more crops developing over a week, with an uncountable number of lesions covering the entire skin surface of the body. In a study of over 750 cases of chickenpox in otherwise healthy children, the average child developed approximately 250 to 500 skin vesicles (Ross et al., 1962). In secondary cases in a household the rash is usually more extensive than in the primary case.

Vesicles develop on the mucous membranes of the mouth in addition to the skin. They occur most commonly over the palate and usually rupture so rapidly that the vesicular stage may be missed. In appearance they resemble the shallow, white 2- to 3-mm ulcers of herpetic stomatitis. The palpebral conjunctiva, pharynx, larynx, trachea, and rectal and vaginal mucosa may also be involved.

Areas of local inflammation such as ammoniacal dermatitis in the diaper area or sunburned skin may have a significant increase in the number of lesions. These vesicles are generally smaller than usual, are usually in the same stage of development, and may become confluent.

In summary, the rash of chickenpox is characterized by (1) a rapid evolution of macule to papule to vesicle to pustule to crust, (2) a central distribution of lesions that appear in crops, and (3) the presence of lesions in all stages in any one anatomical area.

Fever

The temperature curve of a typical case of chickenpox is illustrated in Fig. 34-5. The height of the fever usually parallels the severity of the rash. When the eruption is sparse, the temperature is usually normal or slightly elevated; an extensive rash more likely will be associated with high and more prolonged fevers. Temperatures up to 40.6° C (105° F) are not unusual in severe cases of chickenpox with involvement of almost the entire skin surface.

Other symptoms

Headache, malaise, and anorexia usually accompany the fever. In many cases the most distressing symptom is pruritus, which is present during the vesicular stage of the disease.

Unusual manifestations of chickenpox

Hemorrhagic, progressive, and disseminated varicella. Varicella in an immujocompromised host may be characterized by a hemorrhagic, progressive, and/or disseminated infection and a potentially fatal outcome. Feldman et al. (1975) observed 77 children with cancer at St. Jude Children's Research Hospital who contracted varicella in the pre-antiviral therapy era. No complications were observed among the 17 children no longer receiving anticancer chemotherapy. In contrast, of the 60 children still receiving anticancer chemotherapy, 19 (32%) had evidence of visceral dissemination and four (7%) died. Deaths were associated with varicella pneumonia (all four patients) and encephalitis (two of the four patients). Disseminated varicella occurred more frequently in children with absolute lymphopenia who had fewer than 500 lymphocytes/mm^3.

In a more recent assessment of children with underlying cancer and varicella at the same institution, Feldman and Lott (1987) reported on a total 127 children observed between 1962 and 1986. They found that despite passive immunization and antiviral therapy, fatalities caused

by varicella still occurred. Children with leukemia fared more poorly than children with other malignancies, although the incidence of varicella pneumonia was high in each group, 32% and 19%, respectively. In children with leukemia who had received passive immunization with varicella-zoster immune globulin (VZIG), the incidence of primary viral pneumonia was 15%. Cessation of anticancer chemotherapy during the incubation period did not significantly decrease the incidence of varicella pneumonia.

There are two possible courses of severe varicella in immunocompromised children. In some a fulminant disease with hemorrhagic lesions, pneumonia, and disseminated intravascular coagulation occurs; death usually ensues within a few days, often despite antiviral therapy. In other children a more protracted illness develops, with new crops of vesicles occurring for as long as 2 weeks. At first these children may appear to have mild disease, but as new lesions continue to develop, accompanied by fever, toxicity, abdominal and back pain, and pneumonia, the serious nature of the illness becomes apparent, usually during the second week after onset.

Severe, progressive, fatal varicella infection has also been observed in children treated with high doses of corticosteroids for conditions other than cancer. Gershon et al. (1972) described the development of fulminant varicella in two boys treated with corticosteroids for rheumatic fever; deaths occurred 2 and 4 days after onset of rash. Although children with asthma treated with low doses of steroids apparently are not at risk to develop severe varicella, fatalities have been reported in those receiving high doses (Kasper and Howe, 1991; Silk et al., 1988).

Severe varicella has also been described in patients who have undergone renal (Feldhoff et al., 1981) and bone marrow (Locksley et al., 1985) transplantation and in children with acquired immunodeficiency syndrome (AIDS) (Acheson et al., 1988; Jura et al., 1989; Pahwa et al., 1988). They and other immunocompromised patients are also at high risk to develop varicella or zoster that may be recurrent and/or chronic, although the frequency of this occurrence is unknown (Acheson et al., 1988; Feldhoff et al., 1981; Gershon et al., 1984a; Morens et al., 1980; Patterson et al., 1989). Development of zoster in young adults is a reported sentinel for subsequent development of AIDS

(Colebunders et al., 1988; Melbye et al., 1987).

It has long been thought that immunocompromised children are predisposed to develop severe varicella because their cell-mediated immune response to VZV is deficient. In immunocompromised patients the in vitro lymphocyte response to VZV antigen has been reported to develop more slowly in those with severe disease than in those with an uncomplicated illness (Arvin et al., 1986). Furthermore, lymphocytes from leukemic children with prior varicella show decreased in vitro responses to VZV antigen in comparison to lymphocytes from healthy controls (Giller et al., 1986). This result was attributed to decreased numbers of circulating lymphocytes rather than to impaired antigen presentation. Studies of lymphoid cells from patients with fatal varicella indicated the inability of these cells to inactivate VZV in vitro in contrast to lymphoid cells from control individuals (Gershon and Steinberg, 1979). There is no apparent correlation of poor antibody responses and severe varicella in immunocompromised patients.

Congenital varicella syndrome. The congenital varicella syndrome is extremely rare. Since the 1940s when it was first recognized, approximately 40 cases have been recorded in the world literature (Gershon, 1990; Paryani and Arvin, 1986). Manifestations of the syndrome include a hypoplastic extremity, zosteriform skin scarring, microphthalmia, cataracts, chorioretinitis, and abnormalities of the central nervous system (CNS) (Table 34-1 and Fig. 34-8). There is a spectrum of disease, with most children severely affected but some with only a few stigmata such as chorioretinitis. The incidence of this syn-

Table 34-1. Clinical and laboratory data of 39 infants with the congenital varicella syndrome

Occurrence	(%)
After maternal varicella	87
After maternal zoster	13
Time (weeks) of maternal infection	
Median	12
Range	8-28
Major malformations described	(%)
Cicatricial skin lesions	72
Ocular abnormalities: cataract, chorioretinitis, Horner's syndrome, microphthalmia, nystagmus	62
Hypoplastic limb	46
Cortical atrophy and/or mental retardation	31
Early death	24

Modified from Gershon A. Chickenpox, measles, and mumps. In Remington JS, Klein JO (eds). Infections of the fetus and newborn infant, ed 3. Philadelphia: WB Saunders, 1990.

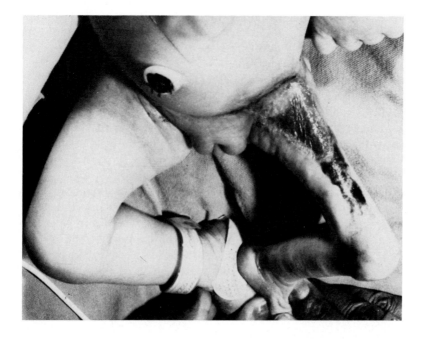

Fig. 34-8. Congenital varicella syndrome illustrating cicatricial skin lesions and hypotrophic left lower limb. (From Srabstein JC et al: J Pediatr 1974;84:239.)

drome following gestational varicella in the first trimester apparently is approximately 2%, with a possible range between 0.5% and 6.5% (Preblud et al., 1986). There have been four small prospective studies of pregnant women with varicella in the first trimester and their offspring. In one (Manson et al., 1960) there were no cases of the congenital varicella syndrome in 70 pregnancies. In another involving 27 women, two infants had cataracts, but none had the full-blown syndrome (Siegel, 1973). In a third study of 23 women there were no infants with abnormalities consistent with the syndrome (Enders, 1984). In the study of Paryani and Arvin (1986), however, of 11 pregnancies complicated by varicella there was one case of the full-blown syndrome in an infant. Thus the incidence of varicella-associated birth defects due to first trimester maternal infection in these studies was three abnormal infants born to 131 women (2%). The congenital varicella syndrome has also very rarely been recorded when maternal varicella has occurred as late as 28 weeks of gestation. Fortunately the syndrome is very rare since there is no practical way to diagnose it in utero or to prevent it. There was one instance in which the congenital defects were identified by fetal ultrasound (Essex-Cater and Heggarty, 1983) and another in which defects were not clearly identified by ultrasound (DaSilva et al., 1990). There is a high correlation (>50%) between hypoplastic extremities and severe brain damage and/or early death. The pathogenesis is not understood, but the rarity of the illness and the pattern of cicatricial skin lesions and damage to the nervous system suggest that the fetus may have experienced varicella followed by zoster in utero. Interestingly, infants with the syndrome have also been reported to develop clinical zoster with a short period of viral latency in postnatal life (Kotchmar et al., 1984). Maternal varicella itself may also be severe during pregnancy, and fatalities have been reported (Paryani and Arvin, 1986).

Severe or fatal varicella in 5- to 10-day-old infants may occur when their mothers have varicella 5 days or less before delivery. It is believed that in infants who develop the illness between 5 to 10 days of age (an incubation period of approximately 10 days), the cellular immune response to VZV has not yet matured. In addition, the size of the inoculum introduced into the infant by the mother's viremia may be large, which might account for the shorter incubation period. Varicella in the newborn may become disseminated such as in a leukemic child with chickenpox. Maternally transmitted antibody may act as a form of passive immunization for the infant, but when the mother has had varicella for less than 5 days before delivery, she has not made or transferred this antibody to her baby. The clinical attack rate of varicella in newborn infants under these conditions has been reported to range from 20% to 50% (Meyers, 1974; Hanngren et al., 1985; Preblud et al., 1986). In infected infants who have been neither passively immunized nor treated with an antiviral drug, the mortality rate is approximately 35% (Meyers, 1974).

Disseminated varicella infection in a newborn infant is characterized by hemorrhagic lesions and involvement of the lungs and the liver. Effects on the newborn infant when maternal varicella occurs near term are shown in Table 34-2.

Bullous varicella. Bullous varicella is an unusual manifestation of the infection characterized by the simultaneous occurrence of typical varicelliform lesions and bullae. Published reports indicate that the bullous lesions are caused by phage group II staphylococci (Melish, 1973; Wald et al., 1973). These staphylococci produce epidermolytic toxin, the cause of staphylococcal scalded skin syndrome. Thus it appears that in bullous varicella the patient may be superinfected by an exfoliative toxigenic *Staphylococcus aureus*, but interestingly VZV has not been cultivated from the bullous fluid itself.

Table 34-2. Maternal varicella near term: effect on the newborn infant (50 cases)

Onset	Effect
Maternal varicella, 5 or more days before delivery; baby's varicella, age 0-4 days	27 of 27 survived
Maternal varicella, 4 days or less before delivery; baby's varicella, age 5-10 days	16 of 23 survived (seven died of disseminated varicella, two had severe disease with survival)

From Gershon AA. In Krugman S, Gershon AA (eds). Infections of the fetus and newborn infant. New York: Alan R Liss, 1975.

Varicella in the adult. Varicella, like many other viral infections, is more likely to be severe in adults than in children. The risk of developing severe varicella in persons more than 20 years of age is 25 times greater than it is in children (Preblud et al., 1984). In general, the fever is higher and more prolonged, the constitutional symptoms are more severe, the rash is more profuse, and complications are more frequent in adults as compared to children. Varicella pneumonia is a significant complication in adults. A prospective evaluation of 114 military personnel with varicella revealed roentgenographic evidence of pulmonary involvement in 16%, although clinical signs were present in only 4% (Weber and Pellecchia, 1965).

Second attacks of varicella. It was once generally accepted that varicella occurs only once in a lifetime. Second attacks of clinical illness are difficult to confirm by laboratory means because most first attacks are diagnosed only clinically. There is a growing body of evidence, however, suggesting that second attacks of varicella may occur (Weller, 1983). Varicella has been observed in persons known to have specific antibodies before onset of illness (Gershon et al., 1984a; Gershon et al., 1988; Gershon et al., 1989; Zaia et al., 1983). Serological evidence of subclinical infection of varicella-immune individuals closely exposed to VZV has also been reported (Arvin, Koropchak, and Wittek, 1983; Gershon et al., 1982; Gershon et al., 1984b; Gershon et al., 1988; Gershon et al., 1989; Luby et al., 1977). Most second attacks have been mild. Second attacks are most common in immunocompromised persons, in those who orginally had subclinical infections, and in children who had varicella in early infancy.

CLINICAL MANIFESTATIONS OF ZOSTER

The incubation period of zoster is unknown because it is impossible to determine the time of reactivation of latent VZV. The predilection of the virus for the posterior nerve root areas accounts for the severe pain and tenderness along the involved nerves and the corresponding areas of skin seen in elderly patients. Fever often is not present.

It is believed that zoster occurs when cellular immunity to VZV is depressed. This depression may be transient such as when otherwise healthy persons develop the illness, or it may be secondary to severe immunosuppression induced by diseases such as malignancy, by anticancer chemotherapy or radiotherapy, or after immunosuppression for organ transplantation.

It is also thought that in immunologically normal as well as in immunocompromised hosts viral reactivation can occur without development of skin lesions (Luby et al., 1977; Gershon et al., 1982; Ljungman et al., 1986; Wilson et al., 1991).

Zoster is usually typified by a characteristic unilateral rash with a dermatomal distribution. The lesions begin as macules and papules and progress through the same stages as the eruption of varicella. The regional lymph nodes may be enlarged and tender. The lesions may appear on the face (involvement of the trigeminal ganglia), the trunk (thoracic ganglia), the shoulders, arms, and/or neck (cervical ganglia), or the perineal area and lower extremities (lumbar or sacral ganglia). When the trigeminal nerve is involved, infection of the maxillary division is associated with lesions of the uvula and tonsillar area; the mandibular division, with lesions of the buccal mucosa; the floor of the mouth and anterior part of the tongue; and the ophthalmic division, with scleral and corneal lesions. Infection of the geniculate ganglion of the facial nerve can result in pain, a vesicular eruption in the auditory canal, and facial paralysis, which usually subsides but may be permanent (Ramsay Hunt syndrome). Severe neuralgia, which may persist for many months after convalescence, is much more common in elderly adults than in children.

Zoster is chiefly a disease of the immunocompromised and of adults, but it can occur in infants and children. A previous clinical or subclinical episode of varicella is a prerequisite.

Disseminated zoster. Disseminated zoster is not uncommon, and it usually occurs in children and adults with marked depression of cell-mediated immunity to VZV. Soon after appearance of the localized lesions the rash becomes generalized, resembling varicella. Fever more likely will be present than in localized zoster. The number of skin lesions outside the dermatomal area ranges from a few to thousands; the extent of the rash reflects the seriousness of the infection. Fatalities may occur when there is extensive visceral involvement if no antiviral therapy is given (Feldman et al., 1973; Shepp et al., 1986; Whitley et al., 1982).

Patients who have undergone bone marrow transplantation are not only at increased incidence to develop zoster, but also to develop severe symptoms. In a study of 1,394 adults who underwent bone marrow transplantation, the incidence of zoster after 1 year was approximately 17% (Locksley et al., 1985). Of these adults, 45% developed disseminated disease, and the overall fatality rate in the group was 6% despite antiviral therapy. There was also a high incidence of postherpetic neuralgia, skin scarring, and bacterial superinfections.

DIAGNOSIS OF VARICELLA
Confirmatory clinical factors

The typical case of chickenpox can be recognized clinically with ease. The characteristic diagnostic features include (1) development of a pruritic papulovesicular eruption concentrated on the face and trunk associated with fever and mild constitutional symptoms; (2) the rapid progression of macules to papules, vesicles, pustules, and crusts; (3) the appearance of these lesions in crops, with a predominant central distribution including the scalp; (4) the presence of shallow white ulcers on the mucous membranes of the mouth; and (5) the eventual crusting of the skin lesions. The knowledge of an exposure to a person with either varicella or zoster is always helpful when present.

Detection of the causative agent

Laboratory diagnosis by methods such as viral isolation are indicated for identification of atypical or unusual types of chickenpox. VZV may be readily isolated from vesicular fluid obtained within the first 1 to 3 days of rash in tissue cultures such as human embryonic lung fibroblasts. VZV antigens may also be detected in vesicles by various immunological means, including direct immunofluorescence with commercially available monoclonal antibodies. Such assays can be performed within an hour's time and can distinguish between VZV and herpes simplex virus (HSV) (Frey et al., 1981; Gleaves et al., 1988; Olding-Stenkvist and Grandien, 1976; Rawlinson et al., 1989; Zeigler, 1984; Zeigler and Halonen, 1985).

Serological tests

Antibody has been detected in serum within days after onset of illness and can be expected to increase in titer over the next 1 to 2 weeks. Consequently, a retrospective diagnosis is possible if acute and convalescent serum specimens are available. The first sample of blood should be collected as soon as possible after the onset of disease; the second should be obtained approximately 10 days later. Enzyme-linked immunosorbent assay (ELISA), which is commercially marketed, is the most frequently used serological test used today (Demmler et al., 1988; Forghani et al., 1978; Gershon et al., 1981; Shanley et al., 1982; Shehab and Brunell, 1983). ELISA may also be used to determine immune status to varicella; if a significant amount of antibody is present in serum, it indicates a prior episode of varicella even in the absence of a history of the illness. The fluorescent antibody to membrane antigen (FAMA) assay, anticomplement immunofluorescence, and radioimmunoassay (RIA) are extremely sensitive but available only on a research basis (Campbell-Benzie et al., 1983; Presissner et al., 1982; Richman et al., 1981; Williams et al., 1974; Zaia and Oxman, 1977). These tests are somewhat better for identification of immunity to varicella but are not necessarily any better than ELISA for making a serological diagnosis of the disease. A newly developed latex agglutination (LA) test, utilizing latex particles coated with VZV antigen, has shown great promise as a sensitive and specific VZV serologic test (Steinberg and Gershon, 1991).

A skin test using VZV antigen has been developed and used to identify individuals who are susceptible to varicella and lack cell-mediated immunity to the virus. This test is very accurate for this purpose in persons under age 40, but it is not available commercially (Florman et al., 1985; Kamiya et al., 1977; LaRussa et al., 1985).

Ancillary laboratory findings

The white blood cell count is not consistent. In most cases it is within the normal range. It is not unusual for adults with primary varicella pneumonia to have leukocytosis with a predominance of polymorphonuclear leukocytes. Mild, transient elevation of liver enzymes commonly occurs in patients with varicella.

DIAGNOSIS OF ZOSTER

Implication of VZV is essential for a definitive diagnosis of zoster because characteristic zosteriform skin lesions have on occasion been observed in HSV infections. In a study of 47 adults with clinical signs and symptoms compatible with zoster, six (13%) yielded HSV from cultures of skin lesions (Kalman and Laskin, 1986). Laboratory diagnosis is made best by demonstration of the virus or viral antigens in vesicular fluid. A fourfold rise in VZV antibody titer 2 to 4 weeks after appearance of lesions provides additional confirmation of the diagnosis, although increases in VZV antibody titer have been described in HSV infections because of shared antigens between these viruses (Schmidt, 1982; Vafai et al., 1990).

DIFFERENTIAL DIAGNOSIS OF VARICELLA

The differential diagnosis of varicella is also discussed in Chapter 36. Varicella may resemble the following conditions.

Impetigo. The skin lesions of impetigo are vesicular at first but rapidly progress to honey-colored crusts. They differ from chickenpox in appearance and distribution. They do not appear in crops, do not involve the mucous membranes of the mouth, and are not accompanied by constitutional symptoms. The lesions commonly involve the nasolabial area because of the tendency for a child to scratch this area with contaminated fingers. Other areas that are easily scratched also become involved.

Insect bites, papular urticaria, and urticaria. Insect bites, papular urticaria, and urticaria are not accompanied by constitutional symptoms. They are papular and pruritic but do not have the typical vesicular appearance and distribution. Vesicles, if present, are pinpoint in size. The scalp and mouth are devoid of lesions.

Scabies. The differential points of scabies are the same as those of insect bites. In addition, the observation of burrows between the fingers and toes and the microscopic identification of *Sarcoptes scabiei* help confirm the diagnosis.

Dermatitis herpetiformis. The lesions in dermatitis herpetiformis are usually symmetrical and consist of erythematous, papulovesicular, and urticarial lesions that are markedly pruritic,

have a chronic course, and heal with residual pigmentation.

Rickettsialpox. Rickettsialpox has the classic triad of signs and symptoms in the following order: (1) the appearance of a primary lesion or eschar on some part of the body, (2) the development of an influenza-like syndrome, and (3) the occurrence of a generalized papulovesicular eruption. The rash of rickettsialpox differs from that of varicella in that the vesicles are much smaller and are superimposed on a firm papule. Crusts do not develop regularly; if they do, they are very small. The diagnosis is confirmed by a specific antibody test.

Eczema herpeticum and other forms of HSV infection. A patient with eczema herpeticum may have a history of contact with a person who had a fever blister; the rash is caused by either primary or reactivated HSV infection. The vesicular and pustular lesions are most profuse over the sites of eczema. The different type of distribution is the most useful differential point. At times it may be necessary to perform laboratory examinations (e.g., direct immunofluorescence, described previously) to identify the causative agent. At one time eczema vaccinatum could also be confused with varicella, but since smallpox vaccine is not routinely used in children, this diagnosis is unlikely.

In the newborn infant HSV and varicella may be confused when only a few vesicular skin lesions are present and there is no history of exposure to either virus. In this instance direct immunofluorescence of skin lesions is helpful. Zosteriform lesions in the neonate due to HSV infection have been reported (Music et al., 1971; Rabalais et al., 1991).

Stevens-Johnson syndrome. With this syndrome there may be a prior history of use of medications and allergy. Annular skin lesions and extensive involvement of mucous membranes should suggest Stevens-Johnson syndrome rather than varicella.

Smallpox. The elimination of smallpox in the 1970s makes this diagnosis extremely unlikely.

COMPLICATIONS OF VARICELLA

Complications of varicella are not common; uneventful recovery is the rule except in immunocompromised persons. The following incidence of serious complications in children aged

1 to 14 years per 100,000 cases of varicella has been recorded: encephalitis, 1.7; Reye's syndrome, 3.2; hospitalization, 1.7; and death, 2.0 (Preblud et al., 1984).

Secondary bacterial infection

The secondary infection of skin lesions is not common enough to warrant the use of prophylactic antimicrobials. Staphylococci or group A β-hemolytic streptococci may gain entry into the lesions and produce impetigo, furuncles, cellulitis, and possibly, erysipelas. Scalded skin syndrome (Melish, 1973; Wald et al., 1973) and toxic shock–like syndrome (Bradley et al., 1991) have both been reported as complications of chickenpox. Although bacterial superinfections can result in septicemia, pneumonia, suppurative arthritis, osteomyelitis, or local gangrene, even in the era before antibiotics were available, there was a low incidence of these complications. Bullous impetigo caused by exfoliative toxigenic *S. aureus*, phage type II, may be considered a secondary bacterial infection. Neutropenia that occasionally follows varicella may predispose to secondary bacterial infections (Koumbourlis, 1988).

Encephalitis

Encephalitis occurs in less than one of every 1,000 cases of varicella and may complicate a mild or a severe infection. Cerebellar involvement with ataxia is the most common form (Peters et al., 1978). If encephalitis occurs as an isolated phenomenon, the prognosis is excellent. The symptoms of CNS involvement usually develop between the third and eighth days after the onset of rash, but at times they may precede the exanthem.

The signs of cerebral involvement include those of meningoencephalitis, with fever, headache, stiff neck, change in sensorium, and occasionally, convulsions, stupor, coma, and paralysis. The cerebral form, in contrast to the cerebellar form, carries a more guarded prognosis, although the prognosis is difficult to assess since in the past varicella encephalitis and Reye's syndrome were often confused with each other. However, in a survey of 59 cases of varicella encephalitis, Applebaum et al., (1953) reported complete recovery in 80%, evidence of brain damage in 15%, and death in 5%. Of 302

cases of varicella encephalitis reported in the United States during 3 years (1963 to 1965), 82 (27.1%) were fatal (McCormick et al., 1969). Other rare CNS complications include transverse myelitis, peripheral neuritis, and optic neuritis (Jemsek et al., 1983). In both cerebellar and cerebral types cerebrospinal fluid (CSF) changes include pleocytosis with a predominance of lymphocytes, an elevated protein value, and a normal glucose value.

Specific antibody has been detected in the CSF of patients with encephalitis caused by VZV (Jemsek et al., 1983) and may be used to confirm the clinical diagnosis. Encephalitis ranging from mild to severe, either accompanying or following zoster with a facial distribution, is a common occurrence. The use of antiviral therapy in patients with CNS complications of varicella or zoster is controversial because the underlying pathology is not well understood. Many physicians elect to treat immunocompromised patients with antiviral drugs but not those who are immunologically normal.

Varicella pneumonia

Varicella pneumonia has been recognized chiefly in otherwise healthy adults and immunocompromised patients of all ages. It is rare in normal children, but it has been seen in certain infants with neonatal varicella. One to 5 days after chickenpox begins, there is an onset of cough, chest pain, dyspnea, tachypnea, and, possibly, cyanosis and hemoptysis. Rales are usually heard over both lung fields. The roentgenogram shows characteristic nodular densities throughout both lung fields (Fig. 34-9). The nodular infiltrates vary in size and occasionally coalesce to form larger areas of consolidation. The leukocyte count may be either normal or slightly elevated.

The course of the pneumonia is variable. It may be extremely mild with little or no cough and no respiratory distress, and roentgenographic evidence of the disease may subside within 1 week. On the other hand, respiratory problems may be severe, with chest pain, hemoptysis, cyanosis, a stormy course of 7 to 10 days, and roentenographic findings that persist for as long as 4 to 6 weeks. Occasionally there is a fatal outcome despite antiviral therapy. Varicella pneumonia may be further complicated by

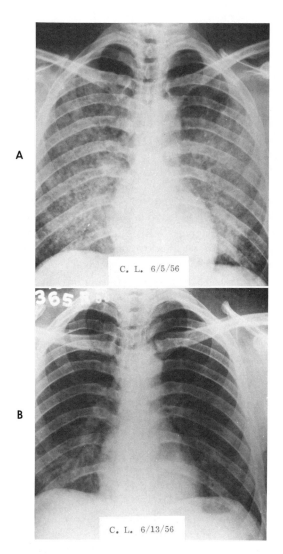

Fig. 34-9. Roentgenograms of the chest of C.L., a 24-year-old man with varicella, characterized on the third day by severe cough, dyspnea, tachypnea, cyanosis, and hemoptysis. **A,** Roentgenogram taken on the fourth day of pneumonia, showing extensive nodular infiltrates throughout both lung fields. **B,** Appearance 8 days later; there was considerable clearing. (From Krugman S, et al. N Engl J Med 1957;257:843.)

pleural effusion, subcutaneous emphysema, pulmonary edema, and adult respiratory distress syndrome (ARDS). Some cases of varicella pneumonia show evidence of other visceral involvement such as varicella hepatitis. Mackay and Cairney (1960) reported roentgenographic evidence of widespread, evenly distributed 1- to 3-mm nodules of calcific density in seven adults who had severe varicella after the age of 19 years. The roentgenograms were taken 3 to 32 years after onset of varicella. A summary of the epidemiological and clinical manifestations of primary varicella pneumonia in the pre-antiviral drug era is given in Table 34-3.

Reye's syndrome

Epidemiological surveys of the infections that have preceded Reye's syndrome demonstrate a large variety of associated agents. In an epidemiological study of this syndrome in Las Cruces, New Mexico, the incidence was estimated as 2.5 per 1,000 cases of varicella, four to nine times greater than its incidence after influenza B (Hurwitz and Goodman, 1982.) Preblud et al. (1984), however, reported an incidence of 3.2 cases per 100,000 cases of varicella. The disease has become even more rare since the administration of aspirin is now contraindicated during chickenpox.

Elevations of liver enzyme levels are not infrequent in otherwise healthy children during varicella (Ey and Fulginiti, 1981; Myers, 1982; Pitel et al., 1980). In the Pitel study of 39 children with varicella, transaminase elevations were greater than normal in 77%. Jaundice rarely develops, and the condition is almost always self-limited. Until these studies were reported, it was not realized that the liver can be involved in uncomplicated varicella. The relationship, if any, between this asymptomatic form of varicella hepatitis and Reye's syndrome is not known, although some children have experienced severe vomiting episodes during the period of abnormal liver enzyme activity. Lichtenstein et al. (1983) obtained liver biopsies from 19 children who had marked elevation of aminotransferase activity with minimal neurological symptoms (lethargy) after varicella (8 children) or an upper respiratory infection (11 children). Microscopic evidence of Reye's syndrome was found in 14 (74%). Therefore Lichtenstein et al. proposed that patients with vomiting, hepatic dysfunction, and minimal neurological impairment after varicella have Reye's syndrome.

Disseminated varicella

For a discussion of disseminated varicella, see p. 593.

Table 34-3. Summary of epidemiological and clinical manifestations of 30 cases of primary varicella pneumonia in the pre-antiviral drug era

Age	Range: 4 to 82 yr		Mean average: 33 yr
	(only two children, 4 and 6 years of age, both with leukemia)		

Sex	Male: 22	Female: 8

Season	January to March: 15 cases	April to June: 14 cases	October to December: 1 case

Day of onset of cough	First: 5	Second: 15	Third: 7	Fourth and fifth: 3

Clinical manifestation	*Severe*	*Moderate*	*Mild*	*None*
Cough	11	8	11	—
Dyspnea	11	7	1	11
Cyanosis	10	0	0	19
Hemoptysis	10	3	1	15
Rales	11	8	1	10
Roentgenographic findings	11	8	11	—

White blood count	Range: 4,000 to 16,200	Mean: 8,600

Complications Hepatitis (4)
Pleural effusion (3)
Pulmonary abscesses (2)
Subcutaneous emphysema (1)
Gastric ulcers (1)

Deaths Pulmonary edema (1)
Pulmonary abscesses and gastric ulcers (1)
Hepatitis (3)
Pulmonary abscesses and Hodgkin's disease (1)
Leukemia (1)

Other rare complications

Retinitis and orchitis have been reported as complications of varicella (Chambers et al., 1989; Wesselhoft and Pearson, 1950). Acute glomerulonephritis has been described in patients either with or without evidence of associated streptococcal infection (Yuceoglu et al., 1967). Myocarditis has also been recorded (Kirk et al., 1987; Lorber et al., 1988; Waagoner and Murphy, 1990).

Varicella arthritis is another rare complication that is usually self-limited. The arthritis is usually monoarticular, with swelling, tenderness, pain, joint effusion, and no erythema. The synovial fluid contains a predominance of lymphocytes and is bacteria free (Mulhern et al., 1971; Priest et al., 1978; Ward and Bishop, 1970). Isolation of VZV from joint fluid obtained from a patient with varicella arthritis has been reported (Priest et al., 1978).

A very rare complication of purpura fulminans and gangrene of the extremities and face has been described (deKoning et al., 1972; Smith, 1967). Another very rare complication of VZV infection is hemiparesis secondary to vasculitis (Fikrig and Barg, 1989; Liu and Holmes, 1990).

PROGNOSIS

Varicella is usually a benign disease of childhood. The typical case clears spontaneously without sequelae or skin scarring. Lesions that are secondarily infected likely will be followed by permanent scars if the deep layers of the skin are involved. The rare case of sepsis, bacterial pneumonia, or osteomyelitis should respond to appropriate antibacterial therapy. Preblud et al. (1985) estimated that there are fewer than 10 deaths caused by varicella in infants under 1 year of age in the United States per year, primarily as a result of pneumonia or encephalitis. This represents a risk of death four times greater than that of older infants and children with varicella. In contrast, the risk of death for adults with varicella is increased by a factor of 25 in comparison to the risk for healthy children (Preblud et al., 1985; Preblud et al., 1984).

Varicella can be a very serious disease in newborn infants, adults, patients receiving high doses of corticosteroids for any reason, and patients treated with chemotherapy or radiotherapy for an underlying malignancy. Children with leukemia are at greatest risk. Varicella pneumonia is potentially fatal. Severe and fatal cases of varicella have been observed in children with underlying AIDS. A newly described syndrome of chronic VZV infection has also been seen in children with AIDS; after recovery from varicella these children may develop scattered, sparse, wartlike lesions from which VZV can be isolated (Jura et al., 1989; Pahwa et al., 1988). Although the natural history of this form of varicella is not yet fully understood, VZV infections seem to smolder in some human immunodeficiency virus (HIV)-infected patients and may eventually result in chronic progressive encephalitis, with a potentially fatal outcome even if treated (Gilden et al., 1988; Pahwa et al., 1988). VZV resistant to acyclovir has developed in some of these patients who were treated for many months (Jacobson et al., 1990; Linnemann et al., 1990; Pahwa et al., 1988).

IMMUNITY

An attack of chickenpox usually confers lasting immunity; second attacks are unusual (Gershon et al., 1984a; Weller, 1983). Varicella-zoster antibody persists for many years after chickenpox. Most immune adults have antibodies detectable by ELISA, FAMA, LA, or RIA.

Transplacental immunity has been studied. In one study 200 mother-infant (cord) serum specimens for VZV antibody were tested by FAMA; 10% of the pairs in this group were seronegative (Gershon et al., 1976). The maternal and cord blood antibody titers were essentially the same. Women born in the United States were more likely to be immune than those born in Latin

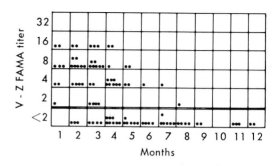

Fig. 34-10. Detection of varicella-zoster antibody in the first year of life in 67 infants. The sensitive fluorescent antibody against membrane antigen *(FAMA)* test was used for the assay. (From Gershon AA, et al. Pediatrics 1976;58:692.)

American countries. Only 5% of U.S.-born women were seronegative, as compared with 16% of a group born in Latin America. A high incidence of susceptibility to varicella in adults from tropical areas also has been noted by others (Nassar and Touma, 1986).

The disappearance of passively acquired antibody in the first year of life is shown in Fig. 34-10. By 6 months of age most infants no longer have detectable VZV antibody. Transplacentally acquired VZV antibody has been detected in the blood of low-birth-weight infants, even those weighing less than 1,500 g (Raker et al., 1978), but not in infants less than 1,000 g at birth (Wang et al., 1983).

Development of mild varicella in young infants despite the presence of transplacental maternal antibody has been reported (Baba et al., 1982). Nine cases of mild to moderate varicella in young infants who had detectable VZV antibody titers before illness were described in this report.

During the course of vaccine trials with the live attenuated varicella vaccine (see p. 608) it was also recognized that the presence of specific serum antibody at the time of exposure to the virus does not necessarily guarantee protection from clinical varicella. Some recipients of varicella vaccine who had underlying leukemia developed mild clinical varicella after an exposure several months after immunization despite serum VZV antibody titers that were predicted as protective (Gershon et al., 1984b; Gershon et al., 1989). In addition, varicella has been reported in persons having detectable VZV antibody after natural infection (Zaia et al., 1983).

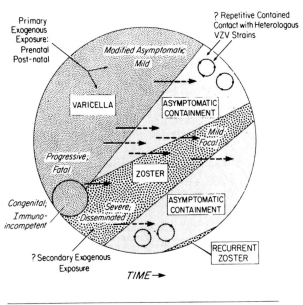

→ Active VZV Replication
- -→ VZV Latent or Persistent
◯ ? Contained Endogenous Activation

Fig. 34-11. Diagrammatic summary of the natural history of infection with varicella-zoster virus. Two variables are depicted: time and clinical severity. In the competent host the containment period is on the order of decades; however, in the immunocompromised person the two clinical processes may merge without an intervening asymptomatic interval. The containment period after congenital varicella is typically of short duration. During the asymptomatic containment period episodes of endogenous viral replication probably occur, and contact with heterologous exogenous strains may stimulate host defenses, usually in the absence of overt disease. (From Weller TH. N Engl J Med 1983;309:1362-1368, 1434-1440.)

These observations have led to reexamination of the mechanism by which immunity to varicella is mediated. Serum antibody may not be fully protective. Either cell-mediated or secretory immunity may also be important in protection (Bogger-Goren et al., 1984; Cooper et al., 1988; Diaz et al., 1989; Gershon and Steinberg, 1980; Giller et al., 1989; Hayward et al., 1986; Ihara, Ito, and Starr, 1986; Rand et al., 1977). It was recognized many years ago that the prognosis of varicella in children with isolated defects in humoral immunity was excellent. In contrast, children with congenital defects in cellular immunity were recognized as at high risk to develop severe infections.

Specific cell-mediated immunity to VZV de-velops after an attack of varicella. Failure to develop a positive cellular immune response correlates with death from varicella (Arvin et al., 1986; Gershon and Steinberg, 1979; Patel et al., 1979). Various types of cell-mediated immune reactions to VZV have been described, including T-cell and macrophage cytotoxicity, antibody dependent cellular cytoxicity (ADCC), and natural killer (NK) cells (Cooper et al., 1988; Diaz et al., 1989; Gershon and Steinberg, 1980; Giller et al., 1989; Hayward et al., 1986; Ihara et al., 1986; Patel et al., 1979; Rand et al., 1977). The exact role of these reactions in protection against VZV infection is under current investigation. A diagram depicting the summary of the natural history of VZV infections is shown in Fig. 34-11.

EPIDEMIOLOGICAL FACTORS

Chickenpox is worldwide in distribution, being endemic in all large cities. Epidemics do not have the periodicity of measles; they occur at irregular intervals determined chiefly by the size and concentration of new groups of susceptible children. All races and both sexes are equally susceptible. Seasonable distribution varies with the particular zone; in temperate areas the incidence rises during the late autumn, winter, and spring. In contrast to varicella, zoster occurs with equal frequency throughout the year.

Varicella is predominantly a disease of childhood, with the highest age incidence between 2 and 10 years. Its occurrence is unusual in adults who have lived in heavily populated urban areas but not uncommon in those who have come from isolated rural areas. Ross et al. (1962) observed a group of 641 adults and 501 children who had intimate household exposures to varicella. The overall attack rates were 1.4% for adults and 78% for children. Of 79 adults with a negative history of varicella, only 8% acquired the disease. In contrast, 87% of 441 children with no history of varicella acquired the disease.

Studies in New York City have indicated that of 92 consecutive adults with no history of varicella, 23 (25%) were actually susceptible (LaRussa et al., 1985). Others have noted a similar percentage of susceptibility in adults from throughout the United States (Alter et al., 1986; Steele et al., 1982).

Nosocomial varicella has become a significant problem, not only because some patients may be at risk to develop a severe infection, but also because of the expense and administrative problems associated with management of a potential hospital outbreak (Krasinski et al., 1986; Weber et al., 1988). Often physicians, nurses, and other personnel susceptible to varicella must be furloughed after an exposure until the potential incubation period ends. In the study of Weber et al. the cost per year at a university hospital was $56,000 for passive immunization of high-risk susceptibles and furloughs of susceptible staff personnel. Similar hospital costs for a year's time were recorded by Krasinski et al. (1986).

Transmission of varicella is rare, however, in the setting of the newborn nursery. Only two instances of such nosocomial spread have been recorded (Gershon et al., 1976; Gustafson et al., 1984).

Although apparent hospital outbreaks of zoster have been described (Schimpff et al., 1972), in many instances they are probably coincidental occurrences since they involve a high proportion of immunocompromised patients. It has been speculated that contact of immunocompromised patients with VZV may induce an immunological alteration of a suppressor nature that predisposes to viral reactivation and development of zoster (Palmer et al., 1985). In addition, some of these apparent cases of zoster are probably second attacks of varicella (Morens et al., 1980).

The age distribution of zoster is different from that of varicella. A study of 108 zoster patients revealed that 69% were 50 years of age or older and less than 10% were children (Miller and Brunell, 1970). In a study of 192 cases the annual incidence of zoster per thousand persons was 0.74 in children under 10 years, 2.5 in persons aged 20 to 50, and 10 in those over age 80 (Hope-Simpson, 1965).

Immunocompromised children are at increased risk to develop zoster compared to healthy children. In a study of children with malignant disease the overall incidence of zoster was 9% (Feldman et al., 1973). This study involved 1,132 patients over a 10-year period. The incidence of zoster in patients with Hodgkin's disease was 22%; it was 10% in children with acute lymphoblastic leukemia, and 5% in children with solid tumors. No specific chemotherapy was associated with increased risk of infection. A similar high incidence of zoster in leukemic children was observed in more recent studies (Brunell et al., 1986; Lawrence et al., 1988).

Chickenpox is one of the most highly contagious diseases, comparable to measles and smallpox in this respect. The infection is spread chiefly by direct contact with a patient with active varicella or zoster. The major source of the virus may be from skin lesions, although respiratory spread can also occur in varicella (Brunell, 1989; Tsolia et al., 1990). It is virtually impossible to culture VZV from the throat even in the early stages of varicella, but viral isolation from skin can be easily accomplished. The chances of viral transmission are increased in patients with the largest number of vesicles (Tsolia et al., 1990). Therefore patients are probably most contagious in the early stages of illness when they have the greatest numbers of moist vesicular skin lesions. That the virus is spread by the airborne route has been documented in hospital outbreak studies in which airflow patterns from patient rooms have been examined (Gustafson et al., 1982; Josephson and Gombert, 1988; Leclair et al., 1980). Presumably as a result of scratching the pruritic skin lesions, VZV gains access to the air. Under hospital conditions indirect contact through the medium of a third person has not been documented, and it is not likely that medical personnel could carry the infection from one place or patient to another.

A patient with chickenpox can transmit the disease to other susceptible persons from 1 or 2 days before onset of rash until all the vesicles have become dry. A mild case will show complete crusting within 5 days and a severe case within 10 days. In contrast to those of smallpox, the dry scabs do not contain infectious virus. Patients with zoster remain infectious to others who have not had varicella as long as new lesions are continuing to develop and the existing ones remain moist.

TREATMENT

Chickenpox in otherwise healthy children is normally a self-limited disease. Symptomatic therapy includes acetaminophen for high fever and constitutional symptoms. A recent comparison of the course of varicella in children who did or did not receive acetaminophen revealed minimal differences in the course of the illness, with the children who were treated having a slightly longer course (Doran et al., 1989). The time to total healing, itching, and activity levels was evaluated in this study, but fever was not evaluated. It seems unlikely that the differences in the course of illness are clinically significant, and the relief of fever afforded by acetaminophen therapy seems worth the theoretical minimal risk. Aspirin should not be given since it may lead to development of Reye's syndrome (Mortimer and Lepow, 1962; Starko et al., 1980). Oral antihistamines and local applications of calamine lotion may help control the itching. Fingernails should be kept short and clean in an attempt to minimize secondary skin infections. For the same reason, daily bathing is also recommended during chickenpox.

Treatment of complications

The following measures are recommended for the treatment of complications of chickenpox.

Bacterial infections. Bacterial infections complicating chickenpox are most often caused by S. *aureus* or group A β-hemolytic streptococci. Infection of a local lesion usually responds to simple measures such as warm compresses. Antimicrobial therapy is indicated for cellulitis, sepsis, or pneumonia. The treatment of severe staphylococcal infections is discussed in detail on p. 469.

Encephalitis. Patients in coma require careful observation and supportive treatment such as parenteral and tube feedings for the maintenance of hydration and adequate nutrition. Corticosteroids have not provided effective therapy for varicella encephalitis. Antiviral therapy may be used but is of no proven value. Cerebellar ataxia is usually a self-limited complication for which specific treatment is unnecessary.

Specific antiviral therapy for varicella and zoster

The antiviral drug acyclovir (9,2-hydroxy-ethoxymethylguanine) has become the drug of choice for specific therapy of VZV infections, but the drug does not prevent or cure latent VZV. Acyclovir is available in topical, oral, and intravenous formulations, but only the latter two are useful against VZV. Only approximately 15% to 20% of orally administered acyclovir is absorbed.

Acyclovir is relatively nontoxic because it interferes mainly with synthesis of viral rather than host DNA; it is not antiviral itself. To interfere with DNA synthesis, acyclovir must be phosphorylated by a virus-induced enzyme, thymidine kinase. This enzyme is present almost exclusively in infected cells; therefore the effect of acyclovir on uninfected cells is minimal.

Strains of VZV can become resistant to acyclovir by no longer producing thymidine kinase since the enzyme is not required for viral synthesis. A few thymidine kinase–negative, acyclovir-resistant strains of VZV have been reported in AIDS patients (Jacobson et al., 1990; Linnemann et al., 1990; Pahwa et al., 1988), but their clinical relevance remains unknown since resistant strains are less invasive than acyclovir-sensitive strains and transmission to non-AIDS patients has not been observed.

The dose of acyclovir used to treat VZV infections is higher than that used to treat HSV infections since VZV is less sensitive to this drug than is HSV. Toxicity of acyclovir includes nausea, vomiting, skin rash, phlebitis (if given intravenously), and precipitation of the drug in the renal tubules in a poorly hydrated patient. Since acyclovir is excreted by the kidneys, lower doses should be used for patients with abnormalities in renal function (Arvin, 1986; Balfour et al., 1983).

In a double-blind, placebo-controlled study of its efficacy acyclovir was administered orally at high dosage in otherwise healthy children (Balfour et al., 1990). These studies were confirmed in a larger collaboration study (Dunkel et al., 1991). A dose of 20 mg/kg of acyclovir four times daily for 5 days was given to 50 children, beginning on the first day of the skin rash. A similar number received placebo. The duration of the disease was shortened by approximately 1 day as evidenced by defervescence and healing of rash, but treated children did not return to school any sooner than placebo recipients, and the rate of complications of varicella was not altered by therapy. Acyclovir did not interfere with development of immunity to VZV (Englund et al., 1990). Since the illness was statistically but not clinically altered significantly by acyclovir, whether to treat children with varicella with acyclovir is problematic. Not only the cost of the drug, but also the fact that long-term adverse effects of ACV are not known for certain and the possibility that drug resistance of VZV may increase with widespread use, must be considered. One possible approach is to give acyclovir to adolescents, who are at greater risk to develop more significant clinical manifestations of varicella, and to secondary cases of varicella in a household since secondary cases usually are more severe than index cases. Early therapy, administered within the first day of onset of rash, apparently is also important and is potentially easier to implement in secondary cases in a household in which the disease will be quickly recognized. There is positive anecdotal experience in administration of acyclovir to adults with varicella (Feder, 1990; Haake et al., 1990).

Orally administered acyclovir has been used with success to decrease the morbidity of otherwise healthy adults with zoster (Cobo, 1988; Huff et al., 1988; McKendrick et al., 1986; Wood et al., 1988). A dose of 4 g per day (800 mg five times a day by mouth for 7 days) has been used. It has been associated with a decrease in acute pain and more rapid healing of skin lesions. In one study there was less acute pain in the group of patients treated with oral acyclovir in comparison to those who received placebo (Huff et al., 1988). Since otherwise healthy children who develop zoster usually have only a mild illness, acyclovir is not often given for zoster in children.

Severe varicella and zoster. Acyclovir, administered intravenously, is the drug of choice for treatment of severe varicella or zoster and for varicella that is potentially life threatening. When administered intravenously to immunocompromised children within 3 days of onset of rash, this drug decreases mortality from varicella (Balfour, 1984; Prober et al., 1982) and prevents viral dissemination (Berger et al., 1981; Feldman et al., 1986; Nyerges et al., 1988). Administering intravenous acyclovir also results in more rapid healing of zoster in normal and immunocompromised patients, ameliorates acute pain, and decreases the likelihood of viral dissemination (Balfour, 1984; Balfour et al., 1983; Peterslund, 1988; Shepp et al., 1988). Acyclovir has been used to treat varicella pneumonia in adults, including pregnant women, with success (Eder et al., 1988; Landsberger et al., 1986; Schlossberg and Littman, 1988). Acyclovir is superior to vidarabine for treatment of VZV infections, mainly because of its lesser toxicity (Feldman et al., 1986; Shepp et al., 1988).

For treatment of immunocompromised patients with varicella or zoster, acyclovir should be administered intravenously at a dose of 750 to 1,500 mg/m² of body surface area per day in three divided doses for 7 to 10 days. For adolescents a dose of 10 mg/kg of body weight every 8 hours may be used. Since the dose for newborn infants with severe varicella is not known, use of the lower dose of 750 mg/m²/day is suggested. Although some investigators have recommended that all infants who develop neonatal varicella despite receipt of passive immunization with VZIG be treated with acyclovir (Haddad et al., 1987; Holland et al., 1986; Sills et al., 1987), the authors prefer to observe these infants carefully and to treat only those appearing to develop a severe infection since more than 90% can be expected to recover with no further treatment (Hanngren et al., 1985; Preblud et al., 1986). Very rare fatalities caused by varicella have been recorded in infants who contracted varicella from their mothers near the time of delivery despite administration of VZIG at an appropriate time and dosage (Bakshi et al., 1986; King et al., 1986). The case reported by King et al., is of special interest because the mother developed the rash of varicella on the second postpartum day.

It is recommended that immunocompromised children who have not been actively or passively immunized be treated with intravenous acyclovir as soon as possible after the diagnosis of varicella has been made, although most patients so treated would recover on their own. Even if the disease appears mild at first, it is impossible to predict which children will develop severe infections. Once the disease has become severe, acyclovir may not be effective. There is no consensus as to whether it is preferable to withhold anticancer chemotherapy (including steroids) after an exposure to varicella and/or after the onset of varicella, with the exception that in steroid-dependent children this medication should not be abruptly withdrawn. Decisions about treatment of these patients should be individualized and made in consultation with the oncologist following the child.

It may seem more compelling to treat all immunosuppressed patients with varicella, since the mortality rate approaches 10%, than to treat all such patients with zoster, which has a lower mortality rate. Among zoster patients, adults with lymphoproliferative cancers and those who have had bone marrow transplantation are at greatest risk for severe disease (Whitley et al., 1982). Since acyclovir is relatively nontoxic, however, an argument can be made to treat most immunocompromised patients with zoster, including children, to decrease morbidity from the illness. In zoster patients who are not especially ill, an attempt to treat with orally administered acyclovir may be made, using, for children, the doses administered for varicella.

Alternative secondary drugs, vidarabine and interferon, are also effective in treatment of varicella and zoster (Arvin et al., 1982; Merigan et al., 1978; Whitley et al., 1982). However, these drugs are more toxic than acyclovir, and they are more difficult to administer. Nausea, vomiting, rash, and tremors have been reported with vidarabine therapy; fever, fatigue, myalgias, and weight loss have been associated with administration of interferon. Administration of both drugs requires hospitalization since they must be given intravenously. VZIG is not useful for therapy of VZV infection.

PREVENTIVE MEASURES

Varicella is usually a benign and uncomplicated disease in children, so no preventive measures are recommended for healthy children who have been exposed. On the other hand, susceptible newborn infants, immunocompromised children, and adults proven susceptible should be protected. Infants whose mothers have the onset of the rash of varicella within 5 days before and 2 days after delivery should also be protected. Indications for the use of VZIG, based on the recommendations of the Committee on Infectious Diseases of the American Academy of Pediatrics and the Advisory Committee on Immunization Practices of the Centers for Disease Control in Atlanta, Georgia, are shown in the box.

Successful passive immunization against varicella was first accomplished with zoster immune globulin (ZIG). ZIG was prepared from plasma of patients convalescing from zoster. A dose of 5 ml of ZIG, given within 72 hours of a household exposure to children with underlying leukemia, modified chickenpox (Brunell et al., 1969; Gershon et al., 1974; Judelsohn et al., 1974; Orenstein et al., 1981).

ZIG has now been supplanted by VZIG, which is prepared from plasma of healthy donors with high antibody titers against VZV. VZIG is similar to ZIG in its ability to modify varicella in high-risk children (Zaia et al., 1983). The dose of VZIG is 1.25 ml/10 kg of body weight, administered intramuscularly, within 3 days of exposure. VZIG may also be effective up to 5 days after exposure, but it is probably not worthwhile to administer it after that interval following exposure.

INDICATIONS FOR USE OF VZIG

1. **No previous history of clinical varicella**
   and

2. **Underlying condition**
   Leukemia, lymphoma
   Congenital or acquired deficiency of cellular immunity *or*
   Immunosuppressive therapy (including prednisone) *or*
   Newborn infant of mother with onset of varicella within 5 days before delivery and 2 days after delivery *or*
   Premature infant more than 28 weeks' gestation whose mother has no prior history of varicella *or*
   Premature infant less than 28 weeks' gestation and/or birth weight under 1,000 g, regardless of maternal history of varicella
   and

3. **Significant exposure**
   Continuous household contact *or*
   Playmate contact greater than 1 hour indoors *or*
   Hospital contact: in same two- or four-bed room or in adjacent beds in large ward; face-to-face contact with an infectious employee or patient *or*
   Newborn contact with infected mother
   and
   Within 3 days of contact (preferably given sooner; in some cases may give up to 5 days after exposure)

Modified from MMWR 1984; 33:84-100.

VZIG has been used successfully to modify varicella in approximately 100 newborn infants whose mothers had varicella at delivery (Hanngren et al., 1985; Preblud et al., 1986). In both studies the attack rate of varicella was approximately 50%, not indicative of a decrease in the attack rate after passive immunization. However, as in immunocompromised children, the illness was clearly modified, with most infants developing mild disease and no fatalities from varicella. An alternative to VZIG is intravenous globulin (Paryani et al., 1984). Neither VZIG nor globulin can be expected to prevent or modify zoster in high-risk patients (Groth et al., 1978; Merigan et al., 1978).

A live attenuated varicella vaccine developed

in Japan by Takahashi et al. (1974) and licensed in Japan, Korea, and several European countries has been undergoing clinical trials in the United States for over 10 years. Despite the success of these studies in healthy children (Arbeter et al., 1982; Arbeter, Starr, and Plotkin, 1986; Arbeter et al., 1986; Arbeter et al., 1984; Brunell et al., 1988; Englund et al., 1989; Johnson et al., 1988), healthy adults (Alter et al., 1985; Arbeter et al., 1986; Gershon et al., 1988; Hardy and Gershon, 1990), and children with underlying leukemia (Gershon et al., 1984b; Gershon et al., 1989), the vaccine has not yet been licensed in the United States.

Administering varicella vaccine in healthy children can be accomplished with only minimal adverse effects and with approximately 90% protective efficacy. Administering varicella vaccine in combination with measles-mumps-rubella vaccine has resulted in excellent antigenic responses to all four viruses (Arbeter et al., 1986; Brunell et al., 1988; Englund et al., 1989). Children with chronic renal insufficiency have also been successfully immunized against chickenpox with few adverse effects except for a mild rash in 5% to 10% (Broyer and Boudailliez, 1985a; Broyer and Boudailliez, 1985b). Approximately 85% of leukemic children have been protected against chickenpox after vaccination. Although 50% develop a vaccine-associated rash in the month after immunization, these rashes can be prevented from becoming serious by administration of high-dose oral acyclovir (Gershon et al., 1984b; Gershon, et al., 1989; Gershon, 1990). Patients who develop a vaccine-associated rash have the potential to spread vaccine-type

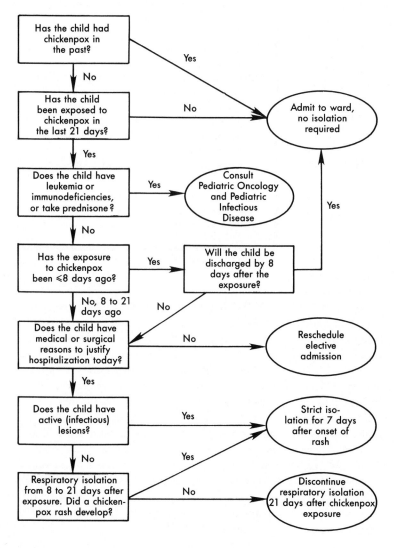

Fig. 34-12. Algorithm for chickenpox exposure. (From Brawley RL, Wenzel RP. Pediatr Infect Dis 1984;3:502-504.)

VZV to others. Contact cases, however, are extremely mild, indicating that the vaccine virus is attenuated (Gershon et al., 1984b; Tsolia et al., 1990). "Breakthrough" cases of wild-type chickenpox in vaccinees subsequently exposed to natural VZV have also been mild cases (Gershon et al., 1989). The incidence of zoster is not increased after vaccination in leukemic children who are ordinarily at high risk to develop reactivation of VZV (Brunell et al., 1986; Lawrence et al., 1988; Sakurai et al., 1982). There is also no evidence of an increased incidence of zoster in healthy children or adults (Gershon et al., 1990; Plotkin et al., 1989). The incidence of zoster is lower after vaccination than after the natural disease in leukemic children (Hardy et al., 1991).

Because the vaccine is so well tolerated, it is likely that it may eventually be administered routinely to normal children if it is found to provide long-lasting protection. A 10-year follow-up study by Asano et al. (1985b) in Japan indicated that positive antibody titers and protective immunity were maintained in healthy children for this period.

ISOLATION AND QUARANTINE

Isolation and quarantine procedures have been drastically modified in recent years for the following reasons: (1) they not only have proved ineffective in the past but also have contributed to unnecessary loss of time from school and other activities; (2) in most instances exposure has occurred before the diagnosis has become apparent; and (3) it makes little sense to prevent an inevitable disease that is generally mild in childhood and postpone it until adulthood when it more likely will be severe and potentially fatal.

Unless there are specific local regulations, isolation and quarantine procedures should be individualized. Most authorities agree that (1) the patient with chickenpox or zoster should be kept at home until all the vesicles have dried, (2) contacts should not be quarantined but merely observed, and (3) efforts to institute isolation precautions within the home to protect siblings are useless and should not be attempted.

On the other hand, rigid isolation precautions should be used for the prevention of chickenpox in high-risk children. Appropriate measures should be instituted to prevent contact with a definite or potential case of chickenpox. If exposure has occurred or is inevitable, use of the preventive measures already described would be indicated. An algorithm for the management of hospital exposures to varicella is shown in Fig. 34-12.

REFERENCES

Acheson DWK, Leen CL, Tariq WU, Mandal B. Severe and recurrent varicella-zoster virus infection in a patient with the acquired immune deficiency syndrome. J Infect Dis 1988;16:193-197.

Alter SJ, Hammond JA, McVey CJ, Myers M. Susceptibility to varicella-zoster virus among adults at high risk for exposure. Infect Contr 1986;7:448-451.

Alter SJ, McVey CJ, Jenski L, Myers M. Varicella live virus vaccine in normal susceptible adults at high risk for exposure (Abstract 457). Interscience Conference on Antimicrobial Agents and Chemotherapy, 1985.

Applebaum E, Rachelson MH, Dolgopol VB. Varicella encephalitis. Am J Med 1953;15:523.

Arbeter A, Starr S, Weibel RE, Plotkin SA. Live attenuated varicella vaccine: immunization of healthy children with the Oka strain. J Pediatr 1982;100:886-893.

Arbeter AM, Baker L, Starr SE, et al. Combination measles, mumps, rubella, and varicella vaccine. Pediatrics 1986;78:742-742.

Arbeter A, Starr SE, Plotkin SA. Varicella vaccine studies in healthy children and adults. Pediatrics 1986; 78(suppl):748-756.

Arbeter AM, Starr SE, Preblud S, et al. Varicella vaccine trials in healthy children: a summary of comparative follow-up studies. Am J Dis Child 1984;138:434-438.

Arvin A. Oral therapy with acyclovir in infants and children. Pediatr Infect Dis 1986;6:56-58.

Arvin A, Koropchak CM, Wittek AC. Immunologic evidence of reinfection with varicella-zoster virus. J Infect Dis 1983;148:200-205.

Arvin AM, Koropchak CM, Williams BR, et al. Early immune response in healthy and immunocompromised subjects with primary varicella-zoster virus infection. J Infect Dis 1986;154:422-429.

Arvin AM, Kushner JH, Feldman S, et al. Human leukocyte interferon for the treatment of varicella in children with cancer. N Engl J Med 1982;306:761-765.

Arvin AM, Pollard RB, Rasmussen L, Merigan T. Selective impairment in lymphocyte reactivity to varicella-zoster antigen among untreated lymphoma patients. J Infect Dis 1978;137:531-540.

Arvin AM, Pollard RB, Rasmussen L, Merigan T. Cellular and humoral immunity in the pathogenesis of recurrent herpes viral infections in patients with lymphoma. J Clin Invest 1980;65:869-878.

Asano Y, Itakura N, Hiroishi Y, et al. Viremia is present in incubation period in nonimmunocompromised children with varicella. J Pediatr 1985a;106:69-71.

Asano Y, Itakura N, Kajita Y, et al. Severity of viremia and clinical findings in children with varicella. J Infect Dis 1990;161:1095-1098.

Asano Y, Nagai T, Miyata T, et al. Long-term protective immunity of recipients of the Oka strain of live varicella vaccine. Pediatrics 1985b;75:667-671.

Baba K, Yabuuchi H, Takahashi M, Ogra P. Immunologic and epidemiologic aspects of varicella infection acquired during infancy and early childhood. J Pediatr 1982; 100:881-885.

Baba K, Yabuuchi H, Takahashi M, Ogra P. Increased incidence of herpes zoster in normal children infected with varicella-zoster virus during infancy: community-based follow up study. J Pediatr 1986;108:372-377.

Bakshi S, Miller TC, Kaplan M, et al. Failure of VZIG in modification of severe congenital varicella. Pediatr Infect Dis 1986;5:699-702.

Balfour H. Intravenous therapy for varicella in immunocompromised children. J Pediatr 1984;104:134-140.

Balfour H, Bean B, Laskin O, et al. Burroughs-Wellcome Collaborative Acyclovir Study Group. Acyclovir halts progression of herpes zoster in immunocompromised patients. N Engl J Med 1983;308:1448-1453.

Balfour H, McMonigal K, Bean B. Acyclovir therapy of varicella-zoster virus infection in immunocompromised patients. J Antimicrob Chemo 1983;12(suppl)B:169-179.

Balfour HH, Kelly JM, Suarez CS, et al. Acyclovir treatment of varicella in otherwise healthy children. J Pediatr 1990;116:633-639.

Berger R, Florent G, Just M. Decrease of the lympho-proliferative response to varicella-zoster virus antigen in the aged. Infect Immunol 1981;32:24-27.

Bogger-Goren S, Bernstein JM, Gershon A, Ogra PL. Mucosal cell mediated immunity to varicella zoster virus: role in protection against disease. J Pediatr 1984;105:195-199.

Bradley JS, Schlievert PM, Sample TG. Streptococcal toxic shock-like syndrome as a complication of varicella. Pediatr Infect Dis 1991;10:77-78.

Broyer M, Boudailliez B. Prevention of varicella infection in renal transplanted children by previous immunization with a live attenuated varicella vaccine. Transplant Proc 1985a;17:151-152.

Broyer M, Boudailliez B. Varicella vaccine in children with chronic renal insufficiency. Postgrad Med J 1985b; 61(S4):103-106.

Brunell P, Ross A, Miller L, Kuo B. Prevention of varicella by zoster immune globulin. J Engl J Med 1969;280:1191-1194.

Brunell PA. Transmission of chickenpox in a school setting prior to the observed exanthem. Am J Dis Child 1989;143:1451-1452.

Brunell PA, Kotchmar GSJ. Zoster in infancy: failure to maintain virus latency following intrauterine infection. J Pediatr 1981;98:71-73.

Brunell PA, Miller L, Lovejoy F. Zoster in children. Am J Dis Child 1968;115:432.

Brunell PA, Novelli VM, Lipton SV, Pollock B. Combined vaccine against measles, mumps, rubella, and varicella. Pediatrics 1988;81:779-784.

Brunell PA, Taylor-Wiedeman J, Geiser CF. Risk of herpes zoster in children with leukemia: varicella vaccine compared with history of chickenpox. Pediatrics 1986; 77:53-56.

Bruusgaard E. The mutual relation between zoster and varicella. Br J Dermatol Syph 1932;44:1-24.

Burke BL, Steele RW, Beard OW, et al. Immune responses to varicella-zoster in the aged. Arch Intern Med 1982;142:291-293.

Campbell-Benzie A, Heath RB, Ridehalgh M, Craddock-

Wilson JE. A comparison of indirect immunofluorescence and radioimmunoassay for detecting antibody to varicella-zoster virus. J Virol Meth 1983;6:135-140.

Chambers RB, Derick RJ, Davidorf FH, et al. Varicella-zoster retinitis in human immunodeficiency virus infection. Arch Ophthalmol 1989;107:960-961.

Cobo M. Reduction of the ocular complications of herpes zoster ophthalmicus by oral acyclovir. Am J Med 1988;85(S2A):90-93.

Colebunders R, Mann J, Francis H, et al. Herpes zoster in African patients: a clinical predictor of human immunodeficiency virus infection. J Infect Dis 1988;157:314-319.

Cooper E, Vujcic L, Quinnan G. Varicella-zoster virus-specific HLA-restricted cytotoxicity of normal immune adult lymphocytes after in vitro stimulation. J Infect Dis 1988;158:780-788.

Croen K, Ostrove J, Dragovic L, Straus S. Patterns of gene expression and sites of latency in human ganglia are different for varicella-zoster and herpes simplex viruses. Proc Soc Natl Acad Sci USA 1988;85:9773-9777.

DaSilva O, Hammerberg O, Chance GW. Fetal varicella syndrome. Pediatr Infect Dis 1990;9:854-855.

Davison AJ, Scott JE. The complete DNA sequence of varicella-zoster virus. J Gen Virol 1986;67:1759-1816.

deKoning J, Frederiks E, Kerkhoven P. Purpura fulminans following varicella. Helv Paediatr Acta 1972;27:177.

Demmler G, Steinberg S, Blum G, Gershon A. Rapid enzyme-linked immunosorbent assay for detecting antibody to varicella-zoster virus. J Infect Dis 1988;157:211-212.

Diaz P, Smith S, Hunter E, Arvin A. T lymphocyte cytotoxicity with natural varicella-zoster virus infection and after immunization with live attenuated varicella vaccine. J Immunol 1989;142:636-641.

Doran TF, DeAngelis C, Baumgardner RA, Mellits ED. Acetaminophen: more harm than good for chickenpox? J Pediatr 1989;114:1045-1048.

Dunkel et al. A controlled trial of acyclovir for chickenpox in normal children. N Engl J Med 1991;325:1539-1544.

Dworsky M, Whitely R, Alford C. Herpes zoster in early infancy. Am J Dis Child 1980;134:618-619.

Eder SE, J.J. A, Weiss G. Varicella pneumonia during pregnancy. Am J Perinatol 1988;5:16-18.

Edson CM, Hosler BA, Poodry CA, et al. Varicella-zoster virus envelope glycoproteins: biochemical characterization and identification in clinical material. Virology 1985;145:62-71.

Enders G. Varicella-zoster virus infection in pregnancy. Progr Med Virol 1984;29:166-196.

Englund JA, Arvine A, Balfour H. Acyclovir treatment for varicella does not lower gpI and IE-62 (p170) antibody responses to varicella-zoster virus in normal children. J Clin Virol 1990;28:2327-2330.

Englund JA, Suarez CS, Kelly J, et al. Placebo-controlled trial of varicella vaccine given with or after measles-mumps-rubella vaccine. J Pediatr 1989;114:37-44.

Essex-Cater A, Heggarty H. Fatal congenital varicella syndrome. J Infect Dis 1983;7:77-78.

Ey JL, Fulginiti VA. Varicella hepatitis without neurologic symptoms or visceral involvement. Pediatrics 1981; 67:285-287.

Feder H. Treatment of adult chickenpox with oral acyclovir. Arch Intern Med 1990;150:2061-2065.

Feldhoff C, Balfour H, Simmons SR, et al. Varicella in children with renal transplants. J Pediatr 1981;98:25-31.

Feldman S, Epp E. Isolation of varicella-zoster virus from blood. J Pediatr 1976;88:265-267.

Feldman S, Epp E. Detection of viremia during incubation period of varicella. J Pediatr 1979;94:746-748.

Feldman S, Hughes W, Daniel C. Varicella in children with cancer: 77 cases. Pediatrics 1975;80:388-397.

Feldman S, Hughes WT, Kim HY. Herpes zoster in children with cancer. Am J Dis Child 1973;126:178-184.

Feldman S, Lott L. Varicella in children with cancer: impact of antiviral therapy and prophylaxis. Pediatrics 1987; 80:465-472.

Feldman S, Chaudhary S, Ossi M, Epp E. A viremic phase for herpes zoster in children with cancer. J Pediatr 1977;91:597-600.

Feldman S, Robertson PK, Lott L, Thornton D. Neurotoxicity due to adenine arabinoside therapy during varicella-zoster virus infections in immunocompromised children. J Infect Dis 1986;154:889-893.

Fikrig E, Barg NL. Varicella associated intracerebral hemorrhage in the absence of thrombocytopenia. Diagn Micro Infect 1989;12:357-359.

Florman A, Umland E, Ballou D, et al. Evaluation of a skin test for chickenpox. Inf Cont 1985;6:314-316.

Forghani B, Schmidt N, Dennis J. Antibody assays for varicella-zoster virus: comparison of enzyme immunoassay with neutralization, immune adherence hemagglutination, and complement fixation. J Clin Micro 1978;8:545.

Frey H, Steinberg S, Gershon A. Varicella-zoster infections: rapid diagnosis by countercurrent immunoelectrophoresis. J Infect Dis 1981;143:274-280.

Gelb LD, Dohner DE, Gershon AA, et al. Molecular epidemiology of live attenuated varicella virus vaccine in children and in normal adults. J Infect Dis 1987; 155:633-640.

Gershon A. Varicella in mother and infant: problems old and new. In Krugman S, Gershon A (eds). Infection of the fetus and newborn infant. New York: Alan R Liss, 1975.

Gershon A. Commentary on VZIG in infants. Pediatr Infect Dis 1987;6:469.

Gershon A. Chickenpox, measles, and mumps. In Remington J, Klein J (eds). Infections of the fetus and newborn infant. Philadelphia. Saunders, 1990, pp 395-445.

Gershon A, Brunell P, Doyle EF, Claps A. Steroid therapy and varicella. J Pediatr 1972;81:1034.

Gershon A, Frey H, Steinberg S, et al. Enzyme-linked immunosorbent assay for measurement of antibody to varicella-zoster virus. Arch Virol 1981;70:169-172.

Gershon A, Raker R, Steinberg S, et al. Antibody to varicella-zoster virus in parturient women and their offspring during the first year of life. Pediatrics 1976;58:692-696.

Gershon A, Steinberg S. Antibody dependent cellular cytotoxicity inactivates varicella-zoster virus in vitro. 11th ICC and 19th ICAAC. Curr Chem Infect Dis 1980;1322.

Gershon A, Steinberg S. Cellular and humoral immune responses to VZV in immunocompromised patients during and after VZV infections. Infect Immun 1979;25:828.

Gershon A, Steinberg S, Borkowsky W, et al. IgM to varicella-zoster virus: demonstration in patients with and without clinical zoster. Pediatr Infect Dis 1982;1:164-167.

Gershon A, Steinberg S, Brunell P. Zoster immune globulin: a further assessment. N Engl J Med 1974;290:243-245.

Gershon A, Steinberg S, Silber R. Varicella-zoster viremia. J Pediatr 1978;92:1033-1034.

Gershon AA, Steinberg S, Gelb L, NIAID Collaborative Varicella Vaccine Study Group. Clinical reinfection with varicella-zoster virus. J Infect Dis 1984a;149:137-142.

Gershon AA, Steinberg S, Gelb L, NIAID Collaborative Varicella Vaccine Study Group. Live attenuated varicella vaccine: efficacy for children with leukemia in remission. JAMA 1984b;252:355-362.

Gershon AA, Steinberg S, LaRussa P, et al and NIAID Collaborative Varicella Vaccine Study Group. Immunization of healthy adults with live attenuated varicella vaccine. J Infect Dis 1988;158:132-137.

Gershon AA, Steinberg S, NIAID Collaborative Varicella Vaccine Study Group. Persistence of immunity to varicella in children with leukemia immunized with live attenuated varicella vaccine. N Engl J Med 1989;320:892-897.

Gershon AA, Steinberg S, NIAID Collaborative Varicella Vaccine Study Group. Live attenuated varicella vaccine: protection in healthy adults in comparison to leukemic children. J Infect Dis 1990;161:661-666.

Gilden D, Rozenman Y, Murray R, et al. Detection of varicella-zoster virus nucleic acid in neurons of normal human thoracic ganglia. Ann Neurol 1987;22:337-380.

Gilden DH, Murray RS, Wellish M, et al. Chronic progressive varicella-zoster virus encephalitis in and AIDS patient. Neurology 1988;38:1150-1153.

Giller RH, Bowden RA, Levin M, et al. Reduced cellular immunity to varicella-zoster virus during treatment for acute lymphoblastic leukemia of childhood: in vitro studies of possible mechanisms. J Clin Immunol 1986;6:472-480.

Giller RH, Winistorfer S, Grose C. Cellular and humoral immunity to varicella zoster virus glycoproteins in immune and susceptible human subjects. J Infect Dis 1989;160:919-928.

Gleaves C, Lee C, Bustamante C, Meyers J. Use of murine monoclonal antibodies for laboratory diagnosis of varicella-zoster virus infection. J Clin Microbiol 1988;26:1623-1625.

Grose C. Varicella-zoster virus: pathogenesis of human diseases, the virus and viral replication, and the major glycoproteins and proteins. Boca Raton: CRC Press, 1987, pp 85-150.

Grose CH. Variation on a theme by Fenner. Pediatrics 1981;68:735-737.

Groth KE, McCullough J, Marker S, et al. Evaluation of zoster immune plasma: treatment of herpes zoster in patients with cancer. JAMA 1978;239:1877-1879.

Guess H, Broughton DD, Melton LJ, Kurland L. Epidemiology of herpes zoster in children and adolescents: a population-based study. Pediatrics 1985;75:512-517.

Gustafson TL, Lavely GB, Brauner ER, et al. An outbreak of nosocomial varicella. Pediatrics 1982;70:550-556.

Gustafson TL, Shehab Z, Brunell P. Outbreak of varicella in a newborn intensive care nursery. Am J Dis Child 1984;138:548-550.

Haake D, Zakowski PC, Haake DL, Bryson YJ. Early treatment with acyclovir for varicella pneumonia in otherwise healthy adults: retrospective controlled study and review. Rev Infect Dis 1990;12:788-798.

Haddad J, Simeoni U, Messer J, Willard D. Acyclovir in prophylaxis and perinatal varicella. Lancet 1987;1:161.

Hanngren K, Grandien M, Granstrom G. Effect of zoster

immunoglobulin for varicella prophylaxis in the newborn. Scand J Infect Dis 1985;17:343-347.

Hardy I, Gershon A. Prospects for use of a varicella vaccine in adults. Infect Dis Clin North Am 1990;4:160-173.

Hardy IB, Gershon A, Steinberg S, et al. The incidence of zoster after immunization with live attenuated varicella vaccine. A study in children with leukemia. N Engl J Med 1991; 325:1545-1550.

Hayakawa Y, Torigoe S, Shiraki K, et al. Biologic and biophysical markers of a live varicella vaccine strain (Oka): identification of clinical isolates from vaccine recipients. J Infect Dis 1984;149:956-963.

Hayward AR, Herberger M, Lazlo M. Cellular interactions in the lysis of varicella-zoster virus infected human fibroblasts. Clin Exp Immunol 1986;63:141-146.

Holland P, Isaacs D, Moxon ER. Fatal neonatal varicella infection. Lancet 1986;2:1156.

Hope-Simpson RE. The nature of herpes zoster: a long term study and a new hypothesis. Proc R Soc Med 1965; 58:9-20.

Huff C, Bean B, Balfour H, et al. Therapy of herpes zoster with oral acyclovir. Am J Med 1988;85(A2A):84-89.

Hurwitz ES, Goodman RA. A cluster of cases of Reye syndrome associated with chickenpox. Pediatrics 1982; 70:901-906.

Hyman RW, Ecker JR, Tenser RB. Varicella-zoster virus RNA in human trigeminal ganglia. Lancet 1983;2:814-816.

Ihara T, Ito M, Starr SE. Human lymphocyte, monocyte and polymorphonuclear leucocyte mediated antibody-dependent cellular cytotoxicity against varicella-zoster virus-infected targets. Clin Exp Immunol 1986;63:179-187.

Jacobson MA, Berger TG, Fikrig S. Acyclovir-resistant varicella-zoster virus infection after chronic oral acyclovir therapy in patients with the acquired immunodeficiency syndrome. Ann Intern Med 1990;112:187-191.

Jemsek J, Greenberg SB, Taber L, et al. Herpes zoster-associated encephalitis: clinicopathologic report of 12 cases and review of the literature. Medicine 1983; 62:81-97.

Johnson CE, Shurin PA, Fattlar D, et al. Live attenuated varicella vaccine in healthy 12- to 24-month old children. Pediatrics 1988;81:512-518.

Josephson A, Gombert ME. Airborne transmission of nosocomial varicella from localized zoster. J Infect Dis 1988;158:238-241.

Judelsohn RG, Meyers JD, Ellis RJ, Thomas EK. Efficacy of zoster immune globulin. Pediatrics 1974;53:476.

Jura E, Chadwick S, SH J, Steinberg S, et al. Varicella-zoster virus infections in children infected with human immunodeficiency virus. Pediatr Infect Dis 1989; 8:586-590.

Kalman CM, Laskin OL. Herpes zoster and zosteriform herpes simplex virus infections in immunocompetent adults. Am J Med 1986;81:775-778.

Kamiya H, Ihara T, Hattori A, et al. Diagnostic skin test reactions with varicella virus antigen and clinical application of the test. J Infect Dis 1977;136:784-788.

Kasper WJ, Howe P. Fatal varicella after a single course of corticosteroids. Pediatr Infect Dis 1991;9:729-732.

King S, Gorensek M, Ford-Jones EL, Read S. Fatal varicella-zoster infection in a newborn treated with varicella-zoster immunoglobulin. Pediatr Infect Dis 1986; 5:588-589.

Kirk S, Marlow N, Quershi S. Cardiac tamponade following varicella. Int J Cardiol 1987;17:221-224.

Kotchmar G, Grose C, Brunell P. Complete spectrum of the varicella congenital defects syndrome in 5-year-old child. Pediatr Infect Dis 1984;3:142-145.

Koumbourlis AC. Varicella infection with profound neutropenia, multisystem involvement, and no sequelae. Pediatr Infect Dis 1988;3:142-145.

Krasinski K, Holzman R, LaCoutre R, Florman A. Hospital experience with varicella-zoster virus. Infect Contr 1986;7:312-316.

Kundratitz K. Experimentelle Ubertragung von Herpes Zoster auf den Mensschen und die Beziehungen von Herpes Zoster zu Varicellen. Monatssbl Kinderheilled 1925;29:516-523.

Landsberger EJ, Hager WD, Grossman JH. Successful management of varicella pneumonia complicating pregnancy. A report of 3 cases. J Reprod Med 1986;31:311.

LaRussa P, Steinberg S, Seeman MD, Gershon AA. Determination of immunity to varicella by means of an intradermal skin test. J Infect Dis 1985;152:869.

Lawrence R, Gershon A, Holzman R, Steinberg S, NIAID Varicella Vaccine Collaborative Study Group. The risk of zoster in leukemic children who received live attenuated varicella vaccine. N Engl J Med 1988;318:543-548.

Leclair JM, Zaia J, Levin MJ, et al. Airborne transmission of chickenpox in a hospital. N Engl J Med 1980; 302:450-453.

Lichtenstein PK, Heubi JE, Daugherty CC, et al. Grade I Reye's syndrome. A frequent cause of vomiting and live dysfunction after varicella and upper-respiratory-tract infection. N Engl J Med 1983;309:133-139.

Linnemann CC, Biron KK, Hoppenjans WG, Solinger AM. Emergence of acyclovir-resistant varicella zoster virus in an AIDS patient on prolonged acyclovir therapy. AIDS 1990;4:577-579.

Liu GT, Holmes GL. Varicella with delayed contralateral hemiparesis detected by MRI. Ped Neurol 1990; 6:131-134.

Ljungman P, Lonnqvist B, Gahrton G, et al. Clinical and subclinical reactivations of varicella-zoster virus in immunocompromised patients. J Infect Dis 1986; 153:840-847.

Locksley RM, Fluornoy N, Sullivan KM, Meyers J. Infection with varicella-zoster virus after marrow transplantation. J Infect Dis 1985;152:1172-1181.

Lorber A, Zonis Z, Maisuls E, et al. The scale of myocardial involvement in varicella myocarditis. Int J Cardiol 1988;20:257-262.

Luby J, Ramirez-Ronda C, Rinner S, et al. A longitudinal study of varicella zoster virus infections in renal transplant recipients. J Infect Dis 1977;135:659-663.

Mackay JB, Cairney P. Pulmonary calcification following varicella. N Z Med J 1960;59:453.

Mahalingham R, Wellish M, Wolf W, et al. Latent varicella-zoster viral DNA in human trigeminal and thoracic ganglia. N Engl J Med 1990;323:627-631.

Manson MM, Logan WPD, Loy RM. Rubella and other virus infections during pregnancy. Reports on public health and medical subjects. London: Her Majesty's Stationery Office, 1960.

Martin JH, Dohner D, Wellinghoff WJ, Gelb LD. Restriction endonuclease analysis of varicella-zoster vaccine virus and wild type DNAs. J Med Virol 1982;9:69-76.

McCormick WF, Rodnitzky RL, Schochet SSJ, McKee AP. Varicella-zoster encephalomyelitis: a morphologic and virologic study. Arch Neurol 1969;9:251-266.

McKendrick M, McGill J, White J, Woos M. Oral acyclovir in acute herpes zoster. Br Med J 1986;293:1529-1532.

Melbye M, Grossman R, Goedert J, et al. Risk of AIDS after herpes zoster. Lancet 1987;1:728-730.

Melish ME. Bullous varicella: its association with the staphylococcal scalded skin syndrome. J Pediatr 1973;83:1019.

Merigan TC, Rand K, Pollard R, et al. Human leukocyte interferon for the treatment of herpes zoster in patients with cancer. N Engl J Med 1978;298:981-987.

Meyers J. Congenital varicella in term infants: risk reconsidered. J Infect Dis 1974;129:215-217.

Miller AE. Selective decline in cellular immune response to varicella-zoster in elderly. Neurology 1980;30:582-587.

Miller L, Brunell PA. Zoster, reinfection or activation of latent virus? Am J Med 1970;49:480.

Morens DM, Bregman DJ, West M, et al. An outbreak of varicella-zoster virus infection among cancer patients. Ann Intern Med 1980;93:414-419.

Mortimer EA, Lepow ML. Varicella with hypoglycemia possibly due to salicylates. Am J Dis Child 1962;103:583.

Mulhern LM, Friday GA, Perri JA. Arthritis complicating varicella infection. Pediatrics 1971;48:827.

Music SI, Fine EM, Togo Y. Zoster-like disease in the newborn due to herpes-simplex virus. N Engl J Med 1971;284:24-26.

Myers M, Duer HL, Haulser CK. Experimental infection of guinea pigs with varicella-zoster virus. J Infect Dis 1980;142:414-420.

Myers M, Stanberry L, Edmond B. Varicella-zoster virus infection of strain 2 guinea pigs. J Infect Dis 1985; 151:106-113.

Myers MG. Viremia caused by varicella-zoster virus: association with malignant progressive varicella. J Infect Dis 1979;140:229-233.

Myers MG. Hepatic cellular injury during varicella. Arch Dis Child 1982;57:317-319.

Myers MG, Connelly B, Stanberry LR. Varicella in hairless guinea pigs. J Infect Dis 1991;163:746-751.

Nassar NT, Touma HC. Brief report: susceptibility of Filipino nurses to the varicella-zoster virus. Infect Contr 1986;7:71-72.

Nyerges G, Meszner Z, Gyrmati E, Kerpel-Fronius S. Acyclovir prevents dissemination of varicella in immunocompromised children. J Infect Dis 1988;157:309-313.

Olding-Stenkvist E, Grandien M. Early diagnosis of virus-caused vesicular rashes by immunofluorescence on skin biopsies. I. Varicella, zoster, and herpes simplex. Scand J Infect Dis 1976;8:27-35.

Orenstein W, Heymann D, Ellis R, et al. Prophylaxis of varicella in high risk children: response effect of zoster immune globulin. J Pediatr 1981;98:368-373.

Ozaki T, Ichikawa T, Matsui Y, et al. Lymphocyte-associated viremia in varicella. J Med Virol 1986;19:249.

Pahwa S, Biron K, Lim W, et al. Continuous varicella-zoster infection associated with acyclovir resistance in a child with AIDS. JAMA 1988;260:2879-2882.

Palmer SR, Caul EO, Donald DE, et al. An outbreak of shingles? Lancet 1985;2:1108-1111.

Paryani SG, Arvin AM. Intrauterine infection with varicella-zoster virus after maternal varicella. N Engl J Med 1986;314:1542-1546.

Paryani SG, Arvin AM, Koropchak C, et al. Do Varicella zoster antibody titers alter the administration of intravenous immune serum globulin or varicella zoster immune globulin. Am J Med 1984;76:124-127.

Patel PA, Yoonessi S, O'Malley J, et al. Cell-mediated immunity to varicella zoster virus in subjects with lymphoma or leukemia. J Pediatr 1979;94:223-230.

Patterson L, Butler K, Edwards M. Clinical herpes zoster shortly following primary varicella in two HIV-infected children. Clin Pediatr 1989;28:854.

Peters ACB, Versteeg J, Lindenman J, et al. Varicella and acute cerebellar ataxia. Arch Neurol 1978;35:769.

Peterslund NA. Management of varicella zoster infections in immunocompetent hosts. Am J Med 1988;85(2A):74-78.

Pitel PA, McCormick KL, Fitzgerald E, Orson JM. Subclinical hepatic changes in varicella infection. Pediatrics 1980;65:631-633.

Plotkin SA, Starr S, Connor K, Morton D. Zoster in normal children after varicella vaccine. J Infect Dis 1989; 159:1000-1001.

Preblud S, Bregman DJ, Vernon LL. Deaths from varicella in infants. Pediatr Infect Dis 1985;4:503-507.

Preblud S, Cochi S, Orenstein W. Varicella-zoster infection in pregnancy. N Engl J Med 1986;315:1416-1417.

Preblud S, Orenstein W, Bart K. Varicella: clinical manifestations, epidemiology, and health impact on children. Pediatr Infect Dis 1984;3:505-509.

Presissner C, Steinberg S, Gershon A, Smith TF. Evaluation of the anticomplement immunofluorescence test for detection of antibody to varicella-zoster virus. J Clin Microbiol 1982:16:373-376.

Priest JR, Groth KE, Balfour HH. Varicella arthritis documented by isolation of virus from joint fluid. J Pediatr 1978;93:990.

Prober C, Kirk LE, Keeney RE. Acyclovir therapy of chickenpox in immunocompromised children—a collaborative study. J Pediatr 1982;101:622-625.

Rabalais GP, Adams G, Yusk J, Wilkerson SA. Zosteriform denuded skin caused by intrauterine herpes simplex virus infection. Pediatr Infect Dis 1991;10:79-80.

Raker R, Steinberg S, Drusin L, Gershon A. Antibody to varicella-zoster virus in low birth weight infants. J Pediatr 1978;93:505-506.

Rand KH, Rasmussen LE, Pollard RB, et al. Cellular immunity and herpesvirus infections in cardiac transplant patients. N Engl J Med 1977;296:1372-1377.

Rawlinson WD, Dwyer DE, Gibbons V, Cunningham A. Rapid diagnosis of varicella-zoster virus infection with a monoclonal antibody based direct immunofluorescence technique. J Virol Meth 1989;23:13-18.

Richman DD, Cleveland PH, Oxman MN, Zaia JA. A rapid radioimmunoassay using 125-I-labeled staphylococcal protein A for antibody to varicella-zoster virus. J Infect Dis 1981;143:693-699.

Ross AH, Lencher E, Reitman G. Modification of chickenpox in family contacts by administration of gamma globulin. N Engl J Med 1962;267:369-376.

Sakurai N, Ihara T, Ito M, et al. Application of a live varicella vaccine in children with acute leukemia. Amsterdam: Exerpta Medica, 1982.

Schimpff S, Serpick A, Stoler B, et al. Varicella-zoster infection in patients with cancer. Ann Intern Med 1972;76:241-254.

Schlossberg D, Littman M. Varicella pneumonia. Arch Intern Med 1988;148:1630-1632.

Schmidt NJ. Further evidence for common antigens in herpes simplex and varicella-zoster virus. J Med Virol 1982;9:27-36.

Shanley J, Myers M, Edmond B, Steele R. Enzyme-linked immunosorbent assay for detection of antibody to varicella-zoster virus. J Clin Microbiol 1982;15:208-211.

Shehab Z, Brunell PA. Enzyme-linked immunosorbent assay for susceptibility to varicella. J Infect Dis 1983; 148:472-476.

Shepp D, Dandliker P, Meyers J. Current therapy of varicella zoster virus infection in immunocompromised patients. Am J Med 1988;85(S2A):96-98.

Shepp DH, Dandliker PS, Meyers JD. Treatment of varicella-zoster virus infection in severely immunocompromised patients: a randomized comparison of acyclovir and vidarabine. N Engl J Med 1986;314:208-212.

Siegel M. Congenital malformations following chickenpox, measles, mumps, and hepatitis. Results of a cohort study. JAMA 1973;226:1521-1524.

Silk H, Guay-Woodford L, Perez-Atayde A, et al. Fatal varicella in steroid-dependent asthma. J Allerg Clin Immunol 1988;81:47-51.

Sills J, Galloway A, Amegavie L, et al. Acyclovir in prophylaxis and perinatal varicella. Lancet 1987;1:161.

Smith H. Purpura fulminans complicating varicella: recovery with low molecular weight dextran and steroids. Med J Aust 1967;2:685.

Starko KM, Ray CG, Dominguez BS, et al. Reye's syndrome and salicylate use. Pediatrics 1980;66:859-864.

Steele R, Coleman MA, Fiser M, et al. Varicella-zoster in hospital personnel: skin test reactivity to monitor susceptibility. Pediatrics 1982;70:604.

Stevens D, Ferrington R, Jordan G, Merigan T. Cellular events in zoster vesicles: relation to clinical course and immune parameters. J Infect Dis 1975;131:509-515.

Straus S, Ostrove J, Inchauspe G, et al. Varicella-zoster virus infections: biology, natural history, treatment, and prevention. Ann Intern Med 1988;108:221-237.

Straus SE, Reinhold W, Smith HA, et al. Endonuclease analysis of viral DNA from varicella and subsequent zoster infections in the same patient. N Engl J Med 1984; 311:1362-1364.

Takahashi M, Otsuka T, Okuno Y, et al. Live vaccine used to prevent the spread of varicella in children in hospital. Lancet 1974;2:1288-1290.

Tsolia M, Gershon A, Steinberg S, Gelb L. Live attenuated varicella vaccine: evidence that the virus is attenuated and the importance of skin lesions in transmission. J Pediatr 1990;116:184-189.

Vafai A, Murray R, Wellish W, et al. Expression of varicella-zoster virus and herpes simplex virus in normal human trigeminal ganglia. Proc Soc Natl Acad Sci USA 1988;85:2362-2366.

Vafai A, Wellish M, Gilden D. Expression of varicella-zoster virus in blood mononuclear cells of patients with postherpetic neuralgia. Proc Natl Acad Sci USA 1988;85:2767-2770.

Vafai A, Wroblewska Z, Graf L. Antigenic cross-reaction between a varicella-zoster virus nucleocapsid protein encoded by gene 40 and a herpes simplex virus nucleocapsid protein. Virus Res 1990;15:163-174.

Waagoner DC, Murphy T. Varicella myocarditis. Pediatr Infect Dis 1990;9:360-363.

Wald EL, Levine MM, Togo Y. Concomitant varicella and staphylococcal scalded skin syndrome. J Pediatr 1973; 83:1017.

Wang E, Prober C, Arvin AM. Varicella-zoster virus antibody titers before and after administration of zoster immune globulin to neonates in an intensive care nursery. J Pediatr 1983;103:113-114.

Ward JR, Bishop B. Varicella arthritis. JAMA 1970;212:1954.

Weber DJ, Rotala WA, Parham C. Impact and costs of varicella prevention in a university hospital. Am J Public Health 1988;78:19-23.

Weber DM, Pellecchia JA. Varicella pneumonia: study of prevalence in adult men. JAMA 1965;192:572.

Weller TH. Varicella and herpes zoster: changing concepts of the natural history, control, and importance of a not-so-benign virus. N Engl J Med 1983;309:1362-1368, 1434-1440.

Weller TH, Coons AH. Fluorescent antibody studies with agents of varicella and herpes zoster propagated in vitro. Proc Soc Exp Biol Med 1954;86:789.

Weller TH, Witton HM. The etiologic agents of varicella and herpes zoster:serologic studies and the viruses as propagated in vitro. J Exp Med 1958;108:869-890.

Wesselhoft C, Pearson CM. Orchitis in the course of severe chickenpox with pneumonitis, followed by testicular atrophy. N Engl J Med 1950;242:651.

Whitley R, Soong S, Dolin R, et al and NIAID Collaborative Study Group. Early vidarabine to control the complications of herpes zoster in immunosuppressed patients. N Engl J Med 1982;307:971-975.

Williams DL, Gershon A, Gelb LD, et al. Herpes zoster following varicella vaccine in a child with acute lymphocytic leukemia. J Pediatr 1985;106:259-261.

Williams V, Gershon A, Brunell P. Serologic response to varicella-zoster membrane antigens measured by indirect immunofluorescence. J Infect Dis 1974;130:669-672.

Wilson A, Sharp M, Koropchak C, et al. Subclinical varicella-zoster virus viremia, herpes zoster, and T lymphocyte immunity to varicella-zoster viral antigens after bone marrow transplantation. J Infect Dis 1991;165:119-126.

Wood MJ, Ogan P, McKendrick MW, et al. Efficacy of oral acyclovir treatment of acute herpes zoster. Am J Med 1988;85(S2A):79-83.

Yuceoglu AM, Berkovich S, Minkowitz S. Acute glomerular nephritis as a complication of varicella. JAMA 1967; 202:113.

Zaia J, Levin M, Preblud S, et al. Evaluation of varicella-zoster immune globulin: protection of immunosuppressed children after household exposure to varicella. J Infect Dis 1983;147:737-743.

Zaia J, Oxman M. Antibody to varicella-zoster virus-induced membrane antigen: immunofluorescence assay using monodisperse glutaraldehyde-fixed target cells. J Infect Dis 1977;136:519-530.

Zeigler T. Detection of varicella-zoster viral antigens in clinical specimens by solid-phase enzyme immunoassay. J Infect Dis 1984;150:149-154.

Zeigler T, Halonen PE. Rapid detection of herpes simplex and varicella-zoster virus antigens from clinical specimens by enzyme immunoassay. Antiviral Res 1985; Suppl 1:107-110.

35

VIRAL INFECTIONS OF THE CENTRAL NERVOUS SYSTEM

Although they occur with far less frequency than infections of the respiratory, gastrointestinal, or genitourinary tracts, central nervous system (CNS) viral infections are often the cause of greater anxiety because of their morbidity and mortality. The varied sites of involvement include the meninges, spinal cord, and brain parenchyma. The clinical syndromes are somewhat arbitrarily divided depending on the principal clinical manifestations. The benign syndrome of headache, fever, nuchal rigidity, vomiting, and other meningeal signs with a cerebrospinal fluid (CSF) pleocytosis fits the aseptic meningitis syndrome. The more virulent clinical picture of obtundation, delirium, agitation, somnolence, seizures, and coma with associated neurologic dysfunction and abnormality reflects inflammation of the brain parenchyma and produces illness far more severe than that of viral meningitis. To a varying degree there may be meningeal involvement with encephalitis or mild parenchymal involvement with meningitis, so the term "meningoencephalitis" is used when there is such overlap. Other less frequent neurological manifestations of viral infection include myelitis, transverse myelitis, cranial nerve palsies, peripheral neuropathies, polyneuritis, Guillain-Barré syndrome, and chronic persistent encephalitis of immunocompromised patients. In this last group are CNS lymphomas, which have been attributed to EB virus activation of lymphocytes in patients with AIDS or with marked immunosuppression for organ or bone marrow transplantation (see Chapter 6).

This chapter focuses principally on viral meningitis and viral encephalitis because they are by far the most common results of viral CNS infection. Although there is some continuing uncertainty regarding pathogenesis, at least two forms of encephalitis can be attributed to viral infection.

The first is the result of direct viral invasion of the CNS with resultant inflammatory changes and neuronal damage. This is often spoken of as primary or acute viral encephalitis. In contrast, postinfectious (or allergic) encephalitis follows an acute viral illness and has a sudden onset of neurological symptoms after a latent phase of varying duration. This is thought to be an autoimmune disorder and, before the widespread use of measles vaccines, was most frequently seen after measles virus infections. However, a variety of other respiratory viruses as well as varicella have been noted to precede it. The pathology of postinfectious encephalitis is distinct from that of acute infection, with demyelination as its hallmark.

VIRAL ENCEPHALITIS

Viral encephalitis may be characterized by (1) a mild abortive infection, (2) a type of illness barely distinguishable from aseptic meningitis, or (3) a severe involvement of the CNS. The last is often characterized by sudden onset, high fever, meningeal signs, stupor, disorientation, tremors, convulsions, spasticity, coma, and death. Case fatality rates vary widely. Sequelae are more common in infants.

Etiology

For a number of reasons, the establishment of definite etiological diagnoses for patients with clinical encephalitis has been difficult. Many cases are never assigned a specific causative agent. The diagnostic techniques may be complex, time consuming, and expensive, requiring the inoculation of a variety of cell culture systems and laboratory animals. The responsible virus may be detectable solely in the brain itself and may not be present, or only very transiently found, in the blood, cerebrospinal fluid (CSF), or other usually available samples. The multiplicity of possible causative agents makes serological diagnosis very difficult unless there are epidemiological or clinical clues that enable the laboratory in search of an antibody rise to focus on a limited number of antigens.

Because the diagnostic tests to establish the etiology of an individual case of viral encephalitis are available only in selected laboratories, and because specimens are frequently not submitted early in the onset of disease, the rates and numbers of cases reported annually are very rough estimates with considerable variation. In an attempt to provide specific diagnoses for all cases of CNS infection, Nicolosi and colleagues (1986) studied all reported CNS infections in Olmstead County, Minnesota, from 1950 to 1981. Their data revealed incidence rates several times higher than those reported annually through the passive system of the Centers for Disease Control (Table 35-1). This was true also for aseptic meningitis.

Because of the availability of vidarabine and acyclovir for chemotherapy, vigorous approaches (including brain biopsy) are pursued if herpes simplex virus is suspected (Chapter 10). However, only a relatively small number of sporadic cases are caused by this agent, perhaps 10% of all encephalitis cases reported (Whitley, 1990).

The common causes of acute viral encephalitis in the United States and among U.S. travelers abroad are as follows:

Togaviruses
  Alphaviruses
    Eastern equine encephalitis (EEE)
    Western equine encephalitis (WEE)
    Venezuelan equine encephalitis (VEE)
  Flaviviruses
    St. Louis encephalitis (SLE)
    Japanese encephalitis (JE)
    Tick-borne
      Powassan
Bunyaviruses
  California group
    LaCrosse
    California encephalitis
    Jamestown Canyon
    Snowshoe hare
  Phlebovirus
    Rift valley fever
Arenaviruses
  Lymphocytic choriomeningitis (LCM)
  Argentinian hemorrhagic fever (Junin virus)
  Bolivian hemorrhagic fever (Machupo virus)
Reoviruses (Orbivirus)
  Colorado tick fever
Rabies (Chapter 20)
Herpes simplex 1 and 2 (Chapter 10)
Enteroviruses (Chapter 5)
  Coxsackie A and B
  ECHO virus
Herpes zoster (varicella-zoster virus) (Chapter 34)
Infectious mononucleosis (Epstein-Barr virus) (Chapter 6)
Cytomegalovirus (Chapter 3)
Human immunodeficiency virus - HIV1 (Chapter 1)
Postinfectious agents
  Measles (Chapter 13)
  Mumps (Chapter 15)
  Rubella (Chapter 23)
  Chickenpox (varicella-zoster) (Chapter 34)
  Influenza (Chapter 21)

Table 35-1. Reported cases of CNS viral infections in United States, 1986-1990*

	1986	*1987*	*1988*	*1989*	*1990*
Aseptic meningitis	11,374	11,487	7,234	10,274	11,852
Encephalitis, primary	1,302	1,418	882	981	1,341
Encephalitis, postinfectious	124	121	121	88	105

*Data from Centers for Disease Control. Summary of notifiable diseases, United States. MMWR 1990;39:53.

This catalog is derived partially from reports to the Centers for Disease Control (CDC) from 1984 to 1991.

Probably the most precise study of etiologies for suspected acute viral encephalitis is that conducted by the NIAID Collaborative Antiviral Study Group. This involved the use of selected diagnostic brain biopsy for cases of presumptive herpes simplex virus (HSV) encephalitis. Of 432 patients suspected of HSV encephalitis, 193 were confirmed by the biopsy; 239 were negative and were carefully evaluated for other causes. Among those discovered, in addition to other nonherpes viral infections were brain tumor, subdural hematoma, systemic lupus erythematosus, brain abscess, vascular disease, and a variety of bacterial and fungal infections (Soong et al., 1991).

In a separate study, Rantala and Uhari (1989) examined the occurrence of encephalitis among children in Finland in an area where no arbovirus infections occur. They found an annual incidence of 8.8 per 100,000 children less than 16 years of age and listed the most common responsible viruses as varicella, mumps, herpes simplex, and measles. Additionally, there were a number of individual cases caused by respiratory and enteric viruses. Reports from other areas of the world would add an even greater number of those viruses involved with arthropod vectors (togaviruses and bunyaviruses) and those associated with hemorrhagic fevers (arenaviruses, filoviruses, Haantan viruses). Although the term "arbovirus" is still used to indicate those agents whose transmission involves the bite of an insect vector, the term retains epidemiological and ecological importance but does not apply to viral taxonomy and classification.

On the basis of differing pathology and the temporal association of the second group with a recent acute infection, encephalitis reporting is usually divided into two categories. The first includes all those infections where direct viral invasion of the CNS is thought to occur; the second, those which are "postinfectious" after a common acute non-CNS infection followed by an immune-reactive demyelinating process. This second category may then include many of the usual childhood infections, the stereotype of which was measles before its control by vaccination. The etiology of more than half of the

annual 1500 reported cases of encephalitis is never determined.

The togaviruses include many of the agents formerly called arboviruses. They possess single-stranded RNA genomes and are enveloped with surface projections or spikes. The genus alphavirus has 20 members, all New World agents with particles 40 to 65 nm in diameter. The flavivirus genus contains nearly 60 members of both Old and New World prevalence with particle size 37 to 50 nm. Most agents pathogenic for humans and detected in the United States are mosquito-borne, but Powassan virus, which is found principally along the U.S.-Canadian border, is carried by Ixodes ticks.

The bunyaviruses are enveloped RNA agents possessing a segmented genome within a lipid envelope. Their diameter ranges from 90 to 120 nm. The four members of the California group listed are all carried by *Aedes* mosquitoes. Rift Valley fever virus is of special interest because of its epizootics in south and east Africa and its spread into Egypt; thus it also poses a risk to American tourists in those areas. Recently Rift Valley fever virus has been detected in West Africa as well, with an outbreak in Mauritania and Senegal involving more than 1,264 cases with 224 deaths (Walsh, 1988). In addition to a unique late-onset retinal vasculitis, it is an occasional cause of encephalitis. Transmission is either by mosquito vector or via aerosol from infected domestic animals.

The arenaviruses include four known human pathogens. They are RNA viruses with round, pleomorphic particles averaging 110 to 130 nm, budding from the cytoplasmic membranes of infected cells. Transmission from infected animal to human occurs through contamination of food by saliva, urine, or feces from infected rodents, aerosolization of rodents' excreta, or, rarely, animal bite. Lymphocytic choriomeningitis is the most commonly encountered within the United States and has been the source of research laboratory outbreaks from contaminated hamster tissues.

All of the remaining viruses listed are discussed in greater detail in other chapters, with the exception of Colorado tick fever virus. It is an unusual member of the Reoviridae family, which chronically infects rodents and may be transmitted to humans by wood ticks, inciting a dengue-like illness. When children are infected they occasionally develop a fatal encephalitis.

Reservoirs of infection for the togaviruses, bunyaviruses, and arenaviruses are found in birds and various animals. The persistence of these agents in nature involves a complicated, fascinating ecosystem. Some of the responsible elements include transovarial viral transmission in the insect, lengthy months of viremia in apparently healthy water birds, and feeding and migratory patterns of insect vectors and of natural bird and mammalian reservoirs.

The properties of the other viruses causing encephalitis and the associated CNS manifestations are described in the chapters noted in parentheses on p. 616.

Pathology and pathogenesis

Virus reaches the CNS following introduction at a distant portal of entry, local replication, and subsequent viremia. The interval between initial infection and eventual CNS involvement may be days or weeks. A number of routes are available but the most likely are (1) extension of virus into neuronal and glial cells adjacent to infected endothelial cells of small capillaries or (2) directly into CSF from the vessels of the choroid plexus via the ependyma. Rabies virus (Chapter 20) in its passage centrally via peripheral nerve pathways is an exception, and some of the herpesviruses may also use similar direct neural transmission under some circumstances (Johnson and Mims, 1968).

In general, invading viruses give rise to similar pathological changes in the CNS. It is usually impossible to distinguish between them on the basis of pathological examination alone. Gross examination of the brain and cord reveals edema and congestion. There may be small hemorrhages. Microscopic examination shows perivascular cellular infiltration and infiltration of the meninges, chiefly with lymphocytes. The principal lesion in the parenchyma consists of neuronal necrosis and degeneration accompanied by neuronophagocytosis. Perivascular cuffing and glial proliferation are common. Destruction of the ground substance of the gray or white matter may be severe. Multiple acellular plaques of necrosis may be seen. The spinal cord may be involved in some types of encephalitis. In general, neuronal lesions and foci of cellular infiltration are widely distributed throughout the brain and spinal cord.

The detection in brain biopsy or autopsy specimens of inclusions within the nucleus or cytoplasm of neuronal or glial cells permits the consideration of a more restricted array of possible etiologies. Herpes simplex, cytomegalovirus, measles, and rabies are those agents most likely to induce inclusion-bearing cells. A few viruses have predilections to localize in selected anatomic sites. Neonatal cytomegalovirus infection may be most marked in the periventricular subependymal matrix; herpes simplex encephalitis in the older infant or child often affects the frontotemporal lobes. Rabies shows a predisposition for the brain stem and cortical gray matter.

Attempts have been made to divide the encephalitides listed on p. 616 and tabulated in Table 35-1 into two groups: (1) those with evidence of direct invasion of the CNS by virus and (2) those considered to involve a postinfectious, autoimmune process. Recent evidence indicates that these are not always necessarily separate and distinct forms, as suggested by their pathological changes; rather, the differences between the two groups may hinge on timing of the onset of encephalitis in relation to the systemic manifestations and differences in the degree of immune response of the host. The demonstration of measles virus antigens and incomplete virions in the brains of patients with subacute inclusion body encephalitis and subacute sclerosing panencephalitis (SSPE) confirmed the participation of active viral replication in the pathogenesis of these rare complications. The sequence of events in acute postinfectious measles encephalitis is less certain, resembling in many ways experimental allergic encephalomyelitis. A study of 19 patients in Peru from 1980 to 1983 (Johnson et al., 1984) revealed myelin basic protein in their CSF and proliferative lymphocytic responses to this protein, strengthening the conclusion that this is an autoimmune process.

Clinical manifestations

There are many types of viral encephalitides, varying from benign forms of meningo-encephalitis that last a few days and are followed by complete recovery to fulminating encephalitis with the clinical manifestations of paresis, sensory changes, convulsions, increased intracranial pressure, coma, and death. Mumps meningoencephalitis is a good example of the usually benign form. Encephalitis caused by herpes simplex virus, on the other hand, is a devastating infection with a high case fatality rate (Chapter 10).

The onset of viral encephalitis may be sudden or gradual and is marked by fever, headache, dizziness, vomiting, apathy, and stiffness of the neck. Ataxia, tremors, mental confusion, speech difficulties, stupor or hyperexcitability, delirium, convulsions, coma, and death may follow. Papilledema may be detected as a sign of increased intracranial pressure, along with palsies of cranial nerves III and VI. In some cases there may be a prodromal period of 1 to 4 days manifested by chills and fever, headache, malaise, sore throat, conjunctivitis, and pains in the extremities and abdomen followed by encephalitic signs just mentioned. Abortive forms with headache and fever only or a syndrome resembling aseptic meningitis may occur. Lymphocytic choriomeningitis virus infection may be accompanied by arthritis, orchitis, and/or parotitis.

The many variations in the clinical patterns of encephalitis depend on the distribution, location, and concentration of neuronal lesions. Ocular palsies and ptosis are uncommon. Cerebellar incoordination is seen. Flaccid paralysis of the extremities resembling that of poliomyelitis is sometimes encountered. Paralysis of the shoulder girdle muscles is described as a singular feature of a tick-borne encephalitis.

The CSF is clear, and manometric readings of pressure vary from normal to markedly elevated. As a rule, pleocytosis of 40 to 400 cells, chiefly mononuclear, is found. The protein and glucose values may be slightly elevated or normal. In eastern equine encephalitis, the CSF may contain 1000 or more cells per cubic millimeter. In the early stages the cells are predominantly polymorphonuclear leukocytes, shifting later to mononuclear elements. In this form of encephalitis the peripheral white blood cell count may be as high as 66,000 with 90% polymorphonuclear leukocytes; in the other types, it is lower, ranging from 10,000 to 20,000, predominantly neutrophils. A general, diffuse, bilateral slowing of background activity is the most usual EEG finding. With accompanying seizures, epileptiform patterns may also be seen. Aside from herpes simplex encephalitis, CT scans and magnetic resonance imaging (MRI) are unhelpful except in postinfectious encephalomyelitis, where high field MRI may show foci of demyelination.

The course of encephalitis varies from that of the fulminating type with hyperpyrexia, ending in death in 2 to 4 days, to that of a mild form in which the fever subsides in 1 or 2 weeks with complete recovery.

Diagnosis

A diagnosis of acute encephalitis is indicated by the clinical findings. The circumstances in which the disease occurs are important. The age and geographic distribution are described later in the discussion of epidemiological factors. The specific type of encephalitis can be determined only by isolation and identification of the virus or by demonstration of the formation of or rise of level of antibody in convalescence. Togaviruses are rarely detected in the CSF, blood, or other materials during life.

On the other hand, enteroviruses, mumps virus, adenoviruses, varicella-zoster virus, and cytomegalovirus may be detected in the CSF and other appropriate materials (see chapters on specific viruses). A serological diagnosis may be reached by means of various antibody tests. Paired serum specimens are usually necessary. The first should be drawn as soon after onset as possible and the second, 2 or 3 weeks later.

A number of diagnostic tests under study and in varying stages of development exploit techniques for the detection of specific viral antigens or early antibodies in CSF. These tests are available in a limited number of laboratories and are still in a research phase. Tests employing immunoglobulin M capture, enzyme-linked immunosorbent assays for eastern and western equine encephalitis, St. Louis encephalitis, and LaCrosse viruses have permitted a specific diagnosis on a single acute phase serum or CSF by the arbovirus reference laboratories of the Centers for Disease Control (1984).

Differential diagnosis

Other diseases of the CNS may be confused with viral encephalitis. Although human *rabies* is extremely rare in the United States, it should be considered (Chapter 20). Several cases of rabies in recent years have been labeled "viral" encephalitis during the patient's illness and the diagnosis of rabies was appreciated only on postmortem examination with the discovery of Negri bodies in the hippocampus or cerebellum.

Tuberculous meningitis or *pyogenic menin-*

gitis may present the picture of encephalitis. In this circumstance, the key lies in the CSF, which may be cloudy, shows pleocytosis, has low glucose and high protein levels, and usually has microorganisms that are evident on smear or culture (Chapter 32). In the case of tuberculous meningitis or tuberculoma, a chest roentgenogram and skin tests with tuberculin may provide additional clues.

Reye's syndrome played a significant role in the diagnosis of acute childhood encephalopathic states following its description in 1963 by the Australian pathologist, Kenneth Reye. Affected children had an acute encephalopathy with hepatic dysfunction that occurred within a few days of a preceding infection, usually influenza virus or varicella. Epidemiological studies in the early 1980s disclosed the close association of ingestion of aspirin during the preceding chickenpox or influenza illness and the metabolic aspects of the syndrome. With widespread public education to the hazards of aspirin administered to children with acute respiratory infections and chickenpox, there was a resultant marked decrease in the numbers of reported cases of Reye's syndrome in the United States (Centers for Disease Control, 1991; Hurwitz, et al., 1987).

Tumor, trauma, and abscess of the brain may be mistaken for encephalitis and are often difficult to differentiate. Roentgenograms of the skull, electroencephalograms, radioisotopic scans, arteriography, and computerized tomography may help in the solution of the problem. *Lead encephalopathy* is distinguished from viral encephalitis (1) by the CSF findings, which consist mainly of increased level of protein, often quite marked, and by no increase or only a slight increase in number of cells, (2) by chemical detection of abnormal amounts of lead in the blood or CSF, (3) by roentgenographic evidence of lead line in the bone, (4) by lead line in the gums if teeth are present, (5) by basophilic stippling and anemia, and (6) by urinary coproporphyrins.

Alcohol, drugs, and other toxins must also be considered in a review of possible causes.

Prognosis

Once viruses reach the CNS, a number of host features render the brain more vulnerable. There are no lymphatic drainage and no sec-

ondary immune organs (lymph nodes) within the CNS. The blood-brain barrier normally impedes the entry of both humoral and cellular immune components. Although the CNS possesses some immunological defenses, they are significantly different from those of other tissues and organs, and their extent has not yet been fully elucidated. It is also important to realize that specific receptor sites or other related membrane functions permit the attachment of given viruses to selected susceptible cells.

The specific virus, the inoculum size, the clinical type of illness, and the age of the patient are some of the factors influencing the outcome of the disease. The decrease in the postchildhood infection category stems mainly from the striking drop in measles in the United States.

Mumps encephalitis carries the lowest mortality, only 1% to 2%. The majority of patients with mumps have CNS involvement, but this is nearly always a benign meningitis. A few patients undergo frank encephalitis, which may result in occasional deaths, but of greater concern is a 25% incidence of CNS sequelae among the survivors (Koskiniemi et al., 1983).

Mortality also varies from epidemic to epidemic. Eastern equine, Japanese, and tick-borne encephalitides are generally associated with higher fatality rates (40% to 75%) than the St. Louis, western equine, and California types. The overall mortality from St. Louis encephalitis is 5% to 30% and from western equine, 7% to 20%. Recovery from either, when it occurs, is usually complete. In young infants with St. Louis or western equine encephalitis, however, permanent injury to the CNS may occur. Seizures, hydrocephalus, and mental retardation have been seen in outbreaks of the St. Louis type, affecting 10% to 40% of infants below the age of 6 months. Similar permanent brain damage was observed in two thirds of the patients surviving eastern equine encephalitis in the Massachusetts epidemic of 1938. The fatality rate is high in Japanese encephalitis.

The fatality rate for measles encephalitis was 12%; for varicella encephalitis it was 28%. The prognosis in general for herpes simplex encephalitis is poor. Death occurs in about one third and serious sequelae occur in about half of the survivors, even in those who received antiviral therapy. The cases of encephalitis caused by enteroviruses are few in number, so it is difficult to estimate the prognosis, although from the available data it appears to be similar to that of mumps except in the neonatal period, when the case-fatality rate is extremely high (exceeding 50%).

Long-term follow-up studies of patients recovering from encephalitis to determine the incidence and severity of sequelae have been limited to small, selected groups of patients. Because so much of CNS development occurs in the early postnatal years, it has always been assumed that adverse events would be recognized more frequently in children. Rantala and colleagues (1991) reviewed the records of 73 children seen at a hospital in Finland between 1973 and 1983 whose diagnostic criteria fit acute encephalitis. Follow-up examinations revealed that 61 of the youngsters had lowered performance and IQs less than randomly selected age-matched controls, but these differences were less severe than anticipated. They concluded that the prognosis for childhood encephalitis, with the exception of that caused by herpes simplex virus, was more optimistic than previously considered. Unfortunately, they did not list the specific viruses responsible. In contrast, significant neurological sequelae following Japanese encephalitis virus infection have been reported in as many as 80% of survivors, especially among children. These involved intellectual, motor, and emotional impairment (Monath, 1988).

Epidemiological factors

The distribution of viral encephalitis varies according to season. Arbovirus encephalitis is a warm weather disease. Epidemics and sporadic cases of the North American forms (St. Louis, California, and the two equine encephalitides) and of Japanese encephalitis begin during the hot summer months and subside during the autumn. Tick-borne encephalitides, unlike the others, attack chiefly forest workers, beginning most frequently in May and June and diminishing over the summer months. Heightened interest in Japanese encephalitis has arisen with increased tourism and commercial travel to areas where epidemics have recently occurred (Peoples Republic of China, Thailand, India, Nepal, Vietnam, Japan, Korea, and Taiwan).

Enteroviral encephalitis occurs predominantly during the summer and fall months. Mumps encephalitis occurs year round, with periodic increases in incidence during the winter and early spring months. The incidence of varicella encephalitis begins to rise in the winter months, peaks in the spring, and declines slowly to lowest levels in the summer and fall. Cases of encephalitis of unknown cause show consistent peaks during the summer months corresponding with those of arbovirus encephalitis. This suggests that some of the undiagnosed cases may be caused by arboviruses, although enteroviruses are also prevalent during the same months.

The age distribution shows that St. Louis, Japanese, and western equine encephalitides all have a predilection for people in the extremes of life. The incidence of St. Louis encephalitis is high in infants and older people and lowest in children from 5 to 12 years of age. Similarly, about 60% of those attacked by Japanese encephalitis are over 50 years of age. In Okinawa and Taiwan, however, the largest proportion of cases has occurred in children. The highest attack rates of western equine encephalitis are likely to be found among male outdoor workers, 20 to 50 years old. High attack rates have also been found in infants. Eastern equine encephalitis attacks primarily the young. In the Massachusetts outbreak of 1938, 70% were under 10 years of age, 25% were below 1 year of age, and only 15% were over 21 years of age.

In general, the incidence is higher in males than in females. There may be an occupational factor in the sex differences observed in western equine and tick-borne encephalitides. The sex ratio in Japanese encephalitis is 124 males to 100 females. Both sexes are equally attacked by eastern equine encephalitis.

Although many of the names of the viruses are derived from their initial geographic sites of detection, surveillance in ensuing years has revealed more variable distribution than was originally appreciated. Western equine encephalitis is found throughout the entire United States and Canada. St. Louis encephalitis has a similar widespread distribution. Eastern equine encephalitis is still confined mainly to the eastern seaboard. Powassan virus, a tick-borne agent, is found mainly along the U.S.-Canadian border. California group viruses, as exemplified by LaCrosse virus, are annually the most prevalent mosquito-borne infection detected in the United States and have been isolated in many states other than California and Wisconsin (first patient with LaCrosse virus), ranging from Utah to North Carolina and from Minnesota to Arkansas.

Geographically, outbreaks and sporadic cases of St. Louis encephalitis have occurred in the central and western states and in western Canada. An epidemic of more than 200 cases occurred in the Tampa Bay area of Florida during the late summer and fall months of 1962; 470 cases were reported in 1964, mainly from Texas, New Jersey, Illinois, Kentucky, Pennsylvania, Colorado, and Indiana. Nearly 1,000 cases occurred in 1975, mainly in the midwestern states.

Small outbreaks of eastern equine encephalitis have occurred in Massachusetts (1938, 1955, 1956, 1971, and 1983) and in Louisiana (1947). During the summer of 1959, New Jersey was struck by a sharp outbreak associated with a high mortality. Cases have occurred sporadically in human beings in Texas, Georgia, Florida, Rhode Island, and Tennessee. The disease in horses and mules is widespread over eastern United States and Canada and areas in Central and South America.

Recent arboviral experiences in the United States have included California serogroup viruses in the upper midwest, St. Louis encephalitis virus in Texas and Louisiana communities bordering the Gulf of Mexico, and eastern equine encephalitis in Florida. Of 62 confirmed cases of LaCrosse infection in 1986, 44 were in children under 18 years of age. In contrast, an outbreak of St. Louis encephalitis in Harris County, Texas, involved 28 cases with five fatalities, all of whom were older than 55 years. Of seven patients with western equine encephalitis virus, four were infants under 6 months of age. In 1991 an outbreak in Arkansas involved 24 cases of St. Louis encephalitis in late July and early August associated with an increase in the population of infected Culex mosquitoes. (Centers for Disease Control, 1987, 1989, 1990, 1991).

The ecological and epidemiological features of these infections are complex, with transmission cycles that may include primary and secondary vertebrate hosts and vectors.

The mode of transmission of St. Louis, Japanese, and eastern and western equine encephalitides is the bite of the mosquito. Mosquitoes become infected by biting wild birds or occasionally certain mammals. Human-to-human transmission does not occur under natural conditions. St. Louis encephalitis and western equine encephalitis are very much alike in respect to ecological and epidemiological factors. Both infect horses in nature, and reservoirs of silent infection have been found in domestic animals and birds. Both are found in wild caught mosquitoes (*Culex tarsalis* and *Culex pipiens*) and can be transferred in the laboratory by the bite of such mosquitoes. Both viruses have been acquired by mosquitoes feeding on birds with occult infection (viremia). The midwestern and western states are seeded with both viruses, which give rise to infection in humans during the summer.

St. Louis encephalitis virus has also been detected in chicken mites (*Dermanyssus gallinae*) during a nonepidemic period. Since transovarian infection has been shown to take place in the mite, the latter may play an important role in maintaining the virus in nature.

Japanese encephalitis virus has been detected in naturally infected mosquitoes (*Culex tritaeniorhynchus*) in Japan, and experimental transmission of infection by mosquitoes has been established. Many animals and wading birds have been suspected of maintaining reservoirs of infection. There is evidence of widespread infection among farm animals, especially pigs.

Eastern equine encephalitis virus has been isolated from naturally infected mosquitoes and birds. Pheasants seem particularly prone to epizootics. The virus has been isolated from chicken mites and chicken lice in an epidemic area. The factors involved in transmission are apparently similar to those found in western equine and St. Louis encephalitides.

The vector for Colorado tick fever is *Dermacentor andersoni*, and the principal host reservoirs are ground squirrels and chipmunks. Powassan virus apparently is transmitted by *Ixodes* ticks, and squirrels and chipmunks may provide the reservoir.

Treatment

It is recommended that all patients suspected of having encephalitis be evaluated promptly to confirm the diagnosis and to rule out other diseases such as partially treated bacterial meningitis, tuberculous meningitis, brain abscess, drug overdosage, toxins, metabolic encephalopathy, or brain tumor. Diagnostic evaluation may include CSF examination, electroencephalogram, CT scan, ultrasound, MRI, and chemical analyses for toxins, drugs, and metabolic aberrations.

Although there has been little to offer in the way of specific treatment for viral encephalitis in the past, evidence (Skoldenberg et al., 1984) indicates that acyclovir or vidarabine may be lifesaving in patients with encephalitis caused by herpes simplex virus (Chapter 10). It is recommended that the diagnosis be established by biopsy of the involved lobe for isolation of herpes simplex virus. Treatment is most beneficial when given early in the course of the disease, before brain damage occurs from necrotic infection or increased intracranial pressure.

The patient with depressed consciousness will be best monitored and managed in a critical care unit where aggressive supporting therapy is available. Increased intracranial pressure, seizures, hyperpyrexia, fluid and electrolyte imbalance, respiratory decompensation, hypotension, and selected organ failures may develop, necessitating prompt awareness and interventions. Some patients may require prolonged assisted ventilation and nutritional support. There is a wide range of individual variation.

Control measures

Active immunization. Effective means of control of postinfectious encephalitis caused by measles, mumps, and rubella viruses have been available for some time. Widespread use of vaccines has significantly reduced the incidence of encephalitis associated with these diseases. On the other hand, the control of arbovirus infections presents many problems. Since man is not part of the infection chain but most often represents an accidental, "dead-end" infection and since outbreaks are unpredictable, a rational basis for mass immunization is hard to demonstrate. In any event, with the exception of Japanese encephalitis, no vaccine suitable for human use is available for the arbovirus infections listed on p. 616. Japanese encephalitis (JE) vaccine, prepared from infected suckling mouse brains, is produced in Japan (Biken JE vaccine) and has been made available to U.S. travelers before departure for endemic areas. It requires three doses subcutaneously at days 0, 7 and 30. Serological studies suggest that the neutralizing antibodies produced are effective in vitro against strains of Japanese encephalitis from both India and Japan.

Arthropod control. Attempts to control the arbovirus encephalitides should be directed against the arthropod vector and reservoirs of infection in order to interrupt the natural cycle of transmission.

In the western states where outbreaks are rural, the intensive use of agricultural insecticides has been followed by reduction in mosquitoes and in human infection rates. In the central states, where outbreaks of St. Louis encephalitis occur in urban-suburban areas, the main vectors are *C. pipiens* and *C. quinquefasciatus* mosquitoes, which are known to multiply in dirty water and in places where there is inadequate drainage. The characteristic pattern observed in many epidemics is a period of heavy rainfall followed by drought, resulting in many pools of stagnant water yielding vast numbers of mosquitoes. Prompt drainage of these areas and application of insecticides (larvicides and adulticides) should interrupt the infection chain and thereby reduce the incidence of human infection.

This discussion has been limited to encephalitis, the major acute manifestation of viral infection of the brain, but it is important to remember that slow viral infections of the CNS have been demonstrated and that the entire field of chronic degenerative disease of the CNS due to viruses or related transmissible agents ("prions") remains to be elaborated further (Prusiner, 1991). Both encephalitis (encephalopathy) and meningitis have been associated with HIV infection, especially in children, where manifestations may progress over a period of months or years (Chapter 1).

VIRAL MENINGITIS

Viral meningitis is usually a benign syndrome of multiple etiologies characterized by headache, fever, vomiting, and meningeal signs. The CSF shows an increase in mononuclear cells, and it yields no bacterial or fungal growth on culture. Recovery occurs in about 3 to 10 days and is nearly always complete. Wallgren (1925), a Swedish pediatrician, recognized and described the meningitis syndrome in the 1920s, delineating its clinical features and differentiating it from bacterial meningitis.

The viruses responsible for the viral meningitis syndrome may also give rise to a more severe involvement of the CNS, such as meningoencephalitis, encephalitis, and encephalomyelitis. The boundary line between viral meningitis and encephalitis is often indistinct and is drawn arbitrarily on clinical grounds. The clinical picture may not always reveal the full extent of CNS involvement.

Etiology and epidemiology

Viral meningitis may be associated with a wide variety of viral agents. Many of these are as follows:

> Mumps
> ECHO virus
> Poliovirus
> Coxsackie virus
> Adenoviruses
> Lymphocytic choriomeningitis
> Herpes simplex
> Herpes zoster
> Epstein-Barr virus (EBV)
> Human immunodeficiency virus (HIV-I)
> Encephalitis: St. Louis, California, eastern equine, and western equine

In spite of improved methods of recognizing these agents, the cause of a large proportion of cases of viral meningitis remains unknown.

Enteroviruses (Chapter 5) have been recognized as significant agents in CNS infections ever since the polioviruses were first known to cause both paralytic and nonparalytic disease. With the marked decrease in circulation of polioviruses, the Coxsackie viruses and ECHO viruses continue to be important causes of viral meningitis. They were probably responsible for approximately three fourths of the cases of viral meningitis reported in the United States (Table 35-1). The characteristics of the enteroviruses and the clinical manifestations produced by them are described in detail in Chapter 5.

In the first 36 weeks of 1991, ECHO virus type 30 was the most common isolate encountered in laboratories throughout New England and the middle and south Atlantic states. In 1990 more than 20% of isolates referred to the Centers for Disease Control were identified as ECHO virus 30. Some of the epidemiology was familiar, with a cluster of cases in a middle school football team involving the coach, the student manager, and several of the players during an

8-day period in September (Centers of Disease Control, 1991).

In attempting to focus on one or another of the many, varied causes of viral meningitis, the physician may be greatly assisted by a careful epidemiological history. Occupational exposure to mouse colonies or a new pet hamster in the home raises the question of lymphocytic choriomeningitis (LCM) virus. Recent travel to endemic or epidemic areas and a history of insect bites may stimulate more careful investigation of current arbovirus infections.

Mumps virus was also a common cause of viral meningitis. It should be considered in unimmunized patients. Mumps meningitis may occur in the absence of parotitis or other manifestations of mumps infection (Fig. 15-3). The diagnosis of mumps and other features of the disease are discussed in Chapter 15. Widespread use of the trivalent measles-mumps-rubella (MMR) vaccine has markedly reduced the numbers of cases of mumps virus infections in the United States in the past decades.

In a 5-year investigation of the causes of certain syndromes of the CNS, Meyer et al. (1960) determined the cause in 305 cases of viral meningitis. In their study the enteroviruses, excluding polioviruses, accounted for 30% of the cases and mumps virus for about 16%. Lymphocytic choriomeningitis (LCM) and herpes simplex virus are less commonly detected as causes of aseptic meningitis.

It is difficult to assess the overall contribution of the arboviruses, but in epidemics of arbovirus encephalitis a sizable number of patients, especially children, will acquire a benign illness with neurological manifestations, predominantly those of viral meningitis, accompanied by no significant change in the sensorium. For example, in the epidemic of St. Louis encephalitis in Houston in 1964, 15 of a total of 26 patients had the mild illness that was confirmed serologically as St. Louis encephalitis virus infection (Barrett et al., 1965). The seasonal distribution of agents associated with viral meningitis is an important clue to their recognition. The enteroviruses and arboviruses predominate during the warm months, whereas mumps virus was present chiefly during the winter and spring months.

Lymphocytic choriomeningitis may be established by the detection of virus in CSF or blood and by a rise in the level of either complement-fixing or neutralizing antibody. The diagnosis of herpes simplex is described on p. 181, of herpes zoster on p. 597, of infectious mononucleosis on p. 92. The recognition of the remaining causes of viral meningitis depends on the distinctive clinical picture of the various diseases, the isolation of the etiologic agent, or the demonstration of an increase in the level of antibody.

Bacterial meningitis may sometimes be a confusing factor. Tuberculous meningitis in the early stages and pyogenic meningitis, particularly that caused by *Haemophilus influenzae*, either early or modified by antibiotic treatment, may resemble aseptic meningitis. The CSF in such cases may show an increase in cells, predominantly lymphocytes. The glucose value is not invariably low and cultures may be sterile. (See Chapter 14.)

Some drugs, especially nonsteroidal antiinflammatory agents, have induced aseptic meningitis in patients who have apparently developed an immediate hypersensitivity to the components. Derbes (1984) reported a woman who underwent four separate episodes of viral meningitis after ingestion of trimethoprim-sulfamethoxizole and a fifth attack after trimethoprim alone.

Kawasaki's syndrome, for which an etiology has yet to be determined, if often accompanied by a viral meningitis that may be responsible in part for the irritability and misery displayed by many of these patients (Chapter 12). Viral meningitis has also complicated Lyme disease (erythema chronicum migrans and arthritis), a disorder now attributed to a spirochete (Chapter 30). Mollaret's syndrome is a recurrent viral meningitis of unknown etiology with repeated episodes of fever and sterile meningitis lasting 4 or 5 days, occurring as frequently as monthly over a 3 or 4 year period.

The introduction into the subarachnoid space of foreign materials such as contrast media (for myelography) or medications (for CNS tumor therapy) may initiate a brisk meningeal pleocytosis with an accompanying clinical syndrome indistinguishable from infectious meningitis. The human diploid cell rabies vaccine (Chapter 20) is far less likely to provoke CNS reactions than were its predecessors, duck embryo or rabbit nervous tissue vaccines.

Usually the attack rates of infection and viral meningitis during enterovirus outbreaks are highest in infants and young children. In the 10 year period from 1970 to 1979, 64% of enterovirus isolates were from children under 10 years of age, 50% from those under 4 years, 29% from those under 1 year (Moore, 1981). Clusters of enterovirus meningitis have been reported among high school football players (Baron et al., 1982; Moore et al., 1983). They experience higher attack rates, suffer greater morbidity, and more frequently require hospitalization than their classmates. The agents most frequently isolated from clinical specimens in the last 7 years are shown in Table 35-2, as well as the total numbers of viral meningitis patients reported to the Centers for Disease Control during those same years.

Pathology

Since most patients with viral meningitis recover completely, few postmorten studies have been reported. A leptomeningitis with inflammatory cell infiltration, polymorphonuclear cells in perivascular sheaths, and mononuclear cells in the choroid plexus has been described.

Clinical manifestations

The onset may be abrupt or gradual. The initial features are headache, fever, malaise, gastrointestinal symptoms, and signs of meningeal irritation. Abdominal pain is a common complaint. Some patients have ill-defined chest pain or generalized muscular pains or aches. Sore throat is occasionally encountered. Nausea and vomiting are common. Stiffness of the neck or back may develop a day or so after the onset. The deep tendon reflexes are normal or show hyperactivity. Muscle power is normal, as a rule, but there may be slight or transitory weakness. A maculopapular rash may accompany the viral

Table 35-2. Reported cases of viral meningitis, U.S.A., 1978-1984

Year	No. cases	Most common agents
1978	6573	ECHO 4, 9
1979	8754	ECHO 7, 11
1980	8028	ECHO 11, Coxsackie B5
1981	9,547	ECHO 9, 30
1982	9,680	ECHO 11, 30
1983	11,740	Coxsackie B5, ECHO 30, 11, 24
1984	8,036	ECHO 9, 30, Coxsackie B5, A9

meningitis syndrome, especially in association with certain types of ECHO and Coxsackie virus infections. The CSF shows pleocytosis with a predominance of lymphocytes. The symptoms and signs usually subside spontaneously and rapidly. The patient is well in 3 to 10 days.

Headache. Headache is one of the most common manifestations and often the initial complaint. It is likely to be severe. Characteristically frontal in location, it may be retrobulbar, occipital, or generalized.

Fever. The temperature ranges from 37.8° C (100° F) to as high as 40° to 40.6° C (104° or 105° F). The fever lasts from 3 to 9 days, with a mean of about 5 days. Sometimes it is biphasic, and this should make one alert for enteroviral infection.

Gastrointestinal symptoms. Gastrointestinal symptoms, including nausea and abdominal pain, are frequent early manifestations. Vomiting may occur at the onset or a day or two later. Diarrhea is more common than constipation.

Pain. Pain occurs in the epigastric or periumbilical areas fairly often. Thoracic pain suggests pleurodynia and Coxsackie virus infection, but mild chest pain may occur in aseptic meningitis caused by ECHO virus type 6 and other agents. Generalized muscular pain in the back and extremities is more likely to appear in enteroviral infections than in mumps meningitis.

Meningeal signs. Signs consisting of stiff neck, stiff back, and tightness of the hamstring muscles are present in the majority of patients. Brudzinski's sign is usually present.

Neuromuscular changes. Deep tendon reflexes are normal or show hyperactivity. Signs of muscle weakness are usually absent or equivocal but myalgia may be prominent. Slight or transitory weakness along with muscle pain and tenderness and abnormal tendon or superficial reflexes point toward the possibility of enterovirus infections. Definite paresis or paralysis has been noted with certain of the enteroviruses (especially ECHO 2, 4, 6, 16; Coxsackie A4, B2, B3; and the newer enterovirus types 70 and 71). This weakness usually recedes more rapidly than with classic poliomyelitis and rarely, if ever, leaves residual paralysis beyond 30 to 60 days from onset. Transitory weakness seldom occurs in other forms of aseptic meningitis. In any patient showing definite or persistent motor weakness or encephalitic signs, a more extensive involvement of the CNS should be considered.

Rash. A macular, maculopapular, or tiny vesicular rash accompanies certain enteroviral infections, particularly ECHO virus types 4, 6, 9, and 16 and Coxsackie virus types A9 and A16. Petechial eruptions have accompanied ECHO type 9 virus infection. The details are described in Chapter 5.

Seizures. Seizures are rarely observed in viral meningitis except in younger patients with high fevers where they may represent febrile convulsions. Their infrequency, however, necessitates a careful consideration of other possible causes. Early bacterial meningitis, a parameningeal inflammatory focus, brain tumor, vascular malformations, local cerebritis, and septic emboli with endocarditis are among the conditions to be considered. Careful observation of the patient's course will be helpful in setting the priority of any further investigative studies.

Laboratory findings. Except for changes in the CSF, the usual clinical laboratory tests are seldom helpful (Clarke and Cost, 1983). The CSF shows a leukocyte count ranging from 10 to 1000 cells mm.[3] The cell count is usually low, the average being under 150 cells. A total cell count over 1500 is not likely but has been seen in ECHO virus and Coxsackie virus infections. Studies of CSF from patients in an epidemic setting have revealed positive cultures for enterovirus even with cell counts less than 10/mm³ (Dagan et al., 1988; Wilfert et al., 1975). In mumps meningitis the cells usually number less than 1000, but counts between 1500 and 4000 have been observed. Mononuclear cells as a rule predominate in all forms of viral meningitis. However, CSF obtained early in the course of illness will frequently display a polymorphonuclear cell preponderance. This will shift rapidly over the next 6 to 8 hours so that a repeat lumbar puncture will yield CSF with more than 50% mononuclear cells.

The shift of CSF polymorphonuclear nuclear cells was shown in most children with viral meningitis caused by enteroviruses to fall below 50% after 24 hours of clinical illness (Amir et al., 1991).

The presence of a CSF eosinophilia suggests a helminthic infestation, lymphocytic choriomeningitis virus, or a number of noninfectious disorders such as Hodgkin's disease (Chesney et al., 1979). In mumps the cells are almost entirely lymphocytes. The total protein content varies from normal to values as high as 100 mg/dl. It may rise even higher in lymphogranuloma venereum and lead poisoning. The glucose content is usually normal or slightly elevated. It is characteristically low in lymphogranuloma venereum and meningitides caused by the tubercle bacillus and other bacteria. Cultures for bacteria and fungi are negative, and the other constituents of the CSF are normal.

Diagnosis

Recognition of the syndrome of viral meningitis is straightforward but can be troublesome (Singer et al., 1980). Headache, fever, vomiting, and signs of meningeal irritation call for a lumbar puncture. The CSF shows characteristic pleocytosis, with predominantly mononuclear elements. The varying causes of this syndrome have been discussed previously. The clinical and epidemiological circumstances often give clues leading to the underlying cause. Since viral infections are the most common causes of viral meningitis, a search should be made for the etiological agent in the CSF, throat, and stool specimens. Serum specimens from the acute and convalescent phases tested for rise in the level of antibody may help in the diagnosis.

CASE REPORT. B.C., a 3 $\frac{8}{12}$-year-old boy, was brought by his parents to the emergency room of Duke Hospital in July 1984 with a history of fever, malaise, drowsiness, irritability, and headache of 3 days' duration. The headache had increased markedly in the past 12 hours. He had vomited after each of several small meals that day and complained of photophobia. Temperature was 39.5° C. There was no rash or conjunctivitis. He had marked nuchal rigidity and positive Kernig and Brudzinski signs. Lumbar puncture disclosed turbid CSF under slightly increased pressure. CSF cell count was 460 WBC/mm³, 75% of which were polymorphonuclear. Gram stain and coagglutination of CSF were negative for bacteria and bacterial antigens respectively. CSF protein was 48 mg/100 ml; glucose was 75 mg/100 ml (blood glucose 110 mg/100 ml). Chloramphenicol and ampicillin were administered intravenously and he was admitted to the hospital.

A second lumbar puncture, performed 8 hours after the initial one, disclosed a white blood cell count of 375/mm³, 35% of which were polymorphonuclear and 65% mononuclear. CSF glucose and protein were essentially unchanged. By the next morning, 18 hours after hospital admission, he was markedly improved, smiling, comfortable, and active. The emergency room CSF culture revealed no bacterial growth and his antibiotic therapy was discontinued. Although his temperature rose again during the second hospital day

to 39° C, he remained alert and increasingly active. The next morning he was discharged home with instructions to his parents to bring him promptly back to the emergency room if his improvement failed to continue. Two days after his discharge, both the CSF and an admission stool specimen submitted to the virology laboratory were positive for enterovirus.

In the case report, the most compelling evidence for a viral, rather than bacterial, etiology was the rapid shift of the CSF distribution of white blood cells in 8 hours from an initial polymorphonuclear to a mononuclear cell preponderance. Even with early antibiotic therapy of pyogenic bacterial meningitis, 48 hours or more will elapse before such a cellular shift occurs. With suspected viral meningitis patients, a prompt second CSF examination after 6 to 8 hours may be of great help in resolving the differential between bacterium and virus.

Rotbart (1990) has attempted to develop a number of more rapid diagnostic approaches to viral meningitis, particularly that caused by enteroviruses. Earlier studies with nucleic acid hybridization assays were unhelpful because of low virus titers in CSF. Using a modified polymerase chain reaction (PCR) assay, he was able to detect enterovirus RNA in CSF of 13 patients whose clinical diagnoses were consistent with enteroviral meningitis. Virus cultures were positive in only 9 of the 13. If this approach can be extended to diagnostic microbiology laboratories, the confirmation of enterovirus meningitis diagnoses could be far more rapid and sensitive than current systems permit. Also, it could be extended to agents other than the enteroviruses.

Differential diagnosis

The various conditions that may be confused with aseptic meningitis are considered in Chapter 14 in the discussion of the differential diagnosis of acute bacterial meningitis. In certain cases of the latter, the CSF may be sterile and contain a predominance of mononuclear cells. This is particularly true of patients with pyogenic meningitis who have previously received antibacterial treatment.

Dagan and colleagues (1988) demonstrated that meningitis, although unsuspected, was frequently present in young infants who were hospitalized with other manifestations of enterovirus infection. When CSF was examined, most of these infants had a pleocytosis but 9% did not. The most frequent isolates in their series were

ECHO viruses 30 and 11 and several Coxsackie B viruses.

Complications

As a rule there are no complications in normal hosts. When they do arise, they are those of the underlying disease.

Prognosis

The prognosis is generally excellent. Recovery is rapid and complete. Few fatalities have been reported. There have been few longitudinal follow-up studies of patients with viral meningitis and it is exceedingly difficult without histological confirmation to be certain whether or not an element of encephalitis supervened.

In two groups of patients, very young infants and children of any age with agammaglobulinemia, viral meningitis may not be a benign illness. The enteroviruses have produced severe infections and some fatalities in newborns and infants in the first months of life (Bacon and Sims, 1976). Longitudinal studies of survivors suggest that language difficulties and smaller head circumference were more common among these infants than among uninfected controls or patients with enterovirus meningitis after the first year of life (Sells et al., 1975; Lepow, 1978; Wilfert et al. 1980). Wilfert et al. (1977) have reported chronic persistent ECHO virus meningitis in patients whose immunological deficit was characterized by absense of surface-immunoglobulin-bearing B lymphocytes. Types 9, 19, 30 and 33 ECHO viruses were recovered repeatedly from CSF for periods from 2 months to 3 years after onset of viral meningitis, and several of these children developed a dermatomyositis-like syndrome. Their CNS manifestations ranged at various times from asymptomatic to meningitic to encephalitic.

Treatment

The main practical problem confronting the clinician is whether or not to treat the patient with antimicrobial agents. The diagnosis of viral meningitis is seldom confirmed by the laboratory in the first days of the patient's illness. Nevertheless, a strong indication of viral cause may be gained from the circumstances in which the disease occurs, that is, in the midst of an outbreak of viral meningitis in the community during the summer or fall months; in the presence of a rash, enanthem, or other features of enteroviral infection; or with exposure to mumps or in the presence of parotitis in the patient. These conditions may suffice to justify withholding antimicrobial treatment. On the other hand, in those situations in which the patient has already received antimicrobial agents in either adequate or inadequate amounts, the physician may choose to continue therapy, observe the patient carefully, and follow laboratory developments until a diagnosis of bacterial meningitis has been excluded (see Chapter 14).

The characteristics of the CSF are not always completely helpful in the decision of whether or not to treat with antimicrobial agents. Early in viral meningitis, polymorphonuclear leukocytes may predominate; conversely, in the early stages of bacterial meningitis the pleocytosis may consist predominantly of lymphocytes. Rapid tests such as coagglutination or latex agglutination may assist in early bacterial diagnosis in the absence of a positive Gram stain before a culture report is available.

The importance of repeated examination of the CSF cannot be overstressed. In as short a time as 8 hours the CSF may markedly change its cellular content (Amir et al, 1991; Harrison and Risser, 1988). Antimicrobial treatment may be started in cases in which the cause is uncertain and be discontinued if the bacterial cultures of the CSF taken *before* treatment prove to be sterile.

Supportive and symptomatic treatment may require analgesics for headaches and pains and antiemetics for vomiting. When the patient is afebrile and asymptomatic, it is important to evaluate muscle power in order to detect the rare instance of residual weakness that may require continuing physiotherapy.

REFERENCES

Adair CV, Ross LG, Smadel JE. Aseptic meningitis, a disease of diverse etiology: clinical and etiologic studies on 854 cases. Ann Intern Med 1953;39:675.

Amir J, Harel L, Frydman E, et al. Shift of cerebrospinal polymorphonuclear cell percentage in the early stage of aseptic meningitis. J Pediatr 1991;119:938-941.

Bacon CJ, Sims DG. Echovirus 19 infection in infants under 6 months. Arch Dis Child 1976;51:631.

Baron RC, Hatch MH, Kleeman K, et al. Aseptic meningitis among members of a high school football team: an outbreak associated with echovirus 16 infection. JAMA 1982;284:1724.

Barrett FF, Yow MD, Phillips CA. St. Louis encephalitis in children during the 1964 epidemic. JAMA 1965;193:381.

Bergman I, Painter MJ, Wald ER, et al. Outcome of children with enterovirus meningitis during the first year of life. J Pediatr 1987;110:705-709.

Centers for Disease Control. Aseptic meningitis surveillance. U.S. Department of Health, Education, and Welfare, Public Health Service, Jan. 1979.

Centers for Disease Control. Aseptic meningitis—Panama. MMWR 1981;30:559.

Centers for Disease Control. Aseptic meningitis in a high school football team. MMWR 1981;29:631.

Centers for Disease Control. Human arboviral encephalitis-United States 1983. MMWR 1984;33:339.

Centers for Disease Control. Eastern equine encephalitis—Florida, eastern United States, 1991. MMWR 1991;40:533-535.

Centers for Disease Control. Reye syndrome surveillance—United States, 1989. MMWR 1991;89:88-90.

Centers for Disease Control. St. Louis encephalitis outbreak—Arkansas 1991. MMWR 1991;40:605-607.

Centers for Disease Control. St. Louis encephalitis—Baytown and Houston, Texas. MMWR 1986;35:693-695.

Centers for Disease Control. Update: St. Louis encephalitis—Florida and Texas, 1990. MMWR 1990;39:756-759.

Charney EB, Orecchio EJ, Zimmerman RA, Berman PH. Computerized tomography in infantile encephalitis. Am J Dis Child 1979;133:803.

Chesney PJ, Katcher ML, Nelson DB, Horowitz SD. CSF eosinophilia and chronic lymphocytic choriomeningitis virus meningitis. J Pediatr 1979;94:750.

Coleman WS, Lischner HW, Grover W. Recurrent aseptic meningitis without sequelae. J Pediatr 1975;87:89.

Cramblett HG, Stegmiller H, Spencer C. California encephalitis virus infections in children. JAMA 1966;198:128.

Dagan R, Jenista JA, Menegus MA. Association of clinical presentation, laboratory findings, and virus serotypes with the presence of meningitis in hospitalized infants with enterovirus infection. J Pediatr 1988;113:975-978.

Derbes SJ. Trimethoprim-induced aseptic meningitis. JAMA 1984;252:2865.

Eglin RP, Swann RA, Isaacs D, Moxon ER. Simultaneous bacterial and viral meningitis. Lancet 1984;2:984.

Ehrenkrantz NJ, Sinclair NC, Buff E, Lyman DO. The natural occurrence of Venezuelan equine encephalitis in the United States. N Engl J Med 1970;282:298.

Farmer K, MacArthur BA, Clay MM. A follow-up study of neonatal meningo-encephalitis due to Coxsackie virus B5. J Pediatr 1975;87:568.

Harrison SA, Risser WL. Repeated lumbar puncture in the differential diagnosis of meningitis. Pediatr Infect Dis 1988;7:143-145.

Haymaker W, Smadel JE. The pathology of viral encephalitis. Washington DC. Army Medical Museum, 1943.

Hurwitz ES, Barrett MJ, Bregman D, et al. Public Health Service study of Reye's syndrome and medications: report of the main study. JAMA 1987;257:1905-1911.

Jarvis WR, Tucker G. Echovirus type 7 meningitis in young children. Am J Dis Child 1981;135:1009.

Johnson RT, Griffin DE, Hirsch RL, et al. Measles encephalomyelitis—clinical and immunologic studies. N Engl J Med 1984;310:137.

Johnson RT, Mims CA. Pathogenesis of viral infections of the nervous system. N Engl J Med 1968;278:23.

Kappus KD, Calisher CH, Baron RC, et al. La Crosse virus infection and disease in western North Carolina. Am J Trop Med Hyg 1982;31:556.

Kelsey DS. Adenovirus meningoencephalitis. Pediatrics 1978;61:291.

Kilham L. Mumps meningocephalitis with and without parotitis. Am J Dis Child 1949;78:324.

Kono R, Miyamura K, Tajiri E, et al. Virological and serological studies of neurological complications of acute hemorrhagic conjunctivitis in Thailand. J Infect Dis 1977;135:706.

Koskiniemi M, Donner M, Pettay O. Clinical appearance and outcome in mumps encephalitis in children. Acta Paediatr Scand 1983;72:603.

Koskiniemi M, Vaheri A, Taskinen E. Cerebrospinal fluid alterations in herpes simplex virus encephalitis. Rev Infect Diseases 1984;6:608.

Lennette EH, Magoffin RL, Knouf EG. Viral central nervous system disease: an etiologic study conducted at the Los Angeles General Hospital. JAMA 1962;179:687.

Lepow ML. Enteroviral meningitis: a reappraisal. Pediatrics 1978;62:267.

Lepow ML, et al. A clinical, epidemiologic and laboratory investigation of aseptic meningitis during the four-year period, 1955-1958. I. Observations concerning etiology and epidemiology. N Engl J Med 1962a;266:1181.

Lepow ML, et al. A clinical, epidemiologic and laboratory investigation of aseptic meningitis during the four-year period, 1955-1958. II. The clinical disease and its sequelae. N Engl J Med 1962b;266:1188.

Levitt LP, Lovejoy FH Jr, Daniels JB. Eastern equine encephalitis in Massachusetts: first human case in 14 years. N Engl J Med 1971;284:540.

Luby JP. St. Louis encephalitis. Epidemiol Rev 1979;1:55.

Marier R, et al. Coxsackievirus B5 infection and aseptic meningitis in neonates and children. Am J Dis Child 1975;129:321.

Medovy H. Western equine encephalomyelitis in infants. J Pediatr 1943;22:308.

Meyer HM Jr, et al. Central nervous system syndromes of viral etiology: study of 713 cases. Am J Med 1960;29:334.

Monath TP. Japanese encephalitis—a plague of the orient. N Engl J Med 1988;319:641-643.

Moore M. Enterovirus surveillance report, 1970-1979. Atlanta: Centers for Disease Control, 1981.

Moore M, Baron RC, Filstein MR, et al. Aseptic meningitis and high school football players. JAMA 1983;249:2039.

Nicolosi A, Hauser A, Beghi E, et al. Epidemiology of central nervous system infections in Olmsted County, Minnesota, 1950-1981. J Infect Dis 1986;154:399-408.

Powell KE, Blakey DL. St. Louis encephalitis, the 1975 epidemic in Mississippi. JAMA 1977;237:2294.

Prusiner SB. Molecular biology of prion diseases. Science 1991;252:1515-1522.

Rantakallio P, Lapinheimu K, Mantyharvi R, Coxsackie B5 outbreak in a newborn nursery with 17 cases of serous meningitis. Scand J Infect Dis 1970;2:17.

Rantala H, Uhari M. Occurrence of childhood encephalitis: a population-based study. Pediatr Infect Dis 1989;8:426-430.

Rantala H, Uhari M, Saukkonen AL, et al. Outcome after childhood encephalitis. Devel Med Child Neurol 1991;33:858-867.

Reye RDK, Morgan G, Baral J. Encephalopathy and fatty degeneration of the viscera: disease entity in childhood. Lancet 1963;2:749.

Rotbart H. Diagnosis of enteroviral meningitis with the polymerase chain reaction. J Pediatr 1990;117:85-89.

Sells CJ, Carpenter RL, Ray CG. Sequelae of central nervous system enterovirus infection. N Engl J Med 1975;293:1.

Silver TS, Todd, JK. Hypoglycorrhachia in pediatric patients. Pediatrics 1976;58:67.

Singer JI, Maur PR, Riley JP, Smith PB. Management of central nervous system infections during an epidemic of enteroviral aseptic meningitis. J Pediatr 1980;96:559.

Skoldenberg B, Forsgren M, Alestig K, et al. Acyclovir versus vidarabine in herpes simplex encephalitis. Lancet 1984;2:707.

Swender PT, Shott RJ, Williams ML. A community and intensive care nursery outbreak of Coxsackie virus B5 meningitis. Am J Dis Child 1974;127:42.

Tsai TF. Arboviral infections in the United States. Infect Dis Clin North Am 1991;5:73-102.

Vianna N, et al. California encephalitis in New York State, Am J Epidemiol 1971;94:50.

Wallgren A. Une nouvelle maladie infectieuse du systeme nerveux central. Acta Paediatr. 1925;4:158.

Whitley RJ. Viral encephalitis. N Engl J Med 1990;323:242-250.

Whitley RJ, Soong SJ, Linneman C, Jr, et al. Herpes simplex encephalitis, clinical assessment. JAMA 1982;246:317.

Wilfert CM, Thompson RJ Jr, Sunder TR, et al. Longitudinal assessment of children with enteroviral meningitis during the first 3 months of life. Pediatrics 1980;67:811.

Wilfert CM, Lehrman SN, Katz SL. Enteroviruses and meningitis, Pediatr Infect Dis 1983;2:333.

Wilfert CM, et al. An epidemic of echovirus 18 meningitis. J Infect Dis 1975;131:75.

Wilfert CM, et al. Persistent and fatal central nervous system ECHO virus infections in patients with agammaglobulinemia. N Engl J Med 1977;296:1485.

36

DIAGNOSIS OF ACUTE EXANTHEMATOUS DISEASES

Under certain circumstances a physician who examines a patient with a rash is charged with a grave responsibility. An error in diagnosis may have a profound effect on the patient, the contacts, and the community. The following examples (effect on the patient, effect on contacts, and effect on the community) will serve as illustrations.

Effect on the patient

The disease of a patient with meningococcemia was mistakenly diagnosed as measles. Specific therapy was not started early; however, a potential fatality was averted when the disease was finally recognized and treated. Another patient with scarlet fever was said to have rubella. Complicating otitis media could have been prevented if the correct diagnosis had been made and appropriate treatment had been instituted.

Effect on contacts

A classic clinical picture of exanthem subitum in an infant was erroneously labeled as rubella. Under normal circumstances this mistake would have been of little consequence. In this instance, however, the patient's mother was 2 months' pregnant and had never had rubella. The error in diagnosis created an unnecessary period of anxiety for the parents who had visions of the future birth of a congenitally malformed infant.

A child with mild measles was said to have rubella. A young sibling contact developed severe measles complicated by pneumonia. This situation could have been prevented by a correct diagnosis that would have dictated the use of immune globulin to attenuate the sibling's disease.

Effect on the community

On March 5, 1947, a 47-year-old businessman was admitted to Bellevue Hospital in New York City because of fever and rash. The initial diagnosis was toxic eruption, and the patient was admitted to a dermatology ward. On March 8 he was transferred to a communicable disease hospital where he subsequently died. The proven cause of his death was smallpox. A small outbreak of the disease was initiated in the general hospital, spreading out from this focus. In the end there were 12 cases of smallpox and two deaths. There were several additional deaths among the 5 million persons who were vaccinated in New York City. The cost in time, effort, and money was incalculable, and the affairs of the entire city and its inhabitants were seriously disrupted. It is unlikely that a similar situation will occur again because smallpox has been eradicated from the world. However, occasionally an adult with severe hemorrhagic varicella may be erroneously diagnosed as having smallpox.

DIFFERENTIAL DIAGNOSIS

The rashes of various exanthematous diseases are so similar in appearance that they may be clinically indistinguishable. On the other hand, each disease has its characteristic total clinical picture that is distinctive. The differential diagnosis of the acute exanthems is based on a number of factors, including (1) the past history of infectious disease and immunization, (2) type of prodromal period, (3) features of the rash, (4) presence of pathognomonic or other diagnostic signs, and (5) laboratory diagnostic tests.

An attack of many of the exanthematous diseases is followed by permanent immunity. Consequently, a past history of measles, for example, might preclude that diagnosis. However, the history is only as reliable as the memory of the patient or the parent or the accuracy of the original diagnosis.

The character and duration of the prodromal period are also important. Some diseases have a prolonged (4 or more days) prodromal period before the rash appears; in others it may be short or absent. In certain diseases the prodrome is characterized by respiratory tract symptoms; in others, influenza-like symptoms predominate.

The character, distribution, and duration of the rash require evaluation. An eruption may be discrete or confluent and central or peripheral in distribution, and it may persist for 1 to 2 weeks or disappear within 1 day.

Pathognomonic and other signs are always helpful diagnostic clues. Koplik's spots, for example, simplify the recognition of measles.

The final diagnosis in many instances cannot be made on clinical grounds alone. Laboratory diagnostic tests must be used for identification of the causative agent or for demonstration of the development of specific antibodies.

CLASSIFICATION OF ACUTE EXANTHEMATOUS DISEASES

The acute exanthematous diseases may be conveniently separated into two categories: those characterized by an erythematous maculopapular or punctiform eruption and those characterized by a papulovesicular eruption. These two types of rash are associated with many conditions other than the acute exanthematous diseases. These diseases and other conditions are given in the accompanying lists.

The following diseases and conditions are characterized by a *maculopapular eruption:*

Measles
Atypical measles
Rubella
Scarlet fever
Staphylococcal scalded skin syndrome

Staphylococcal toxic shock syndrome
Meningococcemia
Typhus and tick fevers
Toxoplasmosis
Cytomegalovirus infection
Erythema infectiosum
Roseola infantum
Enteroviral infections
Infectious mononucleosis
Toxic erythemas
Drug eruptions
Sunburn
Miliaria
Mucocutaneous lymph node syndrome (Kawasaki disease)

The following diseases and conditions are characterized by a *papulovesicular eruption:*

Varicella-zoster infections
Smallpox
Eczema herpeticum
Eczema vaccinatum
Coxsackie virus infections
Atypical measles
Rickettsialpox
Impetigo
Insect bites
Papular urticaria
Drug eruptions
Molluscum contagiosum
Dermatitis herpetiformis

The preceding lists do not include all the conditions associated with a rash.

DIFFERENTIAL DIAGNOSIS OF MACULOPAPULAR ERUPTIONS

The acute exanthems and other conditions listed previously are frequently or occasionally characterized by a maculopapular eruption. These diseases may be differentiated by a complete evaluation of four of the categories described in this discussion of differential diagnosis: (1) prodromal period, (2) rash, (3) presence of pathognomonic or other diagnostic signs, and (4) laboratory diagnostic tests.

Prodromal period

Measles. As indicated in Fig. 36-1, the rash of measles is preceded by a 3- or 4-day prodromal period of fever, conjunctivitis, coryza, and cough.

Atypical measles. The prodromal period of

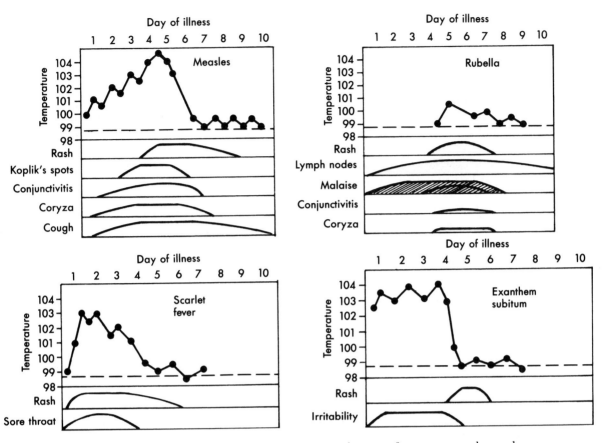

Fig. 36-1. Schematic diagrams illustrating differences between four acute exanthems characterized by maculopapular eruptions.

atypical measles is usually characterized by fever, cough, headache, myalgia, and occasionally pleuritic chest pain preceding the onset of rash by 2 to 4 days.

Rubella. In rubella in children there is usually no prodromal period (Fig. 36-1). The appearance of the rash may be the first obvious sign of illness. Lymphadenopathy that precedes the rash is usually asymptomatic in children. Adolescents and adults may have a variable 1- to 4-day period of malaise and low-grade fever before the rash appears. The temperature may be normal.

Scarlet fever. The rash of scarlet fever occurs within 12 hours of the onset of fever, sore throat, and vomiting. Occasionally the prodromal period may be prolonged to 2 days (Fig. 36-1).

Staphylococcal scalded skin syndrome. Fever and irritability occur at the time of onset of rash

in patients with staphylococcal scalded skin syndrome; there is no prodromal period.

Staphylococcal toxic shock syndrome. High fever, headache, confusion, sore throat, vomiting, diarrhea, and shock may precede or may be associated with the rash of staphylococcal toxic shock syndrome.

Meningococcemia with or without meningitis. The prodrome of meningococcemia with or without meningitis is variable. Usually the rash appears within 24 hours. The initial symptoms are fever, vomiting, malaise, irritability, and possibly a stiff neck.

Epidemic and murine typhus. A 4- to 6-day prodromal period precedes the appearance of the rash of epidemic and murine typhus. It is characterized by high fever, chills, headache, and generalized aches and pains.

Rocky Mountain spotted fever. In patients

with Rocky Mountain spotted fever the onset of rash is preceded by a 3- to 4-day period of fever, chills, headache, malaise, and anorexia.

Erythema infectiosum. In patients with erythema infectiosum no prodromal period is typically present. Usually the first sign of the illness is the appearance of the rash.

Roseola infantum. A 3- or 4-day prodromal period of high fever and irritability precedes the rash of exanthem subitum, which appears as the temperature falls to normal by crisis (Fig. 36-1).

Enteroviral infections. ECHO virus type 16 infection (Boston exanthem) may have a prodromal period resembling that of exanthem subitum, but the fever tends to be lower. Fever and constitutional symptoms in ECHO virus types 4, 6, and 9 and in Coxsackie virus infections may precede but usually coincide with the appearance of the rash.

Mucocutaneous lymph node syndrome (Kawasaki disease). A nonspecific febrile illness with sore throat precedes the rash of mucocutaneous lymph node syndrome by 2 to 5 days.

Toxic erythemas, drug eruptions, sunburn, and miliaria. Toxic erythemas, drug eruptions, sunburn, miliaria, and other noninfectious conditions with a maculopapular eruption do not have prodromal periods.

Rash

Measles. The rash of measles is reddish brown in color, appears on the face and neck first, and progresses downward to involve the trunk and extremities in sequence. As indicated in Fig. 36-2, the eruption is generalized by the third day. The lesions on the face, neck, and upper trunk tend to be confluent; those on the lower trunk and extremities are usually discrete. The eruption fades by the fifth or sixth day, with brownish staining first, followed by branny desquamation. The hands and feet do *not* desquamate.

Atypical measles. The rash of atypical measles associated with previous immunization with killed measles vaccine resembles Rocky Mountain spotted fever more than typical measles. The eruption is characterized by erythematous, urticarial, papular, petechial, and purpuric lesions with a predilection for the extremities, especially the hands, wrists, feet, and ankles; occasionally the lesions may be vesicular.

Rubella. The rash of rubella is pink in color, begins on the face and neck, and progresses downward to the trunk and extremities more

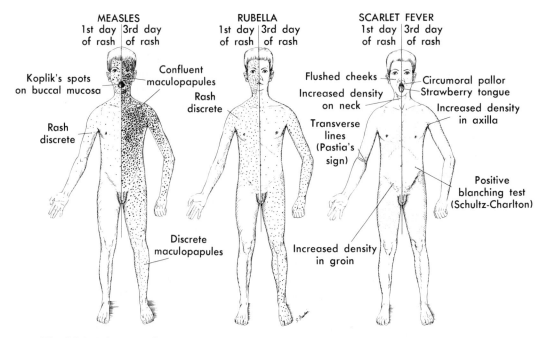

Fig. 36-2. Schematic drawings illustrating differences in appearance, distribution, and progression of rashes of measles, rubella, and scarlet fever.

rapidly than in measles; it becomes generalized within 24 to 48 hours. The lesions are usually discrete rather than confluent, and those that develop first are the earliest to fade. Consequently, on the third day the face is usually clear, and only the extremities may be involved. The eruption usually disappears by the end of the third day, and as a rule it does not desquamate. The striking contrast between the distribution of measles and rubella rashes on the third day of eruption is illustrated in Fig. 36-2.

Scarlet fever. The rash of scarlet fever is an erythematous punctiform eruption that blanches on pressure. It appears first on the flexor surfaces and rapidly becomes generalized, usually within 24 hours. The forehead and cheeks are smooth, red, and flushed, but the area around the mouth is pale (circumoral pallor). The lesions are most intense and prominent in the neck, axillary, inguinal, and popliteal skin folds (Fig. 36-2). Desquamation is characteristic, and in contrast to measles, it involves the hands and feet.

Staphylococcal scalded skin syndrome. In staphylococcal scalded skin syndrome the rash is a generalized, erythematous, scarlatiniform eruption; it has a sandpaper-like texture. The erythema is accentuated in the skin folds, simulating Pastia's lines. The skin is tender. The course of the rash is different from that of scarlet fever. Within 1 to 2 days bullae may appear, and the epidermis may separate into large sheets, revealing a moist, red, shiny surface beneath. In contrast, the pattern of desquamation is different in scarlet fever; it occurs 1 to 2 weeks later and is characterized by fine, branny flakes or thin sheets of skin.

Staphylococcal toxic shock syndrome. The rash of staphylococcal toxic shock syndrome is scarlatiniform in appearance; it occurs most prominently on the trunk and extremities and is associated with edema of the face and limbs and desquamation.

Meningococcemia. In patients with meningococcemia an early, transient maculopapular eruption may precede the petechial, purpuric rash, which often is present when the patient seeks medical attention. In contrast to measles, this early exanthem has no regular, predictable distribution.

Epidemic and murine typhus. The characteristic rash of epidemic and murine typhus is a maculopapular and petechial eruption that has a *central* distribution. The face, palms, and soles are not involved as a rule.

Rocky Mountain spotted fever. The eruption of Rocky Mountain spotted fever is maculopapular and petechial, with a *peripheral* distribution. The palms and soles usually are involved, and occasionally the face also may be affected.

Erythema infectiosum. The afebrile patient with asymptomatic erythema infectiosum develops a characteristic rash that erupts in three stages in the following sequence: (1) red, flushed cheeks with circumoral pallor (slapped-cheek appearance); (2) maculopapular eruption over upper and lower extremities (the rash assumes a lacelike appearance as it fades); and (3) an evanescent stage characterized by subsidence of the eruption, followed by a recurrence precipitated by a variety of skin irritants.

Roseola infantum. The lesions of exanthem subitum are typically discrete rose-red maculopapules that frequently appear on the chest and trunk first and then spread to involve the face and extremities. The eruption usually disappears within 2 days. Occasionally it fades within several hours.

Enteroviral infections. The rashes of ECHO virus and Coxsackie virus infections are often rubella-like in appearance. The lesions are usually maculopapular, discrete, nonpruritic, and generalized. Unlike measles, desquamation and staining do not occur. Petechial lesions suggesting meningococcemia may rarely be noted in ECHO virus type 9 and group A Coxsackie virus type 9 infections.

Mucocutaneous lymph node syndrome (Kawasaki disease). In patients with mucocutaneous lymph node syndrome there is a generalized erythematous rash with elements of macules and papules. The palms and soles are swollen and reddened, eventually peeling after several days or weeks. Dryness with erythema of the lips, mouth, and tongue accompanies bilateral conjunctival injection (see Chapter 12).

Drug eruptions and toxic erythemas. Drug eruptions and toxic erythemas may be characterized by maculopapular eruptions that may simulate any of the diseases listed previously.

Sunburn. Sunburn may be confused with the rash of scarlet fever, particularly if there is a coincident sore throat. The eruption is confined to the area not protected by a bathing suit.

Miliaria. The fine punctiform lesions of miliaria are chiefly confined to the flexor areas. The rash is usually not generalized, and it does not desquamate as a rule.

Presence of pathognomonic or other diagnostic signs

Measles. Koplik's spots are pathognomonic for measles.

Atypical measles. Atypical measles is frequently associated with radiographic evidence of pneumonia and occasionally with pleural effusion.

Rubella. In patients with rubella lymphadenopathy, particularly postauricular and occipital, is a common manifestation, but it also occurs in other diseases.

Scarlet fever. A strawberry tongue and exudative or membranous tonsillitis are typical of scarlet fever.

Staphylococcal scalded skin syndrome. An associated staphylococcal infection such as impetigo or purulent conjunctivitis may be present with staphylococcal scalded skin syndrome. Nikolsky's sign is present.

Staphylococcal toxic shock syndrome. The scarlatiniform eruption of staphylococcal toxic shock syndrome is associated with high fever, toxicity, and a shocklike state.

Meningococcemia. A petechial purpuric eruption associated with meningeal signs would point to meningococcemia.

Epidemic and murine typhus. A maculopapular petechial eruption centrally distributed in a person living in an area where epidemic typhus is endemic is suggestive of the disease.

Rocky Mountain spotted fever. A history of a recent tick bite in a person with a maculopapular, petechial, peripherally distributed eruption is characteristic of Rocky Mountain spotted fever.

Toxoplasmosis. The acquired infection of toxoplasmosis may be characterized by one or more of the following syndromes: (1) fever, pneumonitis, and rash, (2) lymphadenopathy, (3) encephalitis, and (4) chorioretinitis.

Erythema infectiosum. Erythema infectiosum is suggested by the slapped-face appearance in a well child.

Enteroviral infections. The rash of enteroviral infections may be associated with aseptic meningitis. The infections occur most commonly during the summer and fall months.

Infectious mononucleosis. A triad of membranous tonsillitis, lymphadenopathy, and splenomegaly suggests infectious mononucleosis as a possibility.

Laboratory diagnostic tests

Measles. The measles hemagglutination-inhibition (HI) test is the most practical diagnostic test. The pattern of appearance of antibody is shown in Fig. 13-4. A fourfold or greater rise in measles HI antibody is detected during convalescence; the peak titer usually ranges between 1:256 and 1:1024. The blood picture typically shows leukopenia.

Atypical measles. Extraordinary rises in measles HI antibody have been detected within 2 weeks after onset of atypical measles. The titers may exceed 1:100,000.

Rubella. As indicated in Fig. 23-4, a positive throat culture for rubella virus and evidence of a rise in antibody level are helpful diagnostic aids. The blood picture shows either a normal or low white blood cell count.

Scarlet fever. Group A hemolytic streptococci may be cultured from the nasopharynx. There is usually a rise in antistreptolysin O titer.

Staphylococcal scalded skin syndrome. A culture of skin or other sites of infection is positive for phage group II staphylococci in staphylococcal scalded skin syndrome.

Staphylococcal toxic shock syndrome. Cultures of various mucosal surfaces or purulent lesions should be positive for *Staphylococcus aureus*.

Meningococcemia. The microorganism causing meningococcemia may be observed on Gram stain and recovered from the blood, spinal fluid, or petechiae.

Epidemic and murine typhus. The Weil-Felix agglutination reaction with *Proteus* OX-19 is positive. Specific antibody tests are available for epidemic and murine typhus.

Rocky Mountain spotted fever. The Weil-Felix agglutination reaction with *Proteus* OX-19 and OX-2 is positive. Thrombocytopenia, hyponatremia, and hypoalbuminemia are common. Specific Rocky Mountain spotted fever antibody tests are available.

Toxoplasmosis. A rise in *Toxoplasma* antibody

titer during convalescence indicates acute toxoplasmosis.

Erythema infectiosum. No diagnostic test is available for erythema infectiosum at present. In the future serologic tests to confirm parvovirus B-19 infection will become commercially available (see Chapter 18, p. 297).

Roseola infantum. There is no diagnostic test at present. As yet, specific virologic and serologic tests to detect human herpesvirus type 6 are not commercially available (see Chapter 22, p. 379). The blood picture shows leukopenia when the rash appears.

Enteroviral infections. ECHO viruses and Coxsackie viruses may be recovered from stools, throat, blood, or cerebrospinal fluid (CSF). The diagnosis is confirmed by demonstrating a rise in neutralizing antibody titer to the specific virus.

Infectious mononucleosis. In patients with infectious mononucleosis the blood smear is positive for abnormal lymphocytes. The monospot test and heterophil agglutination test are positive. Results of liver function tests such as for aminotransferases are abnormal. Epstein-Barr virus antibody appears during convalescence (see p. 92).

DIFFERENTIAL DIAGNOSIS OF PAPULOVESICULAR ERUPTIONS

The acute exanthems and other conditions listed on p. 632 are usually characterized by a papulovesicular eruption. The following differential criteria are similar to those used for the maculopapular eruptions.

Prodromal period

Varicella. As indicated in Fig. 36-3, a prodromal period is usually absent in patients with chickenpox. The rash and constitutional symptoms, particularly in children, occur simultaneously. In adolescents and adults, however, there may be a 1- or 2-day prodromal period of fever, headache, malaise, and anorexia.

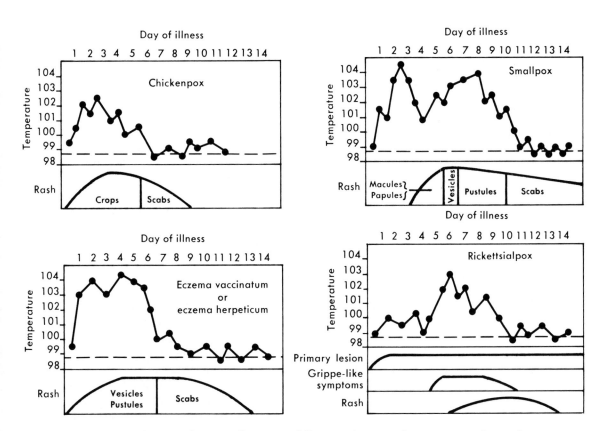

Fig. 36-3. Schematic diagrams illustrating differences between four acute exanthems characterized by papulovesicular eruptions.

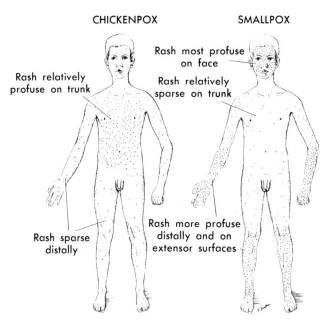

Fig. 36-4. Schematic drawings illustrating differences in distribution of rashes of chickenpox and smallpox.

Smallpox. The smallpox rash is preceded by a 3-day period of chills, headache, backache, and severe malaise (Fig. 36-3). A transient rash with bathing-trunk distribution may occur during the prodrome.

Herpes simplex, herpes zoster, and vaccinia. Herpes simplex, herpes zoster, and vaccinia occur without any prodromal period (eczema vaccinatum and herpeticum, Fig. 36-3).

Rickettsialpox. In patients with rickettsialpox a generalized papulovesicular eruption is preceded by the development of (1) an initial lesion (an eschar) and (2) an influenza-like syndrome (Fig. 36-3).

Rash

Varicella. The rash of chickenpox is characterized by (1) *rapid* evolution of macules to papules to vesicles to crusts, (2) central distribution of lesions, which appear in crops (Fig. 36-4), (3) presence of lesions in all stages in any one anatomic area, (4) presence of scalp and mucous membrane lesions, and (5) eventual crusting of nearly all the skin lesions.

Smallpox. The rash of smallpox is characterized by (1) *slow* evolution of macules to papules to vesicles to pustules to crusts, (2) peripheral distribution of lesions, which are most promi-

nent on the exposed skin surfaces (Fig. 36-4), (3) presence of lesions in the same stage in any one anatomic area, and (4) skin lesions that are more deep seated than those of varicella.

Eczema herpeticum and vaccinatum. In patients with eczema herpeticum and vaccinatum the vesicular and pustular lesions are most profuse on the sites of eczema. Mouth and scalp lesions are generally absent. (See Plate 6.)

Herpes zoster. The lesions of herpes zoster are unilateral and distributed along the line of the affected nerves; vesicles are grouped together and tend to become confluent.

Atypical measles. The papulovesicular lesions of atypical measles may appear on the face and the trunk. During the crusting phase they resemble varicella. This eruption may or may not be associated with the characteristic maculopapular eruption that resembles Rocky Mountain spotted fever in its peripheral distribution.

Rickettsialpox. The primary lesion of rickettsialpox is an eschar that measures 1.5 cm or more in diameter. The generalized papulovesicular eruption is composed of tiny vesicles superimposed on a firm papule. The vesicles are much smaller than those of chickenpox. Many lesions do not crust.

Impetigo. The lesions of impetigo, at first vesicular, become confluent and rapidly progress to the pustular and crusting stage. They do not appear in crops, they commonly involve the nasolabial area and other sites available for scratching, and they do not involve the oral mucous membranes.

Insect bites and papular urticaria. Insect bites and papular urticaria do not have a typical vesicular appearance and do not involve the scalp or mucous membranes.

Molluscum contagiosum. The lesions of molloscum contagiosum are scattered, discrete, firm, small nodular elevations without any surrounding red areolae.

Dermatitis herpetiformis. Dermatitis herpetiformis is characterized by erythematous papulovesicular lesions that are symmetrical in distribution, by a chronic course, and by healing with residual pigmentation.

Laboratory diagnostic tests

Varicella. The virus of varicella is isolated from vesicular fluid or may be identified on smears by indirect immunofluorescence. Detection of specific varicella-zoster antibody during convalescence is accomplished by means of one of the following tests: fluorescent antibody to membrane antigen (FAMA), enzyme-linked immunosorbent assay (ELISA), and latex agglutination (LA) (see p. 597).

Smallpox. The virus of smallpox may be identified by electron microscopy or gel diffusion.

Eczema herpeticum. Herpes simplex virus may be isolated in tissue culture and the viral antigen may be identified in smears by indirect immunofluorescence in eczema herpeticum. A rise in the level of antibodies during convalescence may be demonstrated.

Eczema vaccinatum. The laboratory tests for eczema vaccinatum are the same as those for smallpox.

Herpes zoster. The laboratory tests for herpes zoster are the same as those for chickenpox.

Rickettsialpox. The isolation of *Rickettsia akari* from the blood can be achieved by inoculation of the yolk sac of embryonated eggs. The rise in the level of rickettsialpox and Rocky Mountain spotted fever antibodies occurs during convalescence.

Appendix A

ANTIMICROBIAL DRUGS

The following tables list the currently recommended doses of various antimicrobial drugs, selected from among those in common use. These recommendations are separated into two tables: one applies to newborn infants, the other to older infants and children. This separation is necessary because the immaturity of the newborn infant often results in decreased excretion and/or detoxification of drugs, requiring alterations in dosage regimens to reduce the likelihood of toxicity. The table for older infants and children provides different recommendations for mild and severe infection; that for newborn infants is not divided because infections in this age group, with some exceptions, must all be considered to be severe. All pediatric doses are in milligrams per kilogram of body weight per day, unless otherwise noted. Adult doses are given as the total daily dose, with the intervals assumed to be the same as those for children.

The recommended doses are not absolute; they are only intended as a guide. Individual clinical judgment about the problem, alterations in renal function, patient response, laboratory results, and other factors may dictate modification of these recommendations.

Package insert information should be consulted for such details as diluent for reconstitution of injectable preparations, steps taken to avoid incompatibilities, and similar precautions. The editors are grateful to Christine Rudd, Pharm. D., for her revision of this Appendix.

Antimicrobial drugs for newborn infants

Agent, generic (trade)	Route	Dosage/kg/24 hours	
		<7 days of age	7 to 28 days of age
Penicillin G, crystalline (numerous)	IV, IM	100,000 units in 2 doses	225,000 units in 3 doses
Penicillinase-resistant penicillins			
Oxacillin (Prostaphlin, Bactocill)	IV, IM	50 to 100 mg in 3 doses	100 to 150 mg in 4 doses
Nafcillin (Unipen)	IV, IM	50 mg in 2 doses	75 mg in 3 doses
Broad-spectrum penicillins			
Ampicillin (numerous)	IV, IM	150 mg in 3 doses	200 mg in 4 doses
Mezlocillin (Mezlin)	IV	150 mg in 2 doses	<2 kg: 225 mg in 3 doses
			>2 kg: 300 mg in 4 doses
Ticarcillin (Ticar)	IV, IM	225 mg in 3 doses	300 mg in 4 doses
Aminoglycosides			
Gentamicin (multiple)	IV,* IM	5 mg in 2 doses	7.5 mg in 3 doses
Tobramycin (Nebcin)	IV,* IM	5 mg in 2 doses	7.5 mg in 3 doses
Amikacin (Amikin)	IV,* IM	20 mg in 2 doses	30 mg in 3 doses
Chloramphenicol (Chloromycetin)†	IV	Premature: 25 mg in 2 doses Term: 25 mg in 1 dose	Premature: 25 mg in 1 dose Term: 50 mg in 2 doses
Cephalosporins			
Cephalothin (Keflin)	IV	60 mg in 3 doses	80 mg in 4 doses
Cefazolin (Kefzol, Ancef)	IV, IM	40 mg in 2 doses	60 mg in 3 doses
Cefotaxime (Claforan)	IV, IM	100 mg in 2 doses	150 mg in 3 doses
Ceftazidime (Fortaz, Tazidime, Tazicef)	IV, IM	100 mg in 2 doses	150 mg in 3 doses
Ceftriaxone (Rocephin)	IV, IM	50 mg in 1 dose	75 mg in 1 dose
Other agents			
Imipenem/cilastatin (Primaxin)	IV	40 mg in 2 doses	40 mg in 2 doses
Aztreonam (Azactam)	IV, IM	90 mg in 3 doses	120 mg in 4 doses
Clindamycin (Cleocin)	IV, IM, PO	Term: 15 mg in 3 doses	Premature: <28 days and/or <3.5 kg: 15 mg in 3 doses Premature: >28 days and/or >3.5 kg: 20 mg in 4 doses Term: 20 mg in 4 doses
Metronidazole (Flagyl)	IV, PO	15 mg in 2 doses	30 mg in 2 doses
Vancomycin (Vancocin)	IV*	30 mg in 2 doses	45 mg in 3 doses
Nystatin (Mycostatin)	PO	200,000 to 400,000 units in 4 doses	200,000 to 400,000 in 4 doses
Amphotericin B (Fungizone)	IV‡	0.25 to 1 mg in 1 dose	0.25 to 1 mg in 1 dose
Acyclovir (Zovirax)	IV	30 mg in 3 doses	30 mg in 3 doses (for HSV)

*Intravenous administration over 30 to 60 minutes.
†Use with caution; monitor drug level.
‡See p. 647 under "Comments."

Antimicrobial drugs for pediatric patients beyond the newborn period

Agent, generic (trade)	Route	Dosage/kg/24 hours		Comments
		Mild-moderate infections	Severe infections	
Penicillin G, crystalline, K, or Na (numerous)	IV, IM	50,000 to 100,000 units in 4 doses	100,000 to 250,000 units in 4 to 6 doses	1.68 mEq K or Na per 1,000,000 units; use Na salt for large IV doses
Penicillin G, procaine (numerous)	IM	25,000 to 50,000 units in 1 to 2 doses	Inappropriate	Contraindicated in procaine allergy
Penicillin G, benzathine (Bicillin, Permapen)	IM	<30 lbs: 600,000 units 30 to 60 lbs: 1,200,000 units >60 lbs: 2,400,000 units	Inappropriate	Major use, prevention of rheumatic fever by treatment and prophylaxis of streptococcal infections
Penicillin V, phenoxymethyl penicillin (numerous)	PO	25 to 50 mg in 3 or 4 doses	Inappropriate	1600 units = 1 mg
Penicillinase-resistant penicillins Oxacillin (Prostaphlin, Bactocill)	IV, IM	50 to 100 mg in 4 doses (daily adult dose, 2 to 4 gm)	100 to 200 mg in 4 to 6 doses (daily adult dose, 4 to 12 gm)	
Nafcillin (Unipen, Nafcil)	IV, IM	50 to 100 mg in 4 doses (daily adult dose, 2 to 4 gm)	100 to 200 mg in 4 to 6 doses (daily adult dose, 4 to 12 gm)	
Cloxacillin (Tegopen)	PO	50 to 100 mg in 4 doses (daily adult dose, 2 to 4 gm)	Inappropriate	
Dicloxacillin (Dynapen, Pathocil, Veracillin)	PO	25 to 50 mg in 4 doses (daily adult dose, 2 to 4 gm)	Inappropriate	

Continued.

Antimicrobial drugs for pediatric patients beyond the newborn period — cont'd

Agent, generic (trade)	Route	Dosage/kg/24 hours		Comments
		Mild-moderate infections	*Severe infections*	
Broad-spectrum penicillins				
Ampicillin (numerous)	IV, IM	50 to 100 mg in 4 doses (daily adult dose, 2 to 4 gm)	200 to 400 mg in 4 to 6 doses (daily adult dose, 8 to 12 gm)	Ineffective against penicillin C–resistant staphylococci
	PO	50 to 100 mg in 4 doses (daily adult dose, 2 to 4 gm)	Inappropriate	High incidence of skin rash in patients with infectious mononucleosis
Amoxicillin (Amoxil, Larotid, Polymox)	PO	20 to 40 mg in 3 doses (daily adult dose, 750 mg to 1.5 gm)	Inappropriate	
Amoxicillin and clavulanate potassium (Augmentin)	PO	40 mg per amoxicillin component	Inappropriate	High incidence of nausea, vomiting, diarrhea
Mezlocillin (Mezlin)	IV, IM	200 to 300 mg in 4 to 6 doses (daily adult dose, 16 to 24 gm)	200 to 300 mg in 4 to 6 doses (daily adult dose, 16 to 24 gm)	
Piperacillin (Pipercil)	IV, IM	200 to 300 mg in 4 to 6 doses (daily adult dose, 16 to 24 gm)	200 to 300 mg in 4 to 6 doses (daily adult dose, 16 to 24 gm)	
Ticarcillin (Ticar)	IV	50 to 100 mg in 4 doses (daily adult dose, 4 to 8 gm)	200 to 300 mg in 4 to 6 doses (daily adult dose, 12 to 24 gm)	Contains 5.2 mEq Na/gm
Ticarcillin and clavulanate potassium (Timentin)	IV		200 to 300 mg of ticarcillin in 4 to 6 doses	
Cephalosporins				
Cephalothin (Keflin)	IV	40 to 80 mg in 4 doses (daily adult dose, 2 to 4 gm)	100 to 150 mg in 4 to 6 doses (daily adult dose, 8 to 12 gm)	
Cefazolin (Kefzol, Ancef)	IV, IM	50 mg in 4 doses (daily adult dose, 2 gm)	100 mg in 4 doses (daily adult dose, 4 to 6 gm)	
Cephalexin (Keflex)	PO	25 to 50 mg in 4 doses (daily adult dose, 1 to 2 gm)	Inappropriate	
Cefoxitin sodium (Mefoxin)	IV, IM	80 to 160 mg in 4 doses	80 to 160 mg in 4 doses	

Drug	Route	Dose	Dose	Comments
Cefuroxime (Zinacef, Kefurox)	IV, IM	50 to 100 mg in 3 doses (daily adult dose, 1 to 2 gm)	Inappropriate if CNS infection suspected	
Cefuroxime axetil (Ceftin)		30 to 40 mg in 2 doses (250 to 500 mg/day total)	Inappropriate	
Cefaclor (Ceclor)	PO	40 to 60 mg in 2 to 3 doses	Inappropriate	
Cefadroxil monohydrate (Duracef, Ultracef)	PO	30 mg in 2 doses	Inappropriate	
Cefixime (Suprax)	PO	8 mg in 1 or 2 doses	Inappropriate	Suspension only for otitis media; diarrhea common
Cefprozil (Cefzil)	PO	30 mg in 2 doses	Inappropriate	
Cefotaxime (Claforan)	IV, IM	100 to 150 mg in 4 doses (daily adult dose, 4 gm)	200 mg in 4 to 6 doses (daily adult dose, 8 gm)	
Cefoperazone (Cefobid)	IV	100 mg in 2 to 3 doses (daily adult dose, 2 to 4 gm)	150 mg in 3 doses (daily adult dose, 8 to 12 gm)	
Ceftazidime (Fortaz, Tazicef, Tazidime)	IV, IM	100 mg in 3 doses	150 mg in 3 doses	
Ceftriaxone (Rocephin)	IV, IM	50 to 100 mg in 1 or 2 doses	100 mg in 2 doses	
Clarithromycin (Biaxin)		15 mg in 2 doses	120 mg in 4 doses	
Aztreonam (Azactam)	IM, IV	90 mg in 3 doses	100 mg in 4 doses	
Imipenem-Cilastatin (Primaxin)	IM, IV	60 mg in 4 doses		Adjust dosage with renal insufficiency; seizures associated
Macrolides				
Erythromycin (numerous)	PO	20 to 50 mg in 3 to 4 doses (daily adult dose, 1 to 2 gm)	Inappropriate	
	IV	Inappropriate	20 to 40 mg in 3 to 4 doses (daily adult dose 1 to 4 gm)	
Aminoglycosides				
Gentamicin (Garamycin)	IV, IM	Inappropriate	3 to 7.5 mg in 3 doses (daily adult dose, 3 to 7 mg/kg/day)	Aminoglycosides enter CSF poorly; when used intravenously administer over 30 to 60 minutes Cystic fibrosis patients may require higher doses

Continued.

Antimicrobial drugs for pediatric patients beyond the newborn period — cont'd

Agent, generic (trade)	Route	Dosage/kg/24 hours		Comments
		Mild-moderate infections	Severe infections	
Aminoglycosides — cont'd				
Tobramycin (Nebcin)	IV, IM	Inappropriate	7.5 mg in 3 doses (daily adult dose, 3 to 7 mg/kg/day)	
Amikacin (Amikin)	IV, IM	Inappropriate	15 to 20 mg in 2 or 3 doses (daily adult dose, 15 mg/kg/day)	
Neomycin (Mycifradin)	PO	100 mg in 4 doses		
Clindamycin (Cleocin)	IV, IM	10 to 25 mg in 4 doses (daily adult dose, 600 to 1200 mg)	25 to 40 mg in 4 doses (daily adult dose, 1200 to 2700 mg)	
	PO	8 to 16 mg in 4 doses (daily adult dose, 600 to 1200 mg)	Inappropriate	
Metronidazole (Flagyl)	IV, PO	IV dose: 30 mg in 4 doses (adult dose, 15 mg/kg loading dose then 30 mg/kg in 4 doses) PO dose: 15 to 35 mg in 3 doses (daily adult dose, 2000 mg)	IV dose: 30 mg in 4 doses (adult dose, 15 mg/kg loading dose then 30 mg/kg in 4 doses) PO dose: 15 to 35 mg in 3 doses (daily adult dose, 2000 mg)	
Vancomycin (Vancocin)	IV, PO	IV dose: 40 mg in 4 doses (daily adult dose, 2 gm) PO dose: 10 to 50 mg in 4 doses (daily adult dose, 500 mg)	IV dose: 40 to 60 mg in 4 doses (daily adult dose, 2 gm) PO dose: 10 to 50 mg in 4 doses (daily adult dose, 500 mg)	Oral use for *C. difficile* colitis only
Tetracyclines				
Doxycycline hyclate (Vibramycin, others)	IV	Inappropriate	2-4 mg/kg in 1 dose	Infuse IV over a 2-hour period
	PO	2 to 4 mg in 1 or 2 doses (adult dose 100 mg twice daily)	Inappropriate	Responsible for staining of developing teeth; use only in children over 8 years of age and only when specifically indicated

	Route			
Chloramphenicol				
Succinate	IV	Inappropriate	50 to 100 mg in 3 to 4 doses (daily adult dose, 2 to 4 gm)	Not recommended for intramuscular administration; oral bioavailability superior to intravenous
Palmitate	PO	Inappropriate	50 to 75 mg in 3 to 4 doses (daily adult dose, 2 to 4 gm)	
Sulfonamides				
Sulfadiazine	IV, SC	120 mg in 4 doses	120 to 150 mg in 4 doses	The first dose of sulfadiazine, sulfisoxazole, and triple sulfonamides should be doubled; daily adult dose PO 2 to 4 gm; IV, SC — same as children
Sulfisoxazole (Gantrisin)	IV, SC PO	120 mg in 4 doses 120 mg in 4 doses	120 to 150 mg in 4 doses Inappropriate	
Triple sulfonamides	IV, SC	120 mg in 4 doses	120 mg in 4 doses	
Trimethoprim-sulfamethoxazole (Bactrim, Septra)	PO, IV	8 mg trimethoprim, 40 mg sulfamethoxazole in 2 doses	20 mg trimethoprim, 100 mg sulfamethoxazole in 4 doses	
Urinary antiseptic agents				
Methanamine mandelate (Mandelamine)	PO	50 to 75 mg in 3 to 4 doses (daily adult dose, 2 to 4 gm)	Inappropriate	Should not be used for infants; urine pH must be adjusted to 5 to 5.5
Nitrofurantoin (Furadantin, Macrodantin)	PO	5 to 7 mg in 4 doses (daily adult dose, 200 to 400 mg)	Inappropriate	Should not be used for infants
Antifungal agents				
Nystatin (Mycostatin, Nilstat)	PO	600,000 to 2,000,000 units; total daily dose in 3 to 4 doses		
Amphotericin B (Fungizone)	IV	0.25 to 1 mg in 1 dose	0.5 to 1 mg in 1 dose	Use a slow infusion; usually 1 mg/ml in D5W, 100 cc/kg; do not allow the IV solution to mix with other drugs, since the agent is in an easily disturbed colloid

Continued.

Antimicrobial drugs for pediatric patients beyond the newborn period — cont'd

Agent, generic (trade)	Route	Dosage/kg/24 hours		Comments
		Mild-moderate infections	Severe infections	
Flucytosine (Ancobon)	PO	50 to 150 mg in 4 doses (daily adult dose, 50 to 150 mg/kg/day in 4 doses)	50 to 150 mg in 4 doses (daily adult dose, 50 to 150 mg/kg/day in 4 doses)	Note: Flucytosine is rarely used alone because of the rapidity with which fungi develop resistance.
Fluconazole (Diflucan)	PO/IV		3-6 mg/kg in one dose (daily adult dose 100 to 200 mg in 1 dose)	Route oral in equivalent to intravenous
Griseofulvin (many)	PO	15 mg in 1 dose (daily adult dose, 250 to 500 mg)	15 mg in 1 dose (daily adult dose, 250 to 500 mg)	
Ketoconazole (Nizoral)	PO	5 to 10 mg in 1 or 2 doses (daily adult dose, 200 to 400 mg in 1 dose)	5 to 10 mg in 1 or 2 doses (daily adult dose, 200 to 400 mg in 1 dose)	
Others				
Pentamidine (Pentam 300)	IV, IM	4 mg in 1 dose	Infuse over 1 to 3 hours, monitor blood pressure	
Ciprofloxacin (Cipro)	PO	20 to 30 mg in 2 doses (daily adult dose, 500 mg in 2 doses)	Inappropriate	Not approved for use in children less than 21
	Inhalation	300 mg total dose		For cystic fibrosis
Antivirals				
Acyclovir (Zovirax)	IV	750 mg/m²/day in 3 doses	1.5 gm/m² in 3 doses	Monitor renal function; use higher dose for varicella-zoster infections in high-risk patients
	PO	1 gm in 5 doses / 80 mg in 4 doses	Inappropriate	For genital HSV / For varicella in healthy children
	IV	30 mg in 3 doses		For HSV encephalitis
Amantadine (Symmetrel)	PO	5 to 8 mg in 2 doses (maximum daily dose, 200 mg)	Inappropriate	
Didoxyinosine (Videx)	IV, PO		180 mg/m² in 3 doses	
Ganciclovir (Cytovene)	IV		10 mg in 2 doses	
Ribavirin (Virazole)	Inhalation		6 gm vial by SPAG-2 aerosol generator once daily over 12 to 18 hours	Solution contains 20 mg/ml
Zidovidine (Retrovir)	PO		720 mg/m² in 4 doses	
	IV		480 mg/m² in 4 doses	

Appendix B

ACTIVE IMMUNIZATION FOR THE PREVENTION OF INFECTIOUS DISEASES

The following vaccines have been licensed by the Food and Drug Administration (FDA).

BCG
Cholera
Diphtheria
Haemophilus influenzae, type b
Hepatitis B
Influenza
Measles
Meningococcal
Mumps
Pertussis
Plague
Poliomyelitis
Rabies
Rubella
Smallpox
Tetanus
Typhoid fever
Typhus fever
Yellow fever

Recommendations for the use of these vaccines are reviewed periodically by at least two committees: the Public Health Service Immunization Practices Advisory Committee (ACIP) and the Committee on Infectious Diseases of the American Academy of Pediatrics (AAP). A close liaison exists between representatives of the FDA, ACIP, and AAP. The final recommendations for the use of various vaccines usually represent the consensus of the committees based on their evaluation of the available current data. The acquisition of new knowledge about vaccines and significant changes in the epidemio-logical aspects of the various infectious diseases provide the basis for modifications of the recommendations.

The ACIP is sponsored by the Centers for Disease Control. The recommendations that are developed and revised are published in the Centers for Disease Control *Morbidity and Mortality Weekly Report*. The recommendations of the Committee on Infectious Diseases of the AAP are published by the academy in the so-called *Red Book*. The 1991 report was the twenty-second edition since the first issue in 1938. Revisions of special sections are published periodically in AAP Newsletters.

This appendix is a 1992 update of the ACIP "General Recommendations on Immunization" previously published in the April 7, 1989, *Morbidity and Mortality Weekly Report*.

Recommendations for immunizing infants, children, and adults are based on characteristics of immunobiologics, scientific knowledge about the principles of active and passive immunization, and judgments by public health officials and specialists in clinical and preventive medicine. Benefits and risks are associated with the use of all immunobiologics: no vaccine is completely safe or completely effective. Benefits of immunization range from partial to complete protection against the consequences of disease (which range from mild or asymptomatic infection to severe consequences such as paralysis or death); risks of immunization range from common, trivial, and inconvenient side effects to rare, severe, and life-threatening conditions. Thus recommendations for immunization practices balance scientific evidence of benefits, costs, and risks to achieve optimal levels of

Table B-1. Vaccines available in the United States, by type and recommended routes of administration

Vaccine	Type	Route
BCG (bacillus of Calmette and Guérin)	Live bacteria	Intradermal or subcutaneous
Cholera	Inactivated bacteria	Subcutaneous or intradermal*
DTP (D = diphtheria) (T = tetanus) (P = pertussis)	Toxoids and inactivated bacteria	Intramuscular
HB (hepatitis B)	Inactivated viral antigen	Intramuscular
Haemophilus influenzae b		
Polysaccharide (HbPV)	Bacterial polysaccharide	Subcutaneous or intramuscular†
or	*or*	
Conjugate (HbCV)	Polysaccharide conjugated to protein	Intramuscular
Influenza	Inactivated virus or viral components	Intramuscular
IPV (inactivated poliovirus vaccine)	Inactivated viruses of all 3 serotypes	Subcutaneous
Measles	Live virus	Subcutaneous
Meningococcal	Bacterial polysaccharides of serotypes A/C/Y/W-135	Subcutaneous
MMR (M = measles) (M = mumps) (R = rubella)	Live viruses	Subcutaneous
Mumps	Live virus	Subcutaneous
OPV (oral poliovirus vaccine)	Live viruses of all 3 serotypes	Oral
Plague	Inactivated bacteria	Intramuscular
Pneumococcal	Bacterial polysaccharides of 23 pneumococcal types	Intramuscular or subcutaneous
Rabies	Inactivated virus	Subcutaneous or intradermal‡
Rubella	Live virus	Subcutaneous
Tetanus	Inactivated toxin (toxoid)	Intramuscular§
Td or DT‖ (T = tetanus) (D or d = diphtheria)	Inactivated toxins (toxoids)	Intramuscular§
Typhoid	Inactivated bacteria	Subcutaneous¶
	Live-attenuated bacteria	Oral
Yellow fever	Live virus	Subcutaneous

*The intradermal dose is lower.
†Route depends on the manufacturer; consult package insert for recommendation for specific product used.
‡Intradermal dose is lower and used only for preexposure vaccination.
§Preparations with adjuvants should be given intramuscularly.
‖DT, tetanus and diphtheria toxoids for use in children aged <7 years. Td, tetanus and diphtheria toxoids for use in persons aged ≥7 years. Td contains the same amount of tetanus toxoid as DTP or DT but a reduced dose of diphtheria toxoid.
¶Boosters may be given intradermally unless acetone-killed and dried vaccine is used.

protection against infectious diseases. These vaccine recommendations describe this balance and attempt to minimize the risks by providing specific advice regarding dose, route, and spacing of immunobiologics and delineating situations that warrant precautions or contraindicate their use. They are recommendations for use in the United States because epidemiologic circumstances and vaccines often differ in other countries. Individual circumstances may warrant deviations from these recommendations. The relative balance of benefits and risks can change as diseases are controlled or eradicated. For example, because smallpox has been eradicated throughout the world, the risk of complications associated with smallpox vaccine now exceeds the risk of the disease; consequently, smallpox vaccination of civilians is now indicated only for laboratory workers directly involved with smallpox or closely related orthopox viruses (e.g., monkeypox and vaccinia).

DEFINITIONS
Immunobiologic

Immunobiologics include both antigenic substances such as vaccines and toxoids and antibody-containing preparations, including globulins and antitoxins, from human or animal donors. These products are used for active or passive immunization or therapy. Examples include the following:

Vaccine (Table B-1). A suspension of live (usually attenuated) or inactivated microorganisms (bacteria, viruses, or rickettsiae) or fractions thereof administered to induce immunity and thereby prevent infectious disease. Some vaccines contain highly defined antigens (e.g., the polysaccharide of *Haemophilus influenzae* type b or the surface antigen of hepatitis B); others have antigens that are complex or incompletely defined (e.g., killed *Bordetella pertussis* or live attenuated viruses).

Toxoid. A modified bacterial toxin that has been rendered nontoxic but retains immunogenicity, the ability to stimulate the formation of antitoxin, antibody to toxin.

Immune globulin (IG). A sterile solution containing antibodies from human blood. It is obtained by cold ethanol fractionation of large pools of blood plasma and contains 15% to 18% protein. Intended for intramuscular administration, it is primarily indicated for routine maintenance of immunity of certain immunodeficient persons and for passive immunization against measles and hepatitis A. IG does not transmit hepatitis B virus, human immunodeficiency virus (HIV), or other infectious diseases.

Intravenous immune globulin (IVIG). A product derived from blood plasma from a donor pool similar to the IG pool but prepared so it will be suitable for intravenous use. IVIG does not transmit infectious diseases. It is primarily indicated for replacement therapy in antibody-deficiency disorders.

Specific IG. Special preparations obtained from blood plasma from donor pools preselected for a high antibody content against a specific antigen (e.g., hepatitis B immune globulin [HBIG]), varicella-zoster immune globulin, rabies immune globulin, and tetanus immune globulin. Like IG and IVIG, these preparations do not transmit infectious diseases.

Antitoxin. A solution of antibodies derived from the serum of animals or people immunized with specific antigens used to achieve passive immunity or for treatment.

ROUTE OF IMMUNIZATION

Routes of administration are recommended for each immunobiologic (Table B-1). To avoid unnecessary local or systemic efforts and/or to ensure op-

timal efficacy, the practitioner should not deviate from the recommended routes. Vaccines containing adjuvants must be injected deep into the muscle mass; they should not be administered subcutaneously or intradermally because they can cause local irritation, inflammation, granuloma formation, or necrosis.

DOSAGE

The recommendations on dosages of immunobiologics are derived from theoretical considerations, experimental trials, and clinical experience. Administration of volumes smaller than those recommended such as split doses or intradermal administration (unless specifically recommended) can result in inadequate protection. Use of larger than the recommended dose can be hazardous because of excessive local or systemic concentrations of antigens.

The ACIP strongly discourages any variation from the recommended volume or number of doses of any vaccine. Some practitioners use smaller, divided doses of vaccine, thereby reducing the total immunizing dose. Others use multiple smaller doses that together equal a full immunizing dose (e.g., diphtheria and tetanus toxoids and pertussis vaccine [DTP]) in an effort to reduce reactions. However, the serologic response, clinical efficacy, and/or frequency and severity of adverse reactions of such schedules have not been adequately studied.

AGE AT WHICH IMMUNOBIOLOGICS ARE ADMINISTERED

Several factors influence recommendations concerning the age at which vaccines are administered (Table B-2); they are age-specific risks of disease, age-specific risks of complications, ability of persons of a given age to respond to the vaccine(s), and potential interference with the immune response by passively transferred maternal antibody. In general, vaccines are recommended for the youngest age group at risk whose members are known to develop an acceptable antibody response to vaccination.

SPACING OF IMMUNOBIOLOGICS
Multiple doses of same antigen

Some products require administration of more than one dose for development of an adequate antibody response. In addition, some products require periodic reinforcement (booster) doses to maintain protection. An additional dose of MMR has been recommended to induce immunity that failed to develop after the first dose. In recommending the ages and/or intervals for multiple doses, the ACIP takes into account risks from disease and the need to induce or maintain satisfactory protection (Table B-2).

Intervals between doses that are longer than those recommended do not lead to a reduction in final antibody levels. Therefore it is not necessary to restart an interrupted series of an immunobiologic or to add extra doses.

Table B-2. ACIP recommended schedule of vaccinations for all children

Vaccine	2 Mo	4 Mo	6 Mo	12 Mo	15 Mo	4-6 Yr (before school entry)
DTP		DTP	DTP	DTP		DTP* or DTaP*	DTP or DTaP
Polio		Polio	Polio			Polio*	Polio
MMR						MMR†	MMR‡
Hib							
Option 1§		Hib	Hib	Hib		Hib	
Option 2§		Hib	Hib		Hib		

Vaccine	Birth	1-2 Mo	4 Mo	6-18 Mo
HB				
Option 1	HB	HB‖		HB‖
Option 2		HB‖	HB‖	HB‖

DTP, diphtheria, tetanus, and pertussis vaccine; DTaP, diphtheria, tetanus, and acellular pertussis vaccine; Polio, live oral polio vaccine drops (OPV) or killed (inactivated) polio vaccine shots (IPV); MMR, measles, mumps, and rubella vaccine; Hib, *Haemophilus influenzae* b conjugate vaccine; HB, hepatitis B vaccine.
*Many experts recommend these vaccines at 18 months.
†In some areas this dose of MMR vaccine may be given at 12 months.
‡Many experts recommend this dose of MMR vaccine be given at entry to middle school or junior high school.
§ Hib vaccine is given in either a four-dose schedule (1) or a three-dose schedule (2), depending on the type of vaccine used.
‖Hepatitis B vaccine can be given simultaneously with DTP, polio, MMR, and Hib vaccines at the same visit.

In contrast, giving doses of a vaccine or toxoid at less than recommended intervals may lessen the antibody response and therefore should be avoided. Doses given at less than recommended intervals should not be counted as part of a primary series.

Some vaccines produce local or systemic symptoms in certain recipients when given too frequently (e.g., tetanus and diphtheria [Td or DT] and rabies). Such reactions are thought to result from the formation of antigen-antibody complexes. Good recordkeeping, careful patient histories, and adherence to recommended schedules can decrease the incidence of such reactions without sacrificing immunity.

Different antigens

Experimental evidence and extensive clinical experience have strengthened the scientific basis for giving certain vaccines at the same time. Many of the widely used vaccines can safely and effectively be given simultaneously. This knowledge is particularly helpful when there is imminent exposure to several infectious diseases, preparation for foreign travel, or uncertainty that the person will return for further doses of vaccine.

1. Simultaneous administration

In general, inactivated vaccines can be administered simultaneously at separate sites. However, when vaccines commonly associated with local or systemic side effects (e.g., cholera,

typhoid, and plague) are given simultaneously, the side effects can be accentuated. Whenever possible, these vaccines should be given on separate occasions.

Simultaneous administration of pneumococcal polysaccharide vaccine and whole-virus influenza vaccine elicits satisfactory antibody responses without increasing the incidence or severity of adverse reactions. Simultaneous administration of the pneumococcal vaccine and split-virus influenza vaccine can also be expected to yield satisfactory results. Influenza vaccine should be administered annually to the target population.

In general, simultaneous administration of the most widely used live and inactivated vaccines has not resulted in impaired antibody responses or increased rates of adverse reactions. Administration of combined measles, mumps, and rubella (MMR) vaccine yields results similar to administration of individual measles, mumps, and rubella vaccines at different sites. Therefore there is no medical basis for giving these vaccines separately for routine immunization instead of the preferred MMR combined vaccine.

There are equivalent antibody responses and no clinically significant increases in the frequency of adverse events when DTP, MMR, and oral polio vaccine (OPV) or inactivated polio vaccine (IPV) are administered either simulta-

Table B-3. Guidelines for spacing live and killed antigen administration

Antigen combination	Recommended minimum interval between doses
≥ Two killed antigens	None. May be given simultaneously or at any interval between doses.*
Killed and live antigens	None. May be given simultaneously or at any interval between doses.†
≥ Two live antigens	4-wk minimum interval if not administered simultaneously.

*If possible, vaccines associated with local or systemic side effects (e.g., cholera, typhoid, plague vaccines) should be given on separate occasions to avoid accentuated reactions.
†Cholera vaccine with yellow fever vaccine is the exception. If time permits, these antigens should not be administered simultaneously, and at least 3 weeks should elapse between administration of yellow fever vaccine and cholera vaccine. If the vaccines must be given simultaneously or within 3 weeks of each other, the antibody response may not be optimal.

neously at different sites or separately. As a result, routine simultaneous administration of MMR, DTP, and OPV (or IPV) to all children ≥15 months who are eligible to receive these vaccines is recommended. Administration of MMR at 15 months followed by DTP and OPV (or IPV) at 18 months remains an acceptable alternative, especially for children with caregivers known to be generally compliant with other health-care recommendations. Data are lacking on concomitant administration of *Haemophilus influenzae* b conjugate vaccine (HbCV) or *Haemophilus influenzae* b polysaccharide vaccine (HbPV) and MMR and OPV vaccine. If the child might not be brought back for future immunizations, the simultaneous administration of all vaccines (including DTP, OPV, MMR, and HbCV or HbPV) appropriate to the age and previous vaccination status of the recipient is recommended. Hepatitis B vaccine given with DTP and OPV or given with yellow fever vaccine is as safe and efficacious as these vaccines administered separately.

The antibody responses of both cholera and yellow fever vaccines are decreased if given simultaneously or within a short time of each other. If possible, cholera and yellow fever vaccinations should be separated by at least 3 weeks. If there are time constraints and both vaccines are necessary, the injections can be given simultaneously or within a 3-week period with the understanding that antibody response may not be optimal. Decisions on the need for yellow fever and cholera immunization should take into account the amount of protection afforded by the vaccine, the possibility that environmental or hygienic practices may be sufficient to avoid disease exposure, and the existence of vaccination requirements for entry into a country.

2. **Nonsimultaneous administration**

Inactivated vaccines do not interfere with the immune response to other inactivated vaccines

or to live vaccines except, as noted above, with cholera and yellow fever vaccines. In general, an inactivated vaccine can be given either simultaneously or at any time before or after a different inactivated vaccine or a live vaccine.

There are theoretical concerns that the immune response to one live-virus vaccine might be impaired if given within 30 days of another. Whenever possible, live-virus vaccines not administered on the same day should be given at least 30 days apart (Table B-3).

Live-virus vaccines can interfere with the response to a tuberculin test. Tuberculin testing can be done either on the same day that live-virus vaccines are administered or 4 to 6 weeks afterward.

Immune globulin

If administration of an IG preparation becomes necessary because of imminent exposure of disease, live-virus vaccines can be given simultaneously with the IG product, with the recognition that vaccine-induced immunity might be compromised. The vaccine should be administered at a site remote from that chosen for the IG inoculation. Vaccination should be repeated about 3 months later unless serologic testing indicates that specific antibodies have been produced. OPV and yellow fever vaccines are exceptions, however, and are not affected by administration of IG at any time.

Live, attenuated vaccine viruses might not replicate successfully, and antibody response could be diminished when the vaccine is given after IG or specific IG preparations. Whole blood or other antibody-containing blood products can interfere with the antibody response to measles, mumps, and rubella vaccines. In general, these parenterally administered live vaccines should not be given for at least 6 weeks, and preferably 3 months, after IG administration. However, the postpartum vaccination of susceptible women with rubella vaccine should not be delayed because of receipt of anti-Rho(D) IG (human) or any other blood product during the last trimester of pregnancy or at delivery. These women should be vacci-

Table B-4. Guidelines for spacing the administration of immune globulin (IG) preparations and vaccines

Simultaneous administration: immunobiologic combination	Recommended minimum interval between doses
IG and killed antigen	None. May be given simultaneously at different sites or at any time between doses.
IG and live antigen	Should generally not be given simultaneously.* If unavoidable to do so, give at different sites and revaccinate or test for seroconversion in 3 mo.

Nonsimultaneous administration: immunobiologic administered		Recommended minimum interval between doses
First	Second	
IG	Killed antigen	None
Killed antigen	IG	None
IG	Live antigen	6 wk and preferably 3 mo*
Live antigen	IG	2 wk

*The live-virus vaccines, oral polio and yellow fever, are exceptions to these recommendations. Either vaccine may be administered simultaneously or at any time before or after IG without significantly decreasing the antibody response.

nated immediately after delivery and, if possible, tested in 3 months to ensure that rubella immunity was established.

If administration of IG preparations becomes necessary after a live-virus vaccine has been given, interference can occur. Usually, vaccine virus replication and stimulation of immunity will occur 1 to 2 weeks after vaccination. Thus if the interval between administration of live-virus vaccine and subsequent administration of an IG preparation is <14 days, vaccination should be repeated at least 3 months after the IG product was given, unless serologic testing indicates that antibodies were produced.

In general, there is little interaction between IG preparations and inactivated vaccines. Therefore inactivated vaccines can be given simultaneously or at any time before or after an IG product is used. For example, postexposure prophylaxis with simultaneously administered hepatitis B, rabies, or tetanus IG and the corresponding inactivated vaccine or toxoid does not impair the immune response and provides immediate protection and long-lasting immunity. The vaccine and IG should be given at different sites, and standard doses of the corresponding vaccine should be used. Increasing the vaccine dose volume or number of immunizations is not indicated (Table B-4).

HYPERSENSITIVITY TO VACCINE COMPONENTS

Vaccine components can cause allergic reactions in some recipients. These reactions can be local or sys-temic, including mild to severe anaphylaxis (e.g., hives, swelling of the mouth and throat, difficulty breathing, hypotension, or shock). The responsible vaccine components can derive from (1) animal protein, (2) antibiotics, (3) preservatives, and (4) stabilizers. The most common animal protein allergen is egg protein found in vaccines prepared using embryonated chicken eggs or chicken embryo cell cultures (e.g., yellow fever, mumps, measles, and influenza vaccines). Ordinarily, persons who are able to eat eggs or egg products safely can receive these vaccines; persons with histories of anaphylactic allergy to eggs or egg proteins should not.

Asking persons whether they can eat eggs without adverse effects is a reasonable way to screen for those who might be at risk from receiving measles, mumps, yellow fever, and influenza vaccines. Protocols requiring extreme caution have been developed for testing and vaccinating with measles and mumps vaccines those persons with anaphylactic reactions to egg ingestion. A regimen for administering influenza vaccine to children with egg hypersensitivity and severe asthma has also been developed.

Rubella vaccine is grown in human diploid cell cultures and can safely be given to persons with histories of severe allergy to eggs or egg proteins.

Some vaccines contain trace amounts of antibiotics to which patients may be hypersensitive. The information provided in the vaccine package insert should be carefully reviewed before a decision is made whether the rare patient with such hypersensitivity should be given the vaccine(s). No currently recommended vaccine contains penicillin or its derivatives.

MMR and its individual component vaccines contain trace amounts of neomycin. Although the amount present is less than would usually be used for the skin test to determine hypersensitivity, persons who have experienced anaphylactic reactions to neomycin should not be given these vaccines. Most often, neomycin allergy is a contact dermatitis, a manifestation of a delayed-type (cell-mediated) immune response rather than anaphylaxis. A history of delayed-type reactions to neomycin is not a contraindication for these vaccines.

Bacterial vaccines such as cholera, DTP, plague, and typhoid are frequently associated with local or systemic adverse effects such as redness, soreness, and fever. These reactions are difficult to link with a specific sensitivity to vaccine components and appear to be toxic rather than hypersensitive. On rare occasions, urticarial or anaphylactic reactions in DTP, DP, or Td recipients have been reported. When such events are reported, appropriate skin tests should be performed to determine sensitivity to tetanus toxoid before its use is discontinued.

ALTERED IMMUNOCOMPETENCE

Virus replication after administration of live, attenuated-virus vaccines can be enhanced in persons with immunodeficiency diseases and in persons with suppressed capacity for immune response as occurs with leukemia, lymphoma, generalized malignancy, symptomatic HIV infections, or therapy with alkylating agents, antimetabolites, radiation, or large amounts of corticosteroids. Severe complications have followed vaccination with live, attenuated-virus vaccines and with live-bacteria vaccines (e.g., BCG) in patients with leukemia, lymphoma, or suppressed immune responses. In general, these patients should not be given live vaccines, with the exceptions noted below.

If polio immunization is indicated for immunosuppressed patients, their household members, or other close contacts, these persons should be given IPV rather than OPV. Although a protective immune response cannot be assured in the immunocompromised patient, some protection may be provided. Because of the possibility of immunodeficiency in other children born to a family in which one such case has occurred, no family members should receive OPV unless the immune statuses of the intended recipient and all other children in the family are known.

Patients with leukemia in remission whose chemotherapy has been terminated for at least 3 months can be given live-virus vaccines. Short-term, low-to-moderate dose systemic corticosteroid therapy (<2 weeks), topical steroid therapy (e.g., nasal, skin), long-term alternate-day treatment with low to moderate doses of short-acting systemic steroids, and intra-articular, bursal, or tendon injection with corticosteroids are not immunosuppressive in their usual doses and do not contraindicate live-virus vaccine administration.

The growing number of infants and preschoolers infected with HIV has directed special attention to the appropriate immunization of such children. The evaluation and testing for HIV infection of asymptomatic children presenting for vaccines are not necessary before decisions concerning immunization are made. The inactivated childhood vaccines (e.g., DTP or HbCV) should be given to HIV-infected children regardless of whether HIV symptoms are present. Although OPV has not been harmful when administered to asymptomatic HIV-infected children, IPV is the vaccine of choice if the child is known to be infected. The use of IPV not only eliminates any theoretical risk to the vaccinee but also prevents the possibility of vaccine virus spread to immunocompromised close contacts. Asymptomatically infected persons in need of MMR should receive it. Also, MMR should be considered for all symptomatic HIV-infected children since measles disease can be severe in symptomatic HIV-infected children. Limited studies of MMR immunization in both asymptomatic and symptomatic HIV-infected patients have not documented serious or unusual adverse events. In addition, pneumococcal vaccine is recommended for any child infected with HIV. Influenza vaccine is recommended for children with symptoms of HIV infection (Table B-5).

Table B-5. Recommendations for routine immunization of HIV-infected children—United States

	Known HIV infection	
Vaccine	Asymptomatic	Symptomatic
DTP	Yes	Yes
OPV	No	No
IPV	Yes	Yes
MMR	Yes	Yes*
HbCV	Yes	Yes
HB	Yes	Yes
Pneumococcal	Yes	Yes
Influenza	No†	Yes

DTP, diphtheria and tetanus toxoids and pertussis vaccine, adsorbed—DTP may be used up to the seventh birthday; OPV, poliovirus vaccine live oral, trivalent—contains poliovirus types 1, 2, and 3; IPV, poliovirus vaccine inactivated—contains poliovirus types 1, 2, and 3; MMR, measles, mumps, and rubella virus vaccine, live; HbCV, vaccine composed of *Haemophilus influenzae* b polysaccharide antigen conjugated to a protein carrier; HB, hepatitis B vaccine.
* Should be considered.
† Not contraindicated.

FEBRILE ILLNESS

The decision to administer or delay vaccination because of a current or recent febrile illness depends largely on the severity of symptoms and on the etiology of the disease.

Although a moderate or severe febrile illness is reason to postpone immunizations, minor illnesses such as mild upper-respiratory infections (URI) with or without low-grade fever are not contraindicated for vaccination. In persons whose compliance with medical care cannot be assured, it is particularly important to take every opportunity to provide appropriate vaccinations.

Children with moderate or severe febrile illnesses can be vaccinated as soon as the child has recovered. This precaution to wait avoids superimposing adverse effects of the vaccine on the underlying illness or mistakenly attributing a manifestation of the underlying illness to the vaccine.

Routine physical examinations or measuring temperatures are not prerequisites for vaccinating infants and children who appear to be in good health. Asking the parent or guardian if the child is ill, postponing vaccination in those with moderate or severe febrile illnesses, and immunizing those without contraindications to vaccination are appropriate procedures in childhood immunization programs.

MISCONCEPTIONS CONCERNING CONTRAINDICATIONS TO VACCINATION

Some health-care providers inappropriately consider certain conditions or circumstances contraindications to vaccination. Conditions most often *inappropriately* regarded as routine contraindications include the following:

1. Reaction to a previous dose of DTP vaccine that involved only soreness, redness, or swelling in the immediate vicinity of the vaccination site or temperature of <105° F (40.5° C).
2. Mild acute illness with low-grade fever or mild diarrheal illness in an otherwise well child.
3. Current antimicrobial therapy or the convalescent phase of illnesses.
4. Prematurity. The appropriate age for initiating immunizations in the prematurely born infant is the usual chronological age. Vaccine doses should not be reduced for preterm infants.
5. Pregnancy of mother or other household contact.
6. Recent exposure to an infectious disease.
7. Breastfeeding. The only vaccine virus that has been isolated from breast milk is rubella vaccine virus. There is no good evidence that breast milk from women immunized against rubella is harmful to infants.
8. A history of nonspecific allergies or relatives with allergies.
9. Allergies to penicillin or any other antibiotic, except anaphylactic reactions to neomycin (e.g., MMR-containing vaccines) or streptomycin (e.g., OPV). None of the vaccines licensed in the United States contain penicillin.
10. Allergies to duck meat or duck feathers. No vaccine available in the United States is produced in substrates containing duck antigens.
11. Family history of convulsions in persons considered for pertussis or measles vaccination.
12. Family history of sudden infant death syndrome in children considered for DTP vaccination.
13. Family history of an adverse event, unrelated to immunosuppression, following vaccination.

ADVERSE EVENTS FOLLOWING VACCINATION

Modern vaccines are safe and effective but not completely so. Adverse events have been reported following the administration of all vaccines. These events range from frequent, minor, local reactions to extremely rare, severe, systemic illness such as paralysis associated with OPV. It is often impossible to establish evidence for cause-and-effect relationships when untoward events occur after vaccination because temporal association alone does not necessarily indicate causation. More complete information on adverse reactions to a specific vaccine may be found in the ACIP recommendations for each vaccine.

The National Vaccine Injury Compensation Program established by the National Childhood Vaccine Injury Act of 1986 requires physicians and other health-care providers who administer vaccines to maintain permanent immunization records and to report occurrences of certain adverse events to the U.S. Department of Health and Human Services. Recording and reporting requirements took effect on March 21, 1988. Reportable reactions include those listed in the Act for each vaccine and events specified in the manufacturer's vaccine package insert as contraindications to further doses of that vaccine.

Although there will be one system for reporting adverse events following immunizations in the future, at present there are two separate systems. The appropriate method depends on the source of funding used to purchase the vaccine. Events that occur after receipt of a vaccine purchased with public (federal, state, and/or local government) funds must be reported by the administering health provider to the appropriate local, county, or state health department. The state health department completes and submits the correct forms to CDC. Reportable events that follow administration of vaccines purchased with private money are reported by the health-care provider directly to the FDA.

SOURCES OF VACCINE INFORMATION

In addition to these general recommendations, the practitioner can draw on a variety of sources for specific data and updated information including:

Official vaccine package circulars. Manufacturer-provided product-specific information approved by the FDA with each vaccine. Some of these materials are reproduced in the *Physician's Desk Reference (PDR)*.

Morbidity and Mortality Weekly Report (MMWR). Published weekly by CDC, *MMWR* contains regular and special ACIP recommendations on vaccine use and statements of vaccine policy as they are developed and reports on specific disease activity. Subscriptions are available through Superintendent of Documents, U.S. Government Printing Office, Washington, DC 20402. Also available through MMS Publications, C.S.P.O. Box 9120, Waltham, MA 02254.

Health Information for International Travel. Booklet published annually by CDC as a guide to national requirements and with recommendations for specific immunizations and health practices for travel to foreign countries. Purchase from the Superintendent of Documents (address above).

Advisory memoranda are published as needed by CDC to advise international travelers or persons who provide information to travelers about specific outbreaks of communicable diseases abroad. They include health information for prevention and specific recommendations for immunization. Memoranda and/or placement on mailing list is available from Division of Quarantine, Center for Prevention Services (CPS), CDC, Atlanta, GA 30333.

The Report of the Committee on Infectious Diseases of the American Academy of Pediatrics (Red Book). This report, which contains recommendations on all licensed vaccines, is updated every 2 to 3 years, most recently in 1991. Policy changes for individual recommendations for immunization practices are published as needed by the American Academy of Pediatrics in the journal *Pediatrics*. They are available from American Academy of Pediatrics, Publications Division, 141 Northwest Point Blvd., P.O. Box 927, Elk Grove Village, IL 60009-0927.

Control of Communicable Diseases in Man. This manual is published by the American Public Health Association every 5 years, most recently in 1985 (ed 14). It contains information about infectious diseases, their occurrence worldwide, diagnoses and therapy, and up-to-date recommendations on isolation and other control measures for each disease presented. It is available from the American Public Health Association, 1015 Fifteenth St. N.W., Washington, DC 20005.

INDEX

DATE DUE

DEMCO 38-296